I went back to my sleeping car. I said to myself: Their fate causes these people no suffering. It is not an impulse to charity that has upset me like this. I am not weeping over an eternally open wound. Those who carry the wound do not feel it. It is the human race and not the individual that is wounded here, is outraged here. I do not believe in pity. What torments me tonight is the gardener's point of view. What torments me is not this poverty to which after all a man can accustom himself as easily as to sloth.... What torments me is not the humps nor hollows nor the ugliness. It is the sight, a little bit in all these men, of Mozart murdered.

Wind, Sand and Stars , 1939

Antoine de Saint Exupéry

INFECTIOUS DISEASES OF CHILDREN

INFECTIOUS DISEASES OF
CHILDREN

SAUL KRUGMAN, M.D.
Professor of Pediatrics, New York University School of Medicine;
formerly Chairman, Department of Pediatrics, Director of Pediatrics,
Bellevue Hospital Center, and
Director of Pediatrics, University Hospital,
New York, New York

SAMUEL L. KATZ, M.D.
Wilburt C. Davison Professor and Chairman, Department of Pediatrics,
Duke University School of Medicine,
Durham, North Carolina

ANNE A. GERSHON, M.D.
Professor of Pediatrics, New York University Medical Center
Bellevue Hospital Center,
New York, New York

CATHERINE M. WILFERT, M.D.
Professor of Pediatrics and Microbiology,
Duke University Medical Center,
Durham, North Carolina

EIGHTH EDITION

with 119 illustrations and 8 color plates

THE C. V. MOSBY COMPANY

ST. LOUIS · TORONTO · PRINCETON   1985

MOSBY

A TRADITION OF PUBLISHING EXCELLENCE

Editor-in-Chief: Karen Berger
Assistant Editor: Sandra L. Gilfillan
Editing Supervisor: Peggy Fagen
Manuscript Editor: Debra Ketterer
Designer: Jeanne Genz
Production: Barbara Merritt

EIGHTH EDITION

Copyright © 1985 by The C. V. Mosby Company

Previous editions copyrighted 1958, 1960, 1964, 1968, 1973, 1977, 1981

Printed in the United States of America

The C. V. Mosby Company
11830 Westline Industrial Drive, St. Louis, Missouri 63146

Library of Congress Cataloging in Publication Data
Main entry under title:

Infectious diseases of children.

Rev. ed. of: Infectious diseases of children / Saul
Krugman, Samuel L. Katz. 7th ed. 1981.
    Includes bibliographies and index.
    1. Communicable diseases in children. I. Krugman,
Saul, 1911–   II. Krugman, Saul, 1911–
Infectious diseases of children. [DNLM: 1. Communicable
Diseases—in infancy & childhood.   WC 100 I4186]
RJ401.I52 1985   618.92′9   85-10596
ISBN 0-8016-2795-8

GW/MV/MV 9 8 7 6 5 4 3 2 1

TO
SYLVIA STERN KRUGMAN
WHOSE WARMTH AND WIT
ARE WOVEN INTO THE
FABRIC OF ALL EIGHT
EDITIONS

PREFACE

The first edition of *Infectious Diseases of Children* was published in 1958 in collaboration with the late Dr. Robert Ward. The preface stated that "the purpose of this book is to provide a concise and handy description of certain common infectious diseases of children. It is written primarily for pediatricians, general practitioners, and medical students who deal with children." Since its inception we have attempted to preserve this book as a handy, concise, practical reference without succumbing to the temptation to expand the text into an encyclopedia of all infectious diseases.

This eighth edition has been enhanced by two additional co-authors, Anne A. Gershon and Catherine M. Wilfert. Their valuable contributions to the book stem from their wide experience in the field of infectious diseases and their well-recognized reputations as outstanding educators, clinicians, and investigators.

Recent developments in the field of infectious diseases are reflected in the addition of a new chapter on acquired immunodeficiency syndrome (AIDS) and an all-inclusive chapter on sexually transmitted diseases. In addition, many chapters in the book have had extensive revisions.

The dramatic changes that have occurred since publication of the seventh edition in 1981 are truly incredible. The conceptual and technical advances in molecular and cell biology have been responsible for an unprecedented growth in knowledge about the cell biology of viruses and bacteria that are causative agents of infectious diseases of children. Cloning procedures, molecular DNA hybridization, hybridomas producing monoclonal antibodies, and recombinant DNA techniques have provided alternate approaches for the production of viral and bacterial antigens for vaccine development and new diagnostic methods. For example, it is anticipated that a hepatitis B vaccine prepared by this genetic engineering procedure will be licensed for use in about 2 years.

We are grateful to many colleagues for their contributions to this eighth edition—to Jerome O. Klein for updating his chapter on otitis media, to Laura T. Gutman for preparing the new chapter on sexually transmitted diseases and for revising the chapters on tuberculosis and osteomyelitis, to William Borkowsky for the AIDS chapter, to Keith Krasinski for updating the chapter on urinary tract infections, to Ross E. McKinney for reviewing the recommended doses of antimicrobial drugs and to Sharon Steinberg for editorial assistance.

Saul Krugman
Samuel L. Katz

CONTENTS

COLOR PLATES

1

ACQUIRED IMMUNODEFICIENCY SYNDROME (AIDS)

In 1980, an epidemic of community acquired *Pneumocystis carinii* pneumonitis (PCP) infections in adults without a recognized predisposing immunodeficiency occurred in New York and California. At the same time, an outbreak of Kaposi's sarcoma, a malignancy that is relatively rare in the United States, was also recognized in male homosexuals; the frequency of this illness in these individuals was 50 times the expected rate of 0.02 to 0.06 per 100,000 persons. One fifth of the patients with Kaposi's sarcoma had also developed PCP. It was recognized that these individuals were experiencing an immunodeficiency syndrome that had not been described previously.

Initially, this disorder was found only in male homosexuals. As more cases of opportunistic infections were observed in adults who had previously been normal, it became evident that some heterosexuals also manifested this newly recognized immunodeficiency disease. The syndrome was then termed the *acquired immunodeficiency syndrome* (AIDS).

Adults who had previously been healthy who developed PCP and other opportunistic infections were found to share some common disturbances of immune function. These included lymphopenia, particularly of the helper T-cell subset, and cutaneous anergy to common recall antigens. Upon further examination of presumably high-risk individuals such as sexually promiscuous homosexuals, it was noted that some had laboratory evidence of impaired immunity but no evidence of opportunistic infection or Kaposi's sarcoma. However, these individuals usually had significant lymphadenopathy. As many as 10% subsequently progressed to full-blown AIDS. Thus, lympadenopathy associated with evidence of immune dysfunction in an adult was recognized as a possible prodrome of AIDS.

It was more difficult to establish an AIDS syndrome in infants and children than in adults. Before it could be diagnosed in young immunodeficient patients it was necessary to exclude the possibility of *congenital* immunodeficiency. An additional obstacle in the recognition of AIDS in children was the association of infection with agents such as *P. carinii* and *Mycobacterium avium intracellulare* in individuals not considered to be immunodeficient. Despite these problems, the diagnosis of AIDS has been established in over 120 infants and children by 1985, primarily in New York and California, reflecting the geographic distribution of AIDS in adults. An equal number of children are also believed to have an AIDS prodrome. Since the incidence of AIDS is increasing in young patients, a description of the syndrome and the criteria for its diagnosis in both adults and children is included in this chapter.

CLINICAL MANIFESTATIONS
Adults

Approximately half of the patients have presented with PCP with or without other opportunistic infections. Another third of AIDS patients have presented with Kaposi's sarcoma without *Pneumocystis* infection. The remainder

1

have had either a combination of PCP and Kaposi's sarcoma or other opportunistic infections as the first indication of AIDS. In addition, autoimmune phenomena such as thrombocytopenic purpura, lymphoreticular malignancies such as lymphoma, and squamous carcinomas of the oropharynx, rectum, and cervix have been described. The prodrome of AIDS is associated with lymphadenopathy, weight loss, fever, diarrhea, and mucocutaneous candidiasis. Many adult patients at Bellevue Hospital have presented with severe oral thrush as the first clinical indication of AIDS.

Infants and children

The first description of "pediatric" AIDS and its prodrome was noted in a group of children in Newark, New Jersey (Oleske et al., 1983). The clinical manifestations included interstitial pneumonia, anemia, failure to thrive, hepatosplenomegaly, thrush, and opportunistic infection. Simultaneously, a group of children whose immunodeficiency also was not congenital was reported from New York (Rubenstein et al., 1983). These children exhibited failure to thrive, hepatosplenomegaly, and interstitial pneumonia, but they did not have opportunistic infections. However, recurrent bacterial infections were prominent in their histories, and they had marked lymphadenopathy. These patients proved to be an enigma when attempts were made to classify them as having AIDS, because they lacked documented opportunistic infections. The majority of these children had decreased numbers of T lymphocytes in the peripheral blood, particularly those of the helper phenotype. They also had markedly elevated concentrations of all classes of serum immunoglobulins.

The only possible congenital immunodeficiency consistent with the T-cell findings and the presence of measurable antibody was Nezelof's syndrome. However, in Nezelof's syndrome serum immunoglobulin levels never reach the levels that were observed in these children. The few available biopsy specimens of thymus and lymph nodes demonstrated no T-cell dysplasia, a finding that would have been typical of congenital immunodeficiency. The puzzle was resolved when careful follow-up of these patients revealed that their immunologic function deteriorated progressively, concomitant with the development of documented opportunistic infections. Usually these patients manifested pneumonia due to *P. carinii*, but infection with the protozoan *Cryptosporidium* was also demonstrated in those with chronic diarrhea. Thus it appears that not only is there an AIDS syndrome in the pediatric population but also there is an AIDS prodrome in children.

Why do bacterial infections occur in infants with presumed AIDS despite markedly elevated serum immunoglobulin levels more frequently than in adults with AIDS? Undoubtedly both populations have a similar immune defect, but their past histories are obviously different. Both children and adults with AIDS respond poorly to primary exposure to protein and polysaccharide antigens. Adults with AIDS, however, have had many years of normal immunologic function that preceded their acquired immunodeficiency. Promiscuous homosexuals and drug abusers, furthermore, have had ample natural immunization with infectious agents before developing AIDS, as evidenced by the increased prevalence of antibodies to hepatitis A and B, syphilis, and cytomegalovirus. Infants with AIDS, in contrast, usually have symptoms at 6 months of age. Therefore, their natural exposure to infectious agents is more limited, and, in addition to their developmental inability to respond to polysaccharide antigens, they have an inability to recognize protein antigens.

Although Kaposi's sarcoma is common in adults with AIDS, only two cases have been seen in children with AIDS. Both cases were diagnosed only at postmortem examination.

EPIDEMIOLOGY

The risk factors associated with AIDS among adult patients are also recognized as risk factors for infants and children. These include (1) homosexual contacts, (2) intravenous drug abuse, (3) recipients of blood products (whole blood and its components, including clotting factor concentrates), and (4) sexual contact with a person with AIDS. In addition, individuals of Haitian and Zairean heritage without any of the other risk factors seem to be at an increased risk to develop AIDS. Children with AIDS may have parents who are either drug abusers or who have AIDS or an AIDS prodrome themselves. Vertical transmission of the putative causative agent is presumed to occur when maternal risk factors are present. The reported cases included children who were all born after 1980. Occasionally more than one child in a family was affected. The mean age at diagnosis has been 12 months, with illness first appearing at 5 months of age (Thomas et al., 1984).

In 1983 an infant with *erythroblastosis fetalis* was reported to have developed AIDS after six exchange transfusions during the neonatal period (Ammann et al., 1983). Irradiated blood products from 19 separate donors had been given to the baby. At 4 months of age the infant had hepatosplenomegaly, neutropenia, hemolytic anemia, and thrombocytopenia. His bone marrow was infected with *M. avium intracellulare*. One of the blood donors from whom the child received a platelet transfusion was a 48-year-old male homosexual. Although he was in good health when he donated the blood, 8 months later he developed early signs of AIDS. Seventeen months later the blood donor died with disseminated cytomegalovirus infection, encephalitis of unknown etiology, severe perianal herpes simplex, and salmonella sepsis.

Eighteen adults have been reported to have developed AIDS 15 to 57 months after having received blood transfusions (Curran et al., 1984). These individuals had no other risk factors for AIDS. They received blood products from as few as two and as many as 48 donors. Sixteen received packed cells, 12 received fresh frozen plasma, nine received whole blood, and eight received platelets.

At Bellevue Hospital, we have seen three children with an AIDS prodrome whose only risk factors were multiple transfusions. Two children were transfused because of surgical complications, and one was transfused as a premature infant.

Additional cases of transfusion-associated AIDS in children have been reported in hemophiliacs (Centers for Disease Control, 1982). Two of these children have developed PCP. A 10-year-old and a 7-year-old child who had received 96,000 units and 150,000 units, respectively, of factor VIII developed hypergammaglobulinemia and a deficiency of helper T cells. In a study of 25 adult hemophiliacs investigated at random, five had a deficiency of helper T cells.

Those who received lyophilized factor VIII were more likely to have a helper T-cell deficiency than those who received cryoprecipitate (Lederman et al., 1983; Luban et al., 1983; Menitove et al., 1983).

ETIOLOGY

The cause of AIDS is still controversial. Hypotheses concerning the etiology of AIDS continue to evolve. At one time it was suspected that a variety of well-recognized viruses such as cytomegalovirus, Epstein-Barr virus, hepatitis B virus, and a deltalike hepatitis virus might be causative. Consideration was given to rare agents causing zoonoses such as the African swine fever virus. It was also proposed that "recreational" drugs such as amyl nitrate, multiple infections causing paralysis of the immune system, and the deposition of sperm per rectum might cause the immunodeficiency seen in AIDS, although these mechanisms could not possibly explain the disease in infants. All of these hypotheses now seem unlikely. The existence of the syndrome in infants makes a viral etiology logical.

The most likely cause of AIDS appears to be a retrovirus infection. Retroviruses are single-stranded RNA viruses associated in many species with malignancy and with immunodeficiency in certain animals such as cats. These viruses are usually species restricted in activity. The first association of a retrovirus with human disease was described by American and Japanese investigators (Poiesz et al., 1980; Yoshida et al., 1982).

Seroepidemiologic and nucleic acid hybridization studies have clearly associated a virus, termed *human T-cell leukemia-lymphoma virus* (HTLV-I), with malignancies of mature T lymphocytes in Southern Japan, in the Caribbean, and in Africa (Yoshida, 1983). A second retrovirus, HTLV-II, has been isolated from a single individual with a T-cell tumor (hairy cell leukemia). These viruses cause immortalization of human cord blood T cells and cell syncytia formation in vitro. Initial serologic screening studies of adults with AIDS revealed a low prevalence of antibodies reacting with common retroviral glycoprotein antigens. Subsequent studies using a more sensitive assay for antibodies directed against an HTLV-induced membrane protein indicated, however, that these antibodies were present in 40% of adults with AIDS (Essex et al., 1983). The prevalence of these antibodies in normal adults is less than 1%.

Additional human retroviruses, termed *lymphadenopathy-associated virus* (LAV) by French investigators (Barre-Sinoussi et al., 1983), human T-cell lymphotropic virus—type III (HTLV-III) by American investigators (Gallo et al., 1984; Popovic et al., 1984), and AIDS-associated retroviruses (ARV) by other American investigators (Levy et al., 1984), have been isolated from individuals with AIDS and its prodromes. Serologic evidence of infection with these viruses has been found in 75% to 90% of these patients. Antibodies to these viruses have also been found in 20% to 40% of all homosexuals, 70% of asymptomatic hemophiliacs, and almost 90% of asymptomatic heavy drug abusers (Centers for Disease Control, 1984). Serologic evidence of infection is seen in less than 1% of persons with no risk factors for AIDS. A retrospective analysis of blood specimens from homosexual men attending a clinic for sexually transmitted diseases has detected an increasing prevalence of antibodies to LAV. The rate of seropositivity was 1% in 1978, 25% in 1980, and 65% in 1984 (Centers for Disease Control, 1984).

It remains to be determined whether LAV, HTLV-III, and ARV are identical viruses. However, assuming that they are, they represent the most likely candidates for the cause of AIDS. In addition to being T-cell tropic, they also cause the destruction of infected helper T cells (Popovic et al., 1984). Such a pathogenic effect seems to represent a sine qua non for a putative AIDS agent. A related primate retrovirus has also been implicated as the cause of AIDS in monkeys.

HTLV-III has been isolated from three of eight children with AIDS and from three of four clinically normal mothers of juvenile AIDS patients (Gallo et al., 1984). Seroepidemiologic investigations of mother-child pairs have yet to be reported.

CLINICAL COURSE AND PROGNOSIS

The clinical course of AIDS in adults has been a relentlessly progressive one. Approximately 45% of affected individuals are dead within 1 year of diagnosis. Although most individuals survive their first opportunistic infection, recur-

rences and new infections follow within several months, each one taking its toll. About 60% of adults with AIDS are dead within 2 years of diagnosis, and this percentage increases to 75% after 3 years.

Surveillance data for infants and children accumulated by the Department of Health in New York City have documented that the fate of children with AIDS is no better than that of adults. In a group of 29 children with documented opportunistic infections diagnosed since 1981, 17 (59%) have died. Because 22 of the 29 children have been diagnosed since 1983, the case-fatality rate is consistent with the pattern in adults.

The clinical course of the AIDS prodrome is less predictable. Various studies of adults with the lymphadenopathy syndrome have suggested that anywhere between 0% and 10% of those affected progress to clinical AIDS with the persistence of lymphadenopathy, helper T-cell deficiency, anergy, and, in some, chronic thrush. Obviously a longer period of observation will be required before any definitive statement about their progression is possible.

Even less is known about the outcome of children with an AIDS prodrome. Some children have maintained their lymphadenopathy and immunologic perturbations for as long as 3 years without developing opportunistic infections. However, other children have demonstrated a progressive deterioration of immune function with the onset of opportunistic infection. As for affected adults, continued observation of more children with the AIDS prodrome is required before the true prognosis becomes evident.

DIAGNOSIS AND DIFFERENTIAL DIAGNOSIS

Epidemiologic surveillance criteria for the diagnosis of AIDS in infants and children have been established by the Centers for Disease Control in Atlanta, Georgia. This diagnosis should be considered when biopsy-proven opportunistic infection or Kaposi's sarcoma occurs in a pediatric patient. This diagnosis indicates an underlying deficiency of cellular immunity and, as such, requires exclusion of the following conditions:

1. Recent therapy with an immunosuppressive agent
2. Lymphoproliferative disease

3. Congenital immunodeficiency states
   a. Severe combined immunodeficiency
   b. DiGeorge syndrome
   c. Wiscott-Aldrich syndrome
   d. Neutropenia or defects in killing by and/or mobility of neutrophils
   e. Agammaglobulinemia or hypogamma-globulinemia with increased IgM levels
   f. Ataxia-telangiectasia
4. Severe malnutrition
5. Graft-versus-host disease

In addition, infants with congenital infections (such as toxoplasmosis and cytomegalovirus) need to be excluded.

The New York City Department of Health has adopted another case definition for children with unexplained immunodeficiency who have not had a diagnosed opportunistic infection. Children meeting the criteria of the Centers for Disease Control without the presence of opportunistic infection are probably the pediatric equivalent of the AIDS prodrome in adults. The criteria are as follows:

1. Clinical
   a. Hepatomegaly (with or without spleno-megaly) persisting for longer than 2 months
   b. Lymphadenopathy (palpable nodes in at least three sites persisting for longer than 2 months)
   c. Failure to thrive
   d. At least two of the following:
      i. Persistent oral thrush
      ii. Persistent pneumonitis without a documented pathogen
      iii. History of bacterial sepsis or meningitis
2. Laboratory
   a. Low helper T-cell numbers
   b. Inverted helper T cell:suppressor T-cell ratio (less than 1)
   c. Elevated immunoglobulins (greater than 2 standard deviations above the mean for IgG, and/or IgM, and/or IgA)
   d. Depressed in vitro lymphocyte proliferative response to mitogens (phyto-hemagglutinin, concanavalin A, and, particularly, pokeweed mitogen)
   e. In vitro anergy to antigens to which the child is known to have been exposed (such as tetanus toxoid and diphtheria toxoid)

Pediatric patients with AIDS or a prodrome of AIDS should be evaluated for the presence of AIDS risk factors. Horizontal and vertical mechanisms of transmission should be investigated. When possible, immunologic investigation of the parents should be performed. A combination of clinical, laboratory, and epidemiologic criteria will assist in establishing a diagnosis.

COMPLICATIONS

The presence of multiple infections and elevated immunoglobulins provides an ideal setting for the formation of immune complexes, which may lead to immune complex disease syndromes. For example, there is an increased incidence of immune thrombocytopenia in patients with an AIDS prodrome. Platelets recovered from these patients are coated with immune complexes which hasten their disappearance from the circulation (Morris et al., 1983).

Some children have had a pneumonitis associated with a diffuse lymphocytic interstitial proliferative histologic picture. While the exact cause of the pathology is unknown, markedly elevated gene copies of Epstein-Barr virus (EBV) DNA have been detected in the lung tissue and peripheral blood of a few patients (Andiman et al., 1985). This suggests that the oxygen diffusion difficulties these patients experience may be related to unregulated lymphocytic proliferation triggered by EBV.

TREATMENT

No effective therapy has been found to correct the severe cell-mediated immunodeficiency that results in infection with opportunistic agents. The use of immunostimulants, T-cell growth factors, and bone marrow transplantation has yielded disappointing results. Interferon therapy has proven somewhat effective for Kaposi's sarcoma, but it has not improved immune function. Some investigators have suggested that administration of intravenous gamma globulin has reduced bacterial infections and failure to thrive in some children with AIDS or its prodrome. Unfortunately, controlled studies are lacking.

One is therefore left with attempting to treat individual infections rather than treating the cause of the syndrome. Some infections, however, have proven quite resistant to therapy. Over 20 drug combinations have failed consistently to eradicate Cryptosporidium from the stool. EBV and cytomegalovirus infections are also not readily treated. Other infections such as those due to herpes simplex virus and *Candida* are likely to respond to standard therapies devised for these agents (vidarabine or acyclovir, and ketoconazole, respectively).

The drug of choice for the treatment of *Pneumocystis carinii* pneumonia is trimethoprim-sulfamethoxazole. While treatment of normal individuals with this drug is associated with only rare episodes of thrombocytopenia, individuals with AIDS seem to be unduly sensitive to this drug. Neutropenia occurs frequently despite therapy with folinic acid. The appearance of neutropenia prompts some physicians to change therapy to pentamidine, a drug that is associated with additional serious complications such as hypoglycemia. The frequency of toxicity to trimethoprim-sulfamethoxazole and the lack of evidence of efficacy for prophylaxis of *Pneumocystis* infections are contraindications for prophylactic use of this drug in AIDS patients.

PREVENTION

The epidemiology and risk factors associated with AIDS suggest that the disease is not readily transmissible by ordinary humans. Sexual contact, exposure to blood products, and congenital transmission suggest that the AIDS agent behaves very much like the hepatitis B virus. However, it seems to be even less contagious; for example, there is currently no evidence of transmission of AIDS solely by household or school contact. Inadvertent skin puncture by needles used for phlebotomy of individuals with AIDS has yet to result in transmission of AIDS. A local cryptococcal abscess, however, has been seen when a needle stick occurred after phlebotomy of an AIDS patient with cryptococcal septicemia. Since children with AIDS may be infected with cytomegalovirus, appropriate hand washing precautions should be exercised by those who care for these patients. Care should also be taken when handling clothing, other personal articles, and surfaces soiled with secretions and excretions of affected children.

In March 1983 the U.S. Public Health Service issued interagency recommendations on the

prevention of AIDS. Subsequently, in January 1985, the interagency group recommended routine screening of donated blood and and plasma for antibody to the virus causing AIDS. These two reports are found in Appendix 2.

REFERENCES

Ammann AJ, Cowan MJ, Wara DW, et al. Acquired immunodeficiency in an infant: possible transmission by means of blood products. Lancet 1983;1:956-958.

Andiman W, Eastman RN, Markowitz RI, Miller G. EBV associated chronic lymphocytic interstitial pneumonia in a child with AIDS related complex. J Pediatr 1985; in press.

Barre-Sinoussi F, Cherman JC, Rey F, et al. Isolation of a T-lymphotrophic retrovirus from a patient at risk for acquired immunodeficiency syndrome (AIDS). Science 1983;220:868-871.

Centers for Disease Control. Update on acquired immunodeficiency syndrome (AIDS) among patients with hemophilia A. Morbid Mortal Weekly Rep 1982;31:652-654.

Centers for Disease Control. Antibodies to a retrovirus etiologically associated with acquired immunodeficiency syndrome (AIDS) in populations with increased incidence of the syndrome. Morbid Mortal Weekly Rep 1984;33:377-379.

Curran JW, Lawrence DN, Jaffe H, et al. Acquired immunodeficiency syndrome (AIDS) associated with transfusions. N Engl J Med 1984;310:69-75.

Essex M, McLane MF, Lee TH, et al. Antibodies to cell membrane antigens associated with human T-cell leukemia virus in patients with AIDS. Science 1983;220:859-862.

Gallo RC, Salahuddin SZ, Popovic M, et al. Frequent detection and isolation of cytopathic retroviruses (HTLV-3) from patients with AIDS and at high risk for AIDS. Science 1984;224:500-503.

Lederman MM, Ratnoff OD, Scillian JJ, et al. Impaired cell mediated immunity in patients with classic hemophilia. N Engl J Med 1983;308:79-83.

Levy JA, Hoffman AD, Kramer, SM, et al. Retroviruses from San Francisco patients with AIDS. Science 1984;225:840-842.

Luban NLC, Kelleher JF Jr, Reaman GH. Altered distribution of T-lymphocyte subpopulations in children and adolescents with haemophilia. Lancet 1983;1:503-505.

Menitove JE, Aster RH, Casper JT, et al. T lymphocyte subpopulations in patients with classic hemophilia treated with cryoprecipitates and lyophilized concentrates. N Engl J Med 1983;308:83-86.

Morris L, Distenfeld A, Amorosi E, et al. Autoimmune thrombocytopenic purpura in homosexual men. Ann Intern Med 1983;73:171-178.

Oleske J, Minnefor A, Cooper R Jr, et al. Immune deficiency syndrome in children. JAMA 1983;249:2345-2349.

Poiesz BJ, Ruscetti FW, Gazdar, et al. Detection and isolation of type C retrovirus particles from fresh and cultured lymphocytes of a patient with cutaneous T cell lymphoma. Proc Natl Acad Sci USA 1980;77:7415-7419.

Popovic M, Sarngadharan MG, Read E, et al. Detection, isolation, and continuous modulation of cytopathic retroviruses (HTLV-III) from patients with AIDS and pre-AIDS. Science 1984;224:497-500.

Rubenstein A, Sicklick M, Gupta A, et al. Acquired immunodeficiency with reversed T4/T8 ratios in infants born to promiscuous and drug addicted mothers. JAMA 1983;249:2350-2356.

Stevens CE, Toy PT, Tong MJ, et al. Perinatal hepatitis B virus transmission in the United States: prevention by passive-active immunization. JAMA 198; in press.

Thomas PA, Jaffe HW, Spina TJ, et al. Unexplained immunodeficiency in children. JAMA 1984;252:639-644.

Yoshida M, Miyoshi I, Hinuma Y. Isolation and characterization of retrovirus from cell lines of human adult T cell leukemia and its implications in the disease. Proc Natl Acad Sci USA 1982;79:2031-2035.

Yoshida M. Human leukemia virus associated with adult T-cell leukemia. Gann 1983;74:777-789.

2
CYTOMEGALOVIRUS INFECTIONS

When the human cytomegaloviruses (CMVs) were first reported to replicate successfully in vitro (Rowe et al., 1956; Smith, 1956; Weller et al., 1957), techniques became available to study the events surrounding recognized clinical infections by these agents. Most initial research focused on the known entities of salivary gland inclusion disease and so called cytomegalic inclusion disease (CID), the congenital disseminated form of infection. Another decade passed before it was discovered that CID and other overt clinical entities were but the proverbial "tip of the iceberg," with a far greater number of inapparent infections regularly occurring in neonates as a result of vertical transmission from maternal genital shedding of CMV. Attention shifted then to the elucidation of the epidemiology, virology, and immunology of these common occult infections, which involved as many as 1% to 2% of newborns and 5% to 25% of pregnant women. Longitudinal studies are still in progress to determine the long-term effects of these asymptomatic perinatal infections on infant and child development. The most recent area of CMV morbidity to be appreciated has been its transmission or reactivation in immunosuppressed and immunocompromised patients. As with other agents whose initial association was detected with only a limited clinical syndrome, CMV has emerged as a ubiquitous virus with host interactions ranging over the full spectrum of health and illness.

ETIOLOGY

It had been suspected for many years that CID is caused by a virus. Similarities observed between cytomegalic inclusion cells and those seen in varicella (Goodpasture and Talbot, 1921) and in herpetic lesions (Von Glahn and Pappenheimer, 1925) are remarkable in light of modern evidence classifying CMV with the herpesvirus group. Cole and Kuttner in 1926 established the viral cause of a related infection, salivary gland virus disease of guinea pigs. In 1930, Andrewes described inclusion bodies in tissue cultures inoculated with guinea pig virus. Further progress was delayed until the advent of the tissue culture era. Smith in 1954 was the first to carry out serial propagation of murine CMV in mouse tissue cultures.

The CMV is a DNA agent with an icosahedral capsid composed of 162 capsomeres and an inner core. The virus particles or capsids are surrounded by an envelope, and some cores contain a ringlike internal substructure or tegument (Fig. 2-1). The virus also contains protein and essential lipids. Human CMV appears to be one of the most heat-labile animal viruses studied to date. For example, its half-life at 37° C is approximately 55 minutes, and its Arrhenius constant is less than 55,000 calories/mole from 0° to 44° C (Krugman and Goodheart, 1964). It is grown best in human fibroblastic tissue cultures.

Neutralizing and complement-fixing antibodies are formed in infected infants and their moth-

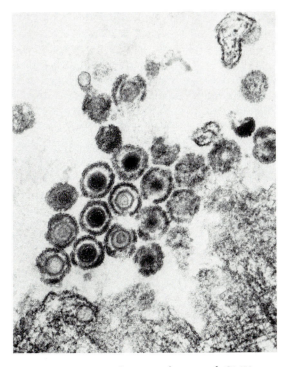

Fig. 2-1. A group of negatively stained CMV particles propagated in human lung fibroblasts. The typical hexagonal capsid (actually icosahedral in three dimensions) of a herpesvirus can be seen, surrounded by a tegument and double-layered envelope. (× 155.000.) (Courtesy Janet D. Smith, Ph.D.)

ers. Moreover, viral antigen may be identified in infected cells by means of fluorescent-labeled antibody (McAllister et al., 1963). It has been suggested that two and possibly three or more serotypes of CMV may exist (Weller et al., 1960; Weller, 1971). CMVs are related to the Epstein-Barr virus (EBV), varicella zoster virus, and herpes simplex virus types 1 and 2. Cultivation of CMV in human fibroblasts reveals characteristic cytomegaly with intranuclear inclusion bodies and paranuclear cytoplasmic "dense bodies."

PATHOGENESIS

A superb medical progress report by Weller (1971) has summarized knowledge of the natural history of CMV infection in humans. The sequence of events following primary infection and subsequent reinfection or activation is shown in Fig. 2-2.

Primary infection

A susceptible (immunologically inexperienced) host may be infected during the prenatal, perinatal, or postnatal period. Prenatal, or congenital, infection is usually acquired via the transplacental route. Viremia during pregnancy may

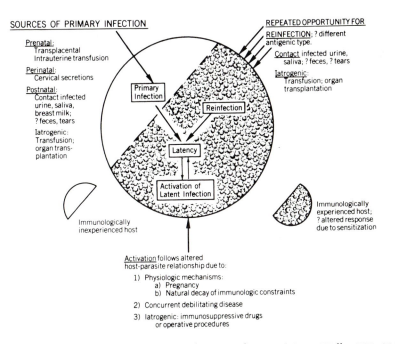

Fig. 2-2. Natural history of human cytomegalovirus infection. (From Weller TH. N Engl J Med 1971;285:203.)

be the most common source of prenatal CMV infection.

Perinatal infection is probably caused by exposure to CMV-infected cervical secretions. The presence of CMV in cervical secretions was well documented by Alexander (1967) and Diosi et al. (1967).

Postnatal infections are most commonly acquired by contact with various secretions that are known to be infected with CMV, such as urine, semen, saliva, breast milk, and tears. The exact route of transmission is unknown; it may be the oral route, the respiratory route, or both. It has been postulated that close contact is essential for the transmission of CMV. Therefore, it is possible that CMV, like infectious mononucleosis and hepatitis B virus, may be transmitted by kissing.

Breast milk is a recognized vector for transmission of CMV to infants, despite the presence of maternal CMV antibody. Acquisition of CMV by the infant from breast milk has been associated with prolonged viral shedding, but rarely do symptoms occur. Caution concerning the potential feeding of fresh banked breast milk that might contain CMV, particularly to seronegative low birth weight infants has been advised (Stagno et al., 1980; Dworsky et al., 1983). Protracted pneumonitis, neutropenia, thrombocytopenia, and hepatosplenomegaly in low birth weight infants due to CMV have been described (Yeager et al., 1972; Whitley et al., 1976; Stagno et al., 1981; Dworsky et al., 1983).

Other exogenous sources of postnatal CMV infection include transfusions with CMV-infected blood and transplantation of organs infected with the virus. These iatrogenic causes of primary CMV infection have been recognized with increasing frequency (Yeager et al., 1972).

Reinfection or reactivation of CMV

The immunologically experienced host may be exposed to exogenous or endogenous sources of infection. Reactivation of latent CMV infections may stem from various physiologic, pathologic, or iatrogenic mechanisms. Pregnancy or concurrent debilitating disease may be associated with an increased incidence of CMV infection. The administration of immunosuppressive drugs or surgical procedures may activate a latent infection.

The birth of a second congenitally infected infant has been reported in a few instances and it is assumed that this is a rare happening (Stagno et al., 1973). Humoral antibody in an immune mother does not prevent maternal excretion of CMV during pregnancy or curtail acquisition of the infection by her infant. Stagno et al. (1977b) found that intrauterine infection with CMV occurred in 3.4% of infants of immune (seropositive) mothers. It is not known whether these infants are at the same risk of developmental impairment as are those of seronegative mothers. However, it seems unlikely.

In a study of 3712 pregnant women by Stagno et al. (1982b), about one third had no evidence of prior immunity to CMV. Infants with symptomatic congenital CMV infections were born only to women in the susceptible group; presumably they had primary infections during pregnancy. Some women with recurrent CMV infections during pregnancy gave birth to congenitally infected infants, but they were asymptomatic at birth and at 1 year of age. It seems likely that the risk of bearing an infected symptomatic infant is increased in women without prior immunologic experience with CMV, although immunity to this virus can only be described as partial. There is at least one report in the literature of an infant with severe CMV born to a mother who had a reactivation CMV infection during pregnancy (Ahlfors et al., 1981).

Whether a vaccine could prevent symptomatic congenital CMV infections if administered to seronegative females, analogous to protection conferred by live attenuated rubella vaccine, remains to be seen.

The rates of CMV excretion increase in the later months of pregnancy. One factor in the failure of immune mothers to restrict spread of CMV to their infants despite the presence of elevated antibody titers may be specific impairment of cell-mediated immunity to CMV, reported by Rola-Pleszczynski et al. (1977), Reynolds et al. (1979), and Starr et al. (1979). On the other hand, since fetal infection is not invariably the result of depressed maternal cellular immunity to CMV, its exact role in modulating transmission of congenital infection is unclear (Faix et al., 1983).

PATHOLOGY

The histologic lesion of CMV infection is characterized by enlarged cells that contain intranuclear and cytoplasmic inclusion bodies. The intranuclear inclusion body appears reddish purple after being stained with hematoxylin and eosin, and is surrounded by a halo. The paranuclear cytoplasmic inclusion or dense body is more granular and more basophilic in appearance.

The inclusion-bearing cells are widely disseminated. Involvement of the following organs has been seen: salivary glands, kidney, liver, lung, brain, pancreas, thyroid gland, adrenal glands, gastrointestinal tract, spleen, thymus, lymph nodes, parathyroid gland, pituitary gland, testis, epididymis, ovary, heart, eye, muscle, bone marrow, skin, and blood vessels. Involvement of the kidneys and lungs induces chronic interstitial nephritis and pneumonitis, with focal areas of infiltration of mononuclear cells in the interstitial tissue. In the liver, focal areas of necrosis may occur. The brain may show necrotizing granulomatous lesions and extensive calcifications (Fig. 2-3). The liver and spleen may have evidence of extramedullary hematopoiesis.

CLINICAL MANIFESTATIONS

The clinical manifestations of congenital and postnatal CMV infections include a broad spectrum. Both types of infection may range from an asymptomatic process associated with viruria and presence of specific antibody to a severe, widely disseminated disease involving virtually every organ in the body. The great majority of CMV infections, however, are totally inapparent.

Congenital infection

The typical clinical manifestations of severe generalized CMV infection are listed in Fig. 2-4. This fulminating illness is characterized by jaundice, hepatosplenomegaly, and petechial rash; it occurs several hours or days after birth in a newborn infant who usually is premature. Early onset of lethargy, respiratory distress, and convulsive seizures may be followed by fatal termination at any time from a few days to a few weeks later.

In infants who survive, jaundice may subside in as few as 2 weeks, or it may persist for months. The hemorrhagic phenomena subside rapidly. The hepatosplenomegaly may increase for the

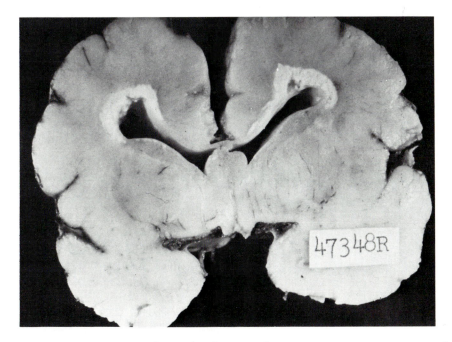

Fig. 2-3. Brain of an infant with congenital CMV infection. Note extensive periventricular necrosis and calcification.

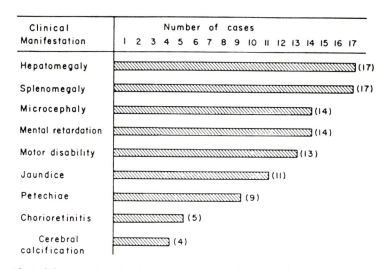

Clinical Manifestation	Number of cases 1 2 3 4 5 6 7 8 9 10 11 12 13 14 15 16 17
Hepatomegaly	(17)
Splenomegaly	(17)
Microcephaly	(14)
Mental retardation	(14)
Motor disability	(13)
Jaundice	(11)
Petechiae	(9)
Chorioretinitis	(5)
Cerebral calcification	(4)

Fig. 2-4. Clinical features in 17 infants with congenital CMV infection. (From Weller TH, Hanshaw JB. N Engl J Med 1962;266:1233.)

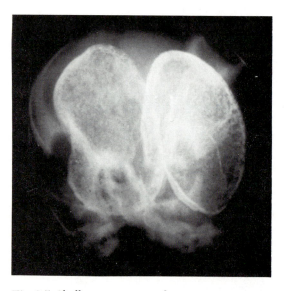

Fig. 2-5. Skull roentgenogram demonstrating massive intracranial calcifications of a 1-week-old infant with severe congenital cytomegalovirus infection.

first 2 to 4 months, persisting for a prolonged period thereafter. Chorioretinitis commonly occurs.

Laboratory findings usually include anemia and thrombocytopenia. The cerebrospinal fluid (CSF) may show pleocytosis and increased concentration of protein. Roentgenograms of the skull may reveal evidence of cerebral calcifications (Fig. 2-5). Examination of a *fresh* urine specimen sometimes reveals the inclusion bodies in cells of the urinary sediment. The virus can be isolated from urine, blood, or saliva. Recovery of virus is a more sensitive technique than cytology, which on occasion may give repeatedly negative results in the face of large quantities of virus isolated from the urine.

As indicated in Fig. 2-4, many affected infants have severe neurologic sequelae. Mental retardation and motor disability are common. In many infants microcephaly either is present at birth or becomes apparent in a few months. Other manifestations of cerebral damage include spasticity, diplegia, epileptiform seizures, and blindness. Deafness has also become apparent with increasing age. An excellent review by Hanshaw (1970) includes a summary of cerebral, ocular, and extraneural abnormalities associated with congenital CMV infection of 260 infants, from birth to 12 months of age. These defects may occur singly or in combination. The malformations caused by CMV appear to be the result of tissue necrosis rather than interference in organogenesis. Hanshaw (1983) also has pointed out that it is difficult to assess which, if any, of these developmental defects are actually caused by CMV.

Extensive overt disease is the exception in congenital CMV infection. More than 95% of congenitally infected infants are totally asymptomatic in the neonatal period (Alford et al., 1975). These inapparent CMV infections have been reported in 0.5% to 2.5% of all newborns. Although infants with occult CMV infections are clinically well at birth, they do have a significant risk of later developmental handicaps. Reynolds et al. (1974), Hanshaw et al. (1975), and Stagno (1977a) have demonstrated bilateral sensorineural hearing loss ranging from moderate to profound, and increased school failure rates associated with lowered IQ in 15% to 20% of congenitally infected CMV patients followed as long as 7 years.

Perinatal infection

Infants may be infected at the time of birth despite the presence of maternal CMV antibody, by passage through the maternal cervix where secretions harbor CMV due to reactivation infection. Perinatal infections, while common, are thought to be of little significance to the infant. About 2% to 5% of all newborn infants are so infected. The infants develop viruria at about 1 month of age, but they remain asymptomatic. All are seropositive both before and during infection.

Infants may also be infected after birth from either a maternal or nonmaternal source. Maternally derived infections are usually contracted through breast milk, presumably via lymphocytes infected with latent CMV. These infections are not accompanied by symptoms or sequelae.

On the other hand, when CMV is acquired by a seronegative infant from a nonmaternal source, a severe infection may occur. Yeager et al. (1972) described two low birth weight infants with CMV infections believed to have been acquired from blood transfusions. Subsequently Yeager (1974) determined that CMV infections occurred in 19 of 77 (25%) of high risk infants who were transfused and in only seven of 74 (11%) of those who were not.

Ballard et al. (1979) have also reported CMV infections in small premature infants who had received multiple blood transfusions in the first weeks of life. At about 6 weeks of age they developed hepatosplenomegaly, gray pallor, respiratory deterioration, lymphocytosis with atypical lymphocytes, and thrombocytopenia. Of 14 such infants, three died. Prospective studies indicated that these infants had acquired CMV infection in the intensive care nursery, most likely a result of multiple blood transfusions (mean of 21 separate blood units per infant). Unpasteurized banked breast milk is also a potential source of infection, especially for low birth weight infants.

Postnatal infection

Postnatal CMV infection in children, as well as infection in adults, is usually inapparent and asymptomatic. The clinical manifestations, when present, may be associated with specific involvement of the liver as well as a mononucleosis-like syndrome.

Evidence of a relation between an illness resembling infectious mononucleosis and CMV has been reported by Kääriäinen et al. (1966a). A significant rise of complement-fixing and neutralizing antibodies to CMV was described in four adult patients and one child, all of whom had a negative heterophil agglutination test. Illness in the four adults was characterized by fever lasting 2 to 5 weeks, cough, headache or pain in the back or limbs, a large number of atypical lymphocytes, and abnormal results of liver function tests. The 22-month-old child exhibited fever; migratory polyarthritis in the knees, fingers, and toes; skin rash with small red spots; and pneumonia. The pneumonia and arthritis cleared completely, and the child was well 2 months after discharge from the hospital. None of 19 patients with heterophil-positive infectious mononucleosis showed a significant rise in titer of complement-fixing antibodies to CMV.

An illness resembling infectious mononucleosis, with fever, rubelliform rash, atypical lymphocytes, but a negative heterophil antibody test, occurred in a 28-year-old woman 3 weeks after open-heart surgery, during which she received fresh blood from 14 donors. CMV was isolated from the urine 40 days after onset of illness, and the complement-fixing antibody rose from a titer of less than 1:4 at onset to 1:512 on the fortieth day. Moreover, a significant rise in complement-fixing antibodies to CMV was demonstrated in the absence of clinical manifestations of disease in eight of 20 successive patients after open-heart surgery accompanied by fresh-blood transfusion.

Systemic severe disease due to CMV is more likely to occur in immunocompromised than in normal persons. In a prospective study of 80 bone marrow transplant recipients, there were 43 episodes of interstitial pneumonia, about one half of which were believed to be due to CMV. Of the 43 patients, 28 died, many from CMV infection (Neiman et al., 1977). Severe CMV infections with fever, pneumonia, and chorioretinitis have been reported in children with underlying leukemia (Cox and Hughes, 1975).

In addition, there is a growing body of clinical and experimental evidence indicating that CMV is itself immunosuppressive. Patients with CMV mononucleosis have depressed in vitro cell-mediated immune responses (Ho, 1981). In a study of CMV infections in a day care center, three of four infants with *Haemophilus influenzae* infections were also simultaneously infected with CMV (Pass et al., 1982). Similarly in a series of 49 recipients of heart transplants, the incidence of bacterial and pneumocystis pulmonary infections was higher in the 11 patients with primary CMV infection after the transplant than in the 19 patients with evidence of CMV infection prior to transplantation (Rand et al., 1978). One of the contributing factors to immunosuppression seen in patients with the acquired immunodeficiency syndrome (AIDS) may be CMV infection.

DIAGNOSIS

The presence of CMV should be strongly considered in a newborn infant with enlargement of the liver and spleen, jaundice, petechial rash, microcephaly, thrombocytopenia, and cerebral calcification. Mental retardation and motor disability (and microcephaly) may become evident in older infants.

In older children and adults the possibility of CMV infection should be kept in mind (1) in instances of pneumonia in immunocompromised patients or in those with chronic debilitating diseases such as malignant tumors and leukemia, (2) in unexplained chronic liver disease, (3) in illnesses similar to infectious mononucleosis in which heterophil antibody tests are normal, (4) in patients receiving organ transplants, and (5) in children with AIDS (Scott et al., 1984).

The diagnosis may be confirmed by one or more of the following procedures: (1) examination of sediment of fresh urine or gastric contents for presence of the typical inclusion bodies located in the exfoliated cells, (2) biopsy of liver for histologic evidence of typical inclusion bodies, (3) identification of virus in tissue cultures inoculated with urine or biopsy specimens, or (4) appropriate use of one of the serologic tests for detection of CMV antibody, such as the neutralizing antibody test, complement fixation (CF) test, or indirect fluorescent antibody test.

As indicated in Fig. 2-6, CMV may persist in urine for prolonged periods of time. Urinary excretion of CMV by 99 infants congenitally infected, of whom 22 were symptomatic, and 33 infants perinatally infected is shown in Fig. 2-6 (Stagno et al., 1983). Symptomatic congenitally infected infants shed the greatest amount of virus. Those with perinatal infections usually began to shed virus between 4 and 8 weeks of age; in one such infant, shedding began at 3 weeks of age. Practically speaking, therefore, culture of urine for CMV during the first 2 weeks of life is necessary to distinguish between congenital and perinatal infection. As can be seen from Fig. 2-6, prolonged viral shedding by all infected infants is the rule. Diagnosis by urine culture thus may be problematic. A positive culture is conclusive in the newly born infant with obvious symptoms of CMV infection. Diagnosis of CMV in the infant asymptomatic at birth who later manifests developmental problems, statistically the most likely situation, however, is virtually impossible, because one cannot distinguish congenital from postnatal CMV infection by urine culture after the neonatal period. In addition, asymptomatic urinary shedding of CMV in infants with other infections has been documented (Florman et al., 1973). Isolation of CMV from cerebrospinal fluid (Jamison and Hathorn, 1978) is obviously significant although rather unusual.

Antibody titers to CMV are also often difficult to interpret. There are few differences in titers from babies with congenital and perinatal infections. Presumably any specific IgM present in an infant's serum is diagnostic of infection. An indirect immunofluorescence test for CMV IgM, described by Hanshaw et al. (1968), was positive only in infants with symptomatic congenital CMV infections. This test has yielded false-positive results in some other laboratories, how-

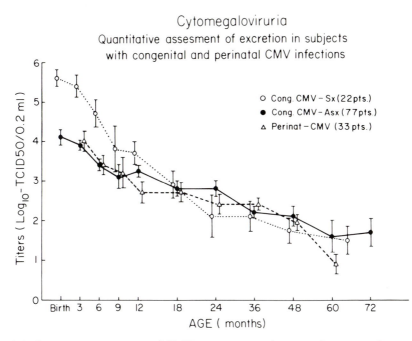

Fig. 2-6. Quantitive assessment of CMV excretion in subjects with congenital symptomatic *(open circles)*, congenital asymptomatic *(closed circles)*, and perinatal *(triangles)* infections. (From Stagno S, et al.: Semin Perinatol 1983;7:31-42. By permission.)

ever, and it is not generally available. A radioimmunoassay (RIA) for CMV IgM has been developed and tested by Griffiths et al. (1982a,b). These investigators have found CMV IgM in 17 of 17 (100%) infants with symptomatic CMV infections; 66 of 76 (87%) infants with asymptomatic infections also had detectable CMV IgM. Unfortunately, however, it is unlikely that this test will ever become widely available because of technical difficulties involved in the assay.

With this same assay, primary and recurrent maternal CMV infections were studied since only mothers with primary CMV developed CMV IgM. CMV IgM was detected by RIA in 6 of 29 (55%) women with primary CMV infection and in none of 18 women with recurrent infection. It was thus possible to identify high-risk pregnancies and infants with a high likelihood of symptomatic congenital CMV (Griffiths et al., 1982a,b). More data, however, are required to be certain that ISM develops only in primary CMV infection. An enzyme-linked immunosorbent assay (ELISA) procedure for CMV IgM has become available and is being evaluated. Obviously, more practical methods for diagnosis of CMV infections are needed.

Diagnosis of CMV syndromes other than congenital infection is usually based on virus isolation from urine as well as antibody titers. Diagnosis may often be difficult because shedding of CMV by normal persons may occur. Lee et al. (1978) have reported detection of CMV in urine specimens prepared for electron microscopic examination by the pseudoreplica technique. Recently CMV has been detected in urine samples using DNA hybridization techniques (Chou and Merigan, 1983). While low levels of CMV DNA could be detected in urine from some patients with asymptomatic shedding of virus, those with *disease* due to CMV were excreting much greater quantities of virus, and, therefore, this assay served to identify patients with illness due to CMV. With this same technique, CMV could also be detected in buffy coat cells from bone marrow transplant patients (Spector et al., 1983). A rise in CMV antibody titer associated with viruria is usually presumptive evidence of infection, if accompanied by suggestive clinical symptoms such as pneumonia or hepatitis. Many new techniques such as ELISA are being developed to measure CMV antibody titers. Since some of these tests report results as an optical density reading rather than as a titer, it is necessary to check with the laboratory for the range of normal values.

DIFFERENTIAL DIAGNOSIS

Congenital symptomatic CMV infection must be distinguished from a variety of infections and diseases that are characterized by jaundice, hepatosplenomegaly, and purpura in the neonatal period.

Congenital rubella syndrome

The consequences of fetal infection with rubella virus during the first trimester of pregnancy, which in the aggregate has been termed the *congenital rubella syndrome*, include features also seen in infants with CMV, such as hepatosplenomegaly, jaundice, petechial and purpuric rashes, thrombocytopenia, microcephaly, and mental retardation. The diagnosis of the rubella syndrome, suggested by a history of maternal infection in the first 3 to 4 months of pregnancy, should be confirmed by virologic and serologic evidence.

Congenital toxoplasmosis

The clinical picture of congenital toxoplasmosis is remarkably similar to that of generalized CMV. Both are characterized by jaundice, hepatosplenomegaly, chorioretinitis, and cerebral calcifications. Petechial and purpuric eruptions, which are common in CMV infections, are rare in toxoplasmosis. When toxoplasmosis involves the central nervous system (CNS), elevated protein levels and pleocytosis are often detected in CSF, findings much less frequently associated with CMV infections. The precise diagnosis may be established by serologic evidence of congenital toxoplasmosis or virologic and serologic evidence of CMV infection.

Erythroblastosis fetalis

The jaundice, purpura, and lethargy in an infant with erythroblastosis fetalis are associated with a positive Coombs' test. The serum alanine aminotransferase (ALT) activity, which is increased in CMV hepatitis, is within normal limits in erythroblastosis fetalis.

Disseminated herpes simplex infection

Although cerebral calcification has generally not been observed in this disease, a few cases have been reported with late appearance of calcium deposition. Skin lesions, which may be found in up to 80% of herpes simplex patients, are rare in CMV infections. Isolation of the virus and serologic studies are required to confirm a diagnosis of herpes simplex virus infection.

Sepsis of the newborn

Sepsis of the newborn may be characterized by lethargy, jaundice, and hepatomegaly. A blood culture usually reveals the causative organism.

Congenital syphilis

The unusual case of congenital syphilis can be differentiated from CMV infection by serologic tests and roentgenographic evidence of syphilitic osteitis.

EPIDEMIOLOGIC FACTORS

CMV infections are worldwide in distribution. Virologic and serologic studies have contributed to knowledge of the epidemiology of CMV infection. Surveys of unselected newborn infants in the United States and England have startlingly revealed a 1% to 2% incidence of viruria, indicative of congenital infection. Surveys of virus shedding in pregnant women from various countries have revealed incidences ranging from 1.9% to 5.6%. It is likely, therefore, that more than 30,000 infants with CMV infection are born each year in the United States. About 10% will manifest symptoms such as deafness and mild mental retardation. These findings suggest that congenital CMV infection is the most common fetal infection of humans.

The incidence of CMV infection is related to age, geographic location, and economic status. Serologic evidence of CMV infection increases with advancing age, reaching levels of 80% in various parts of the world. In general, infection is acquired at an earlier age by children who live under crowded, unhygienic conditions that may be prevalent in slum areas, institutions for mentally retarded children, and certain day-care centers.

The incidence of primary CMV during pregnancy is higher in upper- and middle-income women than in low-income women (Stagno et al., 1982a,b). Similarly, the incidence of congenital CMV is greater in highly industrialized nations than in developing countries. Acquisition of CMV in girls is a natural form of immunization that later prevents symptomatic CMV infection of offspring.

Intrauterine transmission of CMV after primary infection is thought to occur in about 40% of cases (Plotkin et al., 1984). Over 35% of postpartum women excrete reactivated CMV in breast milk, vaginal secretions, urine, or saliva. Approximately 20% of breast fed infants become infected with CMV (Stagno et al., 1983). One study of the risks of seronegative women acquiring a primary CMV infection in 122 pediatric health care workers revealed an annual attack rate of about 3%, similar to that of young women in the community (Dworsky et al., 1983). However, another study of 842 female employees in a pediatric hospital revealed that 5 of 45 (10.9%) intensive care nurses, 2 of 11 (18.2%) IV team nurses, and 3 of 81 (3.7%) ward nurses seroconverted to CMV after 1 year (Friedman et al., 1984).

There is increasing evidence for iatrogenic CMV disease in certain individuals. Some of these infections are undoubtedly reactivation syndromes that occur when immunosuppressive drugs are given to patients for underlying malignancy or organ transplantation. Others are primary infections caused by transfusions containing white blood cells harboring latent CMV, or transplantation of a kidney from a CMV seropositive donor into a CMV seronegative recipient (Ho et al., 1975). The risk of acquiring CMV from transfusion rises as increasing units of transfused blood and numbers of donors are used (Adler, 1983). Other CMV infections may be acquired by person-to-person spread.

The recent development of restriction endonuclease "fingerprinting" techniques has made it possible to document various transmissions of CMV. For example, transmission from mother to fetus has been demonstrated (Huang et al., 1980) as has transmission from infant to mother (Spector and Spector, 1982). On the other hand, two CMV infections in medical staff personnel known to have been exposed to a patient with CMV were shown to have been infected from a different source (Wilfert et al., 1982; Yow et al., 1982). Data from one of these cases are shown in Fig. 2-7. A pregnant physician who contracted CMV while caring for a baby with CMV had her pregnancy terminated. As indicated in Fig. 2-7, DNA of the CMV isolated from the physician-

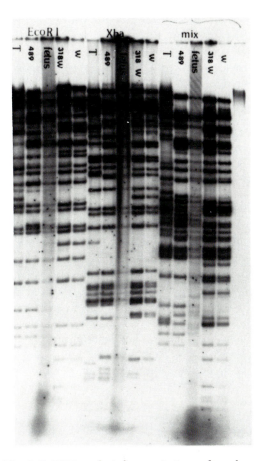

Fig. 2-7. DNA analysis by restriction endonucleases obtained from *T*, Towne (control) strain of CMV; *489*, mother's CMV; *fetus*, fetal CMV; *318W* and *W*, CMV of index case. Fetus and 489 are similar but different from 318W and W.

mother and her fetus were similar but different from the DNA isolated from the index case, indicating that the source of the physician's infection was not her patient.

PROGNOSIS

Infants who survive generalized CMV infection usually have severe neurologic sequelae. Microcephaly, mental retardation, and motor disability are the results of brain damage caused by CMV infection. Of 16 patients followed by Weller and Hanshaw (1962), only two failed to show residual damage. Of 34 patients with congenital symptomatic CMV infections followed for 9 months to 14 years, 10 died, 16 (70%) had microcephaly, 14 (61%) had mental retardation, seven (30%) had hearing loss, eight (35%) had neuromuscular disorders, and five (22%) had chorioretinitis or optic atrophy (Pass et al., 1980).

The many infants who have asymptomatic congenital CMV infection may show no effects until later childhood when some manifest hearing loss and school failure (Reynolds et al., 1974; Hanshaw et al., 1975; Stagno et al., 1977a). Current studies suggest this may occur in as many as 10% of congenitally infected children. With approximately 3.5 million births annually in the United States this could involve 3500 school children each year.

Infants infected in the perinatal period rarely if ever manifest sequelae, with the exception of seronegative premature infants inadvertently infected with CMV by blood or banked breast milk containing latent virus. Some of these infants have developed pneumonia, shock, and hematologic abnormalities thought to be due to CMV (Ballard et al., 1979). The long-term prognosis for these infants is unknown.

Evaluation of the prognosis in immunocompromised older children and adults is often complicated by the underlying condition for which the patient has received immunosuppressive drugs (leukemia, cancer, and organ transplantations). Renal transplant patients who acquire CMV may manifest fever, pneumonia, chorioretinitis, and hepatitis, all caused by CMV itself, as well as severe bacterial, protozoal, and fungal superinfections. Pneumonia caused by CMV in bone marrow transplant patients is usually fatal. The prognosis of primary CMV infection in severely immunocompromised patients is very grave.

In immunocompetent patients with disease resembling infectious mononucleosis the outlook for complete recovery appears to be excellent.

TREATMENT
Preventive measures

While no proved method is available for prevention of severe CMV infections, several approaches are under investigation.

Experimental live CMV vaccines are being evaluated by various investigators. Studies by Elek and Stern (1974) and Plotkin et al. (1976) have revealed that it is possible to prepare a live CMV vaccine that is well tolerated and antigenic. The subject has been well reviewed by Lang

(1980). Preliminary data from Plotkin's studies in immunized renal transplant patients suggest that while infection with CMV is not prevented by prior immunization, the illness may be modified (Plotkin et al., 1984).

Questions that have been raised about a live CMV vaccine include (1) the degree of its attenuation, (2) its potential to become oncogenic, (3) its potential to induce a persistent infection, (4) the duration of immunity, and (5) whether it will protect against disease. Present and future studies will clarify the safety and possibly the efficacy of this vaccine.

Several approaches to prevention of CMV infection in low birth weight hospitalized infants may be taken. Infants to be breast-fed may be given milk from their own mothers only, frozen or pasteurized banked human breast milk, or a prepared formula. Unfortunately, any cellular immunity present in milk that is theoretically of potential benefit to the infant will be destroyed along with the virus by pasteurization or freezing. The infectivity of CMV is lost after freezing (except at very low temperatures, such as $-70°$ C) or heating to $62°$ C (pasteurization). Prevention of CMV infections in infants may also be accomplished by use of blood from seronegative donors only or by use of frozen red blood cells (Yeager et al., 1981; Adler, 1983).

While only CMV seronegative infants are at risk, most hospitals do not test babies for CMV antibodies. Appropriate preventive measures are therefore best carried out for all low birth weight infants unless CMV antibody determinations are performed.

Hyperimmune globulin has been found to reduce the incidence of severe CMV infections in bone marrow transplant patients (Meyers et al., 1983; Condie and O'Reilly, 1984). Interferon prophylaxis has been found to reduce clinical signs of CMV reactivation syndromes in renal transplant patients (Hirsch et al., 1983).

Therapy

No specific treatment is available. The in vitro synthesis of CMV is inhibited by adenine arabinoside (Ara-A). Treatment with Ara-A has resulted in transient reductions of virus shedding but no evidence of clinical improvement. Other experimental approaches have included the administration of interferon and transfer factor.

General supportive measures are indicated, including transfusions of sedimented red blood cells for anemia and transfusions of platelet-rich plasma for thrombocytopenia. Antimicrobial agents are indicated only for patients with concurrent bacterial infections or in instances in which the diagnosis of sepsis of the newborn infant has not been excluded.

REFERENCES

Adler SP. Transfusion-associated cytomegalovirus infections. Rev Infect Dis 1983;5:977-993.

Ahlfors D, Harris S, Ivarsson S, et al. Secondary maternal cytomegalovirus infection causing symptomatic congenital infection. N Engl J Med 1981;305:284.

Alexander ER. Maternal and neonatal infection with cytomegalovirus in Taiwan. Pediatr Res 1967;1:210.

Alford CA, Jr, Reynolds DW, Stagno S. Current concepts of chronic perinatal infections. In Gluck L, editor: Modern perinatal medicine. Chicago; Year Book Medical Publishers, Inc., 1975.

Andrewes CH. Immunity to the salivary virus of guinea pigs studied in the living animal, and in tissue culture. Br J Exp Pathol 1930;11:23.

Ballard RA, Drew WL, Hufnagle KG, et al. Acquired cytomegalovirus infection in preterm infants. Am J Dis Child 1979;133:482.

Benyesh-Melnick M, Dessy SI, Fernbach DJ. Cytomegaloviruria in children with acute leukemia and in other children. Proc Soc Exp Biol Med 1964;117:624.

Brandt JA, Kettering JD, Lewis JE. Immunity to human cytomegalovirus measured and compared by complement fixation, indirect fluorescent-antibody, indirect hemagglutination, and enzyme-linked immunosorbent assays. J Clin Microsc 1984;19:147.

Chou S, Merigan TC. Rapid detection and quantitation of human cytomegalovirus in urine through DNA hybridization. N Engl J Med 1983;308:921-925.

Cole R, Kuttner AG. A filtrable virus present in the submaxillary glands of guinea pigs. J Exp Med 1926;44:855.

Condie RM, O'Reilly RJ. Prevention of cytomegalovirus infection by prophylaxis with an intravenous, hyperimmune, native, unmodified cytomegalovirus globulin. Am J Med 1984;76:134-141.

Cox F, Hughes WT. Cytomegalovirus in children with acute lymphatic leukemia. J Pediatr 1975;87:190.

Diosi P, Babusceac L, Nevinglovschi O, et al. Cytomegalovirus infection associated with pregnancy. Lancet 1967;2:1063.

Dworsky M, Stagno S, Pass RF, et al. Persistence of cytomegalovirus in human milk after storage. J Pediatr 1982;101:440-443.

Dworsky ME, Welch K, Cassady G, et al. Occupational risk for primary cytomegalovirus infection among pediatric health-care workers. N Engl J Med 1983;309:950-953.

Dworsky M, Yow M, Stagno S, et al. Cytomegalovirus infection of breast milk and transmission in infancy. Pediatrics 1983;72:295-299.

Elek SC, Stern H. Development of a vaccine against mental retardation caused by cytomegalovirus infection in utero. Lancet 1974;1:1.

Faix RG, Zweig SE, Kummer JF, et al. Cytomegalovirus-specific cell-mediated immunity during pregnancy in lower socioeconomic class adolescents. J Infect Dis 1983;148:621-629.

Farber S, Wolbach SB. Intranuclear and cytoplasmic inclusions (protozoan-like bodies) in salivary glands and other organs of infants. Am J Pathol 1932;8:123.

Florman AL, Gershon AA, Blackett PR, et al. Intrauterine infection with herpes simplex virus. JAMA 1973;225:129-132.

Friedman HM, Lewis MR, Nemerofsky DM, et al. Acquisition of cytomegalovirus infection among female employees at a pediatric hospital. Pediatr Infect Dis 1984;3:233-235.

Goodpasture EW, Talbot FB. Concerning the nature of "protozoan-like" cells in certain lesions of infancy. Am J Dis Child 1921;21:415.

Griffith PD, Stagno S, Pass RF, et al. Infection with cytomegalovirus during pregnancy: specific IgM antibodies as a marker of recent primary infection. J Infect Dis 1982;145:647-653.

Griffiths PD, Stagno S, Pass RF, et al. Congenital cytomegalovirus infection: diagnostic and prognostic significance of the detection of specific immunoglobulin M antibodies in cord serum. Pediatrics 1982b;69:544-549.

Hanshaw JB. Viruses in circulating lymphocytes. N Engl J Med 1969;280:1353.

Hanshaw JB. Developmental abnormalities associated with congenital cytomegalovirus infection. Adv Teratol 1970;4:64.

Hanshaw JB. Cytomegalovirus. In Remington JS, Klein JO, eds. Infections of the fetus and newborn infant. 2nd ed. Philadelphia: W.B. Saunders Co, 1983.

Hanshaw JB, Betts RF, Simon G, et al. Acquired cytomegalovirus infection. Association with hepatomegaly and abnormal liver function tests. N Engl J Med 1965;272:602.

Hanshaw JB, Steinfeld HJ, White CJ. Fluorescent-antibody test for cytomegalovirus macroglobulin. N Engl J Med 1968;279:566.

Hanshaw JB, Weller TH. Urinary excretion of cytomegaloviruses by children with generalized neoplastic disease: correlation with clinical and histopathologic observations. J Pediatr 1961;58:305.

Hanshaw JB, et al. CNS sequelae of congenital cytomegalovirus infection. Infections of the fetus and the newborn infant. Prog Clin Biol Res 1975;3:47.

Hirsch M, Schooley RT, Cosimi AB, et al. Effects of interferon alpha on cytomegalovirus reactivation syndromes in renal-transplant recipients. N Engl J Med 1983;308:1489-1493.

Ho M. The lymphocyte in infections with Epstein-Barr virus and cytomegalovirus. J Infect Dis 1981;143:857-862.

Ho M, Suwansirkul S, Dowling JN, et al. The transplanted kidney as a source of cytomegalovirus infection. N Engl J Med 1975;293:1109.

Huang ES, Alford CA, Reynolds DW, et al. Molecular epidemiology of cytomegalovirus infections in women and their infants. N Engl J Med 1980;303:958-962.

Jamison RM, Hathorn AW. Isolation of cytomegalovirus from cerebrospinal fluid of a congenitally infected infant. Am J Dis Child 1978; 132:63-64.

Kääriäinen L, Klemola E, Paloheimo J. Rise of cytomegalovirus antibodies in an infectious mononucleosis-like syndrome after transfusion. Br Med J 1966a;2:1270.

Kääriäinen L, et al. Cytomegalovirus-mononucleosis. Isolation of the virus and demonstration of subclinical infections after fresh blood transfusion in connection with open-heart surgery. Ann Med Exp Biol Fenn 1966b;44:297.

Kanich RE, Craighead JE. Cytomegalovirus infection and cytomegalic inclusion disease in renal homotransplant recipients. Am J Med 1966;40:874.

Kluge RC, Wicksman RS, Weller TH. Cytomegalic inclusion disease of newborn: report of a case with persistent viremia. Pediatrics 1960;25:35.

Krugman RD, Goodheart CR. Human cytomegalovirus: thermal inactivation. Virology 1964;23:290.

Lamb SG, Stern H. Cytomegalovirus mononucleosis with jaundice as presenting sign. Lancet 1966;2:1003.

Lang DJ. Cytomegalovirus immunization: status, prospects, and problems. Rev Infect Dis 1980;2:449-458.

Lang DJ, Hanshaw JB. Cytomegalovirus infection and the post perfusion syndrome: recognition of primary infections in four patients. N Engl J Med 1969;280:1145.

Lang DJ, Kummer JF. Cytomegalovirus in semen: observations in selected populations. J Infect Dis 1975;132:472.

Lee FK, Nahmias AJ, Stagno S. Rapid diagnosis of cytomegalovirus infection in infants by electron microscopy. N Engl J Med 1978;299:1266.

McAllister RM, Straw RM, Filbert JE, et al. Human cytomegalovirus. Cytochemical observations of intracellular lesion development correlated with viral synthesis and release. Virology 1963;19:521.

McAllister RM, Wright HT, Jr, Tasem WM. Cytomegalic inclusion disease in newborn twins. J Pediatr 1964;64:278.

Medearis DN Jr. Cytomegalic inclusion disease: analysis of clinical features based on literature and six additional cases. Pediatrics 1957;19:467.

Medearis DN Jr. Observations concerning human cytomegalovirus infection and disease. Johns Hopkins Med J 1964;114:181.

Meyers JD, Leszczynski J, Zaia JA, et al. Prevention of cytomegalovirus infection by cytomegalovirus immune globulin after marrow transplantation. Ann Intern Med 1983;98:442-446.

Neff BJ, et al. Clinical and laboratory studies of live cytomegalovirus vaccine Ad-169. Proc Soc Exp Biol Med 1979;160:32.

Neiman PE, Reeves W, Ray G, et al. A prospective analysis of interstitial pneumonia and opportunistic viral infection among recipients of allogeneic bone marrow grafts. J Infect Dis 1977;136:754-767.

Panjvani ZFK, Hanshaw JB. Cytomegalovirus in the perinatal period. Am J Dis Child 1981;135:56-60.

Pass RF, Stagno S, Myers G, et al. Outcome of symptomatic congenital cytomegalovirus infection: results of long term longitudinal follow-up. Pediatrics 1980;66:758-762.

Plotkin SA, Farquhar J, Hornberger E. Clinical trials of immunization with the Towne 125 strain of human cytomegalovirus. J Infect Dis 1976;134:470-475.

Plotkin SA, Michelson S, Alford CA, et al. The pathogenesis and prevention of human cytomegalovirus infection. Pediatr Infect Dis 1984;3:67-74.

Rand KH, Pollard RB, Merigan TC. Increased pulmonary superinfections in cardiac-transplant patients undergoing primary cytomegalovirus infection. N Engl J Med 1978; 298:951.

Reynolds DW, et al. Maternal cytomegalovirus excretion and perinatal infection. N Engl J Med 1973;289:1.

Reynolds DW, et al. Inapparent congenital cytomegalovirus infection with elevated cord IgM levels. Causal relation with auditory and mental deficiency. N Engl J Med 1974;290:291.

Reynolds DW, Dean PH, Pass RF, et al. Specific cell-mediated immunity in children with congenital and neonatal cytomegalovirus infection and their mothers. J Infect Dis 1979;140:493-499.

Rola-Pleszczynski M, et al. Specific impairment of cell-mediated immunity in mothers of infants with congenital infection due to cytomegalovirus. J Infect Dis 1977; 135:386.

Rowe WP, et al. Cytopathogenic agent resembling human salivary gland virus recovered from tissue cultures of human adenoids. Proc Soc Exp Biol Med 1956;92:4181.

Scott GB, Buck BE, Leterman JG, et al. Acquired immunodeficiency syndrome in infants. N Engl J Med 1984; 310:76-81.

Smith KO, Rasmussen L. Morphology of cytomegalovirus (salivary gland virus). J Bacteriol 1963;85:1319.

Smith MG. Propagation of salivary gland virus of the mouse in tissue cultures. Proc Soc Exp Biol Med 1954;86:435.

Smith MG. Propagation in tissue cultures of a cytopathogenic virus from human salivary gland virus (SGV) disease. Proc Soc Exp Biol Med 1956;92:424.

Spector SA, Rua LA, Spector DH, et al. Rapid diagnosis of CMV viremia in bone marrow transplant patients by DNA-DNA hybridization. Abstract 914 of the Twenty-Third Interscience Conference in Antimicrobial Agents and Chemotherapy, Las Vegas, Nevada, 1983.

Spector SA, Schmidt K, Ticknor W, et al. Cytomegaloviruria in older infants in intensive care nurseries. J Pediatr 1979;95:444.

Spector SA, Spector DH. Molecular epidemiology of cytomegalovirus infections in premature twin infants and their mother. Pediatr Infect Dis 1982;1:405-409.

Stagno S, Brasfield DM, Brown MB, et al. Infant pneumonitis associated with cytomegalovirus, chlamydia, pneumocystis, and ureaplasma: a prospective study. Pediatrics 1981;68:322-329.

Stagno S, Dworsky ME, Tores J, et al. Prevalence and importance of congenital cytomegalovirus infection in three different populations. J Pediatr 1982a;101:897-900.

Stagno S, Pass RF, Dworsky ME, et al. Congenital cytomegalovirus infection. The relative importance of primary and recurrent maternal infection. N Engl J Med 1982b; 306:945-949.

Stagno S, Pass R, Dworsky M, et al. Congenital and perinatal cytomegalovirus infections. Semin Perinatol 1983;7:31.

Stagno S, Pass R, Thomas JP, et al. Defects of tooth structure in congenital cytomegalovirus infection. Pediatrics 1982c;69:646.

Stagno S, Reynolds DW, Pass RF, et al. Breast milk and the risk of cytomegalovirus infection. N Engl J Med 1980; 302:1073-1076.

Stagno S, Reynolds DW, Tsiantos A, et al. Comparative serial virologic and serologic studies of symptomatic and subclinical congenitally and natally acquired cytomegalovirus infections. J Infect Dis 1975;132:568-577.

Stagno S, et al. Congenital cytomegalovirus infection: consecutive occurrence due to viruses with similar antigenic compositions. Pediatrics 1973;52:788.

Stagno S, et al. Auditory and visual defects resulting from symptomatic and subclinical congenital cytomegaloviral and toxoplasma infections. Pediatrics 1977a;59:669.

Stagno S, et al. Congenital cytomegalovirus infection. Occurrence in an immune population. N Engl J Med 1977b;296:1254.

Starr SE, Tolpin MD, Friedman HM, et al. Impaired cellular immunity to cytomegalovirus in congenitally infected children and their mothers. J Infect Dis 1979;140:500-505.

Von Glahn WC, Pappenheimer AM. Intranuclear inclusions in visceral disease. Am J Pathol 1925;1:445

Wahren B, Espmark A, Wallden G. Serological studies on cytomegalovirus infection in relation to infectious mononucleosis and similar conditions. Scand J Infect Dis 1969;1:145.

Weller TH. The cytomegaloviruses: ubiquitous agents with protean clinical manifestations. N Engl J Med 1971;285:203-214.

Weller TH, and Hanshaw, JB. Virologic and clinical observations on cytomegalic inclusion disease. N Engl J Med 1962;26:1233.

Weller TH, Hanshaw JB, Scott DE. Serologic differentiation of viruses responsible for cytomegalic inclusion disease. Virology 1960;12:130.

Weller TH, Macaulay JC, Craig JM, et al. Isolation of intranuclear inclusion agents from infants and illnesses resembling cytomegalic inclusion disease. Proc Soc Exp Biol Med 1957;94:4.

Whitley RJ, Brasfield D, Reynolds DW, et al. Protracted pneumonitis in young infants associated with perinatally acquired cytomegaloviral infection. J Pediatr 1976;89:16-22.

Wilfert CM, Huang ES, Stagno S. Restriction endonuclease analysis of cytomegalovirus deoxyribonucleic acid as an epidemiologic tool. Pediatrics 1982;70:717-721.

Yeager AS. Transfusion-acquired cytomegalovirus infection in newborn infants. Am J Dis Child 1974;128:478-483.

Yeager AS, Grumet FC, Hafleigh EB, et al. Prevention of transfusion-acquired cytomegalovirus infections in newborn infants. J Pediatr 1981;98:281-287.

Yeager AS, Jacobs H, Clark J. Nursery-acquired cytomegalovirus infection in two premature infants. J Pediatr 1972;81:332-335.

Yow MD, Lakeman AD, Stagno S, et al. Use of restriction enzymes to investigate the source of a primary cytomegalovirus infection in a pediatric nurse. Pediatrics 1982;70:713-716.

3

DIPHTHERIA

Diphtheria is an acute infectious preventable disease caused by *Corynebacterium diphtheriae*. The microorganism produces an exotoxin that is responsible for the resulting pathologic process. The disease is characterized clinically by a sore throat and a membrane that may cover the tonsils, pharynx, and larynx. It is occasionally followed by myocarditis and neuritis.

In developed areas of the world diphtheria is so rare today that it is thought to be of little importance, and therefore it is neglected in the differential diagnosis. In many developing countries, however, it is still prevalent, and importation of cases may occur with jet plane speed.

HISTORY

The recognition of diphtheria as a disease probably dates back to the second century. It was in 1826, however, that Bretonneau accurately described the clinical manifestations and gave it its name *la diphthérite*. He distinguished scarlet fever from diphtheria and identified membranous croup as a form of diphtheria. A century of progress culminated in 1923 in the development of a safe and effective vaccine capable of conquering the disease.

The diphtheria bacillus was discovered by Klebs in 1883 and was isolated in pure culture by Löffler. It was called the Klebs-Löffler bacillus, and its etiologic relationship to the disease was demonstrated in 1884. Roux and Yersin in 1888 showed that the bacillus produced an exotoxin that was responsible for the various clinical manifestations of the disease, such as myocarditis and neuritis. In 1893 von Behring reported that the toxin stimulated the production of antitoxin. Schick described his intradermal test for immunity in 1913. In the same year, von Behring used toxin neutralized by antitoxin to induce immunity in animals and humans. A large-scale immunization program to protect children was initiated by Park in 1922. Finally, in 1923 Ramon showed that formalin-treated toxin, currently known as *toxoid*, was superior to toxin-antitoxin as an immunizing agent.

ETIOLOGY

The causative agent of diphtheria, *C. diphtheriae*, has characteristic properties related to its morphologic traits, cultivation, and ability to produce toxin.

Morphology

C. diphtheriae organisms are slender gram-positive rods that measure 2 to 4 μm by 0.5 to 1 μm. They vary in diameter, and the ends are broader than the center, producing a typical club-shaped appearance. In suboptimal media the protoplasm is irregularly distributed in the cells, producing a beaded or bandlike appearance. The metachromatic granules are accumulations of polymerized polyphosphates. The bacteria appear in palisades or as individual cells at sharp angles to each other. These V and L or Chinese-letter formations result from a snapping movement when two cells divide.

Cultural characteristics

C. diphtheriae are facultative aerobes and anerobes. The organism was isolated by Löffler on a medium containing coagulated blood serum, which inhibited the growth of pneumococci and streptococci. Potassium tellurite has a similar effect and is superior to Löffler's medium. By using selective tellurite media, it is possible to differentiate three colonial types of *C. diphtheriae*—gravis, mitis, and intermedius. No constant relationship exists between colonial type and disease severity.

C. diphtheriae is an antigenically heterogeneous species with a large number of serologic types. The different colonial types reflect cell surface differences. Heat-labile K antigens, which are proteins of the superficial cell wall, are responsible for type specificity. These multiple surface antigens are probably the reason the host can be colonized by *C. diphtheriae* despite previous experience with the organism.

The heat-stable O antigen is a group antigen common to the corynebacteria parasitic to humans. The O antigen is a polysaccharide containing arabinogalactans and is responsible for cross-reactivity with mycobacteria and *Nocardia*.

Colonization of mucous membranes can be accomplished by both toxigenic and nontoxigenic strains. The organisms have a cord factor, a toxic glycolipid, considered a necessary adjunct of virulence.

The most important characteristic of the diphtheria bacillus is its ability to produce an exotoxin both in vivo and in vitro. This toxin is responsible for many of the serious clinical manifestations of the disease. It is extremely unstable and is easily destroyed by heat (75° C for 10 minutes), light, and aging. Toxin is produced only by strains of *C. diphtheriae* that are lysogenic for a bacteriophage carrying the tox gene. Thus, a person may harbor *C. diphtheriae* and acquire one of the many phages that convert the bacterium to a toxin producer. Toxin production does not require lytic growth of the phage. The tox gene can be expressed when the phage is vegetatively growing and is present as a prophage or as a superinfecting, nonreplicating exogenote in lysogenic cells.

Diphtheria toxin is maximally produced when iron is the growth rate–limiting substrate. It seems that iron favors the formation of a repressor-iron complex that binds to the phage tox operator locus and prevents toxin formation. When the iron concentration is lowered, dissociation of the complex from the tox operator locus occurs and toxin is produced.

The toxin is synthesized and released extracellularly as a single inactive polypeptide chain. Cleavage of the molecule into two fragments, A and B, and reduction of disulfide bonds must occur to activate the toxin. Fragment B is unstable, is not enzymatically active, and is required for attachment of the activated toxin molecule to receptors of sensitive host cells, which then allows penetration of fragment A into the cell. All human cells have receptor sites that may be glycoproteins for fragment B, and the binding is rapid and irreversible.

Diphtheria toxin receptors on a cell membrane appear to concentrate in a "coated pit," and toxin penetrates cells by endocytosis. This enfolding and vesicle formation provide access of the toxin to the interior of the cell. The subsequent natural acidification of the endosome containing the toxin results in the passage of toxin across the membrane of the endosome to the cytosol. Species such as mice and rats are resistant to toxin and contrary to early ideas do not lack plasma membrane receptors for the toxin. Receptors are present in these species, but the transport process is defective and toxin cannot reach the cytosol of the cell.

Fragment A is extremely stable, enzymatically active, and responsible for the toxic effects, which are achieved by inhibition of cellular protein synthesis. Fragment A inactivates elongation factor 2 (EF-2), which is a protein common to all eukaryotic cells. This protein is essential for translocation of peptidyl transfer RNA on ribosomes. There is a single site on EF-2 that is adenosine diphosphate (ADP)-ribosylated. This is an unusual amino acid now named *diphthamide*.

PATHOGENESIS AND PATHOLOGY

Virulent diphtheria bacilli lodge in the nasopharynx of susceptible persons. As bacterial growth takes place in the secretions and epithelial debris, the toxin is elaborated and absorbed by the local mucous membrane. The toxic effect on the cells causes tissue necrosis, which provides fertile soil for further growth of the organism and production of more toxin. A vicious cycle is set up. As the process extends, more and more tissue is destroyed in ever-increasing circumference and depth.

In addition to the necrosis, an inflammatory and exudative reaction is also induced by the toxin. The necrotic epithelial cells, leukocytes, red blood cells, fibrinous material, diphtheria bacilli, and other bacterial inhabitants of the nasopharynx—all these elements—combine to form the typical membrane. The superficial epithelial cells of the mucosa form an integral part of the membrane and cause it to be adherent; attempts to separate it are followed by bleeding and the formation of a new membrane. It sloughs off during the recovery period.

The toxin produced at the site of the membrane is distributed via the bloodstream to tissues all over the body. The size of the membrane usually reflects the amount of toxin produced—the larger the membrane is, the more toxin is available for absorption. The site of the membrane influences the amount of toxin absorbed; the toxin reaches the circulation more readily from the pharynx and tonsils than from the larynx and trachea. Consequently, laryngotracheal diphtheria produces less toxemia than pharyngotonsillar involvement. On the other hand, the obstruction of the airway by the laryngotracheal membrane may have serious consequences.

All human cells are potentially susceptible to toxin, as they have receptors and EF-2. Differential effects on various tissues are observed and poorly explained. In vitro, endothelial cells are far more sensitive to toxin than myocardial cells, leading to the hypothesis that initial damage may be vascular with ischemic secondary effects compounding the effects of toxin. It is also possible that the rate of protein synthesis is less in myocardium, so the time course of effects could be slower. The maximal pathologic effects of fatty degeneration and fibrosis are seen after the first week, correlating with clinical symptoms of myocarditis that usually develop from 10 to 14 days after onset.

Nervous system manifestations occur from 3 to 7 weeks after onset. Pathologically, peripheral lesions are limited to a few millimeters of segmental degeneration of myelin visible within posterior root ganglia and adjacent anterior and posterior roots with sparing of axis cylinders. Macrophages ingest myelin, but otherwise there is little inflammation. It has been suggested that

Schwann cells are sensitive to toxin and that degeneration of existing myelin in the absence of protein synthesis leads in time to development of segmental lesions. When myelinization is resumed, recovery occurs.

In rare instances virulent diphtheria bacilli may contaminate the skin of a susceptible individual, usually at the site of a wound. The resulting lesion is an ulcer with sharply demarcated edges and a gray membranous base.

CLINICAL MANIFESTATIONS

Diphtheria develops after a short incubation period of 2 to 4 days, with a range of 1 to 5 days. For clinical purposes it is convenient to classify the disease in accordance with the anatomic location of the membrane. The following types of diphtheria may occur: (1) nasal, (2) tonsillar (faucial), (3) pharyngeal, (4) laryngeal or laryngotracheal, and (5) nonrespiratory, including skin wounds and conjunctival and genital lesions. More than one anatomic site may be involved at the same time.

Nasal diphtheria

The onset of nasal diphtheria is indistinguishable from that of the common cold. It is characterized by a nasal discharge and a lack of constitutional symptoms. Fever, if present, is usually low grade. The nasal discharge, which at first is serous, subsequently becomes serosanguineous. In some cases there may be frank epistaxis. The discharge, which may be unilateral or bilateral, becomes mucopurulent and usually excoriates the anterior nares and upper lip, giving rise to an impetigious appearance. The discharge may obscure the presence of a white membrane on the nasal septum. The poor absorption of toxin from this site accounts for the mildness of the disease and the paucity of constitutional symptoms. In the untreated patient the nasal discharge may persist for many days or weeks. This rich source of diphtheria bacilli becomes a menace to all susceptible contacts. The infection can be terminated rapidly by antibiotic therapy.

Tonsillar and pharyngeal diphtheria

The illness usually begins insidiously with malaise, anorexia, sore throat, and low-grade fever. Within 24 hours a patch of exudate or membrane appears in the faucial area. When completely formed, the membrane varies in extent from a small patch on one tonsil to extensive involvement of both tonsils, uvula, soft palate, and pharyngeal wall (Plate 1). It is smooth, adherent, and white or gray in color; in the presence of bleeding it may be black. Forcible attempts to remove it are followed by bleeding.

Pharyngotonsillar involvement is characterized by a variable amount of cervical adenitis and periadenitis. In severe cases the marked swelling produces a so-called bull neck appearance.

The course of the illness depends in large part on the severity of the toxemia. The temperature remains either normal or slightly elevated, but the pulse is disproportionately rapid. In mild cases, the membrane sloughs off between the seventh and tenth days, and the patient has an uneventful recovery. Very severe cases are characterized by increasing toxemia manifested by severe prostration, striking pallor, rapid thready pulse, stupor, coma, and death within 6 to 10 days. In moderately severe cases convalescence is slow, with the course frequently complicated by myocarditis and neuritis (see Complications).

Laryngeal diphtheria

Laryngeal diphtheria most often develops as an extension of pharyngeal involvement. Occasionally, however, it may be the only manifestation of the disease. The illness is ushered in by fever, hoarseness, and cough, which develops a barking quality. Increasing obstruction of the airway by the membrane is manifested by inspiratory stridor followed by suprasternal, supraclavicular, and subcostal retractions. The membrane in some severe cases of laryngeal diphtheria extends downward to involve the entire tracheobronchial tree.

In mild cases or in those modified by antitoxin therapy the airway remains patent, and the membrane is coughed up between the sixth and tenth days. In very severe cases there is increasing obstruction followed by progressive anoxemia, which is manifested by restlessness, cyanosis, severe prostration, coma, and death. A sudden acute and fatal obstruction may occur in a mild case in which a partially detached piece of membrane blocks the airway.

The clinical picture of laryngeal diphtheria is dominated by the consequences of the mechanical obstruction to the air passages caused by the membrane, congestion, and edema. Signs of toxemia are minimal in primary laryngeal involvement, because toxin is poorly absorbed from the mucous membrane of the larynx. In most instances, however, the laryngeal involvement is associated with tonsillar and pharyngeal diphtheria. Consequently, the clinical manifestations are those of both obstruction and severe toxemia.

Unusual types of diphtheria

Diphtheritic infections may occasionally develop in sites other than the respiratory tract. Cutaneous, conjunctival, aural, and vulvovaginal infections may occur (Belsey, 1975). The typical skin lesion is an ulcer with sharply demarcated edges and a membranous base. The conjunctival lesion primarily involves the palpebral part, which is reddened, edematous, and membranous. Involvement of the external auditory canal is usually manifest by a persistent purulent discharge. Vulvovaginal lesions are usually ulcerative and confluent.

DIAGNOSIS

An early diagnosis of diphtheria is essential because delay of administration of antitoxin may impose a serious and preventable risk to the patient. Accurate bacteriologic confirmation by means of culture requires a minimum of 15 to 20 hours; smears are not reliable. Consequently, the initial diagnosis, as a basis for therapy, must be made on clinical grounds alone. Occasionally, a rapidly executed blood smear and heterophil antibody test may point to a diagnosis of infectious mononucleosis and obviate the need for antitoxin.

Bacteriologic diagnosis

An accurate diagnosis of diphtheria is made by the demonstration of diphtheria bacilli cultured from material obtained from the site of infection. Care should be exercised in taking the culture. The swab should be rubbed firmly over the lesion or, if possible, should be inserted beneath the membrane. Then a Löffler slant, a blood agar plate, and a tellurite plate should be streaked with the swab. The slant and plates should be placed in the incubator without delay. After incubation, the organisms on the plates should be identified by an experienced person.

Diphtheria bacilli that are isolated on culture

should be tested for toxigenicity by means of a virulence test. Two guinea pigs are inoculated intracutaneously with a broth suspension of the test microorganisms; one of the animals should be pretreated with diphtheria antitoxin. If the bacilli are toxigenic, an inflammatory lesion will appear at the site of inoculation in 24 hours, and it will become necrotic in 72 hours. The antitoxin-treated animal will show no skin reaction.

DIFFERENTIAL DIAGNOSIS

The differential diagnosis of diphtheria varies with the particular anatomic site of involvement. In all types of possible diphtheria, the patient's immunization history would provide helpful information for the physician.

Nasal diphtheria

The following conditions may simulate nasal diphtheria.

Foreign body in nose. The condition caused by a foreign body in the nose is frequently confused with nasal diphtheria. Both are characterized by a secondary infection with a persistent, profuse nasal discharge that may at times be bloody. The diagnosis is clarified when examination with a nasal speculum reveals evidence of either a foreign body or a diphtheritic type of membrane.

Rhinorrhea. Rhinorrhea due to a common cold, sinus, or adenoid infection may be distinguished from nasal diphtheria by the absence of a membrane and, generally, by the absence of a bloody discharge.

Tonsillar and pharyngeal diphtheria

The following diseases may resemble tonsillar and pharyngeal diphtheria.

Acute streptococcal membranous tonsillitis. During the first few days of the disease the patient usually appears more acutely ill, the temperature is higher, and the membrane is usually confined to the tonsil. The dramatic response to penicillin therapy within 24 hours and the recovery of streptococci on culture usually establish the diagnosis.

Infectious mononucleosis. Infectious mononucleosis is commonly characterized by membranous tonsillitis and splenomegaly in addition to the lymphadenopathy. A blood smear showing a large percentage of abnormal lymphocytes and

a positive heterophil antibody test (p. 65) are helpful diagnostic aids.

Nonbacterial membranous tonsillitis. Nonbacterial membranous tonsillitis is a common pediatric entity of varying causes. The illness is characterized by fever, sore throat, membranous tonsillitis, and a 4- to 10-day course that is not affected by antimicrobial therapy. The white blood cell count is usually low or normal, and cultures from throat specimens reveal normal bacterial flora. This syndrome has been reported as a manifestation of adenovirus infection and acquired toxoplasmosis. Other agents may be responsible for this disease.

Primary herpetic tonsillitis. The lesions of herpes simplex may occasionally coalesce on the tonsil and produce a pseudomembrane. This is usually accompanied by herpetic involvement of other portions of the mucous membrane.

Thrush. Thrush may also simulate a diphtheritic membrane. However, the absence of constitutional symptoms and presence of lesions on the buccal mucosa and tongue usually clarify the diagnosis.

Posttonsillectomy faucial membranes. Posttonsillectomy faucial membranes have an alarming resemblance to the membranes of diphtheria. It is clear the patient has had surgery and the lesions are usually stationary and do not spread.

Laryngeal diphtheria

The following diseases and conditions may simulate laryngeal diphtheria.

Infectious croup. *Infectious croup* is a term that describes two types of acute obstructive laryngitis of which diphtheria is the least common today; the most common type is caused by parainfluenza viruses (p. 260). A negative culture for bacterial pathogens and the absence of a membrane suggest the possibility of viral croup.

Spasmodic croup. Spasmodic croup, or acute subglottic edema, presumed to have an allergic cause, may also simulate laryngeal diphtheria. It appears suddenly, usually at night, and clears up by morning. There is a tendency for the condition to recur for one or two nights.

Epiglottitis. The second most common type of obstructive lower airway diseases is caused by *Haemophilus influenzae* type b. This condition has a typical clinical picture. It is characterized by sudden onset of high fever, drooling because of pain upon swallowing, and dyspnea due to supraglottic obstruction. The epiglottis is markedly swollen and beefy red. This characteristic physical finding establishes the diagnosis, which is confirmed by positive blood and/or throat culture for *H. influenzae* type b.

Foreign body in larynx. If there is a history of aspiration, there is no difficulty in diagnosing the condition caused by a foreign body in the larynx. Frequently, however, aspiration is not witnessed. A history of sudden choking and coughing spells suggests the diagnosis. The presence of the object is usually detected by laryngoscopic and roentgenographic examination.

COMPLICATIONS

Since the advent of antimicrobial therapy, the incidence of secondary bacterial complications has been significantly reduced. Penicillin, which is recommended for eradication of the diphtheria bacillus, prevents the occurrence of secondary streptococcal infections.

The most common and most serious complications are those caused by the effect of the toxin on the heart and central nervous system (CNS).

Myocarditis

Myocarditis occurs frequently as a complication of severe diphtheria, but it may also follow milder forms of the disease. The more extensive the local lesion and the more delayed the institution of antitoxin therapy, the more frequently myocarditis occurs. In most instances the cardiac manifestations appear during the second week of the disease. Occasionally myocarditis may be noted as early as the first week and as late as the sixth week of the disease.

Diminution in intensity of the first heart sound or arrhythmia during the course of diphtheria is usually indicative of myocardial involvement. Abnormal electrocardiographic findings confirm this impression, including elevation of the S-T segment, prolongation of the P-R interval, and evidence of heart block. The myocarditis may be followed by cardiac failure.

Neuritis

Neuritis is also generally a complication of severe diphtheria. The manifestations of neuritis have the following characteristics: (1) they ap-

pear after a variable latent period, (2) they are predominantly bilateral with motor rather than sensory involvement, and (3) they usually clear completely.

Paralysis of soft palate. The most common manifestation of diphtheritic neuritis is paralysis of the soft palate. It occurs during the third week and is characterized by a nasal quality to the voice and nasal regurgitation. The paralysis usually subsides completely within 1 to 2 weeks.

Ocular palsy. Ocular palsy usually occurs during the fifth week and is characterized by paralysis of the muscles of accommodation, causing blurring of vision. Less commonly there may be involvement of the extraocular muscles, causing strabismus. Involvement of the lateral rectus muscle, causing an internal squint, is the most common symptom.

Paralysis of diaphragm. Paralysis of the diaphragm may occur between the fifth and seventh weeks as a result of neuritis of the phrenic nerve. Death will occur if mechanical respiratory aids are not employed.

Paralysis of limbs. Paralysis of limbs may occur between the sixth and tenth weeks. The absence of deep tendon reflexes, the bilateral symmetrical involvement, and the presence of an elevated value of spinal fluid protein make this complication clinically indistinguishable from the Guillain-Barré syndrome.

PROGNOSIS

Before the turn of the century the mortality of diphtheria ranged between 30% and 50%. The advent of diphtheria antitoxin in 1894 and the beginning of large-scale active immunization programs in 1922 resulted in a dramatic reduction in mortality to less than 5%.

In spite of the low fatality rate, the prognosis in the individual case of diphtheria must be extremely guarded. Sudden death may be caused by a variety of unpredictable events, such as (1) the sudden complete obstruction of the airway by a detached piece of membrane, (2) the development of myocarditis and heart failure, and (3) the late occurrence of respiratory paralysis due to phrenic nerve involvement. Patients who survive myocarditis or neuritis generally recover completely. Occasionally, however, diphtheritic myocarditis may be followed by permanent damage to the heart.

The prognosis in a particular case depends on a variety of factors pertaining to the disease, the host, and the environment.

IMMUNITY
Schick test for immunity

The introduction of the Schick test in 1913 provided a valuable tool for the determination of immunity or susceptibility to diphtheria. In this test a person is inoculated intracutaneously with a measured amount of diphtheria toxin. In the absence of antitoxic immunity, the toxin has a damaging effect on the tissue and a positive reaction occurs. Thus, a positive Schick test indicates susceptibility to diphtheria. If antitoxic immunity is present, the toxin is neutralized, and a negative reaction results. A negative Schick test usually indicates immunity to diphtheria. Schick test reagents are available from the Massachusetts State Laboratory.

Passive immunity

Passive immunity may be acquired either by transplacental transfer from an immune mother or by parenteral inoculation with diphtheria antitoxin. Congenitally acquired passive immunity persists for approximately 6 months. Protection after injection of diphtheria antitoxin disappears after 2 to 3 weeks.

Active immunity

Active immunity may be induced either by an attack of diphtheria or, more commonly today, by inoculations with diphtheria toxoid. The toxin is more toxic than immunogenic, and, thus, more reliable immunity is produced by toxoid injections. Persons having diphtheria should therefore be immunized. Recurrent attacks of the disease are not unusual. Some individuals show evidence of immunity probably acquired as a result of an inapparent infection. Immunization with diphtheria toxoid can be relied on to prevent serious or fatal disease. The widespread and routine immunization of infants and children has had a profound effect on the immune status of the population at large (Nelson et al., 1978; Sheffield et al., 1978). Fully immunized individuals may become nasopharyngeal carriers or uncommonly they may develop a mild form of the disease (Munford et al., 1974).

EPIDEMIOLOGIC FACTORS

Diphtheria is worldwide in distribution. The extensive use of diphtheria toxoid since World War II has been associated with a striking decline to fewer than 100 reported cases annually in the United States. The highest seasonal incidence occurs during the autumn and winter months. The age incidence is dependent on the immune status of the population. In most areas where infants and children are routinely immunized, the disease is becoming relatively more common in adults. Most reports of recent outbreaks of diphtheria confirm the predominance of the disease among the poor, who have limited access to health care facilities. The fatalities usually occur among unimmunized children.

Diphtheria is acquired by contact with either a person with the disease or a carrier of the organism. The microorganisms are disseminated by the acts of coughing, sneezing, or even talking. Milk-borne epidemics have been reported. Fomites play a small part in the spread of the disease.

TREATMENT
Antitoxin therapy

Diphtheria antitoxin must be given promptly and in adequate dosage. Any delay increases the possibility that myocarditis, neuritis, or death may occur.

During an infection, diphtheria toxin may be present in three forms: (1) circulating or unbound, (2) bound to the cells, and (3) internalized in cytoplasm. Antitoxin will neutralize circulating toxin, may affect bound toxin, but will not affect internalized toxin that is bound to EF-2. Ideally, if there is no evidence of sensitivity, antitoxin should be given intravenously so that a high concentration will be immediately available for neutralization of toxin.

Studies by Tasman et al. (1958) have revealed the following advantages of intravenous antitoxin therapy: (1) The peak serum antitoxin level is reached within 30 minutes after intravenous inoculation as compared with 4 days after intramuscular inoculation. (2) The excretion pattern of diphtheria antitoxin is essentially the same after intravenous or intramuscular administration. (3) Antitoxin appears in the saliva very rapidly after intravenous inoculation but may be

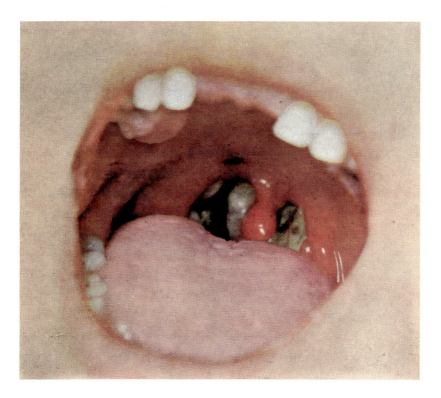

Plate 1
Tonsillar diphtheria. (Reproduced by courtesy of Franklin H. Top, M.D., Professor and Head of the Department of Hygiene and Preventive Medicine, State University of Iowa, College of Medicine, Iowa City, Iowa, and Parke, Davis & Company's *Therapeutic Notes*.)

Table 3-1. Dosage of antitoxin recommended for various types of diphtheria

Type of diphtheria	Dosage	Route
Anterior nasal	10,000 to 20,000 units	Intramuscular
Tonsillar	15,000 to 25,000 units	Intramuscular or intravenous
Pharyngeal	20,000 to 40,000 units	Intramuscular or intravenous
Laryngeal	20,000 to 40,000 units	Intramuscular or intravenous
Combined types	40,000 to 50,000 units	Intravenous
Late cases	40,000 to 60,000 units	Intravenous

delayed for hours or days after intramuscular injection. (4) The comparison of both routes of administration in the treatment of experimental diphtheria in guinea pigs reveals a lower mortality, less myocarditis, and less neuritis in the intravenously treated group.

The administration of diphtheria antitoxin is not a completely benign procedure. It may be followed by an immediate reaction such as acute anaphylactic shock or a delayed type of reaction such as serum sickness. Therefore, the following precautions must be taken before therapy is instituted: (1) history regarding previous horse serum injections or possible allergy should be obtained, (2) skin or eye sensitivity tests should be performed, and (3) a syringe loaded with a 1:1000 solution of epinephrine and a tourniquet should always be ready for emergency use.

Skin test. An injection of 0.1 ml of a 1:100 dilution of diphtheria antitoxin in physiologic saline solution is given intracutaneously. The test is read in 20 minutes and is positive if a wheal 1 cm or more in diameter is present. The use of undiluted antitoxin will invariably cause a false-positive reaction; therefore, dilution is mandatory.

Conjunctival test. One drop of a 1:10 dilution of the serum in physiologic saline solution is instilled inside the lower lid of one eye; 1 drop of physiologic saline solution is used as a control for the other eye. The test is read in 20 minutes and is positive if conjunctivitis and lacrimation are present. If a positive reaction occurs, the eye should be treated with 1 drop of a 1:100 solution of epinephrine.

• • •

If the history and sensitivity tests are negative, the total recommended dose of antitoxin should be given without delay. If intravenous therapy is indicated, antitoxin should be diluted with saline solution in a 1:20 proportion and administered slowly at a rate of approximately 15 drops per minute. The addition of 0.1 to 0.3 ml of a 1:1000 dilution of epinephrine to the solution is a useful precaution. Antitoxin is given undiluted intramuscularly into the buttocks.

The precise dose and route of administration will be determined by the location and extent of the membrane, the degree of toxemia, and the duration of the illness. The patient's age and weight are of no consequence. The dosages shown in Table 3-1 are recommended for the various types of diphtheria.

If a patient has been shown to be sensitive to horse serum, the indications for the diphtheria antitoxin should be reevaluated in the light of this potential risk. If the antitoxin is to be administered, it should be given carefully at 20-minute intervals in gradually increasing doses as follows:

0.1 ml of a 1:20 dilution subcutaneously
0.1 ml of a 1:10 dilution subcutaneously
0.1 ml undiluted subcutaneously
0.3 ml undiluted intramuscularly
0.5 ml undiluted intramuscularly

If no reaction has occurred, the remaining dose should be injected intramuscularly. In the event of a reaction during the course of therapy, the subsequent dose should be reduced. Signs of acute anaphylaxis call for the immediate intravenous injection of 0.2 to 0.5 ml of 1:1000 epinephrine solution.

Antibacterial therapy

Penicillin and erythromycin are effective against most strains of diphtheria bacilli. Penicillin is usually the preferred drug and may be given as aqueous procaine penicillin G, 600,000 units intramuscularly once daily. Patients who are sensitive to penicillin should be given erythromycin in a daily dosage of 50 mg per kilogram of body weight orally; the maximum dose is 1 gm. Antimicrobial therapy is not a substitute for antitoxin therapy but should be given as a supplement to it and is generally continued until three consecutive cultures are negative for *C. diphtheriae*. Since the treatment may be prolonged, penicillin may be given orally instead of parenterally.

Supportive treatment

Bed rest is more important in the management of diphtheria than in most other infectious diseases. It should be enforced for at least 12 days because of the possibility of complicating myocarditis. The patient's activity will subsequently be guided by the results of the daily physical examinations, the serial electrocardiograms, and the presence or absence of complications.

Laryngeal diphtheria. In addition to requiring antitoxin, penicillin, and other supportive measures, patients with laryngeal diphtheria require special treatment for the relief of obstruction to breathing. Intubation and/or tracheostomy may be necessary.

Treatment of complications

Myocarditis and neuritis are the most important complications requiring therapy.

Myocarditis. In general, the management of diphtheritic myocarditis and its sequelae is the same as that employed for any other type of acute myocardial damage. Bed rest and inactivity may be beneficial. Sudden death due to myocardial failure may be precipitated by excessive activity. The administration of digitalis is controversial; however, it should not be withheld if there is evidence of cardiac decompensation.

Diphtheritic neuritis. Palatal and pharyngeal paralysis may be complicated by aspiration because of the tendency for regurgitation and difficulty in swallowing. In these circumstances gastric or duodenal intubation is indicated.

Treatment of diphtheria carriers

A carrier is an individual who has no symptoms and has a negative reaction to the Schick test and yet harbors virulent diphtheria bacilli in the nasopharynx. The eradication of these microorganisms may be extremely difficult and occasionally impossible. The following measures are recommended to be used in sequence until the culture becomes negative:

Aqueous procaine penicillin, 600,000 units daily for 4 days

Penicillin, 200,000 units orally four times daily for 4 days

Erythromycin, 50 mg per kilogram of body weight per day for 1 week

Occasionally, an undetected foreign body in the nose may be responsible for persistence of a carrier state.

PREVENTIVE MEASURES

The dramatic decline in the incidence of diphtheria since 1922 can be attributed for the most part to mass immunization programs and routine immunization of infants and children.

The preferred immunizing agent is diphtheria toxoid. It is usually given in combination with tetanus and pertussis antigens (DTP) (see p. 475).

ISOLATION AND QUARANTINE
Care of patient

The patient is infective until diphtheria bacilli can no longer be cultured from the site of the infection. The duration of this infective period is variable. After the acute stage of the disease has subsided, three consecutive negative cultures are usually required before the patient is released from isolation.

Care of contacts

Intimate contacts should be isolated until the following procedures have been carried out. Cultures of nose and throat specimens should be made, and Schick tests should be performed. Previously immunized children should be given a booster dose of diphtheria toxoid. Contacts with negative cultures and negative Schick tests may be released from isolation. Children with positive cultures and negative Schick tests should be treated as diphtheria carriers. A child with no symptoms and the combination of a positive culture and a positive Schick test should be treated with diphtheria antitoxin, 5000 units intramuscularly, and penicillin. If a child has a positive Schick test and a negative culture, active immunization with toxoid should be carried out.

REFERENCES

Belsey MA. Skin infections and the epidemiology of diphtheria: acquisition and persistence of *C. diphtheriae* infections. Am J Epidemiol 1975;102:197.

Brooks GF, Bennett JV, Feldman RA. Diphtheria in the United States, 1959-1970. J Infect Dis 1974;129:172.

Centers for Disease Control: Surveillance report. U. S. Department of Health, Education, and Welfare, 1978.

Collier RJ. Diphtheria toxin: mode of action and structure. Bacteriol Rev 1975;39:54.

Corwell MJ. Morphological and physiological variations in the descendants of a single diphtheria bacillus. J Bacteriol 1926;11:65.

Dobie RA, Tobey DA. Clinical features of diphtheria in the respiratory tract. JAMA 1979;242:2197.

Fisher CM, Adams RD. Diphtheritic polyneuritis. A pathological study. J Neuropathol Exp Neurol 1956;15:243.

Freeman VJ. Studies on the virulence of bacteriophage-infected strains of *Corynebacterium diphtheriae*. J Bacteriol 1951;61:675.

Freeman VJ, Morse U. Further observations on the change of virulence of bacteriophage-infected avirulent strains of *Corynebacterium diphtheriae*. J Bacteriol 1953;63:407.

Hewitt LF. Diphtheria bacteriophages and their relation to the development of bacterial variants. J Gen Microbiol 1952;7:352.

Hodes HL. Diphtheria. Pediatr Clin North Am 1979;26:445.

Ipsen J. Immunization of adults against diphtheria and tetanus. N Engl J Med 1954;251:459.

Kidman AE, et al.: Blockage of fast axonal transport by diphtheritic demyelination in the chicken sciatic nerve. J Neurochem 1978;30:57.

Klebs E. Ueber Diphtheria. Verh Cong Inn Med 1883;2:139.

Löffler FAJ. Untersuchungen uber die Bedeutung der Mikroorganismen fuer die Entstehung die Diphtherie beim Menschen, bei der Taube und beim Kalbe. Mitt ADK Gesundheitsamte 1884;2:451.

Marcuse EK, Grand G. Epidemiology of diphtheria in San Antonio, Tex., 1970. JAMA 1973;224:305.

McCloskey RV, Green MH, Eller J, et al.: Treatment of diphtheria carriers. Ann Intern Med 1974;81:788.

Moloney PJ. The preparation and testing of diphtheria toxoid. Am J Public Health 1926;16:1208.

Morris RE, Sallinger CB. Diphtheria toxin does not enter resistant cells by receptor mediated endocytosis. Infect Immun 1983;42:812.

Munford RS, Ory HW, Brooks GF, et al. Diphtheria deaths in the United States, 1959-1970. JAMA 1974;229:1890.

Murphy JR, et al. Evidence that the regulation of diphtheria toxin production is directed at level of transcription. J Bacteriol 1978;135:511.

Nathenson G, Zakzewski B. Current status of passive immunity to diphtheria and tetanus in the newborn, J Infect Dis 1976;133:199.

Nelson LA, et al. Immunity to diphtheria in an urban population. Pediatrics 1978;61:703.

Pappenheimer AM Jr, Gill DM: Diphtheria. Science 1973;182:353.

Pappenheimer AM Jr, Murphy JR. Studies on the molecular epidemiology of diphtheria. Lancet 1983;2:923.

Park WH, Zingher A: Active immunization in diphtheria and treatment by toxin-antitoxin. JAMA 1914;63:859.

Parsons EI. Induction of toxigenicity in nontoxigenic strains of *C. diphtheriae* with bacteriophages derived from nontoxigenic strains. Proc Soc Exp Biol Med 1955;90:91.

Ramon G: Sur le pourvoir floculant et sur les proprietes immunesantes d'une toxine diphtherique rendue avatoxique (avatoxine). C R Acad Sci [D] (Paris) 1923;177:1338-1340.

Roux E, Yersin A: Contribution à l'etude de la diphtherie. Ann Inst. Pasteur 1888;2:629-661.

Sayers EG. Diphtheritic myocarditis with permanent heart damage. Ann Intern Med 1958;48:146.

Schick B. Die Diphtherietoxin-hautreaktion des Menschen als Vorprobe der prophylaktischen Diphtherieheilserumninjektion. Munch Med Wochenschr 1913;60:2608.

Sheffield FW, et al. Susceptibility to diphtheria. Lancet 1978;1:428.

Tasman A, et al. Importance of intravenous injection of diphtheria antiserum. Lancet 1958;1:1299.

von Behring E: Zur Behandlung der Diphtherie mit diphtheriecheilserum. Dtsch Med Wochenschr 1893;19:548.

4

VIRAL ENCEPHALITIS

Encephalitis is an inflammatory process of the central nervous system (CNS) in which the major area of involvement is the parenchyma of the brain. Because other portions of the CNS may be simultaneously involved, designations are used to include these additional areas of infection ("meningoencephalitis" if there is significant meningeal inflammation, "encephalomyelitis" when the spinal cord is also affected). The major clinical manifestation of encephalitis is an alteration in the patient's state of consciousness ranging from irritability, agitation, delirium, or disorientation through somnolence, obtundation, and coma. Associated neurologic dysfunction and abnormalities are determined by the anatomic sites of the process and the degree of elevated intracranial pressure. The tempo of the illness is varied; acute catastrophic disease contrasts with some cases of more insidious, slow progression pursuing a subacute or chronic course.

In this chapter the following two forms of virus-associated encephalitis are considered: (1) acute encephalitis resulting from direct invasion of the CNS by a virus, giving rise to inflammatory changes and neuronal damage, and (2) postinfectious encephalitis, the pathogenesis of which is not altogether clear but with the histologic finding of striking perivenous demyelination quite different from that in the acute picture. Although it has been postulated that an autoimmune process is responsible for postinfectious encephalitis, evidence has accumulated

that indicates presence of virus in the CNS, at least in some instances.

Viral encephalitis may be characterized by (1) a mild abortive infection, (2) a type of illness barely distinguishable from aseptic meningitis, or (3) a severe involvement of the CNS. The last is often characterized by sudden onset, high fever, meningeal signs, stupor, disorientation, tremors, convulsions, spasticity, coma, and death. Case fatality rates vary widely. Sequelae are more common in infants.

ETIOLOGY

For a number of reasons, the establishment of definite etiologic diagnoses for patients with clinical encephalitis has been difficult. Many cases are never assigned a specific causative agent. The diagnostic techniques may be complex, time consuming, and expensive, requiring the inoculation of a variety of cell culture systems and laboratory animals. The responsible agent, most often a virus, may be detectable solely in the brain itself and may not be present, or only very transiently found, in the blood, cerebrospinal fluid (CSF), or other usually available samples. The multiplicity of possible causative agents makes serologic diagnosis very difficult unless there are epidemiologic or clinical clues that enable the laboratory in search of an antibody rise to focus on a limited number of antigens. Because of the availability of vidarabine and acyclovir for chemotherapy, vigorous approaches (including brain biopsy) are pursued if herpes simplex virus is suspected (Chapter 11). However, only a relatively small number of sporadic cases are caused by this agent, perhaps 2% to 4% of all encephalitis cases reported.

The common causes of acute encephalitis in the United States and among U.S. travelers abroad are as follows:

Togaviruses
  Alphaviruses
    Eastern equine encephalitis (EEE)
    Western equine encephalitis (WEE)
    Venezuelan equine encephalitis (VEE)
  Flaviviruses
    St. Louis encephalitis (SLE)
    Japanese encephalitis (JE)
    Tick-borne
      Powassan
Bunyaviruses
  California group
    LaCrosse
    California encephalitis
    Jamestown Canyon
    Snowshoe hare
  Phlebovirus
    Rift valley fever
Arenaviruses
  Lymphocytic choriomeningitis (LCM)
  Argentinian hemorrhagic fever (Junin virus)
  Bolivian hemorrhagic fever (Machupo virus)
Reoviruses
  California tick fever
Rabies (Chapter 21)
Herpes simplex 1 and 2 (Chapter 11)
Enteroviruses (Chapter 5)
  Coxsackie A and B
  ECHO virus
Herpes zoster (varicella-zoster virus) (Chapter 33)
Infectious mononucleosis (Epstein-Barr virus) (Chapter 6)
Cytomegalovirus (Chapter 2)
Postinfectious agents
  Measles (Chapter 13)
  Mumps (Chapter 16)
  Rubella (Chapter 24)
  Chickenpox (varicella-zoster) (Chapter 33)
  Influenza (Chapter 22)
Nonviral causes
  Mycoplasma pneumoniae (Chapter 22)
  Toxoplasmosis (Chapter 30)
  Rocky Mountain spotted fever (Chapter 23)
  Naegleria fowleri

This catalog is derived partially from reports to the Centers for Disease Control (CDC) from 1967 to 1984. Reports from other areas of the world would add an even greater number of those viruses involved with arthropod vectors (togaviruses and bunyaviruses) and those associated with hemorrhagic fevers (arenaviruses, filoviruses, Hantaan viruses). A continuing, incomplete reclassification of these many agents based on their biophysical and biochemical properties has drastically altered the former concept of "arboviruses," which now has become a descriptive term for the natural history of the many members of several different virus groups using the common pathway of transmission by the bite of an insect vector.

On the basis of differing pathology and the temporal association of the second group with a recent acute infection, encephalitis reporting is usually divided into two categories. The first includes all those infections where direct viral invasion of the CNS is thought to occur; the second, those which are "postinfectious" after a common acute non-CNS infection followed by an immune-reactive demyelinating process. This second category may then include many of the usual childhood infections, the stereotype of which was measles prior to its control by vaccination. The etiology of more than half of the annual 1500 to 2000 reported cases of encephalitis is never determined.

The togaviruses include many of the agents formerly called arboviruses. They possess single-stranded RNA genomes and are enveloped with surface projections or spikes. The genus alphavirus has 20 members, all New World agents with particles 40 to 65 nm in diameter. The flavivirus genus contains nearly 60 members of both Old and New World prevalence with particle size 37 to 50 nm. Most agents pathogenic for humans and detected in the United States are mosquito-borne, but Powassan virus, which is found principally along the U.S.-Canadian border, is carried by *Ixodes* ticks.

The bunyaviruses are enveloped RNA agents possessing a segmented genome within a lipid envelope. Their diameter ranges from 90 to 120 nm. The four members of the California group listed on this page are all carried by *Aedes* mosquitoes. Rift Valley fever virus is of special interest because of its epizootics in south and east Africa and its spread into Egypt; thus it also poses a risk to American tourists in those areas. In addition to a unique late-onset retinal vasculitis, it is an occasional cause of encephalitis.

Transmission is either by mosquito vector or via aerosol from infected domestic animals.

The arenaviruses include at least 10 agents of which three are known human pathogens. They are RNA viruses with round, pleomorphic particles averaging 110 to 130 nm, budding from the cytoplasmic membranes of infected cells. Transmission to humans is via excretion (saliva, urine, feces) from infected rodents. Lymphocytic choriomeningitis is the most commonly encountered within the United States and has been the source of research laboratory outbreaks from contaminated hamster tissues.

Of the remaining viruses listed on p. 33, all are discussed in greater detail in other chapters, with the exception of Colorado tick fever virus. It is an unusual member of the Reoviridae family, which chronically infects rodents and may be transmitted to man by wood ticks, inciting a dengue-like illness. When children are infected they occasionally develop encephalitis.

Reservoirs of infection for the togaviruses, bunyaviruses, and arenaviruses are found in birds and various animals. The persistence of these agents in nature involves a complicated, fascinating ecosystem. Some of the responsible elements include transovarial viral transmission in the insect, lengthy months of viremia in apparently healthy water birds, feeding and migratory patterns of insect vectors and of natural bird and mammalian reservoirs, and overwintering in snakes by some strains (Reeves, 1974).

The properties of the other viruses causing encephalitis and the associated CNS manifestations are described in the chapters noted in parentheses on p. 33.

PATHOLOGY AND PATHOGENESIS

Virus reaches the CNS following introduction at a distant portal of entry, local replication, and subsequent viremia. The interval between initial infection and eventual CNS involvement may be days or weeks. A number of routes are available but the most likely are (1) extension of virus into neuronal and glial cells adjacent to infected endothelial cells of small capillaries or (2) directly into CSF from the vessels of the choroid plexus via the ependyma. Rabies virus (Chapter 21) in its passage centrally via peripheral nerve pathways is an exception, and some of the herpesviruses may also use similar direct neural transmission under some circumstances (Johnson and Mims, 1968).

In general, invading viruses give rise to similar pathologic changes in the CNS. It is usually impossible to distinguish between them on the basis of pathologic examination alone. Gross examination of the brain and cord reveals edema and congestion. There may be small hemorrhages. Microscopic examination shows perivascular cellular infiltration and infiltration of the meninges, chiefly with lymphocytes. The principal lesion in the parenchyma consists of neuronal necrosis and degeneration accompanied by neuronophagocytosis. Perivascular cuffing and glial proliferation are common. Destruction of the ground substance of the gray or white matter may be severe. Multiple acellular plaques of necrosis may be seen. The spinal cord is involved in most types of encephalitis. In general, neuronal lesions and foci of cellular infiltration are widely distributed throughout the brain and spinal cord.

The detection in brain biopsy or autopsy specimens of inclusions within the nucleus or cytoplasm of neuronal or glial cells permits the consideration of a less vast array of possible etiologies. Herpes simplex, cytomegalovirus, measles, and rabies are those agents most likely to induce inclusion-bearing cells. A few viruses have predilections to localize in selected anatomic sites. Neonatal cytomegalovirus infection may be most marked in the periventricular subependymal matrix; herpes simplex encephalitis in the older infant or child often affects the frontotemporal lobes. Rabies shows a predisposition for the brain stem and cortical gray matter.

Attempts have been made to divide the encephalitides listed on p. 33 and in Table 4-1 into two groups: (1) those with evidence of direct invasion of the CNS by virus and (2) those considered to involve a postinfectious, autoimmune process. Recent evidence indicates that these are not necessarily separate and distinct forms, as suggested by their pathologic changes; rather, the differences between the two groups may hinge on timing of the onset of encephalitis in relation to the systemic manifestations and differences in the degree of immune response of the host. The demonstration of measles virus antigens and incomplete virions in the brains of patients with subacute inclusion body encephalitis and subacute sclerosing panencephalitis (SSPE) confirmed the participation of active viral replication in the pathogenesis of these rare complications. The sequence of events in acute

Table 4-1. Encephalitis reported in the United States, 1977-1983*

Classification	1977	1978	1979	1980	1981	1982	1983	Average fatality rates
Total cases	1533	1429	1588	1402	1516	1500	1847	12%
Indeterminate etiology	1003	1021	1192	952	1056	1090	NA†	15%
Postchildhood infection‡	119	65	84	38	38	36	NA	20%
Herpes simplex	63	77	61	NA	97	138	NA	35%
Other known etiologies§	341	266	177	264	322	197	NA	5%

*Compiled principally from data published by the Centers for Disease Control.
†*NA*, Data not available.
‡Chickenpox, mumps, measles, rubella.
§Arbovirus, enterovirus, adenovirus, EB virus, etc.

postinfectious measles encephalitis is less certain, resembling in many ways experimental allergic encephalomyelitis. A study of 19 patients in Peru from 1980 to 1983 (Johnson et al., 1984) revealed myelin basic protein in their CSF and proliferative lymphocytic responses to this protein, strengthening the conclusion that this is an autoimmune process.

With greatly improved methods currently available for the detection of viruses and their components, a vigorous effort should be made to isolate these agents from CSF and CNS tissues and to carry out careful pathologic examinations. Paradoxically, these new insights into virus-CNS interactions come at a time when cases of measles encephalitis are exceedingly rare, as a result of successful measles immunization programs, so that the numbers of patients to be studied with improved techniques are few indeed (Fig. 13-6).

CLINICAL MANIFESTATIONS

There are many types of viral encephalitides. They vary from benign forms resembling aseptic meningitis that last a few days and are followed by complete recovery to fulminating encephalitis with the clinical manifestations of paresis, sensory changes, convulsions, increased intracranial pressure, coma, and death. Mumps meningoencephalitis is a good example of the usually benign form. Encephalitis caused by herpes simplex virus, on the other hand, although far less common than that caused by

mumps virus, is a devastating infection with a high case fatality rate (Chapter 11).

The onset of viral encephalitis may be sudden or gradual and is marked by fever, headache, dizziness, vomiting, apathy, and stiffness of the neck. Ataxia, tremors, mental confusion, speech difficulties, stupor or hyperexcitability, delirium, convulsions, coma, and death may follow. In some cases there may be a prodromal period of 1 to 4 days manifested by chills and fever, headache, malaise, sore throat, conjunctivitis, and pains in the extremities and abdomen followed by encephalitic signs just mentioned. Abortive forms with headache and fever only or a syndrome resembling aseptic meningitis may occur. Lymphocytic choriomeningitis virus infection may be accompanied by arthritis, orchitis, and/or parotitis.

The many variations in the clinical patterns of encephalitis depend on the distribution, location, and concentration of neuronal lesions. Ocular palsies and ptosis are uncommon. Cerebellar incoordination is seen. Flaccid paralysis of the extremities resembling that of poliomyelitis is sometimes encountered. Paralysis of the shoulder girdle muscles is described as a singular feature of a tick-borne encephalitis.

The CSF is clear, and manometric readings of pressure vary from normal to markedly elevated. As a rule, pleocytosis of 40 to 400 cells, chiefly mononuclear, is found. The protein and glucose values may be slightly elevated or normal. In eastern equine encephalitis, the CSF may contain 1000 or more cells per cubic millimeter. In the early stages the cells are predominantly polymorphonuclear leukocytes, shifting later to mononuclear elements. In this form of encephalitis the peripheral white blood cell count may be as high as 66,000 with 90% polymorphonuclear leukocytes; in the other types, it is lower, ranging from 10,000 to 20,000, predominantly neutrophils.

The course of encephalitis varies from that of the fulminating type with hyperpyrexia, ending in death in 2 to 4 days, to that of a mild form in which the fever subsides in 1 or 2 weeks with complete recovery.

DIAGNOSIS

A diagnosis of acute encephalitis is indicated by the clinical findings. The circumstances in which the disease occurs are important. The age and geographic distribution are described later in the discussion of epidemiologic factors. The specific type of encephalitis can be determined only by isolation and identification of the virus or by demonstration of the formation of or rise of level of antibody in convalescence. Togaviruses are rarely detected in the CSF, blood, or other materials during life. It is generally fruitless and inappropriate to search for them except in CNS tissue removed with sterile precautions at biopsy or necropsy.

On the other hand, enteroviruses, mumps virus, adenoviruses, varicella-zoster virus, and cytomegalovirus may be detected in the CSF and other appropriate materials (see chapters on specific viruses). A serologic diagnosis may be reached by means of various antibody tests. Paired serum specimens are usually necessary. The first should be drawn as soon after onset as possible and the second, 2 or 3 weeks later.

A number of diagnostic tests under study and in varying stages of development exploit techniques for the detection of specific viral antigens or early antibodies in CSF. These tests are available in a limited number of laboratories and are still in a research phase. Recently introduced tests employing immunoglobulin M capture, enzyme-linked immunosorbent assays for eastern and western equine encephalitis, St. Louis encephalitis, and LaCrosse viruses have permitted a specific diagnosis on a single acute phase serum or CSF by the arbovirus reference laboratories of the Centers for Disease Control (1984).

DIFFERENTIAL DIAGNOSIS

Other diseases of the CNS may be confused with viral encephalitis. Although human *rabies* is extremely rare in the United States, it should be considered (Chapter 21). Several cases of rabies in recent years have been labeled "viral" encephalitis during the patient's illness and the diagnosis of rabies was appreciated only on postmortem examination with the discovery of Negri bodies in the hippocampus or cerebellum.

Tuberculous meningitis or *pyogenic meningitis* may present the picture of encephalitis. In this circumstance, the key lies in the CSF, which may be cloudy, shows pleocytosis, has low glucose and high protein levels, and usually has microorganisms that are evident on smear or culture (p. 415). In the case of tuberculous meningitis or tuberculoma, a chest roentgenogram and skin tests with tuberculin may provide additional clues.

The late Australian pathologist, Kenneth Reye, in 1963 called attention to a group of pediatric patients who died with an acute encephalopathy and fatty degeneration of the liver and other viscera. Subsequent experience has further delineated the clinical picture of *Reye's syndrome* and has demonstrated some epidemiologic relationships. In the United States there have been close temporal associations of Reye's syndrome to chickenpox in younger infants and children and to influenza virus infections (some type A strains and type B) in school-age children. The pathogenesis remains unclear, but the initial viral infection apparently triggers an acute metabolic decompensation with marked hepatic and cerebral dysfunction. After a few days of convalescence from a viral illness of normal severity there is a sudden onset of vomiting accompanied promptly by personality changes and rapid progression to delirium and, in many cases, coma. Laboratory studies show elevated hepatic isoenzymes (AST, ALT, LDH) and hyperammonemia. Muscle enzymes may also rise sharply. Except for increased intracranial pressure, the CSF studies are usually normal. Liver biopsy reveals characteristic ultrastructural mitochondrial changes by electron microscopy. Many therapeutic meneuvers have been used, such as peritoneal dialysis, exchange transfusion, hemodialysis, hepatic perfusion, but the common denominator of success has been to monitor and to reduce the raised intracranial pressure and to maintain cerebral perfusion and oxygenation. With heightened awareness of the physiologic aberrations and prompt organized intensive care to support the patient during the critical days, many Reye's syndrome patients now recover fully, and mortality has dropped from more than 50% to less than 20%. The speed of recovery is often as dramatic as the onset of symptoms, with only a few days separating start from finish. Etiology and pathogenesis are still unclear. An epidemiologic association has been confirmed between Reye's syndrome and the use of salicylates (especially aspirin) during the preceding varicella or respiratory virus infection.

Tumor, trauma, and abscess of the brain may be mistaken for encephalitis and are often difficult to differentiate. Roentgenograms of the skull, electroencephalograms, radioisotopic scans, arteriography, and computerized tomography may help in the solution of the problem. *Lead encephalopathy* is distinguished from viral encephalitis (1) by the CSF findings, which consist mainly of increased level of protein, often quite marked, and by no increase or only a slight increase in number of cells, (2) by chemical detection of abnormal amounts of lead in the blood or CSF, (3) by roentgenographic evidence of lead line in the bone, (4) by lead line in the gums if teeth are present, (5) by basophilic stippling and anemia, and (6) by urinary coproporphyrins.

Alcohol, drugs, and other toxins must also be considered in a review of possible causes.

PROGNOSIS

The specific virus, the inoculum size, the clinical type of illness, and the age of the patient are some of the factors influencing the outcome of the disease. The distribution of causes and fatality rates of encephalitis reported from 1972 to 1983 are shown in Table 4-1. There have been no major epidemics of arbovirus-type encephalitis since the 1975 outbreak of St. Louis encephalitis. The decrease in the postchildhood infection category stems mainly from the striking drop in measles in the United States. An increase in reported herpes simplex encephalitis probably represents more aggressive diagnostic efforts because of availability of specific antiviral chemotherapy.

Mumps encephalitis carries the lowest mortality, only 1% to 2%. The majority of patients

with mumps have CNS involvement, but this is nearly always a benign meningitis. A few patients undergo frank encephalitis, which may result in occasional deaths, but of greater concern is a 25% incidence of CNS sequelae among the survivors (Koskiniemi et al., 1983).

During the period covered in Table 4-1 the mortality of arbovirus encephalitis in the United States was approximately 6%. Mortality also varies from epidemic to epidemic. Eastern equine, Japanese, and tick-borne encephalitides are generally associated with higher fatality rates (40% to 75%) than the St. Louis, western equine, and California types. The overall mortality from St. Louis encephalitis is 5% to 30% and from western equine, 7% to 20%. Recovery from either, when it occurs, is usually complete. In young infants with St. Louis or western equine encephalitis, however, permanent injury to the CNS may occur. Seizures, hydrocephalus, and mental retardation have been seen in outbreaks of the St. Louis type, affecting 10% to 40% of infants below the age of 6 months. Similar permanent brain damage was observed in two thirds of the patients surviving eastern equine encephalitis in the Massachusetts epidemic of 1938. Although the fatality rate is high in Japanese encephalitis, the outlook for complete recovery is fairly good for survivors; 3% to 10% show neurologic or psychic abnormalities.

The fatality rate for measles encephalitis was 12%; for varicella encephalitis it was 28%. The prognosis in general for herpes simplex encephalitis is poor. Death occurs in about one third and serious sequelae occur in about half of the survivors, even in those who received antiviral therapy. The cases of encephalitis caused by enteroviruses are few in numbers so that it is difficult to estimate the prognosis, although from the available data it appears to be similar to that of mumps except in the neonatal period, when the case-fatality rate is extremely high (exceeding 50%).

EPIDEMIOLOGIC FACTORS

The distribution of viral encephalitis varies according to season. Arbovirus encephalitis is a warm weather disease. Epidemics and sporadic cases of the North American forms (St. Louis, California, and the two equine encephalitides) and of Japanese encephalitis begin during the hot summer months and subside during the autumn. Tick-borne encephalitides, unlike the others, attack chiefly forest workers, beginning most frequently in May and June and diminishing over the summer months. Heightened interest in Japanese encephalitis has arisen with increased tourism and commercial travel to areas where epidemics have recently occurred (Peoples Republic of China, Thailand, India, Nepal, Japan, Korea, and Taiwan).

Enteroviral encephalitis also occurs predominantly during the summer and fall months. Mumps encephalitis occurs year round, with periodic increases in incidence during the winter and early spring months. The incidence of varicella encephalitis begins to rise in the winter months, peaks in the spring, and declines slowly to lowest levels in the summer and fall. Cases of encephalitis of unknown cause show consistent peaks during the summer months corresponding with those of arbovirus encephalitis. This suggests that some of the undiagnosed cases may be caused by arboviruses, although enteroviruses are also prevalent during the same months.

The age distribution shows that St. Louis, Japanese, and western equine encephalitides all have a predilection for people in the extremes of life. The incidence of St. Louis encephalitis is high in infants and older people and lowest in children from 5 to 12 years of age. Similarly, about 60% of those attacked by Japanese encephalitis are over 50 years of age. In Okinawa and Taiwan, however, the largest proportion of cases has occurred in children. The highest attack rates of western equine encephalitis are likely to be found among male outdoor workers, 20 to 50 years old. High attack rates have also been found in infants. Eastern equine encephalitis attacks primarily the young. In the Massachusetts outbreak of 1938, 70% were under 10 years of age, 25% were below 1 year of age, and only 15% were over 21 years of age.

In general, the incidence is higher in males than in females. There may be an occupational factor in the sex differences observed in western equine and tick-borne encephalitides. The sex ratio in Japanese encephalitis is 124 males to 100 females. Both sexes are equally attacked by eastern equine encephalitis.

Although many of the names of the viruses are derived from their initial geographic sites of detection, surveillance in ensuing years has revealed more variable distribution than was originally appreciated. Western equine encephalitis is found throughout the entire United States and Canada. St. Louis encephalitis has a similar widespread distribution. Eastern equine encephalitis is still confined mainly to the eastern seaboard. Powassan virus, a tick-borne agent, is found mainly along the U.S.-Canadian border. California group viruses, as exemplified by LaCrosse virus, are annually the most prevalent mosquito-borne infection detected in the United States and have been isolated in many states other than California and Wisconsin (first patient with LaCrosse virus), ranging from Utah to North Carolina and from Minnesota to Arkansas.

Geographically, outbreaks and sporadic cases of St. Louis encephalitis have occurred in the central and western states and in western Canada. An epidemic of more than 200 cases occurred in the Tampa Bay area of Florida during the late summer and fall months of 1962; 470 cases were reported in 1964, mainly from Texas, New Jersey, Illinois, Kentucky, Pennsylvania, Colorado, and Indiana. Nearly 1000 cases occurred in 1975, mainly in the midwestern states.

Small outbreaks of eastern equine encephalitis have occurred in Massachusetts (1938, 1955, 1956, 1971, and 1983) and in Louisiana (1947). During the summer of 1959, New Jersey was struck by a sharp outbreak associated with a high mortality. Cases have occurred sporadically in human beings in Texas, Georgia, Florida, Rhode Island, and Tennessee. The disease in horses and mules is widespread over eastern United States and Canada and areas in Central and South America.

The ecologic and epidemiologic features of these infections are complex, with transmission cycles that may include primary and secondary vertebrate hosts and vectors.

The mode of transmission of St. Louis, Japanese, and eastern and western equine encephalitides is the bite of the mosquito. Mosquitoes become infected by biting wild birds or occasionally certain mammals. Human-to-human transmission does not occur under natural conditions. St. Louis encephalitis and western equine encephalitis are very much alike in respect to ecologic and epidemiologic factors. Both infect horses in nature, and reservoirs of silent infection have been found in domestic animals and birds. Both are found in wild caught mosquitoes (*Culex tarsalis* and *Culex pipiens*) and can be transferred in the laboratory by the bite of such mosquitoes. Both viruses have been acquired by mosquitoes feeding on birds with occult infection (viremia). The midwestern and western states are seeded with both viruses, which give rise to infection in humans during the summer.

St. Louis encephalitis virus has also been detected in chicken mites (*Dermanyssus gallinae*) during a nonepidemic period. Since transovarian infection has been shown to take place in the mite, the latter may play an important role in maintaining the virus in nature.

Japanese encephalitis virus has been detected in naturally infected mosquitoes (*Culex tritaeniorhynchus*) in Japan, and experimental transmission of infection by mosquitoes has been established. Many animals and birds have been suspected of maintaining reservoirs of infection. There is evidence of widespread infection among farm animals including horses, pigs, cattle, sheep, goats, and dogs preceding infection of chickens and human beings.

Eastern equine encephalitis virus has been isolated from naturally infected mosquitoes and birds. Pheasants seem particularly prone to epizootics. The virus has been isolated from chicken mites and chicken lice in an epidemic area. The factors involved in transmission are apparently similar to those found in western equine and St. Louis encephalitides.

The vector for Colorado tick fever is *Dermacentor andersoni*, and the principal host reservoirs are ground squirrels and chipmunks. Powassan virus apparently is transmitted by *Ixodes* ticks, and squirrels and chipmunks may provide the reservoir.

TREATMENT

It is recommended that all patients suspected of having encephalitis be hospitalized promptly in order to confirm the diagnosis and to rule out other diseases such as partially treated bacterial meningitis, tuberculous meningitis, brain abscess, drug overdosage, toxins, metabolic encephalopathy, or brain tumor. Diagnostic evaluation may include CSF examination, skull roentgenograms, electroencephalogram, CT scan, and chemical analyses for toxins, drugs, and metabolic aberrations.

Although there has been little to offer in the way of specific treatment for viral encephalitis in the past, recent evidence (Skoldenberg et al., 1984) indicates that acyclovir or vidarabine may be lifesaving in patients with encephalitis caused by herpes simplex virus (Chapter 11). Clinical manifestations of temporal lobe involvement are common and may be supported by electroencephalograms and brain scan. It is recommended that the diagnosis be established by biopsy of the involved lobe for isolation of herpes simplex virus or by identification of herpesvirus antigen with fluorescent-antibody methods before treatment is begun. Treatment is most beneficial when given early in the course of the disease, before brain damage occurs from necrotic infection or increased intracranial pressure.

The use of corticosteroids or glycerol, urea, mannitol, and other hypertonic solutions may effect a temporary drop in intracranial pressure, but the usual rebound effect diminishes their value. The use of urea is contraindicated in the presence of hepatic or renal insufficiency.

Drugs such as chlorpromazine or diazepam may control hyperexcitability and convulsions. Hyperthermia is usually relieved by giving the patient tepid sponge baths or by using a cooling blanket. Intravenous infusions with 75% of maintenance requirements may be necessary to maintain proper balance of water and electrolytes. Severe involvement of the medulla—with impairment of swallowing, accumulation of secretions in the throat, and paralysis of the vocal cords or respiratory muscles—may occur. If gentle aspiration fails to keep the airway open, intubation or tracheostomy may be required. Ventilator support may be necessary for patients with respiratory paralysis that is either peripheral or central in origin.

CONTROL MEASURES
Active immunization

Effective means of control of postinfectious encephalitis caused by measles, mumps, and rubella viruses have been available for some time. Widespread use of vaccines has significantly reduced the incidence of encephalitis associated with these diseases. On the other hand, the control of arbovirus infections presents many problems. Since man is not part of the infection chain but represents an accidental, "dead-end" infection and since outbreaks are unpredictable, a rational basis for mass immunization is hard to demonstrate. In any event, with the exception of Japanese encephalitis, no vaccine suitable for human use is available for the arbovirus infections listed on p. 33. Japanese encephalitis (JE) vaccine, prepared from infected mouse brains, is produced in Japan (Biken JE vaccine) and has been made available to U.S. travelers before departure for endemic areas. It requires two doses subcutaneously at a 1- to 2-week interval. Serologic studies suggest that the neutralizing antibodies produced are effective in vitro against strains of Japanese encephalitis from both India and Japan.

Arthropod control

Attempts to control the arbovirus encephalitides should be directed against the arthropod vector and reservoirs of infection in order to interrupt the natural cycle of transmission.

In the western states where outbreaks are rural, the intensive use of agricultural insecticides has been followed by reduction in mosquitoes and in human infection rates. In the central states, where outbreaks of St. Louis encephalitis occur in urban-suburban areas, the main vectors are *C. pipiens* and *C. quinquefasciatus* mosquitoes, which are known to multiply in dirty water and in places where there is inadaquate drainage. The characteristic pattern observed in many epidemics is a period of heavy rainfall followed by drought, resulting in many pools of stagnant water yielding vast numbers of mosquitoes. Prompt drainage of these areas and application of insecticides (larvicides and adulticides) should interrupt the infection chain and thereby reduce the incidence of human infection.

REFERENCES

Barrett FF, Yow MD, Phillips CA. St. Louis encephalitis in children during the 1964 epidemic. JAMA 1965;193:381.

Calisher CH, Thompson WH. California serogroup viruses, vol. 123. New York: Alan R Liss Inc., 1983.

Centers for Disease Control. Viral hemorrhagic fever: initial management of suspected and confirmed cases. MMWR 1983;32:27S.

Centers for Disease Control. Human arboviral encephalitis-United States 1983. MMWR 1984;33:339.

Charney EB, Orecchio EJ, Zimmerman RA, Berman PH. Computerized tomography in infantile encephalitis. Am J Dis Child 1979;133:803.

Cramblett HG, Stegmiller H, Spencer C. California encephalitis virus infections in children. JAMA 1966;198:128.

Ecklund CM. Human encephalitis of the western equine type in Minnesota in 1941: clinical and epidemiological study of serologically positive cases. Am J Hyg 1946;43:171.

Ehrenkrantz NJ, Sinclair NC, Buff E, Lyman DO. The natural occurrence of Venezuelan equine encephalitis in the United States. N Engl J Med 1970;282:298.

Fothergill LD, Dingle JH, Farber S, Connerley ML. Human encephalitis caused by virus of eastern variety of equine encephalomyelitis. N Engl J Med 1938;219:411.

Griffith JF, Ch'ien LT. Viral infections of the central nervous system. In Galasso GJ (editor). Antiviral agents and viral diseases of man. New York:Raven Press, 1984.

Haymaker W, Smadel JE. The pathology of viral encephalititis. Washington DC. Army Medical Museum, 1943.

Johnson RT. The contribution of virologic research to clinical neurology. N Engl J Med 1982;307:660.

Johnson RT, Griffin DE, Hirsch RL, et al. Measles encephalomyelitis—clinical and immunologic studies. N Engl J Med 1984;310:137.

Johnson RT, Mims CA. Pathogenesis of viral infections of the nervous system. N Engl J Med 1968;278:23.

Kappus KD, Calisher CH, Baron RC, et al. La Crosse virus infection and disease in western North Carolina. Am J Trop Med Hyg 1982;31:556.

Kiley MP, Bowen ETW, Eddy GA, et al. Filoviridae; a taxonomic home for Marburg and Ebola viruses? Intervirology 1982;18-24.

Koskiniemi M, Donner M, Pettay O. Clinical appearance and outcome in mumps encephalitis in children. Acta Paediatr Scand 1983;72:603.

Koskiniemi M, Vaheri A, Taskinen E. Cerebrospinal fluid alterations in herpes simplex virus encephalitis. Rev Infect Diseases 1984;6:608.

Levitt LP, Lovejoy FH Jr, Daniels JB. Eastern equine encephalitis in Massachusetts: first human case in 14 years. N Engl J Med 1971;284:540.

Luby JP. St. Louis encephalitis. Epidemiol Rev 1979;1:55.

Matthews REF. Classification and nomenclature of viruses. In Melnick JL (ed). Intervirology: 4th report of the international committee on taxonomy of viruses. Basel: S. Karger, 1982.

Medovy H. Western equine encephalomyelitis in infants. J Pediatr 1943;22:308.

Neal JB, et al. Encephalitis: a clinical study. New York: Grune & Stratton, Inc., 1942.

Powell KE, Blakey DL. St. Louis encephalitis, the 1975 epidemic in Mississippi. JAMA 1977;237:2294.

Reeves WC. Overwintering of arboviruses. Prog Med Virol 1974;17:193.

Reye RDK, Morgan G, Baral J. Encephalopathy and fatty degeneration of the viscera: disease entity in childhood. Lancet 1963;2:749.

Roos RP, Graves MC, Wollman RL, et al.: Immunologic and virologic studies of measles inclusion body encephalitis in an immunosuppressed host: the relationship to subacute sclerosing panencephalitis. Neurology 1981;31:1263.

Shope RE. Arboviruses. In Lennette EH, Spaulding EH, Truant JP (ed). Manual of clinical microbiology, ed. 2. Washington DC:American Society of Microbiology, 1974.

Skoldenberg B, Forsgren M, Alestig K, et al. Acyclovir versus vidarabine in herpes simplex encephalitis. Lancet 1984;2:707.

Tesh RB, Peters CJ, Meegan JM. Studies on the antigenic relationship among phleboviruses. Am J Trop Med Hyg 1982;31:556.

Vianna N, et al. California encephalitis in New York State, Am J Epidemiol 1971;94:50.

Whitley RJ, Soong SJ, Linneman C, Jr, et al. Herpes simplex encephalitis, clinical assessment. JAMA 1982;246:317.

5

ENTEROVIRAL INFECTIONS

Human illnesses caused by enteroviruses have certain features in common, such as a predilection of viruses for the central nervous system (CNS) and meninges. The various clinical manifestations range in severity from paralytic poliomyelitis and fatal myocarditis to very mild or inapparent infections. As more information has accumulated about the many enteroviruses and their varied clinical manifestations, it is apparent that with few exceptions there is much overlap in the spectrum of illness induced. No single clinical syndrome is restricted to only one virus type.

HISTORY

Sporadic cases of paralytic disease are as old as recorded history. The term *poliomyelitis* was derived from the Greek for gray marrow of the spinal cord and the Latin (itis) for inflammation; the location of the involved cells in the anterior horns of the spinal cord contributed the designation *anterior*. The first isolation of poliovirus was achieved in 1908 by the inoculation of central nervous system tissue into susceptible monkeys via the intracerebral route. In 1949, Enders, Robbins, and Weller reported their classic experiments on the cultivation of poliovirus in tissue cultures of nonneural human cells.

The histories of the other enteroviruses are relatively recent. In 1948, Dalldorf and Sickles isolated an agent from the stool of a patient with paralytic illness from Coxsackie, New York. Subsequently, a large group of antigenically related viruses have been designated *Coxsackie A and*

B. Isolation of ECHO viruses was accomplished from fecal specimens and frequently from patients without overt disease. Their name is an acronym: E—enteric, C—cytopathic, H—human, O—orphan. They have been associated with a wide variety of illnesses and are no longer "orphans." Since 1969, new enterovirus types have been assigned "enterovirus type" numbers rather than being designated Coxsackie or ECHO viruses.

ETIOLOGY

Enteroviruses were so named because of their natural habitat within the gastrointestinal tract. The family of picornaviruses consists of six major groups: polioviruses, ECHO viruses, group A Coxsackieviruses, group B Coxsackieviruses, the new enterovirus serotypes 68 to 71, and hepatitis A virus (Table 5-1). All of these agents infect and multiply in the gastrointestinal tract.

Table 5-1. Picornaviradae

Virus	Serotype
Polioviruses	1 and 2
Coxsackie viruses, group A	1 to 24*
Coxsackie viruses, group B	1 to 6
ECHO viruses	1 to 34†
Enteroviruses	68 to 71
Hepatitis A	?1

*Coxsackie A-23 is the same as ECHO virus type 9.
†ECHO virus type 10 is now a reovirus; ECHO virus type 28 is now a rhinovirus.

Enteroviruses are 30-nm particles composed of a single-strand RNA genome with a protein coat of icosahedral symmetry. The viruses are indistinguishable morphologically, stable at pH 3, and resist inactivation by ether. Assignment of a virus to one of these groups is based on chemical properties, differences in growth in tissue culture systems, pathogenicity for various strains of laboratory animals, and serologic reactivity.

The RNA of enteroviruses is a positive single strand and therefore, by definition, serves as the messenger RNA for the replication cycle of the virus. This messenger RNA codes for a polyprotein containing the amino acid sequence for all structural proteins of the virus. All enteroviruses code for four proteins (VP1, VP2, VP3, and VP4), which constitute the capsid of the virus and are derived by cleavage of the precursor polyprotein. These proteins can be demonstrated by immunoprecipitation of extracts of radiolabeled infected cells with serotype-specific serum and staphylococcal protein. Fig. 5-1 illustrates resolution of the immunoprecipitated capsid proteins of ECHO virus type 30 by sodium dodecyl sulfate-polyacrylamide gel electrophoresis followed by autoradiography. Experiments examining the antigenic relationship of poliovirus strains by immunoprecipitation and neutralization of virus with type-specific sera suggest that the four capsid proteins contain the antigens that determine the serotype of the virus strain. Recent work suggests that VP2 induces specific neutralizing antibodies for several ECHO viruses and Coxsackie B3 (Beatrice et al., 1980), and VP1 is the major group reactive protein (Katze and Crowell, 1980). These specifications are not the same for each group of enteroviruses. VP1 of polioviruses induces neutralizing antibodies.

It is probable that one or more of the capsid proteins are responsible for specific virus-cell interaction. In the case of the enteroviruses, the specificity of the interaction of a viral protein with a cell receptor most likely determines the tissue tropism of the virus. This has been best elucidated with polioviruses (Medrano and Green, 1973) where naked viral RNA can rep-

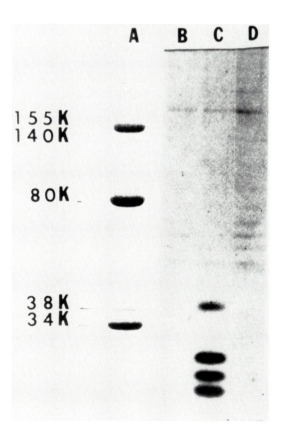

Fig. 5-1. Radioimmunoprecipitation of ECHO virus 30 proteins. Resolution of immunoprecipitated capsid proteins of ECHO virus 30 by sodium dodecyl sulfate–polyacrylamide gel electrophoresis followed by autoradiography. The four protein bands corresponding to VP0, VP1, VP2, and V3 range in molecular weight from Mr 40,000 to Mr 20,000. Reovirus 3 proteins of designated molecular weight are shown in lane A, with appropriate negative controls in lanes B and D. K = 1000. *Lane A*, reovirus 3 marker; *lane B*, ECHO virus 30–infected cell lysate + nonimmune rabbit serum; *lane C*, ECHO virus 30–infected cell lysate + ECHO virus 30–immune rabbit serum; *lane D*, uninfected cell lysate plus ECHO virus 30–immune rabbit serum. (From Wilfert, CM, et al. Pediatr Infect Dis 1983;2:333.)

licate in usually nonpermissive cells once entry into the cell has been accomplished (Holland et al., 1959).

Cell lines permissive to growth of viruses are numerous, and their susceptibility to those viruses pathogenic for humans varies widely. There is no single cell culture system that permits replication of all members of the enterovirus group. Primate epithelial cells are generally used because they support growth of a wide spectrum of enteroviruses. Many strains of the Coxsackie A viruses, however, cannot be isolated in such cell cultures, and suckling mice must be used. Recovery of the virus from the infected tissue or host secretion is the most sensitive means of detecting viral infections, but normally a limited number of cell types is used by each laboratory.

PATHOGENICITY FOR ANIMALS

Grouping of enteroviruses requires mention of their pathogenicity for various species of animals. Coxsackie A viruses grow poorly in cell cultures, whereas newborn mice provide a more reliable system for their detection. The distinction between Coxsackie groups A and B depends on the pathologic lesions produced in mice. Group A viruses cause generalized myositis and flaccid paralysis. Group B viruses cause focal myositis and typical lesions in the infrascapular fat pad and brain. Myocarditis, endocarditis, hepatitis, and necrosis of the acinar tissue of the pancreas can also be produced by group B viruses. Freshly isolated poliovirus and ECHO viruses are not pathogenic for mice, but a strain of poliovirus type 2 has been adapted to these rodents and laboratory strains of ECHO virus type 9 have produced disease in mice. The molecular basis for these differences remains to be defined, but it is probable that the host cell receptor for a virus protein(s) is the limiting determinant.

PATHOGENESIS AND PATHOLOGY OF ENTEROVIRAL INFECTIONS

Enteroviruses gain entry to the host via the mouth. The virus establishes infection in the oropharynx and portions of the gastrointestinal tract where multiplication subsequently occurs. Virus then gains access to adjacent lymph nodes and the bloodstream. With ECHO virus type 9 infections viremia occurs up to 5 days before onset of symptoms (Yoshioka and Horstmann, 1962). The incubation period of enteroviral infections is usually from 1 to 5 days. During the initial replication of virus within the gastrointestinal tract, there may be no overt illness or a nonspecific febrile illness.

Enteroviruses can multiply in peripheral white blood cells in vitro, although there are too few data to make broad generalizations. It has been shown that ECHO virus type 33 multiplies in peripheral mononuclear white blood cells, specifically in monocytes (Gnann et al., 1979). Other studies suggest that these viruses might also replicate in lymphocytes.

Viral invasion of other tissues, such as the meninges or the myocardium, typically occurs from 7 to 10 days after initial exposure to the virus, resulting in the classic biphasic illness such as occurs with poliovirus. Enteroviruses may be excreted in the stool for as long as 6 to 8 weeks after onset of illness. Virus is present for a shorter time in the oropharynx, usually being detected only during the first 5 to 7 days of illness.

Most Coxsackie and ECHO virus infections are transient and nonfatal; therefore, limited histologic information is available. The pathogenic changes of poliovirus in the CNS are most prominent in the spinal cord, medulla, pons, and midbrain. After initial cytoplasmic alterations in the Nissl substance of the motor neurons, nuclear changes develop and pericellular infiltration of polymorphonuclear and mononuclear cells occurs. The final state is destruction with neuron phagocytosis and dropping out of the necrotic cells.

Fatal newborn infection with enterovirus has shown nonspecific but extensive damage of the infected tissues. The ECHO virus infections are associated with hepatic necrosis and evidence of disseminated intravascular coagulation in multiple organs. If the patient has lived long enough, the liver may then show cirrhosis as opposed to the acute process.

CLINICAL ILLNESS

The broad spectrum of clinical disease produced by the enteroviruses overlaps among groups. A listing of the various syndromes are included in Table 5-2. The more common manifestations associated with infection are discussed briefly.

Table 5-2. Clinical manifestations of enterovirus infections

Clinical syndrome	Polio	Coxsackie A	Coxsackie B	ECHO	Enteroviruses 68 to 71
Asymptomatic infection	X	X	X	X	
Nonspecific febrile illness	X	X	X	X	
Respiratory disease		X	X	X	
Exanthems		X	X	X	
Enanthems		X			
Pleurodynia			X		
Orchitis					
Myocarditis			X		
Pericarditis			X	X	
Aseptic meningitis and meningoencephalitis	X	X	X	X	
Disseminated neonatal infection			X	X	
Transitory muscle paresis	X	X	X	X	
Paralytic disease	X	X	X	X	X
Hemorrhagic conjunctivitis		X			X

X, may result from multiple serotypes.

Febrile illness

The great majority of infections with enteroviruses produce no specific clinical manifestations. Although the portal of entry is the gastrointestinal tract, they are not frequently responsible for gastroenteritis. In young children, undifferentiated febrile illness, nonspecific malaise, and myalgias are frequently associated with enterovirus infections. There is nothing unique about this type of clinical presentation. A prospective study of newborn infants in Rochester, New York, demonstrated that during a typical enterovirus season as many as 13% of infants acquired infection with these viruses during the first month of life. Although four fifths of these patients were asymptomatic, most of the symptomatic infants were admitted to the hospital because they were suspected of having bacterial sepsis (Jenista et al., 1984). These observations provide an estimate of the frequency of enteroviral infection of very young infants; it is an impressive seven infections per 1000 live births that occur in the first month of life during the months of seasonal prevalence of these agents. It has come to be appreciated that enteroviral infection is as common as other neonatal infections of widespread clinical concern.

Congenital and neonatal infections

Transplacental and neonatal transmission have been demonstrated with Coxsackie B viruses, resulting in a serious disseminated disease that may include hepatitis, myocarditis, meningoencephalitis, and adrenal cortical involvement (Kibrick and Benirschke, 1958). Coxsackie viruses have also been established as a cause of acute myocarditis of infants. Isolation of Coxsackie B3, B4, and A16 viruses from the myocardium and/or intestine of newborn infants was first reported in the late 1950s.

The onset of illness is sudden with loss of appetite, vomiting, coughing fits, cyanosis, and dyspnea. At first the disease may be mistaken for pneumonia. Marked pallor and tachycardia are characteristic features. Signs of decompensation come on rapidly. The heart and liver become enlarged. No cardiac murmur is heard as a rule. The electrocardiogram shows evidence of severe myocardial damage. In fatal cases the infant shows a gray pallor, goes rapidly into severe prostration and circulatory collapse, and dies. In those who survive, recovery may be equally rapid.

The heart is grossly enlarged and pale; it is dilated and sometimes hypertrophied. Microscopic examination shows myocarditis of varying extent, with little or no evidence of involvement of the pericardium or endocardium. The valves are normal, and the myocardium shows a diffuse cellular infiltration between the muscle fibers. The striations are distinct in some areas, and others show degeneration and necrotic fibers. The infiltration consists of polymorphonuclear leukocytes, lymphocytes, eosinophils, plasma cells, and reticulum cells. The brain and spinal cord of one patient showed focal areas of cellular infiltration and degeneration of glial tissue and ganglion cells (Fig. 5-2). Specific etiology and diagnosis are established by virus isolation and unfortunately may be limited to postmortem tissue specimens unless feces are sampled during life.

Infants infected in the newborn period with ECHO viruses have died with disseminated disease, the predominant feature of the infection being hepatic necrosis (Modlin, 1980). Serologic studies have suggested that maternal antibody protects infants from severe disease, although they may acquire infection as documented by virus excretion (Modlin et al., 1981). It is important not to induce delivery if a pregnant woman near term is suspected of having enteroviral infection, so that maternal antibody formation and subsequent passive transplacental transmission can occur. When poliovirus infections were common, examples of transmission from infected mother to fetus were apparent by the birth of a paralyzed infant.

Heart

Liver

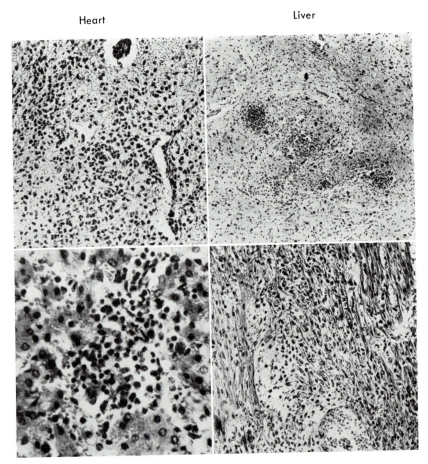

Brain

Fig. 5-2. Histologic appearance of the heart, liver, and brain in Coxsackie virus infection, showing diffuse and focal cellular infiltration. (From van Crevald S, de Jager H. Ann Pediatr 1956;187:100.

Respiratory disease

Mild upper respiratory tract illness has been associated with several of the Coxsackie and ECHO viruses. Very few cases of pneumonia have been attributed to Coxsackie virus infection.

Hemorrhagic conjunctivitis

A pandemic of acute hemorrhagic conjunctivitis was ascribed to enterovirus 70; it occurred from 1969 to 1971 in Africa, Southeast Asia, Japan, and India. The second epidemic in 1981 reached the Americas. Coxsackie A-24 has also been implicated in this syndrome. Severe subconjunctival hemorrhage creates a noticeable and alarming sign. The patient also has swelling, redness, congestion, and tearing and pain in the eye. The prognosis is excellent with complete recovery in approximately 1 week. Unusually, poliolike motor paralysis has accompanied the conjunctivits.

Exanthems and enanthems

Various enteroviruses (particularly ECHO virus types 9 and 16 and Coxsackie viruses A-2, A-4, A-9, A-16, B-3, B-4, and B-5) have been associated with large outbreaks of febrile rash disease. Younger children are more likely to develop exanthems which vary widely in their characteristics. Macular and maculopapular eruptions indistinguishable from rubella have been observed with a number of Coxsackie and ECHO viruses. Petechiae have accompanied some rashes, especially with ECHO virus type 9. The presence of virus has been demonstrated in the skin lesions.

Hand-foot-and-mouth disease. Hand-foot-and-mouth infection is characterized by fever and a vesicular eruption involving chiefly the buccal mucosa and tongue and less frequently the palate, gums, and lips; a maculopapular rash appears on the hands and feet that becomes vesicular, is interdigital on the dorsum of hands and feet, and involves the palms and soles. Robinson et al. (1957) first described this syndrome and its cause as Coxsackie virus A-16. Subsequent reports have confirmed these observations and added Coxsackie viruses A-5 and A-10 as other etiologic agents.

Herpangina. Herpangina is most commonly associated with group A Coxsackie infections and is characterized by sudden onset with high fever lasting from 1 to 4 days. Loss of appetite, sore throat, and dysphagia are common, and vomiting or abdominal pain occurs in about 25% of cases. The hallmark of the infection lies in the throat. Minute vesicles or, if these have ruptured, small, punched-out ulcers appear on the anterior pillars of the fauces, the tonsils, the uvula, the pharynx, and the edge of the soft palate. The gray-white vesicles are 1 to 2 mm in diameter with red areolae. The lesions enlarge for 2 to 3 days, the areolae become more intensely red, and, later, shallow gray-yellow ulcerations not over 5 mm in diameter are seen. The general and local symptoms disappear in 4 to 6 days, and recovery is complete.

The diagnosis of herpangina is suggested by (1) the typical small vesicles or ulcerations limited in number to about 15 or 20 and (2) distribution to the pharyngotonsillar area. Because many different serotypes of the ECHO and Coxsackie viruses can cause identical clinical pictures, virus isolation is necessary to identify the specific etiologic agent. Herpangina is easily confused with herpetic gingivostomatitis (p. 140). Herpangina is likely to occur during the summer or early fall and may also be epidemic, whereas herpes simplex infections occur sporadically in any season. The distinguishing features of herpes simplex infections are swollen red gums, involvement of the buccal mucosa, and the confluent character of the lesions.

Pleurodynia

Pleurodynia is also called epidemic pleurodynia, epidemic myalgia, Bornholm disease, and devil's grip. It is an acute disease caused chiefly by various members of the group B Coxsackie viruses, although occasionally group A viruses may be implicated. The onset is sudden, with severe paroxysmal thoracic pain. Chest pain is pleuritic in type and is aggravated by deep breathing, coughing, or other movements. It is described as stabbing, knifelike, smothering, catching, or like being caught in a vise. About one fourth of the patients have prodromal symptoms beginning 1 to 10 days before the onset of pain and consisting of headache, malaise, anorexia, and vague muscular aches. Abdominal pain occurs in addition to chest pain in about 50% of patients. Pain may be most severe in the substernal region, simulating coronary artery disease. Cough is either nonproductive or productive of a small amount of sputum. It is annoying mainly because of aggravation of pain. In most instances if anorexia, nausea, vomiting, and diarrhea accompany the chest pain they are of short duration.

Fever ranges from 37.2° to 40° C (99° to 104° F). It may last from 1 to 14 days, with the average being 3½ days. A pleural friction rub may be heard in about one fourth of the patients. Tenderness and splinting may be found in the upper abdomen, in the periumbilical area, and on the right side more often than on the left. The tenderness appears most often to be superficial, suggesting involvement of the muscle wall rather than of deeper structures. Laboratory findings, including a roentgenogram of the chest, are normal in most cases, but pleural effusions may be observed.

Orchitis

Although viral orchitis most often is due to mumps, it has accompanied infections with the Coxsackie B viruses.

Myocarditis and pericarditis

Isolated myocarditis and/or pericarditis in older children and adults may result from group B Coxsackie or ECHO virus infections. The spectrum has ranged from benign, self-limited pericarditis to severe, chronic, fatal myocardial disease.

Meningitis-meningoencephalitis

The clinical manifestations of enteroviral CNS infection are not specific. The onset can be gradual or abrupt and the predominant symptoms include fever, headache (when a child is old enough to report it), malaise, and signs of meningeal irritation (Table 5-3). Temperatures as high as 40° C (104° F) can be recorded and fever usually lasts for 3 to 5 days. Infants under 1 year of age often lack meningeal signs. Although the child may have an altered sensorium, focal neurologic findings are rare. Severe illness may be accompanied by seizures, particularly in the youngest infants. Infants who had enteroviral meningitis when less than 1 year of age and who were longitudinally followed demonstrated neurologic deficits that tended to be in the area of

receptive language functions (Sells et al. 1975; Wilfert et al., 1981). Occasionally paralytic illness, indistinguishable from poliomyelitis, occurs due to nonpolio enteroviruses. The spectrum of illness includes motor weakness and encephalitis, but these manifestations are very unusual.

Most patients with enteroviral meningitis recover so that pathologic descriptions are based on only a few cases. There is inflammation of the meninges with perivascular inflammatory cell infiltration. The most acute process is likely to have a predominance of polymorphonuclear cells, whereas mononuclear cells become predominant after a relatively few days.

The physician's assessment of the CNS inflammatory response is judged primarily on the laboratory findings in the cerebrospinal fluid (CSF). The CSF shows a leukocyte cell count ranging from none to several thousand cells per cubic millimeter. Most often the cell count is less than 500. It is common to have a polymorphonuclear cell predominance early in the illness. Cases of viral meningitis with onset of symptoms averaging 1½ days before initial lumbar puncture showed from 68% to 86% polymorphonuclear cells (Feigin and Shackelford, 1973). A second lumbar puncture done after 6 to 8 hours revealed a shift to mononuclear cell predominance in 87% of patients. Thus, serial examination of the CSF can help to differentiate viral from bacterial infection. The rapid shift to lymphocyte predominance during a matter of hours is unusual in

Table 5-3. Clinical signs and symptoms of 103 patients with viral meningitis, Duke University Medical Center, June to September, 1972

Sign or symptom	Number	Percentage
Headache[a]	79	92*
Temperature >38° C (100.4° F)	78	76
Nuchal rigidity	69	67
Nausea and/or vomiting	53	51
Diarrhea	6	6
Cough	6	6
Rash	5	5

*Based on the number of children 5 years of age and older.

bacterial meningitis even with antimicrobial therapy (Feigin and Shackelford, 1973).

The total protein content of the CSF is often within normal limits, but it may be elevated and even markedly so in a small percentage of the patients. Glucose content of CSF is usually normal, but it may be diminished (less than 50% of a simultaneous serum glucose or less than 40 mg/dl) in enteroviral CNS infection (Singer et al., 1980).

Patients with agammaglobulinemia are unable to eradicate enteroviruses from the CNS (Wilfert et al., 1977). Infections have persisted for as long as 8 years. Relentless progressive deterioration in CNS function occurs, frequently accompanied by seizures, transient hemiparesis, and an altered sensorium. Symptoms and signs may wax and wane, but progressive loss of function ultimately is associated with focal defects or cortical atrophy on computed tomographic scan. The final phase of illness is characterized by a dermatomyositis syndrome with virus present in blood and many other tissues.

Poliomyelitis

Poliovirus infections range from asymptomatic to paralytic illness. The ratio of inapparent to paralytic infection is variously estimated to be from 100:1 to 850:1. Even with overt infection, most persons have a mild and brief illness, starting abruptly and lasting from a few hours to a few days. It is characterized by fever, uneasiness, sore throat, headache, nausea, anorexia, vomiting, and pain in the abdomen. One or more of these symptoms may occur. Except for slight redness of the throat, there usually are no physical findings. There are no signs of involvement of the CNS.

Nonparalytic poliomyelitis

Nonparalytic poliomyelitis (meningitis) is characterized by many of the same features just listed and in addition by pain and stiffness of the neck, back, and legs. Headache is more severe, the temperature is higher, and the patient is sicker than with minor illness. Hyperesthesia and sometimes paresthesia may occur. At this stage, the CSF usually shows pleocytosis, with a slight predominance of polymorphonuclear leukocytes. The protein level is slightly elevated. Soon the proportion of lymphocytes rises.

Later the cells diminish as the protein level rises.

Paralytic desease

Poliovirus infection, especially type 1, is responsible for most of the paralytic disease caused by enteroviruses. Occasional cases of transient paralysis and muscle weakness have been noted with other enteroviruses, particularly the group B Coxsackie agents. More recently, enteroviruses 70 and 71 have been associated with paralytic disease and encephalitis (Shindarov et al., 1979; Wadia et al., 1983). With classic paralytic polio, there is a 2- to 6-day incubation period with an initial nonspecific febrile illness. This probably coincides with early replication of virus in the pharynx and gastrointestinal tract. With the subsequent hematogenous spread of virus, central nervous system involvement may result in meningitis and anterior horn cell infection. From 1% to 4% of susceptible patients infected with polioviruses develop central nervous system involvement. The spectrum of paralytic disease is enormously variable and may involve only an isolated muscle group or extensive paralysis of all extremities. Characteristically, the picture is one of asymmetrical distribution, the lower extremities more frequently involved than the upper. Large muscle groups are more often affected rather than the small muscles of the hands and feet. Involvement of cervical and thoracic segments of the spinal cord may result in paralysis of the muscles of respiration. Infection of cells in the medulla and the cranial nerve nuclei results in bulbar polio with compromise of the respiratory and vasomotor centers.

Studies have indicated that tonsillectomy and adenoidectomy predispose to paralytic poliomyelitis in general. Strenuous exercise and fatigue occurring at the onset of the major illness have often been followed by severe paralysis. The relationship of intramuscular injections of vaccines, especially combinations of diphtheria-tetanus-pertussis, and subsequent paralysis in the injected extremity is well established. The mechanisms by which these predisposing factors operate are unknown.

With the return of the patient's temperature to normal, the progress of paralysis ceases, and the subsequent weeks and months reveal a varying spectrum of recovery ranging from full return of function to significant residual paralysis. Atrophy of involved muscles becomes apparent after 4 to 8 weeks. Recovery may be exceedingly slow, and its full extent cannot be judged for 6 to 18 months.

Bulbar poliomyelitis

Bulbar poliomyelitis is characterized by damage to the motor nuclei of the cranial nerves and other vital zones in the medulla concerned with respiration and circulation. It may occur in the absence of clinically recognized involvement of the spinal cord. Tonsillectomy and adenoidectomy within 1 month of onset increase the risk of bulbar involvement. Bulbar poliomyelitis is potentially the most life-endangering form. The incidence of bulbar involvement varies from 5% to 10% of the total number of paralytic cases.

The most ominous form of bulbar poliomyelitis results from spread of infection to the respiratory and vasomotor centers. Damage to the respiratory center causes breathing to become irregular in rhythm and depth. Respirations are shallow and are associated with periods of apnea. The pulse rate and temperature increase. The blood pressure, at first elevated, may drop rapidly to shock levels. The patient becomes confused, delirious, and comatose, and then respiration stops. When the vasomotor center is involved, the pulse becomes extremely rapid, irregular, and difficult to palpate. The blood pressure fluctuates from high to low levels with a small pulse pressure.

On clinical grounds it is impossible to distinguish nonparalytic and preparalytic poliomyelitis from aseptic meningitis of another cause. Since the striking decrease in incidence of poliomyelitis in the postvaccine era, the most commonly recognized causes of aseptic meningitis are Coxsackie and ECHO viruses. Paralytic poliomyelitis has been confused with infectious polyneuritis, or Guillain-Barré syndrome. In contrast to poliomyelitis, the distribution of paralysis in the latter condition is usually symmetrical, and sensory changes including loss of sensation frequently occur. Facial diplegia is also common, and the CSF shows no cells but a high protein content (albuminocytologic dissociation) early in the disease. Recovery is often rapid and complete. Paralysis caused by postdiphtheritic polyneuritis and by transverse myelitis has been mistaken for poliomyelitis. Tick paralysis should

be considered in cases of widespread involvement. Patients with pseudoparalysis caused by pain and tenderness and unwillingness to move an extremity have been referred to a hospital with a diagnosis of poliomyelitis. Subsequent examination has shown osteomyelitis, acute rheumatic fever, trichinosis, scurvy, or congenital syphilis to be the underlying cause. Hysterical paralysis was not uncommon during epidemics.

EPIDEMIOLOGY

The epidemiology of all human enteroviruses is quite similar. The pattern is most clearly defined for the polioviruses because paralytic disease has been so readily identifiable. As early as 1916, the epidemiologic features were defined on the basis of an outbreak that occurred that year in New York City; these features include the following.

1. Poliomyelitis is, in nature, exclusively a human infection, transmitted from person to person without the necessary intervention of a lower animal or insect host.
2. The infection is far more prevalent than is apparent from the incidence of clinically recognized cases, since a large majority of infected persons excrete virus without clinical manifestations. It is probable that during an epidemic a considerable proportion of the population becomes infected, adults as well as children.
3. The most important sources of infection are subclinical and mild abortive cases that ordinarily escape recognition. It is certain that overt paralytic cases are a relatively minor factor in the spread of infection.
4. An epidemic of one to three recognized cases per 1000 immunizes the general population to such an extent that the outbreak declines spontaneously.

Enteroviruses have a worldwide distribution with increased prevalence during the warm months of the year in temperate climates. In the United States, some variation in geographic distribution of infections may be due to importation of viruses from other countries. Epidemics occur between May and October in the United States and other areas of the northern temperate zone. The seasonal prevalence of these viruses is shown in Fig. 5-3. Sporadic infections due to these viruses can occur at any time throughout the year.

The seroepidemiology of enteroviral infections, including polio and hepatitis A viruses, demonstrates an increased transmission of infection at a young age among persons of lower socioeconomic status. Crowding creates intimate living conditions and may also be associated with poor hygiene, which enhances the fecal-to-oral transmission of these agents.

Enteroviral illness is most commonly reported in children 1 to 4 years of age. It is not clear whether the infections occur more frequently in infants or whether recognition and reporting of disease reflects an enhanced concern over any illness at that age. Nevertheless, when specific outbreaks occur within a community, persons of all ages may be infected.

A 2- to 5-year periodicity has been observed with Coxsackie B infections, suggesting that the limited number of serotypes contributes to this pattern. These agents are also able to cause outbreaks of disease when a newly susceptible population is present in the community. When a specific virus circulates frequently, younger infants who have not been exposed previously are more likely to be susceptible and develop disease. Perhaps the numerous serotypes of ECHO viruses have a broader range of age-related attack rates, since a given serotype only circulates through a community sporadically. It is unlikely that any individual would encounter all serotypes of enteroviruses in childhood.

The clinical epidemiology of these infections suggests that respiratory excretion of virus is not as important a means of spread as is fecal-to-oral transmission. Intimate human contact is important in transmission of virus and communicability within households is greatest between children. Diapered infants appear to be more efficient disseminators of infection than other individuals. In the current era of day-care centers and nursery schools, it has already been shown that hepatitis A virus is transmitted in this setting and if present is transmitted to virtually all children in the nursery. It is likely that outbreaks

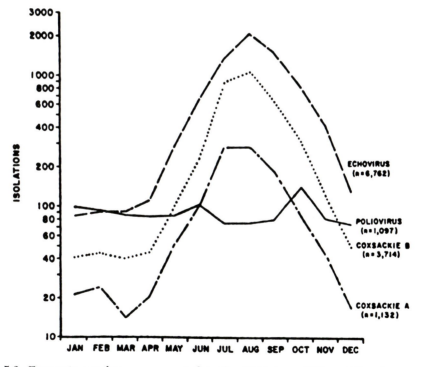

Fig. 5-3. Enterovirus isolations as reported to the CDC from 1970 to 1979. The seasonal distribution of poliovirus isolates is different from other enteroviruses, as these isolates are vaccine virus and reflect immunization practices rather than occurrence of disease. (From Centers for Disease Control. Enterovirus surveillance, summary 1970-1979. U.S. Department of Health and Human Services, November 1981.)

of infection due to other enteroviruses are also occurring in these facilities.

Community outbreaks of enteroviral infection can spread to hospital nurseries. A newborn who acquires virus from his mother or from nursery personnel may spread it throughout the nursery. The viruses can be introduced into intensive care units by patients or personnel. Recognition of such infections imposes a need to institute isolation precautions such as cohorting of infants and personnel to minimize spread of infection.

IMMUNITY

Enteroviruses induce secretory and humoral antibody responses. The humoral responses are initially predominantly IgM antibodies followed by IgA and IgG antibodies which persist for months to years. Coproantibodies, primarily IgA, have been studied as a response to administration of poliovirus vaccines or to natural infection. Local secretory immunoglobulin A production occurs at the site of contact of virus with lymphoid cells. Development of type-specific antibody provides lifelong protection against clinical illness due to the same agent. Local reinfection of the gastrointestinal tract may occur, but this is accompanied by only an abbreviated period of viral replication without clinical illness.

In experimental poliovirus infection specific IgG antibody-producing cells and measurable antibodies can be demonstrated in areas of the central nervous system where virus is replicating. Local central nervous system antibody production is independent of systemic humoral antibody production. Although specific CNS enterovirus antibodies are probably produced primarily within the central nervous system, some passive transfer of serum antibody to the CSF may occur as permeability is increased by inflammation. In viral meningitis, only minimal elevation of CSF globulin has been documented. Evidence for the extreme importance of CNS antibody is deduced from agammaglobulinemic patients who are unable to eliminate enteroviruses from the CNS. Administration of extraordinarily large quantities of parenteral globulin or plasma with specific antibody is necessary to achieve measurable antibody levels in the CSF.

Cellular immunity against enterovirus infection is not well defined. Circulating peripheral white blood cells have been a source of virus isolation during acute illness. Recognition of virus by lymphocytes occurs in experimental models using Coxsackie viruses. The abnormal response of some children with immunodeficiency disease to infection with attenuated polioviruses may offer insights to immune processes normally stimulated by enterovirus infection.

DIAGNOSIS

The clinical illnesses in some instances may permit a presumptive diagnosis of enterovirus infection. However, as shown in Table 5-2, the spectrum of illness is wide. The time of the year may be helpful. In temperate zones, enteroviral infections occur most often in the summer and early autumn. Specimens for virus isolation should be obtained early in the course of illness. The cerebrospinal fluid of patients with viral meningitis and/or meningoencephalitis has been a rich source of enteroviruses, except for the three polio types. Materials such as pleural and pericardial fluid should also be cultured when available.

Specific etiologic diagnosis of enteroviral disease is presently dependent on demonstration of the enterovirus by cell culture techniques. Unfortunately, most of the group A Coxsackie viruses grow poorly in cell cultures, and newborn mice provide a more reliable system for detection of these agents. Various primate and human cell culture systems will support replication of most of the enteroviruses with cytopathic effects revealing their presence. The specimens submitted most often for attempted virus isolations are nasopharyngeal swabs and stool specimens. An enterovirus may be excreted in fecal material for several weeks after the onset of clinical illness. Recovery of an enterovirus from the throat or stool of the patient does not in itself establish this as the etiologic agent of the illness observed. The temporal association of illness, virus recovery, and an antibody rise specific to that agent provide firmer evidence of a causative relationship.

A potentially useful and more practical approach to diagnosis would be the demonstration of viral antigen in clinical specimens, especially CSF. It would be ideal if antigen could be detected by a method capable of providing a specific diagnosis within hours. Recent work has demonstrated the feasibility of detecting enterovirus RNA by hybridization assays employing cell culture-grown virus. The preliminary work shows promise of being specific but is not yet sufficiently sensitive for clinical application. At the present time virus isolation remains the most sensitive means of detecting virus because of the amplification in cell culture.

Acute and convalescent serum samples obtained from 7 to 21 days apart will help to define quantitative changes in antibody titers. Complement fixation, virus neutralization, immunoprecipitation, and, in a few instances, hemagglutination inhibition are the available techniques for assaying enterovirus antibodies. Neutralizing antibodies are type specific, whereas complement fixation demonstrates group-reactive antibodies. In the course of a lifetime, humans sustain multiple infections, occult or overt, with a variety of enteroviruses. A specific infection elicits the production of antibody specific to that virus type but also may prompt an anamnestic response demonstrated by an increase in group-reactive antibody and by parallel rises in antibodies to serotypes of some of the other enteroviruses previously encountered. The concomitant serologic rises in heterologous antibody titer create some problems with serologic surveys, rendering the complement fixation test inadequate to define a specific infection. The isolation of a specific virus provides the opportunity for assessment of the patient's antibody against his own viral agent. In the absence of the recovery of a virus, one faces the problem of seeking specific antibody rises against the whole genus of enteroviruses. Thus the complexity of serology makes the serologic diagnosis of these infections impractical. During an outbreak of enterovirus infection identification of the specific infecting virus makes it possible to assess the sera of patients for the presence of antibody to that serotype. Serologic diagnosis by viral neutralization is a convenient but cumbersome epidemiologic tool for diagnosis in epidemic settings.

TREATMENT

There is no specific treatment for poliomyelitis. There is no evidence that immune serum globulin changes the course of events once signs of the illness have appeared. In fact, most patients already have specific antibodies in the early stages of illness.

Complete bed rest is vital. There is a close correlation between the amount of physical activity early in the major illness and the incidence and severity of subsequent paralysis. It is not possible to discuss here the management of paralytic poliomyelitis in all of its complex details. This is the province of the physician and the physical therapist.

In patients who have difficulty in swallowing and involvement of either the medullary centers or muscles of respiration, the preservation of a clear airway is vital. Respiratory support may include oxygen, endotracheal intubation, and respirator-assisted ventilation. The nurse contributes enormously to the physical needs of the patients, especially those requiring ventilatory assistance. It is often the nursing personnel who help to maintain the patient's morale by showing confidence and efficiency.

Prevention

Because there currently is no specific treatment for enterovirus infections, efforts have focused on means of prevention. The multiple antigenic types, and the usually benign, self-limited course of most ECHO virus and Coxsackie virus infections have resulted in little stimulus to the development of vaccines. The story of the poliovirus vaccines, however, has been one of the most exciting and rewarding sagas in microbiologic history. Prior to the work of Enders and colleagues with successful tissue culture techniques for growth of the polioviruses, there had been several ill-fated vaccines prepared from emulsions of spinal cord removed from monkeys infected with wild-type poliovirus. These preparations were treated with formalin or other inactivating agents. Trials of such "vaccines" in 1935 proved unsuccessful.

Enders' tissue culture techniques lent themselves to the propagation in vitro of sufficient amounts of relatively pure poliovirus, so that controlled formaldehyde inactivation could be used to produce noninfectious virus that retained its antigenicity. Salk and his colleagues pursued this line of research and by 1954 were able to embark on a field trial which established the efficacy of an inactivated poliovirus vaccine in the prevention of paralytic disease. This was a trivalent preparation incorporating the three poliovirus types. After an initial series of two or three injections spaced several weeks to months apart, followed by a booster 6 to 12 months later, there was demonstrable serum antibody to all three polio serotypes. The vaccine was widely used in the United States during the 5 years from 1956 through 1960. The results were dramatic. Previous years had seen from 10,000 to 20,000 cases of paralytic disease reported annually. With the widespread use of the Salk vaccine, this rapidly dropped to 2000 or 3000 cases annually, as increasingly large numbers of susceptible individuals were immunized (Fig. 5-4).

By the early 1960s a second vaccine was available. Strains of poliovirus which Sabin had selected and studied in the laboratory were proven attenuated for monkey and human. Ingestion of these strains resulted in intestinal infection and virus excretion, so that humoral and gastrointestinal tract immunity developed without any illness. Because this vaccine could be administered more conveniently by the oral route, and

because the multiplication in the gastrointestinal tract more closely mimicked natural infection, it offered certain selected advantages, which led to its replacing the injectable Salk vaccine. Over the first 5 years of the 1960s, more than 400 million doses of oral vaccine were distributed in the United States. At the same time, trials also were successfully conducted in European nations, Japan, and other countries. The use of the oral vaccine in the United States was accompanied by a further decrease in the annual reported polio cases (Fig. 5-4), so that beginning in 1966 fewer than 100 have occurred each year. Between 1969 and 1981, with continued use of the oral vaccines, a total of 203 cases of paralytic disease were reported in the United States. In less than 20 years, a disease that had claimed thousands of victims annually and that had been

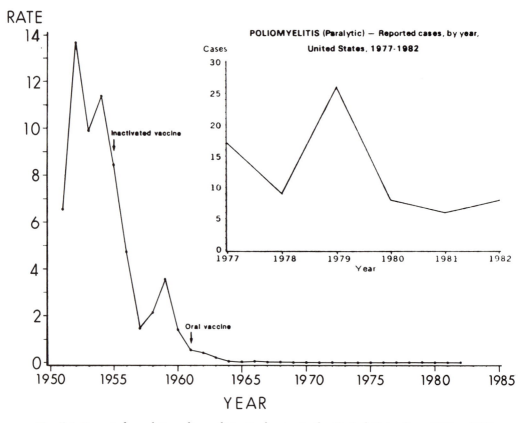

Fig. 5-4. Reported paralytic poliomyelitis attack rates in the United States from 1951 to 1982. (From Morbid Mortal Weekly Rep 1983;31[No.54]:63.)

the source of indescribable community anxiety was reduced to a rarity!

In the complex processes of vaccine development, commercial production, and widespread utilization, a number of unexpected events transpired that merit consideration. After the highly successful field trials of 1954, commercial manufacture of the Salk-type vaccine was licensed. Within a few weeks of its use, paralytic disease was observed in April to June 1955 among children in California and Idaho who had received some of the first lots of commercial vaccine manufactured by the Cutter Laboratories. By the time this had been fully investigated and resolved, it was learned that there were 204 cases of vaccine-associated disease. Seventy-nine were among children who had received the vaccine, 105 were among their family contacts, and 20 were in community contacts. Nearly three quarters of the cases were paralytic, and there were 11 deaths. The agent isolated from these patients was type 1 poliovirus. Laboratory tests on vaccine distributed by Cutter Laboratories revealed viable virulent type 1 poliovirus in 7 of 17 lots (Nathanson and Langmuir, 1963). Revisions of the federal regulations governing vaccine manufacture were promptly promulgated and implemented to prevent recurrence of such a tragic episode.

Manufacturers faced further difficulties in maintaining the fine balance between the complete elimination of the infectious live virus from the production process and the retention of effective antigenicity of the inactivated components. A number of lots of vaccine subsequently proved to be poorly antigenic for type 3 poliovirus. As a result, when community polio outbreaks occurred among well-immunized groups, there were "breakthroughs" with paralytic disease, especially due to type 3 poliovirus, in previously immunized subjects. Such an outbreak was studied in 1959 in Massachusetts, where an analysis of polio cases revealed that 47% (62 of 137) of the patients had previously received three or more inoculations of inactivated vaccine (Berkovich et al., 1961).

In the United States, inactivated vaccine has been used sparingly in the past 20 years. Almost all immunization has been conducted with the oral attenuated product. The average number of cases of paralytic poliomyelitis has been less than 10 per year. A number of European countries, especially those in Scandinavia, have adhered to the use of inactivated vaccine. With successful production of fully potent antigens, their record of achievement in the control of polio had been parallel to that of the United States until 1984. In October 1984 an outbreak of poliomyelitis occurred in Finland. Six patients had paralytic disease caused by type 3 poliovirus. Paralysis occurred in patients who had previously received up to five doses of inactivated poliovaccine. Wild poliovirus type 3 was isolated from 15% of 700 asymptomatic children. The same virus was isolated from sewage specimens collected from sites throughout Finland (WHO, 1985).

The marked decrease in paralytic disease due to "wild" polioviruses has disclosed a small but significant number of cases of oral vaccine recipients who have developed paralytic illness in temporal association to the ingestion of vaccine. In addition to these few cases among recipients of vaccines, there have also been paralytic episodes reported among susceptible family or community contacts of the vaccine recipients. These have been few in number and are difficult to characterize with complete clarity. A small portion of these patients have been found to be immunodeficient children, particularly those with congenital hypogammaglobulinemia. One concern has always been that the attenuated strains of virus might prove genetically unstable in human intestinal passage, so that increased neurovirulence might result from widespread dissemination. This has not been demonstrated. Monovalent oral polio vaccine (MOPV) was used extensively until 1964, when it was supplanted by trivalent vaccine (TOPV). With MOPV the risk of vaccine-associated illness in recipients was estimated to have been 1 per 5 million doses distributed. With TOPV an overall figure of risk to recipients and their contacts has been calculated at 0.28 per million or one case per 3.6 million doses.

The achievements with poliovirus vaccination have been impressive in the United States, Canada, and most of Europe, Australia, and some Asian and African nations. Polio remains an endemic disease in many tropical lands. It is therefore premature to relax the use of poliovirus vaccination in those parts of the world where disease has been nearly eradicated. The possibility of the inadvertent introduction of virulent virus is omnipresent.

REFERENCES

Annual Summary 1980. Morbid Mortal Weekly Rep 1982a; 30:25, 103.

Annual Summary 1980. Morbid Mortal Weekly Rep 1981a; 29:23, 29.

Baron RC, Hatch MH, Kleeman K, et al. Aseptic meningitis among members of a high school football team. An outbreak associated with echovirus 15 infection. JAMA 1982;248:1724.

Beatrice S, Katze MG, Zajac BA, et al. Induction of neutralizing antibodies by the Coxsackie virus B3 virion polypeptide VP2. Virology 1980;104:426.

Berkovich S, Pickering JE, Kibrick S. Paralytic poliomyelitis in Massachusetts, 1959. A study of the disease in a well-vaccinated population. N Engl J Med 1961;264:1323.

Centers for Disease Control. Aseptic meningitis surveillance, annual summary 1976. Atlanta, Ga: U.S. Department of Health, Education, and Welfare, January 1979.

Centers for Disease Control: Enterovirus surveillance, summary 1970-1979. U.S. Department of Health and Human Services, U.S. Public Health Service, November 1981b.

Centers for Disease Control: Poliomyelitis surveillance, summary 1980-1981. Atlanta: U.S. Department of Health and Human Services, U.S. Public Health Service, December 1982b.

Chonmaitree T, Menegus MA, Powell KR. The clinical relevance of CSF viral culture. A two-year experience with aseptic meningitis in Rochester, New York. JAMA 1982; 247:1843.

Dalldorf G, Sickles GM. An unidentified filtrable agent isolated from the feces of children with paralysis. Science 1948;108:61-62.

Enders JF, Weller TH, Robbins FC. Cultivation of the Lansing strain of poliomyelitis virus in cultures of various human embryonic tissues. Science 1949;109:85.

Feigin RD, Shackelford PG. Value of repeat lumbar puncture in the differential diagnosis of meningitis. N Engl J Med 1973;289:571.

Finn JJ, Weller TH, Morgan HR. Epidemic pleurodynia: clinical and etiologic studies based on one hundred and fourteen cases. Arch Intern Med 1949;83:305.

Fox JP, Gelfand HM, LeBlanc DR, et al. Studies on the development of natural immunity to poliomyelitis in Louisiana. I. Overall plan, methods and observations as to patterns of seroimmunity in the study group. Am J Hyg 1957;65:344.

Francis T Jr, et al. An evaluation of the 1954 poliomyelitis vaccine trials, summary report. Am J Public Health 1955;45(Part 2):1-63.

Gard S. Inactivated poliomyelitis vaccine: present and future. In First International Conference on Vaccines Against Viral and Rickettsial Infections of Man, Scientific Publication no. 147, Washington, DC. Pan American Health Organization, World Health Organization, 1967, pp 161-170.

Gnann JW, Hayes EC, Smith JZ, et al. Echovirus 33 replication in human peripheral white blood cells. J Med Virol 1979;3:291.

Holland JJ, McLaren LT, Syberton JT. The mammalian cell virus relationship. IV. Infection of naturally susceptible cells with enterovirus ribonucleic acid. J Exp Med 1959;110:65.

Horstmann DM, McCollum RW, Mascola AD. Viremia in human poliomyelitis. J Exp Med 1954;99:355.

Huebner RJ, et al. Herpangina: etiological studies of a specific infectious disease. JAMA 1951;145:628.

Hughes JR, Wilfert CM, Moore M. Echovirus 14 infection associated with fatal neonatal hepatic necrosis. Am J Dis Child 1972;123:61.

Jenista JA, Powell KR, Menegus MA. Epidemiology of neonatal enterovirus infection. J Pediatr 1984; 104:685.

John CC, Cherry JD. Mild neonatal illness associated with heavy enterovirus infection. N Engl J Med 1966;274:394.

Katze MG, Crowell RL. Immunological studies of the group Coxsackie viruses by the sandwich enzyme-linked immunosorbant assay (ELISA) and immunoprecipitation. J Gen Virol 1980;50:357.

Kibrick S, Benirschke K. Severe generalized disease (encephalohepatomyocarditis) occurring in the newborn period and due to infection with Coxsackie virus, group B. Evidence of intrauterine infection with this agent. Pediatrics 1958;22:857.

Kono R, Sasagawa A, Ishii K, et al. Pandemic of new type of conjunctivitis. Lancet (June 3) 1972;1:1191-1194.

Linnemann CC Jr, et al. Febrile illness in early infancy associated with ECHO virus infection. J Pediatr 1974; 84:49.

Medrano L, Green H. Picornavirus multiplication in human mouse hybrid cell lines. Virology 1973;54:515.

Melnick JL. Portraits of viruses: The picornaviruses. Intervirology. 1983;20:61-100.

Melnick JL, Ledinko N. Development of neutralizing antibodies against the three types of poliomyelitis virus during an epidemic period. The ratio of inapparent infection to clinical poliomyelitis. Am J Hyg 1953;58:207.

Melnick JL, Rennick V. Infectivity titers of enterovirus as found in human stools. J Med Virol 1980;5:205.

Modlin JF. Fatal echovirus 11 disease in premature neonates. Pediatrics 1980;66:775.

Modlin JF, Polk BF, Horton P, et al. Perinatal echovirus infection: risk of transmission during a community outbreak. N Engl J Med 1981;305:368.

Morens DM. Enteroviral disease in early infancy. J Pediatr 1978;92:374.

Nagington J, Wreghitt TG, Gandy G, et al. Fatal echovirus 11 infections in outbreak in special care baby unit. Lancet (September 30) 1978;2:725.

Nathanson N, Langmuir AD. The Cutter incident, I, II, III. Am J Hyg 1963;78:16-81.

Nathanson N, Martin JR. The epidemiology of poliomyelitis: enigmas surrounding its appearance, epidemicity and disappearance. Am J Epidemiol 1979;110:672-692.

Nightingale EO. Recommendations for a national policy on poliomyelitis vaccination. N Engl J Med 1977;297:249.

Nogen AG, Lepow ML. Enteroviral meningitis in very young infants. Pediatrics 1967;40:617.

Ogra PL. Distribution of echovirus antibody in serum, nasopharynx, rectum and spinal fluid after natural infection with echovirus type 6. Infect Immun 1977;2:150.

Ogra PL. Effect of tonsillectomy and adenoidectomy on nasopharyngeal antibody response to poliovirus. N Engl J Med 1971;284:59.

Ogra PL, Ogra S, Al-nakeeb S, et al. Local antibody response to experimental poliovirus infection in the central nervous system of rhesus monkeys. Infect Immun 1973;8:931.

Paul JR. A history of poliomyelitis. New Haven, Connecticut: Yale University Press, 1971.

Robinson CR, Doane FW, Rhodes AJ. Report of an outbreak of febrile illness with pharyngeal lesions and exanthem, Toronto summer 1957: isolation of group A Coxsackie virus. Can Med Assoc J 1957;79:615.

Russell WR. The management of acute poliomyelitis. Monograph series no. 26. Geneva: World Health Organization, 1955, p 137.

Sabin AB. Poliomyelitis: accomplishments of live virus vaccine. In First International Conference on Vaccines Against Viral and Rickettsial Diseases of Man. Scientific Publication no. 147. Washington, DC. Pan American Health Organization, World Health Organization, 1967, pp 171-178.

Sabin AB, et al. Live orally given poliovirus vaccine. Effects of rapid mass immunization on population under conditions of massive enteric infection with other viruses. JAMA 1960;173:1521.

Sells CJ, Carpenter RL, Ray CG. Sequelae of central nervous system enterovirus infection. N Engl J Med 1975; 293:1.

Shindarov LM, Chumakov MP, Voroshilova MK, et al. Epidemiological, clinical and pathomorphological characteristics of epidemic poliomyelitis-like disease caused by enterovirus 71, J Hyg Epidemiol Microbiol Immunol 1979; 23:284-295.

Singer JI, Mauer PR, Riley JP, et al. Management of central nervous system infections during an epidemic of enteroviral aseptic meningitis. J Pediatr 1980;96:559.

Steigman AJ, Lipton MM, Braspenonicke H. Acute lymphonodular pharyngitis: a newly described condition due to Coxsackie A virus. J Pediatr 1962;61:331.

van Creveld S, de Jager H. Myocarditis in newborns, caused by Coxsackie virus. Clinical and pathological data. Ann Pediatr 1956;187:100-112.

Wadia NH, Katrak SM, Misra VP, et al. Polio-like motor paralysis associated with acute hemorrhagic conjunctivitis in an outbreak in 1981 in Bombay, India: clinical and serologic studies. J Infect Dis 1983;147:660.

Wedgwood RJ, Mease PJ, Ochs HD: Successful treatment of echovirus meningoencephalitis and myositis—fascitis with IV immune globulin therapy in a patient with X-linked agammaglobulinemia. N Engl J Med 1981; 304:1278.

Weiner LS, Howell JT, Langford MP, et al. Effect of specific antibodies on chronic Echovirus type 5 encephalitis in a patient with agammaglobulinemia. J Infect Dis 1979; 140:858.

Wenner HA, Lou TY: Virus diseases associated with cutaneous eruptions. Prog Med Virol 1963;5:219.

Wilfert CM, Buckley RH, Mohanakumar T, et al. Persistent and fatal CNS echovirus infections in patients with agammaglobulinemia. N Engl J Med 1977;296:1485.

Wilfert CM, Buckley RH, Rosen FS, et al. Persistent enterovirus infections in agammaglobulinemia. In Schlessinger D, editor: Microbiology 1977, Washington, DC, American society for Microbiology, 1977, p 488.

Wilfert CM, Lauer BA, Cohen M, et al. An epidemic of echovirus 18 meningitis. J Infect Dis 1975;131:75.

Wilfert CM, Lehrman SN, Katz SL: Enteroviruses and meningitis. Pediatr Infect Dis 1983;2:333.

Wilfert CM, Thompson RJ, Sunder T, et al.: Longitudinal assessment of children with enteroviral meningitis during the first three months of life. Pediatrics 1981;67:811.

Wong JY, Woodruff JJ, Woodruff JF. Generation of cytoxic T lymphocytes during Coxsackie virus B-3 infection. I. Model and viral specificity. J Immunol 1977;118:1159.

Woodruff JF, Woodruff JJ: Involvement of T lymphocytes in pathogenesis of Coxsackie virus B3 heart disease. J Immunol 1974;113:1726.

World Health Organization. Outbreak of paralytic poliomyelitis. Weekly Epidem Rec 1985;60:10.

Yolken RH, Torsch VM: Enzyme-linked immunosorbant assay for the detection and identification of Coxsackie B antigen in tissue cultures and clinical specimens. J Med Virol 1980;6:45.

Yolken RH, Torsch VM. Enzyme-linked immunosorbant assay for detection and identification of Coxsackie viruses A. Infect Immun 1981;31:742.

Yoon JW, Austin M, Onodera T, et al. Virus-induced diabetes mellitus. N Engl J Med 1979;300:1173.

Yoshioka I, Horstmann DM. Viremic infection due to echovirus type 9. N Engl J Med 1962;262:224.

6

EPSTEIN-BARR VIRUS INFECTIONS

The Epstein-Barr virus (EBV) was discovered in the 1960s in cell lines derived from Burkitt's African lymphomas (Epstein et al., 1964). Today this virus is well recognized as the etiologic agent of infectious mononucleosis. This syndrome has recently been expanded to include rare chronic and fatal infections that may develop in immunoincompetent hosts. EBV has also been implicated causally in Burkitt's lymphoma, in nasopharyngeal carcinoma, and, most recently, in B-cell lymphomas in immunocompromised patients.

INFECTIOUS MONONUCLEOSIS

Infectious mononucleosis is an acute infectious disease occurring predominantly in children and young adults. It is characterized clinically by fever, exudative or membranous pharyngitis, generalized lymphadenopathy, and splenomegaly. The peripheral blood picture characteristically shows an absolute increase in number of atypical lymphocytes, and the serum has a high titer of heterophil antibody. Specific EBV antibodies are detected early in the illness and persist for years thereafter.

HISTORY

Infectious mononucleosis was first described as "glandular fever" by Pfeiffer in 1889. The term *infectious mononucleosis* was used by Sprunt and Evans (1920) in their description of a clinical syndrome in college students that was characterized by a mononuclear leukocytosis. The first serologic test identifying the association of heterophil antibody and mononucleosis was described by Paul and Bunnell (1932). This nonspecific test was made more specific by the development of differential absorption tests by Davidsohn (1937) and considerably simpler and more rapid by the more recent evolution of slide tests. The association of infectious mononucleosis with EBV was described by Henle et al. (1968) three decades later.

ETIOLOGY

Although discovery of the causative agent of infectious mononucleosis eluded the efforts of many competent investigators for many years, it was generally assumed to be a virus. A report by Henle et al. (1968) provided evidence of a relationship between the herpes-type virus now known as EBV and infectious mononucleosis.

In 1968 Niederman et al. reported the formation of antibodies against EBV by means of an indirect immunofluorescence test. In 24 patients with infectious mononucleosis, antibodies that were absent in pre-illness specimens appeared early in the disease, rose to peak levels within a few weeks, and remained at high levels during convalescence. These antibodies were shown to be clearly distinctive from heterophil antibodies.

Subsequent studies by Niederman et al. in 1970 and Sawyer et al. in 1971 provided additional evidence indicating that EBV is the cause of infectious mononucleosis. The evidence that supports this concept is as follows: (1) EBV antibody is absent prior to onset of illness, appears during illness, and persists for many years thereafter; (2) clinical infectious mononucleosis occurs only in persons lacking antibody, and it fails to occur when antibody is present; (3) EBV has been isolated from the pharynx and saliva of infectious mononucleosis patients during their illness and for many months thereafter (Miller et al., 1973); and (4) cultured lymphocytes from patients who have had infectious mononucleosis will form continuous cell lines in vitro that contain the EBV genome and EBV antigens.

EBV is a member of the herpesvirus group. Mature infectious particles are 150 to 200 nm in diameter, with a lipid-containing envelope surrounding an icosahedral nucleocapsid with 162 capsomeres. The genome is composed of double-stranded DNA. The virus has a very narrow host range, infecting primarily B lymphocytes of human or other primate origin. Its nucleic acid, however, has also been demonstrated in epithelial cells of nasopharyngeal carcinoma tissue. Infected epithelial cells of the buccal mucosa may also be a source of EBV (Neiderman, 1982).

A number of viral antigens have been characterized, including viral capsid antigen (VCA), EB nuclear antigen (EBNA), membrane antigen, and an early antigen (EA) complex of D (diffuse component) and R (restricted component). Antibodies may be demonstrated by complement fixation and virus neutralization, in addition to indirect immunofluorescence (Henle et al., 1979).

PATHOLOGY

The generalized nature of infectious mononucleosis becomes apparent when the pathologic aspects of the disease are studied. Grossly, there may be fairly general enlargement of the lymphoid tissues as manifested by lymphadenopathy, splenomegaly, and pharyngeal lymphoid hyperplasia. Histologically, the focal mononuclear infiltrations are found to involve the lymph nodes, spleen, tonsils, lungs, heart, liver, kidneys, adrenal glands, central nervous system, and skin.

The lymphoid hyperplasia of infectious mononucleosis is nonspecific; pathologically it resembles many other conditions. It is usually a benign lymphoproliferative process. First, EBV-infected B lymphocytes develop a surface membrane antigen that is recognized by T lymphocytes and

that stimulates them to proliferate (Epstein and Achong, 1977). EBV is also a polyclonal activator of B cells that induces them to actively secrete IgG, IgA, and IgM. Rocchi et al. (1977) noted that as many as 0.05% of circulating mononuclear leukocytes in the early acute phase of IM were infected with EBV. EBV remains latent in a smaller number of B lymphocytes following recovery from infectious mononucleosis.

The proliferation of T cells induces generalized lymph node hyperplasia and infiltration of many organs. The characteristic atypical lymphocytes in the peripheral blood in infectious mononucleosis are transformed T lymphocytes, not EBV-infected B cells (Pattengale et al., 1974). Purtilo (1981) has termed these atypical lymphocytes "combatants in an immune struggle." Some of these cells, cytotoxic T cells, have the specific ability to eliminate EBV-infected B cells (Svedmyr and Jondal, 1975). Others nonspecifically eliminate EBV-infected cells (natural killer [NK] cells) (De Waele et al., 1981). Still others suppress activation of EBV-infected B cells (Tosato et al., 1979). It has been proposed that when this complex and finely tuned immunoregulatory mechanism fails, chronic and/or fatal EBV infection results. For example, if cytotoxic or suppressor T cells fail to eliminate infected B cells, excessive lymphoproliferation may occur. If, on the other hand, NK and/or cytotoxic T-cell activity is excessive, extensive B-cell death with resultant agammaglobulinemia may result (Andiman, 1984).

EPIDEMIOLOGY

Although EBV infection is worldwide in distribution, clinical infectious mononucleosis is observed predominantly in developed countries, principally among adolescents and young adults. Seroepidemiologic surveys have revealed a gradual acquisition of antibody with age so that 50% to 90% of persons show a positive antibody reaction by young adult life. The overall incidence of clinical infectious mononucleosis is approximately 50 per 100,000 persons per year in the general population of the United States. The incidence of mononucleosis in susceptible college students is 5460 per 100,000 persons, 100 times higher than in the general population (Evans, 1969; Niederman et al., 1970). The total EBV infection rate is estimated to be higher (11,500 per 100,000 yearly), indicating that as many subclinical infections occur as overt infections. The so-called subclinical infections may be truly apparent infections or an atypical disease such as thrombocytopenia, hemolytic anemia, and/or rash (Andiman, 1979).

The epidemiologic factors that have a significant effect on the host response to EBV infection include age, socioeconomic status, and geographic location. In general, infection during infancy and childhood is apt to be inapparent (Sumaya, 1977). In contrast, clinical infectious mononucleosis is more common in adolescents and young adults. In developing countries of the world where sanitation is poor, exposure to EBV occurs at a very early age. In the United States, infection generally occurs at an early age in low socioeconomic groups who live in crowded conditions with poor hygiene.

Many seroepidemiologic studies have confirmed the well-known fact that infectious mononucleosis is not highly contagious, even in family settings. Henle and Henle (1970) found evidence of spread in three of eight families (37.5%), and Fleischer et al. (1981) found spread in seven of 36 susceptible contacts (19%). However, EBV infection appears to spread more efficiently under the conditions that exist in certain day-care nurseries (Pereira et al., 1969) and orphanages (Tischendorf et al., 1970).

The most likely modes of transmission are oral-salivary spread in children and close intimate contact (kissing) in young adults (Hoagland, 1955; Evans, 1960). Cell-free infectious virus is carried in saliva (Morgan et al., 1979). Miller et al. (1973) have shown prolonged pharyngeal excretion of EBV for periods up to several months after clinical infectious mononucleosis. About 15% of immune individuals excrete EBV in saliva at any one point in time (Henle and Henle, 1970). Presumably this is due to silent reactivation of latent EBV. Patients undergoing immunosuppression appear to develop an increased incidence of reactivation of latent EBV infection and have an increased frequency (over 50%) of oropharyngeal excretion (Strauch et al., 1974). The infection can also be transmitted by transfusion of blood that is contaminated with latent EBV.

CLINICAL MANIFESTATIONS

The incubation period has been estimated to range between 4 and 6 weeks. The accuracy of this estimate, however, is questionable, since in most instances both the source and time of contact are unknown.

The disease may begin abruptly or insidiously with headache, fever, chills, anorexia, and malaise, followed by lymphadenopathy and severe sore throat. The clinical picture is extremely variable in both severity and duration. The disease in children is generally mild; in adults it is more severe and has a more protracted course.

Fever

The temperature usually rises to 39.4° C (103° F) and gradually falls by lysis over a variable period, averaging 6 days. In a severe case it is not unusual for the temperatures to hover between 40° and 40.6° C (104° and 105° F) and to persist for 2 weeks or more. Children are more likely to have low-grade fever, or they may even be afebrile.

Lymphadenopathy

Shortly after the onset of the illness, the lymph nodes rapidly enlarge to a variable size of about 1 to 4 cm. The nodes are typically tender, tense, discrete, and firm to the touch. The symptoms in part depend on the site of enlargement.

Any chain of lymph nodes may become involved. The lymph node enlargement may be generalized, but most commonly it involves the cervical group. In addition to the cervical group, the following lymph nodes also may be affected: axillary, inguinal, epitrochlear, popliteal, mediastinal, and mesenteric. Massive mediastinal lymph node enlargement has been observed in a child in whom primary tuberculosis was originally diagnosed. Mesenteric lymphadenopathy has frequently been confused with acute appendicitis. The lymph node enlargement gradually subsides over a period of days or weeks, depending on the severity and extent of involvement.

Splenomegaly

A moderate enlargement of the spleen occurs in approximately 75% of the cases. In rare instances the enlargement may be followed by spontaneous rupture, causing hemorrhage, shock, and death if it is not recognized. Rutkow (1978) reviewed 107 reports of splenic rupture in infectious mononucleosis and concluded that only 18 were truly spontaneous; most followed trauma.

Tonsillopharyngitis

Sore throat is one of the cardinal symptoms of the disease. The tonsils are usually enlarged and reddened, and more than 50% will show exudate. Thick, white, shaggy membranous tonsillitis is a common finding. In the past an unusually large number of patients who were referred to physicians as having diphtheria because of the appearance of the throat proved to have infectious mononucleosis. The membrane gradually peels off after a period of 5 to 8 days. Petechiae are often seen on the palate.

• • •

The triad of lymphadenopathy, splenomegaly, and exudative pharyngitis in a febrile patient is typical but not pathognomonic of infectious mononucleosis. Other manifestations of the disease include hepatitis, skin eruptions, pneumonitis, myocarditis, pericarditis and central nervous system (CNS) involvement.

Hepatitis

Liver involvement occurs relatively frequently in infectious mononucleosis. Hepatomegaly is common, and moderately abnormal hepatic isoenzymes are found in more than 80% of patients tested. Hyperbilirubinemia, reported in 25% of cases, may result in overt jaundice, which may precede, follow, or occur simultaneously with the lymph node enlargement. Hepatitis frequently provokes such symptoms as anorexia, nausea, and vomiting.

Skin manifestations

Skin eruptions occur in approximately 10% or 15% of all cases of infectious mononucleosis. The most common type is an erythematous maculopapular eruption similar to the rash of rubella. Rashes may also be morbilliform, scarlatiniform, hemorrhagic, urticarial, or nodular. One of our patients had a papulovesicular eruption. Rash has appeared with much greater frequency in patients receiving penicillins, especially ampicillin, early in the course of infectious mononucleosis.

Pneumonitis

A small percentage of patients with infectious mononucleosis may develop a cough that is paroxysmal in type, with a clinical picture and roentgenograms indistinguishable from those of atypical pneumonia. Pleural effusion also may

develop. It has been assumed that this is part of the picture of infectious mononucleosis because of the absence of evidence of other etiologic agents.

Central nervous system involvement

During the past three decades there have been increasing numbers of reports of nervous system involvement in infectious mononucleosis, particularly in the adult age group. These manifestations have also been observed in children. The neurologic pictures have included aseptic meningitis, encephalitis, infectious polyneuritis (Guillain-Barré syndrome), myelitis, Bell's palsy, Reye's syndrome, and acute cerebellar ataxia.

CASE 1. A 10-year-old black boy with generalized lymphadenopathy, splenomegaly, typical blood picture, and positive heterophil antibody titer developed typical encephalitis during the course of his infection. He had headache, vomiting, and drowsiness that progressed to stupor. The cerebrospinal fluid showed pleocytosis with a predominance of lymphocytes and an elevated protein level. His sensorium gradually improved, and he made an uneventful recovery.

CASE 2. A 12-year-old white girl with a classic picture of infectious mononucleosis developed weakness of both lower and upper extremities, with absent reflexes. Spinal fluid findings showed albuminocytologic dissociation characteristic of the Guillain-Barré syndrome. There were no cells and the protein value was 300 mg/dl. The paralysis cleared completely within 6 weeks. The diagnosis of infectious mononucleosis was confirmed by a typical blood smear and positive heterophil antibody test.

In general the neurologic manifestations depend on the site of involvement, which may be anywhere in the nervous system. Although the majority of patients recover completely, a small percentage may have serious sequelae or die.

Chronic mononucleosis syndromes

In 1982 Tobi et al. described seven patients with prolonged atypical illnesses believed to be due to EBV. Fever, weight loss, and lymphocytosis were most frequently reported in these young adults. All had detectable VCA IgM antibody for at least 1 year, strongly indicative of chronic EBV infection. It is unknown whether these infections were primary or due to reactivation of latent EBV. None of these patients had characteristic symptoms of infectious mononucleosis. One other reported patient seemed, at least temporally, to respond to prednisolone (Smith and Denman, 1978). Rarely have cases of classical infectious mononucleosis in apparently normal children evolved into monoclonal or polyclonal lymphomas (Robinson et al., 1980; Abo et al., 1982). These patients may have had undiagnosed immunoregulatory disorders with an abnormal immune response to EBV and resultant chronic or malignant disease.

X-linked immunoproliferative syndrome: Duncan's disease

Bizarre EBV infections in patients with recognized immunologic impairment have also been reported. Severe and often fatal infectious mononucleosis with death occurring after 1 or 2 weeks from hemorrhage, hepatic failure, or bacterial superinfection was described in kindred males (X-linked lymphoproliferative disease [XLP]) by Bar et al. in 1974 and Purtilo et al. in 1977. It has now been recognized that this sex-linked recessive genetic disorder has variable phenotypic expression. Those boys who survive EBV infection may subsequently develop a variety of hematologic complications, such as agammaglobulinemia, hypergammaglobulinemia, agranulocytosis, aplastic anemia, and malignancy (Fig. 6-1). The mean age of 100 of these boys at death was about 6 years (Purtilo et al., 1982). The underlying problem is believed to be variable immunodeficiency to EBV under the control of a defective lymphoproliferative control locus (XLC) on the X chromosome. In children who develop monoclonal B-cell neoplasms or fatal infectious mononucleosis, failure to control proliferation of B cells by cytotoxic T cells and antibodies may be occurring. Agammaglobulinemia, agranulocytosis, and aplastic anemia may be secondary to destruction of antibody-forming B cells by EBV or an excessive suppressor T-cell response, or both (Purtilo et al., 1977). This disease may be difficult to diagnose because many patients have low or undetectable serologic responses to EBV despite infection. Many such patients experience lymphocytosis; EBV DNA can be shown in tissues by molecular hybridization techniques.

EBV infections in transplant patients

It has been known for more than 15 years that EBV persists in latent form for the lifetime of the individual after primary infection with the virus. Clinical reactivation of other latent herpesviruses has long been appreciated, but reactivation of EBV with resultant illness has been recognized only recently. Reactivation with development of clinical symptoms appears to be unusual except in immunocompromised patients. For example, immunosuppressed patients who have undergone renal transplantation are subject to reactivation of EBV, leading to fever, pharyngitis, and lymphadenopathy. Immunocompromised patients may also develop monoclonal or polyclonal malignant lymphoproliferative disorders believed to be caused by EBV. One such patient was treated for some time with acyclovir, with temporary regression of the tumor (Hanto et al., 1982).

Burkitt's lymphoma and nasopharyngeal carcinoma

Burkitt's lymphoma was suspected for many years to have an underlying infectious etiology because of its epidemiologic features, such as its high rate of occurrence in tropical areas of Africa. About 20 years ago EBV was discovered in lymph node biopsy specimens from these patients. It is now hypothesized that development of the tumor requires three stages: (1) infection with EBV at a young age, (2) an environmental cofactor such as hyperendemic malaria that has a profound effect on normal immunoregulation, and (3) a chromosomal change. The latter consists of translocation of the distal part of chromosome 8 to 14; it confers the property of autonomous growth and is found in all Burkitt's lymphoma tumors, which are monoclonal B-cell lymphomas. EBV markers are lacking in the American form of Burkitt's lymphoma. It is postulated that the same genetic translocation occurs either randomly or is induced by a viral infection other than EBV. In either case, however, the outcome of the translocation is the same: development of malignancy (Klein, 1982). A diagram of the hypothesis concerning EBV malignancy, and immunity is shown in Fig. 6-2.

Nasopharyngeal carcinoma is another malignancy associated with EBV; tumor cells carry the virus genome. The disease is common in the Orient but occurs all over the world and may occur in children. IgA to VCA antibody titers correlate directly with extent of the disease, reflecting the growth of the tumor. This phenomenon has diagnostic and prognostic use for these patients.

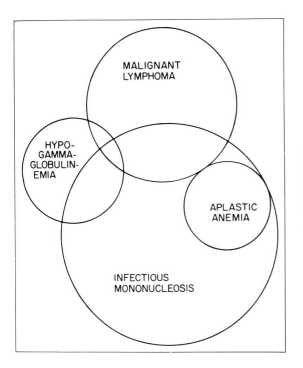

Fig. 6-1. Venn diagram displaying the relative frequency of four major phenotypes of the X-linked lymphoproliferative syndrome. Overlapping of circles indicates simultaneous occurrence of phenotypes. (From Purtilo DT, Sakamoto K, Barnabei V, et al. Am J Med 1982;73:49-56.)

EPSTEIN-BARR VIRUS-INDUCED ONCOGENESIS IN IMMUNE DEFICIENCY

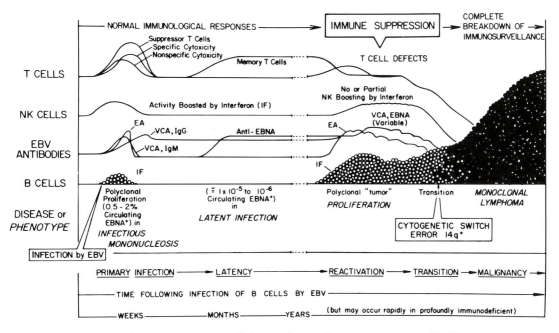

Fig. 6-2. Hypothesis summarizing cellular and humoral Epstein-Barr virus (EBV) responses. Normal immune responses to primary infection are shown at the left. Reactivation of Epstein-Barr virus and resumption of B-cell proliferation in the immune suppressed renal transplant recipient are shown at right. *EA*, early antigen; *VCA*, viral capsid antigen; *EBNA*, Epstein-Barr nuclear-associated antigen; *NK*, natural killer cells. (Reprinted by permission of the publisher from Malignant lymphoproliferative diseases induced by immunodeficient patients, including X-linked; cytogenic, and familial syndromes, by Purtilo DT. Cancer Genet Cytogenet 1981;4:251-268. Copyright 1981 by Observer Science Publishing Co., Inc.)

COMPLICATIONS

Rupture of the spleen. Rupture of the spleen is a serious but, fortunately, rare complication of infectious mononucleosis. It has been attributed to an extensive lymphocytic and mononuclear cell infiltrate that presumably causes a stretching and weakening of the capsule and trabeculae. Consequently, minor trauma such as palpation of the spleen or sudden increases in intraabdominal pressure may precipitate rupture. In rare instances it may be a spontaneous development caused by progressive intrasplenic pathologic change. The presence of this complication should be suspected in any patient who suddenly develops left-sided abdominal pain and signs of peritoneal irritation, hemorrhage, and shock (Rutkow, 1978).

Hematologic complications. The development of epistaxis, petechial and ecchymotic skin lesions, and hematuria suggests a rare complication of infectious mononucleosis. Low platelet counts, prolonged bleeding time, and poor clot retraction confirm the diagnosis of thrombocytopenic purpura. Recovery is the rule. Other rare hematologic complications include hemolytic anemia, aplastic anemia, agranulocytosis and agammaglobulinemia. These complications are most likely to occur in boys with XLP syndrome.

A rare acute hemophagocytic syndrome resembling malignant histiocytosis in infants and children has been linked to EBV infection (Wilson et al., 1981). Patients may present with fever, hepatosplenomegaly, pancytopenia, and disseminated intravascular coagulation; hemophagocytosis is found on examination of bone marrow. The mortality rate ranges from 30% to 40%. Overall the syndrome is poorly understood, except that it may be associated with EBV or other viral infections. Some of these patients appear to be immunodeficient (McKenna et al., 1981; Purtilo et al., 1982).

Cardiac complications. Electrocardiographic changes during the course of infectious mononucleosis have been reported in adults. These are usually the only manifestations of cardiac involvement. However, there have been several reports of pericarditis and myocarditis characterized by severe chest pain and typical electrocardiographic findings (Hudgins, 1976; Butler et al., 1981).

Orchitis. Orchitis may occur rarely in association with infectious mononucleosis. In one case report (Ralston et al., 1960) the testicular involvement was bilateral; in another report (Wolnisty, 1962) it was unilateral. The orchitis subsided in 2 to 4 weeks.

Congenital infection. Occasional infants with birth defects believed to be secondary to congenital EBV infection have been described. One infant manifested bilateral congenital cataracts, cryptorchidism, hypotonia, and mild micrognathia. A "celery stalk" appearance of long bones was noted radiologically, similar to that seen in congenital rubella (Goldberg et al., 1981). A report by Icart et al. (1981) described more than 700 pregnant women with serologic evidence of EBV infection during pregnancy. Their pregnancies were three times as likely to result in early fetal death, premature labor, or delivery of an infant who would become ill. Until further data are available, however, it is difficult to know whether these associations are real or coincidental. One prospective study of 4063 pregnant women during 4108 gestations failed to show any intrauterine EBV infections (Fleischer and Bologonese, 1984).

DIAGNOSIS

The diagnosis of infectious mononucleosis is usually made on the basis of (1) suggestive clinical features, (2) typical blood picture, (3) positive heterophil agglutination antibody test, and (4) ancillary laboratory findings. Younger children may have EBV infection with symptoms not characteristic of infectious mononucleosis and with negative heterophil antibody titers. In such instances measurement of specific EBV serology is required for diagnosis. The diagnosis can be confirmed by the specific tests for various antibodies against EBV antigens (Evans et al., 1975; Rapp and Hewetson, 1978). The sequence of symptoms, atypical lymphocytosis, heterophil antibody, EBV antibody, and EBV oral excretion in a patient with mononucleosis, as seen early in the illness, is illustrated in Fig. 6-3.

Clinical features

A history of fever associated with the triad of lymphadenopathy, exudative pharyngitis, and splenomegaly should suggest infectious mononucleosis as a possibility. The following laboratory tests are not specific but are helpful in establishing the diagnosis.

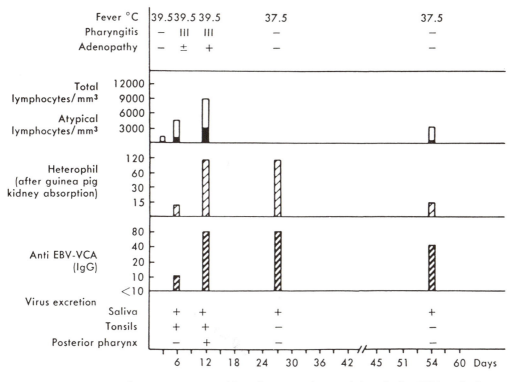

Fig. 6-3. Sequence of symptoms, atypical lymphocytosis, heterophil antibody, EBV antibody (anti-EBV-VCA), and EBV oral excretion in a patient with mononucleosis seen early in the illness. (From Niederman JC, et al. Reprinted by permission of the New England Journal of Medicine 1976;294:1355.)

Blood picture

An absolute increase in the number of atypical lymphocytes is a characteristic finding during some stages of the disease. In a blood smear these cells usually represent 10% or more of the field. These so-called Downey cells vary markedly in size and shape. With Wright stain the cytoplasm is dark blue and vacuolated, presenting a foamy appearance; the nucleus is round, bean shaped, or lobulated and contains no nucleoli. The white blood cell count is variable. During the first week of the disease there may be leukopenia, but most commonly there is leukocytosis with a predominance of lymphocytes. The white blood cell count may be so elevated that the presence of leukemia is suspected.

Atypical lymphocytes are not specific for infectious mononucleosis. They may be observed in a variety of clinical entities, including infectious hepatitis, rubella, primary atypical pneumonia, allergic rhinitis, asthma, and other diseases. Morphologically, the atypical cells in these conditions are indistinguishable from those seen in infectious mononucleosis. However, there does appear to be a *quantitative* difference; in infectious mononucleosis there are usually more than 10% atypical cells in contrast to the other conditions in which the percentage is usually less.

Heterophil antibodies

During the course of infectious mononucleosis, patients acquire a high titer of sheep cell agglutinins (heterophil antibodies) in the serum. Three possible heterophil antibody titer patterns are illustrated in Fig. 6-4.

In a group of 166 patients studied by Niederman (1956), the heterophil antibody test was positive in 38% during the first week, in 60% during the second week, and in approximately 80% during the third week.

Sheep cell agglutinins are not specific for infectious mononucleosis. They occur in a number of other conditions, such as serum sickness, infectious hepatitis, rubella, leukemia, and Hodgkin's disease. Low titers can also be demon-

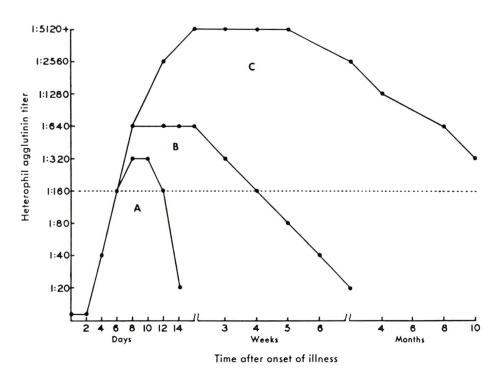

Fig. 6-4. Schematic diagram illustrating three possible patterns of the rise and fall of heterophil agglutinin titers. Titers above the horizontal dotted line are considered significant. Curve *A* shows a rapid rise and fall of agglutinins during a 2-week period. In curve *C* the agglutinin titer rises to higher levels and persists for many months. Curve *B* illustrates an intermediate pattern.

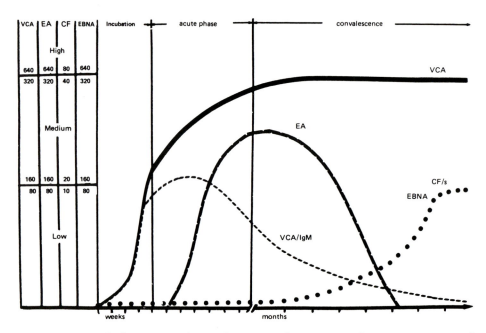

Fig. 6-5. EBV antibody response during the course of IM. *EA*, Early antigen; *VCA*, viral capsid antigen; *EBNA*, EB nuclear antigen; *CF*, complement fixation test. (From de Thé G. In Klein G. Viral oncology. New York:Raven Press, 1980, p 775.

strated in the serum of some normal persons. In general, the agglutinin titer is higher in infectious mononucleosis than in other conditions. In many laboratories a heterophil antibody titer above 1:128 is considered to be significant.

A rapid slide test utilizing equine red blood cells stabilized by formaldehyde has been evaluated as a diagnostic test for infectious mononucleosis. In 1965 Hoff and Bauer reported a high degree of correlation with the standard heterophil antibody test. They described the following advantages: (1) low incidence of false reactions, (2) high degree of specificity for infectious mononucleosis antibody, and (3) great rapidity (2 minutes) and ease of performance. This rapid test has proved to be a valuable diagnostic aid in clinical practice. Other rapid slide tests have become available, utilizing the same principle of the absorbed heterophil agglutination but employing equine or ovine erythrocytes that are citrated or formalinized. All of these have shown a high index of positive correlation with the standard Paul-Bunnell titer of 1:56 or greater (Rapp and Hewetson, 1978).

Antibody titers to specific EBV antigens

Although infectious mononucleosis occurs only in seronegative individuals, IgG antibody to the VCA may already be detectable early in the course of the illness. This antibody usually persists for life. Antibody to the nuclear antigen (EBNA) appears more slowly, taking from 1 to 6 months to become detectable. Thus a positive anti-VCA titer and a negative anti-EBNA titer is diagnostic of acute infectious mononucleosis. The acute illness may also be diagnosed if EBV-specific IgM is present in serum, but this assay is difficult to perform and may yield false-positive reactions due to rheumatoid factors in blood. It is only available on a research basis. A diagram showing the sequence of development and persistence of these antibodies to EBV is shown in Fig. 6-5.

DIFFERENTIAL DIAGNOSIS

Infectious mononucleosis is a great mimic of many other diseases. Lymphadenopathy, splenomegaly, and exudative tonsillitis are common manifestations of a number of entities. The following conditions are often confused with infectious mononucleosis.

Streptococcal tonsillitis or pharyngitis

This is suggested by fever, sore throat, exudative tonsillitis, and cervical adenitis. An increase in number of polymorphonuclear leukocytes, positive culture from a throat swab specimen, and prompt therapeutic response to penicillin all point to a streptococcal cause.

Diphtheria

The membranous tonsillitis of infectious mononucleosis frequently resembles diptheria. The diagnosis is confirmed by positive culture.

Blood dyscrasias

Blood dyscrasias, particularly leukemia, are suggested by the lymphadenopathy, splenomegaly, and increase in number of lymphocytes. Laboratory tests, including bone marrow aspiration, establish the true diagnosis.

Rubella

Rubella is commonly associated with a 2- to 4-day period of malaise and lymphadenopathy preceding the appearance of the rash. Rubella has a milder course, and frequently there is a history of exposure. A definite diagnosis of rubella can be established by evidence of a rise in the level of hemagglutination-inhibition (HI) antibody.

Measles

Measles, which is less frequently confused with infectious mononucleosis, is easily identified by the pathognomonic Koplik's spots. In doubtful cases a diagnosis of measles can be confirmed by demonstration of a rise in the level of measles HI antibody.

Viral hepatitis

This disease may be clinically indistinguishable from infectious mononucleosis with jaundice. Specific serologic tests can confirm a diagnosis of hepatitis A or B.

Cytomegalovirus infection

A mononucleosis-like syndrome characterized by fever, splenomegaly, and atypical lymphocytes has been shown to occur in some patients with acute CMV infection (p. 13). These patients have a negative heterophil agglutination and no evidence of recent EBV infection. Details concerning diagnosis of cytomegalovirus infection are given on p. 14.

Acquired toxoplasmosis with lymphadenopathy

Toxoplasmosis infection may be clinically indistinguishable from infectious mononucleosis. It is characterized by generalized lymphadenopathy, chiefly of the cervical group, and occasionally by pharyngeal involvement and exanthem. The differentiation is based on the EBV and toxoplasma antibody determinations. (Diagnosis of toxoplasmosis is discussed on p. 394.)

• • •

In addition to simulating the diseases just described, infectious mononucleosis with its protean manifestations may simulate Hodgkin's disease, scarlet fever, secondary syphilis, typhoid fever, rickettsial diseases, and many others.

PROGNOSIS

In general the prognosis is excellent. Severe cases of infectious mononucleosis may be followed by long periods of asthenia. Neurologic complications may cause serious sequelae or death, but fortunately these are rare. Spontaneous rupture of the spleen, which also is very rare, is fatal if it is not recognized and treated promptly. Deaths reported in infectious mononucleosis have resulted from CNS complications, splenic rupture, secondary bacterial infection in neutropenic patients, and myocarditis. In 1970 Penman was able to identify a total of only 20 such fatal cases. As has been noted, however, prognosis of the XLP syndrome is poor.

TREATMENT

Infectious mononucleosis is a self-limited disease, and treatment of it is chiefly supportive. Antimicrobial drugs are not effective and do not alter the course of the infection. Bed rest is indicated in the acute stage of the disease. Aspirin is usually adequate to control the pain or discomfort caused by the enlarged lymph nodes and pharyngeal involvement. In severe cases codeine or meperidine (Demerol) may be required.

Corticosteroid therapy has been reported to have a beneficial effect. Symptoms referable to the throat and enlarged lymph nodes improve within 24 hours in many instances. In a well-controlled study of 132 patients with severe uncomplicated mononucleosis, Bender (1967) observed a significant decrease in the duration of fever; it persisted for an average of 1.4 days in the 66 corticosteroid-treated patients as compared with 5.6 days in the 66 matched control patients. Steroids may be considered for treatment of severe cases characterized by marked toxemia, progressive tonsillar enlargement, and evidence of neurologic involvement. Steroids are not recommended for treatment of mild cases of infectious mononucleosis because the long-term effects of intervention in the normal immune response to EBV are unknown. Contact sports should be avoided until the patient's spleen size has returned to normal.

Spontaneous rupture of the spleen requires immediate surgery. Transfusions, treatment for shock, and splenectomy are life-saving measures. Treatment of severe EBV infections in immunocompromised patients with drugs such as acyclovir (Hanto et al., 1982) and transfer factor (Jones et al., 1981) deserves further study.

REFERENCES

Abo W, Takada K, Kamada M, et al. Evolution of infectious mononucleosis into EBV carrying monoclonal malignant lymphoma. Lancet 1982;1:1272-1275.

Andiman WA. Primacy Epstein-Barr virus infection and thrombocytopenia during late infancy. J Pediatr 1976; 89:435-438.

Andiman WA. The Epstein-Barr virus and EB virus infections in childhood. J Pediatr 1979;95:171-182.

Andiman WA: Epstein-Barr virus-associated syndromes: a critical reexamination. Pediatr Infect Dis 1984;3:198-203.

Andiman WA, Markowitz RI, Horstmann DM: Clinical, virologic, and serologic evidence of Epstein-Barr virus infection in association with childhood pneumonia. J Pediatr 1981;99:880-886.

Bar RS, DeLor CJ, Clauben KP, et al. Fatal infectious mononucleosis in a family. N Engl J Med 1974;290:363-367.

Bender CE. The value of corticosteroids in the treatment of infectious mononucleosis. JAMA 1967;199:97.

Butler T, Pastore J, Simon G, et al. Infectious mononucleosis myocarditis. J Infect 1981;3:172-175.

Cleary TG, Henie W, Pickering LK. Acute cerebellar ataxia associated with Epstein-Barr virus infection. JAMA 1980; 243:148-149.

Davidsohn I. Serologic diagnosis of infectious mononucleosis. JAMA 1937;108:289.

de Thé, G. Role of Epstein-Barr virus in human diseases: infectious mononucleosis, Burkitt's lymphoma, and nasopharyngeal carcinoma. In Klein G. New York: Raven Press, Viral oncology. 1980, pp 769-797.

De Waele M, Thielemans C, Van Camp BKG. Characterization of immunoregulatory T cells in EBV-induced infectious mononucleosis by monoclonal antibodies. N Engl J Med 1981;304:460-462.

Downey A, McKinley CA. Acute lymphoadenosis compared with acute lymphatic leukemia. Arch Intern Med 1923; 32:82.

Downey H, Stasney J. Infectious mononucleosis; hematologic studies. JAMA 1935;105:754.

Dunnet WN. Infectious mononucleosis. Br Med J 1963; 1:1187.

Epstein MA, Achong BG. Various forms of Epstein-Barr virus infection in man: established facts and a general concept. Lancet 1973;2:836.

Epstein MA, Achong BG. Pathogenesis of infectious mononucleosis. Lancet 1977;2:1270.

Epstein MA, Achong BG, Barr YM. Virus particles in cultural lymphoblasts from Burkitt's lymphoma. Lancet 1964;1:702-703.

Evans AS. Infectious mononucleosis in University of Wisconsin students. Report of five-year investigation. Am J Hyg 1960;71:342.

Evans AS. Infectious mononucleosis: recent developments. GP 1969;40:127.

Evans AE, et al. A prospective evaluation of heterophile and Epstein-Barr virus-specific IgM antibody tests in clinical and subclinical infectious mononucleosis: specificity and sensitivity of the tests and persistence of antibody. J Infect Dis 1975;132:546.

Fleischer G, Bologonese R. Epstein-Barr virus infections in pregnancy: a prospective study. J Pediatr 1984;104:374-379.

Fleisher GR, Pasquariello PS, Warren WS, et al. Intrafamilial transmission of Epstein-Barr virus infections. J Pediatr 1981;98:16-19.

Ginsburg CM, Henle W, Henle G, et al. Infectious mononucleosis in children. Evaluation of Epstein-Barr virus-specific serological data. JAMA 1977;237:781.

Goldberg GN, Fulginiti VA, Ray CG, et al. In utero EBV (infectious mononucleosis) infection JAMA 1981;246:1579-1581.

Grose C, Henle W, Henle G, Feorino PM. Primary Epstein-Barr virus infections in acute neurologic diseases. N Engl J Med 1975;292:392.

Hanto DW, Frizzera G, Gajl-Peczalska KJ, et al. Epstein-Barr virus induced B-cell lymphoma after renal transplantation. N Engl J Med 1982;306:913-918.

Hellmann D, Cowan MJ, Ammann AJ, et al. Chronic active Epstein-Barr virus infections in two immunodeficient patients. J Pediatr 1983;103:585-588.

Henle G, Henle W. Observations on childhood infections with the Epstein-Barr virus. J Infect Dis 1970;121:303.

Henle G, Henle W, Diehl V. Relation of Burkitt's tumor-associated herpes-type virus to infectious mononucleosis. Proc Nat Acad Sci USA 1968;59:94.

Henle W, Henle GE, Horwitz CA. Epstein-Barr virus specific diagnostic tests in infectious mononucleosis. Human Pathol 1974;5:551-565.

Henle W, Henle G, Lennette ET. The Epstein-Barr virus. Sci Am 1979;241:48.

Hoagland RJ. The transmission of infectious mononucleosis. Am J Med Sci 1955;229:262.

Hoff G, Bauer S. A new rapid slide test for infectious mononucleosis. JAMA 1965;194:351.

Hoffman GS, Franck WA. Infectious mononucleosis, autoimmunity and vasculitis. JAMA 1979;241:2735.

Horwitz CA. Practical approach to diagnosis of infectious mononucleosis. Postgrad Med 1979;65:179.

Hudgins JM. Infectious mononucleosis complicated by myocarditis and pericarditis. JAMA 1976;235:2626.

Icart J, Didier J, Dalens M, et al. Prospective study of Epstein-Barr virus (EBV) infection during pregnancy. Biomedicine 1981;34:160-163.

Joncas J, Mitnyan C. Serological response of the EBV antibodies in pediatric cases of infectious mononucleosis and in their contacts. Can Med Assoc J 1970;6:1260.

Jones JF, Jeter WS, Fulginiti VA, et al. Treatment of childhood combined Epstein-Barr virus/cytomegalovirus infection with oral bovine transfer factor. Lancet 1981;2:122-124.

Klein G. The role of Epstein-Barr virus in the etiology of Burkitt's lymphoma and nasopharyngeal carcinoma. In Rosenberg S, Kaplan H (eds). Malignant lymphomas. New York: Academic Press, 1982, pp 155-173.

McKenna RW, Risdall RJ, Brunning RD. Virus associated hemophagocytic syndrome. Hum Pathol 1981;12:395-398.

Miller G, Niederman JC, Andrews LL: Prolonged oropharyngeal excretion of Epstein-Barr virus after infectious mononucleosis. N Engl J Med 1973;288:229.

Mills MJ. Post-viral haemophagocytic syndrome. J R Soc Med 1982;75:555-557.

Morgan DG, Miller G, Niederman JC, et al. Site of Epstein-Barr virus replication in the oropharynx. Lancet 1979; 2:1154-1157.

Niederman JC. Heterophil antibody determinations in a series of 166 cases of infectious mononucleosis listed according to various stages of the disease. Yale J Biol Med 1956;28:629.

Niederman JC. Infectious mononucleosis: observations on transmission. Yale J Biol Med 1982;55:259-264.

Niederman JC, Evans AS, Subrahmanyan MS, McCollum RW: Prevalence, incidence and persistence of EB virus antibody in young adults. N Engl J Med 1970;282:361.

Niederman JC, McCollum RW, Henle G, Henle W. Infectious mononucleosis: clinical manifestations in relation to EB virus antibodies. JAMA 1968;203:205.

Niederman JC, et al. Infectious mononucleosis: Epstein-Barr-virus shedding in saliva and oropharynx. N Engl J Med 1976;294:1355.

Pattengale PK, Smith RW, Perlin E. Atypical lymphocytes in acute infectious mononucleosis. Identification by multiple T and B lymphocyte markers. N Engl J Med 1974;291:1145.

Paul JR, Bunnell WW. The presence of heterophile antibodies in infectious mononucleosis. Am J Med Sci 1932;183:90.

Penman HG. Fatal infectious mononucleosis: a critical review. J Clin Pathol 1970;23:765.

Pereira MS, Blake JM, Macrae AD: EB virus antibody at different ages. Br Med J 1969;4:526.

Pfeiffer E. Dreusenfieber. Jahrb Kinderheilkd 1889;29:257.

Purtilo DT. Malignant lymphoproliferative diseases induced by Epstein-Barr virus in immunodeficient patients, including X-linked, cytogenetic, and familial syndromes. Cancer Genet Cytogenet 1981;4:251-268.

Purtilo DT, DeFlorio D, Hutt LM, et al. Variable phenotypic expression of an X-linked recessive lymphoproliferative syndrome. N Engl J Med 1977;297:1077-1081.

Purtilo DT, Sakamoto K, Barnabei V, et al. Epstein-Barr virus-induced diseases in boys with the X-linked lymphoproliferative syndrome (XLP) Am J Med 1982;73:49-56.

Ralston LS, Saiki AK, Powers WT. Orchitis as a complication of infectious mononucleosis. JAMA 1960;173:1348.

Rapp CE Jr, Hewetson JF. Infectious mononucleosis and the Epstein-Barr virus. Am J Dis Child 1978;132:78.

Rennie LE, Wroblewski F. The clinical significance of serum transaminase in infectious mononucleosis. N Engl J Med 1957;257:547.

Risdall RJ, McKenna RW, Nesbit ME, et al. Virus-associated hemophagocytic syndrome. Am Cancer Soc 1979;44:993-1002.

Robinson JE, Brown N, Andiman W, et al. Diffuse polyclonal B-cell lymphoma during primary infection with Epstein-Barr virus. N Engl J Med 1980;302:1293-1297.

Rocchi G, et al. Quantitative evaluation of Epstein-Barr-virus-infected mononuclear peripheral blood leukocytes in infectious mononucleosis. N Engl J Med 1977;296:132.

Rutkow IM. Rupture of the spleen in infectious mononucleosis. Arch Surg 1978;113:718.

Sawyer RN, Evans AS, Niederman JC, McCollum RW. Prospective studies of a group of Yale University freshmen. I. Occurrence of infectious mononucleosis. J Infect Dis 1971;123:263.

Simonsen E, Christensen K. Mononucleosis infectiosa, a 5-year material with special reference to the effect of prednisolone treatment. Acta Med Scand 1966;180:729.

Sixby JW, Nedrud JG, Raab-Traub N, et al. Epstein-Barr virus replication in nopharyngeal epithelial cells. N Engl J Med 1984;310:1225.

Smith H, Denman AM. A new manifestation of infection with Epstein-Barr virus. Br Med J 1978;2:248-250.

Sprunt TP, Evans FA. Mononuclear leukocytosis in reaction to acute infections ("infectious mononucleosis"). Bull Johns Hopkins Hosp 1920;31:410.

Strauch B, Siegel N, Andrews LL, Millers G. Oropharyngeal excretion of Epstein-Barr virus by renal transplant recipients and other patients treated with immunosuppressive drugs. Lancet 1974;1:234.

Sullivan JL, Byron KS, Brewster FE, et al. Treatment of life-threatening Epstein-Barr virus infections with acyclovir. Am J Med 1982;13(1A):262-266.

Sumaya CV: Primary Epstein-Barr virus infections in children. Pediatrics 1977;59:16.

Sutton RNP, Marston SD, Almond EJP, Edmond RTD. Aspects of Epstein-Barr virus infection in childhood. Arch, Dis Child 1974;49:102.

Svedmyr E, Jondal M. Cytotoxic effector cells specific for B cell lines transformed by EBV are present in patients with infectious mononucleosis. Proc Nat Acad Sci USA 1975;7:1622-1626.

Tidy HI, Daniel EC: Glandular fever and infective mononucleosis. Lancet 1923;2:9.

Tischendorf P, et al. Development and persistence of immunity to Epstein-Barr virus in man. J Infect Dis 1970;122:401.

Tobi M, Ravid Z, Feldman-Weiss V, et al. Prolonged atypical illness associated with serological evidence of persistent Epstein-Barr virus infection. Lancet 1982;1:61-64.

Tosato G, Magrath I, Koski I, et al. Activation of suppressor T cells during Epstein-Barr-virus-induced infectious mononucleosis. 1979;301:1133-1137.

Turner AR, MacDonald RN, Cooper BA, et al. Transmission of infectious mononucleosis by transfusion of pre-illness plasma. Ann Intern Med 1972;77:751-753.

Wahren B, et al. EBV antibodies in family contacts of patients with infectious mononucleosis. Proc Soc Exp Biol Med 1970;133:934.

Wilson ER, Malluh A, Stagno S, et al. Fatal Epstein-Barr virus-associated hemophagocytic syndrome. J Pediatr 1981;98:260-262.

Wolnisty C. Orchitis as a complication of infectious mononucleosis: report of a case. N Engl J Med 1962;266:88.

7

ERYTHEMA INFECTIOSUM (FIFTH DISEASE)

Erythema infectiosum is a mildly contagious disease of childhood characterized by a typical eruption and usually no fever or other constitutional symptoms. The rash erupts in the following sequence: first, on the face as a bright red erythema of the cheeks with circumoral pallor; second, as a symmetrical rose-red maculopapular eruption of the extremities beginning proximally and then spreading to involve the trunk and distal extremities, with the lesions assuming a lacelike appearance on fading; and, finally, as an evanescent rash that tends to recur if the skin is irritated or traumatized.

The first recognized outbreak of this disease occurred in Germany and was described in 1889 by Tschammer who considered it a modified form of rubella. In 1899 Stricker described another epidemic and gave the disease its present name of *erythema infectiosum*. Since that time it has been reported from many other parts of the world, including the United States.

ETIOLOGY

The cause of erythema infectiosum has always been presumed to be a virus. Reports of a possible association with rubella virus and ECHO virus type 12 (Balfour et al., 1972) have not been confirmed (Lauer et al., 1976). However, a report by Anderson et al. (1984) has provided convincing evidence that the infection is caused by a human parvovirus. They investigated an extensive outbreak of erythema infectiosum that involved about 162 children in a London pri-

mary school. Virologic and serologic studies of 36 typical cases of the disease revealed the presence of parvovirus-specific IgM antibody. Previous studies by Anderson et al. (1982) had revealed that specific IgM antibody is detectable for about 3 months after a primary infection and it is seldom present in asymptomatic controls.

Viruses of the parvovirus family are small (20 nm), single-stranded DNA agents that have cubic symmetry with 32 capsomeres and no envelope. Human infection with parvovirus was first described by Cossart et al. in 1975. They detected the agent in serum obtained from nine healthy blood donors, a recipient of a renal transplant, and a patient with acute hepatitis. Seroepidemiologic studies using such assays as immune electron microscopy (IEM) and counter immunoelectrophoresis (CIE) revealed detectable antibody in 30% to 40% of adults (Cossart et al., 1975; Paver and Clarke, 1976). More recent studies have revealed an association between the parvovirus agent and aplastic crises in children with homozygous sickle cell disease (Pattison et al., 1981; Anderson et al., 1982; Plummer et al., 1985).

It is likely that human parvoviruses, like other human viruses, may cause inapparent (subclinical) or clinical infections. One could speculate that erythema infectiosum is an example of a clinical syndrome caused by the virus, and an aplastic crisis may be induced when an inapparent infection without rash occurs in a patient with chronic hemolytic anemia.

PATHOLOGY

Since no deaths have been reported, the pathologic findings are limited to examination of skin biopsy material. Histologic sections of skin lesions reveal a perivascular lymphocytic infiltration with edema of the dermis.

EPIDEMIOLOGIC FACTORS

The disease appears to be mildly contagious. It does not spread like measles or rubella. Many of the outbreaks have been confined to family, school, and other institutional groups, and some have been community wide. The mode of transmission is unknown. It has been assumed that the spread is from person to person by droplet infection.

Geographic distribution appears to be worldwide. The original cases were reported from Germany and Austria. The disease has been recognized in such widely separated areas as China, Italy, Tunisia, Uruguay, Turkey, Palestine, Cuba, Australia, Japan, and many parts of the United States.

Age distribution indicates that it is primarily a disease of childhood with a concentration of cases in the 2- to 12-year age group. The peak incidence is 7 years (Hidano et al., 1983). The disease also has been observed in infants and adults.

The seasonal distribution is similar to measles and rubella. Most outbreaks occur in late winter and spring with the peak incidence in April.

Sex incidence appears to be equal.

CLINICAL MANIFESTATIONS

The incubation period has not been clearly defined but has an estimated range of 6 to 14 days. The first and usually only apparent sign of illness is the appearance of the rash. Generally, the patient is afebrile and asymptomatic. Fever, if present, is accompanied by slight malaise.

Rash

The most significant feature of the disease is the rash, which is very characteristic in its appearance, distribution, evanescence, and tendency to recur. Typically, it erupts in three stages.

First stage. The rash appears first on the face as an intensely red eruption confined chiefly to the cheeks. A large number of erythematous maculopapules coalesce to form a confluent rash that has raised borders and is erysipeloid. It is hot to the touch but not tender. The circumoral area, which is not involved, presents a contrasting pallor adjacent to the red efflorescent cheeks, which have a slapped appearance. Scattered discrete lesions may be present on the forehead, chin, and postauricular area. The eruption fades rapidly, disappearing from the face within 1 to 4 days.

Second stage. Approximately 1 day after its involvement of the face, the rash appears as maculopapular red spots symmetrically distributed on the upper and lower extremities. Initially these lesions develop on the extensor surfaces of the arms and thighs (proximal parts of the extremities). Within 1 to 2 days they spread to the flexor surfaces, the distal parts of the extremities, and the buttocks and trunk. As the rash progresses, the earlier lesions on the arms and thighs begin to fade centrally, thereby giving rise to a lacelike appearance. The lesions during the second stage persist for several days or for a week or more before they subside. A number of reports emphasize the lack of involvement of the palms and soles. However, in an outbreak of the disease on Long Island, New York, Karelitz (personal communication) observed the eruption on both the palms and soles.

Third stage. After the rash subsides, it may reappear after a variable period of time. The recurrence of the eruption may be precipitated by a variety of skin irritants such as trauma, sunlight, and extremes of hot and cold.

DIAGNOSIS

At the present time the diagnosis is based entirely on the clinical features of the disease. The white blood cell count is usually within normal limits, with a tendency to eosinophilia in some cases. If human parvovirus is proved to be the cause of erythema infectiosum, the diagnosis could be confirmed by detecting parvovirus-specific IgM antibody in acute phase serum specimens obtained within 2 weeks after onset of rash. Anderson et al. (1982, 1984) have reported that specific IgM is detectable for about 3 months after a primary infection with human parvovirus.

DIFFERENTIAL DIAGNOSIS

Differential diagnosis is discussed in Chapter 34.

COMPLICATIONS

Arthritis and arthralgia may occur. The joint manifestations are transient, self-limited, and more common in adults than in children (Ager et al., 1966). Hemolytic anemia has also been reported (Wadlington and Riley, 1968). Encephalitis associated with erythema infectiosum was observed in an 8-year-old boy by Balfour et al. (1970); subsequent recovery was complete. In contrast, Hall and Horner (1977) described the occurrence of progressive severe encephalopathy with permanent neurologic sequelae in a 9-month-old boy who had erythema infectiosum. However, in the absence of a specific diagnostic test it would be impossible to confirm the diagnosis of erythema infectiosum and the associated encephalopathy.

PROGNOSIS

The prognosis is excellent.

Treatment

No treatment is indicated.

REFERENCES

Ager EA, Chin TD, Poland JD. Epidemic erythema infectiosum. N Engl J Med 1966;275:1326.

Anderson MJ, Davis LR, Jones SE, et al. The development and use of an antibody capture radioimmunoassay for specific IgM to a human parvovirus agent. J Hyg 1982;88:309.

Anderson MJ, Lewis E, Kidd IM, et al. An outbreak of erythema infectiosum associated with human parvovirus infection. Personal communication.

Balfour HH Jr, Schiff GM, Bloom JE. Encephalitis associated with erythema infectiosum. J Pediatr 1970;77:133.

Balfour HH Jr, et al. A study of erythema infectiosum: recovery of rubella virus and Echovirus—12. Pediatrics 1972;50:285.

Cossart YE, Field AM, Cant B, et al. Parvovirus particles in human sera. Lancet 1975;1:71.

Fox MJ, Clark JM. Erythema infectiosum. Am J Dis Child 1947;73:453.

Hall CB, Horner, FA. Encephalopathy with erythema infectiosum. Am J Dis Child 1977;131:65.

Herrick TP. Erythema infectiosum. Am J Dis Child 1926;31:486.

Hidano A, Ogihara Y, Oryu F, et al. Epidemiology of an outbreak of erythema infectiosum in Tokyo. Int J Dermatol 1983;22:161.

Lauer BA, MacCormack JN, Wilfert C. Erythema infectiosum. An elementary school outbreak. Am J Dis Child 1976;130:252.

Lawton AL, Smith RE. Erythema infectiosum: clinical study of an epidemic in Branford, Connecticut. Arch Intern Med 1931;47:28.

Pattison JR, Jones SE, Hodgson J, et al. Parvovirus infections and hypoplastic crisis in sickle-cell anemia. Lancet 1981;1:44.

Paver WK, Clarke SKR. Comparison of human fecal and serum parvo-like viruses, J Clin Micro 1976;4:67.

Plummer FA, Hammond GW, Forward K, et al. An erythema infectiosum-like illness caused by human parvovirus infection. N Engl J Med 1985;313:74.

Stricker G. Die neue Kinderseuche in der Umgebung von Giessen (erythema infectiosum). Z Prat Aerztl 1899;40:121.

Tschammer A. Ueber örtliche Rötheln. Jahrb Kinderh 1889;29:372.

Wadlington WB, Riley HD Jr: Arthritis and hemolytic anemia following erythema infectiosum. JAMA 1968;203:473.

Werner GH, et al. A new viral agent associated with erythema infectiosum. Ann NY Acad Sci 1957;67:338.

8

EXANTHEM SUBITUM (ROSEOLA INFANTUM)

Exanthem subitum is a common benign infectious disease of infancy characterized by 3 or 4 days of high fever associated with a paucity of physical findings. The temperature falls to normal by crisis coincidental with the appearance of a morbilliform rash that fades within 2 days. Occasionally the disease is ushered in by a convulsion.

ETIOLOGY

In all probability exanthem subitum is a disease of viral cause. The long incubation period, the leukopenia, the failure to respond to antimicrobial agents, and the failure to recover bacteria from the various body fluids are all indirect evidence for this hypothesis. The successful human transmission of the infection was reported by Kempe et al. in 1950 and by Hellström and Vahlquist in 1951. A report of possible association between rotavirus and exanthem subitum (Saitoh et al., 1981) has not been confirmed (Gurwith et al., 1981).

CLINICAL MANIFESTATIONS
Incubation period

The incubation period is difficult to determine because the contact is rarely known. The experimental disease produced by intravenous injection of serum had an incubation period of 9 days. In the epidemics reported by Cushing (1927) and by Barenberg and Greenspan (1939), this period appeared to range between 10 and 15 days.

Course

The typical course of exanthem subitum is illustrated in Fig. 8-1. The temperature rises abruptly to about 40° to 40.6° C (104° to 105° F). The infant may be anorexic and irritable and usually shows no evidence of coryza, conjunctivitis, or cough. The fever persists for approximately 3 to 4 days and then falls by crisis coincidental with the appearance of the rash. Most infants with this disease do not appear as acutely ill as their temperature chart seems to suggest. Occasionally, they may be listless and irritable during periods of hyperpyrexia. It is not uncommon for the disease to be ushered in by a convulsion.

Fever

The characteristic temperature curve is illustrated in Fig. 8-1. The fever is typically high and continuous, persisting for 3 or 4 days. Administration of aspirin causes a temporary drop that is followed by a rapid rise to the same high levels as before. In some patients the temperature is of the intermittent type, being normal or slightly elevated in the morning and very high in the evening. On either the third or the fourth day it drops precipitously back to normal levels. In rare instances the fever may persist for more than 5 days, but the diagnosis under these circumstances may be questionable. Also, occasionally the temperature may fall by rapid lysis rather than by crisis.

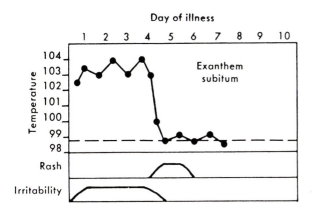

Fig. 8-1. Schematic diagram illustrating typical clinical course of exanthem subitum. Between the third and fourth days the temperature drops to normal and a maculopapular eruption appears.

Rash

As indicated in Fig. 8-1, the appearance of the rash coincides with the subsidence of the fever on the third or fourth day. Occasionally it may not be apparent until after 1 day of normal temperature, or it may even emerge before the fever has subsided. The lesions are discrete, rose-pink macules or maculopapules, 2 to 3 mm in diameter, that fade on pressure, rarely coalesce, and are similar in appearance to those of rubella and modified measles. The rash characteristically appears on the trunk first and then spreads to the neck, upper extremities, face, and lower extremities. Occasionally the rash may be limited to the trunk. The duration of the eruption is usually 1 to 2 days; occasionally it may be evanescent, disappearing in a matter of hours. There is usually no evidence of pigmentation or desquamation.

Other clinical features

The most significant clinical manifestation of exanthem subitum is the striking contrast between the infant's general appearance and the febrile course. In spite of a persistently elevated temperature, the patient may be alert and playful and may not look acutely ill. The physical findings are rather nonspecific. The pharynx is usually mildly inflamed. The tonsils, if present, are usually reddened and occasionally are covered with a follicular exudate. Mild catarrhal otitis media may be present. Lymphadenopathy, particularly of the occipital, cervical, and post-

auricular groups, is a common finding. All these manifestations are caused by the primary infection and not by secondary bacterial invaders.

DIAGNOSIS

A diagnosis of exanthem subitum is made chiefly on the basis of clinical manifestations. As yet, no specific serologic test is available for confirmation of the diagnosis. The white blood cell count is usually low, but as a rule leukopenia does not develop until the third day of illness. Indeed, during the first 2 days there may be leukocytosis with an increase in polymorphonuclear leukocytes. As leukopenia develops, the percentage of lymphocytes and monocytes increases. The development of a rash and leukopenia in an infant who has been febrile for the previous 3 or 4 days should strongly suggest exanthem subitum as the most probable diagnosis.

DIFFERENTIAL DIAGNOSIS

Differential diagnosis is discussed in Chapter 34.

COMPLICATIONS

The most common complication seen in hospital practice is convulsive seizures. Most infants with exanthem subitum are treated at home. Consequently, a more accurate estimate of the incidence of this complication can be obtained from surveys in general practice rather than in hospital practice. In general, the incidence would probably parallel that of febrile convulsions. In all probability, the occurrence of seizures is closely related to the abrupt rise of temperature in an infant who is prone to develop febrile convulsions. Spinal taps have been performed routinely on many patients, with completely normal results.

Encephalitis and other complications of the central nervous system have been reported but are extremely rare. The following case history illustrates the contribution of a virus laboratory in proving that a patient suspected of having a neurologic complication of exanthem subitum actually had another disease—poliomyelitis.

CASE REPORT. R. W., a 19-month-old white infant (patient of Dr. Horace L. Hodes), was admitted to the hospital for fever, facial paralysis, and pooling of secretions in the throat. A lumbar puncture revealed pleocytosis (40 monocytes). His temperature was high (40° to 40.6° C or 104° to 105° F) for 3 to 4 days, after which it fell to normal by crisis. With the subsidence of the fever, a maculopapular eruption appeared. The question of a rare neurologic complication of exanthem subitum was raised. However, a diagnosis of poliomyelitis was established by the recovery of type 1 virus from the patient's stool and the demonstration of a 25-fold rise in the level of neutralizing antibody in his serum during convalescence. In all probability this infant had two diseases, poliomyelitis and exanthem subitum.

PROGNOSIS

The prognosis is uniformly excellent even for those cases complicated by convulsive seizures. The 3-day period of high, unresponsive fever may be a harrowing experience for both the parents and the physician. With subsidence of the fever and appearance of the rash, however, the diagnosis becomes obvious, and a complete recovery ensues for the infant and everyone else concerned.

IMMUNITY

One attack probably confers permanent immunity. As in measles and rubella, second attacks have been reported, but these are extremely rare and usually reflect diagnostic errors. There is ample evidence to indicate that exanthem subitum is a specific entity and has no cross-immunity with either measles or rubella. The rarity of the disease in infants under 6 months of age suggests that the newborn infant probably acquires passive protection from his mother.

EPIDEMIOLOGIC FACTORS

The age incidence is very striking. The vast majority of cases, more than 95%, occur in infants between 6 months and 3 years of age. The disease has occasionally been described in older children and in adults. In 1949 James and Freier reported an outbreak in a maternity hospital with cases in newborn infants, nurses, mothers, and fathers. The lack of a specific diagnostic test makes it difficult to confirm the diagnosis. It is possible that the epidemic reported by James and Freier was an ECHO virus infection rather than exanthem subitum.

Both sexes are equally susceptible.

The disease occurs the year round, with a concentration of cases in the spring and autumn months.

Exanthem subitum is the most common exanthem seen in infants under 2 years of age. It has been estimated that approximately 30% of all children develop the apparent disease. It is conceivable that in the majority of infants it occurs as either an inapparent infection or a febrile illness without rash.

Exanthem subitum does not have the contagious characteristics of measles, rubella, or chickenpox. It is rare for children to acquire the disease from a sibling, even when they are under 3 years of age. Epidemics in foundling homes have been reported, but they are exceptional. For many years patients with illnesses diagnosed as exanthem subitum have been routinely admitted to our general infants' ward. During this period we have not observed a single instance of spread of the infection.

TREATMENT

There is no specific treatment for patients with exanthem subitum. Aspirin may be given for its antipyretic effect. Elixir of phenobarbital may be given to infants with a history of convulsive seizures during either the current or previous illnesses.

Antimicrobial agents do not alter the course of the infection. Since the diagnosis is established only after the patient has recovered, the physician may have a dilemma. Should he treat or not treat with antimicrobial agents? In the following case, treatment may be justifiably withheld if an infant (1) appears well and shows no abnormal physical findings despite continued hyperpyrexia and (2) has a normal or low white blood cell count. On the other hand, treatment may be indicated if high fever is accompanied by one or more of the following manifestations: (1) inflammatory exudate on the tonsils and pharynx, (2) catarrhal otitis media, and (3) leukocytosis.

The management of an infant whose disease is ushered in by high fever and convulsions should be the same as that for any initial febrile convulsion. It has been our policy to perform a diagnostic spinal tap before any antimicrobial agent is given.

REFERENCES

Barenberg LH, Greenspan L. Exanthem subitum (roseola infantum). Am J Dis Child 1939;58:983.

Berenberg W, Wright S, Janeway CA. Roseola infantum (exanthem subitum). N Engl J Med 1949;241:253.

Clemens HH. Exanthem subitum (roseola infantum): report of 80 cases. J Pediatr 1945;26:66.

Cushing HB. An epidemic of roseola infantum. Can Med Assoc J 1927;17:905.

Gurwith M, Gurwith D, Wenman W, et al. Exanthem subitum not associated with rotavirus. N Engl J Med 1981;305:174.

Hellström B, Vahlquist B. Experimental inoculation of roseola infantum. Acta Paediatr 1951;40:189.

James U, Freier A. Roseola infantum; outbreak in maternity hospital. Arch Dis Child 1949;24:54.

Juretić M. Exanthem subitum: a review of 243 cases. Helv Paediatr Acta 1963;18:80.

Kempe CH, Shaw EB, Jackson JR, Silver HK. Studies on the etiology of exanthem subitum (roseola infantum). J Pediatr 1950;37:561.

Neva FA, Enders JF. Isolation of a cytopathogenic agent from an infant with a disease in certain respects resembling roseola infantum. J Immunol 1954;72:315.

Rothman PE, Naidich MJ. Nervous complications of exanthem subitum. Calif Med 1958;88:39.

Saitoh Y, Matsuno S, Mukoyama A. Exanthem subitum and rotavirus. N Engl J Med 1981;304:845.

Zahorsky J. Roseola infantum. JAMA 1913;61:1446.

9

ACUTE GASTROENTERITIS

Acute infectious gastroenteritis is one of the most common infectious diseases of humans. It ranks second to acute respiratory infections as a worldwide cause of morbidity, and in developing areas of the world it is a significant cause of death in infants. It has been estimated that up to 15% of children in developing nations may die of diarrhea before 3 years of age. The usual clinical syndrome is characterized by various combinations of the following symptoms: nausea, vomiting, abdominal cramps, and diarrhea. Fever may or may not be present. The causative agent is most often a bacterium or virus but may be protozoal (Table 9-1).

BACTERIAL GASTROENTERITIS

Disease caused by *Escherichia coli*, *Salmonella*, *Shigella*, *Campylobacter fetus* ss. *jejuni*, *Yersinia enterocolitica*, and *Vibrio cholerae* will be discussed in this chapter. Staphylococcal gastrointestinal disease will be presented in Chapter 27. Most of these bacterial pathogens are identifiable in the laboratory, and fluid replacement as well as appropriate specific therapy may favorably alter the course of illness.

Etiology

Escherichia coli. *E. coli* bacterium was named for Escherich, a pediatrician who isolated it in 1885. *E. coli* organisms are common inhabitants of the intestine and ordinarily cause no clinical symptoms. The organism is a gram-negative bacillus, measuring 2 to 3 μm in length and 0.6 μm in breadth. The bacilli may form chains, and most strains are motile. This facultatively anaerobic organism grows on ordinary laboratory media, and the optimum temperature for growth is 37° C; it is killed at a temperature of 60° C for 30 minutes. Although it is easy to isolate *E. coli*, recognition of pathogenic strains is increasingly complex because of the multiple factors that enable this organism to cause disease. Specific recognition of pathogenic strains is readily accomplished only in research laboratories, and, thus, the laboratory confirmation of gastrointestinal disease due to *E. coli* is not generally available.

E. coli organisms were shown to be serologically heterogeneous by Kauffmann (1951), who divided the species into various somatic groups. In addition to the cell wall (or somatic) O antigens, H (or flagellar) antigens and K (or capsular) antigens were also identified. The serotype is a chromosomally determined characteristic and is therefore stable. Serogroups have been shown to correlate with disease production in newborns despite the inability to demonstrate a universal virulence factor.

E. coli strains that cause diarrhea are now grouped according to their pathogenic mechanism(s). There are enterotoxin-producing *E. coli* (ETEC), enteroinvasive *E. coli* (EIEC), and enteropathogenic *E. coli* (EPEC).

Enterotoxigenic Escherichia coli (ETEC). Enterotoxigenic *E. coli* (ETEC) are those organisms producing plasmid-encoded enterotoxins. These organisms are not identified by serotyping. The initially recognized heat-labile enterotoxin (LT)

Table 9-1. Etiology of acute gastroenteritis

Viruses	Bacteria	Protozoa
Rotaviruses 1 to 3	Salmonellae	*Giardia lamblia*
Norwalk-like agents	Shigellae	*Entomoeba histolytica*
Enteric adenoviruses	*Escherichia coli*	Cryptosporidium
Coronaviruses	*Vibrio cholerae*	
Calciviruses	Other vibrios	
Astroviruses	*Campylobacter fetus*	
Mini-reoviruses	*Yersinia enterocolitica*	
Small round viruses	Staphylococci	

and heat-stable enterotoxin (ST) are the best described and form the foundation of current information about this mechanism of disease production (Table 9-2). LT, like cholera toxin, activates adenylate cyclase, resulting in increased production of cyclic adenosine monophosphate (cAMP). The toxin is detectable in tissue culture or by immunologic tests. At least two ST toxins have now been identified. One activates guanylate cyclase with a resulting increase in cyclic guanosine monophosphate (GMP). A second stable toxin does not activate either adenylate cyclase or guanylate cyclase and does not result in chloride anion secretion. It too is an enterotoxin that acts via a novel pathway, and its role in human disease remains to be further delineated. Many of the ETEC strains are now known to possess specific adhesion factors enabling them to colonize the small intestine. Such colonization factor antigens (CFA/1, CFA/2) contribute to disease production by these toxigenic bacteria. Colonization factors are visualized by electron microscopy as filamentous structures resembling fimbriae.

Enteroinvasive Escherichia coli (EIEC). A second group of *E. coli* produce gastrointestinal disease by virtue of their ability to penetrate and then multiply within the intestinal epithelial cells. These enteroinvasive *E. coli* (EIEC) are like shigellae in this respect. Although these *E. coli* tend to fall into certain serologic groups, the serotype specificity is not essential, and therefore serotyping to identify disease due to these organisms is not a reliable test. The invasive qualities of these organisms and of shigellae are dependent on a transmissible plasmid. Demonstration of the enteroinvasive quality of the organism is possible by tissue culture tests or by the Sereny test, which is the production of keratoconjunctivitis in the guinea pig eye after inoculation of the organism.

Enteropathogenic Escherichia coli (EPEC). All *E. coli* causing diarrhea were originally called enteropathogenic *E. coli* (EPEC) when it was appreciated that certain serotypes could be associated with disease. The terminology has evolved as the pathogenic mechanisms have been elucidated so that enteropathogenic *E. coli* now refers only to those organisms causing disease that do not produce the LT or ST, do not have the genes coding for these toxins, and are not enteroinvasive. This third group of *E. coli*, the EPEC, have been shown to cause diarrhea in volunteers. Some of these organisms have been shown by pathologic studies to adhere to the microvilli of the rabbit ileum. In vitro, adherence to HEp2 cells is a correlate of their ability to adhere in vivo. Biopsies of human intestine shows that the brush border of the small intestine is effaced and the organisms are densely adherent. This ability to adhere also seems to be associated with the presence of a plasmid that is different from that which is necessary for the invasive qualities of EIEC mentioned above.

Recent investigations suggest that there may be additional (other than LT and ST) enterotoxins associated with some strains of EPEC. One such candidate toxin has been shown to cause accumulation of fluid in the gastrointestinal tract of an infant rat model. Other investigators have described a candidate enterotoxin also distinct from LT and ST that produces a cytotoxic effect on monolayers of Vero cells. This cytotoxin is apparently identical to the toxin produced by *Shigella dysenteriae.* Several of these strains belong to the somatic or O antigen serogroups 26, 128, 39, and 157. This observation has stirred a great deal of interest because some strains of *E.*

Table 9-2. Enterotoxins

Organism toxin	V. cholerae cholera toxin	E. coli labile toxin	E. coli stable toxin	Shigella and shigellae toxin (cytotoxin, enterotoxin, neurotoxin)
MW	84,000	73,000	3000 to 6000	68,000 to 72,000
Immunogenic	Yes	Yes	No	Yes
Genetic control of toxin	Chromosomal	Plasmid	Plasmid	?Plasmid
Subunit A and B structure	Yes	Yes	No	Yes
A and B synthe-sized separately and then associated	Yes	Yes		Yes
B subunit binds to cell	Yes	Yes		Yes
Cell receptor	GM_1 ganglioside	GM_1 ganglioside	100,000 MW protein (not GM_1)	Glycoprotein with exposed B-1,4-linked N-acetyl glucosamine
Internalization	By noncoated surface microinvaginations	By noncoated surface microinvaginations	?	?By receptor-mediated endocytosis through coated pits
A subunit with enzymatic activity	Yes	Yes		Yes
Intracellular target site	Inner surface plasma membrane	Inner surface plasma membrane	Inner surface plasma membrane	Cytosol
Action	Modification of plasma membrane enzymes	Modification of plasma membrane enzymes	Modification of plasma membrane enzymes	Modification of factor necessary for protein synthesis
Enzyme affected	Activate adenylate cyclase	Activate adenylate cyclase	Activate guanylate cyclase	Unknown but not EF-2
Mode of action	NAD-dependent ADP ribosylation of GTP binding component of adenylate cyclase		?	A1 catalyzed inactivation of the 60 S ribosomal subunit
Site of action	Small intestine epithelium	Small intestine epithelium	Small intestine epithelium	Intracellular in L1 epithelial cells Small intestine epithelium
Physiologic action	↓ Absorption ↑ Secretion	↓ Absorption ↑ Secretion	↓ Absorption ↑ Secretion	Small intestine— ↑ secretion Large intestine— ? kill cells

coli, such as 0157:H7, have been associated with outbreaks of hemorrhagic colitis and sporadic cases of hemolytic uremic syndrome. The mechanism of the colonization of the small intestine with EPEC is unknown but is a critical factor in disease production.

In summary, there are toxin (LT, ST)-producing *E. coli*, invasive *E. coli*, and pathogenic *E. coli*. Some of the last group are adherent, some produce poorly characterized toxins, and some produce disease by unknown means.

Vibrio cholerae. *V. cholerae* is a gram-negative curved bacillus with a single flagellum responsible for its motility. The name *Vibrio* is derived from the organism's movement, which is apparent as a vibration in live or wet preparations. *V. cholerae* will grow rapidly on certain alkaline-enrichment media such as thiosulfate-citrate-bile (TCBS) agar, which has a pH greater than 6.0. The organisms can be distinguished from other enteric bacteria on TCBS agar, as they form characteristic opaque yellow colonies. There are two major somatic antigenic types of the organism, Inaba and Ogawa, that may cause disease.

V. cholerae elaborates a heat-labile enterotoxin in alkaline growth conditions. The toxin production of this organism is coded for by chromosomal DNA (Table 9-2). This toxin has provided a wealth of information about the structure and function of enterotoxins as well as the pathogenesis of diarrheal diseases. It is now known that this protein exotoxin activates adenylate cyclase and catalyzes the formation of cyclic AMP, which results in the secretion of fluid into the lumen of the gastrointestinal tract. The protein toxin has two component parts, one of which serves as a receptor (B) and binds the toxin to a specific GM_1 ganglioside present on the surface of intestinal cells. The second component part of the toxin (A) penetrates the cell and must gain access to the interior to catalyze the adenosine diphosphate (ADP) ribosylation of a guanosine triphosphate (GTP)-binding protein. This results in activation of adenylate cyclase and conversion of adenosine triphosphate (ATP) to $3',5'$ cyclic AMP. The increased concentration of intracellular cyclic AMP activates electrolyte transport isomotically with water from the extracellular fluid to the lumen of the gastrointestinal tract. Secretion then exceeds fluid absorption.

Increased cyclic AMP also inhibits the transport of sodium and chloride from the lumen of the gut across the brush border and into the cell; that is, absorption is decreased as membrane permeability in the villus cell is diminished. Glucose coupled Na^+ and water transport into cells occurs by an independent mechanism which is unaltered. Thus, oral electrolyte solution can still be absorbed from the intestine.

Salmonellae. Salmonellae are gram-negative, motile aerobic bacilli which do not ferment lactose and sucrose but produce acid when using glucose, maltose, and mannitol. All human species except *Salmonella typhi* produce gas with fermentation. Salmonellae are currently classified into three species: *S. enteritidis*, *S. typhi*, and *S. cholerasuis*. There are greater than 1400 serobiotypes of salmonellae, which are typed by their heat-stable (O) or somatic antigens, and heat-labile (H) or flagellar antigens. They are frequently given names of places, for example, *S. newport*. Serogrouping may be useful epidemiologically and is generally done by state laboratories. *S. typhi* and *S. cholerasuis* species each consist of a single serotype, and all 1400 others are now in the group of *S. enteritidis*. Biotype *S. typhimurium* is responsible for about 20% of all reported infections in the United States, but virtually any serotype can cause human disease. *S. typhi* is a pathogen *only* of humans and in contrast to all other salmonellae is not harbored by other animal species.

Shigellae. In 1896 Shiga isolated a gram-negative nonmotile rod from patients studied in an epidemic of dysentery in Japan and presented evidence for the causal relationship to the microorganism that was named for him. Four years later, Flexner studied cases of dysentery in the Philippines and reported the detection of an organism very similar to Shiga's bacillus. Today there are four main groups of *Shigella* organisms responsible for bacillary dysentery. Each group comprises a number of types that differ serologically: group A, *S. dysenteriae;* group B, *S. flexneri;* group C, *S. boydii;* group D, *S. sonnei*.

The human gastrointestinal tract is the only natural habitat of shigellae. They are slender, motile, gram-negative rods which ferment glucose but not lactose and do not produce H_2S. They are isolated on an agar such as MacConkey's, which allows selection of non-lactose-fermenting organisms. They are readily cultured from fresh stool obtained early in illness and plated soon after collection.

An enterotoxin originally described as limited to *S. dysenteriae* is now known to be produced by all groups of shigellae (Table 9-2). Production of the enterotoxin is iron dependent and thus culture conditions influence its detection. This heat-labile toxin is protease sensitive and cell associated. Experimentally it causes increased fluid secretion in the jejunum of animals and is a cytotoxin in cell culture. The role(s) of toxin in disease production is discussed in Pathogenesis and Pathology.

Yersinia enterocolitica. *Y. enterocolitica* has emerged as a significant pathogen of humans. The genus *Yersinia* includes *Y. pestis*, *Y. pseudotuberculosis*, and *Y. enterocolitica*. It is a small pleomorphic gram-negative rod with rounded ends. The organism is motile at 22° C. It is a nonlactose fermenter but ferments sucrose and splits urea. There are five biotypes and 34 serotypes of *Y. enterocolitica* that inhabit the GI tract of many animals and birds and survive in fresh water. The laboratory usually needs to be alerted to the possibility that this organism is being considered so that appropriate selective media can be used.

Campylobacter fetus. The taxonomy of these bacteria has evolved in recent years resulting in great confusion. The genus of organisms originally known as *Vibrio fetus* is now *Campylobacter fetus*. In 1973, three subspecies were proposed: *fetus*, *jejuni*, and *intestinalis*. Currently, organisms that were designated *C. fetus* ss. *intestinalis* are designated *C. fetus* ss. *fetus*. This subspecies is primarily an animal pathogen but may cause invasive human disease in compromised hosts, including the newborn infant. "Related vibrios" are now termed *C. fetus* ss. *jejuni* and are normal inhabitants of animal GI tracts, but importantly it is the organisms of this genus that cause human gastroenteritis. Thus, there are currently only two subspecies recognized as human pathogens and discussion of *Campylobacter* diarrhea refers to disease caused by *C. fetus* ss. *jejuni*. They are thin, curved gram-negative rods (1.5 to 5 μm by 0.2 to 0.5 μm) that are motile with a polar flagellum and require reduced oxygen tension for growth. They do not ferment or oxidize carbohydrates, and a selective medium such as Novobiocin brilliant green blood agar is necessary for optimal recognition of the organisms when cultured from the stool.

Other bacteria. Other microorganisms that are either implicated less often as causes of gastroenteritis or are less firmly established to be etiologic agents include *Bacillus cereus*, which produces two different enterotoxins, *Aeromonas hydrophilia*, and *Vibrio parahemolyticus*. The latter bacterium requires high salt concentration for growth and is implicated as a cause of food poisoning attributable to shellfish.

Pathogenesis and pathology

The gastrointestinal tract has a number of nonimmunologic defense mechanisms helping to formulate a barrier to human infection. The indigenous flora whose acquisition begins at birth are present in numbers up to 10^{11} organisms per gram of stool in the large bowel. Competition for substrate as well as other alterations of the environment such as decreased pH or production of antibacterial substances probably contribute to which organisms succeed in causing disease. Antibiotics alter the growth of indigenous flora and therefore may contribute to successful colonization by pathogens.

Secretions from saliva to mucin may diminish bacterial adherence to epithelial cells both mechanically and by competitive receptor sites. Normal peristalsis expels organisms that are not adherent. Gastric acid inhibits growth of many bacteria, such as salmonellae. Lysozyme and bile salts are also in the gastrointestinal (GI) tract and can hinder growth of many bacteria.

Immunologic defense mechanisms include secretory IgA, whose production is dependent on antigen exposure to the local intestinal surface. The secretory piece of IgA increases resistance of these antibodies to proteases, and thus this class of antibody best withstands the environment of the lumen of the bowel. Antibody binds toxins and bacteria, thus preventing adsorption, and may be bactericidal in combination with complement and lysozyme.

Gastroenteritis produces diarrhea. Malabsorption, or profuse watery isotonic diarrhea, is caused by dysfunction of the small intestine. Some organisms, and *V. cholerae* is the prototype, cause a profuse malabsorption because of the effects of its enterotoxin on intestinal cells. On the other hand, in dysentery the colon and/or terminal ileum are invaded by bacteria. Shigellae have been the prototype of invasive organisms causing dysentery. The mucosal invasion and disruption is visible as ulceration and results in blood and pus being present in the stool. The symptoms of dysentery include painful cramps and tenesmus as might be expected from the pathology.

Bacterial pathogens must be able to adhere in the intestinal mucosa in order to cause disease, and so the receptor(s) of the bacteria become a critical part of the virulence. The flagellum of V. *cholerae* appears to have adhesins responsible for adherence to the brush border. The organism produces a soluble protease capable of hydrolyzing mucin which may facilitate adsorption. This organism does not destroy the brush border or invade cells, and no histologic lesions are observed.

E. *coli* cause disease by several mechanisms. All E. *coli* producing disease must adhere to the intestinal mucosa. The first recognized surface attachment antigens of ETEC were protein fimbriae (CFA/1 and CFA/2) and are plasmid encoded. However, it has now been shown that adherence of these E. *coli* is more complex. Deletion of the gene coding for pili, thus creating organisms without pili, creates organisms that are still able to adhere.

The LT of ETEC is immunologically identical to cholera toxin and similarly is comprised of two component parts, a receptor subunit and toxin subunit which activates intracellular adenylate cyclase by ADP ribosylation (see Table 9-2). The effects are generally less in magnitude than cholera toxin for reasons that are not clear. Again, these organisms do not destroy the brush border, invade the mucosa, or cause histopathologic lesions.

The second E. *coli* toxin, ST, is not related to LT or to cholera toxin (see Table 9-2). It is a protein but it is a poor immunogen, and it is also stable to proteases. The receptor on GI tract cells is unknown but it is different than that for LT. A measurable increase in cyclic GMP in the small and large intestines occurs as a result of the toxin's effect on guanylate cyclase. It has been suggested that ST alters Ca^{++} channels in cell membranes and with increased Ca^{++} uptake, calmodulin is activated and a series of events finally results in the stimulation of guanylate cyclase. Approximately 40% to 50% of ETEC produce only ST, 30% to 40% produce

ST and LT, and 20% to 30% produce only LT. Disease may be produced by any of these ETEC and is of the malabsorption type.

The enteroinvasive E. *coli* (EIEC) and shigellae must also adhere to mucosal cells via specific surface receptors and require a specific plasmid to be adherent. The structure of the cell wall determines virulence and may protect the organism from phagocytosis and lysis in the absence of specific antibody. These virulent organisms induce their own uptake by epithelial cells. They penetrate the mucosa and multiply in enterocytes of the large intestine. Shigellae produce a toxin that causes increased secretion of fluid in the small intestine (see Table 9-2). A receptor for *Shigella* toxin thought to be a glycoprotein is present on epithelial cells of the small intestine. In the intracellular location of the epithelial cells of the large intestine, the *Shigella* cytotoxin inhibits protein synthesis and probably contributes to the cellular dysfunction and necrosis in the colon with characteristic ulceration. The exudative response of neutrophils and mononuclear cells are apparent microscopically. The superficial ulcerations of the mucosa and submucosa heal with formation of granulation tissue.

Finally, the adherent but noninvasive EPEC colonize the small intestine by undefined receptors. The in vitro adherence to HEp2 cells by these organisms is mediated by nonfimbrial adhesions. The mechanism of disease production by these organisms is unknown. Pathologically, clusters of organisms adhere to the mucosa, and microvilli are destroyed at the site of adherence, which causes visible damage to the brush border of the epithelium. The villi are blunted and hypertrophy of the crypts occurs.

To cause disease salmonellae must adhere to and then penetrate the mucosal cells by endocytosis before reaching the lamina propria. This is characterized as mucosal translocation and bacterial proliferation in the lamina propria and mesenteric nodes. The penetration is very rapid, and macrophage engulfment without killing has been demonstrated. The terminal ileum and cecum are maximally involved, and neutrophilic inflammation is apparent in these locations. Peyer's patches and the mesenteric nodes may be enlarged. Salmonellae seem to survive in an intracellular location, gain access to the reticuloendothelial system, and are thus protected from antibody and some antibiotics. This intracellular location may contribute to prolonged carriage and excretion of the organism.

Although several enterotoxins have been shown to be produced by various salmonellae, their role in disease is not well defined. There are demonstrable water and electrolyte transport abnormalities in experimental *Salmonella* infections. The tissue invasion places the organisms in position to enter the lymphatic and/or the vascular system with access to the reticuloendothelial system. Involvement of tissues outside the GI tract is an unusual occurrence. *S. typhi*, on the other hand, elicits a mononuclear cell response in the lamina propria. *S. typhi* traverses the mucosa and is more likely to cause bacteremia than other *Salmonella* species.

C. fetus ss. *jejuni* and *Y. enterocolitica* produce a dysentery syndrome and are thus similar to shigellae. Pathologically, they generally mimic the mucosal translocation and bacterial proliferation in nodes and lamina propria described for *Salmonella* species. An enterotoxin has been described for *C. fetus* that has an action similar to cholera toxin and LT of ETEC. A stable toxin has been produced in vitro at 26° to 30° C by *Y. enterocolitica*. Both of these organisms must invade the mucosa, and the features contributing to their virulence have not yet been delineated.

Clinical manifestations (Table 9-3)

Escherichia coli. ETEC are an important cause of diarrhea in infants of developing nations. When an etiology is defined, one half of the cases of travelers' diarrhea, usually in adults, are attributable to ETEC. The severity varies from mild to severe, with 10 to 20 stools per day. An inoculum of 100 million to 10 billion organisms produces disease in adults, with an incubation period of several days. Disease is self-limited, lasting 3 to 5 days in a normal host, but if severe dehydration occurs in infants, morbidity is substantial. Disease is a malabsorptive diarrhea with watery stools without blood or white blood cells, and low-grade fever may be present.

EIEC produce dysentery with blood and pus in stools. Two million to 100 million organisms are necessary to produce disease. Symptoms may be rapid in onset with fever, nausea, cramps, and tenesmus. EIEC disease is uncommon in infants.

EPEC, which may be grouped by serotypes, characteristically infect infants and have caused numerous outbreaks of infantile enteritis. These organisms are of particular importance in tropical countries and developing nations with crowding and poor standards of hygiene. Frequent, green, slimy stools are produced usually without blood or WBC.

Cholera. Contaminated food or water transmit *V. cholerae*, and 100 million to 10 billion organisms are necessary to infect humans unless achlorhydria is present, when 100 to 10,000 organisms will cause infection. After a brief incubation period, usually 2 to 3 days (range, 6 hours to 5 days), there is the sudden onset of profuse, painless, watery diarrhea. Severe cases may be characterized by rapid fluid loss in excess of 20 liters per 24 hours. Profound shock and death can occur within a day if fluid replacement is not instituted.

The acutely ill patient usually appears in a shocklike state with his clothes soiled by the excessive fecal discharge. The feces are usually clear, without odor, and contain flecks of mucus that impart a "rice-water" appearance. Vomiting without nausea, described as effortless, usually follows the onset of diarrhea. The skin of the hands may have a characteristic appearance, resembling wrinkled "washer-woman's hands." Fever, if present, is low grade, or there may be hypothermia.

Salmonellae. Infection with salmonellae may cause one of four types of clinical syndrome: (1) acute gastroenteritis, which is most common; (2) enteric fever; (3) septicemia with or without localized infections; and (4) inapparent infection and carrier state. The clinical manifestations of these syndromes often overlap.

Gastroenteritis. Gastroenteritis, or food poisoning, is by far the most common manifestation of *Salmonella* infection, with greater than 200,000 cases reported yearly in the United States. The infection varies in severity from mild to extremely severe forms. The onset of symptoms may vary from a few to 72 hours after the ingestion of contaminated food. The illness is due to infection, not ingestion of preformed toxin. Nausea, vomiting, and diarrhea are associated with severe abdominal cramps. Fever and prostration may be pronounced. Feelings of weakness and chilliness are common. The stools are numerous, watery, and may contain mucus, pus, and blood. Such cases are clinically indistinguishable from other causes of bacillary dysentery. Bloody diarrhea is observed often in young children but rarely in adults. Physical findings are scant. Rose spots and meningismus are sometimes observed. The spleen is seldom enlarged. In about one half of the patients, the temperature falls to normal within 1 or 2 days, and recovery is uneventful. In others, the disease may last 1 week or more. Protracted or recurrent diarrhea occurs and may represent secondary consequences of mucosal invasion and destruction of the epithelium. In very severe infections, the patient may be in shock with cy-

Table 9-3. Differential clinical features of bacterial diarrheas*

	Enterotoxigenic E. coli	Enteroinvasive E. coli	Enteropathogenic E. coli†	Shigellae	Salmonellae	V. cholerae	C. jejuni	Y. enterocolitica
Malabsorption								
Small bowel affected	X		Some strains	X	X	X		
Toxin mediated	X		Some strains	X		X		
Stool								
Large volume	X		X	X		X		
Watery	X		X	X		X		
Colorless	X			X		X		
Mucus								
Duration (untreated)	5 to 10 Days					3 to 6 Days		
Fever 38.8° C (102° F)	0		0					
Age	Any In U.S. travelers		1 year Outbreak in nursery		Any	Any		
Dysentery								
Large bowel affected		X	Some strains	X	X		X	X
Toxin present		0			Yes/?role		Yes/?role	Yes/?role
Stool								
Small-moderate volume		X	X	X	X		X	X
Viscous/slimy		X		X	X		X	X
Bloody/green		X	X	X			X	X
Mucus		X	X	X	X		X	X
WBC		X	X	X	X		X	X
Duration			7 to 14 Days	7 to 14 Days	3 to 7 Days		X	X
Fever 38.8° C (102° F)		X						
Cramps, tenesmus		X		X	X		X	X
Age		Any		Any	Any		Any	Any

*Modified from table prepared by Nelson JD, and Hieber JP.
†EPEC, heterogeneous group of organisms; see text for discussion.

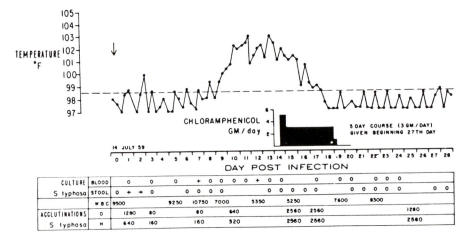

Fig. 9-1. Summary of the clinical course of induced typhoid fever in an adult volunteer. Therapy consisted of two 5-day courses of chloramphenicol separated by a 1-week interval. (From Hornick RB, et al. N Engl J Med 1970;283:686.)

anosis, hypothermia, and circulatory collapse, which precedes death.

In some cases the gastroenteric type of infection is followed by the enteric fever syndrome or the septicemic syndrome or by signs of localization. Metastatic foci are more likely to occur in patients with sickle cell disease, infants less than 6 months of age, or the immunocompromised person.

The leukocyte count is usually 10,000 to 15,000 per cubic millimeter. with perhaps a slight increase in number of polymorphonuclear cells. The leukopenia found in the enteric fever type of infection is seldom seen in the gastroenteric form. Positive blood cultures are more frequent in infants less than 6 months of age and are occasionally found in older persons, especially in severe infections. Stool cultures almost always yield salmonellae during the acute phase of the disease and often for several weeks thereafter. Symptoms subside despite continued colonization with the organism.

Enteric fever. Although infections caused by salmonellae of various types constitute a serious public health problem, those caused by S. *typhi* have become relatively infrequent in the United States. For example, the number of cases of typhoid fever reported in the United States during the last two decades rarely exceeded 500 per year.

The onset of typhoid fever in most cases is gradual, with fever, headache, malaise, and loss of appetite. The typical course in an adult is illustrated in Fig. 9-1. The temperature rises in a steplike manner during 2 to 7 days to an average of about 40° C (104° F) and characteristically remains at about this level for 3 or 4 weeks in the absence of specific antimicrobial therapy. The pulse rate tends to be slow relative to the fever. Diarrhea is present in some patients, although constipation may persist throughout the infection. Either manifestation may be accompanied by abdominal tenderness, distention, and pain. In the early stages of illness, discrete rose-colored spots may be scattered over the trunk, especially the abdomen. The spleen is enlarged in most cases. Severely ill patients may become delirious or stuporous. The white blood cell count as a rule shows leukopenia.

Typhoid fever in the first 2 years of life exhibits certain differences from the picture seen in adults. The diagnosis in infancy is often made by the chance isolation of S. *typhi* from stools or blood. It may resemble bacillary dysentery. The onset is often abrupt, with high fever, vomiting, convulsions, and meningeal signs. The slow pulse rate is not a frequent finding. Rose spots are seen less commonly than in adults. Leukocytosis is the rule and the white blood cell count may be as high as 20,000 to 25,000 but neutrophils rarely exceed 60% to 70%. The spleen is usually palpable. The course of the disease is short, rarely persisting more than 2 weeks. Although previously the mortality in infancy was high (12.5%), probably as a result of dehydration, today, with appropriate therapy, deaths are not common.

Salmonellae other than *S. typhi* may give rise to a disease with all the manifestations of typhoid fever, including persistent fever, gastrointestinal symptoms, rose spots, leukopenia, and positive cultures of blood, stool, and urine specimens.

Septicemia with or without localized infection. Salmonellae are also responsible for a disease characterized by intermittent fever, chills (in adults), anorexia, and loss of weight. The characteristic features of typhoid are absent. Stool cultures are usually negative, although blood cultures yield the causative organism.

A focus of infection is identified in approximately one fourth of the patients with bacteremia. The acute focal process may be directly or indirectly connected with the gastrointestinal tract, causing appendicitis, cholecystitis, peritonitis, or salpingitis. Hematogeneous spread of organisms may result in foci of infection in the brain, skin, lungs, spleen, or middle ear, bone, or joints. Meningitis is caused by a variety of *Salmonella* types and occurs principally in young infants with a high morbidity. The urinary tract can also be infected. In the days before antimicrobial therapy, the outcome was almost always fatal, but in the last decade a high proportion of recoveries has been reported.

Osteomyelitis and pyarthrosis are caused by many serotypes. Almost any bone may be involved, but the long bones, spine, and ribs are most commonly attacked. Pneumonia occurs and usually is accompanied by high fever and often terminates fatally. This manifestation occurs almost exclusively in elderly patients, many of whom suffer from unrelated medical problems.

Inapparent infection and the carrier state. Asymptomatic infection with salmonellae occurs in an estimated 0.2% of people as documented by positive stool cultures in the absence of clinical illness. Some of these persons have had known contact with symptomatic persons or are being investigated because of a recognized source of contaminated food. Persons who have been infected usually excrete organisms for weeks and some do so for months. Carriers of *S. typhi* may excrete organisms for years.

Shigellae. Bacillary dysentery is an acute infection caused by various strains of *Shigella*. The classical clinical picture is one characterized by severe abdominal pain, tenesmus, and constitutional symptoms with frequent stools containing mucus, pus, and blood. Moderately severe cases may have an abrupt onset with fever, abdominal pain, vomiting, and then diarrhea. Stools occur seven to twelve times daily, are watery, green or yellow, and contain mucus and undigested food. Disease may progress with development of all of the features of dysentery. Acute symptoms may persist for 7 to 10 days and meningismus, delirium, and convulsions may accompany *Shigella* dysentery. Morbidity and mortality usually result from severe dehydration. The worst illness occurs most frequently at the extremes of life, in young infants and old, debilitated persons.

Fortunately, mild infections with transient diarrhea or no GI symptoms are a more common manifestation of *Shigella* infection. These persons have simple watery diarrhea or loose stools for a few days with mild or absent constitutional symptoms.

Campylobacter fetus. The spectrum of symptoms is similar to that caused by shigellae. The incubation period for diarrhea is from 1 to 3 days. Organisms are excreted for 2 to 3 weeks or occasionally longer.

Yersinia enterocolitica. Diarrhea is the most common manifestation of infection and is usually watery or malabsorptive in character. However, infection with these organisms can produce a dysentery syndrome, and systemic signs such as arthritis or erythema nodosum are seen. To some extent, these are age related so that infants more commonly manifest infection as febrile diarrhea. Adolescents and older children have acute mesenteric adenitis and/or ileitis and may have findings suggestive of appendicitis. Adults have febrile diarrhea, enterocolitis, arthritis, and erythema nodosum. Acute bacteremia with metastatic foci including liver and spleen is seen in aged adults or immunocompromised hosts.

Diagnosis and differential diagnosis

The bacteria already presented and the viruses to be enumerated in the latter part of the chapter plus *Giardia lamblia* and *Entamoeba histolytica* and *Cryptosporidium* compromise the list of the most common etiologic agents of gastrointestinal infection. The age of the patient, life-style, geographic setting, and broad classification of symptoms provide the clinical framework for the etiologic diagnosis. Examination of stool for the presence of leukocytes and/or blood will provide insight into whether the organism is invasive. Laboratory culture can detect *V. cholerae, Salmonella, Shigella, Campylobacter,* and *Y. enterocolitica*. Laboratory confirmation of *E. coli*-caused disease is not generally accessible because detection of enterotoxin(s) or invasive properties require cell culture, animals, or other specific assays. Serotyping of *E. coli* in diarrheal outbreaks in infants is potentially helpful for recognition of EPEC but probably provides epidemiologic insights more effectively than diagnostic help with an infant.

S. typhi is frequently detected in blood cultures during the first 2 weeks of illness, and when enteric fever is suspected blood must be cultured. Serologic tests may be helpful if they are positive, as they will be in about two of three patients. Usually a single agglutinin titer of 1:320 or greater for antibody to the O antigen alerts the physician to consider typhoid. Recent vaccination, infection with another salmonella, or liver disease may give false-positive agglutinins.

V. cholerae presents diagnostic problems in the United States where it is such a rare pathogen. The unprepared laboratory may miss the diagnosis, so it is essential that the clinician suspect the diagnosis, alert the laboratory, and thus increase the likelihood of a correct diagnosis as described on p. 81.

Similarly, to culture *Y. enterocolitica* or *C. fetus*, the laboratory may need to be alerted to employ specific conditions and/or media to facilitate growth and recognition of the organism in fecal flora (see p. 82).

Prognosis

The prognosis is largely dependent on the age and the nutritional status of the patient and or the presence of an underlying disease. The vast majority of gastroenteritis is self-limited with no complications and complete recovery. The very young, the aged, and those with protein-calorie malnutrition and underlying disease are at risk for complications and/or prolonged illness. Overall, fatality from any of these agents seldom exceeds 1% where health care delivery is adequate. Those with meningitis or endocarditis due to salmonella have a much higher mortality.

Complications

The severity of acute bacterial gastroenteritis is best correlated with fluid and electrolyte loss and the extent of dehydration. Most of these infections are self-limited and localized to the gastrointestinal tract. The availability of fluid replacement has totally altered the morbidity and mortality of cholera. Extracellular volume depletion secondary to the intestinal loss of isotonic fluid; acidosis secondary to bicarbonate loss in stool; and hypokalemia secondary to fecal potassium loss are the major deficits during cholera. Abnormalities in renal function occur secondary to the three initial deficits, and renal failure has even occurred as a result of hypovolemia and shock. Replacement fluids have diminished morbidity for all diarrheal illnesses, and specific antibiotics have contributed to effective therapy of several of these entities. In developing nations where nutrition is poor, diarrheal illnesses often contribute to protein calorie malnutrition and increase growth failure and susceptibility to additional pathogens in the population.

Salmonella infections are common, and suppurative foci such as meningitis, pyarthrosis, and osteomyelitis occur infrequently. The patient may have an altered mental status with a spectrum of effects including delirium, stupor, and aphasia. It is important to ascertain if direct invasion of the CNS has occurred in the presence of such signs. Fortunately, gastrointestinal perforation and hemorrhage are extremely rare even with *S. typhi*, primarily because infections are treated. These complications characteristically occurred after 2 weeks of untreated disease. Relapse may occur in 15% to 20% of treated *S. typhi* patients and does so usually within 10 to 18 days of stopping antibiotics. Chronic carriage of *S. typhi* has been attributed to chronic infection of the gallbladder.

Although the pathogenesis of Reiter's syndrome and hemolytic uremic syndrome are not clear, these entities have been observed in association with *Shigella* infections.

Unusually, *Y. enterocolitica* can cause chronic and recurrent enteric symptoms which respond to antibiotic therapy. Septicemic illness is potentially severe and has been seen in immunocompromised hosts. The nonsuppurative arthritis is usually self-limited and normally lasts a few months.

Immunity

ETEC must be able to adhere to the mucosa to elaborate their toxins and produce disease. Immunization of animals with organisms bearing fimbrial adherence antigens but not elaborating toxin will produce protection to homologous organisms that do elaborate toxin. Apparently, local antibody directed at fimbrial (attachment) factors prevents disease by blocking attachment. A series of epidemiologic observations in humans support the concept of acquired immunity. First, breast milk can confer passive protection to the infant GI tract. Second, that the age-specific incidence, that is, disease, affects primarily infants in the endemic areas suggests that immunity is acquired. Third, adults from areas where organisms are endemic have less disease than travelers from nonendemic areas. Challenge/rechallenge studies in adult volunteers have corroborated the epidemiologic findings with the demonstration of homologous immunity against disease. However, the asymptomatic subjects shed organisms in the same quantity and for the same period of time, suggesting that antibodies are not bactericidal. Despite all these accumulated data, it is still appreciated that a person can experience diarrhea due to ETEC more than once. There are several colonization factors already known, each inducing only homologous antibodies; this is one explanation for several episodes of disease. The LT elaborated by various human *E. coli* is thought to be the same. Serum antibody to LT is easily measured as is GI antibody to toxin after natural infection; thus an explanation for repeated disease is needed. It is known that ST toxin is a poor immunogen, and no local IgA antibodies can be measured with infection. Organisms often elaborate both LT and ST, so repeated disease could be due to ST. Finally, it is also becoming apparent that adherence is more complex than the single protein CFAs. Multiple factors seem to contribute to adherence.

Enteroinvasive E. coli have surface antigens that cross react with those of shigellae and are essential for virulence. Local (secretory IgA) antibody develops within the first week of illness and is probably protective against disease. Circulating antibodies also develop, but it is doubtful if they contribute to protection.

V. cholerae stimulates a complex series of responses on the part of the host. Measurable humoral IgM and IgG bactericidal antibodies can be measured, which wane over the months following infection and correlate in general with resistance to cholera. Systemic antibody to cholera toxin is also demonstrable but without any correlation with resistance to infection. It is suggested that local antibody both to toxin and to the organism is important in protecting the host. Breast milk diminishes occurrence of disease, but infants may still be colonized. Whole killed organisms used as parenteral vaccine provided suboptimal protection with development of humoral immunity to the organism without local antibody to either organism or toxin. Similarly, parenteral administration of toxoid provides no gastrointestinal protection by production of only humoral antibodies against toxin. Challenge/rechallenge studies in adults demonstrate that immunity can be induced. Measurable local antibody to toxin occurred as well as humoral vibriocidal and antitoxin antibodies.

Epidemiology

Many features of the epidemiology of these bacteria have been alluded to in previous portions of this chapter. All of these pathogens are worldwide in distribution and are transmitted by the fecal-to-oral route. Transmission often occurs with a vehicle of contaminated food or water allowing the organisms to multiply. A large inoculum is necessary for virtually all these bacteria, ranging from estimates of 10,000 to 100 billion organisms. Shigellae are the exception, with 10 to 100 organisms transmitting infection. *S. typhi* and *Shigella* are inhabitants of only the human GI tract, whereas the other organisms have animal hosts and can be introduced to man by contact with contaminated materials.

ETEC cause disease primarily in infants less than 18 months of age in developing nations and in adult travelers. Only occasional outbreaks of disease have been associated with contaminated water. EPEC cause outbreaks of disease, especially in infant nurseries via contaminated instruments, health personnel, or other aspects of the environment. EIEC are an uncommon cause of infantile diarrhea and are more often transmitted via contaminated food.

Cholera has occurred in devastating worldwide pandemics, with perpetual endemic disease occurring in India and Bangladesh. A very few cases have been identified in the United

States over the past decade and are related to shellfish in the Gulf of Mexico. Ratios of inapparent infection to clinical disease vary from an estimated 4:1 to 36:1. Carriage and excretion of the organism usually lasts several weeks but may last longer. Thus, quarantine of symptomatic cases does not curtail spread. In endemic areas, cholera is a disease of childhood sparing the infants less than 1 year of age. When epidemics reach previously uninfected countries, all ages are infected.

Humans usually ingest *Salmonella* from contaminated food with meat and poultry products heading the list. Organisms are present on the surface of meat, not in abscesses, and thus any conditions favoring multiplication enhances the possibility of disease production. The animals are infected and perpetuate the infection among themselves, easily contaminating other animals during transport. There are an estimated 2 million cases of *Salmonella* gastroenteritis per year in the United States, but only 1% of these are reported. Nosocomial transmission within hospitals, nursing homes, and institutions result from cross contamination, including personnel, equipment, and aerosol. In those areas where sewage disposal and water purification are inadequate, enteric infections are frequent, and the likelihood of spread enhanced.

Shigella and *S. typhi* are exclusively human pathogens, and communicability of disease depends on human fecal material transmitting infection either through person-to-person contact or via food and water. The highest incidence of *Shigella* is in infants from 1 to 4 years of age. Large outbreaks of infection usually are related to contaminated food or water.

Campylobacter fetus. Many mammalian hosts including domesticated animals and avian species are reservoirs for *C. fetus* ss. *jejuni*. These birds and animals are often not symptomatic. Contaminated food and water have been implicated as vehicles for outbreaks of disease. Person-to-person transmission also occurs, but more frequently contamination results from infected animals. Although the organisms are worldwide in distribution, disease is more common in developing nations and younger infants are affected.

Yersinia enterocolitica. *Y. enterocolitica* causes a spectrum of illness that includes gastroenteritis and affects all age groups. There is some geographical variation in recognized disease in the United States for reasons that are not clear. Outbreaks of disease have been traced to contaminated food. The reservoirs of these organisms are probably animals but this is less well documented than some of the other pathogens described.

General control measures

Interruption of the intestinal-to-oral circuit is essential for diminishing transmission of all of these enteric pathogens. Individual patients should be isolated during the illness. Strict handwashing should be initiated as well as appropriate processing or disposal of all contaminated materials.

For those pathogens such as *S. typhi* and *Shigella* species that are exclusively human pathogens, the incidence of disease can be diminished by (1) sanitary disposal of human feces, (2) purification and protection of water supplies, (3) pasteurization of milk and milk products, (4) strict sanitary supervision of preparation and serving of all foods, (5) proper refrigeration of food and milk, and (6) exclusion of persons with diarrhea from handling food.

Reducing the spread of enteric pathogens with animal reservoirs, for example, salmonellae, is more complex. Any food or drink contaminated with organisms may transmit infection. The huge animal reservoirs are probably responsible for the majority of human *Salmonella* infections in the United States. Poultry and milk products are often implicated either directly or indirectly with contamination of meat processing areas, markets, or kitchens. By-products of the meat packing industry such as fertilizer or bone meal perpetuate infection in animals. Prevention of *Salmonella* infections in humans depends on interrupting transmission. The task of controlling salmonellosis among animals and preventing the spread of infection to people is enormous. Continued surveillance is needed to identify and to eliminate the multiple sources of infection.

Treatment

Infants, children, and adults with gastroenteritis require fluid replacement. Hospitalization may be necessary when a fluid deficit ($\geq 5\%$) has occurred or oral hydration cannot be tolerated. Oral hydration with fluid containing sugar and electrolytes has significantly reduced the morbidity and mortality. *V. cholerae* causes the most rapid losses, and replacement may be an emergency. Since glucose-coupled electrolyte and water transport across the epithelium are unaltered by the various toxins, it is possible to replace fluids orally. A replacement fluid made of ½ teaspoon NaCl, ¼ teaspoon KCl, ½ teaspoon NaHCO₃, 2 tablespoons glucose or 4 tablespoons sucrose, and 1 quart of water is one formulation.

Drugs such as motility inhibitors or analgesics are not recommended because they do not alter the fluid loss and in some situations have been implicated in prolongation of symptoms.

It is well documented that specific *antimicrobial therapy* (Table 9-4) alters the course of typhoid and *Shigella* infections. Additionally, the

Table 9-4. Antimicrobial therapy of gastroenteritis

Organism	Antimicrobial agent*
E. coli	
EPEC	Neomycin or colistin
ETEC	Neomycin or colistin; trimethroprim-sulfamethoxazole
EIEC	Ampicillin; trimethoprim-sulfamethoxazole; parenteral aminoglycoside
Salmonella gastroenteritis	None (ampicillin or trimethoprim-sulfamethoxazole for other sites of infection)
Salmonella typhi	Chloramphenicol; trimethoprim-sulfamethoxazole; ampicillin (not effective for carriers)
Shigellae	Trimethoprim-sulfamethoxazole; ampicillin
Vibrio cholerae	Tetracycline
Yersinia enterocolitica	Trimethoprim-sulfamethoxazole; tetracycline; aminoglycoside
Campylobacter species	Erythromycin; tetracycline
Entomoeba histolytica	Metronidazole
Giardia lamblia	Metronidazole or quinacrine or furazolidone
Cryptosporidium	No effective regimen; furazolidone may suppress symptoms

*See text for details.

period of time shigellae are excreted is shortened and therefore communicability is lessened. In contrast, the course of infections of salmonellae other than *S. typhi* has not been shown to be altered by antibiotics, and excretion of the organisms is not shortened and may be prolonged. Routine antibiotic therapy is of no benefit. On the other hand, many experts recommend therapy of infants (less than 6 months) and immunocompromised patients with *Salmonella* gastroenteritis with appropriate antimicrobials because of the risk of dissemination of organisms. It is hoped that therapy during the acute gastroenteritis will provide protection while the patient develops an immune response to the organism thereby diminishing the risk of bacteremia. Patients with *Salmonella* infections in sites other than the GI tract should also be treated with antimicrobial agents.

EPEC diarrhea in infants is also treated with specific antimicrobial agents. Prior studies suggest that the disease in infants caused by those serogroupable organisms could be shortened by antimicrobial agents. In fact, these are the only organisms for which nonabsorbable drugs like neomycin have proved useful. This may well be related to the noninvasive nature of many of those organisms.

V. cholera, ETEC, *C. fetus*, and *Y. enterocolitica* infections are all treated with antibiotics when the patient is symptomatic and the organism has been identified. Excretion of the organism is shortened and therapy may alter disease. Toxins attach to epithelial cells and generally penetrate membranes. It appears that their effects are permanent, that is, the epithelial cell must be sloughed before effects will cease. Thus, antibiotics may stop organisms from elaborating toxin but do not immediately alter symptoms.

Specific antimicrobial therapy is often administered empirically to the febrile, dehydrated individual with gastroenteritis. Table 9-4 lists the organisms and drugs used for therapy. Trimethoprim-sulfamethoxazole (TMP-SMX) has been effective in treating *Salmonella/Shigella* infections, and *Y. enterocolitica* is likely to be sensitive in vitro. Although a nonabsorbable drug like neomycin has curtailed symptoms of EPEC, it will not do so for invasive organisms. Therefore, when the physician feels obliged to treat the diarrhea, electing to use an absorbable compound like TMP-SMX or ampicillin has a better chance of being effective against the entire spectrum of pathogens. Suspicion of *S. typhi* or *V. cholerae* in areas where these infections are endemic would affect the choice of drug. If the stool culture yields *Campylobacter*, therapy can be changed to erythromycin and if *Y. enterocolitica* is isolated, sensitivities to available antimicrobials can guide therapy.

Immunization

Vibrio cholerae. Parenterally inoculated, killed whole cell vaccine has been available for years. This vaccine stimulates high titers of serum vibriocidal antibodies, but it does not induce antibodies to toxin. In an individual previously primed by gastrointestinal contact with the organism, the vaccine also produces an anamnestic response in gastrointestinal IgA directed against the somatic O antigen. In field trials, homologous protection by vaccine has been induced for about 1 year, with vaccine efficacy approximating 70%. It has become clear that local gastrointestinal immunity against the organism and against the toxin should provide a better, less reactogenic immunogen. Utilizing recombinant DNA technology, an "attenuated" *V. cholerae* organism that lacks the genes for production of the A and B subunits of toxin was created. A plasmid was then constructed and inserted containing the B subunit gene. Thus, a candidate live *V. cholerae* vaccine containing all the cell wall antigens necessary for adherence and the capacity to produce only the B subunit of toxin has been engineered. In theory, this could provide ideal local immunity without toxicity. Initial trials have demonstrated a vaccine efficacy of 90% to rechallenge with virulent organisms. A surprise observation was the induction of diarrhea in volunteers with the vaccine bacterium lacking the gene for subunit A. Unexpectedly, a new cholera toxin was subsequently identified.

Enterotoxigenic Escherichia coli. Humans produce serum IgM and secretory IgA antibodies to the homologous O antigen of an infecting strain of ETEC. These antibodies do not prevent adherence of the organism or action of the toxin. Experience with ETEC in animals has greatly advanced our understanding of disease and its prevention. One can prevent disease by blocking adherence of organisms; for human ETEC infections this requires delineation of all the critical colonizing factors because only homologous

immunity is produced. Purified fimbriae (CFA/2) given orally, has produced a local IgA response which primed the recipient. Later a parenteral inoculation of CFA/2 was given to stimulate a humoral and secretory immune response.

Any effective immunogen should induce a local antibody response to LT and ST. Since the ST is a poor immunogen, such approaches as conjugation of the ST toxoid to the B (receptor) subunit of LT are being investigated.

Salmonella typhi. An acetone-killed whole bacterial cell vaccine for parenteral injection achieved 70% to 90% efficacy, but it induced significant side effects including fever, malaise, and severe local reactions. Since an immune host can kill organisms within macrophages, it is logical to assume specific humoral antibody would provide protection against this invasive organism.

A live attenuated oral typhoid vaccine is being tested and has become available in some countries. This vaccine is the stable mutant of *S. typhi* strain Ty21a. It lacks an enzyme, UDP-galactose-4-epimerase, that normally converts UDP-glucose to UDP-galactose. Since galactose is essential for its lipopolysaccharide, absence of the enzyme forces the organism to utilize exogeneous galactose, thereby accumulating galactose-1-phosphate and UDP-galactose. In the presence of galactose, these organisms lyse spontaneously. The results of initial field trials have shown a high degree of efficacy in the prevention of typhoid fever.

Enteropathogenic Escherichia coli. Recognition of the association of specific O and H serotypes with EPEC led to unsuccessful attempts to immunize with oral preparations of killed bacteria or extracts of bacteria. Recognition of the essential role that adherence plays in disease production as well as the identification of a plasmid encoding for this property, may lead to more successful approaches to prevention of disease.

Shigella. There is no vaccine currently available. Various attenuated organisms were tested in the 1960s and 1970s without demonstration of consistent efficacy. Recognition of the possible role of outer membrane proteins as adhesins, the association of virulence with the smooth lipopolysaccharide, and identification of enterotoxin have led to new strategies. Ty21a, an attenuated oral *S. typhi* organism, has served as the recipient of a shigella plasmid encoding for the lipopolysaccharide of S. sonnei. The resulting strain of bacterium manifests both S. typhi and S. sonnei O antigens. This strain tested in a small number of humans induces no diarrhea; it stimulated antibodies to both antigens in animal experiments.

VIRAL GASTROENTERITIS
Etiology

Viral agents recognized during the past decade have been shown to be responsible for a large proportion of the diarrhea for which an etiologic agent can be defined. Acute viral gastroenteritis affects all age groups and may occur in either sporadic or epidemic form. Most such illnesses are self-limited, and in normal hosts recovery is complete. If severe dehydration occurs, morbidity and mortality may be substantial. Viral agents discussed in detail in this chapter are those associated with clinical symptoms related to viral replication within the gastrointestinal tract.

Rotaviruses. In 1943 an outbreak of diarrhea occurring in infants was reported by Light and Hodes. They isolated the filterable agent in stool specimens that causes diarrhea in calves. They established the incubation period and reproduced diarrhea with serial passage of the agent. The pathology of the bowel, the development of immunity to the agent, and passive protection by the administration of immune serum was described. It was not until 1973, however, when viral particles were visualized in a duodenal biopsy by electron microscopy that the etiologic agent was finally defined as a rotavirus. The original specimens of Drs. Hodes and Light were subsequently examined by electron microscopy and found to contain rotavirus particles. In the last decade, rotaviruses have come to be appreciated as the single most common agent causing endemic diarrhea in infants from 6 to 24 months of age. Rotaviruses are also known to cause diarrhea in foals, lambs, piglets, rabbits, deer, monkeys, and other species. Experimental infection of animals other than the species of origin occurs with most rotaviruses.

Rotaviruses constitute one genus of the family reoviridae (Fig. 9-2). The rotavirus genome consists of 11 segments of double-stranded RNA, and polyacrylamide gel electrophoresis has established a pattern distinguishable from the other genera of reoviridae. Complete rotavirus particles have a double shell of outer and inner capsids and a buoyant density of 1.36 gm/cm^2. At least 12 polypeptides have been detected in rotavirus-infected cells.

It is only relatively recently that one of these viruses has been successfully propagated in cell culture. Reassortants of human and bovine rotaviruses or human and monkey rotaviruses have now been created. On the basis of such experiments it has been learned which segment of the RNA is responsible for restriction of growth in cell culture. Similarly it has become clear that one segment codes for a protein that is responsible for the induction of neutralizing antibodies. Another RNA segment codes for a major internal structural protein that is responsible for subgroup specificity as determined by tests such as complement fixation. To clarify the nomenclature it has been proposed that *serotype* be reserved for reference to the antigen responsible for neutralization. *Subgroup* will be used to designate an antigen defined by complement fixation, enzyme-linked immunosorbent assays (ELISA), or immune adherence hemagglutination. At the present time, it would appear that there are probably four serotypes of rotavirus.

Norwalk group of viruses. Epidemic gastroenteritis occurs in a form that produces an explosive, self-limited disease lasting for 24 to 48 hours. It may be community wide, involving school-age children, family contacts, and adults. Such an outbreak of gastroenteritis occurred in Norwalk, Ohio in 1969. Within a matter of 48 hours, gastrointestinal illness developed in half the students and teachers in an elementary school with a secondary symptomatic attack rate affecting approximately one third of family contacts. A bacteria-free filtrate from a stool specimen produced gastroenteritis in several volunteers, and stools from the infected individuals could be serially passaged in additional volunteers. In 1972 immune electron microscopy with serum from a symptomatic patient demonstrated small, 27-nm particles in an infectious stool filtrate (Fig. 9-2). Morphologically, they resemble picornaviruses, parvoviruses, or, in some preparations, caliciviruses. A listing of the currently identified Norwalk-like agents is included in Table 9-5. Probably at least three serotypes exist. The viruses are not yet classified and have not been propagated in vitro but it is thought they are RNA-containing agents. The Norwalk agent

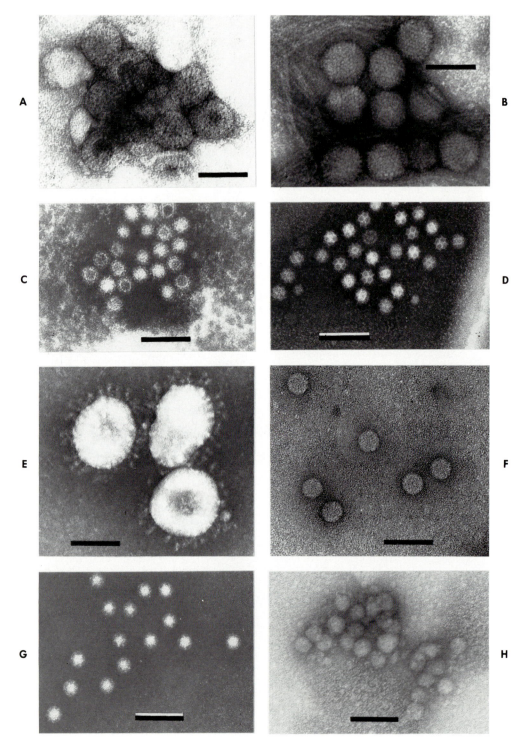

Fig. 9-2. Electron microscope appearance of viruses visualized in stool. All viruses printed with bar representing 100 nm to illustrate differences in size. Courtesy of Dr. S. Miller, Duke University Medical Center. **A,** Rotavirus; **B,** adenovirus; **C,** Mini-reovirus; **D,** calicivirus; **E,** coronavirus; **F,** ECHO virus; **G,** astrovirus; **H,** small round virus. (**A, B, F,** and **H** courtesy Sara E. Miller, Duke University, Durham, North Carolina; **C, D,** and **G** courtesy Maria T. Szymanski, Hospital for Sick Children, Toronto, Ontario, Canada; **E** courtesy D.W. Bradley, Centers for Disease Control, Atlanta, Georgia.)

has been found to be acid stable and relatively heat stable. Studies of the proteins of the Norwalk virion showed a single virion-associated protein with a molecular weight of 59,000 daltons and a single soluble protein with a molecular weight of 30,000 daltons (Tyrell and Kapikian, 1982). Among the mammalian viruses in this size range, the caliciviruses are the only ones that possess a single structural protein of approximately 65,000 daltons. This is suggestive evidence that the Norwalk-like agents could be caliciviruses.

Enteric adenoviruses. The fastidious enteric adenoviruses first described by Flewett in 1975 have now been established as a significant pathogen of diarrheal illness in children (Fig. 9-2). Preliminary characterization of agents isolated from geographically distinct outbreaks indicates

Table 9-5. Norwalk and Norwalk-like agents associated with acute epidemic gastroenteritis in humans*

Agent	*Antigenic relationships*
Norwalk	Distinct
Hawaii	Distinct
Montgomery County	Related to Norwalk agent by IEM and cross-challenge studies
Ditchling	Ditchling and W agents related to each other but appear to be distinct from Norwalk and Hawaii by IEM
W	
Cockle	Distinct from Norwalk by IEM
Paramatta	Distinct from Norwalk by IEM
Colorado	Distinct from Norwalk, Hawaii, and Marin County agents by IEM
Marin County	Distinct from Norwalk, Hawaii, and Colorado agents by IEM or RIA

*Modified from Tyrell DAG, Kapikan AZ (ed): Virus infections of GI tract. New York: Marcel Dekker, Inc., 1982. IEM, immune electron microscopy; RIA, radioimmunoassay.

that they are almost all representatives of the adenovirus serotype 38. These agents do not grow well in the usual cell culture systems, and thus far successful in vitro cultivation has been dependent on the use of Graham 293 cells, a human embryonic kidney cell line containing some of the genome of adenovirus type 5. In these cells, the cytopathic effects produced are typical of adenoviruses.

The estimated frequency of adenovirus as a cause of diarrhea varies. If the study period is selected when rotavirus disease is not occurring, adenoviruses are responsible for a larger proportion of illness, recorded to be as high as 50%. If a prospective study is conducted for several years, 4% to 8% of all the diarrhea observed may be associated with these fastidious adenoviruses. Serologic studies of children indicate that most children have been infected with these agents within the first 2 years of life.

Coronaviruses. The coronaviridiae are pleomorphic, enveloped single-strand RNA viruses with widely spaced 20-nm club-shaped surface projections (Fig. 9-2). These viruses had been well identified as etiologic agents of respiratory and intestinal disease in animals. In 1960, the first of these agents was isolated from a human with a cold and subsequently described in 1965 by Terrell and Bynoe. The agent grew in human tracheal organ culture and was morphologically similar to avian infectious bronchitis virus of the coronaviridiae. The second isolate and prototype strain of human coronavirus (229E) was first isolated in human kidney cell culture in 1962 and reported in 1966 by Hamre and Procknow.

Human coronaviruses were first etiologically associated with upper respiratory tract disease in adults and lower respiratory tract disease in hospitalized children. Coronavirus infections tend to occur in small outbreaks that take place during the late winter and early spring. Sporadic outbreaks at other seasons can also occur. Reinfection with coronavirus is a frequent event as shown by the presence of infection in persons having preexisting neutralizing antibodies.

It was predicted in the middle 1970s that an association of coronavirus with enteric disease of humans would be identified because of the known involvement of these agents with enteric disease in animals. Electron microscopic examination of stool then revealed coronaviruslike particles in human feces. In fecal specimens it has been estimated that there are as many as 10^8 coronavirus particles per gram of feces. The morphology of the particles in the stool suggests that a large number of these particles are defective, implying that the intracytoplasmic maturation may be faulty within the gastrointestinal tract.

These agents seem less likely to be responsible for diarrhea within the first year of life and are more commonly visualized in diarrheal stools of older children and young adults. In the course of epidemiologic studies it has been apparent that human enteric coronaviruses can be excreted over a long period of time. Virus has been excreted for as long as 1½ years and in some of the persistent excretors, chronic gastroenteritis was present. Conclusions concerning the epidemiology are complicated by asymptomatic individuals who can be excreting virus. Endemic diarrheal disease occurs in situations where poor hygiene exists, and acquisition of virus does coincide with the development of gastroenteritis.

Work with coronaviruses isolated from humans has been difficult because these agents grow best in organ cultures, and those in the respiratory tract require the use of ciliated epithelium. They withstand poorly the procedures of virus purification and do not produce easily measurable soluble antigens. The successful cultivation in vitro of several human strains is beginning to advance our knowledge of these viruses. Human coronaviruses have four major structural polypeptides. The surface projections probably consist of two large glycopeptides. There are at least two antigenic groups of mammalian coronaviruses. Coronavirus replication usually occurs in the cytoplasm of infected cells; mature particles bud into the cisternae of the endoplasmic reticulum. These enveloped viruses do not appear to bud from the plasma membrane of infected cells. Frequently there are large vacuoles seen within infected cells; presumably they represent coalescence of endoplasmic vesicles containing coronavirus particles. The end result of virus replication is the lysis of infected cells with the release of large numbers of virus particles.

Other viruses associated with gastroenteritis. The examination of stools by electron microscopy has revealed other morphologically distinct virus particles associated with clinical illness. Caliciviruses, astroviruses, and other small round viruses have been visualized (Fig. 9-2). As many of these viruses do not grow in cell culture systems their morphology serves as the only means of identification.

Astroviruses were first described in 1975 and are 28-nm particles shed in the stool (Fig. 9-2). They have been visualized in the stool of infants with and without gastroenteritis. The characteristic star shape designates the particles as astrovirus. Similar particles have been identified in feces from adults and children and in diarrheal feces from lambs and calves. These agents are able to infect monolayers of human embryonic kidney cells without producing a cytopathic effect. There are no serologic relationships of human, bovine, and lamb astrovirus to each other or to the Norwalk-like agents. The evidence that they cause disease is equivocal. Early serologic studies have demonstrated seroconversion in association with demonstrable infection and fecal excretion. However, feeding of these agents to adult volunteers infrequently produced disease but no antibody rise occurred in the majority of volunteers.

Calici-like particles are small spherical viruses of 30 to 40 nm with an ill-defined border. They too have been visualized in the feces of children and calves with diarrhea. Caliciviruses isolated from humans have not yet been cultured in vitro. In animals these agents are known to infect mucous membranes, particularly the nose, throat, and intestinal tract. They are single-strand RNA viruses and probably have one major structural polypeptide.

Small round viruses (picorna-parvoviruslike viruses) are a heterogeneous collection of 20 to 30 nm round viruses visualized in stools. They have no detectable surface structure and do not grow in vitro in routine cell culture systems. These particles have been visualized in stools from patients who have no clinical symptoms; more information is needed to establish their causative role in gastroenteritis.

Mini–reovirus agents are 30-nm particles with a double capsid shell. They have been visualized in stools from children with diarrhea and in infants who have acquired diarrhea within the hospital setting. Additional information is needed to establish their role as etiologic agents in gastroenteritis.

Pathogenesis and pathology

Transmission of rotavirus from person to person occurs via the fecal-to oral-route. The incubation period as first established by Light and Hodes is 2 to 5 days. Adults are often contacts of symptomatic children and have infections that may be asymptomatic or associated with clinical illness. Virus is excreted in extraordinarily large amounts, with as many as 10^{11} particles per gram of feces. The virus is generally stable in feces even at room temperature, although intestinal proteolytic enzymes may disrupt the morphology of the virus. It is excreted in feces for approximately 8 days after the onset of symptoms.

Rotaviral particles have been visualized by electron microscopy in intestinal epithelial cells, aspirated duodenal secretions, and feces of infected persons. Morphologically, shortening and blunting of the villi of the duodenum and small intestine accompany acute illness. The microvilli of the absorptive cells are distorted and other cells have swollen mitochondria. Virus particles are visualized in the cytoplasm and bud into the cisternae of the endoplasmic reticulum of the enterocytes. Immunofluorescence studies have also demonstrated rotavirus antigens in the cytoplasm of the villus epithelial cells but not in the cells of the crypts or lamina propria. This suggests that the specificity of the virus particle is for the mature or differentiated enterocytes located on the villi. This destruction of the mature enterocyte is associated with decreased production of one or more mucosal disaccharidases. The destroyed infected cells are replaced by immature cells resulting in a deficit in glucose-facilitated sodium transport. Diarrhea then results from decreased absorption secondary to the altered ion transport. In contrast to the toxin-mediated diarrheas, there is no increase in intestinal secretion. Complete recovery has been confirmed by biopsy as early as 4 weeks after the episode of diarrhea. There is no evidence of infection outside the gastrointestinal tract by these viruses, although some patients have reportedly had associated respiratory symptoms. Virus has not been demonstrated in respiratory tissues or gastric contents in association with gastrointestinal symptoms.

The Norwalk-like group of agents are also transmitted by the fecal-to-oral route. Infected volunteers have had detectable virus in their stools during the first 72 hours after the onset of illness. Infection with these agents results in delayed gastric emptying, although the gastric mucosa is morphologically normal. Microscopic broadening and blunting of the villi in the jejunum is apparent. The mucosa remains histologically intact but there is a mononuclear cell infiltration. Viruses have not yet been detected in involved mucosal cells by electron microscopy. Small intestinal enzyme studies showed decreased amounts of the enzymes measured. The incubation period appears to be about 48 hours.

Clinical manifestations

Acute infections due to rotaviruses are characterized by an abrupt onset of severe watery diarrhea which is not characteristically associated with blood or mucus in the stool. Fever and vomiting are often present at the onset of illness. Dehydration and metabolic acidosis are observed in children hospitalized with this infection. Those most severely affected are between the ages of 6 and 24 months. Rotaviruses are responsible for at least one half of the cases of infantile diarrhea requiring hospitalization.

Roughly one third of identified outbreaks of gastroenteritis can be attributed to a Norwalk-like agent. The outbreaks have occurred in schools, recreation camps, cruise ships, nursing homes, and after ingestion of inadequately cooked contaminated shellfish or contaminated water. These agents are transmitted by the fecal-to-oral route. Although respiratory symptoms are very unusual in patients with Norwalk-like infections, the rapidity of spread suggests the possibility of aerosolization of virus. Most patients who sustain these infections have nausea, vomiting, abdominal cramps, and approximately half of them have associated diarrhea (Fig. 9-3). Fever and chills are less common. The symptoms last from 12 to 24 hours and the incubation period appears to be around 48 hours. Usually the stools are not bloody and do not have mucus or lymphocytes. A transient lymphopenia has been observed in volunteers challenged with these agents.

The enteric adenoviruses have been responsible for acute diarrhea in infants less than 1 year of age. Onset of illness is usually manifested by

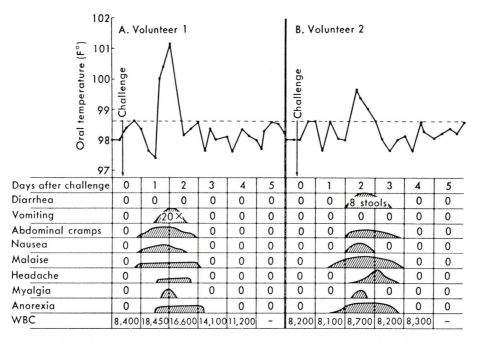

Fig. 9-3. Clinical course in two volunteers following oral administration of stool filtrate containing Norwalk agent. The height of the curve is directly proportional to the severity of the sign or symptom. (From Dolin R, et al. J Infect Dis 1971;123:307.)

diarrhea and the young child may also have respiratory symptoms including cough, rhinorrhea, or wheezing. Pneumonia and conjunctivitis have also accompanied adenovirus gastroenteritis. The illness is usually mild to moderate in severity and occurs throughout the year. The viruses have been visualized in the feces of patients for a period of 2 weeks.

Diagnosis and differential diagnosis

The clinical differentiation of viral from bacterial gastroenteritis is often difficult. Various epidemiologic factors may be helpful. None of these viruses can be identified currently by routine microbiologic techniques. Electron microscopic examination of fecal extracts obtained during the acute illness can demonstrate approximately 10^3 to 10^4 virus particles, a quantity usually present.

Fecal specimens often contain sufficient amounts of virus for successful antigen detection. Commercial enzyme-linked immunosorbent assay and radioimmunoassay techniques have become available for the detection of rotavirus particles in stool. All known rotaviruses share a common antigen thought to be located in the inner capsid, which makes the immunologic detection of these viruses a practical reality. Thus, antisera prepared against one strain will show cross-reactivity with other human subgroups and animal rotaviruses. The sensitivity of the enzyme-linked immunosorbent assay is based on the fact that a single molecule of enzyme can react with a large number of molecules of substrate. Indirect assays employ an unlabeled specific antibody and subsequent measurement of the antibody antigen combination with an enzyme-labeled antiglobulin. Since a single antiglobulin can be used for a number of different antigen assay systems it becomes a more practical tool. The indirect assays are also somewhat more sensitive than direct assays, presumably because a single molecule of antiviral antibody can react with a number of molecules of labeled antiglobulin.

Immune electron microscopy is also the best available procedure for identification of members of the Norwalk-like group of agents. These particles tend to aggregate spontaneously without the addition of serum, and therefore clumps of particles do not necessarily indicate the presence of antibody. Specific coating of the particle with antibody needs to be observed if the immune response is being assessed. Radioimmunoassay is more efficient than immune electron microscopy because it is able to detect soluble antigens as well as particulate antigens. This test is dependent on the availability of appropriate high titered serum, and its use is restricted to research laboratories.

Each of the other viruses discussed has been most frequently demonstrated by the use of electron microscopy of stool. Examination of stool by electron microscopy provides one test for the entire spectrum of viruses causing gastroenteritis.

Complications

Severe dehydration is a consequence of vomiting and diarrhea. In young infants or in elderly debilitated adults dehydration constitutes the most serious complication of gastroenteritis.

Prognosis

In general, the prognosis with any of these viral infections of the gastrointestinal tract is excellent. The illness is self-limited and usually a matter of days in duration.

Immunity

Primary infection with rotavirus produces an initial serum IgM response followed by an IgG response. Specific antibody has been demonstrable in both the stool and serum.

Adults with rotavirus infection show an anamnestic response with elevation of IgG antibodies. Some of the studies in the adult volunteers suggest that protection from rotavirus correlates better with secretory IgA of the small intestine than with serum antibody. It is clear that patients experience more than one infection with rotavirus, and it is not yet clear whether these are always different serotypes.

Specific antibody has been demonstrated in colostrum and milk for as long as 9 months of lactation. In nurseries where rotavirus infection has been endemic, breast-fed infants seem to acquire infection less often than formula-fed infants. Those who are infected excrete less virus and are less often symptomatic. Antibodies in human colostrum and milk are capable of neutralizing rotavirus in vitro. Weaning from breast milk in developing nations is temporally associated with the onset of the diarrhea/malnutrition cycle.

Immunity to the Norwalk-like viruses is a very puzzling feature of the infections that they cause. Challenge of volunteers will produce disease in some persons and not in others. Repeat challenge with a homologous virus within several months of the original infection will not produce clinical illness. Subsequent challenge 2 to 4½ years later produces disease in the same volunteers who had symptomatic illness with the first contact with the virus. Those individuals who were asymptomatic and did not acquire infection with the first contact did not do so with subsequent challenge. Those individuals who acquire clinical infection have demonstrable antibody that wanes but rises after a subsequent challenge a short time later. Volunteers who fail to develop illness have no demonstrable antibody. Individuals who develop illness have higher mean antibody titers in jejunal fluid than do those who remain well. Neither serum nor local intestinal antibody correlates with resistance to Norwalk virus challenge. Thus, those individuals who have demonstrable serum antibody are at risk for symptomatic infection. These findings are not understood, but it is possible that some individuals are resistant to these viruses because of genetically determined factors.

Epidemiology

Sporadic diarrhea occurring predominantly in infants and young children is associated with rotavirus infection. The peak prevalence of rotavirus infection occurs during the cooler months of the year in temperate climates, but in tropical areas cases are identified throughout the year (Fig. 9-4). Populations throughout the world have been studied and serologic evaluation has demonstrated that it is common to acquire antibodies to rotaviruses between the ages of 6 and 24 months.

Virus is excreted in the feces for approximately 8 days and it is stable. It seems likely the virus is readily transmissible by hands and inanimate objects to susceptible individuals. This may occur within a family setting, nursery, or hospital.

Epidemic gastroenteritis due to the Norwalk group of viruses may affect an entire community. It has involved school-age children, family contacts, and adults. Roughly one third of the identified outbreaks of gastroenteritis may be attributed to a Norwalk-like agent. Outbreaks have

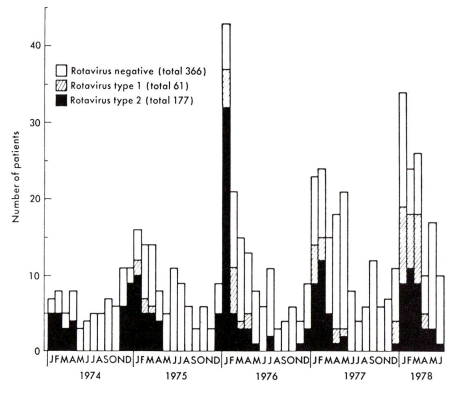

Fig. 9-4. Rotavirus infections in 604 infants and young children who were hospitalized with gastroenteritis. (From Brandt CD, et al. Am J Epidemiol 1979;110(3):243.)

occurred at all times of the year, and antibody surveys suggest that the agent is worldwide in distribution. In the less developed nations antibody is detected in early childhood. In the United States, antibody usually develops during late adolescence and early adulthood.

Coronaviruses are unlikely to be responsible for diarrhea within the first year of life. They have been more commonly visualized in the diarrheal stools of older children and young adults. The prolonged excretion of virus makes it difficult to assess the role of these agents in the etiology of gastroenteritis.

The enteric adenoviruses most often appear to be responsible for acute diarrhea in infants less than 1 year of age. Infections may occur during any month of the year.

Treatment

The general principles of rehydration therapy are the same as those described for bacterial gastroenteritis. Antibiotics are of no value in treating gastroenteritis.

Preventive measures

Careful hygiene and interruption of the fecal-to-oral spread of these agents are as important as bacterial causes of gastroenteritis. Handwashing and other hygienic methods should be employed to prevent direct and indirect transmission of these agents from infected patients.

Prevention of rotavirus would be a major contribution in reduction of the morbidity from gastroenteritis. For immunization to be effective, immunity within the gastrointestinal tract is probably a necessity. Various approaches to immunization that are being considered include a live attenuated human rotavirus vaccine; an attenuated reassortant rotavirus vaccine; a vaccine made from an animal rotavirus strain; and cloning of the human rotavirus genome by DNA technology. Reassortants have already been created, and the work with human rotaviruses in cell culture has recently facilitated the study of these agents. The task of defining protective antigens has made the feasibility of a vaccine a more accessible goal for the future.

REFERENCES

Almeida JD, Waterson AP. The morphology of virus-like antibody interaction. Adv Virus Res 1967;15:307.

Attridge SR, Rowley D. The role of the flagellum in the adherence of V. cholerae. J Infect Dis 1983;147:864-872.

Bishop RF, Davidson GP, Holmes I II, Ruck BJ. Evidence for viral gastroenteritis. N Engl J Med 1973;289:1096.

Blacklow NR, et al. Acute infectious nonbacterial gastroenteritis: etiology and pathogenesis. Ann Intern Med 1972;76:993.

Blaser MJ, Reller LB. Campylobacter enteritis. N Engl J Med 1981;305:1444-452.

Brandt CD, et al. Comparative epidemiology of two rotavirus serotypes and other viral agents associated with pediatric gastroenteritis. Am J Epidemiol 1979;110(3):243-254.

Chang MJ, et al. Trimethoprim-sulfamethoxazole compared to ampicillin in the treatment of shigellosis. Pediatrics 1977;59:726.

Clausen CR, Christie DL. Chronic diarrhea in infants caused by adherent enteropathogenic E. coli. J Pediatr 1982;100:358-361.

Dolin R, et al.: Transmission of acute infectious nonbacterial gastroenteritis to volunteers by oral administration of stool filtrates. J Infect Dis 1971;123:307.

Dolin R, et al. Biological properties of Norwalk agent of acute infectious non bacterial gastroenteritis. Proc Soc Exp Biol Med 1972;140:578.

DuPont HL, Hornick RB. Adverse effects of Lomotil therapy in shigellosis. JAMA 1973;226:1525.

Eidels L, Proia RL, Hart DA. Membrane receptors for bacterial toxins. Microbiol Rev 1983;47:596-620.

Evans DJ, Evans DG. Classification of pathogenic E. coli according to serotype and the production of virulence factors, with special reference to colonization-factor antigens. Rev Infect Dis 1983;5(4):692-701.

Fekety R. Recent advances in management of bacterial diarrhea. Rev Infect Dis 1983;5:246-257.

Flewett TH, Bryden AS, Davies H, Morris CA. Epidemic viral enteritis in a long stay children's ward. Lancet 1975;1:4-5.

Formal SB, Hale TL, Sansonetti PJ. Invasive enteric pathogens. Rev Infect Dis 1983;5(4):702-707.

Goldschmidt MC, DuPont HL. Enteropathogenic Escherichia coli: lack of correlation of serotype with pathogenicity. J Infect Dis 1976;133:153.

Gorbach SL, Khurana CM. Toxigenic Escherichia coli: a cause of infantile diarrhea in Chicago. N Engl J Med 1971;287:791.

Gorbach SL, et al. Travelers' diarrhea and toxigenic Escherichia coli. N Engl J Med 1975;292:933.

Grady GF, Keusch GT. Pathogenesis of bacterial diarrheas. N Engl J Med 1971;285:831.

Gutman LT et al. An inter-familial outbreak of Yersinia enterocolitica enteritis. N Engl J Med 1973;288:1372.

Hamre D, Procknow JJ. A new virus isolated from the human respiratory tract. Proc Soc Exp Biol Med 1966;121:190-193.

Holmes IH et al. Infantile enteritis viruses: morphogenesis and morphology. J Virol 1975;16:937.

Holmgren J. Actions of cholera toxin and the prevention and treatment of cholera. Nature 1981;292:413.

Hornick RB et al. Typhoid fever: pathogenesis and immunologic control. N Engl J Med 1970;283:686, 739.

Jacewicz M, Keusch GT. Pathogenesis of shigella diarrhea. VIII Evidence for a translocation step in the cytotoxic action of Shiga toxin. J Infect Dis 1983;148:844-854.

Kapikian AZ, et al. Visualization by immune electronmicroscopy of a 27-nm particle associated with acute infectious non bacterial gastroenteritis. J Virol 1972;10:1075.

Kapikian AZ, et al. Reovirus-like agent in stools: association with infantile diarrhea and development of serologic tests. Science 1974;185:1049.

Kapikian AZ, et al. Human reovirus-like agent as the major pathogen associated with "winter" gastroenteritis in hospitalized infants, young children and their contacts. N Engl J Med 1976;294:965.

Karmali MA, Fleming PC. Campylobacter enteritis in children. J Pediatr 1979;94:527.

Karmali MA, Petric M, Steele BT, Lin C. Sporadic cases of Haemolytic uraemic syndrome associated with faecal cytotoxin and cytotoxin producing E. coli in stools. Lancet 1983;1:619-620.

Kauffmann F. Enterobacteriacae. Ed 1. Copenhagen: Ejnor Munksgaards Forlag, 1951, p 187.

Kim HW, et al. Human reovirus-like agent infection: occurrence in adult contacts of pediatric patients with gastroenteritis. JAMA 1977;238:404.

Konowalchuk J, Speirs JI, Stavric S. Vero response to a cytotoxin of E. coli. Infect Immun 1977;18:775-779.

Levine MM, Berquist EJ, Nalin DR, et al. E. coli strains that cause diarrhea but do not produce heat-labile or heat stable enterotoxins and are non-invasive. Lancet 1978;1:1119-1122.

Levine MM, Black RE, Clements ML, et al. Duration of infection derived immunity to cholera. J Infect Dis 1981;143:818-820.

Levine MM, Black RE, Clements ML, et al. Evaluation in humans of attenuated V. cholorae El Tor Ogawa strain Texas State-SR as a live oral vaccine. Infect Immun 1984;43:515-522.

Levine MM, Kaper JB, Black RE, Clements ML: New knowledge on pathogenesis of bacterial enteric infections as applied to vaccine development. Microsc Rev 1983; 47:510-550.

Levine MM, Nalin DR, Hoover DL, et al. Immunity to ETEC. Infect Immun 1979;23:729-736.

Light JS, Hodes HL. Studies on epidemic diarrhea of the newborn: isolation of filterable agent causing diarrhea in calves. Am J Public Health 1943;33:1451.

McIver J, Grady GF, Keusch GT. Production and characterization of endotoxin(s) of S. dysenteriae type I. J Infect Dis 1975;131:559-566.

Nelson JD. Duration of neomycin therapy for enteropathogenic Escherichia coli diarrheal disease: comparative study of 113 cases. Pediatrics 1971;48:248.

Nelson JD, Haltalin KC. Accuracy of diagnosis of bacterial diarrheal disease by clinical features. J Pediatr. 1971; 78:519.

Nelson JD, et al. Trimethoprim-sulfamethoxazole therapy for shigellosis. JAMA 1976;235:1239.

Novak R, Feldman S. Salmonellosis in children with cancer: review of 42 cases. Am J Dis Child 1979;133:298.

Pai CH, Sorger S, Lackman L. Campylobacter gastroenteritis in children. J Pediatr 1979;94:589.

Pickering LK, DuPont HL, Olarte J. Single-dose tetracycline therapy for shigellosis in adults. JAMA 1978;239:853.

Riley IW, et al. Hemorrhagic colitis associated with a rare E. coli serotype. N Engl J Med 1983;308:681-685.

Robins-Brown RM, Levine MM, Rowe B, Gabriel EM. Failure to detect conventional enterotoxins in classical enteropathogenic (serotyped) E. coli strains of proven pathogenicity. Infect Immun 1982;138:798-801.

Rudoy RC, Nelson JD. Enteroinvasive and enterotoxigenic Escherichia coli: occurrence in acute diarrhea of infants and children. Am J Dis Child 1975;129:688.

Sac DA, Sac RB. A test for enterotoxigenic Escherichia coli. Infect Immun 1975;11:334.

Saphra I, Winter JW. Clinical manifestations of salmonellosis in man. An evaluation of 7,779 human infections identified at the New York Salmonella Center. N Engl J Med 1957;256:1128.

Schreiber DS, Blacklow NR, Trier JS. The mucosal lesion of the proximal small intestine in acute infections nonbacterial gastroenteritis. N Engl J Med 1973;288:1318.

Scotland SM, Day NP, Rowe B. Production of a cytotoxin affecting Vero cells by strains of E. coli belonging to traditional enteropathogenic serogroups. FEMS Microbiol Lett 1980;7:15-17.

Scragg JN, Rubidge CJ, Applebaum PC. Shigella infection in African and Indian children with special reference to septicemia. J Pediatr 1978;93:796.

Sereny B. Experimental shigella keratoconjunctivitis: a preliminary report. Acta Microbiol Acad Sci Hung 1955; 2:293.

Shore EG, et al. Enterotoxin-producing Escherichia coli and diarrheal disease in adult travelers: a prospective study. J Infect Dis 1974;129:577.

Snow J. On the mode of communication of cholera—1855. In Snow on cholera. A reprint of two papers by John Snow, New York and London. Hofner, 1965.

Thomas DD, Knoop FC. The effect of calcium and prostaglandin inhibitors on the intestinal fluid response to heat stable enterotoxin of E. coli. J Infect Dis 1982;145:141-147.

Thomas DD, Knoop FC. Effect of heat-stable enterotoxin of E. coli on cultured mammalian cells. J Infect Dis 1983;147:450-459.

Tyrrell DAJ, Bynoe MC. Cultivation of a novel type of common cold virus in organ cultures. Br. Med J 1965;1:1467-1470.

Tyrrell DAJ, Kapikian AZ, eds. Virus infections of GI tract, New York: Marcel Dekker, Inc, 1982.

Ulshen MH, Rollo JL. Pathogenesis of E. coli gastroenteritis in man—another mechanism. N Engl J Med 1980;302:99-101.

Vaughan M. Cholera and cell regulation. Hosp Pract June, 1982, pp 145-152.

Vesikari T, Isolauri E, Delem A, et al. Immunogenicity and safety of live oral attenuated bovine rotavirus vaccine Strain RIT 4237 in adults and young children. Lancet (October 8) 1983;2:807.

Vesikari T, Maki M, Isolauri E. Epidemiologic background for the need of rotavirus vaccine in Finland. Preliminary experience of RIT 4237 strain of live attenuated rotavirus vaccine in adults. International Symposium on Enteric Infections in Man and Animals: Standardization of Immunological Procedures, Dublin, Ireland, 1982. Dev Biol Scand, Vol 53, pp 229-236, 1983 (Basel, 1983, S. Karger).

Walker WA. Host defense mechanisms in GI tract. Pediatrics 1976;57:901-916.

Walker WA, Isselbacher KJ. Intestinal antibodies. N Engl J Med 1977;297:767-775.

Watanabe H, Timmis KH. A small plasmid in S. dysenteria 1 specifies one or more functions essential for O antigen production and bacterial virulence. Infect Immun 1984; 43:391-396.

Weissman JP, et al. Shigellosis: to treat or not to treat. JAMA 1974;229:1215.

Yolkin RH, et al. Epidemiology of human rotavirus types 1 and 2 as studied by enzyme-linked immunosorbent assay. N Engl J Med 1978;229:1156.

10

VIRAL HEPATITIS

Hepatitis A
Hepatitis B
Hepatitis D
Non-A, non-B hepatitis
Epidemic non-A, non-B hepatitis

The term *viral hepatitis* refers to a primary infection of the liver most commonly caused by at least six etiologically and immunologically distinct viruses: hepatitis A (HAV), hepatitis B (HBV), hepatitis D (HDV), epidemic non-A, non-B (NANB), and two or more non-A, non-B viruses. Hepatitis D is a defective virus; it requires HBV synthesis for its expression. Hepatitis may also occur as a secondary infection during the course of severe generalized disease caused by a number of viruses such as cytomegalovirus, Epstein-Barr virus, and varicella-zoster virus.

Hepatitis A is synonymous with *infectious hepatitis*, an ancient disease described by Hippocrates and long known as *acute catarrhal jaundice, epidemic jaundice*, and *epidemic hepatitis*. The fulminating form of the disease was called *acute yellow atrophy of the liver*.

Hepatitis B is synonymous with *serum hepatitis*, a disease with a more recent history, the first known outbreak having occurred in 1883 among a group of shipyard workers who were vaccinated against smallpox with glycerinated lymph of human origin (Lürman, 1885). Later, an increased incidence of the disease was observed among patients attending venereal disease clinics, diabetic clinics, and other facilities where multiple injections were given with inadequately sterilized syringes and needles contaminated with the blood of a carrier. The most extensive outbreak occurred in 1942 when yellow fever vaccine containing human serum caused 28,585 cases of hepatitis B infection with jaundice among U.S. military personnel. It was unknown at the time of vaccination that the human serum component of the vaccine was contaminated with HBV. During the past three decades the increasing use of blood transfusions and blood products has played an important role in the wide dissemination of the infection. The various aliases of viral hepatitis type B recorded in the literature include *serum hepatitis, homologous serum jaundice, transfusion jaundice, syringe jaundice*, and *postvaccinal jaundice*.

Non-A, non-B hepatitis was first recognized in the 1970s when specific tests for the identification of type A and type B hepatitis became available. Studies at that time revealed that most cases of transfusion-associated hepatitis were caused by transmissible agents that were neither HAV nor HBV. Subsequent studies by various investigators indicated that at least two immunologically distinct agents were responsible for non-A, non-B hepatitis (Mosley et al., 1977; Tsiquaye and Zuckerman, 1979).

The occurrence of several epidemics of hepatitis A-like illness in Southern Asia and the Middle East revealed the existence of so-called epidemic non-A, non-B hepatitis. These outbreaks were epidemiologically like hepatitis A, but serologic studies revealed no evidence of HAV or HBV infection (Khuroo, 1980; Wong, et al., 1982). It is possible that the epidemic NANB virus may prove to be either a new serotype of HAV or an entirely new virus.

ETIOLOGY

Current concepts of the cause of viral hepatitis stem from human volunteer studies that were conducted in the 1940s. These studies were initiated because of the failure to propagate the causative agents of human hepatitis in laboratory animals. Later the advent of tissue culture techniques in the 1950s provided new methods for the isolation and identification of various viruses. However, intensive efforts by many investigators failed to provide reproducible evidence for the cultivation of the viruses responsible for hepatitis in man. The human volunteer studies in the 1940s and 1950s provided indirect evidence for the existence of at least two hepatitis viruses, A and B.

The specific identification of these viruses was achieved in the late 1960s and early 1970s in the wake of (1) the successful transmission of hepatitis A and B viruses to nonhuman primates and (2) the visualization and detection of these agents by electron microscopy and by various serologic procedures.

Hepatitis A

Before the mid-1960s knowledge of the properties of HAV was derived from human volunteer studies. The agent survived a temperature of 56° C for 30 minutes (Havens et al., 1944) and was inactivated by heating at 98° C for 1 minute (Krugman et al., 1970). It retained its infectivity after storage at − 18° to − 70° C for several years. HAV was more resistant to chlorine than many bacteria found in drinking water.

Oral or parenteral administration of the virus caused hepatitis after an incubation period ranging from 15 to 40 days, averaging approximately 30 days. Extensive studies with the MS-1 strain of HAV confirmed observations by Havens et al. (1944) and by Neefe et al. (1946) indicating that hepatitis A and B viruses are immunologically distinct (Krugman et al., 1967).

In 1966 Deinhardt et al. reported the successful transmission of hepatitis to marmoset monkeys. Later, additional studies by his group (Holmes et al., 1969) and by Lorenz et al. (1970), Mascoli et al. (1973), Provost et al. (1973), and Maynard et al. (1974) confirmed the successful transmission of human HAV to marmosets. In addition, Dienstag et al. (1975b) successfully transmitted HAV to susceptible chimpanzees.

In 1973 Feinstone et al. reported the identi-fication of 27-nm viruslike particles in the stools of adults who had been infected with the MS-1 strain of HAV. These particles were identified by immune electron microscopy (IEM), a method used by Almeida et al. (1969) to detect hepatitis B antigen. These findings were confirmed by Maynard et al. (1974), who induced hepatitis in marmosets by inoculating them with stool filtrates containing the 27-nm particles.

Human hepatitis A virus was further characterized by Provost et al. (1975b), who reported that the 27-nm particles appeared to have the physical, chemical, and biologic characteristics of an enterovirus. It has been designated enterovirus type 72 (Melnick, 1982). An electron micrograph comparing hepatitis A virus with hepatitis B virus is shown in Fig. 10-1. Unlike HBV, it is a simple, nonenveloped virus with a nucleocapsid that has been designated hepatitis A antigen (HA Ag). The HAV capsid consists of 32 capsomeres arranged in icosahedral conformation; it is composed of four virion polypeptides (VP1, VP2, VP3, and VP4). A single-stranded molecule of RNA is present inside the capsid.

Purified HAV is inactivated by formalin, ultraviolet irradiation, heating at 100° C for 5 minutes, or treatment with chlorine (Provost et al., 1975b, Peterson et al., 1982). The purified virus was shown by IEM to be specifically aggregated by hepatitis A antibody (anti-HAV).

Miller et al. (1975) prepared hepatitis A antigen (HA Ag) from infected marmoset liver for use in an immune adherence hemagglutination (IAHA) antibody test. Both HA Ag and anti-HAV can be detected by various established serological methods, including IEM (Feinstone et al., 1973), radioimmunoassay (RIA) (Hollinger et al., 1975), enzyme immunoassay (EIA) (Duermeyer et al., 1978), and immunofluorescence (IF) (Murphy et al., 1978). The RIA and EIA tests are the most practical for serodiagnosis of acute hepatitis A.

In 1979 Provost and Hilleman reported the propagation of human HAV in primary explant cell cultures of marmoset livers and in the normal fetal rhesus kidney cell line (FRhK6). Provost et al. (1981) subsequently isolated HAV directly from acute-phase human stool specimens by in vitro propagation in an FRhK6 line. Other workers demonstrated that HAV could be cultivated in human diploid fibroblasts (Gauss-Muller et al., 1981), in FL (human amniotic) and

Vero cells (Kojima et al., 1981), and in African Green monkey kidney (AGMK) cell cultures (Daemer et al., 1981). HAV propagates in the cytoplasm and is noncytopathic.

Studies to clone the genome of HAV by DNA recombinant technology are currently in progress. Ticehurst et al. (1983) have obtained clones that appear to represent parts of the viral RNA. The goal is to achieve cloning of the full-length HAV genome as has been achieved for poliovirus RNA.

Hepatitis B

The human volunteer studies of the 1940s indicated that hepatitis B was highly infectious by inoculation. These studies suggested that hepatitis B virus caused a parenteral infection characterized by a long incubation period of 50 to 180 days and, unlike hepatitis A virus, was not infectious by mouth.

Studies in the 1960s provided evidence for the existence of two types of viral hepatitis with distinctive clinical, epidemiologic, and immunologic features (Krugman et al., 1967). One type, MS-1, resembled hepatitis A; it was characterized by an incubation period of 30 to 38 days and a high degree of contagion by contact. The other type, MS-2, resembled hepatitis B; it had a longer incubation period of 41 to 108 days. Contrary to the prevailing concept, the MS-2 strain of hepatitis B virus was infectious by mouth as well as parenterally, and the disease in patients was moderately contagious.

The successful transmission of hepatitis B virus to chimpanzees was achieved in the early 1970s (Maynard et al., 1972; Barker, et al., 1973). The chimpanzee has proved to be a highly sensitive animal model for the study of hepatitis B infection.

The discovery of Australia antigen by Blum-

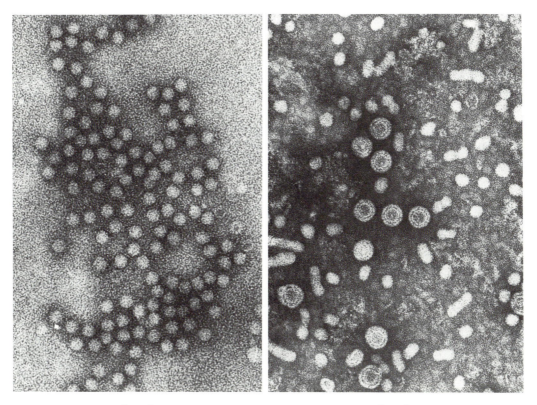

Type A   Type B

Fig. 10-1. Electron micrographs of type A and type B hepatitis viruses. Type A: Note 27-nm particles, uniform in size. Type B: Note 43-nm Dane particles (hepatitis B virus) as well as spherical and filamentous particles 20 nm in diameter (hepatitis B surface antigen). (From Provost PJ, et al. Am J Med Sci 1975;270:87.)

berg et al. (1965) and its subsequent association with hepatitis B had a major impact on the understanding of the etiology and natural history of the disease.

By the early 1970s the agent responsible for hepatitis B had been identified and characterized. Electron microscopic examination of serum obtained from patients with acute or chronic type B hepatitis revealed the following types of viruslike particles: (1) spherical particles, 20 nm in diameter (Bayer et al., 1968); (2) filamentous particles, 100 nm or more in length and 20 nm in diameter (Hirschman et al., 1969); and (3) "Dane particles," about 42 nm in diameter (Dane et al., 1970) (Fig. 10-1). The available evidence indicates that the Dane particle is the complete hepatitis B virion and that the 20-nm spherical particles represent excess virus-coat (HBsAg) material. The HBsAg and Dane particles have been shown to occur free in serum.

Hepatitis B virus (Dane particle). The HBV, a complex 42-nm virion, is a member of a new class of viruses designated "hepadna." The precise nomenclature of HBV is hepadna virus type 1 (Melnick, 1982). Unlike HAV, it has not been successfully propagated in cell culture. Nevertheless, its biophysical and biochemical properties have been well characterized.

A schematic illustration of the structure of HBV and its antigens is shown in Fig. 10-2. The virus is a double-shelled particle; its outer surface component, the hepatitis B surface antigen (HBsAg) is immunologically distinct from the inner core component, the hepatitis B core antigen (HBcAg). The core contains the genome of HBV, a single molecule of partially double-stranded DNA. One of the strands is incomplete, leaving a single-stranded or gap region. Additional components of the core include DNA-dependent DNA polymerase and hepatitis B e antigen (HBeAg).

A simple, direct molecular hybridization test has been developed to detect HBV DNA in serum. Studies by various investigators have revealed that most HBeAg-positive sera have detectable HBV DNA (Lieberman et al., 1983; Scotto et al., 1983).

Hepatitis B surface antigen. The HBsAg particle contains approximately seven polypeptides. Multiple antigenic specificities of HBsAg are associated with these polypeptides. Serologic analysis of HBsAg particles indicates (1) that they share a common group-specific determinant a and (2) that they usually carry at least two mutually exclusive subdeterminants, d or y and w or r (LeBouvier, 1972). The subtypes are the phenotypic expressions of distinct genotype variants of hepatitis B virus. Four principal phenotypes have been recognized: adw, adr, ayw, and ayr. Other complex permutations of these subdeterminants and new variants are listed in Table 10-1. The subtypes are valuable epidemiologic markers of infection. Protection against infection appears to be conferred by antibody against the a specificity.

The buoyant density of HBsAg particles in cesium chloride is 1.20 to 1.22 gm/ml. The particles remain stable after treatment with pepsin, 8 M urea, and ether, after exposure to temperatures ranging between $-20°$ C (for many years) and $100°$ C (for 3 minutes), and after incubation at an acid pH for several hours.

Various tests for the detection of HBsAg and anti-HBs have been developed. These techniques have proved to be very useful for various studies involving (1) the testing of blood donors and blood products, (2) diagnosis of acute and chronic hepatitis as well as the hepatitis B carrier state, (3) epidemiology of hepatitis B infections, (4) various investigations designed to enhance knowledge of the pathogenesis and immunologic aspects of the disease, and (5) the evaluation of active and passive immunizing procedures for the prevention of HBV infections.

HEPATITIS B VIRUS AND ANTIGENS

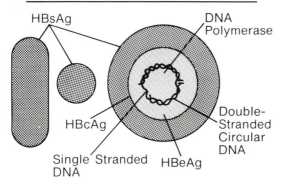

Fig. 10-2. Schematic illustration of the hepatitis B virus (HBV) and its antigens: hepatitis B surface antigen (HBsAg), hepatitis B core antigen (HBcAg), and hepatitis B e antigen (HBeAg).

Tests for HBsAg. The development of tests for the detection of HBsAg has occurred in three phases. The test used by Blumberg et al. (1965), agar gel diffusion (AGD), represented the first phase. The second phase was characterized by the development of assays that were two to ten times more sensitive, such as counterelectrophoresis (CEP) and complement fixation (CF). More recently, the third phase has been characterized by the development of tests that are more sensitive than AGD, such as RIA, EIA, and reversed passive hemagglutination (RPHA). At the present time it is clear that these are the optimal tests for the detection of HBsAg. The identification of HBsAg in tissues or cells has been accomplished by immunofluorescence microscopy, electron microscopy, and IEM.

Tests for anti-HBs. When AGD, CEP, and CF methods were used to detect anti-HBs, it was obvious that these tests were not sensitive enough to detect the antibody in convalescent serum specimens obtained from patients who

Table 10-1. Nomenclature of hepatitis B antigens and antibodies*

HBV	Hepatitis B virus; a 42-nm double-shelled virus, originally known as the Dane particle
HBsAg	Hepatitis B surface antigen; the hepatitis B antigen found on the surface of the virus and on the accompanying unattached spherical (22-nm) and tubular particles
HBcAg	Hepatitis B core antigen; the hepatitis B antigen found within the core of the virus
HBeAg	The e antigen, which is closely associated with hepatitis B infection
anti-HBs	Antibody to hepatitis B surface antigen
anti-HBc	Antibody to hepatitis B core antigen
anti-HBe	Antibody to the e antigen

Subdeterminants of hepatis B surface antigen:

ayw1	(a_1yw)	*adw*$_2$	(a_2^1dw)
ayw2	(a_2^1yw)	*adw*$_4$	(a_3dw)
ayw3	(a_2^3yw)	*adr*	
ayw4	(a_3yw)	*adyw*	
ayr			

*From World Health Organization Expert Committee on Viral Hepatitis: Advances in viral hepatitis, WHO Tech Rep Ser No. 602, 1977.

recovered from type B hepatitis. The development of other more sensitive methods, such as passive hemagglutination assay (PHA) (Vyas and Shulman, 1970), RIA, and EIA, provided techniques that were many times more sensitive. The PHA, RIA, and EIA methods to detect anti-HBs have proved to be very valuable for epidemiologic surveys as well as for diagnostic procedures.

Hepatitis B core antigen. The core component of HBV possesses a subunit structure characterized by icosahedral symmetry. The nucleocapsid consists of one major and one or two minor polypeptides and a unique double-stranded circular DNA; about 30% of the circular genome is single-stranded. When appropriate nucleotides and salts are added, the single-stranded region is made double-stranded by a DNA-dependent DNA polymerase within the nucleocapsid.

The HBV genome or pieces of the genome have been inserted into *Escherichia coli* plasmids (Sninski et al., 1979). This technique has enabled these groups to clone and produce large quantities of HBV genome and to translate parts of the genome into HBcAg and other viral antigens.

The buoyant density of HBcAg in cesium chloride is 1.31 to 1.34 gm/ml. The core antigen remains stable after treatment with ether and after incubation at acid pH. However, it is inactivated by temperatures of 30° C to 60° C for 30 minutes and 100° C for 1 minute.

Tests for HBcAg. Free HBcAg has not been detected in the serum of persons who have acute hepatitis B or who are hepatitis B carriers. This antigen has been detected in the nuclei of hepatocytes and in the core of HBV particles by various methods, including IEM (Almeida et al., 1969) and indirect immunofluorescence (Barker et al., 1973; Brzosko et al., 1973).

Tests for anti-HBc. The following tests have been used for the detection of anti-HBc: immune electron microscopy (Almeida et al., 1969), immunofluorescence (Brzosko et al., 1973), CF (Hoofnagle et al., 1973), and RIA-inhibition (Purcell et al., 1973/1974). The use of these tests has revealed detectable anti-HBc in the serum of patients with acute type B hepatitis (Fig. 10-3, *A*) and in the serum of those

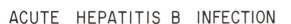

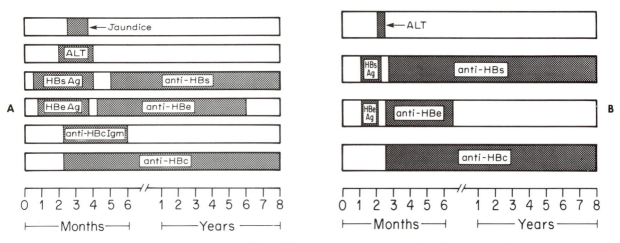

Fig. 10-3. A, Acute hepatitis B followed by recovery, showing results of serial tests for serum alanine aminotransferase (ALT), hepatitis B surface antigen (HBsAg) and its antibody (anti-HBs), hepatitis B e antigen (HBeAg) and its antibody (anti-HBe), hepatitis B core antibody (anti-HBc), and anti-HBc IgM. **B,** Subclinical hepatitis B infection followed by an immune response. Shaded areas denote "abnormal" or "detectable" and white areas denote "normal" or "not detectable." (From Krugman S. Pediatr Rev 1985; 7:3-11).

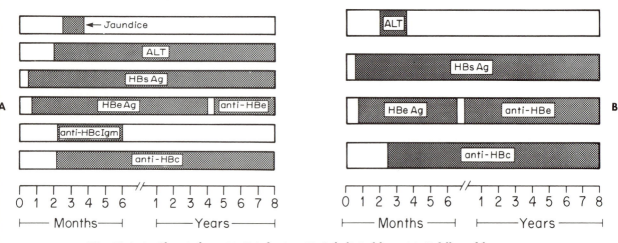

Fig. 10-4. A, Chronic hepatitis B infection. **B,** Subclinical hepatitis B followed by an asymptomatic chronic carrier state. See Fig. 10-3 for key. (From Krugman S. Pediatr Rev 1985; 7: 3-11).

with subclinical hepatitis B followed by an immune response (Fig. 10-3, *B*).

Hepatitis B e antigen. The e antigen-antibody system first described by Magnius and Espmark (1972) is now designated hepatitis B e antigen (HBeAg) and antibody (anti-HBe). This marker of hepatitis B infection is immunologically distinct from HBsAg and HBcAg; it is a low molecular weight polypeptide component of the nucleocapsid (core) of the HBV. The HBeAg is found only in HBsAg-positive sera. In acute type B hepatitis, it is detected shortly after HBsAg and it disappears shortly before HBsAg is no longer detectable (Fig. 10-3).

HBeAg is known to be an excellent marker of infectivity. The persistence of HBeAg may be associated with the occurrence of chronic persistent or chronic active hepatitis (Fig. 10-4, *A*). However, its role as a prognostic indicator for chronic hepatitis has not been confirmed (Aikawa et al., 1978).

The e antibody is most commonly detected in patients who have recovered from type B hepatitis; it has been detected also in the blood of asymptomatic HBsAg carriers who have normal liver function tests.

Delta antigen. The delta antigen-antibody system was first detected by immunofluorescence in liver cell nuclei and in serum of Italian HBsAg carriers who had chronic liver disease (Rizzetto et al., 1977). Studies in chimpanzees have revealed that it is a transmissible agent associated with but distinct from HBV. It is a 35- to 37-nm particle containing an RNA core and a surface component that is HBsAg. Replication of this defective agent is initiated and maintained by the helper function provided by HBV infection. The biologic expression of this new pathogen occurs only if concomitant HBs antigenemia is present.

If a patient acquires HBV and delta simultaneously, the pathogenic potential of the defective agent is limited by the brief hepatitis B viremia in a case of acute hepatitis with recovery. However, delta infection of a chronic HBsAg carrier is more likely to be followed by severe chronic active hepatitis or by fulminant hepatitis. In a large hepatitis outbreak that occurred among indigenous Yucpa Indians in Venezuela, combined HBV and delta infection was characterized by an 18% attack rate of fulminant hepatitis. In ad-

dition, superinfected HBsAg carriers were more likely to develop chronic liver disease (Hadler et al., 1984).

Epidemiologic surveys have revealed that delta infection is worldwide in distribution. Endemic areas have been identified in southern Europe, Africa, the Middle East, and South America. Parenteral drug addicts are at highest risk, but the agent can be transmitted by intimate contact.

Non-A, non-B hepatitis viruses

Various investigators have described the occurrence of acute hepatitis that proved to be neither type A nor type B by specific serologic tests. The causative agent or agents have not been identified. Prince et al. (1974) studied 204 patients who received an average of 15 units of blood during cardiac surgery. Of 51 patients who subsequently developed hepatitis, 15 (29%) had type B and 36 (71%) had non-A, non-B hepatitis. The incubation period and course of non-A, non-B hepatitis were similar to those of type B hepatitis (Fig. 10-5).

Evidence of non-A, non-B hepatitis was observed in an area where viral hepatitis was endemic. Villarejos et al. (1976) studied 12 patients in whom both type A and type B hepatitis were

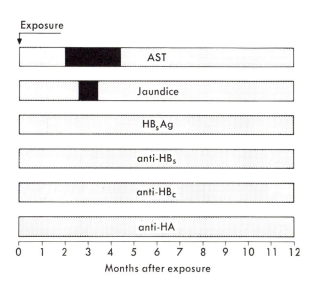

Fig. 10-5. Non-A, non-B acute viral hepatitis. Results of serial tests for alanine aminotransferase, jaundice, HBsAg, anti-HBc, anti-HBs, and hepatitis A antibody (anti-HA). See Fig. 10-3 for key.

excluded by serologic testing. These patients had not received blood tranfusions.

The following evidence supports the speculation that there are at least two non-A, non-B agents: (1) observations of variable clinical and epidemiologic characteristics of non-A, non-B hepatitis and (2) reports of multiple attacks of non-A, non-B hepatitis (Mosley et al., 1977; Tsiquaye and Zuckerman, 1979).

Shimizu et al. (1979) have identified two different ultrastructural alterations in liver cells of chimpanzees inoculated with infectious plasma derived from two patients with non-A, non-B hepatitis. The agent from one patient was associated with the development of tubular particles, 20 to 25 nm in diameter, in the cytoplasm of the hepatocytes. The agent from the other patient was associated with the development of aggregates of 20- to 27-nm particles in the nuclei of the hepatocytes.

Shimizu et al. believe that the cytoplasmic and nuclear structures are specifically associated with non-A, non-B hepatitis and if so may represent important markers of infection. However, they stated that they "cannot exclude the possibility that they might represent hitherto unknown responses of hepatocytes to injury." To date, the relationship of the structures to the specific infectious agents of non-A, non-B hepatitis remains uncertain.

In all areas of the world where non-A, non-B hepatitis has been investigated it has been found to be a major cause of viral hepatitis. In the United States non-A, non-B hepatitis viruses are responsible for more than 90% of posttransfusion hepatitis cases and about 40% of sporadic cases of viral hepatitis. It has been estimated that 0.5% to 8% of U.S. blood donors are asymptomatic carriers of these viruses.

Seroepidemiologic studies of epidemic hepatitis in India and Asia revealed evidence of a non-A, non-B etiology. Evaluation of sera from two extensive water-borne outbreaks revealed no evidence of HAV or HBV infection (Khuroo, 1980; Wong et al., 1980; Tandon et al., 1982). The outbreak in Delhi involved more than 29,000 cases of hepatitis with jaundice caused by sewage-contaminated water. The transmission via the fecal-to-oral route and the absence of chronic infection resemble hepatitis A. On the other hand, the following features are different from HAV infection: (1) longer incubation period (mean, 40 days), (2) age distribution (mean, 27 years), (3) high mortality in pregnant women, and (4) high fetal wastage. This non-A, non-B agent has not been identified as yet.

PATHOLOGY
Acute viral hepatitis

The histologic features of acute viral hepatitis caused by HAV and HBV are indistinguishable. The characteristic findings on biopsy include necrosis and inflammation of the lobule, architectural consequences of the necrosis, and proliferation of the mesenchymal and bile duct elements. Anicteric hepatitis shows the same histologic appearance as icteric but usually with less severity.

During the fully developed stage of hepatitis there is degeneration and death of liver cells, proliferation of the Kupffer cells, mononuclear cell infiltration, and bile duct proliferation. The hepatic cell changes involve the entire lobule, with a concentration of lesions in the centrolobular areas. The cells are usually swollen but occasionally they are shrunken. As the lesions progress there may be a variable degree of collapse, condensation of reticulin fibers, and accumulation of ceroid pigment and large phagocytic cells, first within the lobules and later in the portal tracts.

During the recovery period the following residual changes may be seen: pleomorphic liver cells around central veins, focal inflammatory infiltration of portal tracts, and a mild degree of fibrosis extending from the portal tracts. Liver cell necrosis is slight or absent but ceroid pigment may be found in the portal tracts.

Complete resolution is the usual course of viral hepatitis. In most cases complete regeneration of the liver cells is observed after 2 or 3 months. However, other possible consequences include chronic persistent or chronic active hepatitis, resolution of hepatitis with postnecrotic scarring, cirrhosis, or fatal massive necrosis.

Chronic active hepatitis

Chronic active hepatitis is characterized histologically by accumulations of lymphocytes and plasma cells that are located in the portal tracts and in foci of necrosis scattered throughout the hepatic lobules. Other findings include disruption of the limiting plate of the hepatic lobule adjacent to the portal tract and extension of the inflammatory reaction out of the portal tract into the hepatic parenchyma. The hepatocytes undergoing necrosis in these areas appear to be entrapped by the inflammatory infiltrate (so-called piecemeal necrosis). Small clusters of hepatocytes may be surrounded by the inflammatory process, thereby creating a "rosette" appearance.

The inflammation may vary in severity and distribution. A predominance of plasma cells may be found in patients with lupoid hepatitis.

The pattern of lobular collapse and necrosis bridging portal areas and central veins has been termed *submassive necrosis* or *bridging necrosis* (Boyer and Klatskin, 1970). These findings on biopsy indicate a poor prognosis.

The presence of portal fibrosis is variable. In more severe cases there is a marked deposition of fibrous tissue in the portal areas accompanied by collapse of the hepatic lobular architecture and formation of fibrous tissue "bridges" between adjacent portal areas and central veins. In advanced stages the extensive cirrhosis may mask the chronic inflammatory process, resulting in histologic evidence of cryptogenic or macronodular cirrhosis.

Chronic persistent hepatitis

In chronic persistent hepatitis, the lymphocytic inflammatory infiltration is confined chiefly to the portal tracts. The lobular architecture of the liver is preserved, evidence of hepatocellular damage is minimal or absent, and there is only slight or absent fibrosis. Piecemeal necrosis, very typical in chronic active hepatitis, is lacking in chronic persistent hepatitis.

Fulminant hepatitis

In fulminant hepatitis with death occurring within 10 days, the size of the liver is reduced, and its color is yellow or mottled (acute yellow atrophy). Histologic findings include extensive, diffuse necrosis and loss of hepatocytes, which are replaced by an inflammatory infiltrate—both polymorphonuclear and monocytic cells. The lobular structure of the liver may be collapsed. Occasionally, however, the architecture of the liver may be well preserved. Kupffer cells and histiocytes contain phagocytized material from disintegrated liver cells. Bile thrombi may be seen in the canaliculi. Portal triads that are usually retained are filled with monocytes and lymphocytes as well as polymorphonuclear cells. Occasionally, surviving liver tissue may be seen in the periphery of the lobules.

Regeneration of liver tissue may begin if patients survive for several days. The regeneration appears as clusters of cells scattered randomly throughout the liver. As regeneration advances, these "pseudolobules" of liver parenchyma appear to form adenomalike groups of liver cells unrelated to the normal lobular architecture and lacking central veins.

These patients who survive fulminant hepatitis usually have a remarkable recovery of liver function. Little or no residual liver damage may be seen on liver biopsy, although occasionally a course lobular type of cirrhosis may be noted (Karvountzis et al., 1974).

IMMUNOPATHOLOGY
Hepatitis A

Hepatitis A antigen is detected in the cytoplasm of hepatocytes shortly before onset of acute hepatitis. Viral expression decreases rapidly after the appearance of clinical and histologic manifestations and IgM specific anti-HAV. These findings indicate that hepatocellular damage is caused chiefly by immunologic rather than cytotoxic factors. It is of interest that propagation of HAV in tissue culture is not associated with a cytopathic effect.

Hepatitis B

The pathologic and clinical consequences of hepatitis B infection are related to at least two factors: (1) that HBV is not cytopathogenic and (2) that liver cell necrosis is in great part the result of host defenses.

Cell necrosis is the result of a cellular and immune response to HBV infection. Acute hepatitis B with recovery is associated with an efficient immune response that eliminates virus-infected cells by means of spotty necrosis. Viral antigens (HBsAg and HBcAg) that may be present in the liver before elicitation of the immune response are eliminated at the height of the acute disease. In contrast, chronic forms of hepatitis B are the result of a quantitatively and/or qualitatively ineffective immune response.

Under the conditions of high-grade immunosuppression, such as occurs in kidney transplant recipients, HBV may persist in the liver without any substantial liver cell damage. On the other hand, in chronic active hepatitis the occurrence of piecemeal necrosis may be a consequence of a partially deficient immune state. The available evidence indicates that an immune defect resulting in the incomplete elimination of infected hepatocytes is a cause of chronic HBV infection.

CLINICAL MANIFESTATIONS

The similarities and differences of the clinical manifestations of viral hepatitis types A, B, and non-A, non-B are listed in Table 10-2 and illustrated in Fig. 10-6. The incubation period of type A hepatitis ranges between 15 and 40 days, and the onset of symptoms is usually acute. In contrast, the incubation period of type B hepatitis is longer—50 to 180 days—and the onset is more apt to be insidious. The incubation period of non-A, non-B hepatitis may be the same as both type A and type B hepatitis; it may range

between 15 and 180 days. In general, the clinical features of non-A, non-B hepatitis resemble type B infection more than type A.

The clinical picture shows great variation. In children the disease is generally milder, and its course is shorter than in adults. In children or adults, jaundice may be inapparent or evanescent, or it may persist for many weeks. The course of the disease often may be separated into two phases—preicteric and icteric—although occasionally jaundice may be the initial symptom.

Preicteric phase

Fever, when present, appears during the preicteric phase of the disease; often it is absent or fleeting in young children, but in adolescents and adults it may last for about 5 days. The temperature ranges between 37.8° and 40° C (100° and 104° F) and generally is accompanied by

Table 10-2. Viral hepatitis types A, B, and non-A, non-B—comparison of clinical, epidemiologic, and immunologic features

Features	Type A	Type B	Type non-A, non-B
Incubation period	About 25 days; mean range, 15 to 40 days	About 70 days; mean range, 50 to 180 days	About 60 days, mean range, 15 to 180 days
Type of onset	Usually acute	Usually insidious	Usually insidious
Fever	Common; precedes jaundice	Less common	Less common
Age group affected	Usually children and young adults	All age groups	All age groups
Prodrome: arthritis and rash	Not present	May be present	Unknown
Jaundice	Rare in children; more common in adults	Rare in children; more common in adults	Same as types A and B
Abnormal AST or ALT	Transient—1 to 3 weeks	More prolonged—1 to 8+ months	Usually prolonged
HBsAg in blood	Not present	Present in incubation period and acute phase; occasionally may persist	Not present
Virus in feces	Present during late incubation period and acute phase	May be present but no direct proof	Unknown
Virus in blood	Present during late incubation period and early acute phase	Present during late incubation period and acute phase; occasionally persists for months and years	Same as type B
Carrier state	No	Yes	Yes
Immunity			
Homologous	Present	Present	Present
Heterologous	None	None	Unknown

headache, lassitude, anorexia, nausea, vomiting, and abdominal pain. Urticaria and arthralgia or arthritis occurring during the preicteric phase usually are manifestations of type B hepatitis. The liver may be enlarged and tender, and splenomegaly and lymphadenopathy may be present in some patients.

Icteric phase

Jaundice begins to emerge as the fever subsides; it usually is preceded by the appearance of dark urine (biliuria). In young children the transition to the icteric phase is most often marked by disappearance of symptoms. The patient's appetite returns, and he frequently feels fine when jaundice is most marked. On the other hand, in adults and older children the icteric phase may be accompanied by an exacerbation of some of the original symptoms. It is characterized by anorexia, nausea, vomiting, and abdominal pain. Mental depression, bradycardia, and pruritus, all frequently occurring in adults, are uncommon in children. The liver is enlarged and tender. The spleen is palpable in about 25% of patients. The stools may be clay colored, but this is an inconstant finding. The icteric phase persists from a few days to as long as a month, the average duration being about 8 to 11 days

in children in contrast to 3 to 4 weeks in adults. As jaundice fades, the patient's appetite returns and he feels better. As a rule, convalescence is rapid and uneventful. Excessive weight loss is more common in adults than in children.

In small infants and children under 3 years of age there is evidence that hepatitis may be largely anicteric. In a group of 36 infants with hepatitis A infection in an orphanage, Capps et al. (1952) found only one with overt jaundice. The symptoms in the rest were nonspecific. They included failure to gain weight, loose and light-colored stools, fever, anorexia, respiratory symptoms, lassitude, distention, and vomiting. The probability that most of these infants did indeed have anicteric hepatitis is strengthened by the demonstration of virus in the stools of two of them. This was accomplished by oral administration of fecal suspension to adult volunteers who developed hepatitis with jaundice after 22 and 26 days, respectively.

We studied 45 children and adults for a 6-month period after admission to an institution in which type A hepatitis was endemic. Seventeen of the 45 patients acquired hepatitis, six had minimal jaundice, and 11 did not have jaundice. In this small group there was a 2:1 ratio

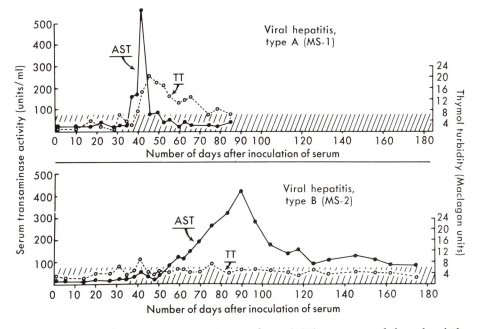

Fig. 10-6. Pattern of serum aspartate aminotransferase (AST) response and thymol turbidity (TT) response during the course of viral hepatitis type A and viral hepatitis type B.

of anicteric to icteric cases. Type B hepatitis infection in children is usually anicteric; the ratio of anicteric to icteric cases may be 10:1 or more.

LABORATORY FINDINGS
Viral hepatitis A

The characteristic laboratory findings and the profile of abnormal liver function are shown in Table 10-2 and Fig. 10-7. After an incubation period of approximately 30 days, there is a spik-ing rise in serum aspartate aminotransferase (AST) and serum alanine aminotransferase (ALT) levels. The duration of abnormal AST and ALT levels in children is brief, rarely exceeding 2 to 3 weeks.

The serum bilirubin value usually becomes abnormal when AST reaches peak levels. The increased level of serum bilirubin may be transient, and the duration may be as short as 1 day, or it may persist for more than 1 month. In

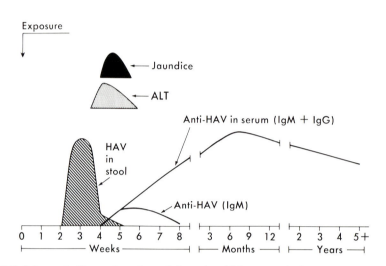

Fig. 10-7. Schematic illustration of serial clinical and laboratory findings in a patient with type A hepatitis. Hepatitis A virus (HAV) is detected in stool during the latter part of the incubation period before onset of the disease. Appearance of hepatitis A antibody (anti-HAV) coincides with disappearance of HAV in stool. IgM-specific anti-HAV is detected at the time of onset of disease; IgG-specific anti-HAV appears about 1 week later. (Modified from Frösner GG. Munch Med Wochenschr 1977;119:825.)

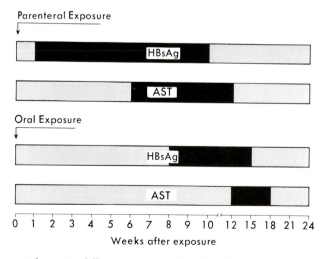

Fig. 10-8. Type B hepatitis following parenteral and oral exposure. Note prolongation of incubation period following oral exposure. See Fig. 10-3 for key.

general, jaundice is transient in children and more apt to be prolonged in adults.

The following tests are available for the detection of hepatitis A antibody: immune adherence hemagglutination (IAHA), RIA, and EIA. As indicated in Fig. 10-7, RIA anti-HAV is detected very early, at the time of onset of disease. Initially, RIA anti-HAV is predominantly IgM; later it is exclusively IgG. The time of appearance of EIA anti-HAV is the same as RIA, and the test appears to be equally sensitive.

Viral hepatitis B

The detection of hepatitis B surface antigen in the blood of a patient with acute hepatitis is indicative of hepatitis B virus infection. The characteristic laboratory findings and the profile of abnormal liver function are shown in Table 10-2 and Figs. 10-3 and 10-6.

Hepatitis B surface antigen may be detected by RIA 6 to 30 days after a parenteral exposure and 56 to 60 days after an oral exposure (Krugman, 1979; Krugman et al., 1979). The antigen may be detected about 1 week to 2 months before the appearance of abnormal levels of ALT and jaundice (Fig. 10-8). In most patients with acute hepatitis B, HBsAg is consistently present during the latter part of the incubation period and during the preicteric phase of the disease. The antigen may become undetectable shortly after onset of jaundice.

The pattern of serum ALT or AST activity is illustrated in Fig. 10-6. After an incubation period of approximately 50 days, the serum ALT values become abnormal, rising gradually over a period of several weeks. The duration of ab-

normal ALT or AST activity may be prolonged, usually exceeding 30 to 60 days.

As indicated in Fig. 10-3, the first antibody to be detectable is anti-HBc. It appears approximately 1 week or more after onset of hepatitis. The anti-HBc titers, predominantly IgM, are usually high for several months. Thereafter, IgM values decline to low or undetectable levels, but anti-HBc persists for many years. (Chau et al., 1983). The commercially available test for anti-HBc IgM is a solid-phase immunoassay; its cutoff assay value was established to differentiate high levels of antibody (positive) from low or undetectable levels (negative). The test is negative in healthy HBsAg carriers and in patients with cirrhosis. It may be positive in those with chronic active hepatitis characterized by marked inflammatory changes without cirrhosis.

The anti-HBc IgM assay should be useful for differentiating recent from remote HBV infections and identifying acute hepatitis B in patients whose HBsAg has declined to undetectable levels before appearance of anti-HBs (window-phase). Antibody to the hepatitis B surface antigen usually appears late, approximately 2 weeks to 2 months after HBsAg is no longer detectable. Anti-HBs is detected in approximately 80% of patients with hepatitis B who eventually become HBsAg negative. In the remainder the levels are too low to be detected. Anti-HBs may be detected in about 5% to 10% of HBsAg carriers.

The results of tests for HBsAg, HBeAg, anti-HBs, and anti-HBc during the course of hepatitis B are shown in Table 10-3 and in Figs. 10-3 and 10-4.

Table 10-3. Detection of hepatitis B surface antigen (HBsAg), antibody to HBsAg (anti-HBs), antibody to hepatitis B core antigen (anti-HBc), hepatitis B e antigen (HBeAg), and antibody to HBeAg (anti-HBe) during the course of type B hepatitis infection.

Time of hepatitis B infection	HBsAg	anti-HBs	anti-HBc	HBeAg	anti-HBe
Late incubation period	+	0	0	+	0
Early in course of acute hepatitis (<1 week)	+	0	+	+	0
Late in course of acute hepatitis (1 to 4 weeks)	+ or 0	+ or 0	+	+ or 0	0 or +
Convalescence from acute hepatitis					
Early (4 to 8 weeks)	0	+ or 0	+	0	+ or 0
Late (>8 weeks)	0	+	+	0	+ or 0

Key: +, present; 0, not present.

COURSE

Various factors may affect the course of hepatitis infection: age, type of virus, and immunocompetence. In general, hepatitis A is a mild or inapparent infection in infants and children. However, it is generally more severe in adults. In contrast, infants infected with HBV are more likely to develop chronic hepatitis B than older children and adults. Unlike hepatitis A, type B and non-A, non-B hepatitis infections are more likely to progress to chronic liver disease.

Acute hepatitis

The duration of illness caused by HAV is variable, ranging from several weeks to several months. The degree of morbidity and duration of jaundice correlate directly with age. Even with prolonged acute illness, lasting several months, complete resolution of hepatitis usually occurs. Most patients with hepatitis A recover completely. Hepatitis B and non-A, non-B hepatitis, on the other hand, are associated with more debility, and about 10% of patients develop evidence of chronic disease, either chronic persistent hepatitis or chronic active hepatitis. In rare instances acute hepatitis may progress to a fulminant fatal outcome.

Chronic persistent hepatitis

Chronic persistent hepatitis is a pathologic diagnosis based on a liver biopsy. It is an inflammatory process involving only the portal areas. This form of hepatitis usually lasts longer than 6 months, and it is more common and less severe than chronic active hepatitis. In general, the patient is asymptomatic and usually has a mild hepatomegaly and moderate elevation of serum aminotransferases without jaundice. Chronic persistent hepatitis may resolve after several years or progress to chronic active hepatitis. These patients may be HBsAg carriers.

Chronic active hepatitis

This form of hepatitis, also referred to as *chronic aggressive hepatitis*, is more likely to progress to cirrhosis. The disease is characterized by chronic and recurrent episodes of jaundice, abnormal levels of serum AST and ALT, and evidence of portal hypertension with ascites if the disease progresses to cirrhosis. Severe episodes of hepatic necrosis may terminate in hepatic failure.

Most patients with chronic hepatitis (persistent and/or active) have not had a past history of acute illness with jaundice. The disease usually follows mild, anicteric forms of hepatitis.

Fulminant hepatitis

The occurrence of hepatic failure within the first few days or within 4 weeks after onset of acute hepatitis indicates a fulminant course. When the course is more prolonged and hepatic failure occurs after 1 to 3 months of illness, the term *subacute hepatitis* is used; it is associated with portal hypertension, ascites, and submassive hepatic necrosis.

Fulminant hepatitis is usually characterized by mental confusion, emotional instability, restlessness, bleeding manifestations, and coma. The progressive jaundice and coma are associated with a shrinking liver. The Fulminant Hepatic Failure Surveillance Study (Trey, 1972) included 142 patients with fulminant viral hepatitis. The survival rate was influenced by the age of the patient. Of 27 patients under 15 years of age, 10 (37%) survived; of 73 patients 15 to 44 years of age, 12 (16%) survived; and of 42 patients 45 to more than 75 years of age, 3 (7%) survived. The overall survival rate was 18%.

Hepatoma

The striking association between chronic hepatitis B infection and primary hepatocellular carcinoma (PHC) has been well established. The relationship is supported by the following factors: (1) geographic distribution of PHC, (2) presence of HBsAg in serum of patients with PHC, (3) detection of HBV markers in tumor tissue and PHC cell lines, (4) occurrence of PHC in certain animals infected with hepadna viruses, and (5) integration of the HBV genome in the tumor cell genome.

Worldwide seroepidemiologic studies have revealed a remarkable correlation between the prevalence of HBsAg carriers and the incidence of PHC (Szmuness, 1978). The highest frequency of carrier and PHC rates has been observed in Southeast Asia and sub-Saharan Africa. Various studies have revealed that the prevalance of HBsAg is significantly higher in patients with PHC than in comparable controls (Szmuness, 1978).

Histochemical and immunochemical methods have revealed the presence of HBsAg and

HBcAg in the liver of patients with PHC. HBsAg has been detected in the tumor as well as the surrounding liver tissue. In addition, cultured cell lines derived from human PHC secrete enormous quantities of HBsAg into supernatant culture media (MacNab et al., 1976). Integration of the HBV genome has been demonstrated by molecular hybridization analysis of DNA extracted from human PHC. These studies revealed HBV DNA sequences integrated into the tumor cell genome (Shafritz and Kew, 1981).

The occurrence of PHC in certain animals has provided additional evidence of an association with chronic hepatitis infection. The tumors have been observed in woodchucks infected with woodchuck hepatitis virus (WHV), a member of the hepadna virus group. The inflammatory hepatic lesion caused by active viral infection is associated with a high frequency of hepatoma formation (Popper et al., 1981).

EXTRAHEPATIC MANIFESTATIONS OF VIRAL HEPATITIS

It is now well recognized that hepatitis B virus infections may be associated with a variety of extrahepatic manifestations. The following sites may be affected: skin, joints, small arteries and arterioles, and renal glomeruli. The underlying pathology is usually a diffuse and widespread immune-complex–type vasculitis. The following syndromes have been identified: (1) serum sickness–like prodrome, (2) polyarteritis nodosa, (3) glomerulonephritis, (4) "essential" mixed cryoglobulinemia, (5) polymyalgia rheumatica, and (6) infantile papular acrodermatitis (Gianotti-Crosti syndrome) (Gocke, 1975).

Serum sickness–like prodrome

Serum sickness–like prodrome is characterized by a transient erythematous maculopapular eruption, polyarthralgia, and occasionally actual arthritis as well as urticaria. These symptoms and signs usually occur during the latter part of the incubation period or early acute phase of the disease, and they last just a few days. During the early phase of the skin and joint manifestations there may be a transient suppression of the complement titer and of C3 and C4 (Alpert et al., 1971). The critical role that the composition of the immune complex plays in the causation of tissue injury has been demonstrated in studies by Wands et al. (1974) on the pathogenesis of

arthritis associated with type B (HBsAg-positive) hepatitis.

Polyarteritis nodosa

The association of polyarteritis nodosa with persistent HBs antigenemia was initially described by Gocke et al. (1970) and Trepo and Thiyolet (1970). The illness usually begins with fever, polyarthralgia, myalgia, rash, and urticaria. The syndrome may evolve over a period of months, and it is characterized by various manifestations of acute vasculitis, including peripheral neuropathies, hypertension, and evidence of renal damage. Biopsy reveals lesions in small arteries characterized by typical fibrinoid necrosis and perivascular infiltration associated with polyarteritis nodosa. About 30% to 40% of patients with polyarteritis nodosa have high titers of HBsAg, but the liver involvement that is present is not the primary problem.

Circulating immune complexes composed of HBsAg and anti-HBs are present during the acute phase of the disease. At this time the whole complement titer and C3 levels are decreased. Immunofluorescent studies of biopsy specimens reveal deposition of HBsAg, IgM, IgG, and C3 in a nodular pattern along the elastic membrane of damaged vessels (Gocke et al., 1971).

A study of HBsAg-positive and HBsAg-negative polyarteritis nodosa revealed that the fatality rate was essentially equal (42% and 44%, respectively) in the two groups after a 3-year follow-up period (Sergent et al., 1976).

Glomerulonephritis

The association of glomerulonephritis with chronic hepatitis B has been studied by various investigators (Combes et al., 1971; Brzosko et al., 1974; Kohler et al., 1974a). They observed typical immune complex deposits along the subepithelial surface of the glomerular basement membrane by electron microscopy. Fluorescent antibody studies showed nodular deposition of HBsAg, immunoglobulin, and C3 in the glomeruli. The glomerulonephritis is usually of the membranous or membranoproliferative type.

Most cases of glomerulonephritis in adults have occurred in patients with existing evidence of chronic active hepatitis and a persistent HBsAg carrier state. However, studies by Brzosko et al. (1974) revealed the presence of HBsAg-antibody complex deposits in renal glomeruli in about 35% of children with clinical nephrosis or glomerulonephritis.

Other possible extrahepatic syndromes

Mixed cryoglobulinemia. Mixed cryoglobulinemia is an immune complex disease characterized by arthralgias, purpura, weakness, vasculitis, and diffuse glomerulonephritis (Meltzer et al., 1966). Levo et al. (1977) described this syndrome in patients who had evidence of HBV infection and circulating immune complexes composed of HBsAg and anti-HBs.

Polymyalgia rheumatica. Polymyalgia rheumatica is another distinct connective tissue disorder that has also been associated with hepatitis B infection (Bacon et al., 1975; Plouvier et al., 1978).

Papular acrodermatitis. The association of infantile papular acrodermatitis (IPA) with hepatitis B infection was first described by Gianotti (1973). A striking epidemic of this disease occurred in Japan involving 153 patients in a pediatric clinic during the 3-year period 1974 to 1977 (Ishimaru et al., 1976; Toda et al., 1978). Of this group, 89% were associated with HBsAg. During the outbreak all of the index cases were 1 year old or younger, but the age ranged from 3 months to 10 years. In about 40% of patients with IPA who were 1 year of age or younger HBs antigenemia persisted for 1 year.

Neonatal hepatitis B infection

Perinatal transmission of HBV from mother to infant during the course of pregnancy or at the time of birth was first reported by Stokes et al. (1954). They observed an infant born by cesarean section to a mother who was a hepatitis B carrier. The infant, who developed hepatitis with jaundice at 2 months of age, later died at age 18 months with advanced fibrosis of the liver.

The availability of tests to detect HBsAg has enabled various investigators to study infants whose mothers had acute hepatitis B or asymptomatic chronic carrier state during pregnancy (Schweitzer et al., 1972; Stevens et al., 1975). Signs of neonatal hepatitis B infection (antigenemia) are usually not present at the time of birth but may be detected between 2 weeks and 5 months of age. About 5% of infants may be infected in utero, and about 95% may be infected at the time of birth. Certain infants escape

infection completely, others develop only persistent antigenemia with no liver disease, others may develop severe chronic active hepatitis, and still others may develop fulminant hepatitis (Fawaz et al., 1975).

Perinatal transmission of hepatitis B infection from mother to infant depends in great part on the presence of HBeAg. Infection is most likely to occur if the mother is HBeAg positive (Stevens et al., 1975). Infants born to HBeAg-positive carrier mothers have a 90% chance of contracting chronic hepatitis B infection and possible subsequent progression to cirrhosis and hepatocellular carcinoma. In contrast, the attack rate of hepatitis B in infants whose HBsAg-positive mothers are anti-HBe–positive is less than 20%. These infants usually recover completely. Chronic hepatitis is rare, but occasionally the infection may be fulminant with a fatal outcome (Delaplane et al., 1983).

Possible routes of transmission from mother to baby include (1) leakage of virus across the placenta late in pregnancy or during labor, (2) ingestion of amniotic fluid or maternal blood, and (3) breast-feeding, especially if the mother has cracked nipples. Studies by Alter (1980) with HBsAg-positive and HBeAg-positive pregnant chimpanzees revealed that cesarean section and postdelivery isolation did not prevent infection of newborn chimpanzees. They became HBsAg positive in spite of these precautions.

Infants who inadvertently receive contaminated blood or blood products during the neonatal period may subsequently develop severe hepatitis B. Dupuy et al. (1975) described their experience with 14 infants 2 to 5 months of age admitted to the hospital with severe or fulminant hepatitis. Of the 14 infants, 11 had serologic evidence of hepatitis B infection. Of the 11 infants with hepatitis B, seven received blood derivatives during the neonatal period and four were exposed to their mothers who were chronic HBsAg carriers. The case fatality rate was very high; eight of the 14 infants died.

DIAGNOSIS

The diagnosis is usually based on clinical and epidemiologic grounds. The occurrence of jaundice in association with a prior febrile episode and anorexia, nausea, and abdominal pain is suggestive of viral hepatitis. The presence of an elevated serum AST or ALT value provides additional evidence. The diagnostic features of viral hepatitis types A, B, and non-A, non-B are listed in Table 10-2. The detection of HBsAg in the serum is indicative of hepatitis B infection. The value of specific serologic tests for the diagnosis of type A or type B hepatitis is dependent on the time the blood is obtained during the course of the disease. The presence of IgM-specific anti-HAV indicates hepatitis A infection. The interpretation of various serologic tests for the diagnosis of hepatitis B infection is shown in Table 10-3.

DIFFERENTIAL DIAGNOSIS

Before jaundice emerges, the following diseases may be considered in the differential diagnosis: infectious mononucleosis, acute appendicitis, gastroenteritis, influenza, and, in some parts of the world, malaria, dengue, and sand fly fever. The diagnosis of these diseases may be established by the detection of specific etiologic agents, by serologic tests, or by the subsequent course.

In the presence of jaundice, the diseases that may be confused with viral hepatitis are congenital or acquired hemolytic jaundice or obstructive jaundice due to blockage of the bile ducts by stone or tumor or, in infants, congenital atresia; hepatocellular jaundice resulting from chemical poisons, cirrhosis, or neoplasm of the liver (primary or metastatic); spirochetal jaundice (Weil's disease); yellow fever; acute cholangitis; and jaundice associated with various other infections such as infectious mononucleosis, brucellosis, amebiasis, malaria, and syphilis. Before considering these diseases in the differential diagnosis it would be important to rule out a diagnosis of hepatitis A (absence of IgM anti-HAV) and hepatitis B (absence of HBsAg and IgM anti-HBc).

Hemolytic jaundice

Hemolytic jaundice can be differentiated from obstructive jaundice by the history, the presence of anemia, positive Coombs' test, presence of urobilin in the stools, and absence of bilirubinuria.

Extrahepatic obstructive jaundice

Calculi and neoplasms are rare in children. In infancy congenital obliteration of the bile ducts may present difficulties at first. The distinction should be clear in the course of the illness as the jaundice progressively deepens and the stools remain chalky or gray. Serum aminotransferase levels are said to be lower than those found in viral hepatitis.

Hepatocellular jaundice

Hepatocellular jaundice or parenchymal jaundice caused by chemical poisons may be difficult to diagnose in the absence of a history of ingestion of toxic agents. The history is also important in the recognition of cirrhosis or neoplasm, both of which are uncommon in children in the United States.

Drug-associated hepatitis

Hepatitis induced by the following drugs may be clinically, biochemically, and morphologically indistinguishable from viral hepatitis: pyrazinamide, isoniazid, zoxazolamine, gold, and cinchophen. A clinical picture similar to the cholestatic form of the disease may be produced by the phenothiazine derivatives (for example, chlorpromazine), methyltestosterone, and contraceptive drugs. Fatal toxic hepatitis has been described in a child receiving indomethacin for rheumatoid arthritis.

Jaundice associated with infections

In this type of jaundice the diagnosis is established by demonstrating the specific etiologic agent or a rise in the specific antibody in convalescence. Jaundice in the neonatal period should suggest bacterial sepsis, syphilis, cytomegalovirus infection, toxoplasmosis, congenital rubella, herpes simplex, or Coxsackie B infections. Neonatal hepatitis associated with these infections is present at the time of birth or several days thereafter. In contrast, hepatitis B is usually detected several weeks to as long as 5 months after birth. The diagnosis is established by detection of HBsAg in the blood.

COMPLICATIONS

Acute viral hepatitis that does not heal completely may progress to chronic persistent hepatitis, chronic active hepatitis possibly complicated by cirrhosis, subacute hepatitis with submassive necrosis, or fulminant hepatitis. Hepatoma is also associated with chronic hepatitis B infection. These complications are discussed on pp. 116 and 117.

Fulminant hepatitis may be complicated by the occurrence of sepsis and hemorrhage into such vital organs as the lungs and the brain.

TREATMENT
Acute viral hepatitis

The management of patients with acute hepatitis involves decisions about (1) the duration of bed rest, (2) the choice of a diet, and (3) the value of various nonspecific drugs. At the present time there is no antiviral agent that has been shown to alter the course of either type A or type B hepatitis.

Bed rest is recommended for patients who are symptomatic during the acute stage of the disease. Studies by Chalmers et al., (1955) provided the basis for a more liberal attitude toward bed rest during the convalescent period. They observed that ad lib activity was preferable to rigidly enforced bed rest for prolonged periods of time.

The liberal attitude toward bed rest described by Chalmers et al., in the 1950s is just as pertinent today in the 1980s. Resumption of normal activity is usually gradual. Progressively decreasing serum aminotransferase and bilirubin levels are helpful guides to increasing activity. It is not necessary to restrict the activity of an asymptomatic patient for the many weeks and months that the transaminase levels are elevated. Generally, children return to normal activity much sooner than adults.

Diet is best regulated by the patient's appetite. While anorexia exists, liquids such as chicken soup and fruit juices should be given. It is recommended that with the return of appetite, a normal diet be given that is nutritious, properly balanced, and palatable. There is no contraindication to fats in moderate amounts.

Drugs such as corticosteroids are not indicated for uncomplicated hepatitis. Although beneficial effects of cortisone have been reported in severe cases in adults, the value of this therapy for HBsAg-positive hepatitis is questionable.

Chronic persistent hepatitis

Since this type of hepatitis is usually a benign, self-limited disorder, normal activity is advised, and dietary restrictions are unnecessary. Corticosteroid or other immunosuppressive forms of therapy are not indicated.

Chronic active hepatitis

Patients with chronic active hepatitis may be permitted to carry out normal activities on an ad lib basis. There is no evidence that bed rest and limitation of activity are of benefit. Alcohol should be avoided. A normal, well-balanced diet is recommended. The value of corticosteroid therapy is controversial. It appears to be more effective for HBsAg-negative than for HBsAg-positive hepatitis. The parenteral administration of human leukocyte interferon and other antivirals for the treatment of patients with chronic hepatitis B infection and chronic active hepatitis is a subject of continued clinical investigation.

Fulminant hepatitis

Sudden onset of mental confusion, emotional instability, restlessness, coma, and hemorrhagic manifestations in a patient with hepatitis requires prompt therapy. The rationale of the treatment is to combat the deleterious systemic effects of liver failure. The major objective of treatment is to reduce the load of nitrogenous products entering the portal circulation. Failure of the compromised liver to remove and detoxify these products is probably responsible for the cerebral dysfunction. The following measures are employed: (1) restriction of protein intake, (2) removal of protein already in the gastrointestinal tract (laxatives and high colonic irrigations), and (3) suppression of bacterial population of the bowel (neomycin sulfate by mouth or nasogastric tube).

The following therapeutic procedures of unproved benefit have been employed: (1) corticosteroids, (2) exchange transfusion, (3) cross-perfusion with human, baboon, or pig liver, and (4) total body perfusion. Studies by the Acute Hepatic Failure Study Group (1977) failed to show any difference in survival rates between groups treated with hepatitis B immune serum globulin (HBIG) as compared with those treated with standard immune globulin (IG). Studies are currently in progress to evaluate the effect of liver transplantation.

PROGNOSIS

Viral hepatitis type A is an infection that is better to have as a child than as an adult. The outlook for complete recovery is excellent, and it ranks as one of the mildest of childhood infections. In young adults in military service the fatality rate was one to two per 1000 cases. In pregnant women and older individuals, particularly women beyond the menopause, it may be higher. Viral hepatitis types B and non-A, non-B may be more severe than hepatitis A infection, particularly in young infants, debilitated patients, and elderly patients.

Sudden onset of mental confusion, emotional instability, restlessness, coma, and bleeding manifestations are ominous signs. This fulminant course usually progresses to a fatal outcome within 10 days. Burnell et al. (1967) collected a group of 191 reported cases of viral hepatitis complicated by "acute massive hepatic necrosis with severe coma"; the mortality was 83%. In general, relapse occurs in from less than 1% to about 20% of adult cases. In a small number of patients, resolution and repair of the liver injury are incomplete. In these patients the ultimate course is chronic hepatitis or cirrhosis. Redeker et al. (1975) studied 72 patients with fulminant hepatitis. The survival rate of those with hepatitis B infection was 34%; it was only 7% in those with non-A, non-B fulminant hepatitis.

EPIDEMIOLOGIC FACTORS
Hepatitis A

The geographic distribution of hepatitis A is worldwide. It is endemic in parts of the world, such as the Mediterranean littoral and parts of Africa, South and Central America, and the Ori-

ent, where its presence creates a danger to susceptible military and civilian persons working or traveling in such areas.

Although no age is immune, the highest incidence in civilian populations occurs among persons under 15 years of age. In military groups the youngest persons are the ones chiefly affected.

Persons of either sex seem to be equally susceptible to infection.

The well-defined autumn-winter seasonal incidence has changed. In recent years no consistent seasonal patterns have been observed. In general, at the present time the incidence of hepatitis is fairly constant throughout the year.

There is abundant evidence favoring transmission through intestinal-oral pathways. Hepatitis A virus is found in the stools of both naturally and experimentally infected persons. The period of infectivity of stool and serum is summarized in Fig. 10-9. In the study referred to in Fig. 10-9, viremia was detectable during the incubation period, 2 to 3 weeks before onset of jaundice; it was also detected on the twelfth day of the incubation period and 3 days after onset of jaundice. Blood obtained 7 days after jaundice appeared was not infectious. Virus was detected in the stools on the twenty-fifth day of the incubation period, 2 to 3 weeks before onset of jaundice, and within the first 8 days after onset of jaundice; it was not detected 19 to 33 days after onset of jaundice. Urine obtained on the first day of jaundice has been shown to be in-

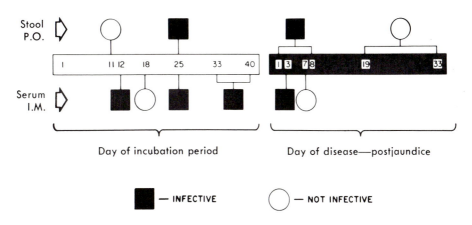

Fig. 10-9. Schematic summary of studies of the period of infectivity of patients with viral hepatitis type A. (Modified from Krugman S, et al. N Engl J Med 1959;261:729; Krugman S, Ward R, and Giles JP. Am J Med 1962;32:717; and Giles JP, et al. Virology 1964;24:107.)

fectious (Giles et al., 1964). The findings of the studies on infectivity of stool (Fig. 10-9) were confirmed in part by Dienstag et al. (1975a), who detected evidence of fecal shedding of hepatitis A antigen early in the course of the infection. These findings indicate that the infection is usually spread during the preicteric phase of the disease and that it is generally not communicable after the first week of jaundice.

Epidemics have long been known to occur in association with poor sanitation in mili-

tary camps. Explosive water-borne, milk-borne, and food-borne epidemics have been reported. Ingestion of raw shellfish from polluted waters is known to have caused many epidemics. There is evidence also for human association as the principal mode of spread. The precise pathways taken by the virus have not been defined. It should be emphasized, however, that human association or contact infection does not preclude the many potential routes of the intestinal-oral circuit. Hepatitis A virus may also be transmit-

Table 10-4. Age distribution of hepatitis A antibody (immunity) in persons living in Pennsylvania and Costa Rica*

	Proportion seropositive			
	Pennsylvania		Costa Rica	
Age (years)	No.	Percent	No.	Percent
1	0/18	0	4/20	20
2	0/17	0	10/20	50
3	0/16	0	8/20	40
4-6	0/22	0	38/60	63
7-9	0/16	0	48/60	80
10-14	0/18	0	19/20	95
15-19	0/20	0	19/20	95
20-29	2/20	10	18/20	90
30-39	6/21	29	18/20	90
40-49	10/17	59	18/20	90
50 +	5/12	42	16/20	80

*From Villarejos VM, et al.: Proc Soc Exp Biol Med 1976; 152:524.

Table 10-5. Antibody to hepatitis A antigen (anti-HAV) in healthy adults from various parts of the world*

Country	Number tested	Number anti-HAV positive[†]	Percent positive (crude)	Percent positive age-standardized
United States	629	251	39.9	44.7
Switzerland	98	23	23.5	28.7
Belgium	133	116	87.2	81.1
Yugoslavia	100	97	97.0	96.9
Israel	112	105	93.7	95.3
Taiwan	123	110	89.4	88.7
Senegal	102	76	74.5	76.2

*From Szmuness W, et al.: Am J Epidemiol 1977;106:392.
[†]IAHA titer $\geq$ 1:10. Direct method; rates for Taiwan and Senegal were standardized to the 1974 Taiwan population distribution; rates for the remaining countries were standardized to the 1970 United States population distribution.

ted like hepatitis B virus through the use of blood or blood products and contaminated needles, syringes, and stylets. However, this potential mode of transmission is very rare, chiefly because viremia is transient in hepatitis A infection, and a carrier state has not been observed.

When hepatitis A occurs in circumscribed situations such as households, day-care centers, orphanages, institutions for mentally handicapped children, military installations, and children's camps, it may smoulder for months or years or may strike in explosive outbreaks. In families secondary cases may occur in about 20 to 30 days.

Seroepidemiologic surveys by various investigators have provided valuable information about the distribution of hepatitis A antibody (anti-HAV) in various population groups (Miller et al., 1975; Szmuness et al., 1976; Villarejos et al., 1976). They observed a striking correlation between the presence of anti-HAV and socioeconomic status. Persons from lower socioeconomic groups were more likely to have detectable antibody (past hepatitis A infection) than those from middle and upper socioeconomic groups. The detection of anti-HAV was strongly correlated with age. In New York City the prevalence increased gradually in adults, reaching peak levels in persons 50 years of age or older. In Costa Rica, however, peak levels were reached by 10 years of age. The comparative age distribution of anti-HAV in open populations in Pennsylvania and Costa Rica is shown in Table 10-4. It is clear that the prevalence of anti-HAV (1) varies among different population groups, (2) increases with age, and (3) is independent of sex and race.

Studies in healthy adult blood donors from various countries of the world revealed striking differences in the prevalence of anti-HAV. As indicated in Table 10-5, the prevalence ranged from a low of 23.5% in Switzerland to a high of 97% in Yugoslavia (Szmuness et al., 1977).

It is likely that the continued improvement of environmental and socioeconomic conditions will decrease the probability of exposure to hepatitis A, thereby changing a predominantly childhood infection to one that is more apt to occur in adults. This changing epidemiologic pattern was typical for poliomyelitis during the first half of the twentieth century in the United States. Poliomyelitis, like hepatitis A, is a more severe and more disabling disease in adults than in children.

Hepatitis B

Early epidemiologic concepts indicated that hepatitis B virus was transmitted exclusively by the parenteral route. It is now clear, however, that other modes of transmission play an important role in the dissemination of the virus. The experimental demonstration of oral transmission and the demonstration that contact-associated transmission is common have clarified previous epidemiologic concepts. The term *contact-associated hepatitis* includes one or more of the following possible modes of transmission: (1) oral-oral, (2) sexual, and (3) intimate physical contact of any type. The antigen has been detected in saliva (Ward et al., 1972), in semen (Heathcote et al., 1974), and in many other body fluids.

The major reservoir of hepatitis B virus is healthy chronic carriers and patients with acute hepatitis. The infection is transmitted to susceptible persons by transfusion of blood, plasma, or other blood products or by the use of inadequately sterilized needles and syringes. Medical and paramedical personnel may be infected by accidental inoculation or ingestion of contaminated materials. Outbreaks have occurred among drug addicts using unsterilized equipment. Tattooing has been responsible for transmitting the infection. Patients and personnel in the following areas have been shown to be at high risk: renal dialysis, intensive care, and oncology units, as well as various laboratories in which potentially contaminated blood and tissues are examined.

Seroepidemiologic surveys to detect the presence of HBsAg and anti-HBs have confirmed the worldwide distribution of the disease. The antigen has been detected in all populations, even in those living in the most remote areas devoid of parenteral modes of transmission. The antigen is most prevalent among persons living under crowded conditions and with poor hygienic standards. This accounts for the endemicity of the disease in institutions for mentally retarded persons and in certain developing countries of the world.

Table 10-6. An estimate of HBsAg prevalences and numbers of persistent carriers in the world*

Geographical region	Population 1970 estimates (millions)	Average prevalence (percent)	Number of carriers (thousands)
United States and Canada	275.3	0.25	688.25
Central and South America	232.1	1.5	3481.5
North and Western Europe	232.3	0.25	580.75
South and Eastern Europe	266.0	1.5	3990.0
U.S.S.R.—European	100.0	1.5	1500.0
U.S.S.R.—Asiatic	143.0	5.0	7150.0
Middle East	70.2	5.0	3510.0
Southern Asia	691.6	5.0	34,580.0
Southeast Asia	300.2	10.0	30,020.0
China	800.0	7.5	60,000.0
Japan	103.4	1.5	1551.0
Australia and New Zealand	19.0	0.25	47.5
Northern Africa	70.1	5.0	3505.0
Central and South Africa	256.8	10.0	25,680.0
WORLD TOTAL	3560.0	—	176,284.0

*From Szmuness W: Progr Med Virol 1978;24:40.

Table 10-7. Prevalence of antibody to hepatitis B surface antigen (anti-HBs) in the populations surveyed for HAV infections*

Country	Number tested	Number anti-HBs positive	Percent positive
United States	1000	108	10.8
Switzerland	98	3	3.1
Belgium	133	7	5.3
Yugoslavia	97	33	34.0
Israel	112	17	15.2
Taiwan	123	96	78.0
Senegal	96	60	62.5

*From Szmuness W, et al.: Am J Epidemiol 1977;106:392.

The HBsAg carrier rate may range from 0.1% to more than 10%; it is dependent on such factors as geographic location, age, and sex. The carrier rate is higher in tropical underdeveloped areas than in temperate developed countries, higher in urban than in rural communities, and higher among males than among females (Table 10-6). As indicated in Table 10-7, the prevalence of anti-HBs in various populations ranges from 3.1% in Switzerland to 78% in Taiwan.

The period of infectivity of patients with viral hepatitis type B is dependent on the presence or absence of a carrier state. As indicated in Figs. 10-4 and 10-10, HBsAg is detectable in the blood during the latter part of the incubation period and for a variable period after onset of jaundice. Infectivity has also been associated with the presence of HBeAg and a high titer of HBsAg. For example, perinatal transmission of hepatitis B infection from HBsAg-positive mothers to their infants is highly likely if they are HBeAg positive. On the other hand, HBsAg-positive and anti-HBe–positive mothers are much less likely to transmit infection.

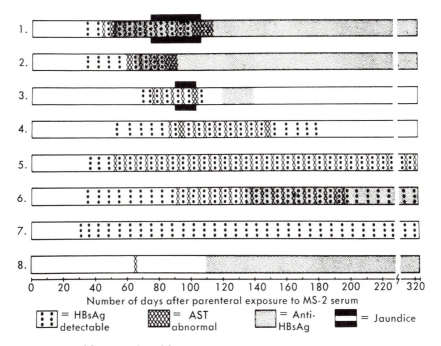

Fig. 10-10. Natural history of viral hepatitis type B. Note variation in response to infection after parenteral exposure as indicated by appearance and persistence of hepatitis B surface antigen (HBsAg), serum aspartate aminotransferase (AST), jaundice, and antibody to HBsAg (anti-HBs).

IMMUNITY

An attack of hepatitis A virus infection is followed by homologous immunity, but it does not protect against subsequent hepatitis B infection. An attack of hepatitis B infection is followed by homologous immunity, but it does not protect against subsequent infection with hepatitis A virus. In general, infection with one subtype (HBsAg/*ad*) protects against subsequent exposure to another subtype (HBsAg/*ay*). The common "*a*" determinant is responsible for this protection. The agents that are responsible for non-A, non-B hepatitis are also immunologically distinct.

Hepatitis A

The immune response to HAV infection is shown in Fig. 10-7. Antibody becomes detectable at the time of onset of clinical illness. Both IgM and IgG anti-HAV appear early in infection. Initially, however, IgM-specific antibody predominates, and it is a useful marker of recent HAV infection.

Hepatitis B

The humoral immune response has been studied by tests for detection of anti-HBc, anti-HBs, and anti-HBe. Cellular immune response has been assessed by various tests, including lymphocyte stimulation and leukocyte migration inhibition (LMI).

The immunologic events during the course of the acute and convalescent phases of hepatitis B, summarized by Vyas et al. (1975), are shown in Fig. 10-11. They divided the sequence of events into three phases. In the first phase, the acute hepatitis is associated with the presence of HBsAg in the serum and the appearance of anti-HBe. The second phase coincides with the disappearance of HBsAg and the appearance of cell-mediated immunity as indicated by a positive LMI test that disappears after 3 to 6 weeks. The third phase begins with the appearance of anti-HBs approximately 2 weeks to 2 months after the disappearance of HBsAg. Not all patients develop detectable anti-HBs.

The antibody to the hepatitis B surface anti-

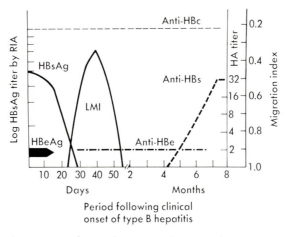

Fig. 10-11. Immunologic events during the course of acute and convalescent phases of icteric hepatitis B infection illustrating appearance of hepatitis B surface antigen (HBsAg), antibody to hepatitis B core antigen (anti-HBc), leukocyte migration inhibition (LMI) response, and antibody to HBsAg (anti-HBs). (From Vyas GN, et al. Am J Med Sci 1975;270:241.)

gen has been shown to be the protective antibody. It is present in high titer in hepatitis B immune serum globulin. Detection of anti-HBs in the serum of a person is indicative of past infection or immunization with hepatitis B vaccine. Persons who have had hepatitis B infection in the past, with or without detectable anti-HBs, show evidence of homologous immunity. Most of these patients have detectable anti-HBc. This immunity is solid for the usual type of exposure. However, it may not be absolute if there is an overwhelming challenge with material that contains large quantities of hepatitis B virus.

CONTROL MEASURES
Hepatitis A

As in other excremental infections, procedures designed to block intestinal-oral pathways should be undertaken in an effort to control the spread of the infection. These measures include scrupulous hand washing before meals and after evacuation of the bowels; proper sterilization of food utensils (boiling in water for at least 1 minute or sterilization by steam under pressure or by dry heat); exclusion of potentially infected food handlers; fly abatement; and other steps to prevent fecal contamination of food, milk, and water supplies. The usual chlorination procedures preceded by filtration and settling of water are thought to be effective in reducing the risk of acquiring hepatitis A. However, the risk may

be increased under conditions of heavy sewage pollution.

Studies demonstrating the presence of virus in stools and blood during the incubation period and icteric phase of infectious hepatitis A are summarized in Fig. 10-10. These findings have a significant bearing on the control of the disease. The disease should be considered potentially infectious in patients for no more than 1 week after onset of jaundice.

The excretion of virus for as long as 2 weeks before the appearance of jaundice could be responsible for spread of the infection before the presence of the disease is suspected. Therefore, isolation and quarantine of patients and contacts are of limited value in controlling the spread of hepatitis A. The problem is made even more difficult by the large number of subclinical cases capable of spreading the infection.

The efficacy of immune globulin (IG) in the prevention of hepatitis A with jaundice has been well established by studies in many parts of the world. Various studies have indicated that IG has a modifying rather than a completely prophylactic effect. Under conditions of intense exposure, the administration of IG may be followed by passive-active immunity.

The efficacy of IG depends on various factors: (1) degree and type of exposure, (2) dose and antibody content, and (3) time interval between exposure and administration. For optimum effect, IG should be given as soon as possible after exposure since the incubation period may be as short as 15 days, and infection may be established about 1 week before onset of disease. The recommended dose of IG and indications for its use are described in detail in Chapter 35, (p. 491).

Hepatitis B

Detection of HBsAg in blood is indicative of the presence of hepatitis B virus. Consequently, it is essential that blood for transfusion be screened for the presence of antigen. Since the most sensitive test (RIA) is not sensitive enough to detect low levels of HBsAg, blood may contain antigen in spite of a negative test.

Effective control of hepatitis B requires careful screening of blood donors. In addition to tests for HBsAg, the following precautions are indicated: (1) use of voluntary donors if possible, since commercial donors are more likely to be drug addicts and chronic carriers; (2) rejection of blood from persons who have had blood transfusions within the previous 6 months; (3) rejection of blood from persons who were intimately exposed to hepatitis within the previous 6 months; and (4) rejection of blood from persons who were responsible for a case of hepatitis in the past. The indications for the use of a single unit of blood should be carefully assessed because of the risk of transmitting hepatitis.

The knowledge that hepatitis B virus is infectious by mouth and by close contact has highlighted the importance of hand-washing techniques and other measures when caring for chronic carriers or patients with acute hepatitis. Outbreaks have occurred among hospital personnel who have been exposed to HBsAg-positive patients with active bleeding.

All equipment that comes in contact with blood or its derivatives should either be sterilized by heat-boiling for at least 10 minutes, autoclaving at 15 pounds pressure, or dry-heat sterilization at 170° C for 30 minutes.

Plasma should not be used if albumin or stable plasma protein solution are suitable substitutes. Irradiation of liquid plasma with ultraviolet light is not an effective method of inactivating hepatitis B virus. Plasma prepared from small pools (10 to 20 donors) is less likely to transmit hepatitis than plasma prepared from large pools (more than 100 donors).

Immune globulin prophylaxis. The efficacy of standard IG for the prevention of hepatitis B has been a controversial subject for many years. Reports of its value have varied from limited protection to none at all. It is likely that this phenomenon has been due in part to the fact that most lots of IG prepared prior to 1972 contained low or undetectable levels of anti-HBs. Since 1972, however, various lots of standard IG have been shown to contain higher titers of antibody (Hoofnagle et al., 1975). Moreover, the development of HBIG with an antibody titer 25,000 to 50,000 times higher than standard IG (Prince et al., 1971) indicates that the efficacy of IG will require further evaluation. Our preliminary trial with HBIG revealed that it was 70% effective (Krugman et al., 1971a). Subsequent studies have confirmed the efficacy of HBIG for the prevention or modification of hepatitis B infection (Grady et al., 1975). Persons who have had a definite exposure to hepatitis B should receive HBIG. The U.S. Public Health Service recommendations for the use of HBIG are described in detail in Chapter 35 (p. 498).

Public health implications of hepatitis B infection. The Committee on Viral Hepatitis of the Division of Medical Sciences, National Academy of Sciences–National Research Council and the Public Health Service Advisory Committee on Immunization Practices prepared a joint statement entitled "Perspectives on Control of Viral Hepatitis, Type B" that was published in the Center for Disease Control *Morbidity and Mortality Weekly Report* (May 7, 1976, Vol. 25, No. 17). The following two sections are extracted verbatim from this report: (1) "Recommendations for minimizing transmission in specific settings" and (2) "Management of high-risk persons and populations."

RECOMMENDATIONS FOR MINIMIZING TRANSMISSION IN SPECIFIC SETTINGS

The risk of acquiring hepatitis B is greatest for persons who frequently encounter hepatitis patients or specimens containing HBsAg. Generally speaking, the highest risk involves a few specific household and hospital settings. Before considering them in detail, and to avoid redundancy, some general comments can be made.

Regardless of the setting, patients and human biological specimens should be managed carefully because some will present an unrecognized hepatitis risk. To protect susceptible patients and staff, blood and other specimens from hepatitis patients and HBsAg-positive persons should be labeled as such and optimally be enclosed in impermeable bags. Charts of these patients should be flagged (e.g., "Hepatitis B," "blood and instrument precautions," etc.). All persons involved, patients and staff, should practice careful handwashing and personal hygiene.

Specific recommendations should be tailored to the particular setting and reflect the unique aspects of each environment:

Household

Within the household, spouses and other intimate contacts of patients with acute hepatitis B or of asymptomatic HBsAg-positive persons appear to have the greatest risk of infection. It is important that all household contacts know how hepatitis B is transmitted and that blood and possibly other body fluids, if HBsAg-positive, might spread HBV infection. In addition to practicing good personal hygiene (especially handwashing), they also need to handle and dispose of blood-contaminated articles carefully and avoid practices which might increase the opportunity for infection such as sharing razors, toothbrushes, towels, washcloths, or other personal items.

Hospitals
General patient care area

Hepatitis B has spread from patients to staff in intensive care units, transplant units, hematology-oncology wards, and general medical-pediatric and surgical wards. Nevertheless, patients with acute hepatitis or HBsAg-positive persons in these environments generally need *not* be placed in isolation: they can be cared for in semi-private or ward accommodations providing blood and instruments are handled with the precautions discussed earlier. When handling blood or blood-contaminated objects from HBsAg-positive patients, staff should wear gloves and possibly other protective clothing as well. During procedures which could result in splattering or splashing infective material, a surgical-type mask or facial covering to protect eyes, nose, and mouth has value. Disposable needles and syringes, proper sterile technique, and adequate sterilization and chemical disinfection procedures are important to control percutaneous spread.

Laboratories

Clinical biochemistry and hematology-serology laboratories, hepatitis research laboratories, and autopsy laboratories are recognized to be settings where hepatitis B transmission occurs. Common exposures are accidentally pricking the skin with instruments contaminated with HBV, pipetting infective fluids, contaminating cuts or scratches with infective blood or splashing it in eyes or mouth. Contamination may result from shaking specimens, homogenizing, opening screw-cap bottles, blowing the last drop of fluid from a pipette, pouring fluids, and centrifuging. Mouth pipetting, smoking, and eating in the laboratory are dangerous practices and should be forbidden. Protective clothing, including gloves and facial coverings (if there is danger of splashing), may be appropriate. This is especially important when performing autopsies on HBsAg-positive persons. Gloves and other protective clothing must be properly used (changed frequently, especially when contaminated or torn) and should not be considered a substitute for careful technique and good personal practices. Work areas should be thoroughly cleaned and disinfected daily. All laboratory accidents resulting in HBsAg exposure must be promptly reviewed with regard to need for environmental decontamination and personal prophylaxis.

Laboratories should specify that potentially infective specimens be properly packaged and labeled. It may be useful for them to have a designated safety officer who keeps records of laboratory accidents, educates personnel in methods of control and prevention, and periodically evaluates and updates safety procedures.

Hemodialysis units

Hemodialysis units present a great risk of hepatitis B for patients and staff. Most infections in patients are subclinical, and a large percentage of them result in persistent HBsAg-positivity. Staff commonly have overt hepatitis, often hampering operations.

HBV can be introduced into the units by patients, staff, or infective blood, plasma, or blood products. Once seeded, HBV can be spread among patients and staff by personal contact or parenteral exposure.

Surveillance

Continuous surveillance of patients and staff for HBV infection is essential. Those who are sero-negative should be tested periodically for HBsAg, anti-HBs, and, possibly, SGOT and/or SGPT. The frequency of testing depends on whether hepatitis B is occurring. If no hepatitis B infections among patients or staff develop in 6-12 months of testing, routine sampling intervals of 2-4 months would be reasonable. If antigen or antibody does appear, HBV spread is probably occurring, and more frequent (e.g., monthly) sampling should be undertaken.

It is useful to screen new hemodialysis patients and staff for HBsAg and anti-HBs before admission to the unit. This provides baseline information on their susceptibility or potential infectiousness and the need to institute precautions.

Records

Detailed records of patient management (e.g., machine and other equipment assignments and dates of use) will be essential to determine whether any infections are related to specific procedures. Records should also include complete descriptions of mishaps (needle punctures, membrane leaks-ruptures, etc.)

Staff

Highest quality aseptic technique is fundamental to prevent HBV spread. Protective clothing should be used but changed on a regular basis and whenever obviously contaminated. It should not be worn outside the unit. Using gloves during procedures where there is contact with blood, such as handling shunts, drawing blood, or cleaning or dismantling dialysis machines, has been shown to decrease the risk of HBV infection. A fresh pair of gloves should be used with each patient. However, gloves are not a substitute for good technique and proper personal hygiene. Surgical-type masks or other facial coverings may decrease the risk of infection when splattering of blood occurs. Abrasions, lacerations, and other breaks in the skin should be bandaged to protect them from contact with infectious material.

Operating procedures

Operating procedures should minimize the amount of close personal contact among patients and staff. Overcrowding is to be avoided, and individual equipment and supplies used whenever possible. Patients and staff should not eat, drink, or smoke in the immediate hemodialysis area.

Susceptible patients should be separated from known HBsAg-positive patients or those whose antigen status is unknown. If practical, staff should be assigned to attend HBsAg-positive or HBsAg-negative patients, but not both, during the same shift. Staff with anti-HBs might preferentially be assigned to HBsAg-positive patients. Until their antigen/antibody status is known, new patients should be managed in areas separate from those being used for chronic hemodialysis.

After each use, equipment which cannot be heat or gas sterilized should be washed to remove adherent material and cleaned with a disinfectant solution. Nonpermeable disposable diaphragms can prevent contamination of equipment such as venous pressure monitors.

Institutions for the mentally retarded

Viral hepatitis, both sporadic and epidemic, has long been known to occur in custodial institutions for the mentally retarded and poses a risk for both patients and staff. The risk of infection appears to increase with the duration of institutionalization. Prac-

tical precautions are needed to reduce transmission of HBV from HBsAg-positive mentally retarded residents to persons such as teachers, classmates, and parents who come in close personal contact. In general and until more definitive information on the infectiousness of persons with HBsAg becomes available, it is important to avoid placing unwarranted limitations or restrictions on HBsAg-positive retarded persons.

Surveillance

Serologic surveys of institutionalized persons are not considered necessary as a routine procedure. However, in institutions where hepatitis B infection has been shown to be endemic, periodic screening of residents will be helpful in identifying high-risk areas, in investigating hepatitis outbreaks, and in evaluating the effectiveness of control measures.

Since persons who are antigen-positive may become negative even after 6 or more months of positivity, each HBsAg-positive person should be retested periodically to determine whether the antigen persists. Once seroconversion to anti-HBs occurs, any specific hepatitis precautions can be removed.

Control measures

Parents and personnel responsible for the care of institutionalized mentally retarded persons must be aware of the need for good hygienic practices. This is especially important after caring for open wounds or having contact with blood or blood-contaminated fluids and before eating or handling food. Personal toiletry articles should not be shared. No special procedures need to observed for laundering clothing or linens, although all blood-contaminated items should be handled with appropriate precautions (gloves, etc.). No other restrictions need be imposed on antigen-positive residents when they participate in routine activities, such as special education programs and in nursery, day care, or foster care facilities.

Physicians, dentists, laboratory workers, and others providing care for known antigen-positive persons should be so advised so that adequate precautions can be exercised during patient contact or specimen handling. Because of the likelihood of contact with unrecognized HBsAg-positive persons or specimens, health workers in institutions should always be alert to the risk of hepatitis B and use appropriate protective measures.

Community placement programs, nursing homes

Because residents of institutions for the retarded more frequently are HBsAg-positive than non-institutionalized populations, they should be tested for HBsAg before transfer to other institutions or discharge to community placement programs or nursing homes. Information on their antigen status will alert health personnel and others who have close contact with them in community programs to use precautions when there is a risk of hepatitis B. HBsAg-positive persons should be given the same consideration for placement programs or nursing homes as those who are negative. Parents and personnel in contact with antigen-positive retarded persons should be informed of the risk of hepatitis B and given instruction in control and prevention. (HBsAg-positive residents in community programs should be managed as are those in institutions; see above.)

MANAGEMENT OF HIGH-RISK PERSONS AND POPULATIONS

Certain persons and groups, particularly those involved in health care, are at greater risk than the general population of acquiring hepatitis B; this is because of occupational and environmental exposures. Since most hepatitis B infections are subclinical and 5%-10% of those infected may develop persistent HBsAg, there may also be an increased risk of hepatitis B for the general population brought into contact with HBsAg-positive individuals in health care settings. Precautions against spreading HBV infection currently depend on awareness of personal risks and use of good hygienic practices.

Management of persons with persistent HBsAg who work in environments and under circumstances where there are many chances for transmitting HBV infection (e.g., regular contact with blood, involvement with parenteral and surgical procedures, etc.) require special consideration. As has been emphasized, the presence of HBsAg is sufficient reason for personal precautions, but not necessarily evidence of a substantial hepatitis risk for contacts or associates. It is extremely important to prevent misunderstanding and unreasonable management of persons or population groups with HBsAg. Since it now appears that individuals who have persisting HBsAg may become negative even after 6 or more months of positivity, each antigen-positive person should be retested periodically (e.g., every 6 months) to determine whether antigen persists.

General recommendations

Persons working where there is a high risk of hepatitis B infection (especially hemodialysis or hematology-oncology units and clinical laboratories) need to be fully aware of the risks and to use good hygienic practices to minimize any chance for infection. It is reasonable to keep such "high risk" population groups under serologic surveillance for hepatitis B infection in order to be able to detect and investigate problems as quickly as possible. On the other hand, there is no need to routinely test health professionals and hospital employees not working in high-risk areas.

Health personnel observed to be HBsAg-positive should not be restricted from patient contact solely on the basis of this serologic finding. Rather, their personal procedures and practices should always reflect an awareness of the potential for transmitting HBV and include rigorous efforts to reduce any chance that transmission might occur. Knowing that contact with blood or serum containing HBV is the likely cause of hepatitis B infections, scrupulous aseptic technique, avoidance of personal hand injuries, and use of gloves in office-based minor surgery, dental procedures, wound dressing, etc. have obvious value.

Health personnel clearly associated epidemiologically with HBV transmission obviously pose a greater risk for patients and associates and must be evaluated carefully with respect to continuing risks. In these instances, more restrictive measures (e.g., limiting or eliminating some types of procedures or contact with patients) may be needed. Obviously, each such episode will have to be dealt with separately and recommendations and control measures tailored to the specific conditions.

Health care personnel (dentists, nurses, physicians, technicians, etc.)

Recent investigations of hepatitis B among contacts of antigen-positive health personnel demonstrate that HBV transmission does occur but seems to be very rare. There appears to be considerable variation in the likelihood that persons with persistent HBsAg will spread infection. The risk depends in part on the kind and extent of contact with susceptibles. In the few instances where epidemiologic evidence linked health workers in specific hospital or dental environments to hepatitis B cases, infection seemed to have been caused by a presumably minute amount of blood or serum which was transferred during routine procedures. Minor hand injuries have generally been thought to be the source of infective blood which then is introduced by oral or percutaneous routes.

Food handlers

There is no evidence that HBsAg-positive food handlers pose a health risk to the general public, and transmission of hepatitis B by food has not been documented. Nonetheless, it is prudent to restrict food handlers with acute hepatitis B from working while ill. Food handlers with persistent HBsAg, like all antigen-positive persons, should be educated about HBV transmission, the need for attention to good personal hygiene, avoidance of hand injuries, etc.

Pregnant women

Women with hepatitis B infection during pregnancy sometimes transmit the infection to their infants. The risk is highest when an acute illness occurs during the third trimester. Infected newborns who may be HBsAg-negative at birth generally become HBsAg-positive 1 to 2 months later in the absence of clinical hepatitis. Most infants who become HBsAg-positive develop persistent HBsAg, and many eventually have histopathologic evidence of inflammatory liver disease. For these reasons, seronegative pregnant women working in high-risk environments should be transferred to work areas where the risk is lower for the duration of pregnancy.

Indochinese refugees. The following guidelines for the management of Indochinese refugees who are chronic HBsAg carriers were published in the October 5, 1979 issue of the Centers for disease Control *Morbidity and Mortality Weekly Report* 1979, (Vol. 28, p. 463).

Preliminary data from screening of Indochinese refugees entering Canada indicate that about 12% of them are positive for hepatitis B surface antigen (HBsAg) *(1)*. Most such individuals are asymptomatic and carry the antigen chronically. The following summarizes CDC's assessment of the current situation with respect to hepatitis B in Indochinese refugees and provides recommendations for dealing with chronic HBsAg carriers.

Assuming a 0.3% prevalence of antigenemia in the U.S. population, there are about 600,000 chronic hepatitis B carriers in this country. The additional number of carriers expected among the Indochinese refugees would increase the pool of carriers in the United States by approximately 4%. Most refugees are arriving in family units. Many are immune to hepatitis B and pose no threat of transmitting the disease. In general, therefore, any increased risk of transmitting hepatitis B to the U.S. population is expected to be small. This risk can be minimized by proper care and management.

Active immunization. The successful cultivation of various viruses in cell culture provided the basis for the development of safe and effective vaccines for the prevention of poliomyelitis, measles, rubella, and mumps. In spite of efforts by many investigators, the successful cultivation of HBV has not been achieved. Nevertheless, progress toward the development of hepatitis B vaccines has been very encouraging.

Two important observations provided the basis for the development of inactivated hepatitis B vaccines: (1) the discovery of Australia antigen (subsequently proved to be HBsAg) by Blumberg et al. (1967) and (2) the demonstration that heated serum containing HBV and HBsAg was not infectious but was capable of stimulating the development of anti-HBs, thereby conferring protection against subsequent exposure to HBV (Krugman et al., 1970, 1971b; Krugman and Giles, 1973). The studies with heat-inactivated serum indicated that immunized persons who were exposed to HBV were more likely than unimmunized persons to be completely protected or to develop a more attenuated, transient infection. In addition, a decreased HBsAg carrier rate was observed in immunized persons. The demonstration of anti-HBs in recipients of vaccine suggested that the noninfectious HBsAg component was the immunizing antigen needed for vaccine production.

The first hepatitis B vaccine to be licensed for use was unique because it was manufactured from human plasma obtained from HBsAg carriers. The manufacturing process involved a series of complex physical and chemical procedures to isolate the 20-nm spherical noninfectious particles. These procedures included concentration of HBsAg by ammonium sulfate precipitation, isopycnic ultracentrifugation in sodium bromide, and rate zonal centrifugation in sucrose. The partially purified HBsAg particles were then treated with pepsin at pH 2 and with 8 M urea to remove extraneous blood plasma and human liver proteins. After gel filtration, the antigen was treated with formalin in a 1:4000 dilution. The final step was formulation of the vaccine to contain 20 μg of HBsAg and 0.5 mg of Al^{3+} as aluminum hydroxide in each 1-ml dose. Thimerosal, in a concentration of 1:20,000, was added as a preservative.

Each of the three steps (pepsin, urea, and formalin) was shown in chimpanzee studies to inactivate HBV. In addition, pepsin inactivated viruses from every known group, such as rhabdoviruses (vesicular stomatitis virus), poxviruses (vaccinia), togaviruses (sindbis), herpesvirus (herpes simplex type 1), coronaviruses (infectious bronchitis virus), and reovirus. The urea treatment inactivated myxoviruses (Newcastle disease virus), picornaviruses (mengovirus), and slow viruses (scrapie agent) as well as the viruses inactivated by pepsin. Formalin inactivated a wide variety of viruses, including non-A, non-B hepatitis (NANB) viruses, parvoviruses, retroviruses, and the delta agent. All of the protein in the final product was accounted for as HBsAg, thereby decreasing the potential risk of an autoimmune response to extraneous protein.

Tests for safety of the vaccine included in vitro and in vivo assays for viral and microbial sterility of the bulk plasma, the purified antigen, and the final product. Each lot of vaccine was tested in chimpanzees to detect possible residual infectivity for HBV or other viral agents.

A second generation hepatitis B vaccine has been developed using HBsAg produced by a DNA recombinant strain of the yeast *Saccharomyces cerevisiae*. The yeast cells contain a plasmid into which the HBV gene for HBsAg is incorporated. The HBsAg synthesized by these cells is purified from an extract of yeast cells by physical and chemical methods. It is treated with formalin and adsorbed to alum. The final product is indistinguishable from native 22-nm HBsAg particles. Side effects and immunogenicity are similar to plasma-derived hepatitis B vaccine.

Immunogenicity. The inactivated hepatitis B vaccine is highly immunogenic for infants and children. It is given intramuscularly in a three-dose schedule at 0, 1, and 6 months. The anti-HBs response exceeds 95%. To date, vaccine-induced anti-HBs has persisted for at least 5 years in 85% to 90% of vaccinees. Since antibody titers would be expected to decline, it is likely that an additional booster dose may be required in the future.

Clinical trials. The efficacy of hepatitis B vaccine has been evaluated in three randomized, placebo-controlled, double-blind trials among (1) 1083 homosexual men in New York City, (2) 1402 homosexual men in five additional cities, and (3) 865 staff members of 43 hemodialysis units in the United States. The vaccine proved to be highly effective in preventing HBV infection and disease. The difference in life table attack rates between the vaccine and placebo groups was highly significant. The P value was <0.0001 in the first study, <0.0004 in the second, and <0.01 in the third. The vaccine recipients were protected against acute hepatitis B,

asymptomatic infection, and the chronic HBsAg carrier state. All vaccine recipients who had an anti-HBs response were protected. The only cases of hepatitis B in the vaccine group occurred in those who did not respond and those who were already infected at the time of entry in the study. However, the vaccine appeared to be partially effective when given after exposure. In the hemodialysis study, the vaccine that contained HBsAg subtype *ad* protected medical staff who were exposed to patients who had HBsAg subtype *ay* infection.

Safety. Experience involving more than 1 million recipients of hepatitis B vaccine has confirmed the safety of the vaccine. There has been no evidence of association with acquired immune deficiency syndrome (AIDS) or any other serious disease.

The benefits of a safe and effective vaccine are obvious. Hepatitis B is an important cause of disability for certain high-risk groups, such as (1) medical and paramedical personnel, especially physicians, dentists, nurses, and patients and staff of hemodialysis centers, (2) laboratory personnel who handle blood specimens, (3) residents and staff of institutions for mentally disabled children, (4) promiscuous male homosexuals, (5) military personnel, (6) spouses of chronic HBsAg carriers, (7) travelers to highly endemic areas, and (8) infants born in highly endemic areas of the world.

Prevention of hepatitis B infection in newborn infants

Pregnant women who are HBsAg positive may transmit hepatitis B to their newborn infants (see p. 118). If the HBsAg-positive mother is HBeAg positive, her infant will have a 90% chance of acquiring hepatitis B infection. In such cases most neonates will be infected at the time of birth; however, about 5% may be infected in utero. It has been shown that 0.5 ml of HBIG given shortly after birth and at 3 and 6 months will prevent about 75% of the chronic infections.

The attack rate of hepatitis B in infants whose HBsAg-positive mothers are anti-HBe–positive is less than 20%. Moreover, as a general rule, these infants recover completely, and chronic hepatitis B is rare. However, on rare occasions, the infection may be fulminant with a fatal outcome. Thus HBIG therapy is recommended for all newborns whose mothers are HBsAg positive, regardless of the mother's HBeAg status.

It has also been demonstrated that administration of HBIG and hepatitis B vaccine given simultaneously at separate sites is immunogenic. HBIG does not inhibit the antibody response to the vaccine. The combined use of HBIG and vaccine will provide immediate as well as long-term protection. At the present time, inactivated hepatitis B vaccine is recommended for high-risk infants, including newborns. Various studies have indicated that administration of HBIG shortly after birth followed by immunization with hepatitis B vaccine is highly effective for the prevention of hepatitis B in those born to hepatitis B carrier mothers (Beasley et al., 1983; Stevens et al., 1985). Therefore, the following guidelines are suggested for the care of HBsAg-positive mothers and their newborns:

1. Screen all high-risk pregnant women for HBsAg during the prenatal period if possible, or soon after admission to the hospital. Screening of women who are not considered to be at high risk should be optional.
2. Newborns of HBsAg-positive mothers should receive 0.5 ml of HBIG intramuscularly within a few hours after birth, if possible.
3. At birth or within 1 week 0.5 ml (10 μg) of hepatitis B vaccine may be given; the second dose of vaccine should be given 1 month after the first dose.
4. At 6 months of age the infant's serum should be tested for HBsAg to determine if HBV infection occurred.
   a. If HBsAg is detected, additional therapy is neither beneficial nor necessary.
   b. If HBsAg is not detected in the infant's serum, give 0.5 ml (10 μg) of hepatitis B vaccine intramuscularly.
5. At 12 to 15 months of age, test for HBsAg, anti-HBc, and anti-HBs to determine the success or failure of treatment. The absence of HBsAg and the presence of anti-HBs with or without anti-HBc indicates success. The presence of HBsAg indicates failure.

The decision to breast-feed or not to breast-feed will depend on various circumstances. A report by Beasley et al. (1975) presented data indicating that breast-feeding did not affect the attack rate of hepatitis B infection in infants born of Taiwanese mothers who were asymptomatic HBsAg carriers. Evidence of hepatitis B infection was detected in 53% of infants who were breast-fed and in 60% of those who were not breast-fed.

Breast milk of hepatitis B carrier mothers has been implicated as a possible cause of newborn infection for two reasons: (1) the possible ingestion of infectious serum that exudes from cracked nipples, a common occurrence, and (2) the possibility that virus may be present in breast milk. Thus breastfeeding must be considered as one of many possible modes of transmission of hepatitis B virus. The infant of an HBsAg-positive carrier mother may be exposed to infection in utero, at the time of birth, during the postpartum period in the hospital, and at home after discharge.

During the delivery an infant is born in a "bath of blood." Therefore, infection may occur as a result of ingestion of hepatitis B virus. In addition, the virus may be inadvertently inoculated by various routine procedures carried out in the delivery room. For example, vigorous suction procedures may cause minor submucosal tears in the infant's mouth and pharynx. During the course of labor certain monitoring procedures involve the use of needles that penetrate the infant's scalp, thereby inoculating the agent. The injection of vitamin K may penetrate skin that is contaminated with virus.

The potential benefits of breast-feeding for infants in developing areas of the world far outweigh the potential risks of hepatitis B infection from breast milk. Artificial milk formulas are too costly and adequate refrigeration facilities are usually not available. The study by Beasley and his colleagues has provided reassuring data to justify the continuation of breast-feeding for infants who live in these areas. On the other hand, in countries where hepatitis B infection is not endemic and artificial milk formulas are safe and available, the potential risks of breastfeeding may exceed its benefits. However, the use of HBIG and hepatitis B vaccine has significantly reduced the risk of neonatal hepatitis B infection. Therefore, the risk of breastfeeding by immunized infants should be negligible, and breastfeeding should not be discouraged.

REFERENCES

Acute Hepatic Failure Study Group. Failure of specific immunotherapy in fulminant type B hepatitis. Ann Intern Med 1977;86:272.

Aikawa T, et al.: Seroconversion from hepatitis B e antigen to anti-HBe in acute hepatitis B virus infection. N Engl J Med 1978;298:439.

Alberti A, et al.: T-lymphocyte cytotoxicity to HBsAg-coated target cells in hepatitis B virus infection. Gut 1977;18:1004.

Allison AC, Blumberg BS: An immunoprecipitin reaction distinguishing human serum protein types. Lancet 1961;1:634.

Almeida J, Rubenstein D, Stott EJ: New antigen-antibody system in Australia-antigen-positive hepatitis. Lancet 1971;2:1225.

Almeida JD, Waterson AP: Immune complexes in hepatitis. Lancet 1969;2:983.

Almeida JD, et al.: Immune electron microscopy of the Australia-SH (serum hepatitis) antigen. Microbios 1969;2:117.

Alpert E, Isselbacher KJ, Schur PH: The pathogenesis of arthritis associated with viral hepatitis. N Engl J Med 1971;285:185.

Alter HJ: The infectivity of the healthy hepatitis B surface antigen carrier. In Bianchi L, Gerok W, Sickinger K, Stalder GA, eds: Virus and the liver, Lancaster, England. M.T.P. Press, Ltd., 1980, p 261.

Bacon PA, Doherty SM, Zuckerman AJ: Hepatitis B antibody in polymyalgia rheumatica. Lancet 1975;2:476.

Bancroft WH, Mundon, RK, Russell PK: Detection of additional antigenic determinants of hepatitis B antigen. J Immunol 1972;109:842.

Barker LF, et al.: Some antigenic and physical properties of virus-like particles in sera of hepatitis patients. J Immunol 1969;102:1529.

Barker LF et al.: Transmission of serum hepatitis. JAMA 1970;211:1509.

Barker LF et al.: Transmission of type B viral hepatitis to chimpanzees. J Infect Dis 1973;127:648.

Bayer ME, Blumberg BS, Werner B. Particles associated with Australia antigen in the sera of patients with leukemia, Down's syndrome and hepatitis. Nature 1968;218:1057.

Beasley RP. Discussion: viral hepatitis: the disease, Am J Med Sci 1975;270:57.

Beasely RP, Hwang L-Y, Lee GYC, et al. Prevention of perinatally transmitted hepatitis B virus infections with hepatitis B immune globulin and hepatitis B vaccine. Lancet 1983;2:1099-1102.

Beasley RP, Shiao IS, Stevens CE, Meng HC. Evidence against breast-feeding as a mechanism for vertical transmission of hepatitis B. Lancet 1975;2:704.

Beasley RP, Stevens CE. Vertical transmission of HBV and interruption with globulin. In Vyas, GN, et al., eds. Viral hepatitis, Philadelphia, 1978, The Franklin Institute Press, p 333.

Berger RL, et al. Exchange transfusion in the treatment of fulminating hepatitis. N Engl J Med 1966;274:497.

Blumberg BS, Alter HJ, Visnich S. A "new" antigen in leukemia sera. JAMA 1965;191:541.

Blumberg BS, Sutnick AI, London WT. Hepatitis and leukemia: their relation to Australia antigen. Bull NY Acad Med 1968;44:1566.

Blumberg BS, et al. A serum antigen (Australia antigen) in Down's syndrome leukemia and hepatitis. Ann Intern Med 1967;66:924.

Boyer, JL, Klatskin G. Pattern of necrosis in acute viral hepatitis. Prognostic value of bridging (subacute hepatic necrosis). N Engl J Med 1970;283:1063.

Brechot C, Pourcel C, Louise A, et al. Presence of integrated hepatitis B virus DNA sequences in cellular DNA of human hepatocellular carcinoma. Nature 1980;286:533.

Brzosko WJ, et al. Duality of hepatitis B antigen and its antibody. I. Immunofluorescence studies. J Infect Dis 1973;127:648.

Brzosko WJ, et al. Glomerulonephritis associated with hepatitis B surface antigen immune complexes in children. Lancet 1974;2:477.

Burnell JM, et al. Acute hepatic coma treated by cross-circulation or exchange transfusion. N Engl J Med 1967;276:935.

Burrell CJ, et al. Expression in *Escherichia coli* of heptatitis B virus DNA sequences cloned in plasma PBR322, Nature 1979;279:43.

Capps, RB, Bennett, AM, and Stokes J, Jr. Endemic infectious hepatitis in an infants' orphanage. I. Epidemiologic studies in student nurses. Arch Intern Med 1952;89:6.

Capps RB, et al. Infectious hepatitis in infants and small children. Am J Dis Child 1955;89:701.

Center for Disease Control. Nomenclature of antigens associated with viral hepatitis, type B. Morbid Mortal Weekly Rep. 1974;23:29.

Chalmers TG, et al. Treatment of acute infectious hepatitis. Controlled studies of the effects of diet, rest, and physical reconditioning on the acute course of the disease and on the incidence of relapses and residual abnormalities. J Clin Invest 1955;34:1163.

Chau KH, Hargie MP, Decker RH, et al. Serodiagnosis of recent hepatitis B infection by IgM class anti-HBc. Hepatology 1983;3:141.

Combes B, et al. Glomerulonephritis with deposition of Australia antigen-antibody complexes in glomerular basement membrane. Lancet 1971;2:234.

Coulepis AG, Locarnini SA, Westaway EG, et al. Biophysical and biochemical characterization of hepatitis A virus. Intervirology 1982;18:107.

Daemer RJ, Feinstone SM, Gust ID, et al. Propagation of human hepatitis A virus in African Green Monkey Kidney cell culture: primary isolation and serial passage. Infect Immun 1981;32:388.

Dane DS, Cameron CH, Briggs M. Virus-like particles in serum of patients with Australia-antigen-associated hepatitis. Lancet 1970;1:695.

Deinhardt, F, et al. Studies on the transmission of human viral hepatitis to marmoset monkeys. I. Transmission of disease, serial passages, and description of liver lesions. J Exp Med 1966;125:673.

Delaplane D, Yogev R, Crussi G, Schulman ST. Fatal hepatitis in early infancy. Pediatrics 1983;72:176.

Desmyter J, et al. Administration of human fibroblast interferon in chronic hepatitis-B infection. Lancet 1976;2:645.

Dienstag JL, Feinstone SM, Kapikian AZ, Purcell RH. Fecal shedding of hepatitis-A antigen. Lancet 1975a;1:765.

Dienstag JL, et al. Experimental infection of chimpanzees with hepatitis A virus. J Infect Dis 1975b;132:532.

Duermeyer W, van der Veen J, Koster B. ELISA in hepatitis A. Lancet 1978;1:823.

Dupuy JW, Frommel D, Alagille D. Severe viral hepatitis type B in infancy. Lancet 1975;1:191.

Edmondson HA. Needle biopsy in differential diagnosis of acute liver disease. JAMA 1965;191:136.

Fawaz KA, Grady GF, Kaplan MM, Gellis SS. Repetitive maternal-fetal transmission of fatal hepatitis B. N Engl J Med 1975;293:1357.

Feinstone SM, Kapikian AZ, Purcell RH. Hepatitis A: detection by immune electron microscopy of a virus-like antigen associated with acute illness. Science 1973; 182:1026.

Findlay GM, Martin NH. Jaundice following yellow fever immunization. Lancet 1943;1:678.

Freeman G. Epidemiology and incubation period of jaundice following yellow fever vaccination. Am J Trop Med 1946;26:15.

Frösner GG. Nachweis von hepatitis-A-infection. Munch Med Wochenschr 1977;119:825.

Gauss-Muller V, Frosner GG, Deinhardt F. Propagation of hepatitis A virus in human embryo fibroblasts. J Med Virol 1981;7:233.

Gianotti F. Papular acrodermatitis of childhood: an Australia antigen disease. Arch Dis Child 1973;48:794.

Giles JP, Liebhaber H, Krugman S, Lattimer C. Early viremia and viruria in infectious hepatitis. Virology 1964;24:107.

Giles JP, et al. Viral hepatitis: relationship of Australia/SH antigen to the Willowbrook MS-2 strain. N Engl J Med 1969;281:119.

Gocke DJ. Extrahepatic manifestations of viral hepatitis. Am J Med Sci 1975;270:49.

Gocke DJ, et al. Association between polyarteritis and Australia antigen. Lancet 1970;3:1149.

Gocke DJ. et al. Vasculitis in association with Australia antigen. J Exp Med 1971;134:330.

Grady GF, et al. Risk of posttransfusion hepatitis in the United States: a prospective cooperative study. JAMA 1972;220:692.

Grady GF, et al. Hepatitis B immune globulin—prevention of hepatitis from accidental exposure among medical personnel. N Engl J Med 1975;293:1067.

Greenberg HB, et al. Effect of human leukocyte interferon on hepatitis B virus infection in patients with chronic active hepatitis. N Engl J Med 1976;295:517.

Hadler SC, DeMonzon M, Ponzetto A, et al. Delta virus infection and severe hepatitis: an epidemic in Yucpa Indians of Venezuela. Ann Intern Med 1984;100:339-344.

Havens WP, Jr. Etiology and epidemiology of viral hepatitis. JAMA 1957;165:1091.

Havens WP, Jr., Paul JR. Prevention of infectious hepatitis with gamma globulin. JAMA 1945;127:144.

Havens WP, Jr, Paul JR. Infectious hepatitis and serum hepatitis. In Horsfall FL, Jr, Tamm I, eds. Viral and rickettsial infections of man. ed. 4. Philadelphia: JB Lippincott Co., 1965.

Havens WP, Jr, Ward R, Drill VA, Paul JR. Experimental production of hepatitis by feeding icterogenic materials. Proc Soc Biol Med 1944;53:206.

Heathcote J, Cameron CH, Dane DS. Hepatitis-B antigen in saliva and semen. Lancet 1974;1:71.

Hilleman MR, et al. Purified and inactivated human hepatitis B vaccine: progress report. Am J Med Sci 1975;270:401.

Hirschman RJ, et al. Virus-like particles in sera of patients with infectious and serum hepatitis. JAMA 1969;208:1667.

Holland PV, et al. Gamma globulin in the prophylaxis of posttransfusion hepatitis. JAMA 1966;196:471.

Hollinger FB, Bradley DW, Dreesman GR, et al. Detection of hepatitis A viral antigen by radioimmunoassay. J Immunol 1975;115:1464.

Hollinger FB, Vorndam V, Dreesman GR. Assay of Australia antigen and antibody employing double antibody and solid-phase radioimmunoassay techniques and comparison with the passive hemagglutination methods. J Immunol 1971;107:1099.

Holmes ZW, et al. Hepatitis in marmosets: induction of disease with coded specimens from a human volunteer study. Science 1969;165:816.

Hoofnagle JH, Gerety RJ, Barker LR. Antibody to hepatitis B virus core in man. Lancet 1973;2:869.

Hoofnagle JH, Gerety RJ, Barker LF. Antibody to the hepatitis B surface antigen in immune serum globulin. Transfusion 1975;15:408.

Horstmann DM, Havens WP, Jr, Deutsch J. Infectious hepatitis in childhood. A report of 2 institutional outbreaks and a comparison of the disease in adults and children. J Pediatr 1947;30:381.

Ishimaru Y, et al. An epidemic of infantile papular acrodermatitic (Gianotti's disease) in Japan associated with hepatitis B surface antigen subtype ayw. Lancet 1976; 1:707.

Jones PO, et al. Viral hepatitis: a staff hazard in dialysis units. Lancet 1967;1:835.

Kaplan PM, et al. DNA polymerase associated with human hepatitis B antigen. J Virol 1973;12:995.

Karmen A, Wrobiewski F, LaDue JW. Transaminase activity in human blood. J Clin Invest 1955;34:126.

Karvountzis GD, Redeker AG, Peters RL. Long term follow-up studies of patients surviving fulminant viral hepatitis. Gastroenterology 1974;67:870.

Katz R, Rodriguez J, Ward R. Posttransfusion hepatitis: effect of modified gamma globulin added to blood in vitro. N Engl J Med 1971;285:925.

Kelsey WM, Scharyl M. Fatal hepatitis probably due to indomethacin. JAMA 1967;199:154.

Khuroo MS. Study of an epidemic of non-A, non-B hepatitis. Am J Med 1980;68:818-824.

Kohler PF, et al. Chronic membranous glomerulonephritis caused by hepatitis B antigen-antibody immune complexes. Ann Intern Med 1974a;81:488.

Kohler PF, et al.. Prevention of neonatal hepatitis B with antibody to HB_s Ag. N Engl J Med 1947b;291:1378.

Kojima S, Shibayoma T, Sato A, et al. Propagation of human hepatitis A virus in conventional cell lines. J Med Virol 1981;7:273.

Krugman S. Viral hepatitis, type B: prospects for active immunization. Am J Med Sci 1975;270:391.

Krugman S. Incubation period of type B hepatitis. N Engl J Med 1979;300:625.

Krugman S, Friedman H, Lattimer C. Viral hepatitis, type A: identification by specific complement fixation and immune adherence tests. N Engl J Med 1975;292:1141.

Krugman S, Giles JP. Viral hepatitis: new light on an old disease. JAMA 1970;212:1019.

Krugman S, Giles JP. Viral hepatitis type B (MS-2 strain): further observations on natural history and prevention. N Engl J Med 1973;288:755.

Krugman S, Giles JP, Hammond J. Infectious hepatitis: evidence for two distinctive clinical, epidemiological and immunological types of infection. JAMA 1967;200:365.

Krugman S, Giles JP, Hammond J. Hepatitis virus: effect of heat on the infectivity and antigenicity of the MS-1 and MS-2 strains. J Infect Dis 1970;122:432.

Krugman S, Giles JP, Hammond J. Viral hepatitis, type B (MS-2 strain): prevention with specific hepatitis B immune serum globulin. JAMA 1971a;218:1665.

Krugman S, Giles JP, Hammond J. Viral hepatitis, type B (MS-2 strain): studies on active immunization. JAMA 1971b;217:41.

Krugman S, Ward R. Infectious hepatitis: current status of prevention with gamma globulin. Yale J Biol Med 1962;34:329.

Krugman S, Ward R, Giles JP. The natural history of infectious hepatitis. Am J Med 1962;32:717.

Krugman S, Ward R, Giles JP, Jacobs AM. Infectious hepatitis: studies on the effect of gamma globulin and on the incidence of inapparent infection. JAMA 1960;174:825.

Krugman S, et al. Viral hepatitis, type B: DNA polymerase activity and antibody to hepatitis B core antigen. N Engl J Med 1974;290:1331.

Krugman S, et al. Viral hepatitis, type B: studies on natural history and prevention re-examined. N Engl J Med 1979;300:101.

LeBouvier GL. The heterogeneity of Australia antigen. J Infect Dis 1971;123:671.

LeBouvier GL. Subspecificities of the Australia antigen complex. Am J Dis Child 1972;123:420.

Levo Y, et al. Association between hepatitis B virus and essential mixed cryoglobulinemia. N Engl J Med 1977;296:1501.

Lieberman HM, La Brecque DR, Kew MC, et al. Detection of hepatitis B virus DNA directly in human serum by a simplified molecular hybridization tests: comparison to HBeAg/anti-HBe status in HBsAg carriers. Hepatology 1983;3:285.

Ling CM, Overby LR. Prevalence of hepatitis B virus antigen as revealed by direct radioimmune assay with I-125 antibody. J Immunol 1972;109:834.

Linnemann CC, Jr, Goldberg S. HB Ag in breast milk. Lancet 1974;2:155.

Lorenz D, et al. Hepatitis in the marmoset, *Saguinus mystax*, Proc Soc Exp Biol Med 1970;135:348.

Lucke B, Mallory T. The fulminant form of epidemic hepatitis. Am J Pathol 1946;22:867.

Lürman A. Eine Icterusepidemie. Berl Klin Wochenschr 1885;22:20.

Magnuis LO, Espmark A. A new antigen complex co-occurring with Australia antigen. Acta Pathol Microbiol Scand 1972;80:335.

Mallory TB. The pathology of epidemic hepatitis. JAMA 1947;134:655.

Mascoli CC, et al. Recovery of hepatitis agents in the marmoset from human cases occurring in Costa Rica. Proc Soc Exp Biol Med 1973;143:276.

Maupas PAG, et al. Immunization against hepatitis B in man. Lancet 1976;1:1367.

Maynard JE. Infectivity studies of hepatitis A and B in non human primates. Proc Int Assoc Biol Stand Symposium on Viral Hepatitis. Milan, Italy: December 16-19, 1974.

Maynard JE, Berquist KR, Krushak DH, Purcell RH. Experimental infection of chimpanzees with the virus of hepatitis B. Nature 1972;237:514.

MacNab GM, Alexander JJ, Lecatsas G, et al. Hepatitis B surface antigen produced by a human hepatoma cell line. Br J Cancer 1976;34:509.

Melnick JL. Classification of hepatitis A virus as enterovirus type 72 and of hepatitis B virus as hepadna virus, type I. Intervirology 1982;18:105.

Meltzer M, et al. Cryoglobulinemia—a clinical and laboratory study. II. Cryoglobulins with rheumatoid factor activity. Am J Med 1966;40:837.

Miller WJ, et al. Specific immune adherence assay for human hepatitis A antibody. Application of diagnostic and epidemiologic investigations. Proc Soc Exp Biol Med 1975;149:254.

Mirick GS, Shank RE. An epidemic of serum hepatitis studies under controlled conditions. Trans Am Clin Climatol Assoc 1959;71:176.

Mirick GS, Ward R, McCollum RW. Modification of posttransfusion hepatitis by gamma globulin. N Engl J Med 1965;273:59.

Mosley JW. The surveillance of transfusion-associated viral hepatitis. JAMA 1965;193:1007.

Mosley JW, et al. Multiple hepatitis viruses in multiple attacks of acute viral hepatitis. N Engl J Med 1977;296:75.

Murphy BL, Maynard JE, Bradley DW, et al. Immunofluorescence of hepatitis A virus antigen in chimpanzees. Infect Immun 1978;21:663.

Neefe JR, Gellis SS, Stokes J, Jr. Homologous serum hepatitis and infectious (epidemic) hepatitis. Studies in volunteers bearing on immunological and other characteristics of the etiological agents. Am J Med 1946;1:3.

Neurath AR, Strick N. Association of HBeAg determinants with the core of Dane particles. J Gen Virol 1979;42:645.

Okochi K, Murakami S. Observations on Australia antigen in Japanese. Vox Sang 1968;15:374.

Peterson DA, Hurley TR, Hoff JC, et al. Hepatitis A virus infectivity and chlorine treatment. In Szmuness W, Alter HJ, Maynard JE, (eds) Proceedings, 1981 International Symposium on Viral Hepatitis. Philadelphia: Franklin Institute Press, 1982, p 624.

Plouvier B, Wattre P, Devulder B. HBsAg in superficial artery of a patient with polymyalgia rheumatica. Lancet 1978;2:932.

Popper H, Shih JW-K, Gerin JL, et al. Woodchuck hepatitis and hepatocellular carcinoma: correlation of histologic with virologic observations. Hepatology 1981;1:91.

Prince AM. An antigen detected in the blood during the incubation period of serum hepatitis. Proc Natl Acad Sci USA 1968;60:814.

Prince AM, et al. Antibody against serum-hepatitis antigen: prevalence and potential use as immune serum globulin in prevention of serum hepatitis infections. N Engl J Med 1971;285:933.

Prince AM, et al. Long-incubation period posttransfusion hepatitis without serological evidence of exposure to hepatitis B virus. Lancet 1974;2:241.

Prince AM, et al. Hepatitis B "immune" globulin; effectiveness in prevention of dialysis-associated hepatitis. N Engl J Med 1975;293:1063.

Propert SA. Hepatitis after prophylactic serum. Br Med J 1938;1:677.

Provost PJ, Giesa PA, McAleer WJ, et al. Isolation of hepatitis A virus in vitro in cell culture directly from human specimens. Proc Soc Exp Biol Med 1981;167:201.

Provost PJ, Hilleman MR. Propagation of human hepatitis A virus in cell culture in vitro. Proc Soc Exp Biol Med 1979;160:213.

Provost PJ, Ittensohn OL, Villarejos VM, Hilleman MR. A specific complement fixation test for human hepatitis A employing CR326 virus antigen. Diagnosis and epidemiology. Proc Soc Exp Biol Med 1975a;148:961.

Provost PJ, Wolanski BS, Miller WJ, Ittensohn OL. Biophysical and biochemical properties of CR326 human hepatitis virus. Am J Med Sci 1975b;270:87.

Provost PF, et al. Recovery of hepatitis agents in the marmoset from human cases occurring in Costa Rica. Proc Soc Exp Biol Med 1973;142:1257.

Purcell RH, Feinstone SM, Kapikian AZ. Recent advances in hepatitis A research. In Greenwalt T, Jamieson GA, eds. Transmissible disease and blood transfusion. New York: Grune & Stratton, Inc., 1975.

Purcell RH, Gerin JL. Hepatitis B subunit vaccine: a preliminary report of safety and efficacy tests in chimpanzees. Am J Med Sci 1975;270:395.

Purcell RH, et al. A complement-fixation test for measuring Australia antigen and antibody. J Infect Dis 1969;120:383.

Purcell RH, et al. Serologic tests for the detection of the internal component of the Dane particle (a virus-like particle antigenically related to hepatitis B antigen) and its antibody. Intervirology 1973/1974;2:231.

Purcell RH, et al. Inactivated hepatitis B vaccine. Am J Med Sci 1975;270:395.

Redeker AG. Viral hepatitis: clinical aspects. Am J Med Sci 1975;270:9.

Redeker AG, Yamahiro HS. Controlled trial of exchange-transfusion therapy in fulminant hepatitis. Lancet 1973; 1:3.

Redeker AG, et al. Hepatitis B immune globulin as a prophylactic measure for spouses exposed to acute type B hepatitis. N Engl J Med 1975;293:1055.

Reesink, HW, et al. Prevention of chronic HBsAg carrier state in infants of HBsAg-positive mothers by hepatitis B immunoglobulin. Lancet 1979;2:436.

Ringertz B, Zetterberg B. Serum hepatitis among Swedish track finders. N Engl J Med 1967;276:540.

Rizzetto M, et al. Immunofluorescence detection of new antigen-antibody system (delta/antidelta) associated to hepatitis B virus in liver and in serum of HBsAg carriers. Gut 1977;18:997.

Schweitzer IL, Wing A, McPeak C, Spears RL. Hepatitis and hepatitis-associated antigen in 56 mother-infant pairs JAMA 1972;220:1092.

Scotto J, Hadchouel M, Herej C, et al. Detection of hepatitis B virus DNA in serum by a simple spot hybridization technique. Comparison with results for other viral markers. Hepatology 1983;3:279.

Seeff LB, Hoofnagle JH. Immunoprophylaxis of viral hepatitis. Gastroenterology 1979;77:161.

Seeff LB, et al. Efficacy of hepatitis B immune serum globulin after accidental exposure. Lancet 1975;2:939.

Sergent J, et al. Vasculitis with hepatis B antigenemia. Long term observations in nine patients. Medicine 1976;55:1.

Shafritz DA, Kew MC. Identification of integrated hepatitis B virus DNA sequences in human hepatocellular carcinoma. Hepatology 1981;1:1.

Shimizu YK, et al. Non-A, non-B hepatitis: ultrastructural evidence for two agents in experimentally infected chimpanzees. Science 1979;205:197.

Smedile A, Lavarini C, Crivelli O, et al. Radioimmunoassay detection of IgM antiboides to the HBV-associated delta antigen; clinical significance in delta infection. J Med Virol 1982;9:131.

Smetana HF. Pathologic anatomy of early stages of viral hepatitis. In Hartmann FW, et al., eds. Hepatitis frontiers. Boston: Little, Brown and Co. 1957.

Sninski JJ, et al. Cloning and endonuclease mapping of the hepatitis B viral genome. Nature 1979;279:346.

Stevens C.E., et al. Vertical transmission of hepatitis B antigen in Taiwan. N Engl J Med 1975;292:771.

Stevens CE, Taylor PE, Tong MJ, et al. Hepatitis B vaccine: an overview. In Vyas GN, Dienstag JL, Hoofnagle JH, eds. Viral hepatitis and liver disease. New York: Grune & Stratton, Inc., 1984.

Stevens CE, Toy PT, Tong MJ, et al. Perinatal hepatitis B virus transmission in the United States: prevention by passive-active immunization. JAMA 1985;253:1740.

Stokes J, Jr, et al. Infectious hepatitis. Length of protection by immune serum globulin (gamma globulin) during epidemics. JAMA 1951;147:714.

Stokes J, Jr, et al. The carrier-state in viral hepatitis. JAMA 1954;154:1059.

Szmuness W. Hepatocellular carcinoma and hepatitis B virus: evidence for a causal association. Prog Med Virol 1978;24:40.

Szmuness W, et al. Distribution of antibody to hepatitis A antigen in urban adult population. N Engl J Med 1976;295:755.

Szmuness W, et al. The prevalence of antibody to hepatitis A antigen in various parts of the world. A pilot study. Am J Epidemiol 1977;106:392.

Szmuness W, et al. Hepatitis B vaccine: demonstration of efficacy in a controlled clinical trial in a high risk population in the United States. N Engl J Med 1980;303:833.

Tandon BN, Joshi YK, Jain SK, et al. An epidemic of non-A, non-B hepatitis in North India. J Med Res 1982;75:739.

Ticehurst JR, Recaniello VR, Baroudy BM, et al. Molecular cloning and characterization of hepatitis A virus with DNA. Proc Nat Acad Sci USA 1983;80:5885.

Toda G, Ishimaru Y, Mayumi M, Oda T. Infantile papular acrodermatitis (Gianotti's disease) and intrafamilial occurrence of acute hepatitis B with jaundice: age dependency of clinical manifestations of hepatitis B virus infection. J Infect Dis 1978;138:211.

Traisman AS, Wheeler RC, Fager DB. Virus hepatitis in infancy. J Pediatr 1950;37:174.

Trepo CH, Thiyolet J. Hepatitis associated antigen and periarteritis nodosa (PAN). Vox Sang 1970;19:410.

Trey C. The fulminant hepatic surveillance study. CMA J 1972;106:525.

Trey C, Burns DG, Saunders SJ. Treatment of hepatic coma by exchange blood transfusion. N Engl J Med 1966;274:473.

Tsiquaye KN, Zickerman AJ. New human hepatitis virus. Lancet 1979;1:1135.

Villarejos VM, et al. Seroepidemiologic investigations of human hepatitis caused by A, B, and a possible third virus. Proc Soc Exp Biol Med 1976;152:524.

Voegt H. Zur Aetiologie de Hepatitis epidemica. Munch Med Wochenschr 1942;89:76.

Vyas GN, Roberts I, MacKay IR, Gust ID. Immunologic mechanisms in hepatitis B assayed by antigen-binding lymphocytes. Am J Med Sci 1975;270:241.

Vyas GN, Shulman NR. Hemagglutination assay for antigen and antibody associated with viral hepatitis. Science 1970;170:332.

Wands JR, et al. The pathogenesis of arthritis associated with acute HB_s Ag-positive hepatitis: complement activation and characterization of circulating immune complexes. Gastroenterology 1974;67:813.

Ward R, Borchert B, Wright A, Kline E. Hepatitis B antigen in saliva and mouth washing. Lancet 1972;2:726.

Ward R, Krugman S, Giles JP. Etiology and prevention of infectious hepatitis. Postgrad Med 1960;28:12.

Ward R, et al. Infectious hepatitis: studies of its natural history and prevention. N Engl J Med 1958;258:407.

Wong DC, Purcell RH, Sreenivasau MA, et al. Epidemic and endemic hepatitis in India: evidence for a non-A, non-B hepatitis virus etiology. Lancet 1980;2:882.

World Health Organization Expert Committee on Viral Hepatitis. Advances in viral hepatitis. WHO Tech Rep Ser No 602, 1977.

Wróblewski R. The clinical significance of alterations in serum transaminases in hepatitis. In Hartman FW, et al., eds. Hepatitis frontiers. Boston: Little, Brown and Co., 1957.

11

HERPESVIRUS INFECTIONS

Herpesvirus hominis (herpes simplex virus)

Herpes simplex viruses are among the most widely disseminated infectious agents of humans. The ubiquity of these viruses is not generally appreciated because they often do not produce overt disease. The various clinical syndromes caused by herpesvirus hominis are, however, common in children.

ETIOLOGY

Herpes simplex virus (HSV) has an estimated diameter of 100 to 180 nm. Electron microscopic studies by Wildy et al. in 1960 revealed that the virus particle (virion) consists of a central core, 75 nm in diameter, containing DNA and a protein coat (capsid), 100 nm in diameter, with the symmetry of an icosahedron (20-sided figure). It resembles cytomegalovirus, varicella-zoster (VZ) virus, and Epstein-Barr virus (EBV) in morphologic appearance.

Herpes simplex virus is readily transmitted to a variety of animals, including the rabbit, mouse, guinea pig, cotton rat, and hamster. While inoculation of animals is now seldom used for diagnostic purposes, it is used for studies of viral latency and the efficacy of antiviral drugs. Inoculation of the chorioallantoic membrane of embryonated eggs produces characteristic plaques or pocks. Tissue cultures infected with the virus show cytopathic effect characterized by degeneration and clumping of the cells and the presence of typical intranuclear inclusion bodies and giant cells.

Two antigenic types of HSV have been identified (Nahmias and Dowdle, 1968; Nahmias et al., 1969). Herpes simplex virus type 1 (HSV-1) has been associated chiefly with nongenital infections of the mouth, lips, eyes, and central nervous system; it may also cause genital and neonatal disease. Herpes simplex virus type 2 (HSV-2) has been most commonly associated with genital and neonatal infections; it may also cause oral disease. About 50% of the DNA of HSV-1 and HSV-2 is homologous. There are also subtypes of HSV-1 and HSV-2 that can be identified by analysis of viral DNA with restriction enzymes (Buckman et al., 1978; Corey, 1982).

PATHOGENESIS

Knowledge accumulated during the past 25 years has clarified the pathogenesis of postnatal HSV infections. The host-parasite relationship is shown in Fig. 11-1. Primary infection of a susceptible host may be inapparent. After the primary infection clears, the virus becomes latent in the ganglion cells of local nerves (Baringer and Swoveland, 1973). Various stimuli such as fever, sunlight, and trauma may cause a recurrent infection. Primary symptomatic postnatal infections may also be characterized by a vesicular eruption, fever, and other constitutional symptoms. Recurrent infections are characterized by a local vesicular eruption and absence of constitutional symptoms.

Neonatal HSV infections rarely occur during the prenatal period due to a maternal HSV viremia. Infections in the perinatal period, however, are not uncommon and seem to be increasing in incidence (Sullivan-Bolyai et al.,

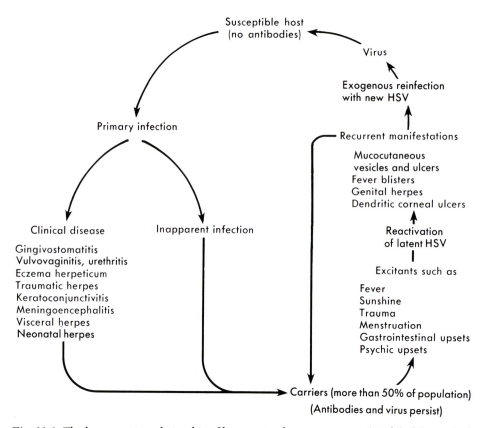

Fig. 11-1. The host-parasite relationship of herpes simplex virus in man. (Modified from Blank H, Rake G. Viral and rickettsial diseases of the skin, eye, and mucous membranes of man. Boston: Little, Brown & Co., 1955.)

1983b). Such infections are most often secondary to maternal genital HSV infection.

PATHOLOGY

The typical lesion caused by HSV in skin is a vesicle; on the mucous membranes it is an ulcer. The epithelium but not the stratum corium is usually involved so that healing followed by scarring is uncommon. Invaded epithelial cells are destroyed by the virus except for an intact superficial cornified layer that covers the vesicle; in the ulcer this upper layer is not present. Cells invaded by HSV demonstrate the following characteristics: coalescence to form multinucleated giant cells, nuclear degeneration, ballooning, and intranuclear inclusions. Cells in deeper tissues characteristically exhibit necrosis. A biopsy of a herpetic vesicle showing eosinophilic intranuclear inclusions and giant cells is shown in Plate 2, *E*.

CLINICAL MANIFESTATIONS OF PRIMARY INFECTIONS

The clinical manifestations of primary herpetic infections are determined by a variety of factors including (1) the portal of entry of the virus and (2) such host factors as age, immune competence, and presence of eczema. The various clinical entities that may be encountered are listed in Fig. 11-1. The most common type of infection in children is acute herpetic gingivostomatitis. The other diseases are relatively uncommon. The incubation period is about 6 days, with a range of 2 to 20 days.

Acute herpetic gingivostomatitis

Primary infection of the mucous membranes of the mouth is the most common HSV infection of childhood. It occurs most often in the 1- to 4-year age group; it may also occur in adoles-

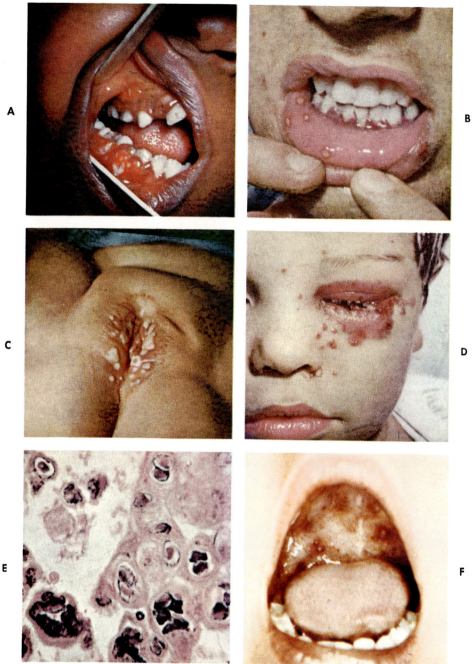

Plate 2

Herpes simplex infections. **A,** Primary herpetic gingivostomatitis in a child. **B,** Same disease in a young adult. **C,** Primary HSVI vulvovaginitis in an infant. **D,** Primary herpetic kerato-conjunctivitis. **E,** Biopsy of herpetic vesicle. Eosinophilic intranuclear inclusions and giant cells. (×800.) **F,** Ulcerative lesions on palate and tongue in hand-foot-and-mouth syndrome caused by Coxsackie A-16 virus. (**A** to **E** from Blank H, Rake G. Viral and rickettsial diseases of the skin, eye, and mucous membranes of man. Boston: Little, Brown & Co., 1955; **F** courtesy James D Cherry, MD)

cents. The illness is ushered in by an abrupt onset of fever (34.4° to 40.6° C; 103° to 105° F), irritability, anorexia, and sore mouth. Along with these severe constitutional symptoms, striking lesions appear on the mucous membranes of the oropharynx. The gums are swollen, reddened, and friable and bleed very easily (Plate 2, *A* and *B*). White 2- to 3-mm plaques or shallow ulcers with red areolae appear on the buccal mucosa, tongue, palate, and fauces. The regional anterior cervical lymph nodes become enlarged and tender. The lesions usually appear in the mouth first. Occasionally, however, they may develop on the tonsils first and subsequently progress forward.

Satellite vesicular lesions around the mouth are not uncommon. Infants with gingivostomatitis who are thumbsuckers can also infect the thumb (or other fingers) by self-inoculation.

The disease varies considerably in severity and duration. It may be extremely mild, with a paucity of lesions, low-grade fever, and minimal constitutional symptoms. Under these circumstances, the patient improves within 5 to 7 days. On the other hand, we have occasionally seen desperately ill hyperpyretic infants with extensive bleeding lesions, evidence of dehydration and acidosis, and a course that does not clear until the tenth to the fourteenth day.

Acute herpetic vulvovaginitis

In contrast to gingivostomatitis, vulvovaginitis is a rare mainfestation of HSV-1 infection in children. However, it is very common in adults, although it is usually caused by HSV-2, which is sexually transmitted. The clinical picture is similar to that of herpetic gingivostomatitis except that the pain is localized to the site of the eruption. One of our patients, a 2-year-old girl, was admitted because of dysuria and refusal to void.

The perineal area is usually reddened, edematous, and studded with painful shallow white ulcers 2 to 4 mm in diameter. Many of these lesions coalesce to form larger ulcers (Plate 2, *C*). The regional inguinal lymph nodes are enlarged and tender. The fever and constitutional symptoms subside within 5 to 7 days, and the lesions become crusted by the tenth to the fourteenth day. Healing is complete without scarring by the end of the third week. Occasionally, vulvovaginitis is associated with gingivostomatitis.

In infants and children who develop vulvovaginitis due to HSV, the virus should be typed because the possibility of child abuse must be considered. The presence of HSV-2 makes child abuse more likely.

Eczema herpeticum (Kaposi's varicelliform eruption)

This manifestation of herpetic infection of the skin was first described by Kaposi in 1887. Eczema herpeticum is characterized by vesicular and crusting eruptions superimposed on atopic eczema or chronic dermatitis. The disease is more likely to be severe if it is primary than if it is secondary. It starts abruptly with high fever (40° to 40.6° C; 104° to 105° F), irritability, and restlessness followed by the appearance of crops of vesicles concentrated chiefly on the eczematous skin. A smaller number of lesions may involve the normal skin. The lesions may appear in crops over a period of 7 to 9 days, and within a few days they rupture and become crusted. Thus, as the disease progresses, the lesions may resemble varicella.

Like other herpetic infections, this disease may vary considerably in severity. It may be either extremely mild or rapidly fatal, especially if it is primary. The extensive area of weeping, oozing skin may be associated with severe fluid loss and with superinfection by resistant microorganisms.

Traumatic herpetic infections

Traumatic herpetic infections of the skin are similar to eczema herpeticum except that they are not generalized but rather are localized to a small area. The site of an abrasion, burn, or break in the skin of a susceptible child may be infected with HSV. The source of the virus may be a sympathetic parent who has "kissed to make well" the injured site to reassure the child. Vesicular lesions that develop at the site of inoculation may be associated with fever, constitutional symptoms, and regional lymphadenopathy.

Acute herpetic keratoconjunctivitis

Primary herpetic infections of the eye are relatively rare. The fever and constitutional symptoms are associated with keratoconjunctivitis and preauricular adenopathy. Usually the infection is unilateral. The cornea has a hazy appearance and the patient may be unable to close the eyelid (Plate 2, *D*). A purulent and membranelike exudate is present. The skin around the eye may be involved by discrete vesicles. There usually is complete clearing of the eye in 2 weeks if the infection is confined chiefly to the conjunctiva. Superficial corneal involvement is characterized by the formation of typical dendritic ulcers. These infections may cause a serious impairment of sight. Deep involvement such as *keratitis disciformis*, *hypopyon keratitis*, as *iridocyclitis* almost always is accompanied by significant scarring.

Acute herpetic encephalitis and meningoencephalitis

Primary infection of the central nervous system (CNS) is an unusual manifestation of herpetic infection. Infection with HSV-2 (often in conjunction with genital HSV) is associated with a self-limited form of meningitis. In contrast, HSV-1 causes a rapidly progressing, fatal type of encephalitis, with death occurring within 1 to 2 weeks in about 70% of patients who are untreated. The clinical manifestations of 113 biopsy-proved cases of HSV-1 encephalitis are noted in Table 11-1. The encephalitis may be localized frequently in the frontotemporal area, simulating a mass lesion, or it may be widespread, involving both cerebral hemispheres. The cerebrospinal fluid (CSF) usually shows pleocytosis

Table 11-1. Historical findings and signs at presentation of 113 patients with biopsy-proved herpes simplex encephalitis*

Characteristics	Number/total	Percent
Historical findings		
Altered consciousness	109/112	97
Fever	101/112	90
Personality change	62/87	71
Headache	89/110	81
Vomiting	51/111	46
Recurrent herpes labialis	24/108	22
Memory loss	14/59	24
Signs and presentation		
Dysphasia	58/76	76
Autonomic nervous system dysfunction	53/88	60
Ataxia	22/55	40
Seizures	43/112	38
Hemiparesis	41/107	38

*Modified from Whitley RJ, et al. JAMA 1982b;247:318.

with a predominance of lymphocytes. Computerized axial tomography can often be used to localize the area of affected brain. The diagnosis is confirmed by recovering the virus from a brain biopsy. In this disease, HSV-1 can rarely be cultured from CSF.

HSV-2 meningitis is usually a relatively benign disease. However, a review of 10 cases, confirmed by a positive CSF culture, revealed evidence of chronic neurologic symptoms lasting up to 10 months in two patients; three patients developed recurrent meningitis (Hevron, 1977).

Neonatal HSV infections

HSV infections in premature and newborn infants are usually caused by HSV-2, the most common cause of maternal genital infections; HSV-1 infections are less common. Transplacental antibodies do not protect an infant from acquiring infection (Nahmias et al., 1971), although antibodies may provide partial protection (Yeager et al., 1980). At the end of the first week of life, an infant may develop fever or hypothermia, progressively increasing icterus, hepatosplenomegaly, and vesicular lesions. Anorexia, vomiting, lethargy, respiratory distress, cyanosis, and circulatory collapse may follow. Untreated, the outcome is frequently fatal. The presence of skin vesicles is helpful in identifying neonatal herpes infection. However, skin lesions may be absent in about 20% of infected infants.

Arvin et al. (1982) have noted that the diagnosis of neonatal HSV should be considered in babies with signs and symptoms of bacterial sepsis and/or meningitis when no bacterial etiology can be identified.

Whitley et al. (1980a,b, 1983) prospectively studied 95 infants with culture-proven neonatal HSV. There were three classifications: disseminated disease (hepatitis, pneumonia, and/or disseminated intravascular coagulation, with or without CNS involvement) (51%), CNS involvement alone (32%), and disease localized to the eye, skin, or mouth (17%). Untreated, the overall mortality was about 70%, with 85% mortality for disseminated, 50% for CNS, and 0% for localized mucocutaneous infections. With antiviral therapy, mortality decreased to 50% and 10% in the first two groups, respectively.

HSV in immunocompromised patients

In the immunocompromised host, herpes simplex infections may show two unusual courses. Disseminated disease may occur with widespread dermal, mucosal, and visceral involvement. Disease may, in contrast, remain localized but with a greatly prolonged course, persisting for periods as long as 9 months with indolent, often painful, ulcerative lesions (Schneidman et al., 1979). These two forms of the infection appear more likely in patients whose T lymphocyte function has been suppressed.

RECURRENT INFECTIONS

Recurrent herpetic infections are more common than primary infections. The most common type of infection is herpes labialis, the well-known fever sore. Other recurrent lesions may appear on any part of the skin or mucous membranes. As indicated before, they are generally mild and not associated with fever and constitutional symptoms. Two exceptions to this general rule are HSV encephalitis, which may be a primary or secondary infection (Whitley et al., 1982a,b), and severe HSV in the immunocompromised, which may be recurrent and yet severe.

DIAGNOSIS

Infection with HSV should be suspected in a patient who develops fever, constitutional symptoms, and a vesicular exanthem or enanthem. The diagnosis can be confirmed by (1) isolation of virus from, or demonstration of viral antigens in, the local lesion, (2) serologic tests showing a significant rise in the level of antibody during convalescence from a primary infection, and (3) histologic evidence of type A intranuclear inclusion bodies and multinucleated giant cells. Electron microscopy can be used to identify icosahedral HSV particles.

Isolation of virus

HSV can be cultivated in a variety of cell cultures, such as primary rabbit or monkey kidney, human embryonic lung fibroblasts (HELF), and diploid human fibroblasts (Wl-38). Inoculation of these cultures produces cytopathic changes associated with intranuclear inclusion bodies and multinucleated giant cells.

Results are usually available within 24 to 48 hours because HSV grows rapidly in tissue cultures. Typing of the virus requires more time and it is costly; therefore, it is not often routinely performed. Culture is superior to Papanicolaou smears for diagnosis of genital HSV, since the

latter is nonspecific and may yield false-negative and false-positive results.

Serologic tests

Paired samples of sera from the acute phase and the convalescent phase should be tested for HSV antibodies. The levels of these antibodies begin to rise by the end of the first week of illness following a primary infection. The demonstration of a significant increase in antibody titer is a helpful confirmatory test. Usually no rise is associated with recurrent disease.

Histologic studies

The demonstration of acidophilic intranuclear inclusion bodies, multinucleated giant cells, and ballooning degeneration of the epithelial cells of a lesion from biopsy material reinforces the diagnosis. Immunofluorescence with specific antiserum can be helpful to confirm such a tissue diagnosis.

DIFFERENTIAL DIAGNOSIS
Acute herpetic gingivostomatitis

Acute herpetic gingivostomatitis can usually be recognized clinically and requires no laboratory confirmation. The following diseases may be confused with it.

Herpangina. The lesions of herpangina, caused by group A Coxsackie virus, are indistinguishable in appearance from those of herpes simplex virus (p. 47). However, the distribution of the lesions enables one to separate these two conditions clinically. In herpangina they are usually confined to the anterior fauces and soft palate; gingivitis does not occur. In herpetic infection, gingivitis is a typical manifestation.

Acute membranous tonsillitis. Acute membranous tonsillitis secondary to streptococcal infection, EBV infection, diphtheria, and other infections may simulate herpetic involvement of the tonsillar area. Invariably, herpetic lesions appear on tongue, buccal mucosa, palate, and gingival tissues. In some cases cultures and blood smears may be helpful diagnostic aids.

Thrush. Thrush is generally not associated with fever and constitutional symptoms. Lesions are polymorphous elevated white plaques without ulceration.

Acute herpetic vulvovaginitis

Any involvement of the skin of the perineal area may simulate herpetic vulvovaginitis. The following conditions are most commonly confused.

Ammoniacal dermatitis with secondary infection. Fever and systemic symptoms are absent as a rule. The lesions extend onto the thighs and diaper area.

Gonorrheal, diphtheritic, and monilial vulvovaginitis. Lesions can be identified by appropriate cultures.

Impetigo. Lesions are usually present elsewhere, particularly on the nares and other sites readily scratched.

Eczema herpeticum

Herpetic infection of eczematous skin lesions must be differentiated from the following conditions.

Eczema vaccinatum. Eczema vaccinatum is extremely difficult to distinguish clinically. This disease is now unusual because smallpox vaccination is rarely used. Virus isolation and serologic studies will identify the cause.

Varicella and smallpox. Varicella and smallpox also must be differentiated from eczema herpeticum (pp. 441 and 460, respectively).

Eczema with secondary infection. The lesions may resemble eczema herpeticum, but fever and constitutional symptoms are usually not present.

Traumatic herpetic infections

Traumatic herpetic infections may be confused with herpes zoster or with secondary bacterial infection of the site that has been traumatized. Virus isolation and serologic tests are required to establish the diagnosis.

Acute herpetic keratoconjunctivitis

Unilateral preauricular adenitis secondary to a membranous conjunctivitis or the so-called Parinaud's syndrome may be caused by Newcastle disease virus, adenovirus type 8 (epidemic keratoconjunctivitis), and tuberculosis. Laboratory procedures must be employed to confirm the diagnosis.

Neonatal HSV

In infants without vesicular lesions HSV may be confused with bacterial sepsis or meningitis. Infants with skin manifestations may appear to have impetigo. Rapid diagnosis of neonatal HSV is important because early treatment with an antiviral drug improves the outcome. If skin lesions are not present, the diagnosis may be made by isolation of HSV from the mouth and conjunctiva, or rarely from urine or CSF.

HSV encephalitis

Many other conditions mimic HSV encephalitis. These include vascular disease, brain abscess, other forms of viral encephalitis (enterovirus, mumps, Epstein-Barr virus, measles, influenza, arbovirus), cryptococcal infection, tumor, toxic encephalopathy, Reye's syndrome, toxoplasmosis, tuberculosis, and lymphocytic choriomeningitis. Therefore, if CAT scanning suggests HSV encephalitis, a brain biopsy is mandatory. This procedure may not only confirm the suspected diagnosis of HSV encephalitis; it has also been helpful in distinguishing it from the other diseases listed above (Whitley et al., 1981).

COMPLICATIONS

Bacterial complications rarely occur in acute gingivostomatitis. Dehydration and acidosis may result from refusal of fluids because of extensive and painful lesions of the mouth.

Eczema herpeticum may occasionally become secondarily infected. This infection may become a potential focus for the development of septicemia.

PROGNOSIS

The prognosis of acute herpetic gingivostomatitis is excellent. Extensive eczema herpeticum, neonatal HSV, and herpes simplex encephalitis are highly fatal and should be treated with an antiviral drug.

IMMUNITY

Many infants are born with HSV antibodies passively acquired from the mother. The passive immunity is not protective and it disappears by 6 months of age. Active immunity develops after an apparent or inapparent primary infection with HSV. Immunity to HSV, however, is incomplete and does not necessarily protect against future exogenous herpetic infections or against recurrent endogenous herpetic infections (Buckman et al., 1979).

In lower socioeconomic groups, most individuals have been infected with HSV-1 before 6 years of age. In contrast, in upper socioeconomic groups, much of the population may escape primary HSV-1 infection in the first decade of life; in these groups young adults may experience primary HSV-1 gingivostomatitis. For HSV-2 infections, as with other sexually transmitted diseases, the highest rate of incidence of disease is during the second and third decades of life.

EPIDEMIOLOGIC FACTORS

Primary infection occurs predominantly in infants and preschool children between the ages of 1 and 4 years. Persons of either sex are equally susceptible. The highest incidence of infection occurs in children of lower socioeconomic groups who live in crowded environments. The disease is worldwide in distribution.

The infection is presumably spread by intimate contact. Virus may be recovered from saliva, skin lesions, urine, and stools, all of which are potential sources of infection. Patients with recurrent lesions may shed infectious virus-antibody complexes.

Juretić (1966) reported an extensive study of the natural history of herpetic infection in 4191 Yugoslavian children. The incidence of clinically apparent infection, primary herpetic gingivostomatitis, was 12.1%. The peak incidence according to age was in the second year of life, and there was no seasonal variation. Adults with herpetic lesions proved to be the chief source of infection. Nine minor epidemics were observed. The incubation period was 2 to 12 days, with a mean of 6.1 days.

Neonatal HSV is usually acquired from a maternal source. Delivery of an infant by cesarean section when the mother has genital lesions will usually prevent infection of the infant if the fetal membranes remain intact or have been ruptured for less than 4 hours prior to delivery. Today most infants who develop neonatal HSV are born vaginally to mothers with no history or knowledge of genital HSV. Investigators in the field recognize the need for a rapid practical screening test for maternal genital HSV. Infants may also on occasion be inadvertently infected via scalp monitors during delivery (Parvey and Ch'ien, 1980), infected breast milk (Sullivan-Bolyai et al., 1983a), in intensive care nurseries (Hammerberg et al., 1983), and from other family members (Yeager et al., 1983). The availability of molecular biologic techniques for viral "finger printing" using restriction endonucleas-

es to evaluate the DNA of HSV isolates has been invaluable in proving many of these transmissions. The newborn is believed to be highly susceptible to HSV infections because of immaturity of cell-mediated immune responses to the virus (Kohl, 1983).

TREATMENT

The treatment of mucocutaneous HSV is chiefly supportive. Antibiotics do not affect the course of any type of herpetic infection. In cases of eczema herpeticum with secondary infection, antimicrobial therapy is indicated after preliminary cultures have been obtained.

Infants require careful observation for possible dehydration. Fluids should be given parenterally if necessary. Citrus fruit juices and other irritating liquids or foods should be avoided. Cold drinks and bland fruit juices such as apricot, pear, and peach juices seem to be fairly well tolerated.

Herpetic keratoconjunctivitis should be treated by an ophthalmologist.

Several forms of antiviral chemotherapy are now available for treatment of severe or life-threatening HSV infections. Interferon (α or type I) is effective for prophylaxis against HSV in high-risk patients and for treatment of severe mucocutaneous HSV infections. It remains unlicensed, however, and it is somewhat toxic when used over long periods of time for prophylaxis or at high dosage for treatment. It is therefore not now the drug of choice for treatment of HSV.

Acyclovir (ACV), a compound that specifically inhibits synthesis of viral DNA with little effect on host DNA synthesis, may well be the most significant antiviral drug against HSV in the future. It has little associated toxicity and is well tolerated. Topical (5% ointment in a polyethylene glycol base) and intravenous forms are licensed in the United States. Topical ACV is only minimally effective for treatment of *primary* genital HSV. It shortens the course from 2 weeks to about 11 days. It also reduces the duration of viral shedding from 7 to 4 days (Corey, 1982). It has no effect on oral HSV. Oral acyclovir results in higher blood levels than does topical use and hastens healing of both primary and recurrent oral and genital HSV (Reichman et al., 1984; Straus et al., 1984; Douglas et al., 1984). This form of ACV may be used to treat moderately severe mucocutaneous HSV infections. When it was given daily for 4 months it suppressed recurrences of HSV in patients with frequent episodes of reactivation. However, there was a rebound phenomenon when ACV was stopped (Douglas et al., 1984). The adult dose for oral ACV is 200 mg five times daily. The drug should not be used for patients in whom the course of HSV is mild or likely to be self-limited. Strains of HSV resistant to ACV are beginning to be described.

Intravenous ACV is licensed for use in immunocompromised patients with severe mucocutaneous HSV. It is used at a dose of 15 mg/kg/day (Hirsch and Schooley, 1983). Acyclovir given intravenously has been successfully used to treat HSV encephalitis (Sköldenberg et al., 1984) and neonatal HSV (Whitley, personal communication). Neonates were given a dose of 30 mg/kg/day divided into three doses.

Adenine arabinoside (Ara-A; vidarabine) has been used for treatment of HSV encephalitis, although it is more toxic than ACV. In a study by Whitley et al. (1981) of 93 patients with brain biopsy-proven HSV encephalitis, the overall mortality rate fell to about 40%, in comparison to a mortality rate of 70% in untreated patients. Survival was most obviously improved in patients under 30 years of age who were treated before onset of coma. Subsequent morbidity was also less in this group than in older, comatose patients, although recovery could take as long as 1 year. The dose of Ara-A employed was 10 mg/kg/day intravenously in 12 hours of fluids, for 10 days. Ara-A is poorly soluble in aqueous media, so that a fairly large fluid volume is usually required to administer the drug.

Ara-A has also been used to treat neonatal HSV (Whitley et al., 1980a,b, 1983). In 59 infants with disseminated or localized CNS HSV infections, the mortality rate was about 40% in comparison with an untreated similar group in which the mortality was about 70%. There was no difference in mortality rate with a dose of Ara-A of 30 mg/kg/day compared to 15 mg/kg/day. The lower dose is therefore recommended and should be given intravenously over 12 hours for a 10-day period.

Since the incidence of progression to CNS or disseminated disease is over 50% in babies presenting with infection localized to the skin or eye, it is mandantory to treat all babies under 1 month of age with documented HSV infection, even if their symptoms are mild.

Certain forms of therapy for HSV infections that were once proposed but have now been discarded include systemic iododeoxyuridine (IDUR), neutral red dye and light, and topical Ara-A for mucocutaneous lesions.

PREVENTIVE MEASURES

Herpetic infections are difficult to prevent. Efforts should be made to protect eczematous infants from persons with herpetic lesions. Infants delivered to mothers with active genital herpes lesions have less risk of neonatal infection if they are delivered by cesarean section before or within 4 hours of rupture of membranes. Newborn infants should not be exposed to personnel with herpes labialis. Smallpox vaccination is not indicated for the prevention of recurrent herpes; it is useless and potentially harmful (Visentine et al., 1978). The advantages of a successful herpes simplex virus vaccine are apparent; attempts to develop one that is safe and of proved efficacy are currently being made. These include a subunit vaccine prepared from glycoprotein D, an antigen of both HSV-1 and HSV-2 that is known to stimulate neutralizing antibodies against both types of virus (Long et al., 1984). Whether this antigen also stimulates cellular immunity (CMI) against HSV and the exact importance of CMI in protection against HSV is being explored.

REFERENCES

Arvin AM, Yeager AS, Bruhn FW, Grossman M. Neonatal herpes simplex infection in the absence of mucocutaneous lesions, J Pediatr 1982;100:715-721.

Baringer JR. Recovery of herpes simplex virus from human sacral ganglions. N Engl J Med 1974;291:828.

Baringer JR, Swoveland R. Recovery of herpes simplex virus from human trigeminal ganglions. N Engl J Med 1973;288:648-650.

Blank H, Rake G. Viral and rickettsial diseases of the skin, eye, and mucous membranes of man. Boston: Little, Brown & Co., 1955.

Buchman TG, Roizman B, Adams G, Stover BH. Restriction endonuclease fingerprinting of herpes simplex virus DNA: a novel epidemiologic tool applied to a nosocomial outbreak, J Infect Dis 1978;138:488-498.

Buchman TG, Roizman B, Nahmias AJ. Demonstration of exogenous genital reinfection with herpes simplex virus type 2 by restriction endonuclease fingerprinting of viral DNA. J Infect Dis 1979;140:295-304.

Cohen GH, Dietzschold B, Ponce-de-Leon M, et al. Localization and synthesis of an antigenic determinant of

HSV glycoprotein D that stimulates the production of neutralizing antibody. J Virol 1984;49:102-108.

Corey L. The diagnosis and treatment of genital herpes. JAMA 1982;248:1041-1049.

Daniels CA, LeGoff S, Notkins AL. Shedding of infectious virus antibody complexes from vesicular lesions of patients with recurrent herpes labialis. Lancet 1975;2:524.

Doane F, Rhodes AJ, Ormsby HL. Rapid diagnosis of herpetic infections by isolation of virus in tissue cultures. Can Med Assoc J 1955;73:260.

Dodd K, Johnston LM, Buddingh GJ. Herpetic stomatitis. J Pediatr 1938;12:95.

Douglas JM, Critchlow C, Benedetti J, et al. A double-blind study of oral acyclovir for suppression of recurrences of genital herpes simplex virus infection. N Engl J Med 1984;310:1551-1556.

Florman AL, Gershon AA, Blackett PR, Nahmias AJ. Intrauterine infection with herpes simplex virus: resultant congenital malformations. JAMA 1973;225:129-132.

Frenkel N, Roizman B. Ribonucleic acid synthesis in cells infected with herpes simplex virus: controls of transcription and of RNA abundance. Proc Natl Acad Sci USA 1972;69:2654.

Granström KO. A contribution to the knowledge of the importance of herpes infections in corneal and conjunctival infections, especially in membranous conjunctivitis. Acta Ophthalmol 1937;15:361.

Hamilton JB. Notes on forms of keratitis presumably due to the virus of herpes simplex. Br J Ophthalmol 1943;27:80.

Hammerberg O, Watts J, Chernesky M, et al. An outbreak of herpes simplex virus type 1 in an intensive care nursery. Pediatr Infect Dis 1983;2:290-294.

Hevron JE. Herpes simplex virus type 2 meningitis. Obstet Gynecol 1977;49:622.

Hirsch MS, Schooley RT. Treatment of herpesvirus infections. N Engl J Med 1983;309:963-970, 1034-1039.

Juretić M. Natural history of herpetic infection. Helv Paediatr, Acta 1966;21:356.

Kaufman HE. Treatment of herpes simplex and vaccinia keratitis with 5-iodo- and 5-bromo-2'-deoxyuridine. In Pollard M, editor: Perspectives in virology. Vol. 3. New York: Harper & Row, 1963, pp 90-107.

Kohl S. Defective infant antiviral cytotoxicity to herpes simplex virus-infected cells. J Pediatr 1983;102:885-888.

Krugman S. Primary herpetic vulvovaginitis; report of case; isolation and identification of herpes simplex virus. Pediatrics 1952;9:585.

Long D, Madara TJ, Ponce-de-Leon M, et al. Glycoprotein D protects mice against lethal challenge with herpes simplex virus types 1 and 2. Infect Immun 1984;37:761-764.

Lynch FW, Evans CA, Bolin VS, Steves RJ. Kaposi's varicelliform eruption: extensive herpes simplex as a complication of eczema. Arch Dermatol Syph 1945;51:129.

Myers MG, Oxman MN, Clark JE. Failure of neutral-red photodynamic inactivation in recurrent herpes simplex virus infections. N Engl J Med 1975;293:945.

Nahmias AJ, Alford CA, Korones SB. Infection of the newborn with herpesvirus hominis. Adv Pediatr 1970;17:185.

Nahmias AJ, Dowdle WR. Antigenic and biologic differences in herpesvirus hominis. Progr Med Virol 1968;10:110.

Nahmias AJ, Josey WE, Naib ZM. Neonatal herpes simplex infection: role of genital infection in mother as a source of virus in the newborn. JAMA 1967;199:132.

Nahmias AJ, Roizman B. Medical progress: infection with herpes simplex viruses 1 and 2. N Engl J Med 1973; 289:667, 719, 781.

Nahmias AJ, et al. Typing of herpesvirus hominis strains by a direct immunofluorescent technique. Proc Soc Exp Biol Med 1969;132:386.

Nahmias AJ, et al. Perinatal risk associated with maternal genital herpes simplex virus infection. Am J Obstet Gynecol 1971;110:825.

Nahmias AJ, Keyserling HL, Kerrick GM. Herpes simplex. In Remington J, Klein J, eds: Infectious diseases of the fetus and newborn infant, ed 2, Philadelphia: W.B. Saunders Co., 1983, pp 636-678.

Parrott RH, et al. Clinical and laboratory differentiation between herpangina and infectious (herpetic) gingivostomatitis. Pediatrics 1954;14:122.

Parvey LS, Ch'ien LT. Neonatal herpes simplex virus infection introduced by fetal-monitor scalp electrodes. Pediatrics 1980;65:1150-1153.

Quilligan JJ, Jr, Wilson JL. Fatal herpes simplex infection in a newborn infant. J Lab Clin Med 1951;38:742.

Rawls WE. Herpes simplex virus types 1 and 2 and herpesvirus simiae. In Lennette E, Schmidt N, eds. Diagnostic procedures for viral, rickettsial, and chlamydial infections, ed 5. Washington DC: American Public Health Association, 1979, pp 309-360.

Reichman RC, Badger GJ, Mertz GJ, et al. Treatment of recurrent genital herpes simplex infections with oral acyclovir, a controlled trial. JAMA 1984;251:2103-2107.

Schneidman DW, Barr RJ, Graham JH. Chronic cutaneous herpes simplex. JAMA 1979;241:592.

Scott TFM, Steigman AJ, Convey JH. Acute infectious gingivostomatitis; etiology, epidemiology and clinical picture of a common disorder caused by the virus of herpes simplex. JAMA 1941;117:999.

Sköldenberg B, Forsgren M, Alestig K, et al. Acyclovir versus vidarabine in herpes simplex encephalitis: randomized multicentre study in consecutive Swedish patients. Lancet 1984;2(7):707-711.

Spruance SL, et al. Ineffectiveness of topical adenine arabinoside 5'-monophosphate in the treatment of recurrent herpes simplex labialis. N Engl J Med 1979;300:1180.

Straus S, Takiff HE, Seidlin M, et al. Suppression of frequently recurring genital herpes. A placebo-controlled double-blind trial of acyclovir. N Engl J Med 1984; 310:1545-1550.

Stadler H, et al. Herpes simplex meningitis: isolation of herpes simplex virus type 2 from cerebrospinal fluid. N Engl J Med 1973;289:1296.

Sullivan-Bolyai JZ, Fife KH, Jacobs RF, et al. Disseminated neonatal herpes simplex virus type 1 from a maternal breast lesion. Pediatrics 1983a;71:455-457.

Sullivan-Bolyai J, Hull HF, Wilson C, et al. Herpes simplex virus infection in King County, Washington. JAMA 1983b;250:3059-3062.

Visentine AM, Nahmias AH, Josey WE. Genital herpes. Perinatal Care 1978;2:32.

Wenner HA. Complications of infantile eczema caused by the virus of herpes simplex. (a) Description of the clinical characteristics of an unusual eruption and (b) identification of an associated filtrable virus. Am J Dis Child 1944;67:247.

Whitley RJ, et al. Adenine arabinoside therapy of biopsy-proved herpes simplex encephalitis. N Engl J Med 1977;297:289.

Whitley R, Lakeman AD, Nahmias A, et al. DNA restriction analysis of herpes simplex virus isolates obtained from patients with encephalitis. N Engl J Med 1982a;307:1060-1062.

Whitley RJ, Nahmias AJ, Soong S, et al. Vidarabine therapy of neonatal herpes simplex virus infection. Pediatrics 1980a;66:495-501.

Whitley RJ, Nahmias AJ, Visintine AM, et al. The natural history of herpes simplex virus infection of mother and newborn. Pediatrics 1980b;66:489-494.

Whitley RJ, Soong S, Hirsch MS, et al, and the NIAID Collaborative Antiviral Study Group. Herpes simplex encephalitis: vidarabine therapy and diagnostic problems. N Engl J Med 1981;304:313-318.

Whitley RJ, Soong S, Linneman C, Jr, et al. Herpes simplex encephalitis. JAMA 1982b;247:317-320.

Whitley RJ, Yeager A, Kartus P, et al. Neonatal herpes simplex virus infection: follow-up evaluation of vidarabine therapy. Pediatrics 1983;72:778-785.

Whitman L, Wall MJ, Warren J. Herpes simplex encephalitis; a report of two fatal cases. JAMA 1946;131:1408.

Wildy P, Russell WC, Horne RW. The morphology of herpes virus. Virology 1960;12:204.

Wise TG, Pavan PR, Ennis FA. Herpes simplex vaccines. J Infect Dis 1977;136:706.

Yeager AS, Arvin AM, Urbani LJ, Kemp JA. Relationship of antibody to outcome in neonatal herpes simplex virus infections. Infect Immun 1980;29:532-538.

Yeager AS, Ashley RL, Corey L. Transmission of herpes simplex virus from father to neonate. J Pediatr 1983;103:905-907.

12

INFANT BOTULISM

Since the first case report in 1976 (Pickett et al.) describing two infants with a clinical illness attributed to in vivo formation of *Clostridium botulinum* toxin, more than 350 similar cases have been found among infants in the United States. Although most of the cases initially came from California, 30 other states have now reported patients with infantile botulism. California, Utah, and Pennsylvania have the highest rates. Additional reports have come from Canada, England, and Australia. These infants have had constipation followed in varying degrees by lethargy, weakness, difficult feeding, general floppiness, descending paralysis, and oculomotor dysfunction; some progress to life-threatening respiratory failure. The detection of clostridial organisms and specific toxin in the infants' stools has led to the term *infant botulism*. This contrasts with the more frequently recognized form of botulism, which is a "food poisoning" resulting from ingestion of food contaminated by preformed toxin.

ETIOLOGY

C. botulinum organisms, serotypes A and B, have been isolated from feces of affected infants. The same fecal specimens contained the specific toxin of the botulinal serotype (Midura and Arnon, 1976). Toxin has not been detected in serum samples. Apparently, ingested vegetative cells or spores germinate in the infant gastrointestinal tract and release their neurotoxin, which causes the clinical manifestations. *C. botulinum* toxin prevents the release of acetylcholine,

blocking neuromuscular synaptic transmission and resulting in flaccid paralysis. No evidence has been found that these infants ingested preformed toxin, the usual mechanism for botulism of adults and older children. Those factors that permit the sequence of toxin formation in the infant gastrointestinal tract are not yet defined. Of the seven distinct serotypes of *C. botulinum* (A to G) only types A, B, and F have been implicated thus far in infant botulism.

PATHOLOGY

Because nearly all identified patients have recovered after provision of supportive therapy, no published autopsy studies are available. However, an investigation of postmortem specimens from 280 California infants who died in the first year of life revealed *C. botulinum* organisms and/or toxin in 10 infants (Arnon et al. 1979). Nine of the 10 deaths had been classified as resulting from sudden infant death syndrome (SIDS). Among the SIDS infants with positive *C. botulinum* organisms and/or toxin, the study reported intrathoracic organ petechiae, alveoli and airways filled with frothy fluid, and extramedullary hepatic erythropoiesis. Arnon has postulated that infant botulism may be one cause of SIDS.

EPIDEMIOLOGIC FACTORS

The age of patients at onset has ranged from 1 week to 11 months, and there has been no sex predilection. Seventy percent of the affected infants have been predominantly breast fed (Morris et al. 1983). There was an interesting association of the type B cases in California with the use of honey as a carbohydrate source in infant feeding (Arnon et al., 1979) and up to 27% of subsequent patients have been fed honey before their illness. The full extent of the disease is not yet known, but it is safe to assume that many mild cases continue to go unrecognized. Less severely affected infants with moderate hypotonia, transient feeding difficulties, and failure to thrive are not hospitalized and escape detection because stool cultures and toxin assays are not performed. In association with their study of a possible relationship between infant botulism and SIDS, Arnon et al. (1978) pointed out the similar age distribution curves of the two conditions in the first 6 months of life.

CLINICAL MANIFESTATIONS

Constipation (no spontaneous stools for 3 or more days) has been the initial manifestation in most cases. Within a few days this may be followed by lethargy, slow feeding, feeble cry, weakness, loss of head and neck control, generalized floppiness, swallowing difficulties, pooling of oral secretions, and, in some, respiratory arrest. On examination there is loss of muscle tone and diminished deep tendon reflexes. Additional cranial nerve findings may include ptosis, sluggish pupillary light reflexes, decreased extraocular motility, lack of facial movement, and decreased gag reflex (Berg, 1977). The symptoms and signs have been variable in degree and duration, responding spontaneously over a period ranging from 10 days to 8 weeks. The most serious complication has been respiratory arrest, occurring in nearly one half of hospitalized patients. For this reason, admission to an intensive care unit where prompt respiratory support can be provided is crucial. Recovery has been gradual and complete, but rare relapses have been observed. The only deaths reported have been caused by respiratory arrests.

DIAGNOSIS

The clinical suspicion of infant botulism should lead to diagnostic studies, initiated while supportive care is underway. Electromyography may demonstrate a somewhat characteristic pattern of brief, low amplitude, overabundant motor reaction potentials (Caly et al. 1977). Confirmation of precise diagnosis requires demonstration of *C. botulinum* and/or heat-labile botulinal toxin in the patient's stool. Appropriate reference laboratories are available (state health department or Centers for Disease Control) if local facilities are unable to perform the isolation and identification techniques. Midura and Arnon (1976) have described the appropriate tests and their application to fecal specimens.

DIFFERENTIAL DIAGNOSIS

Other conditions considered on the initial presentation of these infants have included sepsis, poliomyelitis, myasthenia gravis, brain tumor, failure to thrive, drug or chemical poisoning, metabolic disorders, infantile polyneuropathy, Werdnig-Hoffmann disease, Reye's syndrome, congenital myopathy, and Leigh's disease. With appropriate cultures and screening tests to exclude many of the others, a specific diagnosis should be achieved. CSF and peripheral blood studies in infant botulism have been normal.

TREATMENT

The difficulties that may arise in handling oropharyngeal secretions and the unpredictability of sudden respiratory arrests require the level of supportive care usually available only in an intensive care unit. If the infant's course is a prolonged one, supplementary nutritional support will also become essential. No advantage has been demonstrated from the use of antitoxin, antibiotics, or cholinomimetic drugs. Infants treated with antibiotics have continued to excrete organisms and toxins for weeks after clinical recovery. The use of aminoglycoside antibiotics is specifically contraindicated as they may augment neuromuscular blockade and produce respiratory arrest (L'Hommedieu et al., 1979; Santos et al., 1981). Many unanswered questions may be resolved by future carefully conducted clinical investigative studies.

REFERENCES

Arnon SS, Damus K, Chin J. Infant botulism: epidemiology and relation to sudden infant death syndrome. Epidemiol Rev 1981;3:45-66.

Arnon SS, et al. Infant botulism. JAMA 1977;237:1946.

Arnon SS, et al. Intestinal infection and toxin production by *Clostridium botulinum* as one cause of sudden infant death syndrome. Lancet 1978;1:1273.

Arnon SS, et al. Honey and other environmental risk factors for infant botulism. J Pediatr 1979;94:331.

Berg BO. Syndrome of infant botulism. Pediatrics 1977; 59:322.

Brown LW. Commentary: Infant botulism and the honey connection. J Pediatr 1979;94:337.

Centers for Disease Control. Morbid Mortal Weekly Rep 1979;28:73.

Clay SA, et al. Acute infantile motor disorder: infantile botulism? Arch Neurol 1977;34:236.

Feldman RA, ed. A seminar on infant botulism. Rev Infect Dis 1979;1:611.

L'Hommedieu C, Stough R, Brown L, et al. Potentiation of neuromuscular weakness in infant botulism by aminoglycosides. J Pediatr 1979;95:1965.

Long SS. Botulism in infancy. Pediatr Infect Dis 1984;3:266-271.

Midura TF, Arnon SS. Infant botulism. Identification of *Clostridium botulinum* and its toxins in faeces. Lancet 1976;2:934.

Morris JG Jr, Snyder JD, Wilson R, Feldman RA. Infant botulism in the United States: an epidemiologic study of cases occuring outside of California. Am J Public Health 1983;73:1385-1388.

Pickett J, et al. Syndrome of botulism in infancy: clinical and electrophysiologic study. N Engl J Med 1976;295:770.

Santos JI, Swensen P, Glasgow LA. Potentiation of *Clostridium botulinum* toxin by aminoglycoside antibiotics: clinical and laboratory observations. Pediatrics 1981;68:50-54.

Thompson JA, Glasgow LA, Warpinski JR, et al. Infant botulism: clinical spectrum and etiology. Pediatrics 1980;66:936-942.

Turner HD, et al. Infant botulism in England. Lancet 1978;1:1277.

13

MEASLES (RUBEOLA)

Measles is an acute, highly contagious, ancient viral disease characterized by fever, coryza, conjunctivitis, cough, and a specific enanthem (Koplik's spots) followed by a generalized maculopapular eruption, which usually appears on the fourth day of the disease. The rash and accompanying illness reach a climax on about the sixth day, followed by subsidence in a few days and, in most cases, complete recovery. Serious complications involving the respiratory tract and central nervous system occur in the minority of patients in highly developed countries. In other parts of the world, however, the high mortality and morbidity associated with measles present serious problems. The widespread use of live attenuated measles virus vaccine has been followed by a sharp decline in the incidence of the disease in the United States.

ETIOLOGY

The transmission of measles to monkeys was first reported by Josias in 1898. Anderson and Goldberger (1911) and Blake and Trask (1921) clearly demonstrated that monkeys could be infected with blood or nasopharyngeal secretions from humans with measles. In 1940 Rake and Shaffer reported the adaptation of measles virus to chick embryos. No obvious gross or microscopic changes were detected in the eggs, but passage in monkeys presumably induced a disease resembling measles. These observations have not been confirmed.

In 1954 Enders and Peebles reported the successful isolation of measles virus in human and rhesus monkey kidney tissue cultures. The characteristic cytopathic changes in tissue culture included (1) formation of multinucleated giant cells, (2) vacuolization in the syncytial cytoplasm, and (3) presence of eosinophilic intranuclear and intracytoplasmic inclusion bodies. The cytopathic changes were neutralized by measles convalescent serum. The tissue culture fluid of infected cultures contained complement-fixing antigen. Measles virus has been adapted to a variety of tissue cultures, including human amnion, human embryonic lung, human carcinoma cells (HeLa, HEp2, and KB), and chick embryo cells. The cytopathic effects in tissue culture have provided a basis for virus isolation procedures, for assay of infectivity, and for determination of neutralizing antibody. The property of hemagglutination of simian erythrocytes by infected tissue culture fluids has been utilized as the basis for a convenient serologic test for the diagnosis of measles.

Measles virus has been classified as a paramyxovirus. It is spherical in appearance, measuring 120 to 250 nm in diameter. It has an outer envelope composed of glycoproteins and lipids and an internal core of RNA. Six major proteins have been identified: L, P, NP, H, F, and M (Mountcastle and Choppin, 1977; Graves et al., 1978; Tyrrell and Norrby, 1978; Wechsler and Fields, 1978). The L and P proteins are associated with the nucleocapsid and are involved in the activity of RNA polymerase. NP is the nucleocapsid structural protein. The hemagglutinin, H, is a surface glycoprotein with receptor-binding activity. F is a surface glycoprotein responsible for virus penetration, cell fusion, and hemolysis. M is an internal-membrane protein with a key role in virus assembly.

Measles virus is very sensitive to heat and cold and is rapidly inactivated at 37° C and at 20° C. It is also inactivated by ultraviolet light, ether, trypsin, and B-propiolactone. Formalin destroys infectivity, but it does not alter complement-fixing activity. The virus in the presence of protein is well preserved at low temperature, surviving storage at −15° to −70° C for 5 years and at 4° C for 5 months. In the lyophilized state with a protein stabilizer it is preserved at 4° C for 18 months.

PATHOLOGY

Measles is a generalized infection, and the pathologic lesions are widespread. During the prodromal period there is hyperplasia of the lymphoid tissue in the tonsils, adenoids, lymph nodes, spleen, and appendix. Large (100 μm) multinucleated giant cells can be demonstrated in these tissues and in the pharyngeal and bronchial mucosa.

Suringa et al. (1970) found that Koplik's spots and the skin lesions of measles share the following histologic features: foci of syncytial epithelial giant cells with pale-staining cytoplasm, intercellular and intracellular edema, and parakeratosis and dyskeratosis. There are between three and 26 giant cell nuclei and many contain pink-staining inclusion bodies. Electron microscopy reveals aggregates of "viral" microtubules within the nuclei and cytoplasm of syncytial giant cells. These tubules are indistinguishable from those seen in tissue cultures infected with measles virus. It is clear that the pathologic aspects of the skin lesions and mucosal lesions (Koplik's spots) are the same.

The lungs show evidence of a peribronchiolar inflammatory reaction with a mononuclear cell infiltrate in the interstitial tissues. The large giant cells are occasionally identified here.

The brain and spinal cord in measles encephalomyelitis show gross evidence of edema, congestion, and scattered petechial hemorrhages. Microscopically, the early stage is characterized by perivascular hemorrhages and lymphocytic cell infiltration. Later, there is evidence of demyelination throughout the central nervous system (CNS). Histologically, these lesions are very

similar to those encountered in postvaccinal encephalitis.

CLINICAL MANIFESTATIONS

The clinical course of a typical case of measles is illustrated in Fig. 13-1. After an incubation period of 10 to 11 days the illness is ushered in by fever and malaise. Within 24 hours there is onset of coryza, conjunctivitis, and cough. These symptoms gradually increase in severity, reaching a peak with the appearance of the eruption on the fourth day. Approximately 2 days before the development of the rash, Koplik's spots appear on the buccal mucous membranes opposite the molars. Over a 3-day period these lesions increase in number and spread to involve the entire mucous membrane. The fever subsides and Koplik's spots disappear by the end of the second day of the rash. The coryza and conjunctivitis clear considerably by the third day of the rash. The duration of the exanthem rarely exceeds 5 to 6 days.

Fever

The temperature curve illustrated in Fig. 13-1 is the one most commonly observed. There is a stepwise increase until the fifth or sixth day of illness at the height of the eruption. Occasionally, however, the temperature curve may be biphasic; an initial elevation for the first 24 to 48 hours is followed by a normal period for 1

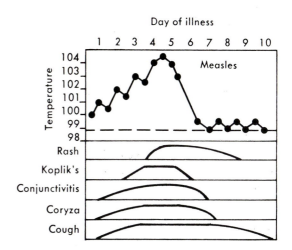

Fig. 13-1. Schematic diagram of clinical course of typical case of measles. The rash appears 3 to 4 days after onset of fever, conjunctivitis, coryza, and cough. Koplik's spots usually develop 2 days before the rash.

day and then by a rapid rise to 39.4° to 40.6° C (103° to 105° F) when the rash is in full bloom. At times, the temperature may reach its peak by the end of the first day and remain elevated at levels of 39.4° to 40.6° C (103° to 105° F) for the remaining prodromal and early rash period. In uncomplicated measles the temperature falls by crisis or rapid lysis between the second and third days after the onset of the exanthem.

Coryza

The coryza of measles is indistinguishable from that of a severe common cold. The early sneezing is followed by nasal congestion and a mucopurulent discharge that becomes most profuse at the height of the eruption. It clears very rapidly after the patient becomes afebrile.

Conjunctivitis

A transverse marginal line of conjunctival injection across the lower lids, described by Stimson in 1928, may be observed in the early prodromal period. Subsequently, this is obscured by an extensive conjunctival inflammation associated with edema of the lids and the caruncles. There is evidence of increased lacrimation, and occasionally the patient complains of photophobia. In severe cases, Koplik's spots may be observed on the caruncle. The conjunctivitis, like the coryza, disappears shortly after the fever has subsided.

Cough

The cough is caused by the inflammatory reaction of the respiratory tract. Like the other catarrhal manifestations, it increases in frequency and intensity, reaching its climax at the height of the eruption. However, it persists much longer, gradually subsiding over a 5- to 10-day period.

Koplik's spots

Approximately 2 days before the rash appears, the pathognomonic Koplik's spots may be detected. These lesions were described by Koplik in 1896 as

small irregular spots of bright red color[;] in the center of each red spot is seen a minute bluish-white speck. There may at first be only two or three or six such rose-red spots, with a bluish-white speck in the center. The combination of a bluish-white speck with a rose-red background on the buccal and labial mucous

membrane is absolutely pathognomonic of the invasion of measles. Sometimes the bluish-white speck is so small and delicately colored that only in a very direct and strong daylight is it possible to bring out the above effect, but the combination is always present.*

Koplik's spots increase to uncountable numbers so that by the end of the first day of rash they usually involve the entire buccal and labial mucosa. The rose-red areas coalesce to form a diffuse erythematous background that is peppered with many pinpoint blue-white elevations. At this stage Koplik's spots resemble grains of salt sprinkled on a red background (Plate 3). By the end of the second day of the rash the spots already begin to slough off, and by the third day of rash the mucous membranes look perfectly normal.

Rash

As indicated in Fig. 13-1, the rash of unmodified measles first makes its appearance 3 to 4 days after the onset of illness. Occasionally, the prodromal period may be as short as 1 day or as long as 7 days.

The exanthem begins as an erythematous maculopapular eruption (Fig. 13-2). It appears first at the hairline and involves the forehead, the area behind the earlobes, and the upper part of the neck. It then spreads downward to involve the face, neck, upper extremities, and trunk. It continues downward until it reaches the feet by the third day. The earlier sites contain many more lesions than those that are affected later. Consequently, the lesions high up on the face and neck tend to be confluent, whereas those low down on the extremities tend to be discrete (Fig. 13-3).

The rash begins to fade by the third day in order of appearance. Therefore, although the face and upper trunk may be clear by the fourth day, an eruption may still be apparent on the lower extremities. The early erythematous lesions blanch on pressure. After 3 or 4 days they assume a brownish appearance (staining). The staining of the skin, which is probably the result of capillary hemorrhages, does not fade on pressure. With the disappearance of the rash, a fine branny desquamation may be noted over the

*Koplik H: The diagnosis of the invasion of measles from a study of the exanthema as it appears on the buccal mucous membrane, Arch Pediatr 1896;13:918.

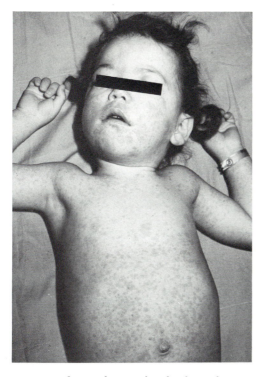

Fig. 13-2. Infant with typical rash of measles. Note confluent maculopapular lesions on face.

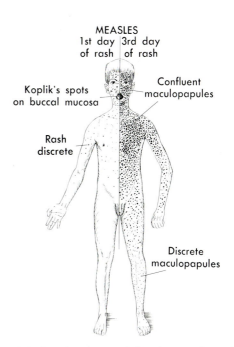

Fig. 13-3. Development and distribution of measles rash.

sites of most extensive involvement. In contrast to scarlet fever, the skin of the hands and feet does not desquamate. Morley (1962) observed extensive desquamation after severe measles in West African children who were protein deficient.

Other manifestations

Anorexia and malaise are usually present during the febrile period. In infants, diarrhea may occur at times. Generalized lymphadenopathy is noted in moderate to severe cases. Like rubella, measles may be associated with enlarged postauricular, cervical, and occipital lymph nodes. Occasionally, a transient prodromal rash may be observed. This eruption may be scarlatiniform or morbilliform and usually disappears within 24 hours. Other manifestations of measles may include giant cell pneumonia without rash (Enders et al., 1959).

Convalescence

The illness reaches its climax between the second and third days of the rash. At this time the temperature is at its peak, Koplik's spots have covered the entire buccal mucous membrane and are beginning to slough, the eyes are puffy and red, the coryza is profuse, and the cough is most distressing. The child looks measly and feels miserable. Within the next 24 to 36 hours the temperature falls by crisis or rapid lysis, the coryza and conjunctivitis clear, and the cough decreases in severity. Within a few days the child feels normal. Fever persisting beyond the third day of rash is usually caused by a complication. The convalescent period of measles is of short duration, although cough may persist for longer periods.

ATYPICAL MEASLES IN CHILDREN PREVIOUSLY IMMUNIZED WITH INACTIVATED MEASLES VIRUS VACCINE

A severe, atypical type of measles was reported by Rauh and Schmidt in 1965, by Nader et al. in 1968, and by Fulginiti et al. in 1967 in children who had received inactivated measles virus vaccine 2 to 4 years previously. The following clinical manifestations have been observed: fever, pneumonitis, pneumonia with pulmonary consolidation and pleural effusion, and an unusual rash for measles. The eruption has been urticarial, maculopapular, petechial, purpuric, and occasionally vesicular with a predilection for the extremities. Edema of the hands and feet, myalgia, and severe hyperesthesia of the skin also have been observed. The appearance and distribution of the exanthem resemble Rocky Mountain spotted fever.

As indicated on p. 158, patients with atypical measles may have extraordinarily high measles hemagglutination-inhibition (HI) antibody titers (1:25,000 to 1:200,000). These levels are sixfold or more higher than those observed following typical measles infection. Serial observations of patients with atypical measles at New York University Medical Center have revealed progressively rising measles HI antibody titers during the first few weeks after onset of illness. For example, test results of one of our patients revealed an HI antibody titer of 1:512 on the fifth day after onset of rash and a titer of 1:120,000 3 weeks later.

CASE REPORT (courtesy Dr. Vincent A. Fulginiti, University of Arizona). D. M., a 6-year-old white girl, was well until April 18, 1967, when she developed high fever (40° to 40.6° C; 104° to 105° F) and headache, followed on April 20 by a maculopapular eruption. The rash was observed first on the ankles; within 2 days it spread to involve most of the lower extremities as well as the trunk, wrists, palms, and neck. The rash became petechial and ecchymotic, and vesicles were noted in a few areas. Other manifestations included irritability, unsteady gait, myalgias, cough, rales over right lower posterior thorax, and edema of the ankles, feet, and hands.

Past history included a trip to the mountains on April 8, at which time a playmate was bitten by a tick. There was possible exposure to measles at school. The patient had received two doses of inactivated measles virus vaccine and one dose of live virus vaccine several years previously.

Laboratory studies revealed a normal white blood cell count and roentgenographic evidence of hilar adenopathy as well as a right-sided pulmonary infiltrate. The rash faded, and the fever subsided after 5 days. The results of serologic tests were as follows:

Date	Proteus OX-2	Proteus OX-19	RMSF-CF	Measles HI
4/22	<10	<10	<4	<4
4/28	<10	<10	<4	≥1024
5/5	<10	<10	<4	≥1024

A sharp rise in measles HI antibody during convalescence and the lack of rise in titer of *Proteus* OX-2 and OX-19 agglutinins as well as complement-fixing antibody to Rocky Mountain spotted fever (RMSF) establish the diagnosis of atypical measles related to sensitization by inactivated measles virus vaccine.

We have observed an adolescent and an adult who had evidence of liver involvement and persistence of the pulmonary lesions for 18 months in addition to the usual manifestations of atypical measles; alanine aminotransferase (ALT) levels ranged between 200 and 300 U/ml. The initial differential diagnosis included type B hepatitis. However, the high measles HI antibody titers (>1:100,000) and previous immunization with inactivated measles vaccine confirmed the diagnosis of atypical measles (Frey and Krugman, 1980).

It has been estimated that 600,000 to 900,000 children were immunized with inactivated measles vaccine between the time of licensure in 1963 until 1967 when it was removed from the market (Halsey, 1978). Consequently, during the 1980s this disease will be seen exclusively in adolescents and adults. It was appropriate for Martin et al. (1979) and Hall and Hall (1979) to describe this problem in detail in the adult medical literature.

The pathogenesis of the atypical measles syndrome is based in great part on the failure of formalin-inactivated measles vaccine to induce antibody to the F protein. Immunity to the F protein is necessary to prevent spread of infection. In addition, hypersensitivity develops to other viral antigens to which immunity had been stimulated previously by the inactivated measles vaccine. Studies of six patients with atypical measles syndrome by Annunziato et al. (1982) revealed that five of six acute sera lacked antibody to F (hemolysin) antigen and five of six contained antibody to H (hemagglutinin) antigen.

SEVERE HEMORRHAGIC MEASLES

Severe hemorrhagic measles (black measles) was not uncommon several decades ago. Recently, however, cases of this type have become rare. The illness may begin with a sudden onset of hyperpyrexia (40.6° to 41.1° C; 105° to 106° F), convulsions, delirium, or stupor that may progress to coma. This is followed by marked

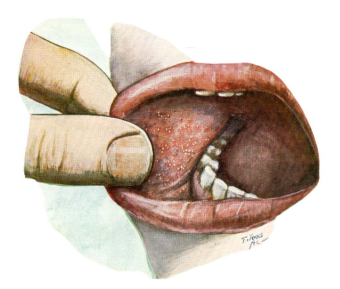

Plate 3
Koplik's spots. (From Zahorsky J, Zahorsky TS. Synopsis of pediatrics. St. Louis. The C.V. Mosby Co., 1953.)

respiratory distress and an extensive confluent hemorrhagic eruption of the skin and mucous membranes. Bleeding from the mouth, nose, and bowel may be severe and uncontrollable. This type of measles is often fatal, probably because it involves disseminated intravascular coagulation (DIC).

Severe hemorrhagic measles should not be confused with the purpuric type of eruption that may occur in fair-skinned children with severe ordinary measles. This type of hemorrhagic eruption is not associated with excessive toxicity, and the illness pursues a more favorable course.

MODIFIED MEASLES

Modified measles most commonly develops in children who have been passively immunized with immune globulin after exposure to the disease. Occasionally, it may also occur in infants whose transplacental passive immunity has only partially waned. The incubation period may be prolonged to 14 or even to 20 days. The illness is an abbreviated, milder version of ordinary measles.

The usual prodromal period of 3 to 4 days may be decreased to 1 or 2 days, or it may even be absent. The fever is generally low grade, but the temperature may be normal. The coryza, conjunctivitis, and cough are usually minimal and may even be absent. Koplik's spots may not be present; if they do appear, they are few in number and disappear within a day or less. The rash

is generally sparse and discrete and in some cases is so mild that it may be missed.

Modification of measles converts a severe 6- to 9-day illness to one that is very mild and of much shorter duration. In contrast to the unmodified disease, it is unusual for modified measles to be followed by complications.

DIAGNOSIS
Confirmatory clinical factors

The development of a generalized maculopapular eruption preceded by a 3- 4-day period of fever, cough, coryza, and conjunctivitis associated with the pathognomonic Koplik's spots points to a clear-cut diagnosis of measles. During the prevaccine era confirmatory laboratory procedures were usually unnecessary.

Isolation of causative agent

Measles virus may be isolated from the blood, urine, or nasopharyngeal secretions during the febrile period of the illness. The agent may be grown in tissue cultures of cells from human kidney, monkey kidney, and human amnion.

Serologic tests

A significant titer of neutralizing, hemagglutination-inhibition (HI), and complement-fixing (CF) antibodies may be detected in serum collected 2 weeks after the onset of illness. Antibodies usually appear within 1 to 3 days after onset of rash. Peak titers are reached 2 to 4

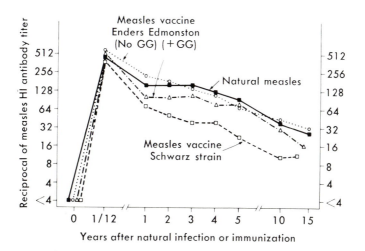

Fig. 13-4. Measles hemagglutination-inhibition (HI) antibody response and persistence. Fifteen-year follow-up. (From Krugman S. J Pediatr 1977;90:1.)

weeks later. Measles neutralizing and HI antibodies may be detected for many years and generally persist for longer periods than CF antibodies. The pattern of development and persistence of measles HI antibody is illustrated in Fig. 13-4. A fourfold or greater increase in antibody titer during convalescence is strongly indicative of measles infection. The measles HI antibody determination is a specific, useful, and practical test for the diagnosis of atypical or subclinical cases of measles.

The peak measles HI antibody titer detected about 1 month after natural measles ranges between 1:64 and 1:4096, with a geometric mean antibody titer (GMT) of 1:512 (Fig. 13-4). However, patients with subacute sclerosing panencephalitis (p. 160) and atypical measles (p. 156) may have measles HI titers that exceed 1:10,000. Serologic studies of three adolescents with classic atypical measles revealed the following HI antibody titers: 1:25,600; greater than or equal to 1:204,800; greater than or equal to 1:204,800. These patients were immunized previously with killed measles vaccine during their childhood.

Other laboratory findings

Uncomplicated measles is typically associated with leukopenia. A characteristic multinucleated giant cell has been identified in sputum and nasal secretions of patients during the prodromal period and in urinary sediment throughout the course of the disease.

DIFFERENTIAL DIAGNOSIS

Differential diagnosis of measles is discussed in Chapter 34.

COMPLICATIONS

The virus of measles is responsible for an inflammatory reaction that extends from the nasopharynx down the respiratory tract to the bronchi. Thus nasopharyngitis with coryza and tracheobronchitis with cough are both manifestations of the natural disease. The more common complications are usually caused by (1) an extension of the inflammation due to the virus, (2) an invasion of damaged tissues by bacteria, or (3) a combination of both. The sites of involvement of complications of measles include the middle ear, the respiratory tract, the central nervous system, the eyes, and the skin.

Otitis media

Infection of the middle ear is one of the most common complications of measles. In the older child it usually begins with earache, and in the infant, with increased irritability and ear pulling. Early in the course of measles the tympanic membranes should be examined frequently for signs such as redness, bulging, and obliteration of the light reflex and landmarks. Particularly in infants the first sign of otitis media may be a purulent discharge from the middle ear. Complicating otitis media is usually responsible for persistence of pyrexia beyond the normal course.

The incidence of otitis media as a complication of measles is affected by factors related to the disease, the host, and the environment. Severe measles is more likely to be complicated than mild forms. Susceptibility is increased in infants as compared with older children and in patients of any age with enlarged adenoids or a history of ear infections. Otitis media was more common in the hospital ward than in the home because of the increased cross-infection rate in the former. During an extensive epidemic in Greenland it was observed that measles was complicated by otitis media in 5% of patients with the disease (Littauer and Sørensen, 1965).

Mastoiditis

Mastoiditis formerly was a common sequela of otitis media. Prompt antibacterial therapy has virtually eliminated this complication.

Pneumonia

Pulmonary complications are as common as otitis media in frequency but more common as a cause of death. During the Greenland epidemic the incidence of pneumonia in patients with measles was 7%. The pneumonia may result from (1) an extension of the viral infection, (2) a superimposed bacterial infection, or (3) a combination of both. It is manifested clinically as either bronchiolitis (in infants), bronchopneumonia, or lobar pneumonia. The presence of a pneumonic complication should be suspected when any child with measles develops respiratory distress associated with persistence or recrudescence of fever. Examination of the chest may reveal dullness to percussion, suppression of breath sounds, bronchial breathing, and localized or generalized rales. A roentgenogram should clarify the diagnosis.

Obstructive laryngitis and laryngotracheitis

Transient mild laryngitis and tracheitis are both part of the normal course of measles. Occasionally, however, the inflammatory process progresses and causes obstruction of the airway. The increased hoarseness, barking cough, and inspiratory stridor associated with suprasternal retractions indicate the development of this complication. These symptoms usually subside when the rash begins to fade. The development of increasing restlessness, dyspnea, and tachycardia points to increasing obstruction that should be relieved by tracheostomy or intubation before extreme cyanosis and other signs of asphyxia occur.

Cervical adenitis

Mild generalized lymphadenopathy is associated with most cases of measles. Formerly, acute cervical adenitis of bacterial cause was not uncommon. Antibacterial drugs have significantly reduced the incidence of this complication.

Acute encephalitis

Acute encephalitis is a serious, potentially crippling and fatal complication that occurs in approximately 0.1% of measles cases. In some epidemics the incidence has been higher; in southern Greenland it approached 0.4%. It occurs most commonly between the second and sixth days after onset of the rash. However, it occasionally develops during the prerash or postrash period.

Fever, headache, vomiting, drowsiness, convulsions, coma, or personality changes may usher in this complication. Frequently there are signs of meningeal irritation such as a stiff neck and Brudzinski's and Kernig's signs. The cerebrospinal fluid (CSF) shows a modest pleocytosis with a predominance of lymphocytes. The protein level is generally elevated; the sugar level is either normal or elevated. In rare instances the CSF may be normal.

The course of encephalitis may be extremely variable. It may be very mild, clearing completely within several days, or it may be a rapidly progressive and fulminating disease, terminating fatally within 24 hours. Between these two extremes there are many variations. In general approximately 60% of patients recover completely; 15% die; and 25% subsequently show manifestations of brain damage, such as mental retardation, recurrent convulsive seizures, severe behavior disorders, nerve deafness, hemiplegia, and paraplegia. The course is unpredictable. It is not unusual for a child to be in a coma for several weeks and subsequently to recover completely without sequelae.

The pathogenesis of measles encephalitis is uncertain. Postulated causes include an invasion of the CNS by measles virus or an allergic type of encephalomyelitis. Available evidence favors the first postulate. (See Chapter 4, p. 34.)

Infants with dehydration and hyperelectrolytemia may present a neurologic picture that closely resembles that of measles encephalitis. Correction of the water and electrolyte disturbance is usually followed by rapid improvement.

Subacute sclerosing panencephalitis

The rare condition of subacute sclerosing panencephalitis (SSPE) can be considered to be a late complication of measles, with an incidence of approximately one per 100,000 cases. It has clinical and pathologic features that are characteristic of a slowly progressing virus infection. The syndrome, first described by Dawson in 1934 and by van Bogaert in 1945, has also been called *subacute inclusion-body encephalitis*.

The early clinical manifestations are characterized by insidious and progressive behavioral and intellectual deterioration, possibly initially manifested by declining school performance. These symptoms are associated with awkwardness, stumbling, and falling. Later the course may be characterized by involuntary myoclonic seizures and increasing mental deterioration and frequently is followed by death within a 6-month period. The confirmatory laboratory findings include (1) an electroencephalogram with paroxysmal spiking at regular intervals and depressed activity between spikes; (2) marked elevation of the CSF globulin, predominantly the IgG fraction of gamma globulin; (3) an exceptionally high serum measles antibody titer; and (4) detectable measles antibody in the CSF.

Pathologic as well as clinical differences have been observed between SSPE and acute encephalitis. The early neuropathologic features of SSPE include perivascular round cell infiltration, neuronal degeneration, and intranuclear and intracytoplasmic inclusion bodies. Later, extensive gliosis and demyelination occur. The demonstration of measles-virus antigen in the brain as well as the serologic findings incriminate the virus itself as the causative agent or, more probably, a defective variant of the virus. Further confirmation of the role of measles virus in SSPE has been provided by electron microscopic demonstration of paramyxovirus nucleocapsids in the inclusion bodies, immunofluorescence with specific measles antiserum of affected cells, and recovery in the laboratory by cocultivation techniques of infectious measleslike virus from brain biopsy or autopsy specimens.

Using immunoprecipitation methods, Hall and Choppin (1981) found a relative lack of antibodies to M protein in serum and CSF of patients with SSPE. However, there were high levels of antibody to other viral proteins. They proposed the following hypothesis: "Since M protein plays an essential part in the assembly of the virus at the cell membrane, a lack of M protein could explain one characteristic of SSPE: the persistence of infection without production of mature, infectious virions." The onset of SSPE occurs many months or many years after an attack of measles. Epidemiologic studies have shown a possible relationship to age of the person. It is usually the youngest male child in the family who develops SSPE, even though older siblings had measles at the same time. Moreover, the initial measles infection is usually very mild. It has been postulated that during the course of a relatively mild or inapparent infection, the virus may survive and persist as a defective virion. The following case report describes a child who had measles at 6 months of age and developed SSPE at 8 years of age.

CASE REPORT. M. R., an 8-year-old girl, was admitted to Bellevue Hospital on November 12, 1966, with a 3-month history of myoclonic seizures and progressive deterioration of behavior manifested by confusion, regression, frequent falls, and bizarre speech. Her growth and development were normal prior to the onset of present illness. She had a history of measles at 6 months of age. During a 9-month period of observation at the hospital, the course of the disease was characterized by gradual mental and motor deterioration. The electroencephalogram was abnormal and characteristic of hypsarrhythmia. Cerebrospinal fluid revealed no cells, normal concentration of sugar, and a protein concentration of 90 mg per 100 ml. The results of measles hemagglutination-inhibition anti-

body tests in serum were as follows: December 1966—1:16,384; March 1967—1:8192; April 1967—1:4096; May 1967—1:2048; August 1967—1:512; and January 1968—1:512. Measles HI antibody was not detected in the cerebrospinal fluid.

A follow-up study of 46 children with natural measles revealed a geometric mean HI antibody titer of approximately 1:128, 1 to 7 years after onset of disease; the titers ranged from a low of 1:4 to a high of 1:2048. In view of this experience, the observation of a measles virus HI antibody titer of 1:16,384 is highly significant in a child who had measles 7 years previously; it suggests an etiologic association (Berman et al., 1968).

Other complications

Purpura, thrombocytopenic and nonthrombocytopenic, may rarely complicate measles. The deleterious effect of measles on pregnancy and on tuberculosis was clearly demonstrated in the southern Greenland epidemic. Of 26 pregnant women with measles, half either aborted or gave birth to premature infants; there were no congenital malformations. There appeared to be a reactivation of previously arrested cases and a striking increase of new cases of tuberculosis as well as an increased mortality of this disease. A positive tuberculin test may temporarily revert to negative during the course of measles. This anergy may persist for as long as 6 weeks. In the majority of cases the tuberculin test becomes positive again within 2 weeks.

Pneumomediastinum and subcutaneous emphysema may occur in rare instances. Bloch and Vardy (1968) described four cases that occurred during an epidemic in a small town in the northern Negev in Israel.

Corneal ulceration is a potentially serious complication that fortunately is very rare. However, nearly all patients have a mild superficial keratoconjunctivitis.

Appendicitis may develop, perhaps as a result of lymphoid hyperplasia in the appendix, and may be so extensive as to obliterate the lumen. In most instances perforation occurs before the complication is recognized.

In certain areas of the world (Africa, India, and Central and South America) where measles is a severe and often fatal disease, the following complications are frequently observed: severe diarrhea and dehydration, kwashiorkor, pyogenic infections of the skin, cancrum oris, and septicemia. Monif and Hood (1970) reported an unusual case of fatal measles that was characterized by severe diarrhea and histologic evidence of ileocolitis probably caused by the virus.

PROGNOSIS

The prognosis of measles has improved significantly during the past three decades. Many of the serious bacterial complications are easily controlled by antimicrobial therapy. In general, the prognosis is better in older children than in infants. A preexisting tuberculous infection may be aggravated. The majority of deaths are the result of severe bronchopneumonia or encephalitis. Modified measles, which is rarely complicated, has an excellent prognosis.

IMMUNITY
Active immunity

One attack of measles is generally followed by permanent immunity. Most so-called recurrent attacks reflect errors in diagnosis. The available evidence suggests that in most cases lasting im-

munity follows an attack of modified measles also. Contemporary studies indicate that comparable lasting immunity will follow immunization with live attenuated measles virus vaccine.

Passive immunity

Neutralizing antibodies for measles virus are present in convalescent serum and in pooled adult serum. These antibodies are contained in the IG fraction that has been employed for passive immunization. Passively acquired measles antibody is detected in cord blood and is usually not measurable after the infant reaches 12 months of age. The results of a longitudinal study of measles immunity during the first year of life are shown in Fig. 13-5.

Studies by Albrecht et al. (1977) revealed the presence of passively acquired measles-neutralizing antibody in serum specimens obtained from 12-month-old infants who had no detectable HI antibody. Previous studies by Krugman et al. (1967) indicated that passively acquired measles HI antibody was not detected after 11 months of age (Fig. 13-5).

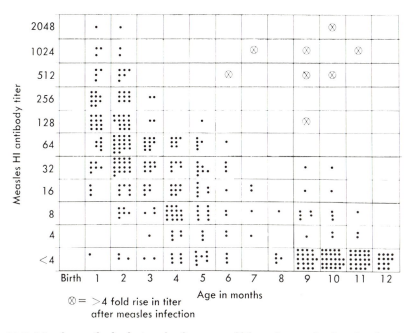

Serial determinations of hemagglutination-inhibition (HI) antibody

⊗ = >4 fold rise in titer after measles infection

Fig. 13-5. Measles antibody during the first year of life—a longitudinal study of 107 infants. Note the disappearance of passive antibody by 12 months of age and the occurrence of eight cases of measles from 6 to 11 months of age. (From Krugman S, Giles JP, Friedman H. PAHO/ WHO Scientific Publication No. 147, May 1967, pp 353-360.)

EPIDEMIOLOGIC FACTORS

Patients with measles harbor the virus in their nasopharyngeal secretions during the acute stage of the disease. Epidemiologic evidence suggests that the patients are contagious for at least 7 days after the onset of the first symptom. Contacts may acquire the infection (1) *directly*, by being sprayed with droplets emanating from a cough or sneeze, (2) *indirectly*, by a third person, or (3) via the *air*. The most common mode of spread is by direct contact. Indirect contact within a house or a hospital ward is also possible. However, it would probably be difficult for a third person to carry measles virus for long distances, particularly if he goes outdoors.

An extraordinary study of an epidemic in Greenland in 1962 may contribute to a better understanding of the *communicability* of measles (Littauer and Sørenson, 1965). A correlation between time of exposure and communicability was observed during this epidemic. It was obvious that the available health facilities would be inadequate to cope with the problems associated with a major outbreak. Accordingly, it was decided that a "guided epidemic" would be the best solution for a potentially critical situation. The area was divided into three quarantinable units: the 800 inhabitants of the town of Umanak, 500 inhabitants of the four most remote settlements, and the 700 inhabitants of the five nearest settlements. The plan involved the deliberate exposure of large groups of susceptible individuals to a person or persons with measles; half the adults and half the children in each household were asked to volunteer for "artificial infection."

The results of this unique plan were very interesting. Approximately 400 persons visited a patient named Josef on the first day of his measles rash. Josef coughed twice in the face of each person. In spite of this exposure, not a single contact acquired measles! Consequently, 3½ weeks later the procedure was repeated, but this time patients in the catarrhal, prerash stage of measles were chosen as the source of infection. Under these circumstances the disease was successfully transmitted to the susceptible contacts.

It is well known that measles virus is present in the nasopharynx during the first day of rash as well as during the catarrhal period of the dis-

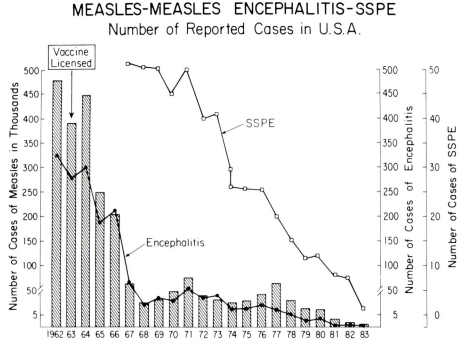

Fig. 13-6. Measles, measles encephalitis, and SSPE: number of reported cases in the United States.

ease. The failure to transmit the infection on the first day of the rash was probably a reflection of the minimal quantity of virus present at that time. The larger quantities of virus present during the catarrhal period were undoubtedly responsible for the communicability of the disease.

During the prevaccine era (before 1963) the *age incidence* varied with the particular environment. In general, measles was a disease of childhood. In congested urban areas, the highest incidence occured in the infant and preschool age groups. In rural and less crowded urban areas, the highest incidence was in children 5 to 10 years of age. In epidemics that occurred in isolated communities, children of all ages were equally affected. In developing countries, measles is most common in infants 1 to 2 years of age. The disease is extremely rare in infants under 3 to 4 months of age because of passively acquired maternal antibodies. If the mother has never had measles, the newborn infant will be susceptible.

Seasonal incidence in the temperate zones is fairly consistent. Measles is essentially a winter-spring disease, with the peak of the outbreak occurring during March and April. In heavily populated areas, epidemics usually occurred at intervals of 2 to 3 years during the prevaccine era. This periodicity was in part caused by the accumulation of a new crop of susceptible children during this interval. The extensive use of live attenuated measles virus vaccine since licensure in 1963 has had a profound effect on the incidence of measles (Fig. 13-6).

Geographic distribution is worldwide. Modern air transportation can carry an infected individual to all parts of the world within the incubation period.

Measles is one of the most highly contagious diseases. The secondary attack rate after an intimate household exposure is over 90%. The reduced intimacy and duration of exposure in a school, bus, or hospital ward are followed by a lower attack rate in susceptible persons—less than 25%.

TREATMENT

Measles is a self-limited disease. The course of uncomplicated infection is not altered by antimicrobial therapy. Treatment is chiefly supportive.

Supportive therapy

Bedrest is advisable and not difficult to enforce during the febrile period. The diet should be either liquid or soft as tolerated. When the child becomes afebrile and the anorexia subsides, regular indoor activity and diet may be resumed.

The measles *cough* is difficult to control. Most cough medicines are not very effective.

The *coryza*, too, is unaffected by treatment and runs a self-limited course. Generally, nose drops are ineffective and unnecessary. The skin around the nares, however, should be protected with petrolatum.

The *conjunctivitis* usually requires no medication. The eyelids should be cleansed with warm water to remove any secretions or crusts. The cornea should be examined for possible ulceration. Corneal complications should be treated by an ophthalmologist. If photophobia is present, bright lights should be avoided; it is depressing and unnecessary to darken the room completely.

Infants with very high fever and children with headache should be treated with appropriate doses of aspirin or other antipyretic drugs.

Prevention of bacterial complications

Antibacterial drugs should not be routinely administered to all children with measles for the purpose of preventing bacterial complications. These agents not only may fail to achieve this goal but also may have the reverse effect and produce superinfections. In many instances the risk of a potential side effect caused by the drug may be greater than the risk of a complication. Consequently, each case of measles should be carefully evaluated before antimicrobial agents are prescribed. The following factors pertaining to the host, the environment, and the disease may influence the decision to administer or withhold these drugs.

Host factors. Age and past experience influence the development of complications. Infants are more prone to develop complications than are older children. Children with a past history of recurrent otitis media are particularly susceptible.

Environmental factors. Patients at home are less likely to acquire a secondary infection than those in hospital wards. The knowledge of a high incidence of streptococcal infections in the patient's environment would influence the decision to give antimicrobial therapy.

Disease factors. A mild case of measles is usually uncomplicated and need not be treated. A severe case, however, would be more likely to be complicated by otitis media or pneumonia.

Treatment of complications

The complications of measles may be treated as follows.

Otitis media. Since hemolytic streptococcus and the pneumococcus are the most common bacterial causes, penicillin will usually provide adequate therapy. Lack of response may indicate an infection caused by *Hemophilus influenzae*, a resistant staphylococcus or coliform bacillus, or an abscess that may require drainage. Treatment of otitis media is discussed in detail on p. 232.

Pneumonia. Bacterial pneumonia may be caused by *Streptococcus pneumoniae*, hemolytic streptocci, *Staphylococcus* species, or *Hemophilus influenzae*. Treatments of these infections are discussed on pp. 185, 378, and 562.

Bronchiolitis. The treatment of infants who develop complicating bronchiolitis is difficult. The details are discussed in Chapter 22.

Obstructive laryngitis and laryngotracheitis. The development of a severe measles croup requires emergency treatment. The child should be hospitalized and placed in a croupette with high humidity and oxygen content. If in spite of this therapy there is increasing restlessness, dyspnea, and tachycardia, a tracheostomy should be performed without delay. It is hazardous to wait for extreme cyanosis and other signs of asphyxia to develop. Treatment of this complication is discussed in detail in Chapter 22.

Encephalitis. Treatment is primarily symptomatic. Convulsive seizures may be controlled by barbiturates. If bulbar involvement is present, the management would be similar to that of bulbar poliomyelitis (p. 53).

The use of large doses of immune globulin (IG) was recommended for treatment, but the value of this procedure was never demonstrated. A careful statistical study was carried out by Greenberg et al. in 1955 comparing 51 children with measles encephalitis treated with IG and 108 children who received no IG. The course of the encephalitis in the IG-treated group did not appear to differ from that of the untreated group.

The use of corticosteroids has been controversial. The very favorable clinical experience reported by Applebaum and Abler in 1956 with 17 treated cases and by Allen in 1957 with ten treated cases appeared to be impressive. Although the number of cases was small (27), the reported incidence of 26 complete recoveries was striking. On the other hand, in 1959 Meade reported comparable results without corticosteroid therapy. He cited a personal observation of over 50 patients, many with respiratory paralysis and status epilepticus, who recovered without sequelae. The evidence for the efficacy of corticosteroids in the treatment of measles encephalitis is not convincing.

An important aspect of the treatment of encephalitis is the supportive medical and nursing care necessary to tide over a comatose child for a period of days and sometimes weeks. This includes careful attention to hydration and nutrition and the prevention and treatment of intercurrent infections.

PREVENTIVE MEASURES
Immune globulin

Measles can be modified or prevented by human IG, which induces passive immunity of approximately 4 weeks' duration. Consequently, it may have to be repeated if reexposure occurs more than 1 month after inoculation. IG is given intramuscularly. Side effects are rare, and it does *not* cause viral hepatitis. The dose for modification of the disease is 0.04 ml per kilogram of body weight; for prevention, 0.2 ml per kilogram of body weight.

Measles virus vaccines

The use of measles virus vaccine for the prevention of measles is discussed in detail on p. 510.

ISOLATION AND QUARANTINE

In general, isolation and quarantine procedures are of limited value in the prophylaxis of measles. Exposure usually occurs before the diagnosis is obvious. Attempts to isolate siblings from each other are useless. The availability of IG and live attenuated measles virus vaccine for household and ward contacts has obviated the need for quarantine.

Isolation of patient

Epidemiologic evidence has indicated that measles is no longer contagious after the fifth day of rash. Consequently, children may return to school or other group activities after this time.

Quarantine of contact

The susceptible contact is a potential source of infection from the eighth day after exposure to as long as the twenty-first day if IG has been administered. Consequently, if quarantine were to be instituted, a child would have to be isolated for almost 2 weeks. Experience has shown that quarantine rarely affects the course of an epidemic. On the contrary, it usually disrupts household and school activities unnecessarily. Once the outbreak has occurred, it would be best to continue normal school and group activities and to rely chiefly on IG and live attenuated measles virus vaccine as prophylactic agents.

REFERENCES

Adams JM. Clinical pathology of measles encephalitis and sequelae. Neurology 1968;18:52.

Albrecht P, Ennis FA, Saltzman EJ, Krugman S. Persistence of maternal antibody in infants beyond 12 months: mechanism of measles vaccine failure. J Pediatr 1977;91:715.

Allen JE. Treatment of measles encephalitis with adrenal steroids. Pediatrics 1957;20:87.

Anderson JF, Goldberger J. Experimental measles in the monkey; a preliminary note. Public Health Rep 1911;26:847.

Annunziato D, Kaplan MH, Hall WW, et al. Atypical measles syndrome: pathologic and serologic findings. Pediatrics 1982;70:203-209.

Applebaum E, Abler C. Treatment of measles encephalitis with corticotropin. Am J Dis Child 1956;92:47.

Barkin RM. Measles mortality: analysis of the primary cause of death. Am J Dis Child 1975;129:307.

Berman PH, Giles JP, Krugman S. Correlation of measles and subacute sclerosing panencephalitis. Neurology 1968;18:91.

Black FL, Yannet H. Inapparent measles after gamma globulin administration. JAMA 1960;173:1183.

Blake FG, Trask JD. Studies on measles. I. Susceptibility of monkeys to the virus of measles. J Exp Med 1921;33:385.

Bloch A, Vardy P. Pneumomediastinum and subcutaneous emphysema in measles. Clin Pediatr 1968;7:7.

Bolande RP. Significance and nature of inclusion-bearing cells in the urine of patients with measles. N Engl J Med 1961;265:919.

Brodsky AL. Atypical measles: severe illness in recipients of killed measles virus vaccine upon exposure to natural infection. JAMA 1972;222:1415.

Brody JA, Detels R. Subacute sclerosing panencephalitis: a zoonosis following aberrant measles. Lancet 1970;2:500.

Christensen PO, et al. An epidemic of measles in Southern Greenland in 1951. Acta Med Scand 1953;144:430, 450.

Connolly JH, Allen IV, Hurwitz LJ, Millar JHD. Measles-virus antibody and antigen in subacute sclerosing panencephalitis. Lancet 1967;1:542.

Dales LG, Chin J. Predicting measles susceptibility. Pediatrics 1984;73:871-873.

Dawson JR Jr. Cellular inclusions in cerebral lesions of epidemic encephalitis. Arch Neurol Psychiatr 1934;31:685.

Degen JA Jr. Visceral pathology in measles: a clinicopathological study of 100 fatal cases. Am J Med Sci 1937;194:104.

Detels R, McNew J, Brady JA, Edgar AH. Further epidemiological studies of subacute sclerosing panencephalitis. Lancet 1973;2:11.

Enders JF, McCarthy K, Mitus A, Cheatham WJ. Isolation of measles virus at autopsy in cases of giant-cell pneumonia without rash. N Engl J Med 1959;261:875.

Enders JF, Katz SL, Milovanovic MJ, Holloway A. Studies on an attenuated measles virus vaccine. I. Development and preparation of the vaccine: techniques for assay of effects of vaccination. N Engl J Med 1960;263:153.

Enders JF, Peebles TC. Propagation in tissue cultures of cytopathogenic agents from patients with measles. Proc Soc Exp Biol Med 1954;86:277.

Enders JF, et al. Measles virus: a summary of experiments concerned with isolation properties and behavior. Am J Public Health 1957;47:275.

Frey HM, Krugman S. Atypical measles syndrome: unusual hepatic, pulmonary, and immunologic aspects. Am J Med Sci 1981;281:51-55.

Fulginiti VA, Eller JJ, Downie AW, Kempe CH. Altered reactivity to measles virus: atypical measles in children previously immunized with inactivated measles virus vaccine. JAMA 1967;202:1075.

Graves MC, Silver SM, Choppin PW. Measles virus polypeptide synthesis in infected cells. Virology 1978;86:254-263.

Greenberg M, Applebaum E, Pellitteri O, Eisenstein DT. Measles encephalitis. II. Treatment with gamma globulin. J Pediatr 1955;46:648.

Hall WW, Choppin PW. Measles-virus proteins in the brain tissue of patients with subacute sclerosing panencephalitis. Absence of M protein. N Engl J Med 1981;304:1152-1155.

Hall WJ, Hall CB. Atypical measles in adolescents: evaluation of clinical and pulmonary function. Ann Intern Med 1979;90:882.

Halsey NA. Current status of measles in the United States 1973-1944. J Infect Dis 1978;137:847.

Jabbour JT, et al. Epidemiology of subacute sclerosing panencephalitis (SSPE). JAMA 1972;220:959.

Josias A. Recherches expérimentales sur la transmissibilité de la rugeole aux animaux. Méd Mod 1898;9:158.

Katz SL, Morley DC, Krugman S. Attenuated measles vaccine in Nigerian children. Am J Dis Child 1962;103:402-405.

Katz SL, et al. Studies on an attenuated measles virus vaccine. VIII. General summary and evaluation of the results of vaccination. N Engl J Med 1960;263:180.

Koplik H. The diagnosis of the invasion of measles from a study of the exanthema as it appears on the buccal mucous membrane. Arch Pediatr 1896;13:918.

Krugman S. Present status of measles and rubella immunization in the United States: a medical progress report. J Pediatr 1971;78:1.

Krugman S. Present status of measles and rubella immunization in the United States: a medical progress report. J Pediatr 1977;90:1.

Krugman S, Giles JP, Friedman H. Studies on immunity to measles. PAHO/WHO Scientific Publication no. 147, May 1967, pp 353-360.

Krugman S, Giles JP, Jacobs AM. Studies on an attenuated measles virus vaccine. VI. Clinical antigenic and prophylactic effects in institutionalized children. N Engl J Med 1960;263:174.

Krugman S, Giles JP, Jacobs AM, Friedman H. Studies with live attenuated measles-virus vaccine: comparative clinical, antigenic and prophylactic effects after inoculation with and without gamma globulin. Am J Dis Child 1962;103:353-363.

Krugman S, Giles JP, Jacobs AM, Friedman H. Studies with a further attenuated live measles-virus vaccine. Pediatrics 1963;31:919.

Krugman RD, et al. Impotency of live-virus vaccines as a result of improper handling in clinical practice. J Pediatr 1974;85:512.

Landrigan PJ, Witte JJ. Neurologic disorders following live measles-virus vaccine. JAMA 1973;223:1459.

Littauer J, Sørensen K. The measles epidemic at Umanak in Greenland in 1962. Dan Med Bull 1965;12:43.

Mallory FB, Medlar EM. Skin lesions in measles. J Med Res 1920;41:327.

Martin DB, et al. Atypical measles in adolescents and young adults. Ann Intern Med 1979;90:977.

McCrumb FR, et al. Globulin-modified live attenuated measles-virus vaccination. Am J Dis Child 1962;103:350-353.

Meade RH III. Common viral infections in childhood: a discussion of measles, German measles, mumps, chickenpox, vaccinia and smallpox. Med Clin North Am 1959;43:1355.

Merz DC, Scheid A, Choppin R. The importance of antibodies to the fusion glycoprotein (F) of paramyxoviruses in the prevention of spread of infection. J Exp Med 1980;151:275.

Monif GR, Hood CI. Ileocolitis associated with measles (rubeola). Am J Dis Child 1970;102:245.

Morley DC. Measles in Nigeria. Am J Dis Child 1962; 103:230.

Mountcasle WE, Choppin PW. A comparison of polypeptides of four measles virus strains. Virology 1977;78:463-474.

Murphy JV, Yunis EJ. Encephalopathy following measles infection in children with chronic illness. J Pediatr 1976;88:937.

Nader PR, Horwitz MS, Rousseau J. Atypical exanthem following exposure to natural measles: 11 cases in children previously inoculated with killed vaccine. J Pediatr 1968;72:22.

Olson RW, Hodges GR. Measles pneumonia: bacterial suprainfection as a complicating factor. JAMA 1975;232:363.

Periés JR, Chany C. Activitée, hémagglutinate et hémolytique, de virus morbilleur. C R Acad Sci [D] (Paris) 1960;251:820.

Rake G, Shaffer MF. Studies on measles. I. The use of the chorio-allantois of the developing chick embryo. J Immunol 1940;38:177.

Rauh LW, Schmidt R. Measles immunization with killed virus vaccine. Am J Dis Child 1965;109:232.

Rosen L. Hemagglutination and hemagglutination-inhibition with measles virus. Virology 1961;13:139.

Scheifele DW, Forbes CE. Prolonged giant cell excretion in severe African measles. Pediatrics 1972;50:867.

Sever JL, et al. Diagnosis of subacute panencephalitis: the value and availability of measles antibody determinations. JAMA 1974;228:604.

Stimson PM. The earlier diagnosis of measles. JAMA 1928;90:660.

Stokes J Jr, et al. Enders' live measles-virus vaccine with human immune globulin. 1. Clinical reactions. Am J Dis Child 1962;103:366, 372.

Suringa DWR, Bank LJ, Ackerman AB. Role of measles virus in skin lesions and Koplik's spots. N Engl J Med 1970;283:1139.

Tompkins V, Macaulay JC. A characteristic cell in nasal secretions during prodromal measles. JAMA 1955;157:711.

Tyrrell DLJ, Norrby E. Structural polypeptides of measles virus. J Gen Virol 1978;39:219-229.

van Bogaert L. Une leuco-encephalite sclerosante subaiguë. J Neurol Neurosurg Psychiatry 1945;8:101.

Wechsler SL, Fields BN. Intracellular synthesis of measles virus-specified polypeptides. J Virol 1978;25:285-297.

Weinstein L. Failure of chemotherapy to prevent the bacterial complications of measles. N Engl J Med 1955; 253:679.

Zahorsky J, Zahorsky TS. Synopsis of pediatrics. St. Louis: The C. V. Mosby Co., 1953.

14

ASEPTIC MENINGITIS

Aseptic meningitis is usually a benign syndrome of multiple etiologies characterized by headache, fever, vomiting, and meningeal signs. The cerebrospinal fluid (CSF) shows an increase in mononuclear cells, and it yields no bacterial or fungal growth on culture. Recovery occurs in about 3 to 10 days and is nearly always complete. Wallgren, (1925), a Swedish pediatrician, recognized and described the aseptic meningitis syndrome in the 1920s, delineating its clinical features and differentiating it from bacterial meningitis.

The viruses and other agents responsible for the aseptic meningitis syndrome may also give rise to a more severe involvement of the central nervous system (CNS), such as meningoencephalitis, encephalitis, and encephalomyelitis (Chapter 4). The boundary line between aseptic meningitis and encephalitis is often indistinct and is drawn arbitrarily on clinical grounds. The clinical picture may not always reveal the full extent of CNS involvement.

ETIOLOGY AND EPIDEMIOLOGY

Aseptic meningitis may be associated with a wide variety of agents and diseases. Many of these are listed as follows:

Viruses
  Mumps
  ECHO virus
  Poliovirus
  Coxsackie virus
  Adenovirus
  Lymphocytic choriomeningitis

  Herpes simplex
  Herpes zoster
  Epstein-Barr virus (EBV)
  Encephalitis: St. Louis, California, eastern equine, and western equine
Bacteria
  Cat-scratch fever
  Syphilis
  Leptospirosis
Miscellaneous
  Toxoplasmosis
  Trichinosis
  Rickettsia
  Mycoplasma pneumoniae
  Lymphogranuloma venereum
  Lyme disease
  Kawasaki's syndrome
  Mollaret's syndrome
Bacterial meningitis
  Tuberculous, in early stages
  Pyogenic, modified by treatment
Noninfectious
  Parameningeal reactions: sinusitis, otitis, mastoiditis, abscess, etc.
  Poisons: lead, arsenic, etc.
  Intrathecal injections: chemotherapeutic agents, contrast media, air
  Vaccines: rabies
  Leukemia and carcinomatosis
Drugs

In spite of improved methods of recognizing these agents, the cause of a large proportion of cases of aseptic meningitis remains unknown.

Enteroviruses (Chapter 5) have been recognized as significant agents in CNS infections ever since the polioviruses were first known to cause both paralytic and nonparalytic disease. With the marked decrease in circulation of polioviruses, the Coxsackie viruses and ECHO viruses continue to be important causes of aseptic meningitis; they were probably responsible for approximately three fourths of the total of more than 11,000 cases of aseptic meningitis reported in the United States in 1983. The characteristics of the enteroviruses and the clinical manifestations produced by them are described in detail in Chapter 5.

In attempting to focus on one or another of the many, varied causes of aseptic meningitis, the physician may be greatly assisted by a careful epidemiologic history. Occupational exposure to mouse colonies or a new pet hamster in the home raises the question of lymphocytic choriomeningitis (LCM) virus. A sexual contact within 1 to 3 weeks with a partner whose inguinal nodes were strikingly enlarged and tender suggests the possibility of lymphogranuloma venereum (LGV), a chlamydial infection. Recent travel to endemic or epidemic areas and a history of insect bites may stimulate more careful investigation of current arbovirus infections. Water-skiing or swimming in a southern fresh water lake or pond in the past 4 or 5 days precedes primary amebic meningoencephalitis due to Naegleria fowleri, an unusual but often severe infection in which the free-living amoebae reach the CNS via the olfactory epithelium (Darby et al., 1979).

Mumps virus was also a common cause of aseptic meningitis. It should be considered in all cases, but especially when mumps is prevalent in the community and during the winter and spring months. Mumps meningitis may occur in the absence of parotitis or other manifestations of mumps infection (Fig. 16-3). The diagnosis of mumps and other features of the disease are discussed in Chapter 16. Widespread utilization of the trivalent measles-mumps-rubella (MMR) vaccine has markedly reduced the numbers of cases of mumps virus infections in the United States in the past decade.

In a 5-year investigation of the causes of certain syndromes of the CNS, Meyer et al. (1960) determined the cause in 305 cases of aseptic meningitis. In their study the enteroviruses, excluding polioviruses, accounted for 30% of the cases and mumps virus for about 16%. Lymphocytic choriomeningitis (LCM) and herpes simplex virus are less commonly detected as causes of aseptic meningitis.

It is difficult to assess the overall contribution of the arboviruses, but in epidemics of arbovirus encephalitis a sizable number of patients, especially children, will acquire a benign illness with neurologic manifestations, predominantly those of viral meningitis, accompanied by no significant change in the sensorium. For example, in the epidemic of St. Louis encephalitis in Houston in 1964, 15 of a total of 26 patients had the mild illness that was confirmed serologically as St. Louis encephalitis virus infection (Barrett et al., 1965). The seasonal distribution of viruses associated with aseptic meningitis is an important clue to their recognition. The enteroviruses and arboviruses predominate during the warm months, whereas mumps virus was present chiefly during the winter and spring months.

Lymphocytic choriomeningitis may be established by the detection of virus in CSF or blood and by a rise in the level of either complement-fixing or neutralizing antibody. The diagnosis of herpes simplex is described on p. 143, of herpes zoster on p. 441, of infectious mononucleosis on p. 64, and of toxoplasmosis on p. 393. The recognition of the remaining causes of aseptic meningitis depends on the distinctive clinical picture of the various diseases, the isolation of the etiologic agent, or the demonstration of an increase in the level of antibody.

Bacterial meningitis may sometimes be a confusing factor. Tuberculous meningitis in the early stages and pyogenic meningitis, particularly that caused by *Haemophilus influenzae*, either early or modified by antibiotic treatment, may resemble aseptic meningitis. The CSF in such cases may show an increase in cells, predominantly lymphocytes. The glucose value is not invariably low and cultures may be sterile. (See Table 15-1.)

A number of case reports call attention to the simultaneous occurrence of bacterial and viral meningitis (Wright et al., 1962; Eglin et al., 1984), but this is a rare coincidence. Some drugs, especially nonsteroidal antiinflammatory agents, have induced aseptic meningitis in patients who have apparently developed an immediate hypersensitivity to the components.

Derbes (1984) reported a woman who underwent four separate episodes of aseptic meningitis after ingestion of trimethoprim-sulfamethoxizole and a fifth attack after trimethoprim alone.

Kawasaki's syndrome, for which an etiology has yet to be determined, is often accompanied by an aseptic meningitis that may be responsible in part for the irritability and misery displayed by many of these patients. Aseptic meningitis has also complicated Lyme disease (erythema chronicum migrans and arthritis), a disorder now attributed to a spirochete. Mollaret's syndrome is a recurrent aseptic meningitis of unknown etiology with repeated episodes of fever and sterile meningitis lasting 4 or 5 days, occurring as frequently as monthly over a 3 or 4 year period.

The introduction into the subarachnoid space of foreign materials such as contrast media (for myelography) or medications (for CNS tumor therapy) may initiate a brisk meningeal pleocytosis with an accompanying clinical syndrome indistinguishable from infectious meningitis. The human diploid cell rabies vaccine (Chapter 21) is far less likely to provoke CNS reactions than were its predecessors, duck embryo or rabbit nervous tissue vaccines.

Usually the attack rates of infection and aseptic meningitis during enterovirus outbreaks are highest in infants and young children. In the 10 year period from 1970 to 1979, 64% of enterovirus isolates were from children under 10 years of age, 50% from those under 4 years, 29% from those under 1 year (Moore, 1981). Clusters of enterovirus meningitis have been reported among high school football players (Baron et al., 1982; Moore et al., 1983). They experience higher attack rates, suffer greater morbidity, and

more frequently require hospitalization than their classmates. The agents most frequently isolated from clinical specimens in the last 7 years are shown in Table 14-1, as well as the total numbers of aseptic meningitis patients reported to the Centers for Disease Control during those same years.

PATHOLOGY

Since most patients with aseptic meningitis recover completely, few postmortem studies have been reported. A leptomeningitis with inflammatory cell infiltration, polymorphonuclear cells in perivascular sheaths, and mononuclear cells in the choroid plexus has been described.

CLINICAL MANIFESTATIONS

The onset may be abrupt or gradual. The initial features are headache, fever, malaise, gastrointestinal symptoms, and signs of meningeal irritation. Abdominal pain is a common complaint. Some patients have ill-defined chest pain or generalized muscular pains or aches. Sore throat is occasionally encountered. Nausea and vomiting are common. Stiffness of the neck or back may develop a day or so after the onset. The deep tendon reflexes are normal or show hyperactivity. Muscle power is normal, as a rule, but there may be slight or transitory weakness. A maculopapular rash may accompany the aseptic meningitis syndrome, especially in association with certain types of ECHO and Coxsackie virus infections, The CSF shows pleocytosis with a predominance of lymphocytes. The symptoms and signs usually subside spontaneously and rapidly. The patient is well in 3 to 10 days.

Headache. Headache is one of the most common manifestations and often the initial complaint. It is likely to be severe. Characteristically frontal in location, it may be retrobulbar, occipital, or generalized.

Fever. The temperature ranges from 37.8° C (100° F) to as high as 40° to 40.6° C (104° or 105° F). The fever lasts from 3 to 9 days, with a mean of about 5 days. Sometimes it is biphasic, and this should make one alert for enteroviral infection.

Gastrointestinal symptoms. Gastrointestinal symptoms, including nausea and abdominal pain, are frequent early manifestations. Vomiting may occur at the onset or a day or two later. Diarrhea is more common than constipation.

Table 14-1. Reported cases of aseptic meningitis, U.S.A., 1978-1984

Year	No. cases	Most common agents
1978	6573	ECHO 4, 9
1979	8754	ECHO 7, 11
1980	8028	ECHO 11, Coxsackie B5
1981	9547	ECHO 9, 30
1982	9680	ECHO 11, 30
1983	11,740	Coxsackie B5, ECHO 30, 11, 24
1984	8036	ECHO 9, 30, Coxsackie B5, A9

Pain. Pain occurs in the epigastric or periumbilical areas fairly often. Thoracic pain suggests pleurodynia and Coxsackie virus infection, but mild chest pain may occur in aseptic meningitis caused by ECHO virus type 6 and other agents. Generalized muscular pain in the back and extremities is more likely to appear in enteroviral infections than in mumps meningitis.

Meningeal signs. Signs consisting of stiff neck, stiff back, and tightness of the hamstring muscles are present in the majority of patients. Brudzinski's sign is usually present.

Neuromuscular changes. Deep tendon reflexes are normal or show hyperactivity. Signs of muscle weakness are usually absent or equivocal but myalgia may be prominent. Slight or transitory weakness along with muscle pain and tenderness and abnormal tendon or superficial reflexes point toward the possibility of enterovirus infections. Definite paresis or paralysis has been noted with certain of the enteroviruses (especially ECHO 2, 4, 6, 16; Coxsackie A4, B2, B3; and the newer enterovirus types 70 and 71). This weakness usually recedes more rapidly than with classic poliomyelitis and rarely, if ever, leaves residual paralysis beyond 30 to 60 days from onset. Transitory weakness seldom occurs in other forms of aseptic meningitis. In any patient showing definite or persistent motor weakness or encephalitic signs, a more extensive involvement of the CNS should be considered.

Rash. A macular, maculopapular, or tiny vesicular rash accompanies certain enteroviral infections, particularly ECHO virus types 4, 6, 9, and 16 and Coxsackie virus types A9 and A16. Petechial eruptions have accompanied ECHO type 9 virus infection. The details are described in Chapter 5.

Seizures. Seizures are occasionally observed in viral meningitis, especially in younger patients with high fevers where they may represent febrile convulsions. Their infrequency, however, necessitates a careful consideration of other possible causes. Early bacterial meningitis, a parameningeal inflammatory focus, brain tumor, vascular malformations, local cerebritis, and septic emboli with endocarditis are among the conditions to be considered. Careful observation of the patient's course will be helpful in setting the priority of any further investigative studies.

Laboratory findings. Except for changes in the CSF, the usual clinical laboratory tests are seldom helpful (Clarke and Cost, 1983). The CSF shows a leukocyte count ranging from 10 to 1000 cells mm³. The cell count is usually low, the average being under 150 cells. A total cell count over 1500 is not likely but has been seen in ECHO virus and Coxsackie virus infections. Studies of CSF from patients in an epidemic setting have revealed positive cultures for enterovirus even with cell counts less than 10/mm³ (Wilfert et al., 1975). In mumps meningitis the cells usually number less than 1000, but counts between 1500 and 4000 have been observed. Mononuclear cells as a rule predominate in all forms of aseptic meningitis. However, CSF obtained early in the course of illness will frequently display a polymorphonuclear cell preponderance. This will shift rapidly over the next 6 to 8 hours so that a repeat lumbar puncture will yield CSF with more than 50% mononuclear cells. The presence of a CSF eosinophilia suggests a helminthic infestation, lymphocytic choriomeningitis virus, or a number of noninfectious disorders such as Hodgkin's disease (Chesney et al., 1979). In mumps the cells are almost entirely lymphocytes. The total protein content varies from normal to values as high as 100 mg/dl. It may rise even higher in lymphogranuloma venereum and lead poisoning. The glucose content is usually normal or slightly elevated. It is characteristically low in lymphogranuloma venereum and meningitides caused by the tubercle bacillus and other bacteria. Cultures for bacteria and fungi are negative, and the other constituents of the CSF are normal.

The CSF in amebic meningoencephalitis due to *Naegleria fowleri* has a lowered glucose with a much higher cell count and polymorphonuclear predominance than the usual aseptic meningitis. In the appropriate epidemiologic setting with failure to visualize or culture bacteria or fungi from such a specimen, a wet mount of CSF under ordinary microscopy may show motile forms with pseudopods (Darby et al., 1979).

DIAGNOSIS

Recognition of the syndrome of aseptic meningitis is straightforward but can be troublesome (Singer et al., 1980). Headache, fever, vomiting, and signs of meningeal irritation call for a lumbar puncture. The CSF shows characteristic pleocytosis, with predominantly mononuclear elements. The varying causes of this syndrome have been discussed previously. The clinical and epidemiologic circumstances often give clues leading to the underlying cause. Since viral infections are the most common causes of aseptic meningitis, a search should be made for the etiologic agent in the CSF, throat, and stool specimens. Serum specimens from the acute and convalescent phases tested for rise in the level of antibody may help in the diagnosis.

CASE REPORT. B.C., a 3 $\frac{5}{12}$-year-old boy, was brought by his parents to the emergency room of Duke Hospital in July 1984 with a history of fever, malaise, drowsiness, irritability, and headache of 3 days' duration. The headache had increased markedly in the past 12 hours. He had vomited after each of several small meals that day and complained of photophobia. Temperature was 39.5° C. There was no rash or conjunctivitis. He had marked nuchal rigidity and positive Kernig and Brudzinski signs. Lumbar puncture disclosed turbid CSF under slightly increased pressure. CSF cell count was 460 WBC/mm^3, 75% of which were polymorphonuclear. Gram stain and coagglutination of CSF were negative for bacteria and bacterial antigens respectively. CSF protein was 48 mg/100 ml; glucose was 75 mg/100 ml (blood glucose 110 mg/100 ml). Chloramphenicol and ampicillin were administered intravenously and he was admitted to the hospital.

A second lumbar puncture, performed 8 hours after the initial one, disclosed a white blood cell count of 375/mm^3, 35% of which were polymorphonuclear and 65% mononuclear. CSF glucose and protein were essentially unchanged. By the next morning, 18 hours after hospital admission, he was markedly improved, smiling, comfortable, and active. The emergency room CSF culture revealed no bacterial growth and his antibiotic therapy was discontinued. Although his temperature rose again during the second hospital day to 39° C, he remained alert and increasingly active. The next morning he was discharged home with instructions to his parents to bring him promptly back to the emergency room if his improvement failed to continue. Two days after his discharge, both the CSF and an admission stool specimen submitted to the virology laboratory were positive for enterovirus.

In the case report, the most compelling evidence for a viral, rather than bacterial, etiology was the rapid shift of the CSF distribution of white blood cells in 8 hours from an initial polymorphonuclear to a mononuclear cell preponderance. Even with early antibiotic therapy of pyogenic bacterial meningitis, 48 hours or more

will elapse before such a cellular shift occurs. With suspected viral meningitis patients, a prompt second CSF examination after 6 to 8 hours may be of great help in resolving the differential between bacterium and virus.

DIFFERENTIAL DIAGNOSIS

The various conditions that may be confused with aseptic meningitis are considered in Chapter 15 in the discussion of the differential diagnosis of acute bacterial meningitis. In certain cases of the latter, the CSF may be sterile and contain a predominance of mononuclear cells. This is particularly true of patients with pyogenic meningitis who have previously received antibacterial treatment.

COMPLICATIONS

As a rule there are no complications in normal hosts. When they do arise, they are those of the underlying disease.

PROGNOSIS

The prognosis is generally excellent. Recovery is rapid and complete. Few fatalities have been reported. There have been few longitudinal follow-up studies of patients with viral meningitis and it is exceedingly difficult without histologic confirmation to be certain whether or not an element of encephalitis supervened.

In two groups of patients, very young infants and children of any age with agammaglobulinemia, aseptic meningitis may not be a benign illness. The enteroviruses have produced severe infections and some fatalities in newborns and infants in the first months of life (Bacon and Sims, 1976). Longitudinal studies of survivors suggest that language difficulties and smaller head circumference were more common among these infants than among uninfected controls or patients with enterovirus meningitis after the first year of life (Sells et al., 1975; Lepow, 1978; Wilfert et al. 1980). Wilfert et al. (1977) have reported chronic persistent ECHO virus meningitis in patients whose immunologic deficit was characterized by absense of surface-immunoglobulin-bearing B lymphocytes. Types 9, 19, 30 and 33 ECHO viruses were recovered repeatedly from CSF for periods from 2 months to 3 years after onset of aseptic meningitis, and several of these children developed a dermatomyositis-like syndrome. Their CNS manifestations ranged at various times from asymptomatic to meningitic to encephalitic.

TREATMENT

The main practical problem confronting the clinician is whether or not to treat the patient with antimicrobial agents. The diagnosis of viral meningitis is seldom confirmed by the laboratory in the first days of the patient's illness. Nevertheless, a strong indication of viral cause may be gained from the circumstances in which the disease occurs, that is, in the midst of an outbreak of aseptic meningitis in the community during the summer or fall months; in the presence of a rash, enanthem, or other features of enteroviral infection; or with exposure to mumps or in the presence of parotitis in the patient. These conditions may suffice to justify withholding antimicrobial treatment. On the other hand, in those situations in which the patient has already received antimicrobial agents in either adequate or inadequate amounts, the physician may choose to continue therapy, observe the patient carefully, and follow laboratory developments until a diagnosis of bacterial meningitis has been excluded (see p. 178).

The characteristics of the CSF are not always completely helpful in the decision of whether or not to treat with antimicrobial agents. Early in viral meningitis, polymorphonuclear leukocytes may predominate; conversely, in the early stages of bacterial meningitis the pleocytosis may consist predominantly of lymphocytes. Rapid tests such as counterimmunoelectrophoresis (CIE), coagglutination, or latex agglutination may assist in early bacterial diagnosis in the absence of a positive Gram stain before a culture report is available.

The importance of repeated examination of the CSF cannot be overstressed. In as short a time as 8 hours the CSF may markedly change its cellular content. Antimicrobial treatment may be started in cases in which the cause is uncertain and be discontinued if the bacterial cultures of the CSF taken *before* treatment prove to be sterile.

Supportive and symptomatic treatment include analgesics for headaches and pains and pillow or blanket roll support under the knees for relief of spasm of extensor muscles of legs and back. When the patient is afebrile and asymptomatic, it is important to evaluate muscle power in order to detect the rare instance of residual weakness that may require continuing physiotherapy.

REFERENCES

Adair CV, Ross LG, Smadel JE.: Aseptic meningitis, a disease of diverse etiology: clinical and etiologic studies on 854 cases. Ann Intern Med 1953;39:675.

Bacon CJ, Sims DG.: Echovirus 19 infection in infants under 6 months. Arch Dis Child 1976;51:631.

Baron RC, Hatch MH, Kleeman K, et al. Aseptic meningitis among members of a high school football team: an outbreak associated with echovirus 16 infection. JAMA 1982;284:1724.

Barrett FF, Yow MD, Phillips CA. St. Louis encephalitis in children during the 1964 epidemic. JAMA 1965;193:381.

Beeson PB, Hankey DD. Leptospiral meningitis. Arch Intern Med 1952;89:575.

Bromberg K, Shank PR, Zinner SH, Peter G. Inability of CIE to detect echovirus in cerebrospinal fluid. Am J Clin Pathol 1983;80:383.

Centers for Disease Control. Aseptic meningitis surveillance. U.S. Department of Health, Education, and Welfare, Public Health Service, Jan. 1979.

Centers for Disease Control. Aseptic meningitis—Panama. MMWR 1981;30:559.

Centers for Disease Control. Aseptic meningitis in a high school football team. MMWR 1981;29:631.

Chesney PJ, Katcher ML, Nelson DB, Horowitz SD. CSF eosinophilia and chronic lymphocytic choriomeningitis virus meningitis. J Pediatrics 1979;94:750.

Clarke D, Cost K. Use of serum C-reactive protein in differentiating septic from aseptic meningitis in children. J Pediatr 1983;102:718.

Coleman WS, Lischner HW, Grover W. Recurrent aseptic meningitis without sequelae. J Pediatr. 1975;87:89.

Darby CP, Conradi SE, Holbrook TW, Chantellier C. Primary amebic meningo-encephalitis. Am J Dis Child 1979;133:1025.

Derbes SJ. Trimethoprim-induced aseptic meningitis. JAMA 1984;252:2865.

Eglin RP, Swann RA, Isaacs D, Moxon ER. Simultaneous bacterial and viral meningitis. Lancet 1984;2:984.

Farmer K, MacArthur BA, Clay MM. A follow-up study of neonatal meningo-encephalitis due to Coxsackie virus B5. J Pediatr 1975;87:568.

Jarvis WR, Tucker G. Echovirus type 7 meningitis in young children. Am J Dis Child 1981;135:1009.

Karzon DT, Hayner NS, Winkelstein W Jr, Barron AL. An epidemic of aseptic meningitis syndrome due to ECHO virus type 6. II. A clinical study of ECHO 6 infection. Pediatrics 1962;29:418.

Kelsey DS. Adenovirus meningoencephalitis. Pediatrics 1978;61:291.

Kilham L. Mumps meningocephalitis with and without parotitis. Am J Dis Child 1949;78:324.

Kono R, Miyamura K, Tajiri E, et al. Virological and serological studies of neurological complications of acute hemorrhagic conjunctivitis in Thailand. J Infect Dis 1977; 135:706.

Lennette EH, Magoffin RL, Knouf EG. Viral central nervous system disease: an etiologic study conducted at the Los Angeles General Hospital. JAMA 1962;179:687.

Lepow ML. Enteroviral meningitis: a reappraisal. Pediatrics 1978;62:267.

Lepow ML, et al. A clinical, epidemiologic and laboratory investigation of aseptic meningitis during the four-year period, 1955-1958. I. Observations concerning etiology and epidemiology. N Engl J Med 1962a;266:1181.

Lepow ML, et al. A clinical, epidemiologic and laboratory investigation of aseptic meningitis during the four-year period, 1955-1958. II. The clinical disease and its sequelae. N Engl J Med 1962b;266:1188.

Marier R, et al. Coxsackievirus B5 infection and aseptic meningitis in neonates and children. Am J Dis Child 1975;129:321.

Meningitis, aseptic or pyogenic (editorial). Lancet 1984; 1:435.

Meyer HM Jr, et al. Central nervous system syndromes of viral etiology: study of 713 cases. Am J Med 1960;29:334.

Moore M. Enterovirus surveillance report, 1970-1979. Atlanta: Centers for Disease Control, 1981.

Moore M, Baron RC, Filstein MR, et al. Aseptic meningitis and high school football players. JAMA 1983;249:2039.

Rantakallio P, Lapinheimu K, Mantyharvi R. Coxsackie B5 outbreak in a newborn nursery with 17 cases of serous meningitis. Scand J Infect Dis 1970;2:17.

Sabin AB, Krumbiegel ER, Wigand R. ECHO type 9 virus disease. Am J Dis Child 1958;96:197.

Sells CJ, Carpenter RL, Ray CG. Sequelae of central nervous system enterovirus infection. N Engl J Med 1975;293:1.

Silver TS, Todd, JK. Hypoglycorrhachia in pediatric patients. Pediatrics 1976;58:67.

Singer JI, Maur, PR, Riley JP, Smith PB. Management of central nervous system infections during an epidemic of enteroviral aseptic meningitis. J Pediatr 1980;96:559.

Swender PT, Shott, RJ, Williams ML. A community and intensive care nursery outbreak of Coxsackie virus B5 meningitis. Am J Dis Child 1974;127:42.

Wallgren A. Une nouvelle maladie infectieuse du systeme nerveux central. Acta Paediatr 1925;4:158.

Wilfert CM, et al. An epidemic of echovirus 18 meningitis. J Infect Dis 1975;131:75.

Wilfert CM, et al. Persistent and fatal central nervous system ECHO virus infections in patients with agammaglobulinemia. N Engl J Med 1977;296:1485.

Wilfert CM, Thompson RJ Jr, Sunder TR, et al. Longitudinal assessment of children with enteroviral meningitis during the first 3 months of life. Pediatrics 1980;67:811.

Wilfert CM, Lehrman SN, Katz SL. Enteroviruses and meningitis. Pediatr Infect Dis 1983;2:333.

Wright HT Jr, McAllister RM, Ward R. "Mixed" meningitis: report of a case with isolation of *Haemophilus influenzae* type B and ECHO virus type 9 from the cerebrospinal fluid. N Engl J Med 1962;267:142.

15

ACUTE BACTERIAL MENINGITIS

Acute bacterial meningitis is a potentially fatal acute infectious disease caused by a variety of bacteria and characterized clinically by fever and several of the following manifestations: headache, vomiting, irritability, convulsions, drowsiness, coma, stiff neck, and bulging fontanelle. Ninety percent of cases occur in children between the ages of 1 month and 5 years; infants aged 6 to 12 months are at greatest risk.

The advent of antimicrobial drugs had a profound effect on the course and prognosis of meningitis; it reduced the mortality of 50% to 90% to less than 20%. It cannot be too strongly emphasized, however, that *undiagnosed* and *untreated* bacterial meningitis is just as fatal and damaging today as it was in the preantibiotic era.

ETIOLOGY

Acute bacterial meningitis can be caused by any one of a variety of pathogenic and nonpathogenic bacteria. The list of microorganisms that have been incriminated as causative agents of purulent meningitis reads like the table of contents of a textbook of microbiology. The major organisms for children of various age groups are as follows:

Infants and children
  Haemophilus influenzae type b
  Streptococcus pneumoniae
  Neisseria meningitidis
Newborn infants
  Group B streptococci
  Escherichia coli
  Listeria monocytogenes

Postsurgery patients
  Staphylococcus species
  Pseudomonas species

For normal hosts the usual etiologic organisms are limited to a few bacterial species that apparently possess "virulence" factors that enable them to successfully invade the central nervous system (CNS). In the immunocompromised host meningitis may be caused by a myriad of different bacteria present in the environment or on normal sites such as skin or mucosal surfaces.

The three most common causes of meningitis in infants and children are *Haemophilus influenzae*, meningococci, and pneumococci. It is estimated that there are about 10,000 cases of *H. influenzae* meningitis per year in the United States. Group B streptococci and the coliform bacilli are the most common causes of neonatal meningitis. Meningococci and pneumococci are the most common causes of bacterial meningitis in adults.

By serologic techniques meningococci have been separated into nine serogroups: A, B, C, D, X, Y, Z, W-135, and 29-E. More than 95% of reported cases have been caused by strains of groups A, B, C, Y, and W-135. The specific polysaccharides of the capsules of A, B, C, X, and Y have been isolated and analyzed chemically. Antibodies against these capsular polysaccharides are important in development of natural immunity to the meningococci and have also been induced by vaccines for groups A, C, Y, and W-135.

Although 84 serotypes of pneumococci have been established on the basis of their capsular polysaccharides, epidemiologic studies indicate that bacteremic disease is attributable to a more limited number. Austrian et al. (1976) showed that 12 types (1, 3, 4, 6, 7, 8, 9, 12, 14, 18, 19, and 23) were responsible for 75% of bacteremic pneumonias in a 10-hospital United States survey of 3600 patients. These figures were for adults, but the limited data available for children show no marked variations. Pneumococcal meningitis appears to be the most serious form of the illness, with the highest case/fatality ratio and the longest average hospital stay in comparison with *H. influenzae* and meningococcal meningitis (Mufson, 1981).

There are six distinct serologic types of *H. influenzae* (a, b, c, d, e, and f) based on the composition of their capsular polysaccharides. Unencapsulated organisms are prevalent, especially in the respiratory tract, and may be isolated from middle-ear fluids of children with otitis media. In children, nearly all *H. influenzae* responsible for systemic disease are encapsulated, and more than 90% are type b. In adults, in contrast, unencapsulated organisms account for more than 50% of invasive disease, indicating that while virulence is associated with the capsule of the organism, the capsule alone does not account for virulence. Antibodies to the capsular antigen polyribose phosphate (PRP) of *H. influenzae* play a role in protection against disease.

Noncapsular antigens of *H. influenzae*, outer membrane proteins, and lipopolysaccharides also induce antibodies that play a role in protection (Hill, 1983). Different organisms have somewhat differing outer membrane proteins as determined by polyacrylamide gel electrophoresis, which also provides a means for classifying *H. influenzae* strains. In a study of 51 organisms from patients treated in St. Louis, nine distinct subtypes were found, based on outer membrane proteins (Barenkamp et al., 1981). Nosocomial outbreaks of disease have been studied by analysis of outer membrane proteins (Barton et al., 1983).

H. influenzae strains have also been classified by biotyping, a classification based on differences in biochemical characteristics of these organisms. There are at least five different biotypes. In a study of 130 *H. influenzae* isolates, one strain accounted for 93% of all isolates (Kil-

ian et al., 1979). In a study involving isolates from a nursery school outbreak, only six of 13 (46%) organisms colonizing contacts of the index case were of the same biotype as the one isolated from the child who was ill (Prober et al., 1982). Thus, biotyping may be a powerful epidemiologic tool for studying *H. influenzae* isolates in addition to analysis of outer membrane proteins.

There is no pathognomonic sign or symptom that will accurately identify the causative agent of a case of purulent meningitis. Petechial or hemorrhagic skin lesions are most characteristic of meningococcal infection, but they may occasionally be associated with other microorganisms. In the final analysis the true cause is determined by analysis and culture of cerebrospinal fluid (CSF).

PATHOGENESIS

Meningitis most commonly results from a bacteremia. Organisms that have colonized the nasopharynx occultly or with minor respiratory symptoms invade and reach underlying blood vessels. This may produce direct involvement of vessels that supply the CNS, especially the highly vascular choroid plexus, or the formation of local thromboemboli which release septic emboli to the vascular system.

Meningococcal, influenzal, and pneumococcal meningitis may also develop by direct extension from a paranasal sinus or from the middle ear to the mastoid and finally to the meninges. Severe head trauma with a skull fracture and/or CSF rhinorrhea may lead to meningitis, usually pneumococcal. This may occur within the first few weeks of injury or be delayed until many months later. This seems to be much less common in children than in adults, as noted by Einhorn and Mizrahi (1978) in a review of 46 pediatric patients with skull fractures that involved rhinorrhea, otorrhea, hemotympanum, or perforated tympanic membranes. Direct inoculation of bacteria into the CSF may occur with congenital dural defects (dermal sinus or meningomyelocele), neurosurgical procedures, penetrating wounds, or extension from a suppurative parameningeal focus. Infants with underlying illnesses such as malignancy, sickle cell disease, and agammaglobulinemia are also predisposed to develop meningitis. Certain population groups such as American Indians, Eskimos, and Blacks are at greater risk as well.

Of the many organisms that colonize the upper respiratory tract and initiate occasional bacteremias, it is notable that pneumococci, meningococci, and *H. influenzae* are the only ones that produce meningitis with some regularity. Among these bacteria, virulence is correlated with a few selected serotypes or serogroups, suggesting that the specific capsular polysaccharides are major determinants in CNS invasiveness. Their chemical constituents are known also to exert an antiphagocytic effect.

PATHOLOGY

The gross appearance of the brain in a patient with meningitis is very striking. The entire surface and base may be covered by a layer of purulent exudate. In meningococcal infections, the exudate is most marked over the parietal and occipital lobes and the cerebellum. In pneumococcal meningitis, the thick purulent fibrinous exudate is confined chiefly to the surface of the brain, particularly the anterior lobes. The basilar portions are involved to a lesser degree. Streptococcal infections are similar to pneumococcal infections, except that the exudate is thinner because it contains less fibrin.

There is also an additional component of vasculitis that may include thrombosis of vessels and/or sinuses, necrosis of vessel walls, and a further compromise of perfusion leading to cerebral edema.

Histologically, the lesion begins with hyperemia and hemorrhages, followed by a purulent inflammatory reaction in the arachnoid and pia mater. The inflammatory exudate consists of masses of polymorphonuclear leukocytes, fibrin, bacterial clumps, and red blood cells.

As the infection extends to the ventricles, thick pus or adhesions may occlude the various foramina or aqueducts and cause obstructive hydrocephalus. Communicating hydrocephalus results as CSF reabsorption by the arachnoid villi is impaired due to occlusion of the sagittal or lateral sinuses, high levels of CSF protein, or obstruction within the basilar cisterns. The exudate may involve the intracranial portion of the optic nerve, with subsequent neuritis and possible blindness. Involvement of the facial and auditory nerves in a like manner may result in facial palsies and permanent deafness. The most frequently affected cranial nerve is the sixth, since its lengthy intracranial course exposes it to direct inflammatory involvement or to compression with increased intracranial pressure.

EPIDEMIOLOGIC FACTORS

There is a characteristic age distribution of the various types of meningitis. *H. influenzae* meningitis is primarily a disease of infancy. The highest incidence is in the first year of life, with most of the cases occurring in children between 3 months and 3 years of age. It rarely occurs in infants less than 3 months of age and is uncommon in children over the age of 5 years. In 1933 Fothergill and Wright showed that the age incidence was inversely proportional to the bactericidal power of the blood for *H. influenzae*. During the first few months most infants are apparently protected by passively acquired antibodies. Neonatal *H. influenzae* infections are rare but they have been reported, presumably because some normal adults lack antibodies to *H influenzae* type b. In the newborn infant, as in the adult, about one half of the cases of invasive disease due to *H. influenzae* are caused by unencapsulated organisms (Dajani et al., 1979). Children begin to synthesize antibodies to *H. influenzae* between 4 and 5 years of age. Adult levels are reached by 7 years of age.

Meningococcal and pneumococcal meningitis have their highest incidence in the first year of life and rarely occur under 3 months of age. Unlike *H. influenzae* infections, they are apt to occur at any age in both children and adults.

Meningitis in newborn and premature infants during the first few months of life is most commonly caused by group B streptococci, *Escherichia coli*, and other gram-negative bacilli. During the period from 1970 to 1977, group B streptococci shifted from being an infrequent cause of neonatal meningitis to be the most commonly isolated pathogen, responsible in some institutions for 50% to 70% of cases (Anthony and Okada, 1977). In the 1980s group B streptococci continue to be the most common cause of meningitis in this age group.

The incidence of acute bacterial meningitis varies according to season. *H. influenzae* meningitis is chiefly an autumn or early winter disease. Pneumococcal and meningococcal infections occur more often during the later winter and early spring; however, these infections may occur during any month of the year.

Over the past 35 years there has been an increase in, or at least an increase in the reporting of, systemic *H. influenzae* disease at medical centers throughout the United States. In addition to meningitis, pyarthroses, epiglottitis, pneumonia, and cellulitis have been reported. Among poor, rural, and Black children *H. influenzae* type b more commonly causes systemic infections. Undoubtedly poor living conditions increase the risk of developing meningitis. The increased incidence in certain ethnic groups and in families, however, as well as the observation that siblings of patients with meningitis have deficient antibody synthesis against *H. influenzae*, have suggested that there is also a genetic vulnerability to the disease (Hill, 1983).

All types of meningitis occur sporadically; only meningococcal infections prevail in epidemic form. Meningococci are transmitted from person to person by nasopharyngeal secretions of a patient or carrier and usually require close contact. Recent epidemics of major import have occurred in Brazil, Finland, Mongolia, and sub-Saharan Africa. Outbreaks among military recruits have been observed in training camps and bases during every period of national mobilization, providing much of the impetus for development and testing of meningococcal vaccines.

The risk of acquiring a secondary case of meningococcal or *haemophilus* disease after a household exposure to the infection is increased by a factor of over 600 compared to the normal population. The risk for haemophilus disease is greatest for infants below 1 year of age and for children between the ages of 1 to 4 years, in whom the incidence of secondary infection is 6% and 2%, respectively (Ward et al., 1979; Nelson, 1982). For meningococcal disease, the incidence of secondary cases is 1% for family members regardless of age (Leedom, 1966).

CLINICAL MANIFESTATIONS

The clinical picture of acute bacterial meningitis depends in large part on the patient's age. The classic manifestations observed in older children and adults are rarely exhibited by infants. In general, the younger the patient, the more obscure and atypical are the symptoms.

Classic meningitis of children and adults

The disease usually begins with fever, chills, vomiting, and severe headache. Occasionally, the first sign of illness is a convulsion that may recur as the disease progresses. Irritability, delirium, and maniacal behavior or drowsiness, stupor, and coma may also develop.

The most consistent physical findings are the presence of moderate to extreme nuchal rigidity associated with Brudzinski's and Kernig's signs. Brudzinski's sign is elicited by rapidly flexing the neck of the supine patient. This maneuver causes brisk flexion of the knees in the presence of meningeal irritation. Kernig's sign is present if there is marked resistance to extension of the knee when the patient is in the supine position with his thigh flexed on his hip and his leg flexed on his knee.

As the disease progresses, the neck stiffness increases, causing the head to be drawn backward. Because of the spasm of the back muscles, the patient assumes a position of opisthotonos.

The reflexes may show extreme variability; usually they are hyperactive. Tache cerebrale may be elicited. This manifestation of vasomotor disturbance is not specific for meningeal irritation and more likely reflects a component of encephalitis. It is elicited by stroking the skin with a dull point or blunt object, causing a red line to appear and persist for several minutes.

The signs and symptoms just described are common to all types of meningitis. There are other manifestations, however, that are peculiar to certain specific infections. Petechial and purpuric eruptions are usually indicative of meningococcemia, although on occasion this has been associated with *H. influenzae* meningitis (Jacobs et al., 1983). Rashes very rarely occur with pneumococcal infections. The rapid development of a hemorrhagic eruption in association with a shocklike state is almost pathognomonic of meningococcemia complicated by the Waterhouse-Friderichsen syndrome. On rare occasions this may occur with other types of sepsis. Joint involvement suggests meningococcal or *H. influenzae* infection.

The presence of a chronically draining ear is commonly associated with pneumococcal meningitis. A history of head trauma also suggests this type of infection. One of our patients had several recurrences of pneumococcal meningitis after a skull fracture.

Patients with *E. coli* meningitis or recurrent meningitis of any type should be examined carefully for the presence of a dimple, sinus, or nevus on the skin over the cervical, thoracic, or lumbar spine. These signs may indicate the presence of a congenital dermal sinus that may communicate with the subarachnoid space.

Meningitis in infancy

Infants between 3 months and 2 years of age rarely develop the classic picture of meningitis. The illness is characterized by fever, vomiting, marked irritability, and frequent convulsions. A high-pitched cry may be present.

A most significant physical finding is a tense *bulging fontanelle*. Nuchal rigidity may or may not be present. Brudzinski's and Kernig's signs are difficult to elicit and to evaluate in this age group.

It is most important to be aware that the highest incidence of meningitis occurs between 6 and 12 months of age. Consequently, any unexplained, persistent febrile illness in an infant should make one suspect the presence of CNS involvement.

Neonatal meningitis

Meningitis in newborn and premature infants is extremely difficult to recognize. The clinical manifestations are vague and nonspecific. In general, if there are overt signs of sepsis, the presence of meningitis should be suspected.

Fever may or may not be present; it is frequently absent. These infants can best be described as "looking and doing poorly." Feedings are usually refused, vomiting occurs frequently, and there may be evidence of either excessive hyperactivity or drowsiness. The fontanelle may be full, tense, or bulging. The neck is usually supple. Respirations are usually irregular. Jaundice is frequently associated with sepsis. Sepsis and meningitis in the newborn are discussed in more detail in Chapter 17.

Recurrent bacterial meningitis

The clinical entity of recurrent bacterial meningitis is a phenomenon that was rarely observed in the preantibiotic era. The use of effective antimicrobial agents has enabled some patients to survive multiple episodes of bacterial meningitis. Recurrent meningitis has been observed in patients with anatomic defects of the CNS and its coverings. The defects may be congenital (meningomyelocele, neurenteric cysts, or midline dermal sinus, either cranial or spinal) or acquired (head trauma with or without an obvious skull fracture). Other causes of recurrent meningitis include parameningeal foci of infection such as chronic mastoiditis, sinusitis, brain abscess, subdural empyema, or epidural abscess of the spine. Defects in immune response may be a rare cause of recurrent meningitis. These include hypogammaglobulinemias, postsplenectomy state, sickle cell and other hemoglobinopathies, leukemia, and lymphoma. After shunting procedures for hydrocephalus, staphylococcal meningitis of a tenacious and often recurrent nature may complicate from 10% to 25% of patients (Sayers, 1976). This often requires complex therapy by intravenous and intraventricular routes plus replacement of the shunt itself.

Relapse of meningitis is to be distinguished from recurrent meningitis. A relapse of meningitis may be associated with improper administration of antimicrobials such as intramuscular chloramphenicol and oral ampicillin during the healing phase of meningitis when the blood-brain barrier is less compromised than during the acute stage. Relapse may also be indicative of an occult focus of infection such as a brain abscess. Relapse has also been associated with infections caused by pneumococci and *H. influenzae* that are relatively resistant to various antimicrobials.

Chronic meningitis (Ellner and Bennett, 1976) due to a large number of infectious agents and noninfectious diseases persists for at least 4 weeks. Among the infections to be considered are bacterial (tuberculous, *Brucella, Leptospiral*), fungal (*Cryptococcus, Candida*, coccidioidomycosis, histoplasmosis), and protozoan (toxoplasmosis, cysticercosis). Noninfectious causes include meningeal leukemia, sarcoidosis, Behçet's syndrome, and uveomeningoencephalitis.

DIAGNOSIS

A diagnosis of acute bacterial meningitis cannot be made on the basis of symptoms and signs alone. The classic picture of fever, headache, vomiting, stiff neck, and Brudzinski's and Kernig's signs may also be due to meningismus or tuberculous or aseptic meningitis. Consequently, a definitive diagnosis can be made only by examination of the CSF. In cases presenting with petechial lesions, smears from these lesions may show meningococci on Gram stain.

Indications for lumbar puncture

A lumbar puncture is indicated if the physician suspects that meningitis is present. Early accurate diagnosis followed by appropriate therapy has a profound effect on the outcome; consequently, it is best to do a spinal tap that yields normal CSF rather than to miss an early diagnosis of meningitis.

In many instances, particularly in infants, fever and convulsions may be the only initial signs of meningitis. It is hazardous to attribute all seizures to febrile convulsions. Experience on a pediatric service where many diagnostic taps have been performed over the years has provided convincing evidence that a properly performed lumbar puncture is a relatively innocuous procedure. Nevertheless, because it is invasive, a lumbar puncture should not be done indiscriminately.

If papilledema is present, and especially if it is accompanied by localizing neurologic signs, radionuclide scanning or computerized axial tomography should be considered prior to the lumbar puncture in order to exclude a brain abscess and avoid the danger of herniation. If such a procedure will significantly delay therapy, however, antibiotics should be instituted before the tap. The subsequent lumbar puncture is conducted under manometric guidance, using a small-gauge needle, with slow removal of the smallest volume of CSF necessary for the diagnostic tests. Consultation with a neurosurgeon before the lumbar puncture should also be considered.

Cerebrospinal fluid findings

Examination of the CSF of a patient with acute bacterial meningitis characteristically reveals (1) a cloudy appearance, (2) an increased white blood cell count with a predominance of polymorphonuclear leukocytes, (3) a low glucose concentration, (4) an elevated protein level, and (5) a smear and culture positive for the causative microorganism.

Cell count. The cell count may be extremely variable, but usually there are well over 1000/mm^3. An analysis of the CSF findings in 68 cases of acute bacterial meningitis seen at Bellevue Hospital revealed an average white cell count of 4400; the lowest was 172 and the highest was 20,000. In 92% of these cases the predominant cell was the polymorphonuclear leukocyte. The remaining 8% of the cases showed not only a predominance of lymphocytes but also a normal CSF glucose value; these findings were similar to those seen in aseptic meningitis.

In rare instances, particularly very early in the illness, the cell count may be normal despite a positive Gram stain or culture of the CSF. Lumbar puncture repeated later may show the characteristic cell count. This phenomenon was illustrated by a 2-month-old male infant admitted to our service with fever and irritability of 1 day's duration. His temperature was 40.2° C (104.4° F) and he appeared acutely ill, but no localizing physical signs were present. The white cell count was 20,400 with 80% neutrophils. Because of the unexplained fever, the leukocytosis, and the excessive irritability, a lumbar puncture was performed. The CSF was clear (it contained six lymphocytes), the glucose value was 86 mg/100 ml, and the protein value was 45 mg/100 ml. The following morning the staff was startled by the culture, which yielded *pneumococcus* type 12. Lumbar puncture repeated 12 hours after the initial one revealed cloudy CSF; 6250 white cells, of which 95% were polymorphonuclear leukocytes; glucose value of 55 mg/100 ml; and protein of 270/100 ml. Antimicrobial therapy was begun, and the patient had an uneventful recovery.

In patients who have received antimicrobial therapy before the first lumbar puncture, the CSF findings are likely to be modified. On the second day of treatment the cell count generally rises. Thereafter it decreases, and there may be a predominance of lymphocytes. The patient with prior antibiotic therapy often poses a more complicated diagnostic challenge because Gram stain and culture may be negative. The CSF glucose will generally remain lowered, the protein elevated, and the white cell count and differential abnormal despite the treatment administered.

Smears. Smears should be made promptly of all spinal fluids. A properly prepared smear examined by an *experienced* person is an invaluable aid for both rapid diagnosis and estimation of prognosis (Feldman, 1977). Countless microorganisms in the presence of relatively small numbers of leukocytes may indicate a poor defense response. Pneumococci are relatively easy to identify on smear, but identification of *H. influenzae* and meningococci is more difficult. One usually should not accept the report of a smear until it is confirmed by culture. A smear from a previously treated patient may contain microorganisms that fail to grow on culture because they are no longer viable.

Culture. Culture should also be performed routinely on all spinal fluid specimens, even those that are clear and show no increase in cell count. Clear acellular CSF may yield a positive culture, as in the patient described above. This occurs most frequently with pneumococci. Accurate identification of the causative microorganism is a prerequisite for the proper management of acute bacterial meningitis.

Glucose. The CSF glucose level is typically low in most cases of acute bacterial meningitis. However, it may be normal in the early stages of the disease and in cases treated before the initial lumbar puncture. Usually a glucose of less than half the blood glucose level is considered abnormal. The return of the glucose level to normal is generally a good early index of response to therapy, although the reverse is not necessarily true.

Protein. Protein concentration is usually increased, but this in not a helpful diagnostic aid early in the course of the disease. Rising protein levels in spite of adequate therapy may be caused by neurologic sequelae.

Other laboratory procedures

A blood culture should be made routinely in every patient who possibly has meningitis. Occasionally, the blood culture is positive when the spinal fluid culture is negative. *Nasopharyngeal and throat cultures*, although not as specific as the blood culture, may provide a helpful clue to the diagnosis in some cases. The *peripheral white blood cell count* is typically high, with a predominance of neutrophils. In some patients with meningitis, however, it may be low. Leukopenia does not necessarily rule out a serious bacterial infection; it may in fact be a poor prognostic sign. *Bacterial antigens* in CSF may be identified by countercurrent immunoelectrophoresis (CIE) and by latex agglutination and staphylococcal coagglutination (Dajani et al., 1979). Kits for these tests are commercially available for the following pathogens: *H. influenzae,*

S. pneumoniae, and *N. meningitidis* (A, B, C, and Y). Latex and coagglutination are more sensitive than CIE. These tests are not meant to replace the CSF culture but merely as an adjunct to it. False-negative and rare false-positive tests may occur. A positive antigen test is therefore meaningful, but a negative test cannot be relied on. The main advantage of these tests is the rapidity with which they may be carried out. The limulus lysate test may also be performed on CSF; this lysate agglutinates in the presence of endotoxin produced by gram-negative organisms. The limulus lysate assay is of no value for testing serum.

In addition to agglutination, CIE, and limulus tests, several experimental assays have been studied in an attempt to identify rapidly a bacterial etiology in patients with meningitis. CSF concentrations of lactic acid and of isoenzymes (lactic dehydrogenase, glutamic oxaloacetic transaminase, and creatine phosphokinase) have been elevated variably but with insufficient specificity to ensure clinical reliability.

DIFFERENTIAL DIAGNOSIS

Acute bacterial meningitis may be simulated by many other diseases that involve the meninges either directly or indirectly. The typical spinal fluid findings of purulent meningitis and other conditions are listed in Table 15-1. As indicated previously, acute bacterial meningitis is characterized by an increase in the number of cells, predominantly polymorphonuclear leukocytes, and by low glucose and high protein concentrations. In exceptional instances, however, the spinal fluid findings do not conform to this typical picture.

Tuberculous meningitis

Tuberculous meningitis may be clinically indistinguishable from acute bacterial meningitis. The diagnosis is established by (1) the CSF showing an increase in number of cells, usually from 50 to 500, predominantly lymphocytes, a low glucose concentration, and a culture negative for the usual pathogenic organisms but subsequently positive for tubercle bacilli; (2) a positive tuberculin skin test; and (3) roentgenograms of the chest showing evidence of a tuberculous lesion. A smear of the spinal fluid should be carefully examined for tubercle bacilli

Table 15-1. Spinal fluid findings of acute bacterial meningitis compared with other diseases

Disease	Number of cells	Glucose level	Protein level
Acute bacterial meningitis	Increased (polymorphonuclear)	Low	High
Tuberculous meningitis	Increased (lymphocytes)	Low	High
Aseptic meningitis	Increased (lymphocytes)	Normal	High or normal
Brain abscess or tumor	Normal or increased (lymphocytes)	Normal	High
Lead encephalopathy	Normal or increased (lymphocytes)	Normal	High
Meningismus	Normal	Normal	Normal

because of the urgency of diagnosis. A thorough description of tuberculous meningitis is given in Chapter 31.

Aseptic meningitis

Aseptic meningitis is discussed in detail in Chapter 14. The spinal fluid typically shows an increase in lymphocytes and a normal glucose level. In some instances the spinal fluid early in the disease may show a large number of cells that are predominantly polymorphonuclear. This is observed particularly in enteroviral infections. The true diagnosis is established by the results of the culture of the spinal fluid and the various procedures referred to in Chapter 14.

Brain abscess

Brain abscess may follow trauma, otitis media, or septic embolization in children with cyanotic congenital heart disease. The symptoms are usually not as acute as those of meningitis. The nuchal rigidity, if present, is less pronounced. Focal neurologic signs and papilledema may be present. The spinal fluid may either be normal or show an increase in number of cells and a normal glucose value. The culture of the CSF specimen is negative. Rupture of the abscess into the subarachnoid space or ventricles will cause a fulminant purulent meningitis.

Brain tumor

The findings of brain tumor are similar to those of brain abscess except that the course is more insidious, fever is usually absent, and the patient is not acutely ill.

Meningismus

Meningismus is characterized by symptoms and signs of meningeal irritation and a *normal* spinal fluid. It is usually associated with pneu-

monia, acute otitis media, acute tonsillitis, and other infectious diseases.

Lead encephalopathy

Lead encephalopathy in infants and children may simulate meningitis. The spinal fluid shows a normal glucose level, an increased protein concentration, and lymphocytes that are either slightly increased or normal in number. Helpful diagnostic aids include (1) a blood smear showing basophilic stippling, (2) roentgenographic evidence of a line of increased density at the metaphyseal ends of the long bones in growing children, (3) coproporphyrinuria, and (4) an increased blood lead level.

COMPLICATIONS

The incidence of complications has been reduced by the early institution of therapy.

Peripheral circulatory collapse and other general phenomena

Peripheral circulatory collapse is one of the most dramatic and most serious complications of meningitis. It is most frequently associated with meningococcemia but may accompany other types of infection. Profound shock usually develops early in the course of the illness and, if untreated, progresses rapidly to a fatal outcome. Disseminated intravascular coagulation (DIC) with marked thrombocytopenia and hypofibrinogenemia may be an associated finding (McGehee et al., 1967). Other laboratory determinations in DIC will include decreases in prothrombin and in coagulation factors II, V, and VIII, plus the presence of fibrin split products and altered erythrocyte morphology. Gangrene of fingers, toes, and other parts of the body may occur in fulminating hemorrhagic meningococcal meningitis. With meningitis and sepsis, metabolic acidosis and tissue hypoxia become important factors to be combated. Many patients also develop the syndrome of inappropriate antidiuretic hormone (IADH) secretion, leading to water retention and sodium loss in the urine, which further complicates fluid management.

Arthritis

Arthritis may be associated with meningococcal infection. It usually involves many joints. *H. influenzae* type b is the most common cause of pyarthrosis in children less than 2 years of age and may produce monoarticular involvement usually of a large weight bearing joint.

Neurologic complications

Neurologic complications include increased intracranial pressure, involvement of the cranial nerves, arteritis and phlebitis, and hydrocephalus.

Increased intracranial pressure. Pressure may be due to the inflammatory process itself, IADH and inadequate fluid management, or a focal complicating lesion such as a brain abscess, subdural effusion, or empyema.

Cranial nerve involvement. Extension of the meningeal infection may involve the second, third, sixth, seventh, and eighth cranial nerves. Damage to the auditory nerve is usually followed by permanent deafness.

Arteritis and phlebitis. Severe vascular involvement of arteries, veins, or venous sinuses may lead to continued focal seizures and to persistent hemiparesis.

Hydrocephalus. Hydrocephalus of either the communicating or obstructive type was common before specific therapy was available. Today it is occasionally seen in patients in whom treatment has been either suboptimal or delayed, and more often in younger infants.

Subdural effusion and empyema

Subdural effusion as a complication of meningitis has been reported with increasing frequency since 1950. It most often follows *H. influenzae* and pneumococcal infections, but it may also occur with meningococcal and other types of meningitis. It develops in patients who have received both early and optimal therapy. The pathogenesis of this complication is unknown. One hypothesis attributes it to a thrombophlebitis of the bridging veins that traverse the subdural space. It may possibly be caused by factors similar to those responsible for pleural effusions complicating pulmonary infections.

The subdural effusion appears during the acute stage of the illness and is usually sterile. In a small percentage of cases the fluid is purulent and contains the microorganism responsible for the meningitis. A true empyema is much rarer than subdural effusion but can cause similar signs. The presence of a subdural collection of fluid should be suspected in any infant with meningitis who does not respond to therapy and shows evidence of (1) prolonged fever, (2) recurrence or persistence of a bulging fontanelle, (3) convulsions, (4) focal neurologic signs such as paralysis, or (5) increasing head circumference. The diagnosis is made by transillumination, computed axial tomography, and/or ultrasound.

Complications of Haemophilus influenzae meningitis

Cellulitis, abscess formation, arthritis, mastoiditis, pneumonia with empyema, pericarditis, and endocarditis may complicate severe *H. influenzae* infections of infants.

Case report. A 14-month-old boy previously in good health was admitted to Duke University Medical Center with a 3-day history of fever, irritability, anorexia, and lethargy. Physical examination revealed a critically ill boy who was difficult to arouse. His temperature was 39.5° C (103.1° F). The left ear and posterior auricular region were red, warm, and swollen. The neck was stiff, and the right upper chest was dull to percussion; on auscultation, rales were heard. The right knee was swollen, warm, and held in a fixed position. A lumbar puncture revealed cloudy fluid with 1640 white cells (83% polymorphonuclear leukocytes), a glucose level of 2 mg/100 ml, and a protein level of 42 mg/100 ml. Numerous gram-negative rods were seen on microscopic examination of CSF. The peripheral blood white cell count was 14,700/mm³ with 70% polymorphonuclear cells. The chest film revealed a right middle lobe pneumonia and a right pleural effusion. Cultures of blood, CSF, and knee and pleural aspirates subsequently yielded *H. influenzae* type b. Despite prompt treatment with ampicillin and chloramphenicol and supportive therapy in the intensive care unit, the patient died 2 days after admission. Final diagnoses were overwhelming sepsis with meningitis, pneumonia, empyema, arthritis, cellulitis, and mastoiditis.

PROGNOSIS

The prognosis of a particular case of meningitis depends on a variety of factors, including (1) the patient's age, (2) the microorganism, (3) the severity of the infection, (4) the duration of the illness before onset of therapy, and (5) the sensitivity of the microorganism to the antimicrobial drugs.

The younger the patient, the more serious the prognosis. The highest mortality occurs in meningitis of the newborn infant. Infections caused by group B streptococci, coliform, and other gram-negative bacilli are more difficult to cure than meningococcal, *H. influenzae*, and pneumococcal infections. A fulminant type of infection complicated by DIC always carries an ominous prognosis. If treatment is inadequate or is instituted late in the course of the disease, irreversible damage may occur. Infections due to resistant organisms are either fatal or followed by serious sequelae.

With adequate antimicrobial and appropriate supportive therapy the chances for survival today are excellent. The mortality of meningococcal meningitis has been reduced from 50% to between 5% and 10%. *H. influenzae* and pneumococcal meningitis formerly had a hopeless prognosis, with a mortality that approached 100%. Today the fatality rate is 10% or less in cases of *H. influenzae* meningitis and approximately 15% in cases of pneumococcal meningitis. There has been a dramatic reduction in the incidence of severe neurologic sequelae after all types of meningitis amenable to antimicrobial therapy.

Even with prompt and adequate therapy, however, infants and children who survive bacterial meningitis are more apt to have seizures, hearing deficits, school problems, and lower intelligence in comparison to their peers who did not have meningitis. Therefore, although today there is adequate antimicrobial therapy for most forms of meningitis, the importance of *prevention* is now well recognized, and various programs have been developed for prophylaxis (Sell et al., 1972a,b; Sell, 1983).

TREATMENT

The treatment of bacterial meningitis is a medical emergency. Any unnecessary delay may make the difference between life and death or between a brain-damaged and a normal child or adult. Consequently, as soon as the clinical and spinal fluid findings suggest this diagnosis, treatment should begin *immediately*. The physician should institute antimicrobial therapy aimed at the most likely type of meningitis based on the patients's age and other historical and clinical data.

An intravenous infusion should be started as soon as the lumbar puncture has been completed. This procedure will facilitate the administration of antimicrobial agents, fluids, anticonvulsant drugs, and other therapy.

Antimicrobial therapy

A guide for the antimicrobial treatment of acute bacterial meningitis follows:

Haemophilus influenzae (ampicillin plus chloramphenicol)
1. Ampicillin
   a. Initial dose, 50 mg per kilogram of body weight intravenously, followed by
   b. Daily dose, 200 to 300 mg per kilogram of body weight per 24 hours given every 6 hours intravenously
2. Chloramphenicol*
   a. Initial dose, 50 mg per kilogram of body weight intravenously
   b. Daily dose, 100 mg per kilogram of body weight per 24 hours given every 6 hours intravenously (maximum dose 4 gm per day)
3. Cefotaxime 200 mg per kilogram of body weight per 24 hours given every 6 hours intravenously (may be substituted for *1* and *2*)

Meningococcus (penicillin or ampicillin)
1. Aqueous crystalline penicillin G
   a. Infants (under 2 years): 100,000 to 200,000 units per kilogram of body weight
   b. Children and adults: 100,000 to 400,000 units per kilogram of body weight per 24 hours given every 4 hours intravenously
2. Ampicillin: same dosage as for *H. influenzae*.

Pneumococcus (penicillin or ampicillin; chlor-

---

*Chloramphenicol dosage (see text): premature infants, 25 mg per kilogram of body weight per 24 hours; full-term infants (4 weeks of age), 50 mg per kilogram of body weight per 24 hours.

amphenicol or vancomycin for resistant strains)

1. Penicillin: same dosage as for *Meningococcus*
2. If resistant to penicillin: chloramphenicol, dosage same as for *H. influenzae*
3. If multiply resistant: vancomycin 40 mg per kilogram of body weight per 24 hours given every 6 hours intravenously

Group B streptococcus (penicillin and an aminoglycoside)

1. Aqueous penicillin G or ampicillin: same dosage as for meningococcus
2. Gentamicin
   a. Newborn infants: 5 to 7.5 mg per kilogram of body weight per 24 hours given intravenously or intramuscularly every 8 to 12 hours

Staphylococcus (methicillin, oxacillin sodium, nafcillin sodium, or vancomycin)

1. Methicillin: 200 to 300 mg per kilogram of body weight per 24 hours given every 6 hours intravenously
2. Oxacillin sodium or nafcillin sodium: 100 to 200 mg per kilogram of body weight per 24 hours given every 6 hours intravenously or intramuscularly (maximum dose 6 gm per day)
3. Vancomycin (as for *pneumococcus*) if patient is allergic to penicillin or organism is resistant to methicillin

Escherichia coli (aminoglycoside)

1. Gentamicin
   a. Newborn infants: 5 to 7.5 mg per kilogram of body weight per 24 hours given intravenously every 12 hours
   b. Older infants and children: 5 to 7.5 mg per kilogram of body weight per 24 hours given intravenously every 8 hours
2. Amikacin
   a. Newborn infants: 15 to 30 mg per kilogram of body weight per 24 hours given intravenously every 8 to 12 hours
   b. Older children: 15 to 30 mg per kilogram of body weight given intravenously every 8 hours
3. Kanamycin: 15 to 30 mg per kilogram of body weight per 24 hours given intravenously or intramuscularly every 12 hours in equally divided doses
4. Ampicillin: same dosage for *Meningococcus*

Pseudomonas aeruginosa (amikacin and mezlocillin)

1. Amikacin: same dosage as for *E. coli*

2. Mezlocillin (combined therapy with gentamicin): 300 mg per kilogram of body weight per 24 hours given intravenously every 6 hours

Unknown (premature and newborn infants)

1. Gentamicin: 5 to 7.5 mg per kilogram of body weight per 24 hours given intravenously every 8 to 12 hours, or amikacin 15 to 22 mg per kilogram of body weight per 24 hours given intravenously every 8 to 12 hours, plus
2. Penicillin: 100,000 units per kilogram of body weight per day until specific organism is identified

Unknown (older infants and children)

1. Ampicillin plus chloramphenicol: same as dosage for *H. influenzae*

In the mid 1960s, ampicillin alone was introduced as broad spectrum treatment for meningitis in infants and children until the results of the CSF culture were known. Subsequently, however, organisms resistant to commonly used antimicrobials have emerged as a significant clinical problem. Pneumococci relatively resistant to penicillin were first described, and then multiply resistant strains not susceptible to a variety of antibiotics were recognized. In 1974, strains of *H. influenzae* resistant to ampicillin were reported; the incidence of resistance now varies between 13% to 36% with a national average of 25%. The case-fatality rate is higher in every age group when meningitis is caused by resistant organisms (Hill, 1983). It is crucial that pediatricians be cognizant of this problem. It is similarly important that all bacterial isolates from CSF be tested for susceptibility to various antimicrobials in vitro. Lumbar punctures should be performed on children treated for 24 to 48 hours who have not responded to therapy because of the possibility of resistant organisms.

The indications for a posttreatment lumbar puncture should be individualized. While the CSF may not yet have become normal after completion of therapy, the culture and Gram stain should be negative, there should be less than 10% polymorphonuclear cells, and the glucose should be greater than 20 mg/100 ml. If any of these criteria are not met, the patient should be reevaluated and additional therapy considered. Most patients with meningitis will require therapy for at least 7 days. They should be afebrile for 5 to 7 days before stopping therapy.

Immediate treatment for meningitis in infants

beyond the newborn age and in children should be (1) ampicillin 50 mg per kilogram of body weight intravenously, and (2) chloramphenicol 50 mg per kilogram of body weight intravenously, as bolus doses. Treatment should be continued at doses of 200 to 300 mg per kilogram of body weight per day of ampicillin (in six divided doses) and 100 mg per kilogram of body weight per day of chloramphenicol (in four divided doses), intravenously. Both drugs should be given until the organism and its susceptibility to antimicrobials is known. At that time, one or the other drug may be eliminated or a different drug may be used, as indicated on p. 183. Since *H. influenzae* may be resistant to ampicillin by means other than by elaboration of beta-lactamase and to chloramphenicol by elaboration of acetyltransferase, disk sensitivities should be performed to determine whether the organism is resistant.

Meningococcal meningitis. Penicillin is the preferred drug; ampicillin is also effective. The recommended dosage schedule is outlined on p. 183. Patients who are allergic to penicillin can be treated with chloramphenicol; it is given intravenously in the dosage of 100 mg per kilogram of body weight for at least 3 days and by mouth thereafter if tolerated. The oral dose of chloramphenicol is 75 mg per kilogram of body weight in three doses. Chloramphenicol should not be given intramuscularly because its absorption is variable by this route.

Haemophilus influenzae type b meningitis. Chloramphenicol is recommended in combination with ampicillin for initial therapy until the susceptibility of the organism has been determined. The recommended dosage is given on p. 183. Feldman (1978a) demonstrated that the combination of ampicillin and chloramphenicol when tested against strains of *H. influenzae* type b was either synergistic or additive, but never antagonistic. Barrett et al. (1972) reviewed the results of therapy in 116 patients who received ampicillin alone and 112 who received chloramphenicol alone or in combination with other antibiotics. The mortality and incidence of neurologic sequelae, including subdural effusions, were similar in the two treatment groups. All of the strains they had studied were ampicillin sensitive. Chloramphenicol has the additional advantage of CSF levels that approximate 50%, whereas ampicillin during acute inflammation

reaches only 30% of blood values and declines thereafter to the 5% range. Chloramphenicol has been shown to be bactericidal against *H. influenzae* (Rahal and Simberkoff, 1979).

As can be seen from Fig. 15-1, the most frequent invasive disease caused by *H. influenzae* is meningitis (Dajani et al., 1979). The organism may also cause epiglottitis, pneumonia, empyema, arthritis, cellulitis, bacteremia, pericarditis, and osteomyelitis. Meningitis caused by this organism is most frequently seen in infants, but it has also been described in adults. In general, the greater the concentration of bacteria in CSF at diagnosis, the poorer the prognosis (Feldman, 1977).

While current treatment for *H. influenzae* meningitis is ampicillin and/or chloramphenicol, third generation cephalosporins such as cefotaxime and moxalactam may be used if an organism resistant to both of the preferred drugs is encountered (Kaplan et al., 1983). Moxalactam has been associated with bleeding due in part to decreased production of vitamin K in the gastrointestinal tract. If moxalactam is used, therefore, vitamin K should also be administered. Moxalactam is not active against pneumococci, and, therefore, it cannot be used alone for initial therapy of meningitis. In contrast, cefotaxime is acceptable when used alone since pneumococci as well as gram-negative organisms are susceptible to this drug (McCracken and Nelson, 1982). The second generation cephalosporin cefuroxine has also been used to treat bacterial meningitis (Schaad et al., 1984).

Infants between the ages of 2 to 6 weeks have been reported to have meningitis caused by diverse organisms including *H. influenzae*, group B streptococci, pneumococci, *E. coli*, and *L. monocytogenes;* the combination of ampicillin and cefotaxime has been suggested as initial therapy for this age group of infants (Baumgartner et al., 1983). Cefamandol is effective against *H. influenzae* in vitro, but it should not be used to treat infections due to these organisms. It does not penetrate well into CSF, and patients have developed meningitis while being treated with this drug for other conditions (Aronoff et al., 1981; Azimi and Chase, 1981).

Pneumococcal meningitis. Penicillin is the preferred drug for pneumococcal meningitis; the recommended dosage is shown on p. 184. Sodium penicillin G should be substituted for potassium penicillin G when large doses of aqueous crystalline penicillin are given to premature and newborn infants to prevent potassium toxicity. Ampicillin is also effective therapy.

Pneumococci relatively resistant to penicillin were first reported in the early 1970s. Such strains have minimal inhibitory concentrations (MICs) of 0.1 to 1.0 μg/ml to penicillin. By the late 1970s, resistant strains with MICs of greater than 1 μg/ml were reported; these organisms are often resistant to other antibiotics such as chloramphenicol, erythromycin, and sulfonamides (Jacobs et al., 1978; Kaplan and Feigin, 1983). Relapsing and fatal cases of meningitis due to these organisms have been described (Naraqi et al., 1974; Paredes et al., 1976; Appelbaum et al., 1977). These observations necessitate testing of all pneumococci from CSF isolates for susceptibility to penicillin. Penicillin-sensitive pneumococci have inhibition zones of equal to or greater than 20 mm with a 1-μg oxacillin disk.

Neonatal meningitis. Meningitis during the first month of life is usually caused by group B streptococci or gram-negative bacilli, most commonly *E. coli*. Additional causes include *L. monocytogenes*, *Aerobacter aerogenes*, *Pseudomonas aerogenosa*, and *Proteus vulgaris*. Initial therapy should include ampicillin and an amino-glycoside, as outlined on p. 211. Modification of this therapy should be determined by (1) the patient's clinical response, (2) identification of the causative agent, and (3) the results of sensitivity tests. Neonatal meningitis caused by gram-negative organisms carries a poor prognosis; 15% to 20% of cases are fatal, and less than one half of the survivors are normal at discharge. Administration of aminoglycosides directly into the cerebral ventricles did not improve the outcome of this disease (McCracken et al., 1980). Moxalactam has also proven no better than ampicillin and an aminoglycoside despite excellent penetration of this drug into CSF (McCracken, 1984).

Chloramphenicol for premature and newborn infants. The administration of chloramphenicol to premature and newborn infants requires special precautions. Chloramphenicol is rapidly absorbed from the gastrointestinal tract and is rapidly excreted in the urine after degradation in the liver. In premature and newborn infants the physiologic handicaps of an immature liver and kidney have a profound effect on the metabolism of the drug. Decreased hepatic glucuronide conjugation and poor renal excretion combine to promote the accumulation of toxic levels of chloramphenicol. Sutherland et al. (1959) demonstrated this phenomenon in a full-

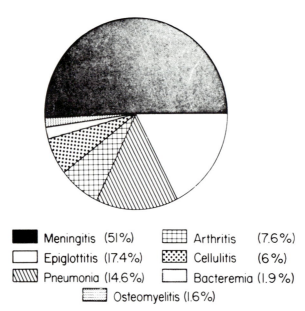

Fig. 15-1. Relative frequencies of different clinical entities due to *H. influenzae* infection. (From Dajani AS, Asmar BI, Thirumoorthi MC. J Pediatr 1979;94:358.)

term newborn infant who received a daily dose of 100 mg per kilogram of body weight for 3 days. Blood levels determined 8, 76, and 100 hours after the last dose were 183, 230, and 201 µg/ml, respectively. (Levels of 10 to 25 µg/ml are usually considered optimal.) Clinical manifestations of chloramphenicol toxicity were first noted 3 days after the last dose, and the infant died 2 days later.

The situation in older, more mature infants presents a striking contrast. Kelly et al. (1951) determined serum levels in two such infants who received a daily dose of 132 mg per kilogram of body weight for 3 days. The peak levels during the course of therapy did not exceed 25 to 35 µg/ml of serum. Eight hours after the last dose of chloramphenicol, the blood levels had decreased to 3 and 8 µg/ml.

Burns et al. (1959) described the clinical manifestations of chloramphenicol toxicity in premature infants ("gray baby syndrome"). The first signs were vomiting or regurgitation and refusal to suck. Within a few hours there ensued rapid shallow respirations, abdominal distention, cyanosis, and diarrhea. Within 24 hours the infants were desperately ill, with an ashen color, flaccidity, and subnormal temperature. Death usually occurred within 1 to 2 days after onset of symptoms. In the infants who survived, improvement was noted within 24 to 36 hours after cessation of chloramphenicol therapy. Toxic symptoms in premature infants were induced by a daily dose of 100 to 165 mg per kilogram of body weight. A daily dose of 25 mg per kilogram of body weight did not produce toxic manifestations. When chloramphenicol is the indicated antibiotic for treatment of a newborn, it should be used in a setting where laboratory backup can provide accurate blood levels so that the dosage can be adjusted to maintain a therapeutic level but remain below a toxic concentration.

Acute bacterial meningitis of unknown cause. One or more of the following factors may be responsible for a failure to identify the causative agent: (1) previous treatment with antimicrobial agents, (2) lack of personnel trained in microbiology, and (3) lack of adequate laboratory facilities. Under these circumstances the meningitis should be treated with the antibiotics recommended on p. 184. This therapy is aimed at the most common causes of acute bacterial meningitis in infants and children.

Cerebrospinal fluid shunt infections. Cerebrospinal shunts usually become infected with staphylococci, including *S. epidermis* as well as *S. aureus*. Gram-negative infections also occur. Most of these infections are indolent rather than acute and fulminant as in other forms of bacterial meningitis. Fever is often absent. While some patients have been cured by long-term antibiotic therapy (6 weeks), most of these infections require removal of the shunt for cure. Recommended initial therapy before the infecting organism is known is vancomycin plus an aminoglycoside (p. 184) (Nelson, 1984). Some patients with this form of meningitis are treated by instillation of antibiotics directly into the cerebral ventricles as well as by the intravenous route.

General supportive therapy

Intravenous therapy should be instituted promptly to provide an open line for antimicrobial drugs and to combat potential shock. The patient should be monitored very carefully during the acute phase of the illness. Frequent determinations of the pulse and respiratory rates and blood pressure should be performed. Urine output measurements are essential for early detection of shock. Studies for DIC such as platelet count, prothrombin time, fibrin split products, factors V and VIII, and partial thromboplastin time may reveal abnormalities.

Measures to combat acutely increased intracranial pressure may be needed. Dexamethasone, glycerol, mannitol, and other agents all have their proponents. If a decision is made to intubate the patient in order to provide mechanical ventilation and to ensure adequate oxygenation with a patent airway, hyperventilation may be used to assist in lowering increased intracranial pressure. The patient should be monitored for IADH by frequent measurement of serum and urine sodium levels and osmolarity.

If shock occurs, intravenous therapy with dextrose-electrolyte solutions, plasma, plasma expanders, or blood would be indicated to combat hypovolemia. Drug therapy may be required to increase cardiac output and peripheral perfusion. A catheter should be inserted for measurement of central venous pressure as a guide to therapy. Sympathomimetic amines may be used to support the circulation of the patient in shock, after attention has first been given to volume replacement. Dopamine and isoproterenol are the preferred agents, in that order of preference, and should be administered with careful monitoring of blood pressure, central venous pressure, and electrocardiogram. Steroids have not been shown to influence the outcome of bacterial meningitis (Kaplan and Feigin, 1983). Heparin therapy and/or fresh frozen plasma may be considered for patients with DIC.

The treatment schedule and various procedures should be so organized that the patient is not being continuously disturbed and unnecessarily handled. Occasionally, there is a tendency to forget that an acutely ill patient requires rest.

Subdural effusions in infants are treated by aspiration only if there are pressure signs or symptoms, or if an empyema rather than an effusion is suspected. In most instances, an effusion clears within 1 or 2 weeks. Persistent or increasing amounts of fluid may indicate presence of a membrane, which may rarely require surgical intervention.

PREVENTION AND CONTROL
Meningococcal infections

Rifampin prophylaxis should be given to persons of all ages who have intimate contact with patients with meningococcal meningitis or meningococcemia. The dose is 10 mg per kilogram of body weight twice daily by mouth for 2 days, with a maximum dose of 1200 mg a day.

The development of meningococcal polysaccharide vaccines has provided safe and effective immunizing agents for the prevention of meningococcal meningitis. There is as yet, however, no vaccine against type B meningococci. The indications and need for meningococcal vaccine will depend in great part on the local epidemiologic circumstances; these are discussed in detail on p. 176.

Haemophilus influenzae infections

There is a significant risk of secondary cases of *H. influenzae* type b disease among young children who are household contacts and among infants and children who are nursery and day-care center contacts of primary patients (Ward et al., 1979). Secondary illnesses are most likely to develop within 4 days of the primary case, but they may occur as late as 60 days after exposure. Exposed children under 4 years of age

should be given rifampin 20 mg per kilogram by mouth once a day for 4 days. To prevent secondary cases in young children, all contacts, including adults, must be treated. The dose for adults is 600 mg per day for 4 days. The index patient should also be given rifampin for 4 days, prior to discharge from the hospital, because ampicillin and chloramphenicol do not eradicate the carrier state, although they cure the illness (Nelson, 1982). In study of 1112 rifampin-treated household and day-care contacts there were no secondary cases, but four of 765 exposed children who received placebo became infected (Band et al., 1984). While it is clear that rifampin prophylaxis should be used in a household setting where there has been invasive disease, its use in day-care centers remains controversial. This is because the attack rate following this type of exposure may be lower, and the policy itself may be difficult to implement since everyone must be treated in order to eradicate the carrier state from the group. Emergence of strains of *H. influenzae* resistant to rifampin after prophylaxis have been reported, but this does not seem to be a frequent occurrence (Murphy et al., 1981; Band et al., 1984).

Immunity to *H. influenzae* is complex. Antibodies that are bactericidal in vitro do not seem to play a role in protection against disease; high levels of these antibodies have been reported in children in the early stages of meningitis. In contrast, antibodies to the somatic antigens of the organism, outer membrane proteins, and lipopolysaccharides, as well as antibodies to the capsular polysaccharide, PRP, play a significant role in protection (Edmonson et al., 1982). These antibodies may be important in inducing opsinization of organisms by white blood cells. Outer membrane proteins and PRP are currently being developed as potential vaccines against *H. influenzae*. PRP is immunogenic and protective for children over 18 months of age (Peltola et al., 1984). PRP administered along with a protein carrier such as diphtheria toxoid is immunogenic in younger children because this converts PRP from a thymic-independent into a thymic-dependent antigen to which young children can respond (Hill, 1983). Outer membrane proteins are immunogenic for young children, and they induce protective antibodies, but different organisms have somewhat different types of outer membrane proteins. Efforts are therefore underway to develop a vaccine from these proteins that would offer protection against the most common types of *H. influenzae*. Purified PRP has been licensed as a vaccine for children from 18 months to 5 years of age (see p. 486). In the meantime studies on conjugated PRP and other *H. influenzae* type b vaccines are still in progress.

Prophylaxis with antimicrobial agents is not indicated for patients with other types of acute bacterial meningitis. Pneumococcal vaccine is discussed in detail on p. 522.

REFERENCES

Abildgaard CF, et al. Meningococcemia associated with intravascular coagulation. Pediatrics 1967;40:78.

Ammann AJ, Addiego J, Wara DW, et al. Polyvalent pneumococcalpolysaccharide immunization of patients with sickle-cell anemia and patients with splenectomy. N Engl J Med 1977;297:897-900.

Anderson EL, Smith EWP, Katz SL. Ampicillin-resistant strains of *Hemophilus influenzae*, type b in North Carolina. N C Med J 1976;37:487.

Anthony BF, Okada DM. The emergence of group B streptococci in infections of the newborn infant. Ann Rev Med 1977;28:355.

Appelbaum PC, Scragg JN, Bowen AJ, et al. Streptococcus pneumoniae resistant to penicillin and chloramphenicol. Lancet 1977;2:995-997.

Aronoff SC, Thomford W, Bertino JS, et al. Development of meningitis during therapy with cefamandole. Pediatrics 1981;67:727-728.

Artenstein MS, et al. Prevention of meningococcal disease by group C polysaccharide vaccine. N Engl J Med 1970;282:417.

Austrian R, et al. Prevention of pneumococcal pneumonia by vaccination. Trans Assoc Am Phys 1976;89:184.

Azimi PH, Chase PA. The role of cefamandole in the treatment of *Haemophilus influenzae*, in infants and children. J Pediatr 1981;98:995-1000.

Band JD, Fraser DW, Ajello G, et al. Prevention of *H. influenzae* infection. JAMA 1984;251:2381-2386.

Barenkamp SJ, Munson RS, Granoff DM. Subtyping isolates of *haemophilus influenzae* type b by outer-membrane protein profiles. J Infect Dis 1981;143:668-676.

Barrett FF, et al. A 12 year review of the antibiotic management of *Hemophilus-influenzae*-meningitis. J Pediatr 1972;81:370.

Barton LL, Granoff DM, Barenkamp SJ. Nosocomial spread of haemophilus influenzae type b infection documented by outer membrane protein subtype analysis. J Pediatr 1983;102:820-824.

Baumgartner ET, Augustine RA, Steele RW. Bacterial meningitis in older neonates. Am J Dis Child 1983;137:1052-1054.

Bøe J, Huseklepp H. Recurrent attacks of bacterial meningitis: "new" clinical problem: report of 5 cases. Am J Med 1960;29:465.

Burns LE, Hodgman JE, Cass AB. Fatal circulatory collapse in premature infants receiving chloramphenicol. N Engl J Med 1959;261:1318.

Chad ZH, Pearson EL, Reece ER, Powell KR. *Haemophilus influenzae* type b meningitis: occurrence in three siblings over a two-year period. Pediatrics 1980;66:9-13.

Chartrand SA, Cho CT. Persistent pleocytosis in bacterial meningitis. J Pediatr 1976;88:424.

Converse GM, Gwaltney JM Jr, Strassburg DA, Hendley JO. Alteration of cerebrospinal fluid findings by partial treatment of bacterial meningitis. J Pediatr 1973;83:220.

Coulehan JL, Hallowell C, Michaels RH, et al. Immunogenicity of a *Haemophilus influenzae* type b vaccine in combination with diphtheria-pertussis-tetanus vaccine in infants. J Infect Dis 1983;148:530-533.

Dajani AS, Asmar BI, Thirumoorthi MC. Systemic *Haemophilus influenzae* disease: an overview. J Pediatr 1979;94:355-365.

Davis SD, Hill HR, Feigl P, Arnstein EJ. Partial antibiotic therapy in *Hemophilus influenzae* meningitis: its effect on cerebrospinal fluid abnormalities. Am J Dis Child 1975;130:802.

Edmonson D, Granoff DM, Barenkamp SJ, et al. Outer membrane protein and investigation of recurrent *Hemophilus influenzae* type b disease. J Pediatr 1982;100:202-208.

Einhorn A, Mizrahi EM. Basilar skull fractures in children. Am J Dis Child 1978;132:1121.

Ellner JJ, Bennett JE. Chronic meningitis. Medicine 1976;55:341.

Feigin RD, Baker CJ, Herwaldt JA, et al. Epidemic meningococcal disease in an elementary-school classroom. N Engl J Med 1982;307:1255-1257.

Feigin RD, et al. Prospective evaluation of treatment of *Hemophilus influenzae* meningitis. J Pediatr 1976;88:542.

Feldman WE. Concentrations of bacteria in cerebrospinal fluid of patients with bacterial meningitis. J Pediatr 1976;88:549.

Feldman WE. Relation of concentrations of bacteria and bacterial antigen in cerebrospinal fluid to prognosis in patients with bacterial meningitis. N Engl J Med 1977;296:433.

Feldman WE. Effect of ampicillin and chloramphenicol against *Hemophilus influenzae*. Pediatrics 1978a;61:406.

Feldman WE. Effect of prior antibiotic therapy on concentrations of bacteria in CSF. Am J Dis Child 1978b;132:672.

Fothergill LD, Wright J. Influenzal meningitis: the relation of age incidence to the bactericidal power of blood against the causative organism. J Immunol 1933;24:273.

Fraser DW, Darby CP, Koehler RE, et al. Risk factors in bacterial meningitis. J Infect Dis 1973;127:271-277.

Friderichsen C. Nebennierenapoplexie bei kleinen Kindern. Jahrb Kinderheilkd 1918;87:109.

Galaid EI, Cherubin CE, Marr JS, et al. Meningococcal disease in New York City, 1973 to 1978. Recognition of groups Y and W-135 as frequent pathogens. JAMA 1980;244:2167-2171.

Gartner JC, Michaels RH. Meningitis from a pneumococcus moderately resistant to penicillin. JAMA 1979;241:1707-1709.

Ginsburg CM, McCracken GH Jr, Rae S, Parke JC Jr. *Haemophilus influenzae* type b disease: incidence in a day care center. JAMA 1977;238:604.

Glode MP, et al. An outbreak of *Hemophilus influenzae* type B meningitis in an enclosed hospital population. J Pediatr 1976;88:36.

Goldschneider I, Gotschlich EC, Artenstein MS. Human immunity to the meningococcus. I. The role of humoral antibodies. II. Development of natural immunity. J Exp Med 1969;129:1307.

Gottschlich EC, Goldschneider I, Artenstein MS. Human immunity to the meningococcus. IV. Immunogenicity of group A and group C meningococcal polysaccharides in human volunteers. J Exp Med 1969;129:1367.

Granoff DM, Squires JE, Munson RS, Suarez B. Siblings of patients with haemophilus meningitis have impaired anticapsular antibody responses to *Haemophilus* vaccine. J Pediatr 1983;103:185-191.

Hansen EJ, Robertson SM, Gulig PA, et al. Immunoprotection of rats against haemophilus influenzae type b disease mediated by monoclonal antibody against a haemophilus outer-membrane protein. Lancet 1982;1:366-367.

Hill JC. From the National Institute of Allergy and Infectious Diseases. Summary of a workshop on *Haemophilus influenzae* type b vaccines. J Infect Dis 1983;148:167-175.

Hunter KW, Fischer GW, Hemming VG, Wilson SR. Antibacterial activity of a human monoclonal antibody to *Haemophilus influenzae* type b capsular polysaccharide. Lancet 1982;2:798-799.

Jacobs RF, Hsi S, Wilson CB, et al. Apparent meningococcemia: clinical features of disease due to *Haemophilus influenzae* and *Neisserie meningitidis*. Pediatrics 1983; 72:469-472.

Jacob J, Kaplan RA. Bacterial meningitis: limitations of repeated lumbar puncture. Am J Dis Child 1977;131:46.

Jacobs MR, Koornhof HJ, Robins-Browne RM, et al. Emergence of multiply resistant pneumococci. N Engl J Med 1978;299:735-740.

Jubelirer DP, Yeager AS. Simultaneous recovery of ampicillin-sensitive and ampicillin-resistant organisms in *Haemophilus influenzae* type b meningitis. J Pediatr 1979; 95:415.

Kaplan SL, Feigin RD. Treatment of meningitis in children. Pediatr Clin North Am 1983;30:259-269.

Kaplan SL, Mason EO Jr, Kvernland SJ, et al. Moxalactam treatment of serious infections primarily due to *Haemophilus influenzae* type b in children. Pediatrics 1983;71:187-191.

Kelly RS, Hunt AD Jr, Tashman SG. Studies on the absorption and distribution of chloramphenicol. Pediatrics 1951;8:362.

Kenny JF, Isburg CD, Michaels RH. Meningitis due to haemophilus influenzae type b resistant to both ampicillin and chloramphenicol. Pediatrics 1980;66:14-16.

Kahn W, et al. *Hemophilus influenzae* type B resistant to ampicillin. JAMA 1974;229:298.

Kilian M, Sørensen I, Frederiksen W. Brochemical characteristics of 130 recent isolates from *Haemmophilus influenzae* meningitis. J Clin Microsc 1979;9:409-412.

King SD, Ramlal A, Wynter H, et al. Safety and immunogenicity of a new *Haemophilus influenzae* type b vaccine in infants under one year of age. Lancet 1981;2:705-709.

Koch R, Carson MJ. Meningococcal infections in children. N Engl J Med 1958;258:639.

Leedom JM, Inler D, Mathies AW, et al. The problem of sulfadiazine-resistant meningococci, Antimicrob Agents Chemother 1966;6:281-292.

Lewin EB. Partially treated meningitis. Am J Dis Child 1974;128:145.

Maguire GR, Myers MG. Antimicrobial selection for meningitis in young infants. Am J Dis Child 1979;133:1132.

Markowitz SM. Isolation of an ampicillin-resistant non-B-lactamase producing strain of *Haemophilus influenzae*. Antimicrob Agents Chemother 1980;17:80-82.

Mathies AW, et al. Experience with ampicillin in bacterial meningitis. Antimicrob Agents Chemother 1965;5:610.

McCracken G. New developments in the management of children with bacterial meningitis. Pediatr Infect Dis 1984;3:532-534.

McCracken GH, Mize SG, Threlkeld N. Intraventricular gentamicin therapy in gram negative bacillary meningitis of infancy. Report of the Second Neonatal Meningitis Cooperative Study group, Lancet 1980;1:781-791.

McGehee WG, Papaport SI, Hjort PF. Intravascular coagulation in fulminant meningococcemia. Ann Intern Med 1967;67:250.

McKay RJ Jr, Morissette RA, Ingraham FD, Matson DD. Collections of subdural fluid complicating meningitis due to *Haemophilus influenzae* (type b); a preliminary report. N Engl J Med 1950;242:20.

Medeiros AA, O'Brien TF. Ampicillin-resistant *Haemophilus influenzae* type b possessing a tem-type β-lactamose but little permeability barrier to ampicillin. Lancet 1975;1:716.

Miller JW, et al. Resistance to sulfadiazine of *Neisseria meningitidis*. JAMA 1963;186:139.

Mufson MA. Pneumoccal infections. JAMA 1981;264:1942-1948.

Munford RS, et al. Eradication of carriage of *Neisseria meningitides* in families. J Infect Dis 1974;219:644.

Murphy TV, McCracken GH, Zweighaft, Hansen EJ. Emergence of rifampin-resistant *Haemophilus influenzae* after prophylaxis. J Pediatr 1981;99:406-409.

Naraqi S, Kirkpatrick GP, Kabins S. Relapsing pneumococcal meningitis: isolation of an organism with decreased susceptibility to penicillin G. J Pediatr 1974;85:671-673.

Nelson J. Cerebropsinal fluid shunt infections. Pediatr Infect Dis 1984;3:530-532.

Nelson JD. How preventable is bacterial meningitis? N Engl J Med 1982;307:1265-1267.

Paredes A, Taber LH, Yow MD, et al. Prolonged pneumococcal meningitis due to an organism with increased resistance to penicillin. Pediatrics 1976;58:378-381.

Parke JC, Schneerson R, Robbins JB. The attack rate, age incidence, racial distribution and case fatality ratio of *H influenzae*, type b meningitis in Mecklenburg County, NC. J Pediatr 1972;81:765-769.

Peltola H, Käyhty H, Sivonen A, Mäkelä PH. *Haemophilus influenzae* type b capsular polysaccharide vaccine in children: a double-blind field study of 100,000 vaccinees 3 months to 5 years of age in Finland. Pediatrics 1977; 60:730.

Peltola H, Käyhty H, Virtanen MV, Makela PH. Prevention of *Hemophilus influenzae* type b bacteremic infections with the capsular polysaccharide vaccine. N Engl J Med 1984;310:1561-1566.

Pincus DJ, Morrison D, Andrews C, et al. Age-related response to two *Haemophilus influenzae* type b vaccines. J Pediatr 1982;100:197-201.

Prober CG, Ipp MM, Bannatyne RM. *Haemophilus influenzae* type b in a nursery school: the value of biotyping. Pediatrics 1982;69:215-218.

Radetsky MS, Istre GR, Johansen TL, et al. Multiply resistant pneumococcus causing meningitis: its epidemiology within a day-care centre. Lancet 1981;2:771-773.

Rahal JJ, Simberkoff MS. Bactericidal and bacteriostatic action of chloramphenicol against meningeal pathogens. Infect Agents Chemother 1979;16:13.

Rapkin RH. Repeat lumbar punctures in the diagnosis of meningitis. Pediatrics 1974;54:34.

Savers MP. Shunt Complications. Clin Neurosurg 1976; 23:393.

Schaad UB, Krucko J, Pfenninger J. An extended experience with cefuroxime therapy of childhood bacterial meningitis. Pediatr, Infect Dis 1984;3:410-416.

Schiffer MS, MacLowry J, Schneerson R, Robbins JB. Clinical, bacteriological and immunological characterization of ampicillin-resistant *Haemophilus influenzae* type B. Lancet 1974;2:257.

Schneerson R, Robbins JB. Induction of serum *Hemophilus influenzae* type b capsular antibodies in adult volunteers fed cross-reacting *Escherichia coli* 075:K100:HS. N Engl J Med 1975;292:1093.

Sell SH. Long term sequelae of bacterial meningitis in children. Pediatr Infect Dis 1983;2:90-93.

Sell SH, Merrill RE, Doyne EO, et al. Long term sequelae of *Hemophilus influenzae* meningitis. Pediatrics 1972a; 49:206-211.

Sell SH, Webb WW, Pate JE, et al. Psychological sequelae to bacterial meningitis: two controlled studies. Pediatrics 1972b;49:212-217.

Shapiro ED. Prophylaxis for contacts of patients with meningococcal or *Haemophilus influenzae* type b disease. Pediatr Infec Dis 1982;1:132-141.

Smith AL. Antibiotics and invasive *Hemophilus influenzae*. N Engl J Med 1976;294:1329.

Smith DH, et al. Bacterial meningitis: a symposium. Pediatrics 1973;52:586.

Sutherland JM, et al. Toxicity of chloramphenicol for the newborn infant. Am J Dis Child 1959;98:648 (abstract).

Swartz MN, Dodge PR. Bacterial meningitis—a review of selected aspects. N Engl J Med 1965; 272:725,779,842, 898,954,1003.

Thornsberry C, Kriven LA. Ampicillin resistance in *Haemophilus influenzae* as determined by a rapid test for beta-lactamase production. Antimicrob Agents Chemother 1974;6:653.

Toews WH, Bass JW. Skin manifestations of meningococcal infection. Am J Dis Child 1974;127:173.

Tomeh MO, et al. Ampicillin-resistant *Haemophilus influenzae* type b infection. JAMA 1974;229:295.

Uchiyama N, Greene GR, Kitts DB, Thrupp LD. Meningitis due to *Haemophilus influenzae* type b resistant to ampicillin and chloramphenicol. J Pediatr 1980;97:421-432.

Ward JI, Fraser DW, Baroff LJ, Plikaytis BD. *Haemophilus influenzae* meningitis—a national study of secondary spread in household contacts. N Engl J Med 1979;301:122.

Ward JI, Siber GR, Scheifele DW, Smith DH. Rapid diagnosis of *Hemophilus influenzae* type b infections by latex particle agglutination and counterimmunoelectrophoresis. J Pediatr 1978;93:37.

Ward JI, Tsai TF, Filice GA, Fraser DW. Prevalence of ampicillin and chloramphenicol-resistant strains of *Haemophilus influenzae* causing meningitis and bacteremia. J Infect Dis 1978;138:421.

Waterhouse R. A case of suprarenal apoplexy, Lancet 1911;1:577.

Whitecar, JP Jr, Reddin JL Spink WW. Recurrent pneumococcal meningitis. N Engl J Med 1966;274:1285.

Wilson HD, Haltalin KC. Ampicillin in *Hemophilus influenzae* meningitis. Am J Dis Child 1975;129:208.

Winkelstein JA. The influence of partial treatment with penicillin on the diagnosis of bacterial meningitis. J Pediatr 1970;77:619.

Wood PR, McKee KT, Lohr JA, Hendley JO. *Haemophilus influenzae* meningitis in school-aged children. JAMA 1982;247:1162-1163.

16

MUMPS (EPIDEMIC PAROTITIS)

Mumps is an acute contagious disease caused by a paramyxovirus that has a predilection for glandular and nervous tissue. Mumps is characterized most commonly by enlargement of the salivary glands, particularly the parotid glands. One or more of the following manifestations of mumps may be associated with or may occur without parotitis: meningoencephalitis, orchitis, pancreatitis, and other glandular involvement. Inapparent infection occurs in a significant percentage of persons (30% to 40%).

ETIOLOGY

Mumps is caused by a specific virus belonging to the parainfluenza subgroup of the paramyxoviruses. It ranges in size from 90 to 135 nm. It is infective for monkeys and chick embryos and produces cytopathic effects in a variety of tissue cultures of primary monkey kidney, human embryonic kidney, and human diploid fibroblast. Infectivity is lost as a result of heating at 55° to 60° C for 20 minutes and after exposure to formalin or to ultraviolet light. Infectivity is maintained for years at temperatures of −20° to −70° C.

Mumps virus has an antigenic relationship to other members of the myxovirus group, including Newcastle disease virus and parainfluenza viruses.

PATHOLOGY

The mumps-infected parotid gland is rarely available for pathologic examination. The interstitial tissue shows edema and infiltration with lymphocytes. There is degeneration of the cells of the ducts, with accumulation of necrotic debris and polymorphonuclear leukocytes in the lumina. Inclusion bodies are not seen.

Mumps orchitis is characterized by edema and a perivascular lymphocytic infiltrate that progresses to involve the interstitial tissue. There is focal hemorrhage and destruction of germinal epithelium, producing plugging of the tubules by epithelial debris, fibrin, and polymorphonuclear leukocytes.

PATHOGENESIS

The current concept of the pathogenesis of mumps stems from experience gained from a variety of epidemiologic, immunologic, clinical, and experimental studies. The virus probably enters through the nose or mouth. Proliferation takes place in either the parotid gland or the superficial epithelium of the respiratory tract. This is followed by viremia, with subsequent localization of virus in glandular or nervous tissue. The parotid gland is most often involved. Mumps virus has been isolated from human saliva, blood, urine, and cerebrospinal fluid (CSF) during the acute phase of the illness. The salivary glands, brain, and spinal cord of experimentally infected monkeys also have yielded virus. The concept of mumps as a generalized infection has been well documented.

CLINICAL MANIFESTATIONS

For a long time the terms *mumps* and *epidemic parotitis* were used interchangeably. Mumps was recognized as primarily an infection of the salivary glands. The isolation of the virus and the development of the serologic specific tests, however, have contributed to a better understanding of the pathogenesis and a clarification of the clinical picture of the disease.

Infection with mumps virus usually develops after an incubation period of 16 to 18 days. In approximately 30% to 40% of the patients the resulting infection is inapparent. The remaining 60% to 70% of the patients develop an illness of variable severity with symptoms that depend on the site or sites of infection. In the majority of instances, clinical mumps is characterized only by parotitis, either unilateral or bilateral. Additional relatively common manifestations include submaxillary and sublingual gland infection, orchitis, and meningoencephalitis. Pancreatitis, oophoritis, thyroiditis, and other glandular infections are relatively rare. These various manifestations of mumps may precede, accompany, follow, or occur without parotitis.

Salivary gland involvement

The classic illness is ushered in by fever, headache, anorexia, and malaise. Within 24 hours the child complains of an "earache" localized near the lobe of the ear and aggravated by chewing movements of the jaw. The following day the enlarged parotid is noticeable and rapidly progresses to its maximum size within 1 to 3 days. The fever usually subsides after a variable period of 1 to 6 days, with the temperature returning to normal before the glandular swelling disappears.

The normal parotid gland is not palpable. It is horseshoe in shape, with the concave portion adjacent to the lobe of the ear (Fig. 16-1). An imaginary line bisecting the long axis of the ear and passing through the ear lobe divides the gland into two relatively equal parts. These anatomic relationships are not altered by the enlarging parotid gland. As the swelling progresses, the lobe of the ear is displaced upward and outward. During the phase of rapid parotid enlargement, the pain and tenderness may be very severe. These symptoms subside after the swelling has reached its peak. The enlarged parotid gradually decreases in size over a period of 3 to 7 days. Thus the swelling may be present for possibly 6 to 10 days. Usually one parotid gland enlarges first and within a few days the other enlarges. Occasionally both sides swell simultaneously. Approximately 25% of all patients have unilateral parotitis.

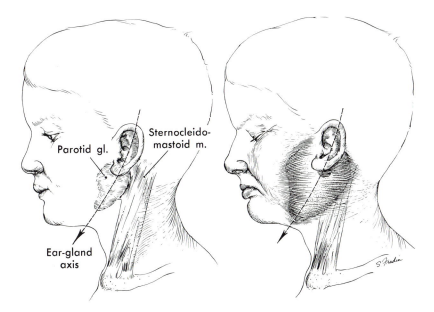

Fig. 16-1. Schematic drawing of parotid gland infected with mumps compared with normal gland. An imaginary line bisecting the long axis of the ear divides the parotid gland into two equal parts. These anatomic relationships are not altered in the enlarged gland. An enlarged cervical lymph node is usually posterior to the imaginary line.

The submaxillary swelling, when present, may be seen and palpated beneath the mandible just anterior to the angle of the jaw and directly beneath the anterior portion of the masseter muscle (Fig. 16-2). During the early stages the edema surrounding the submaxillary gland may spread over the mandible onto the cheek and downward toward the neck. When submaxillary mumps occurs without parotitis, it is clinically indistinguishable from cervical adenitis.

Sublingual mumps is usually bilateral and begins as a swelling in the submental region and on the floor of the mouth. Of the three salivary glands, the sublinguals are the least commonly involved.

The clinical picture of mumps just described is the classic one. The disease, however, is extremely variable. Occasionally, the appearance of local glandular swelling and tenderness may be the only manifestation of infection. Fever and constitutional symptoms may be absent.

Frequently the orifices of the ducts show inflammatory changes. The openings of Stensen's (parotid) and Wharton's (submaxillary) ducts may be reddened and edematous.

Patients with extensive salivary gland involvement may develop edema in the presternal area. It has been postulated that this is caused by an obstruction of the lymphatic vessels by the enlarged salivary glands.

Epididymo-orchitis

Epididymo-orchitis is the second most common manifestation of mumps infection in the adult male. It usually follows parotitis, but it may precede it or occur as an isolated manifestation of mumps. An epididymitis is invariably associated with the orchitis. Unilateral involvement occurs in 20% to 30% of males who develop the disease after puberty. The incidence of bilateral orchitis is low—approximately 2%. Under epidemic conditions the incidence of orchitis may be higher. In 1959 Philip et al. described an epidemic of 363 cases of mumps in a "virgin" population on St. Lawrence Island in the Bering Sea. The incidence of orchitis in males over 10 years of age was approximately 35%; bilateral orchitis occurred in approximately 12%. Orchitis develops within the first 2 weeks of infection, most commonly during the first week. In rare instances it may be delayed to the third week. As indicated in the following case report, mumps orchitis may occur in the absence of salivary gland involvement.

CASE 1. M. R., a 33-year-old man, was admitted to the Bellevue Hospital Infectious Disease Unit on December 5, 1958. He had a history of fever, chills, and right testicular swelling of 4 days' duration. Physical examination revealed a temperature of 102° F, and an enlarged, tender right testicle. The salivary glands were not palpable. The diagnosis of mumps

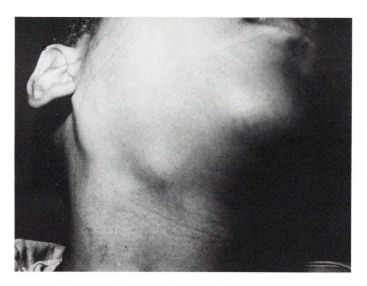

Fig. 16-2. Patient with mumps showing right parotid and submaxillary swelling. Note displacement of ear and characteristic location of both glands.

orchitis was confirmed by a significant rise in the level of mumps complement-fixing antibody during convalescence; the antibody titer was 1:32 on December 10 and ≥1:128 on December 22, 1958.

Orchitis begins abruptly with fever, chills, headache, nausea, vomiting, and lower abdominal pain. The systemic reaction usually parallels the extent of gonadal involvement. The temperature may vary from normal to 41.1° C (106° F). The duration of fever rarely exceeds 1 week. It persists for 3 days or less in approximately 20% of cases, 4 days or less in 50%, and 5 days or less in 80%. The temperature falls by crisis in approximately half the cases and by lysis in the remainder.

With the appearance of the fever, the testis begins to swell rapidly and becomes very painful and tender. It may increase in size very slightly or to as much as four times that of the normal gland. As the fever subsides, the pain and swelling disappear. The tenderness, however, persists for a longer period. As the testis decreases in size, a change of consistency is noted—loss of turgor. In about half of the cases this is sub-

sequently followed by atrophy. However, at least half of the involved glands do return to normal.

One of the most important concerns of men with mumps orchitis is the fear that sexual impotence and sterility will follow. Most orchitis is unilateral. Even with bilateral involvement it would be rare to have complete atrophy of both glands. The extensive experience with mumps orchitis in World Wars I and II failed to demonstrate that impotence and sterility are frequent consequences of this infection.

Meningoencephalitis

Central nervous system (CNS) involvement is another common manifestation of mumps. Symptomatic disease has been estimated to occur in about 10% of all cases. In a study by Bang and Bang (1944) 62% of 371 patients with mumps parotitis had cells in the CSF. Of this group 106 (28%) had CNS symptoms. Mumps meningoencephalitis usually follows the parotitis by 3 to 10 days. However, it may precede or even occur in the absence of salivary gland involvement (Fig. 16-3).

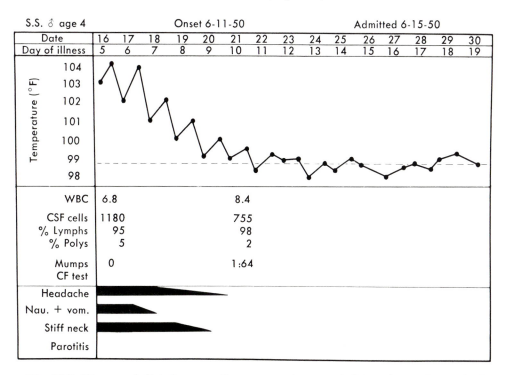

Fig. 16-3. Diagram of clinical course of mumps meningoencephalitis without salivary gland involvement. Pleocytosis with predominance of lymphocytes was found. The diagnosis was established by the development of complement-fixing antibody between the fifth and tenth days of illness.

The illness is characterized by fever, head-ache, nausea, vomiting, nuchal rigidity, change in sensorium, and, only rarely, convulsions. Brudzinski's and Kernig's signs can be elicited. The CSF shows pleocytosis, with a predominance of lymphocytes, normal glucose content, and elevated protein level. Although the glucose content is usually normal, cases with hypoglycorrhacia have been reported (Wilfert, 1969). The temperature usually falls by lysis over a period of 3 to 10 days. As the fever subsides, the symptoms clear, and recovery is usually uneventful. The infection follows the course of benign aseptic meningitis (Chapter 13) and usually has no sequelae.

Pancreatitis

This is a severe but uncommon manifestation of mumps infection. There is a sudden onset of severe epigastric pain and tenderness associated with fever, chills, extreme weakness, prostration, nausea, and repeated bouts of vomiting. The symptoms gradually subside over a period of 3 to 7 days, and the patient usually recovers completely.

Other clinical manifestations

The development of fever, nausea, vomiting, and lower abdominal pain in the female with mumps points to *oophoritis*. When the right ovary is involved, the signs and symptoms may be indistinguishable from those of acute appendicitis.

Many other glands may be involved in the infection. *Thyroiditis, mastitis, dacryoadenitis,* and *bartholinitis* are rare manifestations of mumps. In general, except for the symptoms due to the local swelling, the course is essentially the same as for any other mumps infection.

DIAGNOSIS
Confirmatory clinical factors

The following factors should point to mumps as a diagnostic possibility: (1) a history of exposure to mumps 2 to 3 weeks before onset of illness, (2) a compatible clinical picture of parotitis or other glandular involvement, and (3) signs of aseptic meningitis.

In the classic case of so-called epidemic parotitis, confirmatory laboratory procedures are usually unnecessary. In the absence of parotitis or in the presence of recurrent parotitis, how-

ever, the specific diagnostic aids whose descriptions follow may have to be utilized.

Isolation of causative agent

Mumps virus can be recovered from the saliva, mouth washings, or urine during the acute phase of parotitis and from the CSF early in the course of meningoencephalitis. The isolation may be made by inoculating the amniotic cavities of 8-day chick embryos or susceptible cell cultures. The isolation of mumps virus is not a routine laboratory procedure.

Serologic tests

There are at least four serologic tests that are used to demonstrate the development of specific mumps antibody: complement fixation (CF), hemagglutination-inhibition (HI), enzyme-linked immunosorbent assay (ELISA), and virus neutralization. The CF and ELISA tests are the most practical and most reliable of these diagnostic procedures.

The formation of mumps CF antibody after infection is shown in Fig. 16-4. The antibody becomes detectable in the blood by the end of the first week, and by the end of the second week a fourfold or greater rise in antibody titer can be demonstrated. When a diagnosis of mumps is suspected, acute and convalescent sera should be tested simultaneously. A fourfold or greater rise in the level of antibody confirms the diagnosis. This test is particularly useful for the diagnosis of mumps meningoencephalitis without parotitis, as is illustrated in Fig. 16-3.

Ancillary laboratory findings

The serum amylase level is elevated in mumps parotitis as well as in pancreatitis. The levels seem to parallel the parotid swelling. The values reach a peak during the first week, gradually returning to normal by the second and third weeks. Serum amylase determinations are abnormal in about 70% of cases of mumps parotitis. The finding of normal serum amylase levels may aid in the identification of obscure swellings about the jaw that resemble parotid involvement.

The white blood cell count may be normal or slightly elevated. Usually there is a slight predominance of lymphocytes, but at times the reverse is true.

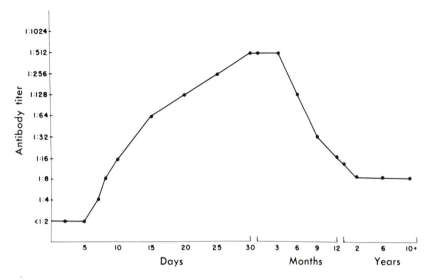

Fig. 16-4. Schematic curve illustrating development of mumps complement-fixing antibody. A significant rise in the level of antibody can be demonstrated in the serum by the end of the second week of illness. The acute and convalescent serum specimens should be tested simultaneously.

DIFFERENTIAL DIAGNOSIS
Parotitis

Mumps parotitis may be simulated by various conditions affecting the parotid glands or neighboring lymph nodes.

Anterior cervical or preauricular adenitis. Involvement of the lymph nodes, with surrounding edema, may simulate mumps parotitis. The parotid gland can usually be identified by its characteristic location, consistency, and outline. Its anatomic relationship to the ear is illustrated in Fig. 16-1. A line bisecting the long axis and lobe of the ear passes through the center of the gland. It has a brawny consistency with a well-defined posterior border and ill-defined anterior and inferior borders. In contrast, an enlarged lymph node has a well-defined, discrete border, is firm, and does not have the characteristic anatomic relationship to the ear. The appearance of the opening of Stensen's duct does not help very much. An elevated serum amylase level would point to parotid involvement. A mumps antibody test will clarify the diagnosis.

Suppurative parotitis. In suppurative parotitis the skin over the gland is usually red and hot, and the gland is exquisitely tender. Pus may be expressed from Stensen's duct by massaging the gland. An increase in the number of polymorphonuclear leukocytes is usually present. Although aerobic bacteria such as *Staphylococcus aureus* are the most common cause of acute suppurative parotitis, occasionally anaerobic bacteria *(Bacteroides, Fusobacterium,* and *Peptostreptococcus)* may be responsible (Brook and Finegold, 1978).

Recurrent parotitis. Recurrent parotitis, a condition of unknown and probably varied causes, is characterized by frequent recurrent swellings of the parotid gland. Infection and hypersensitivity to certain drugs such as iodides and phenothiazines may have a role in the causation of this disease. Roentgenographic studies of the duct system reveal evidence of sialectasia in some cases. The individual attack may be clinically indistinguishable from mumps parotitis. The submaxillary and sublingual glands, which are frequently associated with mumps parotitis, are not involved in recurrent parotitis. The history of previous attacks and a negative or unchanging CF test will clarify the diagnosis.

Calculus. A calculus that obstructs Stensen's duct causes a swelling of the parotid gland that is usually intermittent.

Coxsackie virus infection. In 1957 Howlett et al. described a syndrome of parotitis and herpangina caused by Coxsackie virus.

Parainfluenza 3 virus infection. In 1970 Zollar and Mufson reported acute parotitis in two children associated with detection of parainfluenza 3 virus and a significant rise in the level of homologous antibody.

Mixed tumors, hemangiomas, and lymphangiomas of the parotid. Mixed tumors, hemangiomas, and lymphangiomas of the parotid are responsible for chronic enlargement of the gland and are confused with mumps only during the early stages.

Mikulicz's syndrome. In Mikulicz's syndrome there is chronic bilateral parotid and lacrimal gland enlargement, usually associated with dryness of the mouth and absence of tears.

Uveoparotid fever. Uveoparotid fever is a manifestation of sarcoidosis, which may be confused with mumps.

Meningoencephalitis

Mumps meningoencephalitis without parotitis is clinically indistinguishable from aseptic meningitis caused by Coxsackie virus, ECHO virus, lymphocytic choriomeningitis virus, and a variety of other agents (Chapter 13). The specific mumps CF test usually establishes the diagnosis.

COMPLICATIONS
Deafness

Deafness is a very rare but serious complication of mumps. There is usually a sudden onset of vertigo, tinnitus, ataxia, and vomiting followed by permanent deafness. In most cases it is unilateral. The cause has been ascribed to neuritis of the auditory nerve.

CASE 2. R. S., a 29-year-old man, was admitted to Bellevue Hospital on November 25, 1959. About 4 weeks prior to admission he was exposed to his son who had mumps. On November 18 there was an abrupt onset of fever, left testicular swelling, nausea, vomiting, vertigo, tinnitus, and right-sided deafness. These symptoms progressed until the time of admission, when he was unable to walk because of ataxia and unable to hear with his right ear.

Physical examination revealed left testicular swelling and tenderness, total perceptive hearing loss on the right, and staggering gait to the right. Vestibular tests confirmed a markedly hypoactive right labyrinth. There was no salivary gland involvement.

The blood count, urinalysis results, serum amylase level, and CSF were normal. Reaction to the mumps CF test was positive with a titer of 1:128 on November 25, 1959 and 1:256 on December 3, 1959.

Testicular swelling and all other symptoms and signs except the deafness subsided by the end of the

second week of illness. The patient had been on bed rest because of the orchitis. When he became ambulatory on December 5 he had difficulty in walking because of left foot drop. It became apparent that he had left peroneal neuritis. Examination on December 28 revealed persistence of the deafness and improvement of the neuritis.

The clinical and laboratory findings supported a diagnosis of mumps orchitis without parotitis complicated by acute labyrinthitis, deafness, and peroneal neuritis.

Other neurologic complications

Other neurological complications, also very rare, include *facial neuritis, myelitis,* and *postinfectious encephalitis*. The latter, like measles encephalitis, may be fatal or complicated by serious sequelae. This type of encephalitis occurs very infrequently. Recent experimental studies in rodents infected with mumps virus have shown the late development of aqueductal stenosis and hydrocephalus as sequelae of the infection. Several case reports have linked previous mumps to the later onset of aqueductal stenosis. Whether mumps virus has a causal role in hydrocephalus remains speculative but merits the acquisition of further data (Bray, 1972). Herndon et al. (1974) demonstrated that ependymal cells were shed into the CSF in patients with mumps meningoencephalitis, another indication of ventricular involvement.

Myocarditis

Myocarditis as a complication of mumps has occasionally been observed in adults. Electrocardiographic findings indicate that the incidence may be 15%. The development of dyspnea, tachycardia, or bradycardia during the first 2 weeks of illness associated with T-wave changes and prolongation of the P-R interval should suggest this diagnosis. The myocarditis is usually followed by an uneventful recovery. More rarely, *pericarditis* also may occur.

Arthritis

Arthritis also has been described as a rare complication of mumps. It usually appears as migrating polyarthritis involving the larger and smaller joints and clears spontaneously.

Diabetes mellitus

It has been suggested that some cases of diabetes mellitus may be associated with a previous mumps virus infection (Sultz et al., 1975).

The relationship of mumps virus to diabetes mellitus has been studied epidemiologically and experimentally for many years without clear resolution of the possible role of the virus in the pathogenesis of this disease.

Hepatitis

Hepatitis has been reported as a rare complication of mumps. From the available descriptions, however, it is difficult to determine whether it is truly a complication or possibly a coincident development of viral hepatitis.

Hematologic complications

Unusual hematologic complications have included thrombocytopenia and hemolytic anemia. These have been severe but self-limited (Graham et al., 1974).

PROGNOSIS

In general, the prognosis of mumps is excellent. Fatalities are very rare. Meningoencephalitis is usually benign and is rarely followed by sequelae. In spite of high incidence of testicular atrophy following orchitis, sterility is extremely rare. In a small percentage of cases, permanent deafness may complicate the disease.

IMMUNITY

One attack usually confers lifelong immunity. Mumps may recur, but the rate (4%) that is cited for second attacks probably reflects errors in diagnosis. Acute cervical adenitis and recurrent parotitis are likely to be erroneously diagnosed as mumps. A survey of 100 patients referred to a communicable disease hospital with a diagnosis of mumps revealed that 5% of the group had cervical adenitis. Permanent immunity is conferred by an attack of any type of mumps infection, including unilateral parotitis, meningoencephalitis without parotitis, or orchitis without parotitis. Indeed, even clinically inapparent infections also confer a lasting immunity. Infants born of mothers who have had mumps have passive immunity that lasts for several months.

A number of tests are available to measure the

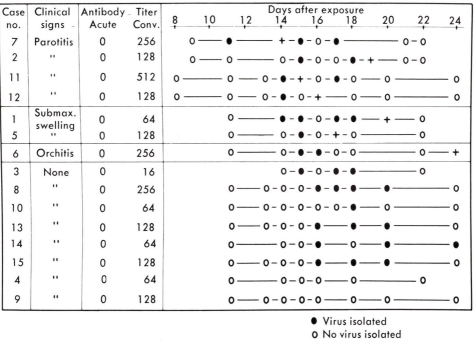

Fig. 16-5. Isolation of virus from saliva of patients with apparent and inapparent mumps infection. Virus was detected from 1 to 6 days before onset of salivary gland involvement. Virus was also readily isolated from six to eight patients with inapparent infection. Significant antibody levels developed in all 15 patients who were studied. (From Henle G, et al. J Exp Med 1948;88:223.)

immune status of a person. These include HI, CF, ELISA, and virus neutralization. It will be noted in Fig. 16-4 that the titer of mumps complement-fixing antibody persists at a low level for many months or years after infection. In a small percentage of cases the antibody level may fall below the detectable range. However, a positive CF test usually indicates past infection.

Several studies have correlated the results of serologic tests with patients who have past histories of a clinical case of mumps. Analysis of the data indicates that 30% to 40% of all susceptible persons exposed to mumps develop the infection in an inapparent form. These conclusions were confirmed experimentally by Henle et al. in 1948 (Fig. 16-5). Of a group of 15 susceptible subjects who were deliberately exposed to mumps, four developed parotitis, two developed submaxillary swelling, and one developed orchitis. The remaining eight subjects developed an inapparent infection as indicated by the isolation of virus and the rise in mumps complement-fixing antibody.

EPIDEMIOLOGIC FACTORS

During the prevaccine era mumps was an endemic disease in most urban populations. In institutions where crowding favored virus transmission, epidemics occurred frequently. Most cases of mumps occurred in the 5- to 10-year age group, with approximately 85% of the infections among children under 15 years of age. It was uncommon in infancy. The age group affected by mumps was older than those groups affected by measles, chickenpox, and pertussis. Consequently, there were epidemics among adolescents in boarding schools and among adults in the armed forces. The disease has occurred in persons of all ages ranging from 1 day to 99 years.

Following the widespread use of live attenuated mumps vaccine during the 1970s, the incidence of mumps declined in all age groups but most dramatically in the 5- to 9-year age group. Thus, during the late 1970s there was an increase in the relative proportion of mumps cases occurring among adolescents and young adults (Hayden et al., 1978). This situation has improved during the 1980s.

Mumps is probably acquired via the oropharynx. The source of infection may be saliva or other virus-containing secretions of an infected person. *Transmission* occurs by direct contact or by droplet infection.

The available epidemiologic evidence suggests that the *period of infectivity* is from several days before the onset of symptoms to the subsidence of the salivary gland swelling. In the average case this represents a period of about 7 to 10 days.

The study of experimentally induced mumps infection by Henle et al. (1948) (Fig. 16-5) has contributed significant data clarifying the period of infectivity. In the patients who developed parotitis 14 to 19 days after exposure, mumps virus was isolated from the saliva as many as 1 to 4 days before onset of parotitis. One patient who developed only submaxillary swelling on the twentieth day yielded mumps virus from the saliva 6 days before. It is of interest that six of the patients with inapparent infection secreted mumps virus in the saliva between the fifteenth and twenty-fourth days after exposure. This is a striking example of how an inapparent case of mumps may be the potential source for the spread of mumps infection. In a later study in 1958, Utz et al. isolated mumps virus in urine as early as the first day of salivary gland involvement and as late as the fourteenth day of illness.

Based on experience with other live attenuated vaccines, it is likely that live attenuated mumps virus vaccine could abort an epidemic in progress. The high incidence of inapparent cases and the infectivity of patients before onset of parotitis both combine to limit the effectiveness of quarantine or isolation. In the past the patient was isolated until the swelling of the salivary gland has subsided. In our opinion, too much time and effort should not be wasted on outmoded rigid isolation and quarantine procedures.

TREATMENT

Mumps is a self-limited infection, the course of which is not altered by use of any of the antimicrobial drugs. Treatment is symptomatic, and supportive measures are used. Aspirin or codeine will usually control the pain caused by glandular swelling. Warm applications seem to help some patients; others prefer cold. Topical ointments are useless. Parenteral administration of fluids is indicated for the support of patients with persistent vomiting associated with pancreatitis or meningoencephalitis.

PREVENTIVE MEASURES

Passive protection

Standard immune globulin (IG) is ineffective. The efficacy of mumps-immune globulin is also questionable. During an epidemic of mumps in Alaska, Reed et al. (1967) evaluated the effect of mumps-immune globulin. The attack rate of mumps was 46% among 56 susceptible individuals who received globulin; it was 45% among 185 susceptible persons who did not receive globulin. In addition, under the conditions of this study there was no evidence that the mumps-immune globulin prevented orchitis or meningoencephalitis.

Active immunization

An inactivated mumps vaccine of uncertain value was available in the past. It has now been replaced by the live attenuated mumps vaccine. Live attenuated mumps virus vaccine was licensed for use in the United States in January 1968. Current recommendations for the use of this vaccine are described in detail on p. 519.

REFERENCES

Appelbaum E, Kohn J, Steinman RE, Shearn MA. Mumps arthritis. Arch Intern Med 1953;90:217.

Bang HO, Bang J. Involvement of the central nervous system in mumps. Bull, Hyg 1944;19:503.

Bilger F, Zimmer A, Lachowiecki J. Traitement de la douleur dan l'epididymité aiguë par l'infiltration du sympathique lombaire. Progr Med, p 9, January 1, 1938.

Blitz D, Eisenoff HM. The clinical evaluation of mumps in an orphanage. NY J Med 1951;51:2765.

Bray PF. Mumps—a cause of hydrocephalus? Pediatrics 1972;49:446.

Brook I, Finegold SM. Acute suppurative parotitis caused by anaerobic bacteria: report of two cases. Pediatrics 1978;62:1019.

Buynak EB, et al. Combined live measles, mumps, and rubella virus vaccines. JAMA 1969;207:2259.

Candel S. Epididymitis in mumps, including orchitis: further clinical studies and comments. Ann Intern Med 1951;34:20.

De Meis JJ, Walker DL. Demonstration of antigenic relationship between mumps and hemagglutinating virus of Japan. J Immunol 1957;78:465.

Enders JF, Cohen S, Kane LW. Immunity in mumps. J Exp Med 1945;81:119.

Evans AS. Newcastle disease neutralizing antibody in human sera and its relationship to mumps virus. Am J Hyg 1954;60:204.

Gellis SS, McGuinness AC, Peters M. A study on the prevention of mumps orchitis with gamma globulin. Am J Med Sci 1945;210:661.

Graham DY, Brown CH, Benrey J, Butel JS. Thrombocytopenia: a complication of mumps. JAMA 1974;227:1162.

Habel K. Vaccination of human beings against mumps; vaccine administered at the start of an epidemic. I. Incidence and severity of mumps in vaccinated and control groups. Am J Hyg 1951;54:295.

Hayden GF, et al. Current status of mumps and mumps vaccine in the United States. Pediatrics 1978;62:965.

Henle G, Deinhardt F. Propagation and primary isolation of mumps virus in tissue culture. Proc Soc Exp Biol Med 1955;89:556.

Henle G, Henle W, Wendell KK, Rosenberg P. Isolation of mumps virus from human beings with induced apparent or inapparent infections. J Exp Med 1948;88:223.

Herndon RM, Johnson RT, Davis LE, Descalzi LR. Ependymitis in mumps virus meningitis. Arch Neurol. 1974; 30:475.

Howlett JG, Somlo F, Kalz F. A new syndrome of parotitis with herpangina caused by the coxsackie virus. Can Med Assoc J 1957;77:5.

Johnson CD, Goodpasture EW. The etiology of mumps. Am J Hyg 1935;21:46.

Kempf JE, Spaeth R. Prophylaxis of epidemic parotitis: antibody response following injection of mumps in varying dosage. J Lab Clin Med 1954;43:647.

Lyon RP, Bruyn HB. Mumps epididymoorchitis. Treatment by anesthetic block of the spermatic cord. JAMA 1966; 196:736.

Philip RN, Reinhard KR, Lackmann DB. Observations on a mumps epidemic in a "virgin" population. Am J Hyg 1959;69:91.

Reed D, et al. A mumps epidemic on St. George Island, Alaska JAMA 1967;199:113.

Stokes J Jr, Enders JF, Maris EP, Kane LW. Immunity in mumps. Experiments on the vaccination of human beings with formolized mumps virus. J Exp Med 1946;84:407.

Sultz HA, Hart BA, Zielezny M. Is mumps virus an etiologic factor in juvenile diabetes mellitus? J Pediatr 1975;86:654.

Utz JP, Szwed CF, Kasel JA. Clinical and laboratory studies of mumps. II. Detection and duration of excretion of virus in urine. Proc Soc Exp Biol Med 1958;99:259.

Utz JP, et al. Clinical and laboratory studies of mumps. I. Laboratory diagnosis by tissue-culture technics. N Engl J Med 1957;257:497.

Vicens CN, Nobrega FT, Joseph JM, Meyer MB. Evaluation of tests for the measurement of previous mumps infection and analysis of mumps experience by blood group. Am J Epidemiol 1966;84:371.

Weibel, RE, Buynak EB, McLean AA, Hilleman, MR. Persistence of antibodies after administration of monovalent and combined live attenuated measles, mumps, and rubella virus vaccines. Pediatrics 1978;61:5.

Weibel RE, et al. Live attenuated mumps-virus vaccine. 3. Clinical and serologic aspects in a field evaluation. N Engl J Med 1967;276:245.

Wilfert CM. Mumps meningoencephalitis with low cerebrospinal fluid glucose, prolonged pleocytosis and elevation of protein. N Engl J Med 1969;280:855.

Zollar LM, Mufson MA. Acute parotitis associated with parainfluenza 3 virus infection. Am J Dis Child 1970;119:147.

17

SEPSIS IN THE NEWBORN

The neonatal host in its immaturity and new environment is susceptible to invasion and rapid spread of organisms so that septicemia, with or without meningitis, occurs at a rate and a tempo more striking than at any other period of life. Reliable statistics of the annual number of cases are not available because sepsis of the newborn is not a reportable disease. Data from individual institutions provide estimates of between one and ten per 1000 live births. With more than 3.5 million births annually, there could be as many as 5000 to 35,000 infants affected. The clinical expression of illness is usually nonspecific so that antemortem diagnosis depends on a high index of suspicion. There are those infants whose infection is acquired prenatally or during the delivery process, and the organisms frequently are those of the maternal genital tract. There is also a second group who are born prematurely or with major medical and/or surgical problems, necessitating prolonged hospitalization and multiple invasive procedures. In contrast to the first group, the latter group is more likely to develop nosocomial infections with opportunistic organisms.

The natural history of sepsis in the newborn infant is affected by multiple factors such as premature rupture of the membranes, maternal infection, and the imperfections of the newborn infant's capacity to resist infection. The changing spectrum of etiologic agents, the subtlety of the clinical signs of illness, and the persistent high mortality despite advances in antimicrobial therapy emphasize the complexity of the subject and warrant its consideration as an entity.

ETIOLOGY

In the first decades of the twentieth century, prior to the availability of antimicrobial agents, gram-positive bacteria were apparently the predominant causative agents of neonatal sepsis. In particular, β-hemolytic streptococci (presumably group A) were the most frequently identified pathogens. In the 1940s and 1950s gram-negative organisms, predominantly *Escherichia coli*, were implicated in the vast majority of cases of neonatal sepsis. A pandemic of staphylococcal disease in the late 1950s and early 1960s involved nursery populations, with the severity of infections ranging from localized pustules to fulminant sepsis. In the mid-1970s a "new" organism, group B β-hemolytic *Streptococcus (Streptococcus agalactiae)* emerged as the predominant pathogen in the newborn period.

A report from Yale (Freedman et al., 1981) illustrates the increasing predominance of *S. agalactiae* or group B β-hemolytic streptococci in the late 1970s (Table 17-1). *E. coli* remains the second most common pathogen. When the organisms are separated according to the age of the infant when the culture was obtained, group B streptococci are responsible for 41% of all positive cultures in the first 48 hours of life (Table 17-2). The organism in this setting is acquired from the maternal flora. *E. coli* may also be acquired from the maternal flora as evidenced by

Table 17-1. Organisms isolated from blood cultures in newborns*, 1966 to 1978, Yale-New Haven Hospital†

Organism	1966 to 1969	1970 to 1973	1974 to 1978	Total
β-hemolytic streptococci				117
Group A	1	1		
Group B	7	26	64	
Group D				
Enterococci	2	4	7	
Nonenterococci (S. bovis)			4	
Nongroupable			1	
Escherichia coli	34	37	51	122
Klebsiella-enterobacter	36	4	16	56
Staphylococcus aureus	1	11	12	24
Haemophilus species		3	8	11
Pseudomonas species	5	4	9	9
Mixed	5	4	6	15
Other	5	7	18	30
TOTAL	96	101	187	384

*<30 days of age.
†Modified from Freedman RM, Ingram DL, Gross I, et al. A half-century of neonatal sepsis at Yale, 1928-1978. Am J Dis Child 1981;135:140.

finding these organisms in 26% of the positive cultures obtained in the first 48 hours. Together, group B streptococci and *E. coli* were responsible for two thirds of early onset sepsis (Table 17-2). Other enteric gram-negative organisms and staphylococci were found in positive cultures obtained after the first 48 hours. Some of these organisms may be acquired from the mother, but many may be selected over time in the nursery setting.

Thirty to forty percent of septicemia and more than 80% of meningitis caused by *E. coli* in newborns is with organisms that have the K1 antigen. Only 15% of *E. coli* in the gastrointestinal flora is K1-antigen positive. The excess of K1 in meningitis relative to septicemia has suggested that this antigen is important in bacterial localization. Furthermore, the K1 antigen is identical to the polysaccharide of meningococcus B, another organism causing meningitis. The polysaccharide consists of a neuraminic acid α 2 → 8 homopolymer. Organisms with K1 antigen exhibit decreased alternative pathway-mediated opsonization and are phagocytosed poorly in the absence of antibody. Of great interest is the recent observation that two polysialosyl glycopeptides (GM3 and GD3) of human fetal brain react with antibodies against meningococcus B capsules. The cross-reactivity of brain tissue with

Table 17-2. Organisms isolated by age of infant when blood culture obtained, 1966 to 1978, Yale-New Haven Hospital*

Organism	Culture <48 hours	Culture >48 hours
β-hemolytic streptococci	89	28
Group B	71	19
Enterococci	7	6
Others	4	3
Escherichia coli	49	73
Klebsiella-Enterobacter	11	45
Staphylococcus aureus	7	17
Haemophilus species	10	1
Pseudomonas species	2	7
Mixed	7	8
Other	12	19
TOTAL	187	198

*Modified from Freedman RM, Ingram DL, Gross I, et al. A half-century of neonatal sepsis at Yale, 1928-1978. Am J Dis Child 1981;135:140.

the capsule of the organism may predispose to infection if the host is tolerant to this antigen (Finne et al., 1983; Soderstrom et al., 1984).

The non-antibody-mediated bactericidal activity of human serum has been suggested to be an important nonspecific defense mechanism against gram-negative invasive infections. Conversely, the serum resistance of gram-negative organisms is potentially an important virulence factor for the organism. Serum sensitivity is related to the 0 antigenicity, which is a function of repeating sugars. These polysaccharides produce smooth colonies of organisms. The organisms lacking these sugars form rough colonies and are more serum sensitive. Four somatic antigens (018, 07, 01, and 016) accounted for about two thirds of 65 K1 *E. coli* isolates from the cerebrospinal fluid (CSF) of newborns (McCracken et al., 1974). Smooth strains of these serotypes that are serum resistant are also invasive in animals, and it has been suggested that this results from their inability to activate the classic complement pathway. Thus, composition of the capsular polysaccharide (K) and the 0 antigen are determinants of complement activation and serum sensitivity and therefore contribute to the virulence of these organisms for the newborn.

Similarly, type III GBS organisms are more often implicated in meningitis than other serotypes of GBS. The capsular polysaccharide antigens of both types III and IA GBS contain sialic acid, which inhibits alternative complement pathway activation in the absence of specific antibody. The sialic acid is essential to the tertiary molecular conformation of the capsule, which is apparently critical to the serologic specificity of the polysaccharide and to complement activation. Thus, for both K1 *E. coli* and type III GBS, the sialic acid of the capsule is important in circumventing the host response.

PATHOLOGY

In most cases of sepsis of the newborn infant, the infection becomes rapidly generalized, often leaving little evidence of an external focus. Inflammatory processes may develop in any organ or part of the body, resulting in meningitis, pneumonia, empyema, pericarditis, myocarditis, endocarditis, peritonitis, hepatitis, urinary tract infection, otitis, osteomyelitis, pyarthrosis, and miliary abscesses in the soft tissues.

Group B streptococcal disease readily demonstrates the characteristic features of such overwhelming bacterial infection. Large numbers of organisms can be found in virtually every tissue from central nervous system (CNS) to lungs, liver, and spleen. The inflammatory response is often minimal even at the time of death, which frequently occurs in 2 to 3 days. In this specific setting the pathologic features tend to substantiate in vitro observations of decreased chemotaxis of polymorphonuclear leukocytes and marrow depletion in the newborn.

Meningitis is the most important lesion or complication of sepsis in the newborn infant. Infants in this age group with gram-negative meningitis have areas of hemorrhagic necrosis of the CNS. In those infants who tend to survive somewhat longer, the inflammatory response is apparent even in fatal disease. Late onset group B streptococcal disease, frequently manifest as meningitis, is accompanied by a significant inflammatory response. Furthermore, the abnormal CSF is easily accessible for Gram stain, culture, and other analyses, which may provide a prompt etiologic diagnosis. In addition to the inflammatory reaction in the meninges, a widespread, devastating infectious vasculitis results in severe cortical changes in most cases examined postmortem.

PATHOGENESIS
Local factors

The time of presentation may afford valuable insight into the etiology of neonatal sepsis. The infant who demonstrates infection in the first few days of life is most likely infected by organisms acquired from the maternal gastrointestinal or genitourinary tract. The infections of the immediate postpartum period probably result from colonization of the gastrointestinal and respiratory tracts and skin, with all mucous membranes and the umbilical cord also affording sites for potential entry of bacteria. *Neisseria gonorrhoeae* have been observed for years to colonize and to invade the conjunctivae unless the infant has received adequate local prophylaxis. More recently these organisms have also been identified in the gastric aspirates of newborns. Identification of staphylococcal skin colonization and recognition of invasive illness have long plagued nurseries with questions concerning the acceptable rates and level of colonization.

The infant who develops infection later, particularly the neonate requiring intensive supportive care, most likely has disease caused by organisms acquired from the environment. Although essential, the invasive life-supportive measures of the intensive care nursery further compromise the neonate with indwelling endotracheal tubes, oral-duodenal feeding tubes, central hyperalimentation lines, cutaneous monitoring devices, and peripheral intravenous lines. Each of these measures bypasses or breaches normal barriers to infection and affords the opportunity for introduction of organisms into areas usually sterile.

Host factors

The humoral defenses of the newborn play a significant role in the pathogenesis of neonatal sepsis. Transplacental transmission of IgG antibodies confers an incomplete spectrum of passive antibody protection to the infant. The neonate receives no globulins of the IgA or IgM classes. Because the normal newborn has not usually been challenged with appropriate antigens, these antibodies are not yet being synthesized, although the fetus is capable of synthesizing IgM and IgA early in intrauterine life. It has been demonstrated that specific antibodies of the IgM class are more efficient (than IgG) in bactericidal and opsonic activities against gram-negative bacteria, and thus the infant lacks optimal humoral protection at birth.

The ability to recognize and respond to specific antigens develops sequentially during gestation and probably for the first several years of life. Infants do not reliably form antibodies to most polysaccharides until 18 to 24 months of age. In contrast, protein antigens are recognized and induce a response. As with any such generalization there are known exceptions, but it is an accepted concept that the newborn has an immature ability to respond to the capsular polysaccharides of many invasive bacterial pathogens.

The complex complement system plays an integral role in host defense against infection. Complement's protective functions are particularly directed against extracellular pathogens, including gram-positive pyogenic bacteria and gram-negative enteric organisms. The organisms that can resist phagocytosis in the absence of antibody tend to be capable of acting as invasive pathogens. GBS and K1 *E. coli* have been discussed as significant pathogens in this age group. Complement and/or antibody opsonize bacteria, which allows phagocytosis to occur.

Complement activation is classically initiated by antigen-antibody interactions (Fig. 17-1). The components "fix" or join the cascade in the sequence 1, 4, 2, 3, 5, 6, 7, 8, 9. The second, or alternative, pathway seems to be triggered by formation of C3b (Fig. 17-1), the major fragment of C3. Generation of C3b continuously occurs at a low level unless a microorganism or other target particle enters the picture and fixes C3b. Then, amplification of fixation occurs with C3b plus B (Bb) acting as an enzyme. Either activation of the classic pathway or alternative pathway fixes C3b to the bacterium and results in its opsonization. Activation of the complement cascade by either pathway also promotes vasodilation by release of C3a and C5a, releases the major chemotactic factor which is a split product of C5, and fixes late-acting components to the organism, which then induces lysis. This is the functional overall scheme, but the newborn complement system is immature, and measurable deficiencies are likely to contribute to the vulnerability of the infant.

First, whole complement activity (CH_{50}) is subnormal in about one half of term infants. All components except C8 and C9 are present in lower concentrations than in normal adults. The lower mean values do not indicate that every baby will have abnormal complement activity. Preterm infants have lower whole complement activity and lower component concentrations than term infants. Components of the alternative pathway are also reduced in comparison to normal adult values. Factor B concentrations have varied from 35% to 60% of adult values and have been abnormal in 15% to 30% of infants tested. Properdin, with values approximating 50% to 70% of adult values, is also significantly lower in serum of preterm infants compared to term infants. Properdin protects the factor B (in enzymatic form, Bb) (Fig. 17-1) from inactivation and, thus, preterm infants may further diminish effective factor B function by inactivation of the enzyme Bb.

Attempts to assay cord blood for diminished activation of complement more often show abnormalities in the alternate pathway. Opsonization and hemolysis mediated by the alterna-

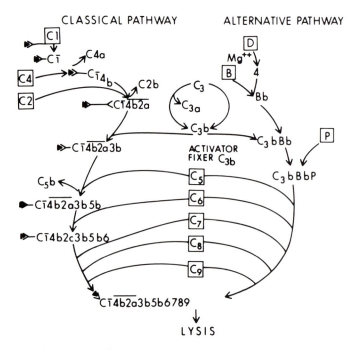

Fig. 17-1. Complement cascade. Classical pathway is activated by antigen-antibody interactions. C3 plays a pivotal role. Native proteins are designated by boxes. Cleavage products are designated by lower case letters. ■, antigen; ●●, complement-fixing antibody.

tive pathway are abnormal in 15% to 75% of term infants. Either or both of the complement pathways may be abnormal. Very few sera are functionally normal by adult criteria. The multicomponent and dual pathway deficiencies of newborns probably contribute to their inability to handle bacterial infections. Since they lack IgM antibody and activate the classic pathway less well, the alternate pathway that functions in the absence of specific antibody becomes more crucial. The newborn is likely to be defective in the alternate pathway. In addition, K1 *E. coli* and group B streptococci are poor activators of the alternative complement pathway as described above. In conjunction with defective phagocytosis, the complement alterations predispose to severe bacterial infections.

Phagocytosis has been examined in multiple studies and as our knowledge has expanded, the complexity of the process of phagocytosis and killing of microorganisms becomes more apparent. Generally speaking, newborn polymorphonuclear cells can ingest particles as well as adult cells in vitro unless the concentration of serum in the test tube is decreased. Measurable deviations from normal function of cells from new-

borns as compared to mature polymorphonuclear cells probably contribute to the response to infection of the newborn infant and are briefly mentioned here. Decreased oxidative metabolic responsiveness as measured by chemiluminescence and decreased bactericidal activity have been reported, and these abnormalities are increased in a stressed newborn. When the number of organisms used in the test system is increased, these defects are exaggerated. Defective locomotion or chemotaxis of newborn polymorphonuclear cells has been a consistent finding. Studies of newborn chemotaxis have examined the mechanisms of altered function (Anderson et al., 1981). Newborn polymorphonuclear cells do sense chemotactic factors normally but have diminished modulation of cell adhesiveness which contributes to the diminished locomotion. Newborn polymorphonuclear cells have morphologically immature microtubular structures, the organelle involved in movement.

The newborn is essentially devoid of secretory immunity in the first weeks of life, during which time the baby is colonized with microorganisms for the first time. The availability of preformed secretory immunity present in colostrum and breast milk provides potential passive protection in a number of ways. Specific antibody, particularly IgA, is present in colostrum and breast milk and contains significant activity against agents such as K1 *E. coli*, without any predictable correlation with specific antibodies of the mother's serum. Such IgA is mainly effective in the infant's gastrointestinal tract. There is also a growth factor favoring *Lactobacillus bifidus*, lysozyme that cleaves the peptidoglycans of bacterial cell walls, and lactoferrin. The last binds iron and is bacteriostatic for *E. coli*. This effect is enhanced by the presence of specific antibody.

Finally, human milk has significant numbers (1 to 2×10^6) of leukocytes which are 80% mononuclear phagocytes. The milk mononuclear phagocyte synthesizes lysozyme, C3, and C4. These cells have IgG Fc receptors and C3b receptors. Thus, these cells may phagocytize opsonized particles via the Fc receptor. The milk macrophage kills bacteria and fungi, can modulate lymphocyte mitogenic reactivity after exposure to plant lectins, can mediate lymphokine activity, and can synthesize inflammatory proteins. These attributes suggest a functional role for these cells in protection of the newborn.

CLINICAL MANIFESTATIONS

The subtlety of the clinical signs of illness is the hallmark of sepsis of the newborn infant. The manifestations are likely to be vague, nonspecific, and sharply contrasted to the traditional sudden onset with high fever, chills, leukocytosis, and prostration characteristic of septicemia in older children and adults. In the newborn infant and especially in the premature infant, the first intimation of infection may be lethargy, inability to tolerate feedings, temperature instability, or the nurse's observations that "this baby is not doing well." To the astonishment of physicians beginning their pediatric experience, such infants and those who exhibit regurgitation, or irritability—without fever and without meningeal signs or signs of systemic disease—may yield a postive blood culture.

It is obvious that sepsis does not account for all cases in which newborn infants fail to do well, feed poorly, regurgitate, or seem irritable. Additional clues that should make one suspect sepsis may be found by careful examination of the mother's record. Predisposing factors include prenatal and perinatal complications such as maternal infection, prematurity, premature and prolonged rupture of membranes, and difficult delivery. Of these, infection of the mother may be the most important. In any case, the presence of the aforementioned vague and nonspecific signs in the infant plus obstetric complications, especially maternal infection, call for a blood culture even in the face of a completely normal physical examination of the infant.

Onset of sepsis in the newborn may occur at any time during the first month of life. Supportive and corrective surgical measures have succeeded in sustaining the life of very small premature infants and those with congenital anomalies. This population of infants may receive prolonged hospitalization, and, because of the underlying condition as well as invasive procedures, they are at high risk of infection. Early onset of illness—for example, in the first 2 days of life—is closely associated with perinatal complications such as premature delivery, premature rupture of the membranes, maternal bleeding, toxemia, infection, cesarean section, and precipitous delivery.

A study of full-term infants in Cook County Children's Hospital (Voora et al., 1982) showed that 100 babies or 1% of all babies born over an 18 month period had a temperature of 37° to 38° C (98.6° to 100.4° F) during the first 4 days of life. Forty-eight of these babies had other symptoms compatible with sepsis. Ten percent or 10 of the 100 febrile infants had culture-proved bacterial disease. Eight of the 10 had other signs, and two had no other signs. Only one infant of 9900 afebrile term infants had culture-proved bacterial disease. Thus, an elevated temperature is likely to be a manifestation of infection in term infants, and sepsis is increasingly probable if other signs or symptoms are also present. This study excluded preterm infants and term infants requiring immediate intensive care for reasons other than fever. The former group of infants may exhibit fever, temperature instability, or subnormal temperatures in response to bacterial infection. In premature infants with sepsis, subnormal temperatures and irregular fluctuations are observed as often as fever.

Gastrointestinal signs

Lack of interest in feeding, poor sucking, or failure to tolerate feedings by gastrointestinal intubation are common signs of sepsis. Vomiting and diarrhea are observed in about one third of the patients. Abdominal distention, also a frequent finding, is probably secondary to paralytic ileus related to generalized infection. Jaundice is common in sepsis of the newborn infant and may be the initial sign in some patients. Usually hyperbilirubinemia is indirect, and in the first few days of life it may be difficult to distinguish from "physiologic" jaundice or hemolytic disease.

Respiratory signs

Cyanosis, irregular breathing, dyspnea, and/or apnea occur frequently in premature infants and infants born after difficult delivery and may be unrelated to sepsis. It is frequently impossible to distinguish respiratory distress syndrome from overwhelming sepsis, especially that due to group B streptococci.

Central nervous system signs

Although meningitis has been considered the most frequent complication of sepsis in the newborn, the two processes evolve simultaneously so often that they should be thought of together. The initial signs are frequently the same. Fullness of the fontanelle may be observed in some infants. The conventional signs of meningitis seen in older children, such as stiff neck, hyperactivity of reflexes, and Brudzinski's sign, are infrequent in the newborn. Because of the nonspecific character of the initial features of both meningitis and sepsis of the newborn infant, examination of the CSF is crucial in establishing the diagnosis.

Complications and sequelae of neonatal meningitis include subdural effusion, brain abscess, hydrocephalus, encephalopathy, and cerebral infarcts. Poor outcome is directly correlated with the presence of ventriculitis, persistence of positive CSF cultures, a CSF cell count >10,000/100 ml, and a CSF protein >500 mg/100 ml.

Cutaneous and mucous membrane

Skin or mucous membrane manifestations associated with sepsis are present in a minority of patients but provide visible evidence of infection. A recognizable focus of infection may be impetigo, cellulitis or a subcutaneous abscess, mastitis, omphalitis, or conjunctivitis. Occasionally evidence of embolic bacterial disease in the form of icthyma gangrenosa (infectious vasculitis) is present. Nonspecific cutaneous pathology suggestive of infection includes petechiae and purpura.

Miscellaneous manifestations

The bacteremic infant should be investigated for possible localized infection. Group B streptococci commonly cause pneumonia and meningitis and frequently are observed to produce otitis media, or they may disseminate to bones, joints, or the urinary tract. These organisms less often cause infections in other tissues. *E. coli* and other gram-negative organisms gain access to the blood from the gastrointestinal tract and may disseminate to any of multiple locations including the CNS, urinary tract, bones and joints, liver, and peritoneal cavity.

DIAGNOSIS

The early recognition of sepsis in the newborn infant hinges on suspecting it in the face of a variety of subtle or seemingly unlikely nonspecific signs and symptoms. Rapid identification of the septic infant is important for effective therapy. Recognition of a potentially infected mother prior to delivery of her infant should alert the obstetrician and pediatrician to the possible danger to the infant.

Ideally, the mother should be evaluated and appropriate specimens obtained if she is suspected of having an infection. This should include Gram stain and bacterial cultures of materials such as amniotic fluid and urine. A positive maternal blood culture may also result in useful information with regard to care of the infant. The identification of a potentially infected mother should include histologic examination of the placenta and umbilical cord at the time of delivery. The presence of funisitis (extravascular white blood cells on histologic examination of the cord) signifies colonization of the amniotic fluid. In the absence of infection, neither immaturity nor prolonged rupture of membranes causes inflammation of the cord. All too often one is remiss in obtaining and using these valuable data, which assist in identifying an infant at greater risk of infection.

The presence of prematurity, prolonged rupture of membranes, or malodorous amniotic fluid suggests that the infant be thoroughly evaluated and appropriate cultures obtained. Examination of a tracheal aspirate during the first 8 hours of life has provided useful information for the infant at risk of infection, who manifests cardiorespiratory symptoms and has an abnormal chest roentgenogram. The presence of polymorphonuclear cells and a single type of organism on Gram stain often correlates with subsequent culture results (Sherman et al., 1980). The stomach and the external auditory canal are accessible sites to sample because amniotic fluid should be present. The presence of three to five polymorphonuclear leukocytes per high-powered field in the gastric aspirate and/or a swab from the external auditory canal has been correlated with the period of time that membranes were ruptured and the subsequent in-

cidence of positive cultures. The presence of cells in these sites should alert the pediatrician to possible sepsis.

The most reliable indirect indicator of bacterial infection is the peripheral white cell count. An absolute neutrophil count outside the normal range (see Fig. 17-2) with a ratio of immature to total neutrophils higher than the established norm for age (Fig. 17-3) indicates bacterial infection. Preterm infants are more likely to have neutropenia than term infants.

Other indirect measurements including C-reactive protein, ESR, haptoglobin, IgM, leukocyte alkaline phosphatase, buffy coat smear, nitroblue tetrozolium dye reduction test, and endotoxin detection by limulus lysate test are unreliable individual tests. Identification of infecting bacteria by Gram stain and culture of available body fluids is essential. It should be emphasized that bacterial flora of the asymptomatic healthy neonate are indistinguishable from those of the infant with suspected infection.

Blood cultures from the infant should be obtained from a peripheral vein after skin cleansing with iodine and alcohol. Infant blood cultures from peripheral veins have a lower incidence of contamination than do cord blood cultures. Quantitative cultures performed on babies with *E. coli* bacteremia have demonstrated that one half of the infants had colony counts of less than 50 organisms per milliliter. When colony counts

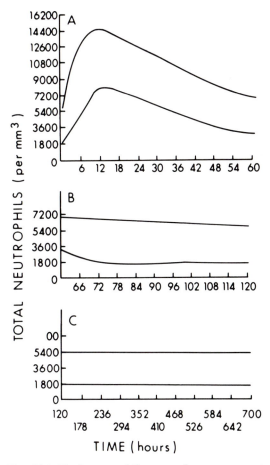

Fig. 17-2. Total neutrophil count reference range: **A,** first 60 hours of life, **B,** 60 to 120 hours of life, and **C,** 120 hours to 28 days. (Modified from Manroe BL, Weinberg AG, Rosenfeld CR, Browne R. J Pediatr 1978;95:89.)

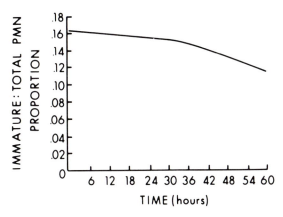

Fig. 17-3. Reference range for the proportion of immature to total neutrophils in the first 60 hours of life. (Modified from Manroe BL, Weinberg AG, Rosenfeld CR, Browne R.: J Pediatr 1978;95:89.)

were in excess of 1000/ml, the incidence of associated meningitis increased, and the mortality was high (Dietzman et al., 1974). These quantitative studies prompted additional work to define the quantity of blood necessary to detect bacteremia in infants. Employing a rabbit model with *E. coli* and simulating the colony counts defined in infants, several interesting observations have been made. Two milliliters of blood placed in a commercial 50-ml bottle of trypticase soy broth allowed detection of all positive bacteremias (Fischer et al., 1974). If the colony count exceeded five organisms per milliliter of blood, then the bacteremias would be detected in 0.2 ml of blood when cultured in broth bottles. No quantity of blood from an infant is too small to culture for suspected bacteremia.

Fortunately, antigen detection by methods such as counterimmunoelectrophoresis (CIE), latex agglutination, or coagglutination with *Staphylococcus* A can provide specific diagnoses of group B streptococci, *H. influenzae* type b, many *S. pneumoniae*, and *N. meningitidis* (A, B, C, X, Y, Z), within minutes to an hour of running the test depending upon the method chosen. Antigen detection is often possible even when organisms are not viable. Testing serum, CSF, and concentrated urine can detect the antigens of group B streptococci in the vast majority of newborn patients infected with this organism. Antigen detection is a useful adjunct to culture but should not take the place of culture. Negative antigen determinations do not rule out bacterial infection.

DIFFERENTIAL DIAGNOSIS

It is most important to realize that the newborn infant responds similarly to a variety of stresses, regardless of their nature or location. Therefore, one should be aware of the possibility of sepsis in the newborn infant with any clinical deterioration, unless the setback is readily explained otherwise and corrected promptly.

PROGNOSIS

Despite advances in antimicrobial therapy, the outlook for infants with neonatal septicemia remains poor. Furthermore, it is unlikely that newer antibiotics will further reduce the mortality or morbidity of established infection. Currently, drugs are available to which organisms are sensitive and which reach all tissues, including the central nervous system. All too often the immature immune function of the neonate is unable to effectively eradicate the infection, and irreversible damage is sustained. Collected experiences over the past four decades show an overall decline in case fatality rates from approximately 90% to 35%, which is probably due to improved supportive measures and optimal antimicrobial therapy.

Important factors influencing the outcome of sepsis in the newborn infant are the etiologic agent, the prompt recognition and initiation of optimal therapy, complications of sepsis, and multiple ill-defined host factors. Early diagnosis and the initiation of specific antimicrobial therapy are helpful in improvement of the prognosis. Unfortunately, even prompt, early therapy has not been able to prevent the mortality or eliminate morbidity.

Meningitis is the most serious focus of infection in respect to both mortality and sequelae. Meningitis due to gram-negative organisms still carries a mortality of about 32%, and one third of the survivors have sequelae. Mortality is greater for preterm infants than for full-term infants. Gram-positive organisms causing meningitis are primarily group B streptococci, and mortality varies from 50% with early onset disease to 25% with late onset disease. Long-range sequelae are present in an estimated 35% of the survivors.

EPIDEMIOLOGIC FACTORS

In an analysis of 2735 consecutive autopsies of newborn infants in 1971, Naeye et al. found the ratio of males to females to be 1.28:1.00 which differs significantly from the 1.05 ratio for all live births in the United States. A nearly equal ratio of males to females was found for most disorders in stillborn infants, whereas diseases arising after birth showed a strong male disadvantage. Interestingly, there is a highly significant preponderance of male newborn infants with septicemia. A comparable sex ratio (1.81:1.00) is also found in neonatal meningitis. The highest ratio of males to females was associated with infections caused by gram-negative bacteria. In 1965 Washburn et al. postulated a genetic origin for these sex differences, which relates to the female's possession of two X chromosomes in contrast to the male's possession of a single X chromosome.

Data obtained from infants with K1 *E. coli* meningitis or group B streptococci have added to our knowledge of the epidemiology of infection in the newborn. Infants with early onset group B streptococcal disease have organisms of the same serotype as those obtained from maternal vaginal secretions, cervical cultures, or gastrointestinal tract. Mothers of affected infants are virtually all positive for the causative organisms. In addition, it is well recognized that many more women are colonized than have infected infants. As many as 100 to 350 colonized mothers will be observed for each infected infant. Similar data have been obtained from infants with K1 *E. coli* meningitis, and it appears that infants acquire these organisms at birth from their mothers. Invasive infection occurs in those infants whose mothers have no specific antibodies to the organism.

Babies with late onset group B streptococcal disease, usually manifest as meningitis, have a wide variety of serotypes. Group 3 organisms still predominate, but the mothers of these babies are not necessarily colonized by the same organism. Longitudinal surveillance studies have demonstrated sequential increases in colonization rates of newborn babies from the first day of life through the 72 hours of normal hospital stay. It has also been demonstrated that newborn infants may become environmentally colonized, that is, by persons other than their mothers, with K1 *E. coli* during their nursery stay.

Clusters and outbreaks of neonatal infection have been recorded within the nursery setting. Antibiotics are an essential part of the supportive therapy in the nursery, but their use selects for survival of resistant organisms. Outbreaks of infection in intensive care nurseries have occurred with gram-negative organisms, including *Klebsiella* species, *Pseudomonas* species, *Serratia marsescens*, and *Citrobacter diversus*. It is important to remember that many of our supportive measures are of necessity invasive to the newborn and may carry a previously unrecognized risk of infection. Thus, hyperalimentation, enteral feeding tubes, and even breast milk (Donowitz et al., 1981) have been associated with nosocomial infection.

TREATMENT

The therapy of any newborn infant suspected of having sepsis must be initiated as rapidly as possible. After all of the appropriate cultures are obtained, therapy can be initiated as outlined in Table 17-3. If gram-positive organisms are visualized in CSF or buffy coat, it is imperative to treat for group B streptococci. If gram-negative organisms are seen, therapy with ampicillin and kanamycin or gentamicin should be initiated, as outlined in Table 17-3. If no organism can be identified, then it is best to start therapy with a combination of a penicillin (ampicillin or crystalline penicillin), which will be effective against group B streptococci, *Listeria*, and the enterococci, and an aminoglycoside (either gentamicin or kanamycin), which will be effective against the Enterobacteriaceae. Use of

Table 17-3. Antibiotic therapy of newborn sepsis*

Organism	*Initial antibiotics*
Group B streptococci	Penicillin + aminoglycoside
Group D streptococci (enterococci)	Ampicillin + aminoglycoside
Listeria monocytogenes	Ampicillin
Staphylococci, coagulase positive	Nafcillin or methicillin
Staphylococcus epidermidis	Vancomycin
Enterobacteriaceae (*Escherichia coli, Klebsiella, Enterobacter, Serratia*)	Ampicillin + aminoglycoside
Proteus species	
Indole negative (mirabilis)	Ampicillin
Indole positive	Kanamycin or gentamicin
Pseudomonas species	Gentamicin + carbenicillin
Unknown	Ampicillin + gentamicin

*Drug dosages for newborns are tabulated in Appendix 1. The above recommendations for initial treatment should be modified by the knowledge of any epidemiologic factors that have altered local resistance patterns. Sensitivity studies of bacterial isolates are essential for determination of optimal continuing therapy.

these two drugs together enhances killing of GBS and may be synergistic against the enteric gram-negative bacteria, *Listeria*, and enterococci. The wise selection of these agents will be based on knowledge of the organisms present in the nursery where the infant is being treated. Antimicrobial sensitivity studies will further guide therapy in these infections, particularly when the etiologic agent is a gram-negative bacterium and its susceptibility to various antimicrobial agents must be determined.

The morbidity and mortality of gram-negative sepsis and/or meningitis have prompted attempts to study different therapeutic approaches to these infants. It is recognized that group B streptococcal organisms are almost always eradicated from the CSF within 24 hours of initiating therapy, although recurrences have been reported. In contrast to this, gram-negative organisms are persistently present in the CSF for several days. In the Neonatal Collaborative Study (McCracken and Mize, 1976) the mean time necessary to sterilize the CSF was about 3 days. The collaborative study completed a protocol examining the effects of parenteral therapy alone versus parenteral therapy plus intrathecal gentamicin administered in the lumbar area for several days. The study did not define any difference in the duration of positive CSF culture, morbidity, or mortality in the two groups of infants.

There is evidence to indicate that aminoglycoside levels do not reach therapeutic range within the ventricular fluid. It is now known that about 70% of infants with gram-negative meningitis may have ventriculitis. Therefore, inadequate levels of antibiotic in the ventricular CSF could also produce persistently positive cultures. To attempt to improve the outcome of this illness, a second Neonatal Collaborative Study was conducted to compare systemic antibiotics (ampicillin and gentamicin) with systemic antibiotics plus intraventricular gentamicin (2.5 mg daily for 1 to 7 days). Unfortunately, the group that received intraventricular antibiotic had a higher mortality than the group that was given systemic drugs only (McCracken et al., 1980). A retrospective review of gram-negative meningitis compared with the prospective use of intraventricular amikacin instilled via a Rickham reservoir showed a lowered mortality with intraventricular drug. Thus, under the su-

pervision of one surgeon and with careful attention to the pharmacokinetics, an intraventricular drug may be a safe adjunct to therapy (Wright et al., 1981).

Although pediatricians have become familiar with chloramphenicol in the treatment of *H. influenzae* meningitis, it is not recommended for therapy of bacterial infection in the newborn period. The variable pharmacokinetics in the neonate necessitate measurement of serum drug levels to avoid severe and even fatal toxicity. Chloramphenicol is bacteriostatic rather than bactericidal against most enteric gram-negative rods, and this could increase the incidence of relapse of meningitis. Finally, emergence of resistance during 10 days of therapy has been described.

Third-generation cephalosporins are proliferating in number. The CSF penetration of moxalactam and ceftriaxone have been shown. They and cefotaxime have a similar spectrum of activity against gram-negative enteric bacilli but are less effective than penicillin/ampicillin against GBS and other gram-positive organisms. Problems with bleeding have been attributed to moxalactam secondary to reduced levels of vitamin K. Moxalactam has also proved no better than ampicillin and an aminoglycoside despite excellent penetration of this drug into CSF (McCracken, 1984). The role of these new drugs and others will depend on the pharmacokinetics, proven efficacy against susceptible organisms, and lack of toxicity. At the present time there is no evidence that these drugs offer any therapeutic advantage over penicillin/aminoglycoside therapy when the bacterium is sensitive to the agents used.

The clinical observations of marked neutropenia and depletion of bone marrow granulocyte stores in septic newborns, which correlated with poor outcome, led to animal studies and small trials in humans of granulocyte transfusions as adjunctive therapy for sepsis. The two small and different studies demonstrate enhanced survival of septic newborns receiving granulocyte transfusions (Laurenti et al., 1981; Christensen et al., 1982). Peripheral WBC were increased and usually a single transfusion was sufficient, implying that the newborn quickly became able to provide adequate numbers of functioning phagocytes. In view of all of the deficiences of the newborn described above, antibody and complement provided by transfusion may also be beneficial. Many centers now employ transfusion or exchange transfusion for the sick newborn on the basis of the available data. However, it remains to be established by larger controlled trials if granulocyte transfusions are indeed important adjunctive therapy.

PREVENTION

Investigation of preventive measures has occurred because treatment, even with the earliest postnatal initiation, has not satisfactorily eliminated morbidity and mortality. To date, for epidemiologic and microbiologic reasons, these have focused mainly on group B streptococcal disease with some promising results.

Antibiotics have been used in a number of prophylactic maneuvers. The sensitivity of group B streptococci to penicillin led to an expectation that prenatal identification of maternal carriers might permit antibiotic eradication of the organisms. With genital and rectal carrier rates among pregnant women ranging from 10% to 35%, this poses a numerically formidable task. When it was discovered that the organisms were transmitted sexually, it was then necessary also to contemplate treatment of male sexual partners with positive urethral cultures. This approach has proved neither practical nor efficacious. Recolonization rates as high as 65% have been observed between the time of treatment and the time of delivery.

Yow et al. (1979) have demonstrated that the intrapartum administration of intravenous ampicillin (500 mg within 6 hours of delivery) prevented the transmission of group B streptococci from colonized mothers to their infants in all of 34 cases studied. Of 24 untreated control mothers whose cultures were positive, 14 delivered colonized infants. Although the study is too small to demonstrate prevention of sepsis, the administration of intrapartum antibiotic might be considered for the woman in premature labor who is known to be colonized. Further investigations of this approach were accomplished at the University of Chicago (Boyer et al., 1972); 2.8% of neonates born to treated women were colonized with GBS, whereas 36% of the control group were colonized, and four cases of early onset disease occurred in the neonates of the control group and three cases of GBS puerperal sepsis in the control mothers.

Two randomized studies were conducted to determine if administration of penicillin at birth could prevent GBS disease. At Cook County Hospital about 1200 infants weighing over 2000 gm were enrolled (Pyati et al., 1983). Early onset disease was diagnosed in 10 of 589 penicillin-treated babies and in 14 of 598 control infants. Twenty-one of the 24 septic infants had positive blood cultures before penicillin was administered, suggesting infection was established at or before birth. In the second study in Dallas, 16,082 infants with birth weights of at least 2000 gm were given a single dose of penicillin within 1 hour of birth (Siegel et al., 1980). GBS disease occurred at a significantly lower rate of 0.6 per 1000 live births compared to 1.7 per 1000 in 15,976 untreated infants. These two studies confound the issue, so no unqualified statement can be made concerning prophylactic penicillin shortly after delivery. It seems unlikely that penicillin administered in a single dose after delivery will alter the course of an infection that has been established prior to delivery.

Baker and Kasper (1976; Baker et al., 1981) have actively sought an immunologic approach. Their studies indicated that those infants at highest risk of group B streptococcal disease were delivered to mothers who not only were culture positive for the organism but also were antibody negative. The apparent susceptibility of the newborn to invasive GBS disease resulted from lack of transmission of maternal type-specific antibody. Attempts are underway to prepare safe, immunogenic vaccines from the streptococcal type-specific polysaccharide in hopes of inducing antibodies early in pregnancy in women identified as seronegative. In these initial studies, type III polysaccharide is immunogenic and safe in adults (Baker et al., 1978).

An interesting sidelight to this approach has been the observation by Fischer et al. (1978) that there is a cross-reaction between type III group B streptococci and *Streptococcus pneumoniae* type 14. This is because the type 14 pneumococcus capsule is structurally identical to the nonsialidated core antigen of type III GBS. The native polysaccharide of type III GBS is different antigenically because of the terminal sialic acid residues. The type 14 *Pneumococcus* can stimulate an anamnestic response to type III GBS but fails to induce a primary response in an unprimed person and is therefore of little use as an immunogen in seronegative persons.

Diminishing the severe consequences of sepsis/meningitis will probably depend on prevention of disease. Immunization of women with appropriate GBS and K1 *E. coli* antigens would provide passive transplacental and colostrum/milk protection to the infant who cannot be immunized. Important concerns with the possible cross-reactivity of K1 *E. coli* and CNS gangliosides must be investigated, and demonstration of protective efficacy will require a controlled, large-scale trial.

REFERENCES

Anderson DC, Hughes BJ, Smith CW. Abnormal motility of neonatal polymorphonuclear leukocytes. J Clin Invest 1981;68:863.

Anthony BF, Okada DM, Hobel CJ. Epidemiology of the group B streptococcus: maternal and nosocomial sources for infant acquisitions. J Pediatr 1979;95:431.

Baker CJ. Nosocomial septicemia and meningitis in neonates. Am J Med 1981;70:698.

Baker CJ, Barrett F. Group B streptococcal infections in infants: importance of various serotypes. JAMA 1974;230:1158.

Baker CJ, Edwards MS, Kasper DL. Immunogenicity of polysaccharides from type III GBS. J Clin Invest 1978;61:1107.

Baker CJ, Edwards MS, Kasper DL. Role of antibody to native type III polysaccharide of GBS in infant infection. Pediatrics 1981;68:544.

Baker CJ, Kasper DL. Correlation of maternal antibody deficiency with susceptibility to neonatal group B streptococcal infection. N Engl J Med 1976;294:753.

Berman PH, Banker BQ. Neonatal meningitis: a clinical and pathological study of twenty-nine cases. Pediatrics 1966;38:6.

Black SB, Levine P, Shinefield HR. The necessity for monitoring chloramphenicol levels when treating neonatal meningitis. J Pediatr 1978;92:235.

Boyer E, et al. Ampicillin prophylaxis of GBS transmission in high risk parturient women (abstract). Pediatr Res 1982;16:280.

Christensen RD, Rothstein G, Anstall HB, Bybee B. Granulocyte transfusions in neonates with bacterial infection, neutropenia, and depletion of mature marrow neutrophils. Pediatrics 1982;70:1.

Cross AS, Gemski P, Sadoff JC, et al. The importance of the K1 capsule in invasive infections cased by *E. coli*. J Infect Dis 1984;149:184.

Cross AS, Zollinger W, Mandrell R, et al. Evaluation of immunotherapeutic approaches for the potential treatment of infections caused by K1-positive *Escherichia coli*. J Infect Dis 1983;147:68.

Davis JP, et al. Vertical transmission of group B streptococcus. Relation to intrauterine fetal monitoring. JAMA 1979;242:42.

Dietzman DE, Fischer GW, Schoenknecht FD. Neonatal *E. coli* septicemia-bacterial counts in blood. J Pediatr 1974;85:128.

Donowitz LG, Marsik FJ, Fisher KA, Wenzel RP. Contaminated breast milk: a source of *Klebsiella bacteremia* in a newborn intensive care unit. Rev Infect Dis 1981;3:716.

Eads ME, Levy NJ, Kasper DL, et al. Antibody-independent activation of C1 by type 1a group B streptococci. J Infect Dis 1982;146:665.

Edwards MS, Baker CJ, Kasper DL. Opsonic specificity of human antibody to the type III polysaccharide of group B streptococcus. J Infect Dis 1979;140:1004.

Edwards MS, Kasper DL, Jennings HJ, et al. Capsular sialic acid prevents activation of the alternative complement pathway by type III, group B streptococci. J Immunol 1982;128:1278.

Edwards MS, Nicholson-Weller A, Baker CJ, Kasper DL. The role of specific antibody in alternative complement pathway mediated opsonophagocytosis of type III, group B streptococcus. J Exp Med 1980;151:1275.

Eisenfeld L, Ermocilla R, Wirtschafter D, Cassady G. Systemic bacterial infections in neonatal deaths. Am J Dis Child 1983;137:645.

Finne J, Leinonen M, Makela PH. Antigenic similarities between brain components and bacteria causing meningitis. Implications for vaccine development and pathogenesis. Lancet (August 13) 1983;2:355-357.

Fischer GW, Crumrine MH, Jennings PB. Experimental *E. coli* sepsis in rabbits. J Pediatr 1974;85:117.

Fischer GW, Lowell GH, Crumrine MH, Bass JW. Type 14 pneumococcal antiserum is opsonic in-vitro and protective in-vivo for group B streptococcus type III. Pediatr Res 1978;12:491.

Freedman RM, Ingram DL, Gross I, et al. A half-century of neonatal sepsis at Yale, 1928-1978. Am J Dis Child 1981;135:140.

Goldmann DA. Bacterial colonization and infection in the neonate. Am J Med 1981;70:417.

Hill H. Phagocyte transfusion—ultimate therapy of neonatal disease (editorial). J Pediatr 1981;98:59.

Krause PJ, Maderazo EG, Scroggs M. Abnormalities of neutrophil adherence in newborns. Pediatrics 1982;69:184.

LaGamma EF, Drusin LM, Mackles AW, et al. Neonatal infections. An important determinant of late NICU mortality in infants less than 1,000 g at birth. Am J Dis Child 1983;137:838.

Laurenti F, Ferro R, Isacchi G, et al. Polymorphonuclear leukocyte transfusion for the treatment of sepsis in the newborn infant. J Pediatr 1981;98:118.

Manroe BL, Weinberg AG, Rosenfeld CR, Browne R. The neonatal blood count in health and disease. I. Reference values for neutrophilic cells. J Pediatr 1978;95:89.

McCracken G. New developments in the management of children with bacterial meningitis. Pediatr Infect Dis 1984;3:532-534.

McCracken GH Jr, Mize SG. A controlled study of intrathecal antibiotic therapy in gram-negative enteric meningitis in infancy. Report of the neonatal meningitis cooperative study group. J Pediatr 1976;89:66.

McCracken GH Jr, Mize SG, Threlkeld N. Intraventricular gentamicin therapy in gram negative bacillary meningitis in infancy. Lancet 1980;1:787.

McCracken GH Jr, et al. Relational between *Escherichia coli* K1 capsular polysaccharide antigen and clinical outcome in neonatal meningitis. Lancet 1974;2:246.

Miller ME, Stiehm ER, eds. Host defenses in the fetus and neonate. Pediatrics [Suppl] 1979;64:705.

Mills EL, Thompson T, Bjorksten B, et al. The chemiluminescence response and bactericidal activity of polymorphonuclear neutrophils from newborns and their mothers. Pediatrics 1979;63:429.

Naeye RL, et al. Neonatal mortality, the male disadvantage. Pediatrics 1971;48:902.

Overall JC Jr. Neonatal bacterial meningitis: analysis of predisposing factors and outcome compared with matched control subjects. J Pediatr 1970;76:499.

Pass MA, Gray BM, Khare S, Dillon HC Jr. Prospective studies of group B streptococcal infections in infants. J Pediatr 1979;94:437.

Pichichero ME, Todd JK. Detection of neonatal bacteremia. J Pediatr 1979;94:958.

Pitt J. K1 antigen of *E. coli*. Epidemiology and serum sensitivity of pathogenic strains. Infect Immun 1978;22:219.

Pluschke G, Achtman M. Degree of antibody dependent activation of the classical complement pathway by K1 *E. coli* differs with 0 antigen type and correlates with virulence of meningitis in newborns. Infect Immun 1984; 43:684.

Pyati SP, Pildes RS, Jacobs NM, et al. Early penicillin in infants weighing two kilograms or less with early onset group B streptococcal disease. N Engl J Med 1983; 308:1383.

Robbins JB, et al. *Escherichia coli* K1 capsular polysaccharide associated with neonatal meningitis. N Engl J Med 1974;290:1216.

Sarff CD, McCracken GH Jr, Schiffer MS, et al. Epidemiology of *Escherichia coli* K1 in healthy and diseased newborns. Lancet 1975;1:1099.

Sherman MP, Goetzman BW, Ahlfors CE, Wennberg RP. Tracheal aspiration and its clinical correlates in the diagnosis of congenital pneumonia. Pediatrics 1980;65:258.

Shigeoka AO, Santos JI, Hill HR. Functional analysis of neutrophil granulocytes from healthy, infected and stressed neonates. J Pediatr 1979;95:454.

Siegel JD, McCracken GH Jr, Threlkeld N, et al. Single-dose penicillin prophylaxis against neonatal group B streptococcal infections: a controlled trial in 18,738 newborn infants. N Engl J Med 1980;303:769.

Soderstrom T, Hansson G, Larson G. The *E. coli* K1 capsule shares antigenic determinants with the human gangliosides GM3 and GD3. Lancet (March 15) 1984;2:725-726.

Squire E, Favara B, Todd J. Diagnosis of neonatal bacterial infection: hematologic and pathologic findings in fatal and nonfatal cases. Pediatrics 1979;64:60.

Voora S, Srinivasan G, Lilien LD, et al. Fever in full term newborns in the first four days of life. Pediatrics 1982; 69:40.

Washburn TC, Medearis DN, Childs B. Sex differences in susceptibility to infections. Pediatrics 1965;35:57.

Wilfert CM. The neonate and gram negative bacterial infections. In Krugman S, Gershon AA, eds. Infections of the fetus and the newborn infants. New York: Alan R. Liss, Inc., 1975, p 167.

Wright PF, Kaiser AB, Bowman CM, et al. The pharmacokinetics and efficacy of an aminoglycoside administered into the cerebral ventricles in neonates: implications for further evaluation of this route of therapy in meningitis. J Infect Dis 1981;143:141.

Yow MD, et al. Ampicillin prevents intrapartum transmission of group B streptococcus. JAMA 1979;241:1245.

18

OSTEOMYELITIS AND PYOGENIC ARTHRITIS

Although osteomyelitis and pyogenic arthritis occur at all ages, infants and children make up a very large portion of the cases that come to medical attention. Changes in the anatomy and physiology of the structures involved impose differing clinical presentations at varying ages. Because the goals of therapy are to assist the patient in regaining total functional integrity and to ensure full growth potential throughout skeletal maturation, it is essential that diagnosis and proper treatment are established as soon as possible. The sooner that treatment is begun, the more likely a full recovery. Osteomyelitis and pyarthrosis may occur as totally separate entities in many patients; in some children they coexist, as the former leads to the latter. In the following pages they are arbitrarily taken up separately for purposes of clarity.

OSTEOMYELITIS

Osteomyelitis is an inflammatory disease of bone structure that occurs secondary to invasion by bacteria, fungi, or, rarely, viruses. It is a term that has not traditionally been applied to infections of the sinus and mastoid bones, although these too should properly be included. Osteomyelitis is most frequent in childhood, and in Baltimore in the 1920s approximately 0.5% of hospital admissions for children were to provide therapy for acute hematogenous osteomyelitis. In the antibiotic era, the prevalance of osteomyelitis by discharge diagnosis was 3.3% during World War II and 1.18% from 1963 to 1966

at Massachusetts General Hospital (Waldvogel et al., 1970).

The most common form of osteomyelitis in children is acute hematogenous osteomyelitis as a result of localization in a bony focus of bacteria introduced during bacteremia. The child is usually acutely ill at the onset of symptomatic disease. Approximately 10% of children with osteomyelitis have bony involvement due to extension of an acute contiguous focus or direct introduction of the infection from an exogenous source. The adjacent focus may be a soft tissue infection, infected sinuses, or teeth. Direct inoculation occurs most commonly with a penetrating wound or at surgery. There is a strong predominance of males in acute osteomyelitis.

Etiology

Using moderately aggressive diagnostic methods it has been possible to identify the responsible organism in nearly 85% of reported cases. Cultures of blood, needle aspirate, or purulent drainage and bone biopsy reveal *Staphylococcus aureus* as the most frequent cause. Gram-negative enteric bacilli (*Escherichia coli, Pseudomonas, Klebsiella, Proteus,* and *Salmonella*) as a group make up a smaller portion. The accumulated results of six studies reported in the 1970s are summarized in Table 18-1. In newborns, group B streptococci have become increasingly common. Although not shown in the table, isolates from newborns have also included gonococci and *Serratia marcescens.* In the less common cases of osteomyelitis, resulting from extension from a contiguous focus, multiple isolates are sometimes seen. These include staphylococci, gram-negative enterics, and occasional anaerobes. Other compromised hosts (immunocompromised patients, those with hemoglobinopathy, heroin addicts, hemodialysis patients) may become infected with a variety of unexpected organisms, so that the need for a specific bacteriologic diagnosis is crucial to selection of proper therapy.

Pathogenesis

The bones are well-defended structures within which it is difficult to establish an infection. With an experimental animal model, organisms must be introduced to an area that has also been injured, as with a blow or by injection of a sclerosing material, if an infection is to result. Anatomic changes with development of the long bones of infants and children may be correlated with the pattern of the infection. In infancy until the age of about 18 months there is a communication between the arterial supply of the metaphysis to the epiphysis. Venous channels perforate the cartilaginous growth plate, which therefore provides no barrier to extension of the infection from the metaphysis to the epiphysis. There are two important consequences to this communication. First, extension of the infection to the epiphysis readily leads to secondary involvement of the adjacent joint. Septic arthritis is therefore a common presentation of hematogenous osteomyelitis in infants and may involve any joint. Second, involvement of the epiphysis commonly leads to disturbances in growth of the involved bone. Fig. 18-1 demonstrates the roentgenographic findings of a 6-week-old infant with group B streptococcal osteomyelitis of the head of the humerus, and Fig. 18-2 depicts the anatomic structure of the bone at this age.

During childhood, from approximately 18 months through the early teens, the epiphyseal growth plate has formed and persists. It provides a functional barrier to the spread of infection from the metaphysis toward the epiphysis. The blood supply to the two regions of bone are separated, a further impediment to involvement of the epiphysis. Consequently, for children of this age, growth of long bones is less likely to be altered following recovery from acute osteomyelitis than if it had occurred in infancy.

Table 18-1. Bacterial agents in acute osteomyelitis of childhood: summary of the isolates from 372 children with acute osteomyelitis in the 1970s*

Author	Number of patients	Staphylococcus aureus	Group A streptococcus	Group B streptococcus	Gram-negative enterics	Salmonella	Hemophilus influenzae	Streptococcus pneumoniae	Other	Multiple isolates	No culture or no growth
Tetzlaff et al. (1978)	39	33	6	—	5	—	—	—	—	9	4
Jacobs (1978)	79	51	7	—	1	—	1	1	—	2	20
Edwards et al. (1978)†	21	6	—	8	4	—	—	1	—	—	2
Medlar and Crawford (1978)	44	30	4	—	4	—	—	1	—	—	5
Dich et al. (1975)	163	100	13	—	14	2	5	2	3	11	24
Blockey and Watson (1970)	26	23	2	—	—	—	1	—	1	—	—
CUMULATIVE TOTAL	372	243	32	8	28	2	7	5	4	22	55

*Note that 65% yielded S. aureus and 15% failed to reveal an etiologic agent.
†Data restricted to the newborn period.

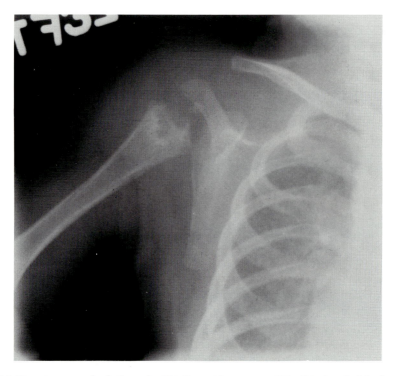

Fig. 18-1. Roentgenograph of a 7-week-old infant with osteomyelitis of the head of the humerus, showing destruction of areas of metaphysis and epiphysis. Pyarthrosis was also present initially.

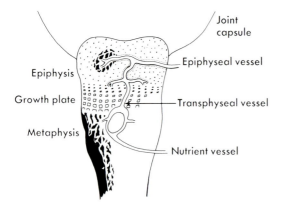

Fig. 18-2. Schematic diagram of the major structures of the bone of an infant prior to maturation of the epiphyseal growth plate. Note the transphyseal vessel, which connects the vascular supply of the epiphysis and metaphysis, facilitating spread of infection between these two areas.

Fig. 18-3. Schematic diagram of the major structures of the bone of a child. Joint capsule A inserts below the epiphyseal growth plate, as in the hip, elbow, ankle, and shoulder. Rupture of a metaphyseal abscess in these bones is likely to produce pyarthrosis. Joint capsule B inserts at the epiphyseal growth plate, as in other tubular bones. Rupture of a metaphyseal abscess in these bones is likely to lead to a subperiosteal abscess but seldom to an associated pyarthrosis.

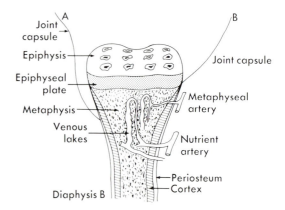

The metaphyseal cortex of a child is thinner than that of the adult, and the periosteum is less tightly adherent to the underlying cortical bone. The metaphyseal area directly adjacent to the epiphysical cartilage contains capillary extensions of the nutrient artery. These capillaries form loops below the growth plate and enter large sinusoidal veins, which then lead to the venous drainage system. It is in this area that infections are usually initiated. Penetration of the cortex from extension of a metaphyseal abscess is common, and subperiosteal collections of pus ensue. Since the nutrient artery courses through the periosteum, the resultant pressure compromises the vascular supply to the bone with resultant ischemia of the bone. This provides the setting for the development of sequestra, areas of devascularized bone that form a nidus for chronic infection.

Because the spread of infection in childhood originates in the metaphysis and spreads laterally, secondary involvement of the adjacent joint, leading to septic arthritis, is usually limited to those joints in which the metaphysis is intracapsular. These include primarily the ankle, hip, shoulder, and elbow. In Fig. 18-3 is depicted the bone of a child; areas through which infection commonly spreads are indicated.

Clinical manifestations and diagnosis

The majority of children with acute osteomyelitis have suffered involvement of the long tubular bones, especially of the lower extremities. The femur and tibia predominate in most series, and those bones plus the fibula, humerus, and radius comprise approximately 80% of infected sites in most series. Multiple sites are involved in approximately 15% of cases of acute hematogenous osteomyelitis.

The early diagnosis of acute osteomyelitis depends primarily on clinical observations. Since early institution of therapy is essential if injury to bony integrity is to be avoided, rapid diagnosis is critically important. Medical therapy alone is usually successful if begun within 48 hours of onset of acute symptoms.

Presenting signs and symptoms of osteomyelitis include the following:

Bone pain and limp or disuse of the limb	100%
Fever	90%
Joint pain	75%
History of recent injury or unusual exercise	35%

Most children visit a physician within 1 or 2 days of onset of first symptoms. At this time, specific roentgenographic changes that would indicate osteomyelitis are usually absent; so the physician must not rely on such findings for a diagnosis. Findings that are helpful in establishing the diagnosis, in addition to those mentioned previously, include point tenderness over a bone. Evidence of a source of infection may be lacking. However, many children have a source or predisposition to bacterial infection, such as furunculosis, infected burn, or recent childhood viral disease (especially measles or chickenpox). Other specific diseases and conditions that predispose to the development of chronic or acute osteomyelitis are discussed later. The majority of children with acute osteomyelitis were previously healthy and vigorous children.

Common conditions that are confused with acute osteomyelitis include child abuse and trauma, cellulitis, rheumatoid arthritis, sickle cell crisis, toxic synovitis, acute paralysis, and generalized bacteremic or viremic diseases. Jacobs (1978) reported that only 37% of children with osteomyelitis were correctly diagnosed at the first visit to the physician, while 70% of children with septic arthritis had a correct diagnosis made at first visit.

Bacteriologic findings. It is important to isolate the bacterium that is causing the infection, since therapeutic decisions depend on identification as well as detailed sensitivity characteristics. Blood cultures should be drawn promptly at the time the diagnosis is first suspected and before antimicrobial therapy is instituted. In addition, apparent sources of sepsis such as a furuncle should be cultured and isolates saved. If the adjacent joint is involved, a joint tap should be done. Needle biopsy or surgical biopsy with drainage of the involved bone should be strongly considered in all children but especially in those who may be expected to have unusual isolates (see Treatment). Table 18-2 depicts the bacteriologic recovery rate in two recent series. Once the immediate clinical samples for culture have been obtained, therapy may be begun, and secondary diagnostic studies may be planned and obtained. The skills and advice of an orthopedic surgeon who is familiar with this disease in children should be fully utilized.

Roentgenographic findings. Roentgenographic changes of the bone may occur late; if therapy

Table 18-2. Bacteriologic findings in patients with acute osteomyelitis. Clinical specimens that yielded bacterial isolates in children with acute osteomyelitis in two medical institutions

	Jacobs, 1978 (79 patients)	Nelson, 1978* (245 patients)
Total blood cultures positive	25%	44%
Total wound, joint, or bone cultures positive	59%	70%
Total with no etiologic agent isolated	25%	16%

*Personal communication kindly furnished by John D. Nelson, M.D.

is begun very early such changes may never become apparent. The earliest findings on roentgenography pertain not to the bone but to adjacent tissues. Displacement of fat lines, blurring of the planes between muscles, evidence of subcutaneous edema, and swelling of the area adjacent to a metaphysis may be appreciated early in the first week after onset of symptoms.

Dich et al. (1975) showed that the most common abnormality was a destructive lesion of bone. Of the 76 children from whom data were available, five first showed a lesion within 6 days of first symptom, 17 first showed a lesion from days 7 to 10, and 31 first showed a lesion between days 11 and 20. New bone formation and periosteal reactions were also common findings and usually were noted after the first week following onset of symptoms.

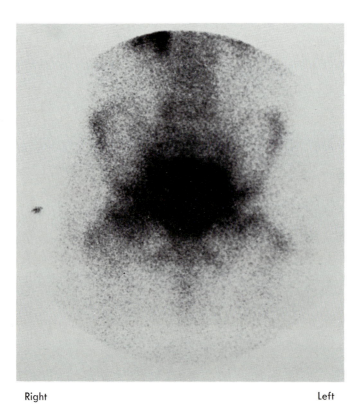

Right   Left

Fig. 18-4. Image intensified technetium pyrophosphate bone scan of the hips and pelvis of a 10-year-old boy with 1 day of point tenderness over the head of the right femur and blood cultures positive for *Staphylococcus aureus*. Roentgenographic areas of radiolucency never appeared.

Other radiologic findings may be helpful. A bone scan with technetium pyrophosphate usually shows increased radionucleotide uptake in the involved area, although decreased uptake has been reported, possibly due to an early decrease in blood flow to the infected area. In children whose therapy is begun very early in the course of illness, an abnormal scan may be the only indication of bony involvement other than physical examination, since the direct roentgenographic examination may never reveal an osteolytic lesion. Fig. 18-4 demonstrates increased uptake in the right femoral head of a child who never developed roentgenographic lesions of osteomyelitis. A gallium citrate scan may also show the areas of involvement to be abnormal, although gallium scans are often avoided in children because of exposure to relatively large amounts of radiation. Technetium bone scans may be helpful in the child who appears to have multiple sites of involvement. In an ill child, a previously unrecognized focus may be identified for which drainage of involved areas is indicated. An abnormal scan indicates an inflammatory process and is not specific for bacterial disease. It may also be abnormal in collagen-vascular disease, in situations with adjacent inflammation such as cellulitis, in trauma, and with neoplasms. The bone scan may also be normal in acute osteomyelitis. A normal scan does not, by itself, rule out this diagnosis.

Other diagnostic tests. Other diagnostic studies are often helpful. Assay of joint fluid for bacterial antigen by counter immunoelectrophoresis (CIE), especially for *Hemophilus influenzae* type b and pneumococcal antigen, may establish a diagnosis. A gel diffusion and an enzyme-linked immunosorbent assay for antibodies to *S. aureus* teichoic acid may indicate the presence of septicemic staphylococcal disease. However, this assay is far more likely to be positive in adults than in children. Le and Lewin (1978) have shown that in 11 children with staphylococcal osteomyelitis or pyogenic arthritis, only four (46%) had detectable levels of antiteichoic acid antibody. A negative reaction is therefore not helpful in ruling out this disease.

The Westergren erythrocyte sedimentation rate (ESR) has traditionally been used to support the diagnosis of osteomyelitis as well as to follow the course of therapy. It is usually significantly elevated at or soon after the time of diagnosis and frequently reaches peaks that are above 100 mm/hour during the first week or two of illness. In the series of Dich et al. (1975) the mean ESR at the onset of therapy was 70 mm per hour. In most instances, it may be expected to decline within a week or two of therapy, and most adequately treated patients have normal sedimentation rates within approximately 1 month. A persistently high ESR or a rising one is an indication for thorough evaluation for persistent foci of disease.

Other diagnostic tests are less helpful. The total white blood cell count is usually elevated at initial examination or shortly thereafter and shows a preponderance of early forms. Anemia is common at the time of presentation.

Osteomyelitis in infants. Osteomyelitis in infants has several features that differentiate it from the disease in older children. First, the isolates are highly variable. While *S. aureus* is most common, *E. coli*, streptococci, *Pseudomonas* species and *Neisseria gonorrhoeae* are all also common. Second, multiple bony sites are commonly involved.

The diagnosis of osteomyelitis in infancy may be difficult. Presenting signs include failure to use the affected extremity, swelling of the limbs, regional adenopathy, and fever. The infants often do not have obvious sepsis or extensive apparent systemic complaints. Predisposing factors such as complications of delivery, prematurity, or recognized foci of disease may also be absent.

Roentgenographic findings that are most commonly made at initial evaluation are deep soft tissue swelling, localized rarefaction, and subperiosteal new bone formation. Concomitant septic arthritis is present in the majority of infants with osteomyelitis, in sharp contrast to its infrequent occurrence in older children.

Many infants with osteomyelitis have some degree of residual deformity. Failure of the involved epiphysis to form is the most severe consequence, resulting in asymmetrical growth and impaired function.

Osteomyelitis due to group B β-hemolytic streptococci (GBS) is a recently recognized condition that is almost entirely restricted to the newborn period. Unlike those with other forms of neonatal osteomyelitis, infants with GBS usually have a good outcome and have a single bone involved. The symptoms are present within the first 6 weeks of life, and the head of the humerus is the most frequent site of involvement (see Fig. 18-1). The children usually lack signs of systemic toxicity, although a blood culture positive for GBS is usually found. It has been hypothesized that the infection involves the head of the humerus because of trauma to that area during delivery.

Osteomyelitis in children with chronic granulomatous disease (CGD). Osteomyelitis in children with CGD is often first seen as a subacute or chronic process and is frequently associated with a bacterial infection in adjacent structures. For example, chronic pulmonary disease may lead to osteomyelitis of a rib by contiguous spread. In the report by Wolfson et al. (1969) eight of 28 children with CGD had roentgenographic evidence of osteomyelitis. The organisms causing osteomyelitis in these children are the same as those that cause other infections in children with CGD: *E. coli*, *S. aureus*, and *Salmonella*, *Pseudomonas*, *Klebsiella*, *Serratia*, *Candida*, *Aspergillus*, and *Nocardia* species. All organisms in this group produce catalase, which is probably central to the pathogenesis of this condition.

Unlike other children with subacute or chronic osteomyelitis, children with CGD most frequently have involvement of the small tubular bones of the hands and feet, the ribs, and the vertebral bodies. The roentgenographic appearance may resemble tuberculous dactylitis or Pott's disease, since the changes indicate a chronic condition with minimal adjacent inflammatory response. Medical therapy may result in full recovery, but drainage may also be required.

Osteomyelitis in children with sickle cell disease. Children with hemoglobin SS, SC, and S-thalassemia appear to be at a very greatly increased risk of osteomyelitis when compared with the general population. Engh et al. (1971) reviewed the courses of 70 patients with sickle cell disease between 1958 and 1969 and noted that 20 (29%) had had at least one hospitalization for osteomyelitis.

Osteomyelitis in children with sickle cell syndromes has several unusual features. First, *Salmonella* sp are remarkably common and in most series comprise well over half the cases. Other gram-negative enteric rods, such as *E. coli*, are also unusually common. Second, multiple bony sites of involvement are usual. In the series of 70 cases of Engh et al., six had multiple involvement. Third, the early signs and symptoms of osteomyelitis in children with sickle cell syndromes are identical with those of a sickle crisis, posing a very serious difficulty in the early identification of the infectious process. This is particularly true in children with acute febrile illness and dactylitis. Finally, rigorous efforts to isolate the infecting organism are justified and may involve aspiration of the bone, biopsy of the bone, stool and urine culture for *Salmonella* sp, and blood culture.

Complications

Acute osteomyelitis. Complications of acute osteomyelitis include all the effects of septicemia. In the preantibiotic era, 32% of children with acute osteomyelitis and bacteremia died, as did 10% who were not shown to be bacteremic. In the current era, death during the acute bacteremic phase still may occur. A list of possible complications of acute osteomyelitis includes:

1. Complications from secondarily infected sites.
   a. Endocarditis
   b. Brain abscess
   c. Multiple bony foci
   d. Other soft tissue abscesses
2. Failure to resolve; relapsing osteomyelitis
3. Impaired growth of limb
4. Pathologic fracture
5. Complications of treatment
   a. Drug reaction
   b. Disuse atrophy
   c. Surgical complications
   d. Hospital-acquired sepsis
6. Nephritis
7. Disseminated intravascular coagulation (DIC)

Progression from acute osteomyelitis to chronic osteomyelitis remains a problem even in children who have received vigorous and early therapy. Many centers report that approximately 10% of cases of acute disease become chronic. This may lead to the development of pathologic fracture and growth arrest or hypertrophy of the involved area. Other sequelae of chronic osteomyelitis include the nephritis characteristic of antigen-antibody complex disease and amyloidosis. Sinus tracts may undergo malignant degeneration.

Immediate other complications are those inherent in the therapy. Moderate to severe drug reactions are common. Nosocomial infections from lengthy courses of intravenous therapy may occur.

Subacute and chronic osteomyelitis. The major forms of chronic osteomyelitis are subacute osteomyelitis, Brodie's abscesses, and diskitis. Children with chronic osteomyelitis seldom have acute systemic signs of disease. They are usually afebrile, have a normal white blood cell count and differential, and may have a normal ESR. The anemia of chronic infection may be the major accessory indication of the disease.

Local findings for subacute osteomyelitis frequently include pain and tenderness, soft tissue swelling, and draining sinuses. Roentgenographic findings indicate sclerosis, lytic lesions, and adjacent soft tissue inflammation. The extent of the disease may be very difficult to define, and exploration at surgery often shows far more widespread bony destruction than had been anticipated.

Subacute osteomyelitis is usually the sequela of a traumatic injury, acute osteomyelitis, or chronic disabling neuromuscular disease, that has led to decubitus ulcers, recurrent orthopedic procedures, and placement of foreign bodies.

The range of infecting organisms in these conditions is much wider than with acute osteomyelitis and particularly includes gram-negative enteric rods. For this reason, special efforts in isolating the pathogen are warranted.

In addition to the usual pathogens seen in osteomyelitis, several other organisms and diseases cause radiologically similar lytic or sclerotic lesions in bones. These include *Mycobacterium tuberculosis* (see Chapter 33), congenital lues, cat-scratch disease, vaccinia, blastomycosis, eosinophilic granuloma, and sarcoidosis. Children with unexplained bony lesions, from whom biopsy specimens are available, should be examined for these conditions.

Brodie's abscesses are cystic lesions of the bone that are secondary to chronic asymptomatic infection with *S. aureus*. The patient seldom has had an acute stage of disease, and the differential diagnosis is often between that and a tumor. The biopsy may indicate a granulomatous response consistent with the chronicity of the condition.

Diskitis involves an infection of the intervertebral disk, usually in the lumbar region. It is most commonly due to *S. aureus* and most commonly found in preschool-age children. A preceding upper respiratory tract infection is common. Presentations include tenderness of the back, stiffness, refusal to walk, and limping. Roentgenographic findings begin slowly, often after many weeks of illness, and begin with narrowing of the disk space. Computerized tomographic findings may be helpful in determining the extent of the condition.

Intervertebral disk space infection may result from or lead to osteomyelitis of the adjacent vertebral bodies. Therapy should resemble that of other forms of osteomyelitis, including attempts to isolate an organism, appropriate antimicrobial therapy, and protection from trauma or stress.

Finally, there has been a recent report of a condition called by Bjorksten et al. (1978) *chronic recurrent multifocal osteomyelitis and pustulosis palmoplantaris*. Characteristics of the syndrome primarily include swelling and pain in the involved bone, fever, and bony lytic lesions. The clavicles and metaphyses of tubular bones are most often affected. Pustules on palms and soles may accompany exacerbations, and the course waxes and wanes over several years. The lesions are granulocytic, and the outlook is for recovery in most cases.

Treatment

The treatment of acute and chronic osteomyelitis remains controversial, and a variety of therapeutic regimens are in current use. Important considerations include the following:

1. Surgical exploration and drainage. Most physicians agree that not all children with acute osteomyelitis will benefit from a drainage procedure. If the disease is promptly recognized and appropriate antimicrobial therapy begun shortly after the onset of symptoms, the patient may do very well without drainage and with medical therapy alone. Patients for which a surgical exploration should be carefully considered include those with persistent fever, prolonged bacteremia, evidence of abscess formation, such as the development of fluctuance, and persistent or severe pain. Children with osteomyelitis should receive their evaluation and care from an orthopedic surgeon as well as a pediatrician whenever possible, and the surgical assessment is best made as soon as the condition is suspected.

In addition to providing drainage for an established abscess, surgical assistance is often needed in order to obtain a specimen from the involved area for culture. A direct aspirate from the involved area is always desirable if an isolate has not already been obtained, as from a blood culture. In the following instances, culture from material of the involved area is especially desirable:

a. Neonates and infants, in whom the etiologies are usually varied
b. Children with chronic osteomyelitis
c. Children with altered host defenses in which the etiologies are also varied; including children with CGD, immunosuppression, and sickle cell disease
d. Children with extension of a wound to the underlying bone

It is important to ask the microbiology laboratory to retain recovered isolates from children with osteomyelitis, so that appropriate bacteriologic studies may be done during therapy. The isolates should be stocked for approximately 6 months following therapy in case a relapse occurs.

2. Immobilization. There is ample experimental and clinical evidence that immobilization of an infected area promotes more rapid healing, decreases pain and morbidity, and prevents further damage to a weakened skeletal structure. Bracing, casting in a bivalve cast, traction, and full casting are methods of accomplishing this goal. Cooperation between the surgical and medical staff will allow the involved areas to be inspected while immobilized and protected.

3. Antimicrobial therapy. Data from several sources indicate that duration of antimicrobial therapy is one of the major variables influencing success or failure of treatment of acute osteomyelitis. Dich et al. (1975) found a 19% failure rate in 37 patients who received parenteral antimicrobial therapy for fewer than 21 days, while only one case among 48 who received longer courses failed therapy. Consequently most recommendations for therapy suggest a course of 3- to 6 weeks duration for acute disease.

During the initial stages of therapy, the chosen drug(s) should be administered parenterally to ensure adequate delivery of medication. Recent studies have documented adequate treatment of many patients with an initial course of parenteral therapy and completion of the full therapeutic course with oral antimicrobial agents. Such a regimen should be undertaken only after a child is afebrile and with beginning resolution of the process. In addition, the hospital must be capable of accurate assay of serum concentration of the antimicrobial agent(s) in use and must be capable of determining the minimum inhibitory concentration (MIC) and minimum bactericidal concentration (MBC) of the bacterial isolate. In these circumstances, a child may be switched from parenteral to oral therapy, often during the first or second week of therapy.

A goal for oral therapy may be that the serum concentration of the drug in use be approximately 16-fold the MBC of the isolate. Since many drugs are erratically absorbed, serum concentrations should be assayed at least twice during the early part of oral therapy and regularly thereafter. Under these conditions, failure of therapy for acute osteomyelitis is very uncommon. If compliance cannot be assured, the patient may require hospitalization through the entire course.

Choice of antimicrobial therapy for acute hematogenous osteomyelitis due to *S. aureus* has usually included a semisynthetic penicillin such as methicillin or nafcillin. In addition, an aminoglycoside may be administered during the initial week of therapy. Although there are no human studies to indicate an improved outcome following combined therapy, studies in rabbits (Norden, 1978) showed decreased bone destruction and more rapid elimination of viable organisms during combined therapy. For a similar reason, infants with osteomyelitis due to group B streptococci may receive penicillin plus an aminoglycoside initially.

Alternatives to semisynthetic penicillin that have been reported to have a high rate of success include clindamycin (Feigin et al., 1975) and cefazolin. Oral therapy may employ cephalexin, dicloxacillin, or cloxacillin.

Courses of therapy may be prolonged if there is evidence of chronic osteomyelitis or failure of excellent response during the acute phase of the treatment. A traditional method of assessing the course is through serial determinations of the Westergren ESR. Falling levels are usually found in patients with uncomplicated courses, while a plateau of a high level or rising level often occurs in patients with inadequate drainage or other focal disease.

Therapy of bacterial or mycobacterial chronic osteomyelitis often requires surgical debridement of nonviable tissue. The optimal duration of antimicrobial therapy for children with chronic osteomyelitis has not been determined and is often extended to months or, occasionally, years.

PYOGENIC ARTHRITIS

Bacterial infection of the joints may occur as a primary complication of bacteremia or may represent a secondary spread from an adjacent osteomyelitis. It occurs as a monoarticular disease in approximately 90% of instances. As with osteomyelitis, large joints are most commonly involved; the knee, hip, ankle, and elbow joints comprise almost 90% of the affected sites.

Etiology

The infecting organism varies with the age of the patient. In the newborn, many organisms cause bacterial arthritis, and there is not a single predominant isolate. S. aureus, group B streptococci, N. gonorrhoeae, gram-negative enteric rods, and Salmonella sp are among the major considerations. By the age of 3 months, H. influenzae type b begins to emerge as a predominant isolate and remains so for children under the age of 2 years. Thereafter, S. aureus, group A streptococci, and S. pneumoniae are most prevalent. In all ages N. gonorrhoeae must be considered (see later).

Clinical manifestations

Children with pyarthrosis often present with a pseudoparesis and swelling of the involved limb. Fever, tenderness to motion of the joint, and heat around the joint support the diagnosis. Many children with septic arthritis have not had an apparent other focus of infection, but minor trauma to the involved joint is a common part of the history. In a report of the experience with bacterial arthritis and osteomyelitis in New York, a correct diagnosis of bacterial arthritis was made at the initial visit to the doctor in 70% of instances, while a correct diagnosis of osteomyelitis was made initially in only 37% of instances (Jacobs, 1978).

As noted in the section concerning osteomyelitis, pyarthrosis may represent an extension of pyogenic osteomyelitis. In newborns this is a very common event, and in children beyond the age of 2 years this also occurs with disease involving the bones of the hip, elbow, shoulder, and knee. Consequently, each child with bacterial arthritis should be evaluated for the possibility of associated osteomyelitis.

Gonococcal arthritis occurs predominantly in the newborn period and again in sexually active adolescents. In infancy it often involves multiple joints. Bacteremic disease of the infected mother may accompany this form of the disease in the infant. The local disease is very destructive, and subsequent permanent disability of the involved joint(s) may occur. The disease is best treated by prevention, which entails screening of pregnant women for gonorrhea during the latter stages of pregnancy. In the teenager, gonococcal arthritis is similar to the syndrome seen in adults. It usually occurs in persons who have an asymptomatic genitourinary focus of N. gonorrhoeae and may be accompanied by characteristic skin lesions on the dorsum of the hands and feet early in the course of illness. Aspirate taken from the affected joint is frequently sterile. Tenosynovitis may be part of the presenting complaint.

Many common viral illnesses have an associated arthralgia or arthritis, including rubella, erythema infectiosum, arbovirus disease, infectious mononucleosis, and hepatitis.

Diagnosis

Aspiration of the joint fluid yields a positive culture in approximately 65% of previously untreated children. A blood culture is positive in about 40% of instances. These two studies in combination will yield an isolate in about 75% of instances. In children with gonococcal arthritis, culture of a distant mucosal site (endocervical, pharyngeal, or rectal) may be the sole means of establishing the diagnosis.

In the evaluation of joint fluid for suspected pyarthrosis, the following assays should be performed:

1. Glucose determination
2. Culture and direct smear for gonococci, other aerobic and anaerobic organisms, tubercle bacilli, and other organisms if specifically indicated
3. Cytology. Two to 5 ml should be collected in a heparinized tube and standard white blood cell count made using normal saline for the diluent. White blood cell count and differential using Wright's stain

4. Mucin clot test for hyaluronidase. Joint fluid is placed in a test tube, and an equal amount of 1% acetic acid is added. Integrity of the clot judged by eye after gentle shaking and tapping of tube
5. Rheumatoid factor and rheumatoid cells or LE cells
6. Assay for antigens of *H. influenzae* type b, meningococci, pneumococci, and group B streptococci

There is considerable overlap in findings of children with rheumatoid arthritis or other collagen-vascular disease and children with septic arthritis. Low glucose concentration, elevated white blood cell count with predominance of polymorphonuclear leukocytes, and a poor mucin clot are characteristic of both. Although evidence of bacterial disease by culture or antigen assay establishes the diagnosis, it should be noted that persons with collagen-vascular disease are predisposed to the development of septic arthritis and should be evaluated for such an underlying disorder. In children who have received antimicrobial therapy prior to aspiration of the joint, antigen assay for bacterial antigens may successfully establish the diagnosis.

Treatment

Therapy of pyarthrosis involves initial drainage of the joint, either by needle aspiration or by open drainage. Because the arterial supply to the femoral head courses through the ligamentum teres, compression and inflammation within the capsule surrounding the hip may lead to necrosis of the femoral head. For this reason, pyarthrosis of the hip is treated by open drainage. In other joints, the decision between open drainage and needle aspiration may be made on the basis of the severity of the signs of disease. If there is rapid reaccumulation of fluid following an initial aspiration, open drainage will probably be necessary. Pyarthrosis due to *S. aureus* will usually require open drainage. However, there are clinical observations suggesting that flexion deformity and ankylosis more frequently follow open drainage than therapy with needle drainage. For this reason, each case of pyarthrosis must be individually evaluated for the most conservative therapy.

Antimicrobial therapy may be administered parenterally. There is good distribution of all major antimicrobial agents through inflamed synovial tissue and fluid. Local instillation of drugs plays no role. The duration of therapy for children with pyarthrosis that is not associated with osteomyelitis is usually approximately 2 weeks for *H. influenzae* type b or *S. pneumoniae* and 3 weeks for other agents, especially *S. aureus*.

REFERENCES
Osteomyelitis

Adyokannu AA, Hendricks RG. *Salmonella* osteomyelitis in childhood. A report of 63 cases seen in Nigerian children of whom 57 had sickle cell anemia. Arch Dis Child 1980;55:175.

Barrett-Connor E. Bacterial infection and sickle cell anemia. An analysis of 250 infections in 166 patients and a review of the literature. Medicine 1971;50:97.

Bjorksten B, et al. Chronic recurrent multifocal osteomyelitis and pustulosis palmoplantaris. J Pediatr 1978;93:227.

Blockey MH, Watson JT. Acute osteomyelitis in children. J Bone Joint Surg 1970;52:77.

Bryson YJ, Connor JD, LeClere M, Giammona ST. Brief clinical and laboratory observation. High-dose oral dicloxacillin treatment of acute staphylococcal osteomyelitis in children. J Pediatr 1979;94:673.

Bujak JS, Kwon-Chung KJ, Chusid MJ. Osteomyelitis and pneumonia in a boy with chronic granulomatous disease of childhood caused by a mutant strain of *Aspergillus nidulans*. Am J Clin Pathol 1974;61:361.

Cabanela ME, Sim FH, Beabout JW, Dahlin DC. Osteomyelitis appearing as neoplasms. Arch Surg 1974;109:68.

Cloward HB. Metastatic disc infection and osteomyelitis of the cervical spine, surgical treatment. Spine 1978;2:194.

Constant E, Green RL, Wagner DK. Salmonella osteomyelitis of both hands and the hand-foot syndrome. Arch Surg 1971;22:148.

Cox F, Hughes WT. Gallium 57 scanning for the diagnosis of infection in children. Am J Dis Child 1979;133:1171.

Dich VQ, Nelson JD, Haltalin KC. Osteomyelitis in infants and children. A review of 163 cases. Am J Dis Child 1975;129:1273.

Edwards MS, Baker CJ, Granbery WM, Barrett FF. Pelvic osteomyelitis in children. Pediatrics 1978;61:62.

Edwards MS, et al. An etiologic shift in infantile osteomyelitis: the emergence of the group B streptococcus. J Pediatr 1978b;93:578.

Engh CA, Hughes JL, Abrams RC, Bowerman JW. Osteomyelitis in the patient with sickle-cell disease. J Bone Joint Surg 1971;53A:1.

Espinoza LR, Spilberg I, Osterland CK. Joint manifestations of sickle cell disease. Medicine 1974;53:295.

Feigin RD, et al. Clindamycin treatment of osteomyelitis and septic arthritis in children. Pediatrics 1975;55:213.

Fitzgerald RH, Kelly PJ, Snyder RJ, Washington JA. Penetration of methicillin, oxacillin and cephalothin into bone and synovial tissues. Agents Chemother 1978;14:723.

Fowles JV, et al. Tibial defect due to acute haematogenous osteomyelitis. Treatment and results in twenty-one children. J Bone Joint Surg 1979;61B:77.

Fox L, Sprunt K. Neonatal osteomyelitis, Pediatrics 1978;62:535.

Gerszten E, Allison MJ, Dalton HP. An epidemiologic study of 100 consecutive cases of osteomyelitis. South Med J 1970;63:365.

Givner LB, Luddy RE, Schwartz AD. Etiology of osteomyelitis in patients with major sickle hemoglobinopathies. J Pediatr 1981;99:411.

Harris NH, Kirkaldy-Willis WH. Primary subacute pyogenic osteomyelitis. J Bone Joint Surg 1965;47B:526.

Jacobs JC. Acute osteomyelitis. Medical management in children. NY State J Med 1978;78:910.

Johnston RM, Miles JS. Sarcomas arising from chronic osteomyelitic sinuses. A report of two cases. J Bone Joint Surg 1973;55A:162.

Kahn DS, Pritzker KPH. The pathophysiology of bone infection. Clin Orthop 1973;96:12.

Lazarus GM, Neu HC. Agents responsible for infection in chronic granulomatous disease of childhood. J Pediatr 1975;86:415.

Le CT, Lewin EB. Teichoic acid serology in staphylococcal infections of infants and children. J Pediatr 1978;93:572.

Mackowiak PA, Jones SR, Smith JW. Diagnostic value of sinus-tract cultures in chronic osteomyelitis. JAMA 1976; 239:2772.

Medlar RC, Crawford AH. Acute hematogenous osteomyelitis. The long-term follow-up in children. Orthop Rev 1978;7:145.

Morrey BF, Bianco AJ, Rhodes KH. Hematogenous osteomyelitis at uncommon sites in children. Mayo Clin Proc 1978;53:707.

Nelson JD, Howard JB, Shelton S. Oral antibiotic therapy for skeletal infections of children. I. Antibiotic concentrations in suppurative synovial fluid. J Pediatr 1976; 92:131.

Norden CW. Experimental osteomyelitis. V. Therapeutic trials with oxacillin and sisomicin alone and in combination. J Infect Dis 1978;137:155.

Norden CW, Kennedy E. Experimental osteomyelitis. II. Therapeutic trials and measurement of antibiotic levels in bone. J Infect Dis 1971;124:565.

Ogden JA, Lister G. The pathology of neonatal osteomyelitis. Pediatrics 1975;55:474.

Prober CG, Yeager AS. Use of the serum bactericidal titer to assess the adequacy of oral antibiotic therapy in the treatment of acute hematogenous osteomyelitis. J Pediatr 1979;95:131.

Ragnhildsveit E, Ose L. Neonatal osteomyelitis caused by group B streptococci. Scand J Infect Dis 1976;8:219.

Roberts PH. Disturbed epiphysial growth at the knee after osteomyelitis in infancy. J Bone Joint Surg 1970;52B:692.

Sartoris DJ, Moskowitz PS, Kaufman RA, et al. Childhood diskitis: computed tomographic findings. Radiology 1983; 149:701.

Seeler RA, Jacobs NM. Pyogenic infections in children with sickle hemoglobinopathy. J Pediatr 1977;90:161.

Steigbigel RT, Greenman RL, Remington JS. Antibiotic combinations in the treatment of experimental Staphylococcus aureus infection. J Infect Dis 1975;131:245.

Sullivan DC, Rosenfield MS, Ogden J, et al. Problems in the scintographic detection of osteomyelitis in children. Radiology 1980;135:731.

Teates CD, Williamson BRJ. "Hot and cold" bone lesion in acute osteomyelitis. Am J Roentgenol Radium Ther Nucl Med 1977;129:517.

Tetzlaff TR, McCracken GH, Nelson JD. Oral antibiotic therapy for skeletal infections of children. II. Therapy of osteomyelitis and suppurative arthritis. J Pediatr 1978; 92:485.

Tetzlaff TR, et al. Antibiotic concentrations in pus and bone of children with osteomyelitis. J Pediatr 1978;92:135.

Wald ER, Mirro R, Gartner SC. Pitfalls in the diagnosis of acute osteomyelitis by bone scan. Clin Pediatr 1980; 19:597.

Waldvogel FA, Medoff G, Swartz MN. Osteomyelitis: a review of clinical features, therapeutic considerations and unusual aspects. N Engl J Med 1970;282:198,260,316.

Watanakunakorn C, Glotzbecker C. Enhancement of the effects of anti-staphylococcal antibiotics by aminoglycosides. Antimicrob Agents Chemother 1974;6:802.

Weissberg ED, Smith AL, Smith DH. Clinical features of neonatal osteomyelitis, Pediatrics 1974;53:505.

Wolfson JJ, et al. Bone findings in chronic granulomatous disease of childhood. J Bone Joint Surg 1969;51A:1573.

Yuille TD. Limb infections in infancy presenting with pseudoparalysis. Arch Dis Child 1975;50:953.

Suppurative arthritis

Dan M. Septic arthritis in young infants: clinical and microbiologic correlations and therapeutic implications. Rev Infect Dis 1984;6:147.

Goldenberg DL, Brandt KD, Cohen AS, Cathcart ES. Treatment of septic arthritis. Comparison of needle aspiration and surgery as initial modes of joint drainage. Arthritis Rheum 1975;18:83.

Howard JB, Highgenboten CL, Nelson JD. Residual effects of septic arthritis in infancy and childhood. JAMA 1976;236:932.

Jacobs BW. Synovitis of the hip in children and its significance. Pediatrics 1971;47:558.

Keiser H, Ruben FL, Wolinsky E, Kushner I. Clinical forms of gonococcal arthritis. N Engl J Med 1968;279:234.

Miller JH, Gates GF. Scintigraphy of sacroiliac pyarthrosis in children. JAMA 1977;238:2701.

Nelson JD. The bacterial etiology and antibiotic management of septic arthritis in infants and children. Pediatrics 1972;50:437.

Nelson JD, Koontz WC. Septic arthritis in infants and children: a review of 117 cases. Pediatrics 1966;38:966.

Pittard WB, Thullen JD, Fanaroff AA. Neonatal septic arthritis. J Pediatr 1976;88:621.

Smith JW, Sanford JP. Viral arthritis. Ann Intern Med 1967;67:651.

Wadlington WB, Riley JHD. Arthritis and hemolytic anemia following erythema infectiosum. JAMA 1968;203:131.

19

OTITIS MEDIA

Surveys of office practices of physicians who provide care to children show that otitis media is the most frequent reason, after well-baby and well-child care, for office visits. Analysis of data from a prospective study in greater Boston of otitis media in 2500 children examined at frequent intervals from birth indicates that by 3 years of age approximately 70% of children have had at least one episode and 33% have had three or more episodes of acute otitis media (Teele et al., 1980). In addition to episodes of acute otitis media, children may have fluid in the middle ear that persists for weeks or months without apparent signs or symptoms. The fluid may produce impairment of hearing of variable duration in the first years of life when perception of language is of critical importance in development of speech and of patterns of learning.

ETIOLOGY

The microbiology of otitis media has been documented by appropriate cultures of middle ear fluids obtained by needle aspiration (Bluestone and Klein, 1981) (Table 19-1). The findings of bacteriologic studies performed in the United States and Scandinavia are remarkably consistent: *Streptococcus pneumoniae* is the most frequent agent in all age groups. *Haemophilus influenzae* is now an important pathogen in all age groups, group A β-hemolytic streptoccus has been a significant pathogen in some studies from Scandinavia but not in studies done in the United States, and *Staphylococcus aureus*, gram-negative enteric bacilli, and anaerobic bacteria

are infrequent causes of otitis media (Table 19-1). Recent studies suggest *Branhamella catarrhalis* may also be an etiologic agent of concern.

Because *S. pneumoniae* is the most important cause of otitis media, investigators have carefully studied the types responsible for infection of the middle ear. The results indicate that relatively few types are responsible for most disease. The eight most common types in order of decreasing frequency are types 19, 3, 6, 23, 14, 1, 18, and 7. All are included in the pneumococcal vaccine licensed in the United States in February 1978.

Otitis media due to *H. influenzae* is associated with nontypable strains in the vast majority of

Table 19-1. Bacterial pathogens isolated from middle ear fluid of children with acute otitis media*

Microorganism	Percent of children with pathogen
Streptococcus pneumoniae	35
Haemophilus influenzae	20
Streptococcus, Group A	8
Branhamella catarrhalis	3
Staphylococcus aureus	2
Gram-negative enteric bacilli	1
Mixed	2
None or nonpathogens	29

*Reports from centers in the United States, Finland, and Sweden, 1953 to 1975, including 3583 children.

patients. In approximately 10%, the otitis is due to type b; some of these children appear to be very toxic and may have bacteremia and meningitis. Until recently *H. influenzae* appeared to be limited in importance to otitis media in preschoolage children, but several studies indicate that this organism is a significant cause of otitis media in all age groups (Grönroos et al., 1964; Howie et al., 1970; Herberts et al., 1971; Schwartz et al., 1977).

Gram-negative enteric bacilli are responsible for about 20% of cases of otitis media in young infants (to 6 weeks of age), but these organisms are rarely present in the middle ear effusion of older children. Other than the greater prevalence of otitis media due to gram-negative bacilli and the presence of other organisms responsible for neonatal sepsis, such as group B streptococci and *S. aureus*, the bacteriology of otitis in the infant up to 6 weeks of age is similar to that in older children (Table 19-2) (Bland, 1972; Tetzlaff et al., 1977; Berman et al., 1978; Shurin et al., 1978).

Recent studies in Cleveland (Shurin et al., 1983) and Pittsburgh (Kovatch et al., 1983) indicate a significant increase in isolation of *B. catarrhalis*. During the period 1980-1981, *B.*

catarrhalis was isolated from 27% and 19% of children with acute otitis media, respectively. Approximately three fourths of the isolates produced beta-lactamase and were therefore resistant to ampicillin. If these results are corroborated, we may need to reconsider usage of ampicillin (or amoxicillin) as the drug of choice for otitis media.

Although epidemiologic data suggest that virus infection is associated with acute otitis media (Henderson et al., 1982), middle ear fluids obtained for cultures of viruses rarely yield an agent (Klein and Teele, 1976). Respiratory syncytial virus and influenza virus have been isolated from middle ear fluids from some children with infection during epidemic periods.

Evidence of virus infection by means of enzyme immunoassay techniques (ELISA) to identify viral antigens was found in middle ear fluids obtained from approximately one fourth of children with acute otitis media by Klein et al. (1982). Respiratory syncytial virus antigen was most frequently identified; influenza virus and rotavirus antigens were identified but were uncommon.

Only one report of isolation of a mycoplasma (*Mycoplasma pneumoniae*) from middle ear fluid of a child with acute otitis media has been published (Sobeslavsky et al., 1965).

Chlamydia trachomatis infection results in a mild but prolonged pneumonitis in infants that may be accompanied by otitis media. *C. trachomatis* has been isolated from middle ear fluids of such infants (Tipple et al., 1979).

PATHOGENESIS

The pathogenesis of otitis media must be approached with the understanding that the disease involves a system having contiguous parts; these include the nares, nasopharynx, eustachian tube, middle ear, and mastoid antrum and air cells ((Fig. 19-1). The middle ear resembles a flattened box, which is approximately 15 mm from top to bottom, 10 mm wide, and only 2 to 6 mm deep. The lateral wall includes the tympanic membrane and the medial wall the oval and round windows. The mastoid air cells lie behind, and the orifice of the eustachian tube is in the superior portion of the front wall.

The eustachian tube connects the middle ear with the posterior nasopharynx, and its lateral one third lies in bone and is open. The medial

Table 19-2. Bacterial pathogens isolated from 169 infants with otitis media during the first 6 weeks of life*

Microorganism	Percent of infants with pathogen
Respiratory bacteria	
Streptococcus pneumoniae	18.3
Hemophilus influenzae	12.4
S. pneumoniae and *H. influenzae*	3.0
Staphylococcus aureus	7.7
Streptococcus, groups A and B	3.0
Branhamella catarrhalis	5.3
Enteric bacteria	
Escherichia coli	5.9
Klebsiella-Enterobacter	5.3
Pseudomonas aeruginosa	1.8
Miscellaneous	5.3
None or nonpathogens	32.0

*Reports from Honolulu, Hawaii (Bland, 1972); Dallas, Texas (Tetzlaff et al., 1977); Denver, Colo. (Berman et al., 1978); and Huntsville, Ala. and Boston, Mass. (Shurin et al., 1978).

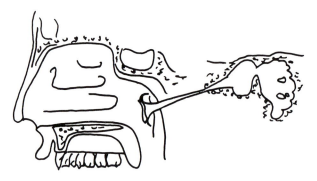

Fig. 19-1. The position of the eustachian tube relative to the nasopharynx and the middle ear. The eustachian tube is a double-horned organ with the proximal two thirds lying in cartilage and the distal one third in bone. The segments are connected by the narrow isthmus, the site most vulnerable to obstruction. Thus the system consists of the nares, nasopharynx, eustachian tube, middle ear, and mastoid air cells.

two thirds are in cartilage, and the walls are in apposition except during swallowing or yawning. In the young infant the eustachian tube is both shorter and proportionately wider than in the older child; the cartilaginous and osseous portions of the tube form a relatively straight line. In an older child, the angle of the tube is more acute. These anatomic differences may predispose some infants to early and repeated illness.

The eustachian tube has at least three important physiologic functions with respect to the middle ear: protection of the ear from nasopharyngeal secretions, drainage into the nasopharynx of secretions produced within the middle ear, and ventilation of the middle ear to equalize air pressure within the box with pressure in the external ear canal. When one or more of these functions is compromised, the result may be obstruction of the tube, accumulation of secretions in the middle ear, and, if pyogenic organisms are present, development of suppurative otitis media. Dysfunction of the eustachian tube because of anatomic or physiologic factors appears to be the most important feature of the pathogenesis of infection of the middle ear.

CLINICAL MANIFESTATIONS

Otalgia (ear pain), otorrhea (ear drainage), hearing impairment affecting one or both ears, and fever suggest infection of the middle ear. However, many children with otitis media do not have these signs. Infants may manifest only general signs of distress, including irritability, bouts of crying, diarrhea, and feeding problems.

Acute otitis media is usually defined by the presence of middle ear effusion accompanied by a sign or symptom of acute illness.

Hyperemia of the tympanic membrane caused by injection of blood vessels is an early sign of otitis media. But redness of the tympanic membrane may be caused by inflammation elsewhere in the system since the mucous membrane is continuous from the nares and eustachian tube and lines the walls of the middle ear cleft. Thus, a "red ear" alone does not establish the diagnosis of otitis media.

Fluid in the middle ear persists for variable periods of time after onset of the acute episode. At the conclusion of antimicrobial therapy, approximately two thirds of children still have fluid in the middle ear. The fluid in the middle ear persists in about 40% of children at 1 month, 20% at 2 months, and 10% at 3 months after onset of acute otitis. Children should be observed until fluid has cleared.

DIAGNOSIS
Clinical

Pneumatic otoscopy provides an assessment of mobility of the tympanic membrane. The normal tympanic membrane moves inward with positive pressure and outward with negative pressure (Fig. 19-2). The motion observed is proportional to the pressure applied by gently squeezing and then releasing the rubber bulb attachment on the head of the otoscope. Normal mobility of the tympanic membrane is indicated when positive, then negative pressure is applied

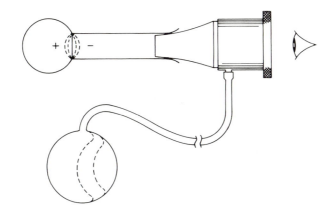

Fig. 19-2. Use of the pneumatic otoscope. The normal tympanic membrane moves inward with positive pressure in the ear canal and outward with negative pressure. The presence of effusion or negative pressure dampens movement of the tympanic membrane.

and the membrane moves rapidly inward and outward like a sail in a brisk wind. Either presence of fluid in the middle ear or high-negative middle ear pressure dampens tympanic membrane mobility.

Tympanometry uses an electroacoustic impedance bridge to record compliance of the tympanic membrane and middle ear pressure. After a small probe is inserted into the external canal by means of a snug-fitting cuff, a tone of fixed characteristics is delivered by an oscillator-amplifier via the probe. The compliance of the tympanic membrane is measured by a microphone, while the external canal pressure is varied by a pump manometer. The tone is delivered at a given intensity as the air pressure in the canal is varied over a positive and negative range. The recording that results—the tympanogram—reflects the dynamics of the middle ear system, including the tympanic membrane, middle ear, mastoid air cells, and eustachian tube. The technique is reliable, simple, and readily carried out by nonprofessional personnel. However, there are technical problems in applications of presently available instruments to young children, particularly those under 7 months of age. Tympanometry is of particular value in diagnosis of ambiguous cases of otitis media, in screening for ear disease, and in training of students and young physicians.

Microbiology

The results of bacterial cultures of the nasopharynx and oropharynx correlate poorly with those of middle ear fluids. Thus cultures of the upper respiratory tract are of limited value in specific bacteriologic diagnosis of otitis media. If the child is toxic or has localized infection elsewhere, culture of blood and/or the focus of infection should be performed.

Needle aspiration of middle ear effusion provides immediate and specific information about the bacteriology of the infection. Although the consistent results of investigations of the bacteriology of acute otitis media provide a guide to the most likely pathogens, S. pneumoniae and H. influenzae needle aspiration should be considered in selected children. These children include those who are critically ill at first visit and those who fail to respond adequately to initial therapy and remain toxic and febrile 48 to 72 hours after onset of therapy. Also included are patients with altered host defenses who may be infected with an unusual agent, such as those with malignancy or immunosuppressive disease, newborn infants, and those with chronic otitis media.

The technique begins with cleansing of the external auditory canal. Methanol (70%) is placed in the canal for 1 minute. Under direct vision, an 18- or 20-gauge, 1½-inch needle attached to a 5-ml syringe is used to pierce the tympanic membrane in its inferior segment. (A Senturia ear specimen collector, which couples a suction tram and Luer-Lok adapter for standard or disposable needles, is available from Storz Instrument Co., St. Louis, Mo.) If fluid is present, it is withdrawn by gentle suction. One drop is placed on a clean glass slide for microscopic examination by Gram stain. The remainder is inoculated into a tube containing beef heart infusion broth with 1% defibrinated horse blood or some other suitable liquid medium for bacteriologic study.

When spontaneous perforation occurs, the exudate in the ear canal is contaminated with flora from the canal. Culture should be obtained, after cleansing the canal with alcohol, by needle aspiration of fluid emerging from the area of perforation or preferably from within the middle ear.

COMPLICATIONS

Suppurative complications of acute infection of the middle ear are now uncommon. Contiguous spread of infection, however, may be responsible for mastoiditis, petrositis, labyrinthitis, brain abscess, and meningitis.

Of more concern, at present, is impairment of hearing associated with fluid in the middle ear. Loss of hearing has been documented in children with acute otitis media and with persistent middle ear effusion (Bluestone, et al., 1973; Kokko, 1975). Olmsted et al. (1964) studied children 2½ to 12 years of age with acute otitis media. Of 82 children included in the study, 33% had no loss of hearing, 40% had loss of hearing (greater than 15 dB) initially, which disappeared in 1 to 6 months, 12% had loss of hearing throughout the 6-month period, and 15% had loss of hearing initially but were lost to the study between 1 and 4 months after the acute episode of otitis media.

The significance of hearing loss associated with acute infection or persistent middle ear effusion is uncertain. Retrospective studies suggest that chronic middle ear disease with effusion occurring during the first few years of life has adverse effects on development of speech and language, hearing, intelligence, and performance in school (Holm and Kunze, 1969; Kaplan et al., 1973; Lewis, 1976; Needleman, 1977; Zincus et al., 1978).

Recent data from a prospective study of Boston children observed from birth showed that children with recurrent acute otitis media who had also experienced a prolonged middle ear effusion scored less well on standard tests of language administered at 3 years of age than did children who had little or no history of middle

ear disease (Teele et al., 1984). The association of prolonged time spent with middle ear effusion and effect of development of speech, language, and cognitive abilities remains controversial because of the many variables to be considered. Many questions remain to be answered. Is there a critical period when children with otitis media are most vulnerable to effects on speech and language? How does the quality of parent-child language interaction affect the association of otitis media and problems in development of speech and language? How does day care affect the incidence of otitis media and the development of speech and language? What role does recurrent otitis media play in relationships of the child with parent and siblings? Most important, if the infant with otitis media suffers near and long-term sequelae, how can such effects be prevented?

EPIDEMIOLOGY

The incidence of otitis media is highest in children aged 6 to 24 months. Subsequently, the incidence of otitis media declines with age except for a limited reversal of the downward trend between 5 and 6 years of age, the time of entrance into school. Otitis media is uncommon in children 7 years of age or older.

Otitis media is more frequent in males than in females. Clusters of cases occur in families; children who have significant experience with middle ear infections are more likely to have siblings or parents with histories of significant middle ear infections than those who have no episodes of otitis media.

The seasonal incidence of infections of the middle ear parallels the seasonal variations in prevalence of upper respiratory tract infections. The incidence of episodes of otitis media increases during outbreaks of viral infections of the respiratory tract in children, which usually occur in winter and spring.

TREATMENT
Acute otitis media

The choice of antimicrobial agents for treatment of children with otitis media is based on the following information: First, *S. pneumoniae* and *H. influenzae* are the most frequent agents isolated from middle ear fluids of children with acute otitis media. Second, *S. pneumoniae* is susceptible to penicillins, cephalosporins, erythromycin, clindamycin, and trimethroprim-sulfamethoxazole (TMP-SMZ). *H. influenzae* is susceptible to ampicillin, amoxicillin, the sulfonamides (including TMP-SMZ) and chloramphenicol. High concentrations of penicillin V, erythromycin, and clindamycin are required for the inhibition of *H. influenzae*. Penicillin G is less active than ampicillin against *H. influenzae*. Third, relatively high concentrations of antimicrobial agents considered for treatment of this infection are achieved in middle ear fluids of children with otitis media (Table 19-3). Fourth, the results of in vivo sensitivity tests corroborate in vitro data, that is, *S. penumoniae* is eradicated from middle ear fluid by penicillins and erythromycin. Ampicillin or amoxicillin and combinations of penicillin V or erythromycin and a sulfonamide are effective in sterilizing middle ear infection due to *H. influenzae*. Penicillin V, intramuscular benzathine penicillin G, or erythromycin alone is inadequate to eradicate *H. influenzae* from the middle ear.

Ampicillin or amoxicillin is the current drug of choice since it provides efficacy in vitro and in vivo against *S. pneumoniae* and *H. influenzae*. For the child who is believed to be allergic to penicillin, erythromycin combined with a sulfonamide, TMP-SMZ, and cefaclor are alternative regimens.

Strains of nontypable *H. influenzae* producing a penicillinase that inactivates ampicillin and amoxicillin (as well as penicillin G, penicillin V, and carbenicillin) have been noted in recent years. About 15% to 30% of strains of nontypable *H. influenzae* isolated from middle ear fluid of children with otitis media at different centers in the United States have been reported to produce penicillinase. The overall incidence of resistant strains in children with otitis media is low (15% to 30% of the approximately 20% of cases of otitis media that are associated with nontypable *H. influenzae*); thus, a change in consideration of ampicillin or amoxicillin for initial therapy is not necessary at this time.

An increase in the incidence of beta-lactamase–producing *H. influenzae* or increased incidence of *B. catarrhalis* (the majority of strains are beta-lactamase producers) may require reconsideration of this recommendation in the future. However, at present if the child does not respond a resistant strain of *H. influenzae* or *B. catarrhalis* may be the cause. Therapy should be changed to TMP-SMZ, erythromycin combined with a sulfonamide, or cefaclor.

Nasal and oral decongestants, administered either alone or in combination with an antihistamine, are currently among the most popular medications for the treatment of otitis media with effusion. The common concept is that these drugs reduce congestion of the respiratory mucosa and relieve the obstruction of the eustachian tube that results from inflammation caused by respiratory infection. The results of clinical trials, however, indicate no significant evidence of efficacy of any of these preparations used alone or in combination for relief of signs of disease or decrease in time spent with fluid in the middle ear after acute infection (Collip, 1961; Fraser et al., 1977; Olson et al., 1978).

Table 19-3. Concentrations of orally administered antimicrobial agents in serum (S) and middle ear fluids (MEF) of children with acute otitis media

Agent	Dosage (mg/kg)	Concentration ($\mu g/ml$)*			Reference
		S	MEF	MEF/S	
Penicillin V	13	8.1	1.8	0.22	Kamme et al., 1969
Ampicillin	10	4.3	1.2	0.28	Lahikainen et al., 1977
Amoxicillin	10	4.8	2.2	0.46	Howard et al., 1976
Erythromycin estolate	7.5	3.9	1.3	0.33	Howard et al., 1976
Sulfonamide (trisulfapyrimidines)	30	13.4	8.3	0.62	Howard et al., 1976

*Measured at 0.5 to 2 hours after administration.

Chronic otitis media with effusion

Appropriate management of the child with chronic otitis media remains controversial. The major goal is to establish and to maintain an aerated middle ear that is free of fluid and has a normal mucosa and, thus, to achieve normal hearing. Current therapies include prolonged courses of antimicrobial agents, courses of decongestants alone or in combination with antihistamines, short courses of steroids, myringotomy, adenoidectomy, and use of tympanostomy (ventilating) tubes. All of these therapies, with the exception of placement of tympanostomy tubes, are of uncertain value for the child with chronic otitis media. Investigations of these drugs or procedures (except for tubes) suggests that any one may be effective in some children but does not result in a beneficial effect for many children.

Tympanostomy tubes, resembling small collar buttons placed in the tympanic membrane, provide drainage of middle ear fluid and ventilate the middle ear. The effect in children who have impaired hearing because of the presence of fluid is restoration of normal hearing. Placement of the tube is treating the effect and not the cause of the persistent effusion. The criteria for placement of ventilating tubes, management of tubes once they are placed, and long-term benefits, if any, are uncertain. The indications for placement of tympanostomy tubes as outlined by Dr. Charles Bluestone, Director of Otolaryngology at Children's Hospital in Pittsburgh, include persistent middle ear effusions that are unresponsive to adequate medical treatment, persistent tympanic membrane retraction pockets with impending cholesteatoma, and persistent negative pressure with significant hearing loss (Bluestone and Shurin, 1974).

PREVENTION

A study in Rochester, New York suggested that chemoprophylaxis may be of value in the prevention of signs of acute infection in children with recurrent otitis media (Perrin et al., 1974). A significant decrease in new episodes of otitis occurred in children receiving sulfisoxazole compared with children receiving a placebo. Other studies (Maynard et al., 1972; Biedel, 1978; Schwartz et al., 1982; Liston et al., 1983; Schuller, 1983) corroborate the results of the

Rochester study. These studies do not provide conclusive evidence of the validity of chemoprophylaxis, but the data are persuasive that children who are prone to recurrent episodes of acute infection of the middle ear are benefited. While we await definitive studies of chemoprophylaxis, it is reasonable to consider the following program:

1. Enrollment criteria—children who have had three documented episodes of acute otitis media in 6 months or four episodes in 12 months
2. Drugs and dosage—sulfisoxazole offers the advantage of demonstrated efficacy, safety, and low cost; amoxicillin is a reasonable alternative; the drugs can be administered once a day in one half the therapeutic dosage (sulfisoxazole 50 mg per kilogram of body weight amoxicillin 20 mg per kilogram)
3. Duration—about 6 months, usually during the winter and spring seasons when respiratory tract infections are most frequent
4. Observation—children should be examined at approximately 1-month intervals when free of acute signs to determine if middle ear effusion is present; management of prolonged middle ear effusion should be considered separately from prevention of recurrences of acute infection

Prevention of disease by use of bacterial vaccines has been considered because of the limited number of pathogens responsible for otitis media. Since the vast majority of *H. influenzae* strains responsible for otitis media are nontypable and current investigational vaccines are prepared from type b capsular polysaccharide, there is no immediate prospect for a vaccine against this organism. A polyvalent pneumococcal vaccine is effective in prevention of bacteremia and pneumonia due to types of *S. pneumoniae* present in the vaccine.

Use of pneumococcal vaccine for prevention of recurrences of otitis media in Finnish and American children under 2 years of age resulted in fewer spisodes of type-specific infection, but the experience of immunized children with acute otitis media was not significantly different than that of children who received only control materials (Makela et al., 1981; Sloyer et al., 1981; Teele et al., 1981). Although some episodes of acute otitis media may be prevented (particularly in children 2 years of age and older, who respond more uniformly to the polysaccharide antigens), the reduction may not be sufficient to significantly alter the experience of children with infections of the middle ear.

REFERENCES

Berman SA, Balkany TJ, Simmons MA. Otitis media in infants less than 12 weeks of age: differing bacteriology among inpatients and outpatients. J Pediatr 1978;93:453.

Biedel CW. Modification of recurrent otitis media by short-term sulfonamide therapy. Am J Dis Child 1978;132:681-683.

Bland RD. Otitis media in the first six weeks of life: diagnosis, bacteriology, and management. Pediatrics 1972; 49:187.

Bluestone CD, Beery QC, Paradise JL. Audiometry and tympanometry in relation to middle ear effusions in children. Laryngoscope 1973;83:594.

Bluestone CD, Klein JO. Otitis media in infants and children. Philadelphia: W.B Saunders Co., 1981.

Bluestone CD, Shurin PA. Middle ear disease in children. Pathogenesis, diagnosis, and management. Pediatr Clin North Am 1974;21:379.

Collip PJ. Evaluation of nose drops for otitis media in children. Northwest Med 1961;60:999.

Fraser JG, Mehta M, Fraser PM. The medical treatment of secretory otitis media: a clinical trial of three commonly used regimens. J Laryngol Otol 1977;91:757.

Grönroos JA, et al. The etiology of acute middle ear infection. Acta Otolaryngol 1964;58:149.

Groothuis JR, et al. Otitis media in infancy: tympanometric findings. Pediatrics 1979;63:435.

Henderson FW, Collier AM, Sanyal MA, et al. A longitudinal study of respiratory viruses and bacteria in the etiology of acute otitis media with effusion. N Engl J Med 1982;306:1377-1383.

Herberts G, Jeppsson PH, Nylen O. Acute otitis media. Pract Otorhinolaryngol 1971;33:191.

Holm VA, Kunze LH. Effect of chronic otitis media on language and speech development. Pediatrics 1969;43:833.

Howard JE, Nelson JD, Clahsen J, Jackson LH. Otitis media of infancy and early childhood. Am J Dis Child 1976; 130:965.

Howie V, Ploussard J, Lester R. Otitis media: a clinical and bacteriologic correlation. Pediatrics 1970;45:29.

Kamme C, Lundgren K, Rundcrantz H. The concentration of penicillin V in serum and middle ear exudate in acute otitis media in children. Scand J Infect Dis 1969;1:77.

Kaplan GJ, et al. Long-term effects of otitis media. A ten-year cohort study of Alaskan Eskimo children. Pediatrics 1973;52:577.

Klein BS, Dollette FR, Yolken RH. The role of respiratory syncytial virus and other viral pathogens in acute otitis media. J Pediatr 1982;101:16-20.

Klein JO, Teele DW. Isolation of viruses and mycoplasmas from middle ear effusions: a review. Ann Otol Rhinol Laryngol 1976;85:140.

Kokko E. Chronic secretory otitis media in children. Acta Otolaryngol 1974; Suppl 327:7.

Kovatch AJ, Wald ER, Michaels RH. β-Lactamase-producing Branhamella catarrhalis causing otitis media in children. J Pediatr 1983;102:261-264.

Lahikainen EA, Vuori M, Virtanen S. Azidocillin and ampicillin concentrations in middle ear effusion. Acta Otolaryngol 1977;84:227.

Lewis N. Otitis media and linguistic incompetence. Arch Otolaryngol 1976;102:387.

Liston TE, Foshee WS, Pierson WD. Sulfisoxazole chemoprophylaxis for frequent otitis media. Pediatrics 1983; 71:524-530.

Makela PH, Leinonen M, Pukander J, et al. A study of the pneumococcal vaccine in prevention of clinically acute attacks of recurrent otitis media. Rev Infect Dis 1981; 3(S):124.

Maynard JE, Fleshman JK, Tschopp CF. Otitis media in Alaskan Eskimo children. JAMA 1972;219:597-599.

National Health Survey. Hearing and related medical findings among children: race, area, and socioeconomic differentials, Publication No. (HSM) 73-1604, Rockville, MD. Department of Health, Education, and Welfare, 1972.

Needleman H. Effects of hearing loss from early recurrent otitis media on speech and language development. In Jaffee B, ed. Hearing loss in children. Baltimore: University Park Press, 1977.

Olmsted RW, et al. The pattern of hearing following acute otitis media. J Pediatr 1964;65:252.

Olson AL, Klein SW, Charney E, et al. Prevention and therapy of serous otitis media by oral decongestant: a double-blind study in pediatric practice. Pediatrics 1978; 61:679.

Paradise JL, Bluestone CD. Toward rational indications for tonsil and adenoid surgery. Hosp Prac 1976;11:79.

Perrin JM, et al. Sulfisoxazole as chemoprophylaxis for recurrent otitis media. A double-blind crossover study in pediatric practice. N Engl J Med 1974;291:664.

Schuller DE. Prophylaxis of otitis media in asthmatic children. Pediatr Infect Dis 1983;2:280-283.

Schwartz RH, Puglise J, Rodriguez WJ. Sulfamethoxazole prophylaxis in the otitis media-prone child. Arch Dis Child 1982;57:590-593.

Schwartz R, Rodriguez J, Khan WN, Ross S. Acute purulent otitis media in children older than 5 years: incidence of Haemophilus as a causative organism. JAMA 1977; 238:1032.

Shurin PA, Marchant CD, Kim CH, et al. Emergence of beta-lactamase-producing strains of Branhamella catarrhalis as important agents of acute otitis media. Pediatr Infect Dis 1983;2:34-38.

Shurin PA, Pelton SI, Donner A, Klein JO. Persistence of middle-ear infusion after acute otitis media in children. N Engl J Med 1979;300:1121.

Shurin PA, et al. Bacterial etiology of otitis media during the first six weeks of life. J Pediatr 1978;92:893.

Sloyer JL Jr, Ploussard JH, Howie VM. Efficacy of pneumococcal polysaccharide vaccine in preventing acute otitis media in infants in Huntsville, Alabama. Rev Infect Dis 1981;3(S):119.

Sobeslavsky O, et al. The etiological role of *Mycoplasma pneumoniac* in otitis media in children. Pediatrics 1965; 35:652.

Teele DW, Klein JO, and The Greater Boston Collaborative Study Group. Use of pneumococcal vaccine for prevention of recurrent acute otitis media in infants in Boston. Rev Infect Dis 1981;3(S):113.

Teele DW, Klein JO, Rosner B. Otitis media and development of speech and language. Pediatrics (in press), 1984.

Teele DW, Klein JO, Rosner B. Epidemiology of otitis media in children. Ann Otol Rhinol Laryngol (Suppl) 1980;68:5.

Tetzlaff TR, Ashworth C, Nelson JD. Otitis media in children less than 12 weeks of age. Pediatrics 1977;59:827.

Tipple MA, Beem MO, Saxon EM. Clinical characteristics of afebrile pneumonia associated with *Chlamydia trachomatis* infections in infants less than 6 months of age. Pediatrics 1979;63:192.

Zinkus PW, Gottlieb MI, Schapiro M. Developmental and psycho-educational sequelae of chronic otitis media. Am J Dis Child 1978;132:1100.

20

PERTUSSIS (WHOOPING COUGH)

Pertussis is no longer a common infection of childhood in the United States. The disease persists in unimmunized populations of the world as a highly contagious and potentially fatal disease of infants. It is caused by *Bordetella pertussis*, first described by Bordet and Gengou in 1906. The illness is characterized by a catarrhal period of nonspecific respiratory symptoms that progresses to a stage of paroxysmal cough accompanied by the typical inspiratory whoop and vomiting. Whooping cough may be complicated by potentially serious involvement of the lower respiratory tract and the central nervous system (CNS).

ETIOLOGY

B. pertussis is the causative agent of whooping cough. The disease has been produced in chimpanzees and in humans by experimental inoculation of the organism. Man appears to be the only natural host for this bacterium. *B. parapertussis* and *B. bronchiseptica*, the other two members of the genus *Bordetella*, have been associated with disease in a few instances.

Bordetella organisms are small, gram-negative coccobacilli, 0.2 to 0.3 μm by 0.5 to 1.0 μm, appearing singly, in pairs, and in small clusters. Upon primary isolation, the bacterial cells are uniform in size, but in subcultures they become quite pleomorphic. Filamentous and thick bacillary forms are common. Bipolar metachromatic staining may be demonstrated with toluidine blue. The only motile member of the genus is *B. bronchiseptica*, which possesses lateral flagella. Capsules are produced but can be demonstrated only by special stains and not by capsular swelling.

Unlike *Haemophilus* species, *Bordetella* organisms have no specific growth requirement for hemin (X factor) and coenzyme I (V factor). Primary isolation does require, however, the addition of charcoal, ion-exchange resins, or 15% to 20% blood to neutralize the growth-inhibiting effects of such substances as unsaturated fatty acids, colloidal sulfur, sulfides, or peroxides. Modified Bordet-Gengou medium (potato-glycerol-blood agar) is recommended for this purpose. Colonies of *B. pertussis* on this medium are smooth, convex, glistening, almost transparent, and pearl-like in appearance. All three species produce a zone of hemolysis that varies with cultural conditions.

B. pertussis freshly isolated from patients in the catarrhal stage of pertussis are smooth colony-forming organisms (phase I or X mode). Adaptation by passage to other media, such as blood or chocolate agar, results in irreversible transition through intermediate forms (phases II and III) to the rough colony-producing form (phase IV). This phase variation is presumably a result of genetic alteration of the organism. Although some properties of phase I and phase IV organisms remain indistinguishable, several characteristics have been lost by phase IV organisms. These are lost in parallel with the ability to induce sensitivity to histamine, protective antibodies in animals, and lymphocytosis. The loss of these properties correlates with the loss of virulence for animals and thus provides additional markers for strain degradation. The mechanisms of phase transition or degradation are not understood, but plasmid functions do not seem to be involved.

The terms *cultural* and *antigenic modulation* have been used to describe a change in phenotype of the organism; it occurs in almost all members of a population of *B. pertussis* as a result of environmental features, for example, medium containing a high level of $MgSO_4$. The modulation is readily reversible, and a single colony may undergo the transition from phase I or X mode to C mode. Phenotypically, the C mode organisms are like phase IV organisms and have lost the properties enumerated above, which are correlated with virulence for animals. Both phase variation and cultural modulation will result in altered antigenicity as measured by the agglutinogen.

Antigens

Experimental protection against infection with *B. pertussis* in the mouse and in human illness is conferred by the immunologic response to the bacterium. The protective antigen(s) of *B. pertussis* was unknown when extensive serologic investigations described the classic antigens of the genus *Bordetella*. The single, heat-stable surface 0 antigen common to smooth strains of *B. pertussis*, *B. parapertussis*, and *B. bronchiseptica* and to rough strains of *B. pertussis* and *B. bronchiseptica* was recognized. This 0 antigen is a protein easily extractable from cells, and it is found in the supernatant fluids of cell cultures but is not responsible for stimulating protection against infection.

The antigenic differences among species and among strains of each of the species are determined by the heat-labile or capsular antigens of Kauffman. The serotype is often indicated by numbers, for example, *B. pertussis* 1.2.4. Eldering (1957) postulated the existence of 14 K antigens, designated as *factors* on the basis of agglutinin absorption tests. Factors 1 through 6 are found only in strains of *B. pertussis*. Factor 7 is common to all strains of the three species of *Bordetella* organisms. Factor 14 is specific for *B. parapertussis*, and factor 12 is specific for *B. bronchiseptica*.

The serotypes per se of *B. pertussis* do not determine virulence, and antibodies to the capsular antigens do not protect against infection.

However, these antigens have been essential in vaccine production, as they provide a method of assaying for the alterations occurring with phase variation and cultural modulation of the strains. Factor 1 antigen is present in all strains of *B. pertussis*, and it has been suggested that the agglutinating antigen (agglutinogen) of the organism is primarily factor 1. Isolated agglutinogen is nontoxic and does not protect animals against *B. pertussis* infection. Agglutinins or antibodies to agglutinogen are a measurable response in immunized persons or those persons sustaining natural infection. These antibodies are reflective of immunity, although these antibodies alone are not protective.

Pertussis toxin or histamine-sensitizing factor (HSF)–lymphocytosis promoting factor (LPF)–islet-activating protein (IAP)

B. pertussis produces an exotoxin. The histamine-sensitizing factor has been known for years, but only with the purification of a single protein from the *B. pertussis* envelope has it become clear that this one protein is also the lymphocytosis-promoting factor and the islet-activating protein. The homogeneous protein has a molecular weight of 117,000; it is a hexamer of five dissimilar peptides and is thermostable. The largest peptide (S1) with a molecular weight of 28,000 is thought to be the toxin or A moiety. The other four peptides, designated S2 to S5 by descending molecular weight, form the B or receptor oligmer. Two dimers (S2-S4 and S3-S4) plus a monomer (S5) comprise the B moiety essential for attachment to target cells. The entire protein that diffuses into the culture medium is a bacterial exotoxin. The purified protein can experimentally induce histamine sensitization, hypoglycemia, inability to respond to epinephrine, and leukocytosis.

Pertussis toxin, that is, the A protomer, affects the adenylate cyclase system by nicotinamide-adenine dinucleotide (NAD)-dependent adenosine diphosphate (ADP) ribosylation of a membrane protein which is believed to be an inhibitory guanosine triphosphate (GTP)-binding subunit of the cylase. This is analogous to the mechanism of action of diphtheria and cholera toxins with different target proteins. In vitro, accumulation of cyclic adenosine monophosphate (cAMP) is shown in affected cells. This results in insulin release if pancreatic beta cells are the experimental system. Normally this is prevented by epinephrine bound to alpha-adrenergic receptors. In isolated rat heart cells and C6 glioma cells, the accumulation of cAMP in response to toxin has also been shown. Toxin prevents the usual cholinergic decrease of cAMP. Thus pertussis toxin alters regulation of adenylate cyclase.

The striking lymphocytosis observed in association with clinical pertussis has been duplicated in the mouse with the HSF-LPF-IAP protein. It has been proposed that lymphocyte migration from small vessels is hindered by the absorption of the protein onto lymphocyte surfaces. The entrapment of lymphocytes in the vascular and lymphatic compartments creates the lymphocytosis. Specific antiserum can prevent or block histamine sensitization, islet cell activation, and lymphocytosis. Clinical and experimental data demonstrate that once toxin fixes to cells, the biologic activities cannot then be affected by antiserum.

Hemagglutinins

B. pertussis has two hemagglutinins, one of which is a filamentous protein with an estimated molecular weight of 130,000. This hemagglutinin (F-HA) is derived from fimbriae on the organism; it is present on phase I organisms and absent from avirulent phases III and IV organisms. The host cell receptor is thought to be the cholesterol of the cell membrane. The organisms adhere to the cilia of epithelial cells in the respiratory tract, to ependymal cells in the mouse, and to erythrocytes.

The second hemagglutinin, HSF-LPF-IAP–HA, or toxin-HA, is a round molecule and has only one twentieth of the hemagglutinating activity of the F-HA. There is no recognized role in clinical disease of the hemagglutinating properties of this protein. This hemagglutinin adheres to sialic acid–containing receptors and is expressed only by phase I organisms. The hemagglutinin portion of the molecule may therefore be important in adherence of toxin to cells. Sialoproteins, including haptoglobin and ceruloplasmin, can compete for the toxin-HA, thereby inhibiting attachment to cell receptors in the respiratory tract.

Heat-labile toxin (HLT)

HLT is considered to be a cytoplasmic protein and may occur in the bacteria as a precursor requiring activation to induce toxicity. A homogeneous protein form of HLT has not been isolated. HLT is released by cell lysis and it is destroyed when heated to 56° C for 15 minutes. It is dermonecrotic and when given intraperitoneally or intravenously it is lethal for mice. It is a poor antigen unless converted to toxoid by formaldehyde treatment of lysed cells (not intact cells). Toxoid-stimulated antibody does not protect mice against intracerebral challenge or children against infection. HLT is not known to stimulate antibody production in humans, and its role in the pathogenesis of human illness is unknown.

Lipopolysaccharide (heat-stable toxin)

The lipopolysaccharide or endotoxin of the cell wall is heat stable, with a general similarity to endotoxins of Enterobacteriaceae but with some suggested differences in macromolecular structure. It can be chemically fractionated into two different polysaccharides, each terminated by a molecule of 3-deoxy-2-octulosonic acid. Two distinct lipid fragments, lipid A and lipid X, are present and contain glucosamine, fatty acids, and esterified phosphate in similar proportions. Lipid X, the minor lipid, has 2-methyl, 3-hydroxydecanoic and tetradecanoic acids that are absent from lipid A. Lipid X seems to be responsible for the acute toxicity of this endotoxin. The lipopolysaccharide does not induce formation of antibodies with protective activity.

Adenylate cyclase

In addition to the exotoxin, all three *Bordetella* species possess an extracytoplasmic adenylate cyclase that is activated by calmodulin, the eukaryotic cell calcium-dependent regulatory protein. This extracellular cyclase gains access to the interior of cells and causes a massive increase in cAMP, which prevents the cell from performing normal regulatory functions. In vitro, the enzyme does not alter phagocytosis, but it does alter chemotaxis and inhibit the oxidative burst of the polymorphonuclear neutrophil leukocytes (PMNs). The extracellular adenylate cyclase has been shown to be necessary for virulence in a mouse model. The role of this enzyme in the pathogenesis of disease remains to be determined.

Tracheal cytotoxin

A second extracellular toxin has been demonstrated to inhibit DNA synthesis and in vitro to duplicate the in vivo ciliostasis and extrusion of ciliated cells from hamster tracheal ring cultures. The role in human disease and cytopathology is unclear.

PATHOLOGY

The specific pathology attributable to *B. pertussis* is limited to the respiratory tract. Pathologic descriptions from fatal disease have been supplemented by ultrastructural analysis of tracheal organ culture and mouse models of infection. The selective adherence of phase I bacteria to ciliated epithelial cells has been studied in detail. Aggregates of bacilli are seen adherent to the cilia of the tracheal and bronchial epithelium. In the model systems diminished ciliary activity can be measured after bacterial attachment. The extrusion of ciliated cells from the epithelial surface has been observed experimentally and in human infections. In pathologic specimens, the bronchial epithelium shows necrosis of midzonal and basilar layers with neutrophilic infiltrates. Peribronchial infiltrates and interstitial pneumonia are common postmortem findings. Patchy areas of atelectasis and emphysema frequently result from obstruction by a mucous plug in a bronchus. Superinfection with other organisms may occur with additional pneumonia and inflammatory exudate of alveoli. Bronchiectasis was a common sequel to this infection. The brain may show various nonspecific changes, including hypoxic damage and microscopic cerebral hemorrhages in patients dying with convulsions.

PATHOGENESIS

Following inhalation of infected droplets, the organisms colonize the respiratory tract. The specificity of attachment of *B. pertussis* to ciliated respiratory epithelial cells is attributable to the F-HA. Such adherence is essential for production of disease, as specific antibody can prevent damage to ciliated cells in vitro or prevent disease in an animal model.

It is presumed that the incubation period and initial mild symptoms of rhinitis, cough, sneezing, and, sometimes, conjunctivitis during the first 1 to 2 weeks of the illness are caused by local multiplication of the organisms in the respiratory tract. Diminished ciliary activity would result in poorer clearance of bacteria and secretions with their resulting accumulation in the respiratory tract. Multiplication of organisms and local toxin production would be facilitated, and toxin would then contribute to necrosis and sloughing of ciliated cells. It is also tempting to speculate that the lack of bacteremia and invasion of other tissues by *B. pertussis* is related to the lack of receptors for the organism on other cells. It is known that bacterial multiplication in other tissue does not occur.

The characteristic systemic manifestations of the paroxysmal phase of disease are most likely due to circulating HSF-LPF-IAP or toxin. The cough, the CNS manifestations, and even the rarely observed hypoglycemia, as well as the leukocytosis and lymphocytosis, may be attributable to the effects of exotoxin. The persistence of cough and lymphocytosis is explainable as a result of the fixation of toxin in cells. Additionally, bacteria are less readily detectable in the respiratory tract during the paroxysmal stage than in the earlier catarrhal phase. Therefore, it is conceptually easy to attribute the multiple systemic manifestations of disease to a circulating exotoxin with its array of defined biologic activities. Antibody to the toxin prevents the lymphocytosis and, in the mouse, also provides protection against disease. Whooping cough results from local bacterial colonization of the respiratory tract and subsequent systemic circulation of bacterial exotoxin. The mechanism(s) by which the toxin exerts its effects and the correlation of the in vitro biologic activities to human illness remain to be elucidated.

CLINICAL MANIFESTATIONS

The clinical syndrome of pertussis is readily defined by the presence of the paroxysmal cough and associated whoop, but the illness is of variable severity, and the milder respiratory syndromes caused by *B. pertussis* are impossible to distinguish on clinical grounds alone. As many as 20% of pertussis infections have been estimated to be atypical illnesses, and these affected patients are infectious to others.

Following inhalation of infected droplets, the organisms colonize the respiratory tract. Symptoms almost always begin within 10 days after exposure to *B. pertussis*, although the incubation period can vary from 5 to 21 days. The clinical illness is divided into three separate stages for descriptive purposes. The catarrhal or prodromal stage lasts from 1 to 2 weeks. During this period of time, the child exhibits only mild symptoms of an uncomplicated upper respiratory infection. Physical examination does not reveal any serious objective findings. The second stage usually lasts from 1 to 6 weeks and is characterized by progression to a paroxysmal cough. A characteristic paroxysm is one in which five to 20 forcible hacking coughs are produced in 15 to 20 seconds, often terminated with the production of mucus or associated vomiting. There is no time for breathing between coughs, and the paroxysm may be sufficiently prolonged to induce anoxia. The final inspiratory breath, which takes place through the narrowed glottis, produces the characteristic whoop. These early stages of illness are frequently associated with leukocytosis of 12,000 to 100,000 mm^3 with a lymphocytosis of 60% or higher (see p. 242).

The third stage of illness is that of convalescence. Coughing may persist for several months after the initial onset of illness. An understanding of the pathogenesis of the cough is of potential therapeutic importance, since the clinical course of the disease and the morbidity are not appreciably altered by administration of specific antimicrobial agents.

The morbidity and mortality associated with pertussis have resulted primarily from compromise of the central nervous system during the acute illness and from secondary bacterial infection, usually involving ears, sinuses, or the lower respiratory tract. The neuropathology of infants dying with pertussis and CNS involvement is nonspecific and indistinguishable from changes produced by anoxia. CNS compromise is clearly not a result of actual invasion by *B. pertussis*.

DIAGNOSIS

Having once watched a typical paroxysmal attack and heard the whoop, the physician has little trouble in recognizing subsequent cases. The bursts of short, rapid coughs on one expiration followed by the high-pitched inspiratory crow are the hallmarks of no other disease. Even in the absence of the typical whoop, as in infants, the clinical diagnosis is strongly suggested by the paroxysmal nature of the cough, the red or cyanotic appearance, and the associated vomiting.

During the catarrhal stage it is usually impossible to differentiate pertussis on clinical grounds from the common cold, bronchitis, or acute respiratory tract disease caused by various agents. A history of contact with a known case or a cough that becomes aggravated after 1 week should cause suspicion.

The definitive diagnosis depends on isolation of *B. pertussis* (or, less commonly, *B. parapertussis* or *B. bronchiseptica*) from the patient. The isolation rate of the organism from the respiratory tract is greatest during the catarrhal stage (Fig.20-1), and organisms are not usually detectable for longer than the first 4 weeks of illness. Appropriate specimens for cultivation from patients are obtained from a nasopharyngeal swab. Mucus collected from the posterior nasopharynx with a thin swab produces more consistent results than the use of cough plates.

Isolation of *B. pertussis* from clinical specimens is dependent on careful transport and efficient processing of the materials obtained for culture. If the specimen will not be planted for 1 to 2 hours, the swab should be placed in 0.25 to 0.50 ml of casamino acids solution with a pH of 7.2 to prevent drying of the swab. When the specimen will be shipped to another laboratory or when holding time exceeds 2 hours, other organisms may overgrow *B. pertussis*. Therefore, swabs should be placed in modified Stuart's medium (SBL) or Mishulow's charcoal agar. These media are better able to maintain the viability of organisms and to support the growth under the conditions of transport, but there is a decreased recovery rate of *B. pertussis* from transport media as compared to direct inoculation. Modified Bordet-Gengou agar is recommended for primary isolation of the organism. The addition of 0.25 to 0.5 unit/ml of penicillin to a second plate is useful in inhibiting the growth of the gram-positive flora of the respiratory tract without affecting growth of *B. pertussis* organisms.

In addition to a specific pattern of biochemical reactions, serologic identification of *B. pertussis* will confirm the isolation. A slide agglutination test can be performed with a standard inoculum of organisms and specific antiserum, which is available commercially.

Fluorescent antibody (FA) staining has been used to identify *B. pertussis* upon direct smears of nasopharyngeal swabs and for identification of organisms growing on Bordet-Gengou plates. The FA examination of nasopharyngeal swab material is often unreliable even in experienced hands. The FA procedure cannot substitute for cultural isolation of the organism, but it can offer the advantage of more rapid laboratory identification of organisms after isolation. The Analytical Bacteriology Section of the Centers for Disease Control and many of the state bacteriology laboratories are prepared to culture and/ or examine secretions by FA techniques for *B. pertussis*.

At present, assessment of antibodies in the serum is accomplished by measuring agglutinins. There are few laboratories in the United States prepared to perform tests for *B. pertussis* agglutinin titers. The current microagglutination tests give titers that have not been correlated with protection against disease. Since these agglutinins are not the protective antibodies, they give only an indirect assessment of immunity, although they do assess experience with *B. pertussis* as an infection or as a vaccine. After infection, there may be only a slight rise in agglutinins, and it tends to occur weeks into the illness. An acute and convalescent pair of sera are needed to define an antibody rise that is indicative of recent contact with antigen.

A generally available, specific, and reliable assessment of the humoral response(s) to infection or immunization with *B. pertussis* is badly needed. Assays of antibody to F-HA and LPF-HSF-IAP have been developed, and data are currently being obtained in association with immunization or natural disease to assess their value. An ELISA assay measuring IgM, IgG, or IgA antibodies to F-HA has shown 96% sensitivity of recognition of culture-positive patients and has identified additional patients who were culture negative. Thus, it is anticipated that these antibodies will reflect immunity in a more accurate manner.

The white blood cell count may contribute to the diagnosis (Fig. 20-1). High counts with a predominance of lymphocytes are characteristic of whooping cough. At the end of the catarrhal phase, white blood cell counts of 20,000 to 30,000/mm^3, with 60% or more lymphocytes, are suggestive of the disease. It is important to remember that infants may respond to any infection with lymphocytosis. In any case, however, counts in excess of 30,000/mm^3, with 70% to 90% lymphocytes, are highly suggestive of

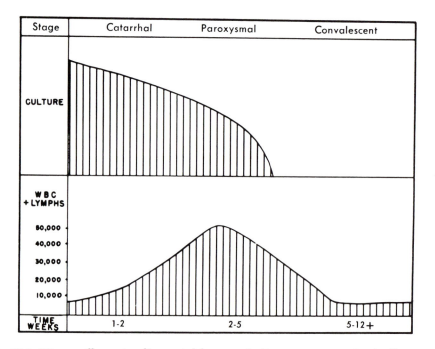

Fig. 20-1. Diagram illustrating diagnostic laboratory findings in pertussis. *Bordetella pertussis* may be recovered usually during catarrhal and early paroxysmal stages (first 4 weeks of illness). The white blood cell count is usually elevated during the paroxysmal stage (second to fifth weeks). Lymphocytes predominate.

pertussis. In some instances, levels of 100,000 or more may be reached.

DIFFERENTIAL DIAGNOSIS

Spasmodic coughing attacks are not pathognomonic of pertussis. *Bronchiolitis* or a spectrum of *pneumonias* in infants may cause confusion, especially since these conditions may also occur as complications of whooping cough. A history of contact or one of gradual onset of catarrhal symptoms progressing to the paroxysmal or spasmodic phase may be helpful. Recently, careful study of infantile pneumonias documented disease in association with *Chlamydia trachomatis*, CMV, *Pneumocystis carinii*, ureaplasma, and combinations of these agents. A pertussis syndrome has been described with *adenoviruses*, and these agents can be present simultaneously with *B. pertussis*. In infants the pulmonary lesion of *cystic fibrosis* not infrequently leads to paroxysmal coughing attacks resembling pertussis. The family history, the presence of chronic digestive disturbances with steatorrhea, the absence of trypsin from the stool or duodenal contents, and an increased concentration of sodium and chloride in the sweat will indicate the correct diagnosis. The pressure of enlarged tracheobronchial lymph nodes, usually tuberculous in origin, may give rise to a paroxysmal cough resembling pertussis but without whoop. The roentgenogram and positive tuberculin test should clarify the diagnosis. A *foreign body* in the air passages may be confused with pertussis, but the mode of onset and endoscopic and roentgenographic examinations should reveal the source of trouble.

COMPLICATIONS
Respiratory tract complications

The most common and usually the most severe complication is pneumonia. It is responsible for 90% of the deaths of children under 3 years of age, and it is especially serious in infants under 1 year of age. Interstitial bronchopneumonia, the most common form, is usually caused by secondary invaders, although *B. pertussis* has been shown on occasion to be the predominant microorganism. A few instances of pneumococcal lobar pneumonia have been described. Generally speaking, pneumonia makes its appearance during the height of the paroxysmal stage. Respirations are rapid and often disproportion-

ate to the fever, which does not reach high levels as a rule. Physical signs may be widespread and obvious, or they may be absent or equivocal. In either case, the roentgenogram will show typical changes. Atelectasis is a common complication of whooping cough. Frequently it is recognized only by roentgenographic examination. It may be patchy and widespread, or it may involve an entire lobe or segment of a lobe. Bronchiectasis, activation of latent tuberculosis, and otitis media occur as complications in infants.

Central nervous system complications

Convulsions may indicate a serious complication of whooping cough. The underlying cause of convulsions may be brain damage related to asphyxia from severe paroxysms, diffuse encephalopathy possibly caused by circulating toxin and leading to cortical atrophy, or petechial hemorrhages.

Other complications

Hemorrhages that are mechanical in origin result from increased venous pressure and congestion associated with paroxysms. Epistaxis and subconjunctival hemorrhages are fairly common. Petechiae and purpuric spots in the skin have been observed.

Ulceration of the frenum under the tongue may be observed in infants whose lower incisors traumatize it when the tongue protrudes during paroxysms. Other complications include hernia, prolapsed rectum, and nutritional disturbances. Loss of weight from starvation and dehydration may present serious problems.

PROGNOSIS

A progressive decline in the case fatality rate of pertussis has occurred in the last 40 years; the overall fatality rate is now less than 10 per 1000 cases. There are probably several reasons for the decline in case fatality rate. Widespread immunization not only prevents infection but also reduces its severity. Improved respiratory support, parenteral nutrition, and antibiotics may also be diminishing the fatality rate. The severity of pertussis has largely been forgotten. The greatest danger from this disease occurs in infancy. When the outlook for an individual patient is assessed, the presence of complications has an important bearing on future health as well as on immediate survival.

EPIDEMIOLOGIC FACTORS

Whooping cough is worldwide in distribution. No place, race, color, or nationality is exempt. The attack rate for black persons is the same as for white persons, but the mortality is higher in blacks. In many developing countries, pertussis presents a major health problem; the disease is severe, highly prevalent, and carries a high mortality (Morley et al., 1966).

Pertussis has not usually been a disease with marked seasonal variations, in contrast to several other childhood infections. Unlike that of other respiratory tract infections, the incidence of whooping cough rises during the spring and summer months, and it is maintained during June, July, and August, followed by a decrease during the autumn months.

In the United States, the number of reported cases has declined from approximately 120,000 in 1950 to 1895 in 1982. Reported deaths declined from approximately 1100 in 1950 to 12 in 1970. The case fatality ratio has been constant from 1970 to 1984. Twenty-six percent of all cases occur in infants under 1 year of age, and the decline in case fatality has been associated with a gradual increase in the age of patients sustaining infection.

A peculiar characteristic of whooping cough, quite different from that of the other contagious diseases of childhood, is the special predilection for infants and young children. Little or no immunity is transferred from the mother to the newborn infant. In the prevaccine era or in unimmunized populations, 40% of all deaths from whooping cough occurred in the first year of life. Approximately two thirds of all cases occurred in children under the age of 7 years. Pertussis has a very low incidence among young adults. This has been shown by military experience in World War I and World War II. Severe attacks have been described in elderly people. In the vaccine era, epidemics of pertussis have occurred in hospital personnel caring for pediatric patients. An outbreak reported by Kurt et al. (1972) involved 11 adults and one reported by Linnemann et al. (1975) involved eight physicians and five nurses.

An outbreak of pertussis in Oklahoma in 1983 typifies the current epidemiology of this infection in the United States. Three hundred thirty cases were identified and the largest numbers were reported from June to August. Approxi-mately 40% of cases were in infants less than 1 year of age. Those babies less than 6 months of age were at greatest risk. Sixty-one persons had received no immunizations, 40 of them being less than 7 months of age. Forty-one persons had received a single dose of vaccine and 20 of them were less than 7 months of age. Twenty-eight youngsters contracted pertussis after receiving two DTP injections. Thirty-seven persons with a history of four DTP infections and five persons with a history of five injections had disease. Even though immunization was not 100% efficacious in preventing disease, if the child contracted *B. pertussis*, the severity of infection was less when the child had been immunized. Babysitting or extended family settings provided the means for interhousehold spread. It was ascertained that only an estimated 50% of infants 3 months to 18 months in the affected county were up to date in their immunizations. Once again, failure to immunize contributed to an outbreak of a preventable disease.

Another singular feature of whooping cough is the distribution according to sex. The morbidity and mortality of pertussis are higher for females than for males. It has been observed that the sex difference increases with age up to the tenth year. The opposite is characteristic of other common infectious diseases of childhood. The peculiar sex ratio in pertussis is an observation of long standing, confirmed the world over. It holds true for different races, for urban and rural areas, and for epidemic and endemic occurrence.

Man is the only known source of *B. pertussis*. The mode of transmission is direct contact with an infected person, most often a symptomatic individual. It is apparently accomplished by the transfer of material from the patient's nasopharynx by coughing, sneezing, and talking to the susceptible contact. Indirect spread by contaminated objects is uncommon. The higher attack rates that follow exposure in family groups as compared with nonfamily contacts suggests the greater effectiveness of intimate and repeated association in the spread of the disease. The high secondary attack rates of 90% or more in susceptible family members indicate that pertussis is highly communicable and perhaps comparable to measles and chickenpox in this respect.

For purposes of control, the period of communicability is considered to extend from 7 days after exposure to 3 weeks after onset of typical paroxysms. A patient with whooping cough is most likely to spread infection during the catarrhal period, before the occurrence of paroxysmal cough indicates the true nature of the disease. This correlates with the number of colonies of *B. pertussis* that may be isolated from the nasopharynx. The number is highest during the catarrhal stage and declines rapidly, so that after about the fourth week of illness, organisms are seldom recovered.

Immunization seems to have altered the epidemiology somewhat. In recent years during epidemics, persons with modification or absence of clinical illness have been shown to excrete *B. pertussis*. These persons are thought to be partially immune as a result of prior immunization, suggesting that asymptomatic carriers may be more common in the vaccine era. Prolonged presence of organisms during convalescence is extremely rare.

IMMUNITY

Naturally occurring whooping cough usually confers protection against subsequent clinical illness. Although second attacks of pertussis are rare, bacteriologically proved instances of both first and second attacks have been observed. Second attacks have usually involved an adult exposed in a family setting. In the present era when most young adults have been immunized in childhood, several outbreaks of pertussis have caused symptomatic disease in adults exposed within the hospital setting (Kurt et al., 1972; Linnemann et al., 1975). These observations suggest that immunity to disease wanes with time after the original infection or immunization. Moreover, a small number of immunized persons have been shown to be colonized and excreting *B. pertussis* in the absence of symptoms. Thus the vaccine appeared to protect against illness but not against colonization.

Mice provide an animal model that allows study of the host response to infection. The pathology of experimental *B. pertussis* respiratory infection of mice is similar to the disease of infants, as is the duration of excretion of bacteria, the lymphocytosis, and higher mortality in infant mice. Moreover, the interval after infection to the onset of histamine sensitization and the persistence of sensitization parallel the catarrhal and paroxysmal stages in the child. Mice that recover from respiratory infection are then resistant to intracerebral challenge. Sera obtained from mice or infants longer than 4 weeks after onset of illness can provide protection to the homologous species. We must rely on such a model to help dissect which antigen(s) is essential for the production of immunity.

It has been known for a long time that phase 1 *B. pertussis* are essential for the production of an effective vaccine. These organisms are virulent for mice, and recent creation of mutant *B. pertussis* strains has shown that virulence is associated with the exotoxin and possibly with the extracellular adenylcyclase.

Phase 1 organisms have fimbriae that are essential for colonization. Antibody to F-HA protects mice against lethal aerosol but not intracerebral challenge with *B. pertussis*. Antibody directed against F-HA should provide protection against infection by preventing adherence of these bacteria to respiratory epithelial cells. Local or respiratory tract antibody should be important in preventing colonization, and in the mouse such local antibody does develop after infection. Nevertheless, infant mice receiving only passive humoral anti-F-HA antibody have been protected from subsequent intranasal challenge. Also, parenteral administration of F-HA induces systemic anti-F-HA antibodies which protect these animals against disease after lethal aerosol challenge.

The single best predictor of *B. pertussis* vaccine potency and efficacy has been the intracerebral challenge of mice with *B. pertussis* (Standfast, 1958). Purified, detoxified pertussis toxin confers protection against intracerebral challenge.

The exotoxin has the capacity to enter the systemic circulation and produce multiple effects on different tissues. The exotoxin can be treated with formalin to eliminate toxicity and it is an immunogenic protein. Antibody, that is, antitoxin, can protect mice against lethal challenge with *B. pertussis* intranasally, intraperitoneally, and intracerebrally. It seems reasonable to expect that circulating antibody to the exotoxin will be important to protect the host.

Current whole cell *B. pertussis* vaccines contain the F-HA, exotoxin, and agglutinogens and induce antibodies to these antigens. Less is known about the tracheal cytotoxin and the extracellular adenylcyclase. It is known that anti-body to the lipopolysaccharide in the presence of complement determines the bactericidal activity of serum against *B. pertussis*, but this bactericidal activity is not correlated with protection against intracerebral challenge of mice.

Epidemiologic observations indicate that immunity to pertussis is specific. In areas where pertussis has not occurred for 5 years, persons of all ages have been susceptible to infection. At the present time there is no practical, reliable means of assessing immunity to whooping cough.

Several other aspects of the host response to *B. pertussis* are being investigated. Muse et al. (1979) demonstrated that antibody enhances opsonization of phase I *B. pertussis* organisms by alveolar macrophages. The intracellular killing rate was similar for both phase I and phase IV organisms. Therefore, it is probably important that antibody be present within the respiratory tract during active infection.

The need to develop an efficacious pertussis vaccine with fewer side effects has sparked interest in this organism. A great deal has been learned about the organism, its exotoxin, and other virulence factors. It is of critical importance that the antigens essential for successful induction of immunity is defined.

TREATMENT
General treatment

Most cases in children are mild, and the patient can usually be cared for at home. Generally speaking, patients with severe disease, especially infants, are better off in a hospital.

Supportive measures such as careful suction to remove tenacious secretions, hydration, nutrition, and electrolyte balance are of great importance in hospitalized patients. Oxygen therapy with increased humidity appears to be beneficial. Administration of human pertussis immune serum globulin has not been established as a useful adjunct to therapy or prevention of disease.

Specific treatment

B. pertussis is sensitive to erythromycin in vitro, and administration eliminates the organism from the nasopharynx and, therefore, shortens the period of communicability. There is some evidence to suggest that if erythromycin

is administered early during the catarrhal stage, the paroxysmal manifestations may be shortened. Ampicillin, tetracycline, or chloramphenicol are considered adequate alternative antimicrobial agents. Secondary bacterial infection may necessitate additional appropriate therapy directed at the responsbile pathogen.

It is recommended that contacts of an infected individual who are under 4 years of age and previously immunized against pertussis should receive a booster dose of vaccine. They should also receive erythromycin, since immunity conferred by vaccine is not absolute. Unimmunized contacts and immunized contacts older than 7 years should receive chemoprophylaxis with erythromycin for approximately 10 days after the contact with the patient has ceased, since immunized persons may asymptomatically harbor organisms and treatment may curtail spread of infection. Human pertussis immune serum globulin may be administered to exposed infants under the age of 2 years who have not been immunized, but protection afforded by this measure is not reliable. The best protective measures for young infants are adequate immunization and avoidance of contact with pertussis.

ACTIVE IMMUNIZATION

Protection of the young infant against pertussis is important because the greatest number of severe complications and highest morbidity occur in this age group. Passive protection is not achieved by the quantity of antibody that traverses the placenta. Routine primary immunization is begun at about 2 months of age unless pertussis is prevalent in the community, in which case immunization should be begun earlier. (See Chapter 35, p. 476.)

Immunization has been successful in the prevention of disease, and widespread usage of vaccine has been associated with the continued decline of reported cases of pertussis in countries where immunization is mandated.

Additional evidence for vaccine efficacy has unfortunately accrued as a result of diminished immunization in several countries, including Denmark and the United Kingdom. In Denmark, an upswing in the number of cases from a few hundred to thousands per year has occurred several years following alterations in immunization requirements, including the use of smaller quantities of antigen. In Great Britain, diminished public acceptance of immunization since 1974 has resulted in pertussis reaching epidemic proportions beginning in 1977-1978. It is estimated that vaccine acceptance has declined from 70% to 80% before 1974 to less than 40%. The resulting epidemic is occurring in younger children who have not received pertussis vaccine. The epidemic in 1982 was the largest since 1957, with 47,508 cases reported from January to September. Studies suggest that current vaccine is 90% effective in prevention of pertussis.

The effectiveness of the vaccine in young children temporarily discouraged the development of purified immunogens. Increased concern with the reputed reactogenicity of the formalinized whole organism vaccine has renewed the study of the organism and pathogenesis of infection. The factor(s) that produces toxicity or contributes to postvaccination encephalopathy have not been defined, and thus it is impossible to test vaccines for this activity. To date, the mouse weight gain test has been employed in the United States as the most accurate animal assessment of potential toxicity of vaccine for humans. More importantly, the definition of F-HA and pertussis toxin have greatly advanced our understanding of the antigens of *B. pertussis* necessary to induce protection. Thus, purified proteins can be administered without other extraneous material from the organism.

Studies conducted in Japan with partially purified vaccine containing F-HA and pertussis toxin are far less reactogenic in children. Thus far, only those children older than 6 to 12 months have been tested. Efficacy data on vaccinees who are household contacts of *B. pertussis* suggest the more purified vaccine does provide protection. It seems probable that a safer, more effective vaccine is on the horizon.

Vaccine-associated encephalopathy is estimated to occur once in 110,000 doses in the United States (Hinman and Koplan, 1984). The National Childhood Encephalopathy Study in the United Kingdom estimated that persistent neurologic damage occurred at a rate of 1:310,000 immunizations (95% confidence limits; 1:5,310,000 to 1:54,000 immunizations) (Alderslade et al., 1981; Miller et al., 1981; Miller et al., 1982; Bellman et al., 1983). The estimated incidence of CNS complications of natural disease has ranged from 1.5% to 14% in hospitalized patients. One third of these die or have severe deficits. The morbidity of prolonged illness and necessity for hospitalization with natural disease make it clear that the risks of immunization are far less than those associated with the natural disease.

REFERENCES

Alderslade R, Bellman MH, Rawson NSB, et al. The National Childhood Encephalopathy Study. In Whooping Cough: reports from the Committee on Safety of Medicines and the Joint Committee on Vaccination and Immunization. London: Department of Health and Social Security, 1981, pp 79-169.

Altemeier WA III, Ayoub EM. Erythromycin prophylaxis for pertussis. Pediatrics 1977;59:623.

Ames RG, et al. Comparison of therapeutic efficacy of 4 agents in pertussis. Pediatrics 1953;11:323.

Ashworth LAE, Robinson A, Irons LI, et al. Antigens in whooping cough vaccine and antibody levels induced by vaccination of children. Lancet (October 15) 1983;2:878-881.

Baraff LJ, Wilkins K, Wehrle PF. The role of antibiotics, immunizations, and adenoviruses in pertussis. Pediatrics 1978;61:224.

Bellman MH, Ross EM, Miller DL. Infantile spasms and pertussis immunization. Lancet 1983;1:1031-1033.

Blom J, Hansen GA, Poulsen FM. Morphology of cells and hemagglutinogens of *Bordetella* species: resolution of substructural units in fimbriae of *Bordetella pertussis*. Infect Immun 1983;42:308-317.

Broome CV, Fraser DW, English WJ. Pertussis—diagnostic methods and surveillances. In Manclark CR, Hill JC, eds. International symposium on pertussis. Washington, DC: U.S. Department of Health, Education and Welfare, 1979. Publication No. (NIH) 79-1830.

Byers RK, Moll FC. Encephalopathies following pertussis vaccine. Pediatrics 1948;1:437.

Centers for Disease Control: Epidemiologic notes and reports: pertussis outbreak—Oklahoma. Morbid Mortal Weekly Rep 1984, pp 2-4, 9-10.

Church MA. Evidence of whooping-cough-vaccine efficacy from the 1978 whooping-cough epidemic in Hertfordshire. Lancet 1979;2:188.

Connor JD. Evidence for an etiologic role of adenoviral infection in pertussis syndrome. N Engl J Med 1970; 283:390.

Eldering G, Hornbeck C, Baker J. Serological studies of *Bordetella pertussis* and related species. J Bacteriol 1957;74:133-136.

Goldman WE, Klapper DC, Baseman JB. Detection, isolation and analysis of a released Bordetella product toxic to cultured tracheal cells. Infect Immun 1982;36:782.

Gordon JE, Hood RI. Whooping cough and its epidemiological anomalies. Am J Med Sci 1951;222:333.

Granston M, Granston G, Lindfosm A, Askelof P. Serologic diagnosis of whooping cough by an enzyme-linked immunosorbent assay using fimbrial hemagglutinin as antigen. J Infect Dis 1982;146:741.

Hinman AR, Koplan JP. Pertussis and pertussis vaccine: reanalysis of benefits, risks and costs. JAMA 1984; 251:3109-3113.

Katada T, Ui M. Islet-activating protein: a modifier of receptor-mediated regulations of rat islet adenylate cyclase. Biol Chem 1981;256:8310.

Klenk EL, Gwaltney JM, Bass JW. Bacteriologically proved pertussis and adenovirus infection. Am J Dis Child 1972;124:203.

Kurt TL, Yeager AS, Guenette S, Dunlop S. Spread of pertussis by hospital staff. JAMA 1972;221:264.

Linnemann CC Jr, et al. Use of pertussis vaccine in an epidemic involving hospital staff. Lancet 1975;2:540.

Manclark CR, Hill JC, ed. International symposium on pertussis. Washington, DC: U.S. Department of Health, Education, and Welfare, 1979. Publication No. (NIH), 79-1839.

Medical Research Council Investigation. The prevention of whooping cough by vaccination. Br Med J 1951;1:1463.

Miller DL, Alderslade R, Ross EM. Whooping cough and whooping cough vaccine: the risks and benefits debate. Epidemiol Rev 1982;4:1-24.

Morley D, Woodland M, Martin WJ. Whooping cough in Nigerian children. Trop Geogr Med 1966;18:169

Morris D, McDonald JC: Failure of hyperimmune gamma globulin to prevent whooping cough. Arch Dis Child 1957;32:163.

Muse KE, Findley D, Allen L, Collier AM. In vitro model of *Bordetella pertussis* infection: pathogenic and microbial interactions. In Manclark CR, Hill JC, eds: International symposium on pertussis. Washington, DC: U.S. Department of Health, Education, and Welfare, 1979. Publication No. (NIH) 79-1830.

Nelson JD. Antibiotic treatment of pertussis. Pediatrics 1969;44:474.

Nelson JD. The changing epidemiology of pertussis in young infants. Am J Dis Child 1978;132:371.

Nelson KE, et al. The role of adenoviruses in the pertussis syndrome. J Pediatr 1975;86:335.

Pittman M. Protective activity of whooping cough convalescent serum and serum IgA level in mice infected with *B. pertussis,* Lancet 1976;2:156.

Pittman M. Pertussis toxin: the cause of harmful effects and prolonged immunity of whooping cough: a hypothesis. Rev Infect Dis 1979;1:401.

Rich AR. On the etiology and pathogenesis of whooping cough. Bull Johns Hopkins Hosp 1932;51:346.

Standfast AFB. The comparison between field trials and mouse protection test against intranasal and intracerebral challenges with *Bordetella pertussis*. Immunology 1958; 1:135-143.

Tamura M, Nogimore K, Murai S, et al. Subunit structure of islet-activating protein, pertussis toxin, in conformity with the A-B model. Biochemistry 1982;21:5516-5522.

Ui M, Katada T, Yajima M. Islet-activating protein in Bordetella pertussis: purification and mechanism of action. In Manclark CR, and Hill JC, eds. International symposium on pertussis. Washington, DC: U.S. Department of Health, Education, and Welfare, 1979. Publication No. (NIH) 79-1830.

Weiss AA, Hewlett EL, Myers GA, Falkow S. Tn5-Induced mutations affecting virulence factors of *Bordetella pertussis*. Infect Immun 1983;42:33-41.

Winter JL. Studies in pertussis immunity. III. Immunization of children with live and killed vaccine. Proc Soc Exp Biol Med 1956;92:832.

21

RABIES (HYDROPHOBIA; RAGE; LYSSA)

Human rabies is a rare, fatal encephalomyelitis caused by a rhabdovirus that is usually transmitted to man by the bite of a rabid animal. In the United States the average annual incidence of human rabies declined from 40 cases during the 1940s to about two cases per year since 1960. Rabies in *domestic* animals has shown a similar decrease. In 1946 there were more than 8000 cases of rabies in dogs, compared with 120 cases in 1977. Therefore the likelihood of human exposure to rabies by domestic animals has decreased greatly, although bites by dogs and cats still give rise to the overwhelming majority of antirabies treatments.

Of 2736 confirmed cases of wildlife rabies in 1977, the distribution was skunks, 59.6%; bats, 23.3%; raccoons, 10.3%; foxes, 4.5%; and mongooses, 1.4%. These data originate in state and federal laboratories of the United States but reflect the worldwide epizootic in wildlife hosts, extending from the Arctic circle to the tropics in both hemispheres. Wild animals constitute the most important source of infection for both man and domestic animals in the United States today.

The general treatment of the bite and the question of whether or not to immunize those persons bitten or scratched by animals suspected of being rabid constitute one of the most difficult problems a physician has to face. Until recently, all available methods of systemic treatment were complicated by numerous instances of adverse reactions, a few of which resulted in death or permanent disability. Furthermore, the decision must be made immediately after exposure because the likelihood that any prophylactic measure will contribute to the prevention of rabies diminishes rapidly as the interval between exposure and treatment increases.

Although occasionally a case of rabies may develop in persons who receive antirabies treatment, evidence from laboratory and field experience in many parts of the world indicates that postexposure prophylaxis can be highly effective when appropriately used.

ETIOLOGY

Rabies virus was the first virus to be transmitted experimentally to a laboratory animal.

Physical and chemical properties

The virus measures about 80 to 180 nm in diameter. It survives storage at 4° C for weeks and in the frozen state for much longer periods in the absence of carbon dioxide. Therefore in dry-ice cabinets it must be stored in sealed glass ampules. It keeps for years in the dried state at 4° C.

Electron microscopy shows that rabies virus is bullet shaped and has a symmetrical structure like a beehive. The single-stranded nucleic acid core is surrounded by a double membrane. Chemical analysis shows that rabies virus is a lipid-containing ribonucleoprotein, which brings about the formation of an inclusion body in the cytoplasm of infected cells; the inclusion body is composed of protein and a small amount of RNA. The general biologic characteristics of rabies are similar to those of subgroup II of the myxoviruses, but on the basis of electron microscopy it has been classified as a rhabdovirus.

Rabies virus also contains specific antigenic material as shown by fluorescent antibody staining methods. It is the only RNA virus inhibited by one DNA inhibitor—arabinosylcytosine (Ara-C). Other DNA inhibitors such as actinomycin D, mitomycin, and 5-fluoro-2′-deoxy-β-uridine (FUDR) enhance rabies virus.

Rabies virus is killed by temperatures of 56° C in 1 hour and 60° C in 5 minutes. It is quickly inactivated by sunlight and ultraviolet light. The virus is resistant to phenol, thimerosal (Merthiolate), and the common antimicrobial agents. It is inactivated by β-propiolactone, ether, formalin, mercury bichloride, and nitric acid.

Host range

Rabies virus has an extensive host range; all warm-blooded animals are susceptible. Introduction of virus by virtually any route usually gives rise to infection, but the intracerebral inoculation with virus from canines almost invariably produces fatal encephalomyelitis. Widely distributed in infected animals, virus is found in the central nervous system (CNS), saliva, urine, lymph, milk, and blood. The salivary glands of infected dogs have yielded high titers of virus; lesser quantities have been detected in the lacrimal glands, pancreas, kidney, adrenal glands, and breast tissue. In man, rabies virus has been recovered from various parts of the CNS, including the olfactory bulbs, horn of Ammon, frontal and occipital cortices, and medulla. It has also been recovered from both cervical and abdominal sympathetic ganglia, salivary glands, adrenal glands, myocardium, walls of both small and large intestines, and mesenteric lymph nodes, and traces of the virus have been found in cervical lymph nodes, tonsillar and pharyngeal tissue, nasal mucosa, pools of liver-spleen-kidney tissues, and lungs. Duffy et al. (1947) established the diagnosis of rabies in a 13-month-old boy by detecting virus in his saliva. Although the number of isolations of rabies virus from human saliva is limited, it is not often looked for; therefore a physician should remember the possibility of its being present in saliva when handling a patient.

The term *street virus* is used to designate strains freshly isolated in the laboratory. Such strains are characterized by incubation periods that vary from 10 days to several months, depending to some extent on the amount of virus injected, and by the production of either prolonged excitation and viciousness (furious type) or depression and paralysis with early onset (dumb type) or, as occurs in most infected dogs, some manifestations of both types. Street virus rabies is almost always associated with the presence of Negri bodies.

The term *fixed virus* refers to strains transferred in series from brain to brain, usually in the rabbit, characterized by a short and constant incubation period of 4 to 6 days, absence of Negri bodies, and diminished ability to spread centrifugally. The Pasteur strain of fixed virus has been maintained in rabbits since its original isolation in 1882 and is the strain generally used for human vaccination (Semple type).

Rabies virus has also been propagated in both chick and duck embryos and in tissue cultures of mouse and chick embryos and hamster kidney, as well as a human diploid cell line (WI-38). After many serial transfers were made in the chick embryo, the Flury strain became attenuated, that is, lost its pathogenicity for animals injected intramuscularly but retained its immunogenic capacity. This modified living virus is being used for immunization of dogs. A killed virus vaccine prepared from duck embryos has been used in man since 1957; its main advantages are the absence of CNS tissue in the vaccine and decreased incidence of the neuromyelitic accidents that may follow injections of Semple vaccine. The duck embryo vaccine has been replaced by an inactivated human diploid cell rabies vaccine (see p. 530).

Immunologic properties

Both neutralizing and complement-fixing antibodies are formed in the course of rabies infection, and they may develop as a result of vaccination. Only one antigenic type of rabies virus has been demonstrated. At least five other viruses serologically related to rabies have been isolated from bats, shrews, midges, mosquitoes, and humans in certain areas of Africa. They are antigenically distinguishable from rabies virus. Hyperimmune rabies serum containing high titers of neutralizing antibody has been prepared from horses immunized repeatedly. It has been used along with rabies vaccine for passive immunization of exposed individuals. Sensitivity to equine proteins has resulted in serum sickness in nearly 40% of adult recipients; anaphylactic reactions have also been reported. In the United States and in some other nations the equine product has been virtually replaced by human rabies immune globulin (HRIG), a concentrate of cold ethanol fractionated plasma from hyperimmunized human donors (Hattwick et al., 1974). The HRIG is of at least comparable efficacy and is not accompanied by adverse reactions other than local pain at the site of injection and slight febrile response.

PATHOLOGY

The principal changes produced by rabies virus are found throughout the CNS; these consist mainly of neuronal necrosis, most pronounced in the thalamus, hypothalamus, substantia nigra, pons, and medulla. The cranial nerve nuclei are severely damaged, and mononuclear cell infiltration is likely to be greater here than elsewhere. The spinal cord shows neuronal changes, especially in the posterior horns.

The most distinctive feature of the pathologic changes is the presence of Negri bodies, which are pathognomonic of rabies. These specific inclusion bodies are found in the cytoplasm of nerve cells and consist of acidophilic structures about 2 to 10 μm in diameter, are sharply demarcated, and are usually round or oval; they occur most abundantly in the hippocampus (horn of Ammon), basal ganglia, pons, and medulla.

Changes similar to those in the brain may be found in the sympathetic ganglia and dorsal root ganglia of the spinal cord. The salivary glands may show degenerative changes of the acinar cells and neurons; Negri bodies may be found in the latter.

PATHOGENESIS

Available evidence indicates that rabies virus multiplies initially in the muscle at the inoculation site and subsequently replicates in peripheral nerves and dorsal root ganglia as it makes its way from the neuromuscular junction via the axoplasm to the CNS. The mechanisms of this central migration remain undefined. After multiplication in neurons centrally, the virus then travels peripherally along nerve pathways to invade many distal tissues and organs. Both humoral and cell-mediated immunity are involved in the host defenses mobilized against the infection. Viremia does not appear to play a significant role in pathogenesis so that humoral antibody may be limited in its effectiveness. Interferon is elaborated by the host as another defense against further virus replication and spread.

CLINICAL MANIFESTATIONS

The incubation period is usually between 1 and 2 months, but wide ranges from 10 days to 1 year have been observed; it is likely to be short after multiple severe lacerations and the introduction of large doses of virus.

The illness may begin, as it does in other kinds of encephalitis, with prodromal symptoms of malaise, fever, headache, anorexia, nausea, sore throat, drowsiness, irritability, and restlessness. The patient may complain of hyperesthesia, paresthesia, or anesthesia in the area of the bite and along the course of the involved peripheral nerves.

Progress of the infection is associated with increased anxiety and hyperexcitability accompanied by mounting fever. Delirium, involuntary twitching movements, and generalized convulsions are often seen. Maniacal behavior may alternate with periods of lethargy. Violent spasmodic contractions of the muscles of the patient's mouth, pharynx, or larynx when he attempts to drink or when he merely sees water are the striking characteristics that gave rabies its common name—*hydrophobia*. These painful spasms may be set off by relatively mild stimuli such as noise or light touch. The patient may drool profusely from the mouth in order to avoid the act of swallowing, which is associated with painful spasm.

Within a few days the patient's condition worsens, the pulse rate increases, respirations become more labored or irregular, and the temperature rises steadily. Periods of responsiveness become less frequent, and muscular spasms may give way to paralysis. Peripheral vascular collapse, coma, and death quickly follow. The disease runs its entire course usually in no more than 5 to 6 days and usually ends fatally.

In 5% to 20% of patients, the clinical picture of rabies may be that of an ascending, symmetrical, flaccid paralysis without hyperexcitability or spasmodic muscle contractions. This resembles the Guillain-Barré syndrome so that, in the absence of known history of rabies virus exposure, such patients may go through the entire course of illness with no suspicion of the diagnosis of rabies until the characteristic findings are observed at autopsy (Baer, 1975).

The cerebrospinal fluid (CSF) is usually normal; its pressure is normal or slightly increased. The fluid is clear, and in most cases the number of cells is not increased. In patients with pleocytosis, the cell count rarely exceeds 100, and the cells are mostly mononuclear leukocytes. There may be a slight increase in the level of protein.

The white blood cell count shows a slight increase in number of leukocytes that may reach 20,000 to 30,000, with a predominance of polymorphonuclear leukocytes. Abnormal urinary findings may include albumin, casts, reducing substances, and acetone.

CASE 1. An 11-year-old boy was bitten on the forehead by a dog 32 days before onset of the disease; the wound was cauterized, but no antirabies vaccine was given. The patient's illness began with headache, drowsiness, anorexia, and malaise that progressed in 2 days to delirium accompanied by fever and vomiting. Delirium associated with visual hallucinations and delusions of persecution were the outstanding and persistently recurring features. He was often manic and struck and bit attendants. Except for transient difficulty in swallowing and slurring of speech on the fourth and fifth days, there was a striking absence of localizing neurologic signs. The CSF was normal. The temperature was sustained between 38.9° and 40.3° C (102° and 104.5° F) for a week. On the tenth day, irregular respirations were observed with periods of apnea lasting as long as 45 seconds. He died on the twelfth day from respiratory and circulatory failure. Postmortem touch preparations of the hippocampus showed typical Negri bodies, and rabies virus was isolated from various parts of the brain and other tissues.

DIAGNOSIS

For the most part, rabies is easily recognized. The characteristic history is that of an animal bite followed in several weeks or months by the onset of overwhelming encephalitis; the CNS signs include those of excitement, anxiety, maniacal behavior, and delirium associated with spasmodic contractions of muscles concerned with swallowing and speech. Clinical laboratory findings are generally of little help.

Tetanus may be confused with rabies. Excitement accompanied by spasms of the laryngeal and pharyngeal muscles is not so common in tetanus and is virtually constant in rabies. Tetanus is characterized by trismus and spasmodic contractions of the muscles of the body.

Diagnosis of rabies can be established by detection of rabies virus in saliva obtained during life or in the CNS, salivary glands, or other tissues obtained postmortem. Direct fluorescence of corneal smears and of skin biopsies from the back of the neck reveal rabies-specific antigens early in the patient's clinical course. At autopsy, direct fluorescence of cells of horn of Ammon is a sensitive test (Plotkin and Koprowski, 1979).

PROGNOSIS

Rabies was considered to be 100% lethal until recent years.

CASE 2. Probable human rabies with survival. On October 10, 1970, in Lima, Ohio, a 6-year-old boy was bitten on his left thumb by a bat while he was asleep. The bat was captured by the boy's father and submitted to the Ohio Health Department, where rabies was confirmed on examination of the brain by fluorescent antibody (FA) technique. On October 14 a 14-day course of treatment with duck-embryo vaccine (DEV) was begun on the boy.

The boy showed no symptoms until October 30, when he complained of neck pain, and during the next several days he bacame lethargic and showed malaise and anorexia. His condition worsened and on November 4 he entered a local hospital with a temperature of 40° C (104° F). During the next 10 days, the boy's temperature dropped, but he became more lethargic. On November 13 stiffness of the neck developed, and the CSF yielded 125 white blood cells. During the next several days, the boy's condition deteriorated; he showed total aphasia, weakness of left arm, bilateral Babinski's signs, and coma. A tracheostomy was done because of respiratory difficulty, tachypnea, and increased pharyngeal secretions. The patient was in and out of coma for a week and then gradually began to improve. In December his condition continued to improve and he was able to walk with assistance and speak in short sentences. As of October 1971, the patient was reported to be normal.

Efforts to establish the diagnosis included biopsy of the brain, which was negative for rabies virus by culture and FA tests. There were no detectable serum antibodies to St. Louis encephalitis, eastern or western equine encephalomyelitis, or leptospirosis. Serum complement-fixing antibody titer to California virus was 1:8 on October 13, and biweekly determinations through December 3 remained the same. Serum neutralizing antibody titers against rabies were 1:300 on November 13, rose to 1:37,000 on November 27, and remained between 1:39,000 and 1:47,000 during December and January. The question arose, Could the 14-day course of treatment with DEV be responsible for these high antibody titers? In answer it can be said that after a 14-day course of treatment with DEV, rabies antibody titers rarely exceed 1:500 and therefore that rabies titers of the magnitude seen in this patient strongly support the diagnosis of rabies. Indeed, the only aspect of this patient's course not compatible with rabies infection is recovery. The clinical management of this patient included the continuous monitoring of cardiac and pulmonary functions, the prevention of hypoxia by prophylactic tracheostomy, and intensive pulmonary assistance. These measures may have contributed to the arrest of clinical illness and eventual recovery.

EPIDEMIOLOGIC FACTORS

Geographic distribution of rabies is known to include most of the world except the British Isles, the Scandinavian countries, the Netherlands, Switzerland, Australia, New Zealand, and the Hawaiian Islands. It is common in Africa and Southwest Asia and is particularly prevalent in India. In the United States the average number of reported cases in man has dropped from 22 per year during the period from 1946 through 1950 to about 2 per year since 1960.

Rabies occurs in any *climate* and in any *season*.

Rabies is no respecter of *age*. The incidence is high in children, probably because of their increased chance of exposure resulting from their friendliness toward animals and their inability to defend themselves against attack.

The *natural reservoirs* of rabies are wild and domestic animals. From the ecologic viewpoint, two types of rabies can be distinguished: (1) the natural form of the disease, occurring in wild animals such as foxes, skunks, raccoons, wolves, coyotes, jackals, mongooses, weasles, squirrels, and bats and (2) the domestic form occurring in dogs, cats, and cattle.

In 1977 and again in 1979 the Mexico-Texas border near Laredo experienced problems with packs of rabid stray dogs responsible for at least two cases of rabies among children who were bitten. Public health groups mobilized vaccination clinics for tens of thousands of domestic dogs plus control programs for stray animals.

During the last two decades in the United States there has been a great decline in the importance of dogs as vectors of rabies. Today the most important source of infection for both man and domestic animals is found in wild animals, especially skunks, foxes, bats, and raccoons.

In general the *attack rate* in persons bitten by rabid animals is hard to estimate; it depends on the extent and location of the bites and the dose of virus entering the wound. Lacerations of the head and neck are followed by higher attack rates than those of the feet and ankles. The amount of virus reaching the nerves is influenced by several additional factors: (1) lack of virus in saliva of 50% of rabid dogs; (2) protection afforded by clothing so that little or no virus enters the wound; and (3) removal or inactivation of virus by soap and water, benzalkonium (Zephiran), or other agents.

Winkler (1968) has pointed out the possibility of airborne respiratory infection acquired in caves inhabited by large numbers of infected bats. Although transmission by inhalation is probably very rare, it must be considered in patients with compatible clinical illnesses who have a history of visits to bat-infested caves. Spelunkers may be listed among those with "high-risk" vocations or avocations for whom preexposure prophylaxis is justified.

A highly unusual case was reported (Houff et al., 1979) of human-to-human transmission of rabies. This resulted from a corneal transplant to a healthy recipient from a donor who had died of a CNS illness with progressive ascending paralysis similar to Guillain-Barré syndrome. One month after the transplant procedure the recipient developed an acute fatal meningoencephalitis, which only at autopsy was recognized as rabies. Studies of the donor's and recipient's eyes then demonstrated the presence of rabies virus in both.

Attack rates in persons bitten by rabid animals and the effect of specific prophylactic measures are shown in Table 21-1. Sabeti et al. (1964) described the results of treatment of individuals bitten in Iran by wolves proved to be rabid. The evidence is clear that the combination of hyperimmune serum and vaccine was superior to vaccine alone, especially in cases of head bites, which are known to be associated with shorter incubation periods and higher attack rates than in those in which the head and neck are not involved.

Table 21-1. Attack rates in human beings bitten by animals proved to be rabid—effect of specific preventive measures

Authors	Persons bitten		Number of rabies deaths	Mortality (percent)	Type of prophylaxis
	Number	On head			
Sabeti et al., 1964*	96	Yes	38	40	Vaccine alone
	71	No	6	8.4	
TOTAL	167		44	26	
	50	Yes	3	6	Serum and vaccine
	24	No	0	0	
TOTAL	74		3	4	
Veeraraghaven et al., 1964*	153	†	77	50	No vaccine
	581	†	49	8.4	Vaccine

*Cited by Johnson HN: Rabies virus. In Horsfall FL, Jr, Tamm I, eds: Viral and rickettsial diseases of man. ed. 4. Philadelphia: J. B. Lippincott Co., 1965, pp 826 and 832.
†No data.

In 1964 Veeraraghaven et al. (cited by Johnson, 1965) compared the attack rates in persons bitten by proved rabid animals in India during 1946 to 1962, when a total of 581 persons exposed in this manner were given a complete course of antirabies vaccine; of these, 49 (or 8.4%) died. By contrast, of 153 persons who were not vaccinated, 77 (or 50%) died (Table 21-1).

With the new human diploid cell strain rabies vaccines, first studied in humans in 1971 (Wiktor et al. 1977), there have now been several convincing studies of efficacy in postexposure rabies prophylaxis. Bahmanyar et al. (1976) described the successful protection of eight groups totaling 45 persons severely bitten in Iran by six dogs and two wolves proved to be rabid. A total of only six doses of vaccine was administered to each patient plus an initial injection of antirabies serum prepared in mules. None developed rabies despite deep wounds of the extremities and in some cases the face and head. In Germany, all of 31 persons bitten by animals proved to be rabid were protected from rabies by a similar vaccine schedule (Kuwert et al., 1976).

PREVENTIVE MEASURES

The most recent development in the evolution of rabies vaccines, which began with Pasteur in 1885, has been the preparation of a new antigen from virus grown in human diploid cell cultures (WI-38), inactivated and concentrated. This ma-

terial is highly immunogenic, free of serious reactions, and effective in postexposure prophylaxis as described previously. It has also been reliable in stimulating high antibody titers when administered in a three-dose schedule to "high-risk" individuals before exposure (Plotkin and Wiktor, 1979).

For full information on rabies prophylaxis see Chapter 35, p. 530.

REFERENCES

Anderson LJ, Nicholson KG, Tauxe RV, et al. Human rabies in the United States, 1960 to 1979: epidemiology, diagnosis, and prevention. Ann. Intern Med 1984;100:728-735.

Baer GM, editor. The natural history of rabies, 2 volumes, New York:Academic Press, Inc., 1975.

Bahmanyar M, et al. Successful protection of humans exposed to rabies infection. Postexposure treatment with the new human diploid cell rabies vaccine and antirabies serum. JAMA 1976;236:2751.

Bhatt DP, et al. Human rabies: diagnosis, complications and management. Am J Dis Child 1974;127:862.

Center for Disease Control: Current trends—human diploid cell strain rabies vaccine. Morbid Mortal Weekly Rep 1978a;27:333.

Centers for Disease Control: Rabies surveillance report—annual summary 1977. U.S. Department of Health, Education, and Welfare, Public Health Service, September 1978b.

Cheetham HD, Hart J, Coghill NF, Box B. Rabies with myocarditis. Two cases in England. Lancet 1970;1:921.

Corey L, Hattwick MAW. Treatment of persons exposed to rabies. JAMA 1975;232:272.

Crick J, Brown F. Efficacy of rabies vaccine prepared from virus grown in duck embryo. Lancet 1970;1:1106.

Debbie JG: Rabies. Prog Med Viral 1974;18:241.

Duffy CE, Wooley PV, Nolting WS. Rabies: a case report with notes on the isolation of the virus from saliva. J Pediatr 1947;31:440.

Garner WR, Jones DO, Pratt E. Problems associated with rabies pre-exposure prophylaxis. JAMA 1976;235:1131.

Greenberg M, Childress J. Vaccination against rabies with duck-embryo and Semple vaccines. JAMA 1960;173:333.

Habel K. Rabies prophylaxis in man. Peidatics 1957;19:923.

Hafkin B, Hattwick MAW, Smith JS. A comparison of a WI-38 vaccine and duck embryo vaccine for preexposure rabies prophylaxis. Am J Epidemiol 1978;107:439.

Hattwick MA, Hochberg FH, Tandrigan PJ, Gregg MB. Skunk-associated human rabies. JAMA 1972;222:44.

Hattwick MA, et al. Recovery from rabies; a case report. Ann Intern Med 1972;76:931.

Hattwick MAW, et al. Postexposure rabies prophylaxis with human rabies immune globulin. JAMA 1974;227:407.

Houff SA, et al. Human-to-human transmission of rabies virus by corneal transplant. N Engl J Med 1979;300:603.

Johnson HN. The significance of the Negri body in the diagnosis and epidemiology of rabies. Ill Med J 1942;81:382.

Johnson HN. Rabies virus. In Horsfall JL Jr, Tamm I, eds. Viral and rickettsial infections of man. ed. 4. Philadelphia: J.B. Lippincott Co., 1965.

Kuwert EK, Marcus I, Hoher PG. Neutralizing and complement-fixing antibody responses in pre- and post-exposure vaccinees to a rabies vaccine produced in human diploid cells. J Biol Stand 1976;4:249.

Miller A, Nathanson N. Rabies: recent advances in pathogenesis and control. Ann Neurol 1977;2:511.

Mozar HN, et al. Myelopathy after duck embryo rabies vaccine. JAMA 1973;224:1605.

Pasteur L. Methode pour prevenir la rage apres morsure. C R Acad Sci 1885;101:765.

Pasteur L, Chamberland Roux and Thullier: Sur la rage. C R Acad Sci 1881;98:457.

Pawan JL. Rabies in the vampire bat of Trinidad with special reference to the clinical course and the latency of infection. Ann Trop Med Parasitol 1936;30:410.

Plotkin SA, Koprowski H. Phobia of hydrophobia justified. N Engl J Med 1979;300:621.

Plotkin S, Wiktor TJ. Rabies vaccination. Annu, Rev Med 1978;29:583.

Plotkin SA, Wiktor T. Vaccination of children with human cell culture rabies vaccine. Pediatrics 1979;63:219.

Rubin RH, et al. A case of human rabies in Kansas. J Infect Dis 1970;122:318.

Rubin RH, et al. Immunoglobulin response to rabies vaccine in man. Lancet 1971;2:625.

Rubin RH, et al. Adverse reactions to duck embryo rabies vaccine. Ann Intern Med 1973;78:643.

Sabeti A, Bahmanyar M, Ghodssi M, Baltazard M. Traitement des mordus par loups enragés en Iran. Ann Inst Pasteur 1964;106:303.

Sabin AB, Ruchman I. Spread of virus in an unvaccinated case of human rabies. Proc Soc Exp Biol Med 1940;44:572.

Semple D. On the nature of rabies and antirabic treatment. Br Med J 1919;2:333.

Shope RE, Baer G, Allen WP. Summary of a workshop on the immunopathology of rabies. J Infect Dis 1979;140:431.

Turner GS, et al. Human diploid cell strain rabies vaccine. Lancet 1976;1:1379.

Wiktor TJ, Plotkin SA, Koprowski H. Development and clinical trials of the new human rabies vaccine of tissue culture (human diploid cell) origin. Dev Biol Stand 1977;40:3.

Wilson JM, Hettiarachchi J, Wijesuriya LM. Presenting features and diagnosis of rabies. Lancet 1975;2:1139.

Winkler WG. Airborne rabies virus infection. Bull Wildl Dis Assoc 1968;4:37.

22

ACUTE RESPIRATORY INFECTIONS

ETIOLOGY

Throughout the world, infections of the respiratory tract and those of the gastrointestinal tract compete as the most significant causes of total morbidity and mortality among infants and children. The definition of a relatively small number of etiologic agents responsible for gastroenteritis (Chapter 9) has led to some optimism regarding eventual control and prevention. Oral rehydration therapy offers a means of simple acute treatment, highly effective in the reduction of morbidity and mortality. In contrast, the enormous multiplicity of agents—viral, bacterial, fungal, and others—identified as the pathogens of respiratory infections provokes no such optimism for these illnesses. Despite the development of abundant new antibiotics, their impact has necessarily been only on that smaller portion of acute respiratory disease caused by bacteria and the even tinier segment attributed to fungi.

Acute respiratory tract infections have been studied in the past with the principal emphasis on their immediate morbidity and mortality. Acute lower respiratory tract infections are listed as the third most common cause of death in infants and children 1 month to 14 years of age in developed nations (Forfar, 1984). In recent years a series of investigations have indicated that some acute infections of infancy and childhood may predispose to recurrent episodes of lower respiratory tract illness and chronic pulmonary changes in later life. Even among children, chronic respiratory disease, often initiated by acute respiratory tract infections, may be responsible for 50% of all school absenteeism attributed to chronic illness (Dees, 1977).

Acute respiratory tract infections are by far the most common acute illnesses encountered in the United States. Although the death rate due to these infections is generally low, the incidence of disease is very high. Longitudinal studies of these illnesses indicate that children have an average of six episodes per year. Acute respiratory infection leads all other acute conditions in terms of loss of productive effort in both school and industry.

Acute respiratory tract illnesses comprise a spectrum of clinical entities ranging from the mild afebrile common cold to severe pneumonia. In between are pharyngitis, laryngitis, croup (laryngotracheobronchitis), bronchitis, and bronchiolitis. Some of the etiologic agents are associated with specific clinical syndromes; for example, rhinoviruses are most often associated with the common cold, respiratory syncytial virus with pneumonia and bronchiolitis of infants, parainfluenza viruses with croup, and *Mycoplasma pneumoniae* with atypical pneumonia.

This formidable problem is complicated by the profusion and heterogeneity of the etiologic agents. More than 200 nonbacterial agents etiologically related to acute respiratory infections have been identified and will be described later. Since only a relatively few etiologic agents are susceptible to antimicrobial treatment, whereas others, mostly viral, are not, the clinician is challenged to be precise. From a practical point of view, it is often difficult to confirm a viral etiology during the acute phase of illness when precision is most needed. By the same token, successful culture of bacteria from the nasopharynx does not establish those bacteria as etiologic agents. It has been estimated that far more than 90% of acute respiratory tract infections are caused primarily by nonbacterial agents.

The purpose of this chapter is initially to describe various etiologic agents—viruses, *Mycoplasma* species, bacteria, chlamydiae, and fungi—associated with acute respiratory tract illness and to estimate the contribution made by each agent to the various clinical syndromes. A second section is concerned with clinical manifestations and treatment of acute respiratory tract infections.

Viruses

In 1940 only a handful of viruses had been established as etiologic agents of respiratory tract diseases of humans; today the total number is well over 200. *Respiratory syncytial* (RS) *virus* appears to be the most important cause of respiratory tract infection in infants, with involvement of the lower respiratory tract—bronchitis, bronchiolitis, and pneumonia. *Parainfluenza viruses* are the most important causes of croup and contribute to other infections of the respiratory tract, both upper and lower. Primary infections with either RS virus or the parainfluenza viruses are likely to be severe, whereas subsequent reinfections with the same virus are not uncommon but tend to be milder.

Although the importance of *influenza viruses* varies from year to year, depending on periodic occurrence of epidemics, it is clear that other agents are responsible for most nonepidemic respiratory tract illnesses. The contribution of *adenoviruses* is curious in that, although they played a prominent role in epidemics of respiratory tract disease in military recruits (especially types 4 and 7), they are responsible for only a small portion of respiratory tract illnesses among college students of comparable age and for no more than about 5% to 10% of respiratory tract infections in children.

Rhinoviruses are chiefly responsible for the common cold; more than 113 distinct serologic types have been reported. Three or more *coronaviruses* contribute to the cause of common

colds in adults. *Group A Coxsackie virus* type 21 (formerly Coe virus) and other members of this group have been implicated in respiratory tract illness. *Group B Coxsackie viruses* have been linked with acute febrile respiratory tract illness, with pleurodynia, and with influenzalike illness. *ECHO viruses* of many types have been associated with respiratory tract infection. *Varicella-zoster virus* is known to give rise to severe pneumonia in patients, usually adults, with chickenpox. It may also cause serious pneumonia in children or adults who are immunocompromised (Chapter 33). The relationship of herpesvirus hominis to acute tonsillopharyngitis with vesicles or ulcers has been recognized for some time (p. 140). At its onset, measles appears to be an upper respiratory tract infection; later manifestations include croup, bronchitis, bronchiolitis, and pneumonia. Measles virus may cause giant-cell pneumonia in the absence of the other typical findings of measles. *Lymphocytic choriomeningitis virus* may occasionally be associated with respiratory tract manifestations, including pneumonia. In infectious mononucleosis, sore throat with tonsillopharyngitis is a prominent feature, and the clinical picture of atypical pneumonia is seen in a small number of patients.

In Table 22-1 the viruses most frequently associated with respiratory tract infections are presented in tabular form with the clinical syndromes they cause.

Orthomyxoviruses and paramyxoviruses. The orthomyxoviruses implicated in human respiratory infections include influenza virus types A, B, and C. Paramyxoviruses include parainfluenza virus types 1, 2, 3, and 4; measles virus; and respiratory syncytial virus (RSV). These viruses have the following biophysical characteristics. They are of medium size, ranging from 100 to 300 nm and are generally pleomorphic. They possess a nucleic acid core consisting of RNA. They possess essential lipids, and they are inactivated by ether and acids. They possess the capacity to produce hemagglutination, hemadsorption, and virus elution. Their cytopathic effect, if present, consists of the formation of giant cells or syncytia and cell lysis. Respiratory viruses are generally transmitted via aerosolized droplets shed by infected individuals. These are deposited on surface respiratory tract mucosal cells to which virus may attach and then pene-

Table 22-1. Viruses in acute respiratory tract disease of man

	Serotypes		
Group of agents	Number	Number associated with respiratory illness	Clinical syndromes
Respiratory syncytial virus	1?	1?	Bronchiolitis; pneumonia; bronchitis; upper respiratory tract infection
Parainfluenza virus	4	4	Croup; bronchitis; bronchiolitis; pneumonia
Influenza virus	3	2	Influenza; croup; upper respiratory tract infection; pneumonia
Coronavirus	3 or more	3+	Common colds in adults
Nonpolio enteroviruses	68	Variable	Febrile pharyngitis (pediatric age group); colds in military recruits; herpangina; pleurodynia
Rhinovirus	113+	113+	Common colds
Adenovirus	40	Many	Both upper and lower respiratory tract disease in children, infants, and military recruits; bronchiolitis obliterans; pertussis syndrome

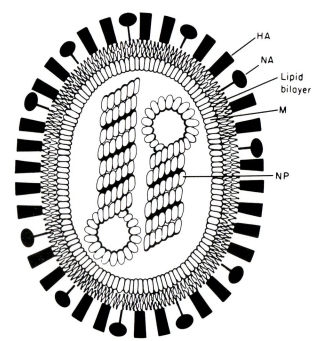

Fig. 22-1. Schematic diagram of the arrangement suggested for the structural components in the influenza virion. The two types of surface projections, hemagglutinin subunits consisting of HA polypeptides and neuraminidase subunits consisting of NA polypeptides, are on the external surface of a lipid bilayer; the mode of their attachment to the bilayer is unknown. On the internal surface of the bilayer is a layer of the membrane polypeptide M, and within this are the ribonucleoprotein composed of NP polypeptides and the viral RNA. The location of the P polypeptides is uncertain. (From Compano, RW, and Choppin PW. Compr Virol 1975; 4:198.)

Table 22-2. Designation of influenza type A strains prevalent in the United States

Prototype strain designation	Surface antigens		Years of prevalence
	HA	NA	
A/PR/34	HO	N1	1934-1946
A/FM/47	H1	N1	1947-1956
A/Japan/57	H2	N2	1957-1968
A/Hong Kong/68	H3	N2	1968-1972
A/England/72	H3	N2	1972-1974
A/Port Chalmers/73	H3	N2	1974-1975
A/Victoria/75	H3	N2	1975-1978
A/New Jersey/76	Hsw1	N1	1976-1977
A/Texas/77	H3	N2	1977-1978
A/USSR/77	H1	N1	1977-1979
A/Brazil/78	H1	N1	1978-1979
A/Bangkok/79	H3	N2	1979-1981
A/Philippines/82	H3	N2	1982-1983
A/Chile/83	H1	N1	1983-1984

trate the lining cells of a susceptible host. Contact with contaminated materials and direct digital inoculation of the conjunctiva or nasal mucosa may provide an alternate route for rhinovirus infections (Hendley et al., 1973). For most viruses inhalation of infected aerosols appears to be the route of major importance.

Influenza viruses. Influenza viruses A, B, and C were first described in 1933, 1940, and 1949, respectively. They are orthomyxoviruses that are classified on the basis of their ribonucleoprotein antigen. The single-stranded RNA genome is found in eight segments. The viruses are pleomorphic and usually spherical particles, 80 to 100 nm in diameter (Fig. 22-1). The surface of the virus is covered by two types of projections 10 nm long, one possessing hemagglutinin activity (HA) and the other neuraminidase activity (NA). The HA spike is responsible for the agglutination of erythrocytes by the virus. The NA spike is responsible for the receptor-destroying activity of type A and B viruses.

Influenza viruses vary in their antigenic stability. Type A virus is least stable and is characterized by frequent antigenic changes, type C virus is most stable, and type B is intermediate between A and C. The classification of influenza viruses before 1972 was based on the type of ribonucleoprotein antigen and the subtype was dependent on the hemagglutinin antigen, such

as A_2. However, when it became obvious that neuraminidase undergoes antigenic variation that is independent of hemagglutinin variation, it was proposed that the influenza virus strain be designated by the antigenic type of its hemagglutinin and neuraminidase—for example, A/Hong Kong/68 (H3N2) (Table 22-2). This designation indicates that the virus was isolated from a person in Hong Kong in 1968 and that it contains HA type 3 and NA type 2 antigens.

The hemagglutinin is the specific envelope antigen and the differences in this antigen among various strains of virus can be identified by hemagglutination-inhibition (HI) tests. The virus is neutralized by antibody to the hemagglutinin. In contrast, neuraminidase antibody does not neutralize the virus, but it does modify infection, probably by its effect on the release of virus from the cells.

In each of the last four decades, major variants emerged whose dominant antigens were relatively new to most people. It appeared therefore that one factor relating to the cyclic occurrence of influenza A epidemics was the periodic change in dominant antigenic composition of the virus that vitiated the previously existing specific immunity. Another factor was the periodic waxing and waning of herd immunity.

Since the breadth of antibody is dependent upon experience with strains of varied composition, inexperienced children exhibit the highest incidence of infection by any and all strains and also most limited reflection of viral antigens. With the passage of time, antibody to succeeding dominants is acquired, but large gaps develop in the immunity of the community to viral antigens which prevailed when the older segments of the population were young. These gaps invite a rearrangement of viral antigens to enter the population and provide the opportunity for rapid passage and development of epidemic potency.*

Because influenza A viruses have been isolated from horses, pigs, and many species of birds, the prevailing theory of the constantly shifting antigens suggests that genetic reassortments occur with strains of influenza in these animal and avian reservoirs.

---

*Francis, T., Jr.: Problems of acute respiratory disease, Yale J. Biol. Med. 34:191, 1961-1962.

The preceding description also fits influenza virus B but to a lesser degree. Comparatively little is known about influenza virus C; outbreaks of disease from it are usually limited to young children and to persons in military installations. In contrast to influenza viruses A and B, influenza virus C seems to have a single stable antigen. Antibody appears early in life and persists in persons in older age groups, in whom the disease is seldom seen.

Influenza virus reaches the respiratory tract via droplet infection. After a short incubation period of 1 to 2 days it is possible to detect virus in the nasopharynx. Viremia is probably a very rare occurrence. The neuraminidase of the virus decreases the viscosity of the mucous covering of the respiratory tract, thereby exposing the cellular receptors and facilitating the spread of virus-containing fluid to the lower respiratory tract. If specific antibody is present at the portal of entry the infection may be aborted. This can be achieved by high levels of serum antibody and/or the presence of local secretory antibody (IgA).

Pathologic changes include evidence of inflammation of the upper respiratory tract with destruction of ciliated epithelial cells. If the infection has progressed to involve the lungs, the findings include interstitial inflammation, necrosis of the bronchiolar and alveolar epithelium, and alveoli filled with RBCs, WBCs, and hyaline membranes. Secondary bacterial infection may be caused by staphylococci, pneumococci, or *H. influenzae*.

Parainfluenza viruses. Parainfluenza viruses comprise four antigenic types, namely, 1, 2, 3, and 4, which appear to be very stable and have not exhibited the continuing antigenic variation so characteristic of influenza A viruses. Parainfluenza viruses have certain biophysical characteristics in common with the influenza viruses, but they also have some unique characteristics not shared by influenza viruses, including the ability to hemolyze certain kinds of red blood cells and to fuse cell membranes. Unlike the influenza viruses they possess a single surface spike for both HA and NA. They are pleomorphic with diameters 150 to 200 nm; their genome is nonsegmented negative stranded RNA coding for six structural proteins.

Most parainfluenza viruses are readily detected and grown in primary or continuous tissue cultures of monkey and human kidney. Cytopathogenic effects may be scant or lacking in first passage, but the presence of virus can be recognized by adding guinea pig RBCs to the culture and observing adsorption of the red cells to the kidney monolayer (hemadsorption technique).

Parainfluenza viruses isolated from patients multiply very poorly in embryonated chickens' eggs, but tissue culture isolates of each of the four types have been adapted to growth in the amniotic and allantoic cavities.

Clinical syndromes associated with parainfluenza viruses. Parainfluenza virus types 1, 2, and 3 have been recovered from 40% of 2359 infants and children with croup, bronchitis, bronchiolitis, or pneumonia and from 6% of 3377 children with mild rhinitis, pharyngitis, or bronchitis or a combination of the three (Parrott et al., 1962). Parainfluenza virus type 1 has been found chiefly in association with croup and is a major cause of severe croup in young children. Altogether, types 1, 2, and 3 constitute the agents most commonly associated with croup.

Serologic studies indicate that primary infection with parainfluenza virus type 1 usually takes place in the first 3 to 5 years of life. Most adults have circulating antibodies. The presence of antibody, however, does not preclude reinfection. Severity of illness is related to previous experience with the virus and, accordingly, to age. Thus primary infection is usually expressed as febrile respiratory illness, and about one third of the patients have involvement of the lower respiratory tract. Reinfection results in either mild upper respiratory tract disease or no disease. Mild afebrile coldlike illness was observed in adult human volunteers given parainfluenza virus types 1 and 3 experimentally via the nose and throat. Most of the volunteers had specific neutralizing antibody before they were given virus, and there was no difference in serum antibody levels between those in whom illness developed and those who escaped illness. The presence of serum antibody did not prevent illness, but the illness was mild and confined to the upper respiratory tract.

In later studies conducted with human volunteers, all of whom had neutralizing antibody to parainfluenza virus type 1 detectable in the serum, Smith et al. in 1966 showed that the presence or absence of neutralizing antibody

(IgA) activity in the nasal secretions was critical in determining whether or not the volunteer would be reinfected after challenge with parainfluenza virus type 1 (Table 22-3). Although an inactivated type 1 parainfluenza virus vaccine stimulated the production of neutralizing antibody in the serum of adult volunteers, the response in their nasal secretions was minimal. The implications of these important studies are (1) that the presence of secretory IgA antibodies in the nasal secretions is a better index of resistance than the level of serum antibody and (2) that a live attenuated virus vaccine offers a better chance than inactivated virus vaccine to stimulate the production of neutralizing antibodies in nasal secretions and resistance, especially if it were administered intranasally.

Respiratory syncytial virus. RSV is now established as the most important single agent responsible for respiratory disease in early life. RS virus was first isolated in 1956 from a chimpanzee with coryza by Morris et al., who named it chimpanzee coryza agent (CCA). The next year Chanock and Finberg recovered the first strains in human beings from children with pneumonia, described the characteristic syncytial cytopathic changes, and suggested the term *respiratory syncytial virus* (1957).

Properties of RSV. RSV is a highly pleomorphic enveloped negative-stranded RNA virus that matures at the limiting membrane of the infected cell. Its internal component shows helical symmetry, and its outer envelope is studded with spikelike glycoprotein projections. The inner helix seems to have a diameter of 13.5 nm. It has been suggested that RSV and pneumonia virus of mice (PVM) may compose a third subgroup of myxoviruses distinct from the orthomyxoviruses and the paramyxoviruses (Joncas et al., 1969).

RSV is relatively unstable at temperatures of 37° C and above. Also approximately 90% of its infectivity is lost after slow freezing. However, when frozen rapidly and stored at −70° C, the virus remains stable. RSV is rapidly destroyed at pH 3 and also by exposure to a 20% solution of ether for 18 hours at 4° C. In contrast to myxoviruses, RSV has not been grown in embryonated eggs nor has hemagglutination or hemadsorption been demonstrated.

On the other hand RSV has experimentally been shown capable of infecting a number of

Table 22-3. Response of volunteers to inoculation with parainfluenza virus type 1*

	Presence or absence of virus neutralizing activity in nasal secretions at time of challenge	
	Present	*Absent*
Number of men inoculated	29	51
Virus recovery	2†	33
Upper respiratory tract illness associated with type 1 virus	4†	29
Upper respiratory tract illness not associated with type 1 virus	7	2

*Data from Smith CB, et al. N Engl J Med 1966;**275**:1145.
†$p < 0.01$.

animals, including the chimpanzee, baboon, monkey, ferret, mink, chinchilla, guinea pig, hamster, and mouse. Signs of illness developed only in the chimpanzee and cebus monkey. RSV can be recovered in high titer from the nasal turbinates of infected ferrets.

Tissue culture. RSV multiplies in cultures of several primary, diploid, and heteroploid human cells, including HeLa and HEp-2 cells. The virus also grows in primary simian and bovine kidney cell cultures. In addition to causing the characteristic formation of syncytial areas in the cell cultures, the virus causes some of the cells to become rounded and to degenerate independently without fusing with other cells in the monolayer.

Antigenic composition. There is no antigenic relationship between RSV and conventional myxoviruses. Whether there is more than one distinct serotype of RSV seems unlikely. Hierholzer and Hirsh (1979) have identified a strain responsible in 1977 for an outbreak in Massachusetts. This crossreacts with a prototype RSV by complement fixation but not at all by neutralization.

Role of immunologic factors in pulmonary disease in infants. Early untoward experiences with inactivated RSV vaccines led some investigators to postulate an immune reaction in the pathogenesis of bronchiolitis/pneumonia (Chanock et al., 1969). If an immunologic reaction between serum antibody and RSV antigen plays a key role in the pathogenesis of RSV disease, the stress should be placed on the development of methods to stimulate production of local respiratory tract secretory antibody (Chanock et al., 1970). Suggested mechanisms of pathogenicity include an IgE-mediated reaction, an immunecomplex reaction, or an antibody-dependent cell-mediated cytotoxicity reaction. Jacobs et al. (1971), in Bristol, England, suggested that the presence of maternal antibody to RSV did not notably affect the incidence or severity of RSV infections in the offspring.

Although full protection against RSV infection is not conferred by transplacental IgG antibodies, nonetheless infants with higher levels of maternal antibody are less often infected, or less severely ill if infected, than are those with low serum antibody titers (Glezen et al., 1981). Reinfections are less severe than primary infections and may represent a combination of acquired immunity and an increase with age in the diameters of affected air passages (Henderson et al., 1979).

Clinical syndromes associated with RSV. RSV has been etiologically linked with five clinical syndromes, including mild upper respiratory tract illness, croup, bronchitis, bronchiolitis, and pneumonia. Of these, bronchiolitis and pneumonia are the most important, especially in the first 6 months of life. Parrott et al. (1973), who collected data over an 8-year period at the Children's Hospital in Washington, D.C., isolated RSV from 29.6% of patients with pneumonia. Studies essentially confirming these results have been reported from other parts of the United States and from Australia. Primary infection with RSV, like infection with parainfluenza virus, tends to be more severe than reinfection, which in adults takes the form of mild upper respiratory tract illness.

Estimates of the morbidity attributable to RSV in the first year of life are hospitalization rates of 10 per 1000 infants and clinic or emergency room visits of 110 per 1000. Beyond the prevalence of acute disease in infancy is the question of the role these earlier episodes play in the development of chronic obstructive airway disease later in childhood. On prospective followup 25% to 50% of infants with bronchiolitis

had recurrent wheezing episodes (Rooney and Williams, 1971). Pullam and Hey (1982) demonstrated continuing abnormalities of pulmonary function 10 years after acute illness. A sequential followup study of 29 children for 8 years after RSV infection in infancy (Hall et al., 1984) revealed that half the group had abnormally low oxyhemoglobin levels for 3 to 4 years, and 21% for the full 8 years. Spirometry measurements confirmed the presence of peripheral airway obstruction.

Outbreaks of illness caused by RSV among infants and children tend to occur annually for sharply defined periods in either mid-winter or spring. This annual epidemic pattern is unlike that of influenza virus A, which tends to recur at intervals of 2 or 3 years, that of influenza virus B, with its 4- to 6-year cycle, or that of parainfluenza virus type 3, which is virtually endemic, being easily detectable in the community almost every month of the year.

Adenoviruses. The adenoviruses were first discovered in 1953 by Rowe et al., who unmasked several agents from adenoids removed from healthy children and grown in tissue culture. Today adenoviruses form a clearly defined group of viruses represented by at least 40 antigenic types isolated from human beings and a number of other types recovered from primates, dogs, cows, mice, and avian species. Adenoviruses are 80 nm in diameter; possess double stranded linear DNA; have an icosahedral structure with 252 capsomeres; are resistant to the action of ether and acid but are heat labile, being destroyed at 56° C for 30 minutes; and share a common, but not identical, soluble complement-fixing antigen. Neutralizing antibody responses are type-specific. The viruses carry many antigenic determinants including those associated with the hexons, pentons, and fibers of the virion. They can be divided into seven subgroups on the basis of the molecular characterization of their DNA. They contain 10 structural polypeptides and replicate and produce inclusions within the nuclei of infected cells. The most favorable cultures in vitro have been human lines of epithelial origin (HeLa, KB, HEp2), primary human embryonic kidney, and fetal diploid lines.

Primary infection with adenoviruses usually occurs in early life, either as an asymptomatic infection or as acute upper respiratory tract disease accompanied by pharyngitis and sometimes conjunctivitis. Adenovirus types 1 through 7, 14, and 21 may be implicated. Occasionally fatal pneumonia in very young infants has been described associated with types 3, 4, 7, and 21. We have seen a fatal case in an infant 9 months old whose lungs revealed necrotizing bronchitis and pneumonia and intranuclear inclusions characteristic of adenoviral infection. Adenovirus type 3 was detected in the lung suspension and was also isolated from the patient's lung tissue.

Outbreaks of respiratory illness caused by adenoviruses have occurred in school-age children living closely together in institutions such as boarding schools and camps.

Although they are usually considered primarily as respiratory tract pathogens, adenoviruses produce viremia, and disease may arise in distant sites. Table 22-4 lists some of the clinical syndromes attributed to adenovirus infections. Outbreaks of keratoconjunctivitis due to adenovirus types 8, 11, or 19 have been associated with nosocomial infections caused by ophthalmic instruments and solutions. Acute paroxysmal cough with lymphocytosis indistinguishable from *Bordetella pertussis* infection has been attributed to adenoviruses. Mufson and Belshe (1976) have reviewed the association of adenoviruses, especially types 11 and 21, with a syndrome of dysuria, frequency, hematuria, and viruria.

Among college students and other adult civilians the incidence of adenoviral infection is

low. Young military recruits, on the other hand, were especially prone to epidemics of acute respiratory disease and atypical pneumonia often with rubellalike rash caused chiefly by adenovirus type 4 and, to a lesser extent, types 3 and 7. All in all, the contribution of adenovirus to respiratory illness in civilians of all ages is probably between 5% and 10% of cases. Among military recruits it was generally higher, ranging from about 8% to as high as 50% of cases in epidemics, until the use of enteric adenovirus vaccines in the first weeks of recruit training terminated these armed forces outbreaks.

Picornaviruses. A family of similar viruses consisting of the rhinoviruses and the enteroviruses (poliovirus, Coxsackie virus, and ECHO virus subgroups) has been designated picornaviruses (*pico*, very small, RNA). They measure between 20 and 30 nm and are characterized by a nucleic acid core of single-stranded RNA, absence of essential lipid as shown by resistance to the action of ether, and cationic stabilization to thermal inactivation.

Rhinoviruses. Rhinoviruses may be isolated from the upper respiratory tract and are the principal cause of mild upper respiratory illness in adults.

Rhinoviruses share many of the properties of enteroviruses, including particle diameter of 20 to 30 nm, RNA core, resistance to ether, and in general, cytopathic effects in tissue culture. In primary cultures of monkey or human embryonic kidney cells, or in human embryonic lung cell lines, rhinoviruses grow best at slightly lower temperatures (33° C) and more acidic pH than enteroviruses. Rhinoviruses differ sharply from the enteroviruses in their sensitivity to acid; all strains of rhinovirus are completely or almost completely inactivated at pH 3 to 5, and enteroviruses are not. From studies published so far, there seem to be at least 113 different serologic types of rhinoviruses.

Epidemiologic investigations indicate that rhinoviruses cause common colds and upper respiratory tract infections in adults and children and occasionally lower respiratory tract illnesses in children. British workers, using volunteers, have shown that a number of strains will produce colds. Virus can be isolated from nasopharyngeal washings in the first 3 to 5 days of illness.

Enteroviruses. The properties of enteroviruses and their role in causing diverse clinical

Table 22-4. Adenovirus infections

Respiratory tract	*Other sites*
Upper respiratory infection (URI)	Keratoconjunctivitis
Exudative pharyngotonsillitis	Hepatitis
Adenoidal-pharyngeal-conjunctival (APC) fever	Intussusception
	Diarrhea
Bronchitis	Interstitial nephritis
Pertussis syndrome	Hemorrhagic cystitis
Bronchiolitis	Rash disease
Pneumonia	Meningoencephalitis
Bronchiolitis obliterans	Myocarditis

syndromes, including aseptic meningitis, paralysis, pleurodynia, febrile exanthem, and myocarditis in newborn infants, are described in Chapter 5. The contribution of enteroviruses to the cause of respiratory illness is less clear. Of the many nonpolio enteroviruses, only Coxsackie A-21 appears to be primarily a respiratory pathogen. Many other Coxsackie and ECHO viruses cause acute respiratory infections, as noted before, but these are not the major segment of their pathogenic potential (Chapter 5).

Group A Coxsackie viruses, notably types 2, 3, 4, 5, 6, 8, and 10, have been etiologically linked with herpangina, an acute illness characterized by fever, vomiting, sore throat, and the appearance of small vesicles or punched-out ulcers in and around the throat (Chapter 5). Steigman et al. (1961) reported the isolation of group A Coxsackie virus type 10 from patients with a summer febrile disease that they called acute lymphonodular pharyngitis characterized by the appearance of discrete raised nonulcerative lesions on the anterior pillars, soft palate, and uvula. Another clinical syndrome associated with group A Coxsackie virus type 16 was observed in Toronto in 1957 and in California in 1961. The illness was characterized by a vesicular enanthem on the buccal mucosa, tongue, gums, and palate; another feature, unlike herpangina, was a papulovesicular exanthem involving the hands, feet, legs, and buttocks in about 25% of the patients; the name *hand-foot-and-mouth disease* is often used to designate this syndrome.

In addition to being the cause of epidemic pleurodynia, which has certain characteristics of a respiratory disease, such as cough and chest pain (p. 47), *group B Coxsackie viruses* 4 and 5 have been implicated in febrile respiratory tract illness accompanied by cough and nasal discharge. These agents have also been associated with influenza-like illness. Suggestive evidence linking enteroviruses with cases of pneumonia, bronchiolitis, and bronchitis in infants under 2 years of age has been reported.

ECHO viruses may sometimes give rise to human infections characterized by upper respiratory tract and enteric tract diseases, and common coldlike illnesses. ECHO viruses have not been found in association with pneumonia. ECHO virus types 1 to 4, 6 to 9, 11, 16, 19, 20, 22, and 25 are known to be responsible for a mild upper respiratory tract illness.

Herpesviruses. Herpesvirus hominis (herpes simplex types 1 and 2 virus), herpesvirus varicellae (varicella-zoster virus), cytomegalovirus, and EBV are the five members of the herpesvirus group (Chapters 2, 6, 11, 33) for which humans serve as the usual hosts and reservoirs. The herpesvirus group is included in this discussion of respiratory viruses because (1) herpes simplex virus is one of the common causes of acute pharyngitis with vesicles or ulcers, (2) varicella-zoster virus may cause pneumonia complicating chickenpox, particularly in adults and immunocompromised patients of all ages, (3) involvement of the lungs with pneumonia occurs in cytomegalovirus infection, and (4) EBV is a cause of acute tonsillopharyngitis in infectious mononucleosis. Andiman et al. (1981) reported a study of 15 children with pulmonary infiltrates in whose sera they detected antibody to EBV indicative of current or recent infection with that virus. Eight of the 15 had evidence of coexistent infection with a second pathogen—viral, bacterial, or mycoplasmal. They speculated that EBV might be a primary or coprimary etiologic agent or that it was reactivated in the presence of infection with the other pathogen.

Lymphocytic choriomeningitis virus. Lymphocytic choriomeningitis virus (LCM), a member of the arenavirus group, is included in this discussion because it may cause human infection characterized by onset with respiratory manifestations such as cough and sore throat, by an influenza-like syndrome, or occasionally, by severe systemic involvement, including pneumonia.

LCM virus is one of 12 arenaviruses, only four of which have been shown to be pathogenic for man (Junin, Machupo, Lassa, and LCM). They are ether-sensitive enveloped viruses containing single-stranded, segmented, linear RNA. The membranous envelope shows surface spikes, and the agent is pleomorphic with diameters of 60 nm to 280 nm. All the arenaviruses are characterized by persistent tolerant infections in their natural hosts, which are a variety of rodents. LCM virus is enzootic in mice, guinea pigs, and hamsters.

Infected gray house mice excrete virus in the saliva and urine, thus providing the most likely source of human infection. There is no evidence of person-to-person spread. The virus is preserved in the frozen state at $-70°$ C and by lyophilization. LCM virus may be isolated from the spinal fluid, blood, and urine by injecting these materials into mice, newborn hamsters, guinea pigs, or tissue culture. Complement-fixing, neutralizing, and indirect fluorescent antibodies (FA) are detected in convalescent sera within 30 days.

Mycoplasma pneumoniae

For many years the agent of cold agglutinin-positive primary atypical pneumonia was thought to be a virus. In 1962 it was shown to be a human mycoplasma, *M. pneumoniae*, capable of colonial growth on artificial medium. There is evidence that this organism, in addition to causing primary atypical pneumonia (both cold agglutinin-positive and occasionally cold agglutinin-negative) in adults, is an important pathogen for pneumonia and wheezing associated respiratory infections (Henderson et al., 1979) in children.

The mycoplasma are ubiquitous, free-living organisms found in many insects, animals, and plants. Unlike bacteria they are unable to synthesize a cell wall, but they are able to grow on cell-free media. Characteristically they grow down into nutrient agar and produce a "fried egg" appearance with dark centers and light periphery. Only one species, *M. pneumoniae*, has been proved to cause significant disease in humans, but there is evidence that other related family members *(Ureaplasma urealyticum* and *M. hominis)* play a role in human urogenital tract disease. *M. pneumoniae* is filamentous, pleomorphic, 10×200 nm, moderately motile and has an electron-dense core at one end with a terminal differentiated structure for attachment to host cell membranes by neuraminic acid receptors. On human ciliated respiratory tract mucosal cells, the organism remains extracellular but exerts a toxic effect that interferes with ciliary function and mucosal cell metabolism. *M. pneumoniae* is resistant to cell wall–active antibiotics such as penicillin but is sensitive to the tetracyclines and erythromycin.

Much of our knowledge of human respiratory infections with *Mycoplasma* emanates from studies begun during World War II of atypical pneumonia among military recruits. The responsible agent(s) was thought to be a virus. Eaton et al. (1944) reported the recovery of an agent from filtered sputum or lung suspensions obtained from patients with cold agglutinin-positive primary atypical pneumonia. The patients' specimens had been inoculated into embryonated eggs, which failed to show definite pathologic changes. Material from inoculated eggs passed to hamsters and cotton rats induced pneumonia that could be prevented by convalescent patients' serum. In 1957 Liu confirmed Eaton's work by providing unequivocal evidence of infection of human beings with the Eaton agent. Using the FA technique, he demonstrated the agent in the bronchial epithelium of the chick embryo.

Marmion and Goodburn (1961) reported the observation of small coccobacillary bodies on the bronchial epithelium of the infected chick embryo corresponding to the distribution of the agent as visualized by Liu's FA technique. This steady accumulation of evidence pointing away from the agent's being a virus culminated in 1962 with the achievement of Chanock et al. in growing the agent on artificial medium consisting of PPLO agar medium supplemented by horse serum and yeast extract. Growth failed to occur in the absence of horse serum. This latter requirement and the morphologic and staining properties of the colonies that formed on the agar plates indentified the organism as belonging to the genus *Mycoplasma* (Fig. 22-2). The FA technique was used to distinguish the colonies specifically as Eaton agent. With the use of paired serum specimens from patients with *M. pneumoniae* pneumonia, it was observed that acute-phase serum failed to stain the colonies, whereas convalescent-phase serum diluted 1:40 gave rise to intense fluorescence of the colonies (Fig. 22-3). Similarly, immune sera were prepared in rabbits against prototype strains of *M. pneumoniae* grown in eggs; these immune sera produced intense staining of Eaton agent colonies but not other mycoplasma colonies obtained from various sources.

To complete the etiologic postulates, Chanock et al. (1963) infected human volunteers experimentally. Of 27 volunteers with no detectable antibody, three developed pneumonia; four, febrile respiratory tract illness without pneumo-

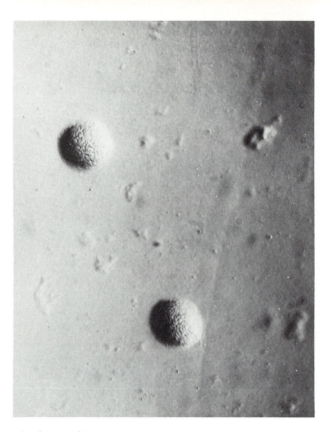

Fig. 22-2. Typical colonies of *M. pneumoniae* on agar plate. (×600.) (From Chanock RM, et al. In Pollard M (ed). Perspectives in virology, vol. 3. New York. Harper & Row, Publishers, 1963.)

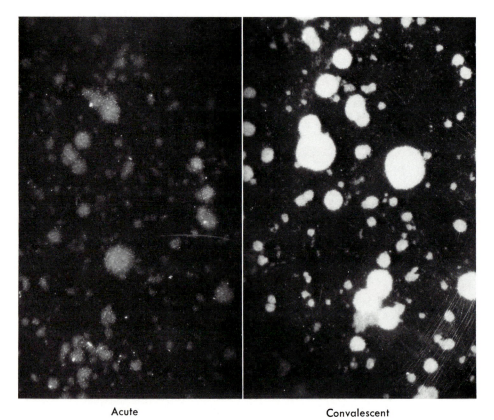

Acute   Convalescent

Fig. 22-3. Agar colonies stained with acute- and convalescent-phase sera from patient with *Mycoplasma pneumoniae* pneumonia. Acute-phase serum fails to stain colonies of *M. pneumoniae*, which indicates absence of antibody; convalescent-phase serum produces intense fluorescence of colonies, indicating presence of antibody. (From Chanock RM, et al. In Pollard M (ed). Perspectives in virology, vol. 3. New York. Harper & Row, Publishers, 1963.)

nia; nine, myringitis with or without bullae and hemorrhage; and four, afebrile respiratory tract illness. All 27 volunteers acquired antibody. Febrile respiratory tract illness without pneumonia developed in other groups of volunteers after administration of *M. pneumoniae* artificially propagated on agar. Of 30 volunteers given these materials, 27 showed development of antibody.

Associated clinical syndromes. In addition to causing a major portion of primary atypical pneumonia, *M. pneumoniae* can also give rise to inapparent infection, mild upper respiratory tract infection, bronchitis, bronchiolitis, bronchopneumonia, and myringitis bullosa. The incidence of *M. pneumoniae* infection in the children in any given locality may fluctuate widely over a period of years. For example, during 1957 to 1959 in Washington, D.C., *M. pneumoniae* was associated with 10% of all pediatric lower respiratory tract illnesses studied at the Children's Hospital, whereas 3 years later only 1% of these conditions were associated with *M. pneumoniae* (Chanock et al., 1963). *M. pneumoniae* plays a major role in respiratory tract disease of school-age children and young adults. Chanock (1965) reported serologic evidence of *M. pneumoniae* infection in 55% of 530 marine recruits with pneumonia and in 28% of 141 recruits with febrile upper respiratory tract infections. Evans and Brobst (1961) found similar evidence of *M. pneumoniae* infection in 25% of 91 university students hospitalized for pneumonia. It should be noted that, although in most persons with cold agglutinin–positive pneumonia serologic evidence of *M. pneumoniae* infection can be obtained, the converse is not true; for example, a sizable proportion of patients with *M. pneumoniae* pneumonia fail to develop cold agglutinins. Thus Chanock observed that among 239 marines with *M. pneumoniae* pneumonia, cold agglutinins formed in only 46% during convalescence.

Inflammation of the tympanic membrane was observed by Mufson et al. (1961) in four of 50 cases in a military outbreak of *M. pneumoniae* pneumonia. Myringitis with bullae and hemorrhage was observed in nine of 27 volunteers infected experimentally with *M. pneumoniae*. *M. pneumoniae* is not known to invade beyond the lining mucosal cells of the respiratory tract, but disease may also be apparent at distant sites.

Table 22-5. Clinical manifestations of infection with *Mycoplasma pneumoniae*

Respiratory tract	*Other sites of involvement*
Coryza	Erythema multiforme, other rashes
Pharyngitis	Meningoencephalitis, cerebellar ataxia
Tracheobronchitis	Guillain-Barré syndrome
Bullous myringitis	Myocarditis, pericarditis
Pneumonia	Autoimmune hemolytic anemia, thrombocytopenia
Pleural effusion	Migratory polyarthritis, hepatitis

The many clinical manifestations associated with infection are collected in Table 22-5.

Rickettsiae

C. burnetii (formerly *Rickettsia burneti*) is the cause of Q fever, an acute illness characterized by sudden onset of fever, chills, headache, malaise, and weakness that progresses to cough, chest pain, and the picture of atypical pneumonia. The properties of *C. burnetii* and the clinical manifestations of Q fever are described in Chapter 23.

Chlamydiae

A number of investigators have studied the role of *Chlamydia trachomatis* in the etiology of pneumonia among infants during the first months of life (Schachter et al., 1975; Beem and Saxon, 1977). The organism had previously been considered mainly an oculogenital pathogen responsible for neonatal conjunctivitis and for nongonococcal urethritis of adult males. Infants born of mothers with positive uterine cervical cultures have a great likelihood of chlamydial colonization and subsequent development of inclusion conjunctivitis and pneumonia. The full spectrum and epidemiology of this lower respiratory tract infection remain the object of current research. *C. psittaci* is another species of the genus, long recognized for its association with human respiratory disease contracted from a variety of avian sources. Pneumonia or milder respiratory illness has been reported among owners or dealers in pet birds.

The chlamydiae are small, intracellular, obligate parasites now considered to be a group of bacteria. They possess a cell wall, contain both RNA and DNA, replicate by binary fission, and are inactivated by some antibiotics (erythromycin, chloramphenicol, tetracyclines, and sulfonamides). The genus *Chlamydia* is divided into two species, *C. trachomatis* and *C. psittaci*. The two subgroups differ in morphology, staining qualities with iodine, antigenic structure, and their usual hosts. *C. psittaci* infects animals and birds with occasional spillover to man. Human infections are characterized by a febrile interstitial pneumonia, ornithosis, acquired by inhalation of dried excreta or secretions from infected birds. Originally only psittacine birds (parrots and parakeets) were thought to be the reservoir, but it is now appreciated that many other species of domestic and wild birds may harbor the organisms. In sheep and cattle *C. psittaci* is a major cause of abortions.

C. trachomatis is further subdivided into those agents associated with lymphogranuloma venereum (LGV) and the TRIC (trachoma-inclusion conjunctivitis) group. It is this latter group that has received increasing attention recently as a cause of pneumonia in infants (Beem and Saxon, 1977). Other clinical syndromes due to TRIC infections include trachoma, neonatal inclusion conjunctivitis, and genital tract infections (nongonococcal urethritis, cervicitis, salpingitis, and epididymitis).

Chlamydiae grow in the yolk sac of the embryonated chicken's egg but more conveniently in cell culture systems. A variety of cells will successfully propagate *C. psittaci*, but the conditions for in vitro growth of *C. trachomatis* are more fastidious. A favorite technique utilizes the McCoy mouse fibroblast cell line pretreated with 5-iodo-2'-deoxyuridine (idoxuridine). Serologic assays for specific chlamydial antibodies are done by immunofluorescent methods with monoclonal antibody. Giemsa stains of infected conjunctival epithelial cells show the inclusion bodies of *C. trachomatis* under the oil-immersion lens. *C. trachomatis* may be responsible for 30% of pneumonias necessitating hospitalization in the first 6 months of life (Harrison et al., 1978). In a prospective study of 244 infants, 25% of whose mothers had cervical cultures positive for *C. trachomatis* antenatally, the exposed infants subsequently had twice the rate of pneumonia and recurrent otitis media in the first 6

months of life (Schaefer et al., 1985). Ancillary laboratory findings in pneumonia of infants include a peripheral eosinophilia and an elevation of IgG and IgM.

Bacteria

It is not easy to assess the present-day quantitative role of bacteria in acute respiratory tract disease. The estimate that the primary cause is nonbacterial in more than 90% of acute respiratory tract infections does not negate the importance of bacteria as both primary and secondary invaders. Patients with lower respiratory tract infections of severity sufficient to require hospitalization are more apt to have bacterial disease than those whose illnesses permit ambulatory care. At the extremes of life, in the newborn and geriatric patient, bacterial pneumonia may be more common with higher morbidity and mortality. Group A β-hemolytic streptococcus is the most common bacterial cause of acute tonsillopharyngitis with exudate or membrane (p. 375). A less common but very important cause is *Corynebacterium diphtheriae* (p. 24), which also must be considered in the differential diagnosis of croup. *Hemophilus influenzae* type b appears to be chiefly responsible for acute epiglottitis (p. 276). Its association with pneumonia and empyema in the pediatric age group has been increasingly apparent in recent years (Ginsburg et al., 1979).

In the face of the multiplicity of different agents, especially viruses, capable of causing any one respiratory syndrome, it is difficult to measure the present-day role of bacteria in the cause of acute respiratory tract disease. To make a precise etiologic diagnosis, the physician must have access to clinical diagnostic laboratories capable of isolating and identifying nonbacterial and bacterial agents. The differential diagnosis between viral and nonviral illness is often made on clinical grounds that are imprecise, even though they may include a white blood cell count and differential, an examination of the polymorphonuclear cells for toxic granulations, an erythrocyte sedimentation rate (ESR), and occasionally the clinical response to a "therapeutic trial" of antibiotic therapy. Early in the course of some lower respiratory tract infections a specific bacteriologic diagnosis may be made when appropriate specimens are available for Gram stain and culture (sputum, pleural fluid, blood) or antigenic analysis by techniques such as counter current immunoelectrophoresis (CIE).

Despite these obstacles to precise definition of etiology, it is clear that bacteria continue to figure prominently in both primary and secondary roles in acute upper and lower respiratory tract illnesses. For example, an inestimable number of cases of streptococcal infections occur annually in the United States; pneumonias complicating epidemic influenza are mostly bacterial and are chiefly responsible for the deaths that follow influenza; and staphylococcal pneumonia with its various complications continues to present a formidable problem, especially in early life.

Hemolytic streptococci. Group A hemolytic streptococci are the main *bacterial* cause of upper respiratory tract infections, including tonsillopharyngitis with exudate or membrane and febrile nasopharyngitis in infants. Today these organisms are seldom responsible for laryngitis (croup) or pneumonia. The characteristics of hemolytic streptococci and the epidemiologic, immunologic, and pathologic aspects and clinical manifestations of streptococcal infections are discussed in Chapter 28.

Staphylococci. The chief contribution of staphylococci to respiratory tract illness is the causation of severe pneumonia. Bacterial tracheitis attributed to staphylococcal infection has reemerged as a recognized clinical entity in recent years (Nelson, 1984). The properties of staphylococci and the pathogenesis, pathologic and immunologic aspects, and clinical manifestations of staphylococcal infections are presented in detail in Chapter 27.

Pneumococci. For many years the pneumococci were primarily or secondarily responsible for the bulk of bacterial pneumonias in children and adults. The incidence of pneumococcal pneumonia dropped sharply in the late 1930s and early 1940s after the introduction of sulfonamides and penicillin and the extensive use of these antimicrobial agents in the treatment of acute upper respiratory tract infections.

Streptococcus pneumoniae in its virulent form is a gram-positive, lancet-shaped cell surrounded by a polysaccharide capsule that contains an M protein specific for each serologic type and a carbohydrate (C substance) common to all. The capsule, acting as a protective shell against phagocytes, provides a significant factor in the virulence of the organism; pneumococci without capsules are avirulent. Type-specific antibody combines with capsular polysaccharide, thereby promoting phagocytosis, and it is also responsible for the Neufeld quellung reaction.

Pneumococci are grown on various bacteriologic media including blood agar and beef infusion broth with 0.5% dextrose and 5% to 10% blood or serum. Pneumococcal cultures are differentiated from other streptococcal species by their bile solubility and their inhibition by optochin (ethylhydrocupreine hydrochloride). On blood agar the colonies are smooth, glistening, 0.5 to 1.5 cm in diameter and α-hemolytic. Encapsulated pneumococci give a mucoid appearance to their colonies.

At least 83 specific antigenic types of pneumococci have been described. The most frequent types encountered in adults with pneumonia are types 8, 4, 1, 14, 3, 7, 12, 6, 18, 9, 19, and 23, in descending order of frequency, as reported by Austrian et al. (1976) in their collaborative study of more than 3600 patients in the United States. Among children, the serotypes most commonly identified with disease are 19, 23, 14, 3, 6, and 1. Gray et al. (1980) noted similar distributions of pneumococcal types in children with bacteremia, meningitis, and otitis media with one addition, type 18.

Pneumococci are common inhabitants of the normal upper respiratory tract. Factors that may predispose to invasive pneumococcal infection include: (1) preceding viral infections, (2) bronchial obstruction and atelectasis, (3) alteration of mucociliary function by allergy, irritants, and other agents, (4) pulmonary congestion with cardiovascular problems, and (5) splenectomy, agammaglobulinemia, lymphocytic leukemia, and sickle cell disease.

Among infants and children pneumococci cause pneumonia, otitis media, mastoiditis, and sinusitis as a direct result of infection in the respiratory tract. More distant foci of pneumococcal illness include meningitis and infrequently cellulitis, peritonitis, arthritis, osteomyelitis, endocarditis, and pericarditis. Occult bacteremia is relatively common in children under 2 years of age, while fulminant, overwhelming septicemia may occur in patients with functional or anatomic absence of the spleen.

Most pneumococci remain highly sensitive to penicillin with minimum inhibitory concentrations (MIC) of 0.05 μg/ml or less. In 1977, resistant strains of *S. pneumoniae* were recovered from South African children with pneumonia, meningitis, and/or bacteremia. These organisms were resistant to penicillin, ampicillin, methicillin, erythromycin, cephalothin, tetracycline, aminoglycosides, and chloramphenicol. The only antibiotics to which these virulent organisms were sensitive were rifampin, vancomycin, and bacitracin (Jacobs et al. 1978). A high nasopharyngeal carrier rate was detected among contacts of the patients. MICs to penicillin were from 1 to 8 μg/ml. Cates et al. (1978) isolated a penicillin-resistant pneumococcus type 14 (MIC 4 μg/ml) from an immune-deficient girl in Minnesota, but this organism fortunately was sensitive to erythromycin, chloramphenicol, trimethoprim-sulfamethoxazole, and clindamycin. Other resistant *S. pneumoniae* organisms have been recovered from ill children in California and Texas. The epidemiology and incidence of penicillin-resistant pneumococci in the United States are currently unknown. It is therefore prudent to examine the penicillin sensitivity of *S. pneumoniae* isolated from patients with invasive disease and to consider the possibility of resistant organisms in patients who fail to respond to penicillin therapy. The mechanism of penicillin resistance currently is not known but does not appear to be due to penicillinase.

Hemophilus influenzae. *H. influenzae* is a small, gram-negative, pleomorphic bacillus found in encapsulated or nonencapsulated forms. Virulent *H. influenzae* possess a type-specific capsular polysaccharide. Six distinct antigenic types, a through f, have been identified by capsular swelling (Neufeld quellung reaction) and precipitin or agglutination tests. More than 90% of serious *H. influenzae* infections in infants and children are caused by type b. Nonencapsulated strains are nontypable and have been associated with otitis media, sinusitis, and chronic bronchitis. Nonencapsulated *H. influenzae* is found frequently in nasopharyngeal cultures of normal children and adults. Respiratory tract disease due to *H. influenzae* type b takes the form of epiglottitis, pneumonia (often with empyema), mastoiditis, sinusitis, and otitis media (Chapter 19). Nonrespiratory illness includes meningitis (Chapter 15), orbital cellulitis, buccal cellulitis, arthritis and osteomyelitis (Chapter 18), pericarditis, and, rarely, endocarditis. Im-

munity to the organism is associated with the development of type-specific bactericidal anticapsular antibodies that can be detected and quantitated in the serum.

Culture of *H. influenzae* in the laboratory requires enriched media containing a heat-stable (X) factor and heat-labile (V) factor. Antigen detection with antiserum against the capsular polysaccharide (polyribosyl-phosphate, or PRP, of type b) has been helpful in detecting organisms rapidly in infected body fluids such as sputum, blood, pleural fluid, urine, and CSF.

As with the pneumococci, changes in antibiotic sensitivity have altered the considerations of chemotherapy of *H. influenzae* infections. Since 1974, strains of ampicillin-resistant *H. influenzae* have been recovered from patients throughout the United States and other nations. From 5% to 25% of isolates from children with invasive disease produce β-lactamase (penicillinase) and are therefore resistant to ampicillin therapy. Chloramphenicol has become the initial drug of choice for infants and children with systemic *H. influenzae* infections. To complicate matters further, a few strains of chloramphenicol-resistant *H. influenzae* have been detected in Europe and the United States, but they are still sufficiently rare to remain only a worry on the horizon. It seems important to test both ampicillin and chloramphenicol sensitivity of clinical isolates from blood, CSF, joint fluid, and other sources associated with invasive infections. Some of the cephalosporins have been subjected to clinical study, with favorable results reported with cefotaxime in invasive *H. influenzae* infections (Chapter 15 and Appendix 1).

Bordetella pertussis. *B. pertussis*, a common respiratory tract pathogen, is mentioned here because the manifestations in the catarrhal stage of pertussis are those of an upper respiratory tract infection, and often the true cause is unsuspected. Moreover, the severity of pertussis and the mortality in infancy, usually from complicating pneumonia, are not generally appreciated. The characteristics of *B. pertussis* and the clinical manifestations of pertussis are discussed in Chapter 20.

Corynebacterium diphtheriae. Despite widespread immunization practices, *C. diphtheriae* may occur as the pathogen responsible for membranous tonsillitis and laryngitis. It is mentioned here to emphasize the importance of early recognition of diphtheria because delay in treatment with antitoxin may jeopardize the patient's life. The cause and other aspects of diphtheria are discussed in Chapter 3.

Legionella pneumophila. As the result of an outbreak of pneumonia in 1976 following a national convention of the American Legion in Philadelphia, a new disease has been identified, studied retrospectively and prospectively, associated etiologically with a previously unrecognized bacterium, and correlated with a wide spectrum of clinical manifestations. Legionnaires' disease has occurred both in outbreaks and sporadically since initial recognition and examination of sera dating back to 1973. The clinical manifestations range from mild febrile pneumonia to the adult respiratory distress syndrome and may be accompanied by extrapulmonary involvement, including encephalopathy, rhabdomyolysis, and gastrointestinal and renal dysfunction. Cases have been reported throughout the United States and also from England and Spain.

The organism responsible for legionnaires' disease is a gram-negative bacillus, *Legionella pneumophila*, that is exceedingly fastidious and difficult to grow in vitro. As a result most diagnostic studies rely on serologic techniques for antibody increases and/or on direct demonstration of the organism in infected tissues, using special stains. Sputum, pleural fluid, bronchial washings, and lung biopsies or aspirates can all be examined by immunofluorescence and by a modification of the Dieterle spirochete stain (Lattimer et al., 1978). Both in vitro and in vivo the organism may be sensitive to erythromycin, which has been used with some success among patients.

Only a few cases have been described among children (Ryan et al., 1979). Because the illness occurs with enhanced morbidity and mortality in the aged and in the immunocompromised, more cases may be recognized in pediatric populations with underlying disorders such as cancer, immunodeficiency, and hematologic malignancies (Sturm et al., 1981; Kovatch et al., 1984).

Miscellaneous agents

Various mycotic infections, including *aspergillosis*, *candidiasis*, *coccidioidomycosis*, and *histoplasmosis*, are relatively common in certain parts of the world and may be manifested by an influenzalike illness or by atypical pneumonia. *Pneumocystis carinii* may cause an invasive pneumonia with bilateral alveolar disease. The acquired forms of *toxoplasmosis*, caused by the protozoon parasite *Toxoplasma gondii*, include a syndrome characterized by fever, maculopapular rash, and pneumonia (Chapter 30). These infections have been noted more frequently as opportunistic respiratory pathogens among immunosuppressed hosts. Atypical pneumonia may accompany Q fever cuased by *Coxiella burnetii* (Chapter 23).

Many other organisms play an etiologic role in respiratory tract infection; many of them are listed in Table 22-5. In patients who are immune compromised or in normal hosts exposed to special geographic or ecologic settings, fungi must be considered in the differential diagnosis. These include *Blastomyces*, *Cryptococcus*, *Histoplasma*, *Mucor*, *Coccidioides*, *Candida*, and *Aspergillus*. Other bacteria, such as *Yersinia pestis* and *Francisella tularensis*, may cause plague and tularemia respectively in patients who have been exposed to infected animal hosts *(F. tularensis)* or fleas from infected animals *(Y. pestis)* while camping or hunting. In recent years the gram-negative rods and Enterobacteriaceae have assumed an increasingly important role in pneumonias of children with immune suppression due to underlying disease or therapeutic protocols and in patients on broad-spectrum antibiotics for other reasons. Aspiration pneumonias may have a predominance of mixed anaerobic bacteria. Infections with *Mycobacterium tuberculosis* are discussed in Chapter 31. More exotic etiologies must always be considered in the compromised host. Parasites including *Ascaris*, *Pneumocystis*, *Toxoplasma*, and *Strongyloides* have all been reported to cause pneumonias in such patients. Stagno et al. (1981) called attention to the role in pneumonia of infancy of a group of pathogens less often considered. These were *cytomegalovirus*, *Chlamydia*, *Pneumocystis*, and *Ureaplasma urelyticum*.

CLINICAL SYNDROMES

The purpose of this section is to describe the clinical signs and symptoms and treatment of acute respiratory tract infections. For the sake of clarity, these illnesses have been grouped

Table 22-6. Acute respiratory tract disease—clinical syndromes and etiologic agents

Clinical syndrome	Etiologic agents		
	Viral	Bacterial	Other
Common cold; coldlike illness; upper respiratory tract infection; coryza; rhinitis; rhinopharyngitis; acute catarrhal tonsillopharyngitis	Respiratory syncytial virus Parainfluenza viruses Rhinoviruses Nonpolio enteroviruses Adenoviruses Coronaviruses		*Mycoplasma pneumoniae*
Febrile nasopharyngitis (in infants)		Streptococcus, Group A Pneumococcus	*Mycoplasma pneumoniae*
Acute tonsillopharyngitis with exudate or membrane	Adenoviruses EB virus	Streptococcus, Group A *Corynebacterium diphtheriae*	
Acute tonsillopharyngitis with vesicles or ulcers	Herpesvirus hominis (herpes simplex virus) Group A Coxsackie viruses		
Acute laryngitis; laryngotracheobronchitis (croup)	Parainfluenza viruses Influenza viruses Adenoviruses Rhinoviruses Respiratory syncytial virus Measles virus	*Corynebacterium diphtheriae*	
Acute epiglottitis (croup)		*Hemophilus influenzae* type b	
Bronchiolitis	Respiratory syncytial virus Parainfluenza viruses Adenoviruses Influenza viruses		*Mycoplasma pneumoniae*
Pneumonia	Respiratory syncytial virus Parainfluenza viruses Measles virus Adenoviruses Influenza viruses Cytomegalovirus Lymphocytic choriomeningitis virus Varicella-zoster virus	Staphylococcus Pneumococcus Hemolytic streptococci *Hemophilus influenzae* Enterobacteriaceae *Pseudomonas aeruginosa* *Klebsiella pneumoniae* Anaerobes (with aspiration) *Mycobacterium tuberculosis* and atypicals *Nocardia* *Legionella pneumophila* *Chlamydia trachomatis* *Chlamydia psittaci* Others	*Mycoplasma pneumoniae* *Ureaplasma urealyticum* *Pneumocystis carinii* *Coxiella burnetii* (Q fever) *Toxoplasma gondii* Fungi (*Candida, Aspergillus, Coccidioides, Histoplasma, Blastomyces, Cryptococcus,* etc.)
Influenza-like illness	Influenza viruses Parainfluenza viruses Adenoviruses Lymphocytic chroiomeningitis virus		

somewhat arbitrarily into nine clinical syndromes and are listed together with their various etiologic agents in Table 22-6. We are aware that this arbitrary division, made largely on anatomic grounds, is often inexact; for example, "pure" bronchiolitis without some extension of the process into the peribronchial tissues is probably a rare event. Nevertheless, the clinical picture of bronchiolitis is so distinct from that of pneumonia that it warrants separate discussion.

From a practical point of view, the question of whether or not to treat a patient with antimicrobial agents confronts every physician responsible for the care of persons with respiratory tract infections. The use of antimicrobial agents in viral infections is worthless and may be harmful because the sensitive bacteria will be eliminated, thereby promoting the growth of resistant organisms that may become the secondary bacterial invaders. On the other hand, the same antibiotics may be lifesaving when administered to a patient with severe bacterial pneumonia. The difficulties in making a precise etiologic diagnosis have been discussed already.

Common cold; coldlike illness; upper respiratory tract infection; coryza; rhinitis; rhinopharyngitis; acute catarrhal tonsillopharyngitis with or without conjunctivitis; febrile nasopharyngitis (in infants)

These illnesses are grouped together under the same syndrome because their clinical manifestations overlap widely, and it would be difficult and serve little purpose to make a clinical distinction between them. Moreover the causes, albeit multiple, are mostly viral.

Clinical manifestations. This syndrome is characterized by varying degrees of nasal congestion and discharge, conjunctivitis, sore throat, cough, and redness of the pharynx and tonsils without exudate. The incubation period is short; the average length is about 2 days, with a range of 1 to 6 days. The first symptom in some persons is a scratchy feeling or soreness of the throat. In others the cold starts with a nasal discharge that is typically thin, clear, and profuse; it may be mucoid or serous. Concomitantly, there is a feeling of fullness in the nasopharynx. Swelling of the nasal mucosa soon blocks one or both nostrils. Sneezing attacks are frequent. The eyes water. Some patients have a nonproductive

cough. Headache or an uncomfortable feeling of fullness in the head is common. There may be slight fever, but the temperature rarely exceeds 38.3° C (101° F). Chilly sensations, malaise, and muscular aches are not uncommon at the beginning, but these are seldom prominent, nor do they persist in uncomplicated colds.

Examination shows variably inflamed and swollen nasal and pharyngeal mucous membranes. The nasal passages may be occluded. The senses of smell and hearing may be impaired. Enlarged nodules of lymphoid tissue may be seen on the posterior pharyngeal wall. The nasal discharge often becomes mucopurulent in 2 or 3 days, and at this time a postnasal drip may be evident. The cervical lymph nodes may be slightly enlarged or tender. Some persons are likely to develop cold sores due to herpes simplex. Uncomplicated colds seldom last more than a week.

The cause of the vast majority of colds and coldlike illnesses is viral. Over 150 different viruses have been implicated, including rhinoviruses (113 or more types), coronaviruses, respiratory syncytial (RS) virus, parainfluenza viruses, adenoviruses, and Coxsackie viruses A and B. In infants under 6 months of age, Group A streptococcus may cause febrile nasopharyngitis, and pertussis in the catarrhal stage acts like an upper respiratory tract infection.

Complications. The common cold may be complicated by an extension of the viral infection or by bacterial infections that include otitis media, sinusitis, tonsillitis, cervical adenitis, laryngitis, bronchitis, bronchiolitis, and pneumonia. Infants and children are particularly likely to develop otitis media. The eardrums should therefore be examined for this complication. Secondary infections may be caused by any pathogenic bacteria in the upper respiratory passages. Appropriate antimicrobial therapy has reduced the seriousness of these complications.

Diagnosis. The typical clinical pattern makes the diagnosis easy in most cases. Rhinitis, coryza, sneezing, scratchiness of the throat, and cough, all in the absence of pronounced constitutional symptoms, point to the common cold. There is no practical laboratory test by which the diagnosis can be confirmed. Similar clinical pictures may be presented by various other conditions. *Allergic rhinitis* may be clinically indistinguishable from the common cold. The presence of eosinophils in the nasal smear and the response to antihistamine drugs may serve to differentiate it. *Influenza* can be distinguished by the prominence of associated constitutional symptoms and by specific diagnostic tests. *Pertussis* in the catarrhal stage may be confused with the common cold. Preeruptive *measles* may be mistaken for a cold. *Nasal diphtheria* and *foreign bodies* in the nose may rarely be mistaken for the common cold. *Streptococcosis* in infants under 6 months of age is characterized by nasopharyngitis associated with a thin mucopurulent discharge and irregular fever. This infection is difficult to distinguish from the common cold except by culture and by its lengthier persistence.

Treatment. Treatment of colds is entirely symptomatic. Antimicrobial agents do not influence the cold itself and should be reserved for bacterial complications such as otitis media, pneumonia, and the like. The occasional case of streptococcal nasopharyngitis should, of course, be treated with penicillin. The prophylactic use of antimicrobial agents is unwarranted. The local or systemic use of decongestants such as ephedrine or phenylephrine to shrink the nasal mucosa and prevent middle ear infection is of questionable value. It may be helpful for infants before feeding or at bedtime, but the effect is transitory and a rebound effect may occur.

Rest in bed is advisable if the patient has fever or feels ill. It will also serve to isolate him in order to reduce his chances of (1) spreading infection to others and (2) acquiring a secondary bacterial infection. Fluids should be given in liberal amounts. Aspirin may offer some symptomatic relief. The diet is best governed by the patient's appetite.

Control measures. There is no effective method of control. Although isolation of the individual patient lowers the risk of his spreading the disease, this procedure is not practicable on a large scale. It is prudent to keep visitors and other people with colds away from infants and small children.

Acute otitis media

Among the most frequent suppurative infections of infancy and childhood are those of the middle ear. These are discussed fully in Chapter 19.

Acute tonsillopharyngitis with exudate or membrane

Acute tonsillopharyngitis with exudate or membrane is characterized by fever, sore throat, tonsillar and pharyngeal reddening and edema, and the presence of an exudate or membrane. A varying degree of cervical lymph node enlargement may be present. The most common cause is Group A streptococcus (p. 375). A less common but very important cause is *Corynebacterium diphtheriae* (p. 24). Membranous tonsillitis is also a frequent manifestation of infectious mononucleosis (p. 61) and is often seen in military recruits, infants, and children up to age 3 years with adenovirus infection. Since Group A hemolytic streptococcus is the most common cause of this syndrome, antistreptococcal therapy (discussed in detail on p. 378) would be indicated for most patients with this condition. Chaudhary et al. (1985) conducted a randomized trial comparing 10 days of penicillin alone with a similar treatment course to which rifampin was added in the final 4 days. While there were no bacteriologic failures (0/40) among the penicillin-rifampin group, there were 11 among the 39 who received only penicillin.

If the diphtheria bacillus is suspected or proved to be the responsible agent, therapy with diphtheria antitoxin in addition to penicillin or erythromycin (p. 28) should be instituted. Antibiotics are of no value in the treatment of infectious mononucleosis or adenovirus infection.

Acute tonsillopharyngitis with vesicles or ulcers

Acute tonsillopharyngitis with vesicles or ulcers is characterized by fever, sore throat, and vesicles or shallow white ulcers 2 to 4 mm in diameter on the anterior fauces, palate, and buccal mucous membrane. It is most commonly caused by a virus, either herpes simplex virus or Group A Coxsackie virus. A primary infection with herpes simplex virus is usually characterized by stomatitis and gingivitis rather than tonsillopharyngitis. (See Chapter 11.) Gingivitis is not associated with herpangina, which is caused by Group A Coxsackie virus. This syndrome is discussed in detail in Chapter 5. Antimicrobial agents are of no value in the treatment of these infections.

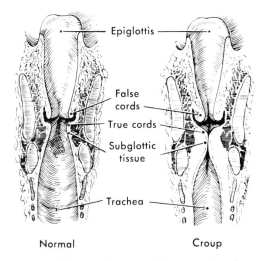

Normal   Croup

Fig. 22-4 Schematic diagram of larynx and trachea in viral croup as compared with normal appearance.

Acute laryngitis; laryngotracheitis; laryngotracheobronchitis; acute epiglottitis—croup

Inflammatory obstruction of the airway produces the characteristic clinical picture in all forms of infectious croup. The severity and extent of the infectious process determine the sites of obstruction in the laryngotracheobronchial tree.

Mild laryngitis is characterized by hoarseness and a barking or croupy cough, which is likely to be worse at night. Low-grade fever, loss of appetite, and malaise may be the only constitutional signs. Difficulty in breathing is slight or absent; the condition responds promptly to appropriate treatment and subsides in a few days.

Acute laryngitis (croup). A more severe type of laryngitis begins in the same fashion but progresses rapidly to the stage of obstruction. The site of obstruction is usually the subglottic area. Hoarseness is more marked. Breathing becomes rapid and labored, with inspiratory stridor and inspiratory retraction of the suprasternal notch, the supraclavicular spaces, the substernal region, and even the intercostal spaces. The child grows restless, often in spite of high humidity and oxygen levels. For a few moments he may scramble about the crib desperately seeking relief and then lie still briefly, only to be roused again by air hunger. The cycle is repeated until the patient becomes exhausted. Cyanosis is sometimes evident in the nail beds and lips. If the obstruction is unrelieved, the patient's color becomes ashen gray, and he sinks into a relaxed, shocklike state as death approaches.

In patients whose infection is limited to the laryngeal area, auscultation of the chest reveals little beyond inspiratory stridor and generally diminished aeration. The pharynx is inflamed, and laryngoscopic examination shows little supraglottic involvement except in *Haemophilus influenzae* epiglottitis (discussed later). The main site of obstruction lies below the vocal cords where the soft subglottic tissues bulge to meet in the midline (Fig. 22-4). The mucosa appears deep red and velvety. A gummy mucopurulent exudate or dry yellow crusts add to the obstruction of the airway.

Acute laryngotracheitis and laryngotracheobronchitis (croup). In severe acute laryngitis the infection may descend rapidly to the trachea and sometimes the bronchi; this increases the patient's struggle for air, prostration, and fever. In laryngotracheobronchitis an expiratory wheeze and various types of bronchitic rales are heard on auscultation of the chest. Aeration of the lungs may be good at one moment and impaired the next. The findings of localized areas of suppressed to absent breath sounds, bronchial breathing or bronchophony, and dullness to percussion indicate atelectasis resulting from the complete plugging of a bronchus with thick, tenacious exudate. If a main bronchus becomes plugged, air hunger, cyanosis, and restlessness are increased. The heart and mediastinum may be shifted to the affected side. In the event of obstructive emphysema caused by partial blocking of a bronchus, the heart and mediastinum may be displaced to the opposite side. These various signs and the alarming dyspnea usually disappear after aspiration of the plugged bronchus.

The progression of symptoms and signs of acute laryngotracheitis has been described by Forbes (1961) as developing in the following four stages:

Stage I
  Fever
  Hoarseness of voice
  Croupy cough
  Inspiratory stridor when disturbed

Stage 2
  Continuous respiratory stridor
  Lower-rib retraction
  Retraction of soft tissue of the neck
  Accessory muscles of respiration come into operation
  Respiration becomes labored
Stage 3
  Signs of anoxia and carbon dioxide retention
  Restlessness
  Anxiety
  Pallor
  Sweating
  Rapid respiration
Stage 4
  Intermittent cyanosis
  Permanent cyanosis
  Cessation of breathing

In patients with mild disease and those whose airway has been improved by treatment, croup rarely progresses beyond Stage 1.

Parainfluenza virus types 1 and 3 are the principal viral agents responsible for croup; adenoviruses, parainfluenza type 2, and RS virus are less frequent contributors. During epidemics, influenza or measles viruses may be frequent causes of croup.

Acute epiglottitis (croup). Acute epiglottitis is bacterial in etiology and nearly always caused by *H. influenzae* type b. The site of the obstruction is *supraglottic*, in contrast with acute viral laryngotracheitis, in which the obstruction is *subglottic*.

There is an abrupt onset of fever, dysphagia, toxicity, and difficult obstructive breathing. The voice is not hoarse, but it may have a "strangled" character. Cough, when present, is not croupy. The illness may progress rapidly to severe prostration and death within a few hours if left untreated.

The typical picture is that of a febrile prostrate child with drooling and air hunger. The noisy breathing has been described by Forbes (1961) as "an expiratory snore due to vibration of the flabby swollen tissue of the epiglottis and aryepiglottic folds." Examination of the throat shows a cherry-red, swollen, hard epiglottis that is easily visualized. If one suspects clinically that a child has epiglottitis, examination of the pharynx with a tongue depressor should be postponed until the properly experienced personnel and equipment are at hand (as quickly as pos-

sible) to proceed with immediate intubation (or in some centers tracheostomy) in case the examination precipitates further or even complete airway obstruction. The same supporting personnel should accompany the patient to the radiology suite if a lateral neck film is to be obtained (Mills et al., 1979).

A marked polymorphonuclear leukocytosis is common. *H influenzae* type b organisms are usually grown in cultures of the nose, throat, and blood. The polyribosyl-phosphate capsular antigen of the organism can be rapidly identified by CIE of serum and/or urine. The distinctive appearance of the epiglottis, the fulminating course, and the high risk of fatal outcome demand immediate establishment of an adequate airway by nasotracheal intubation. Antimicrobial therapy should be started promptly.

Diagnosis. The typical pictures of severe epiglottitis or croup are not soon forgotten. Croup begins as an ordinary upper respiratory tract infection. The child then acquires a hoarse voice and a barking cough. This is followed by dyspnea, inspiratory stridor, and retraction of the soft spaces of the thoracic cage. If obstruction is not relieved, the patient shows increasing restlessness, cyanosis, progressive air hunger, and prostration, ending in death.

First and foremost, it is important to identify *H. influenzae* epiglottitis because it is a medical emergency that requires immediate therapy. The sudden onset of choking-type of breathing associated with an expiratory snore, fever, drooling, no hoarseness, and the presence of a beefy swollen epiglottis makes this diagnosis. Confirmation is obtained by culture of nose, throat, and/or blood.

It is also important to consider the possibility of a diphtheritic laryngitis, especially in unimmunized persons. This diagnosis is suggested by the presence of a faucial membrane and evidence of subglottic obstruction. However, even in the absence of a membrane in the pharynx, progression of inspiratory stridor over a 1- to 2-day period in a toxic patient may indicate the presence of a diphtheritic laryngitis without evidence of pharyngeal involvement. The diagnosis may be confirmed by culture of the throat and tracheal aspirates.

Croup with subglottic involvement is most commonly caused by one of the respiratory viruses, especially parainfluenza viruses. The etiologic diagnosis of viral croup is usually made by excluding other causes. Attempts to identify the specific cause by virus isolation may not help in the immediate management of the patient. However, these procedures would be helpful for epidemiologic purposes.

Differential diagnosis

Spasmodic croup. Spasmodic croup may simulate infectious croup in many respects. It has been distinguished from infectious croup by (1) the absence or mildness of signs of inflammation, (2) the typical remissions during the daytime, and (3) the history of previous attacks lasting for 2 or 3 days followed by uneventful recovery. Cramblett (1960) described a child with three typical attacks of acute spasmodic croup at 4, 11, and 29 months of age. Each attack was associated with an infection from a virus—parainfluenza virus type 2 in the first attack, influenza A virus in the second, and ECHO virus type 11 in the third.

Foreign bodies. An awareness of the capacity of foreign bodies to reproduce the obstructive phenomena is essential. If there is a history of sudden onset of choking, paroxysmal coughing, and absence of signs of infection, it can be expected that fluoroscopic and roentgenographic examinations and endoscopy will clarify the diagnosis.

Retropharyngeal abscess. Retropharyngeal abscess may be mistaken for infectious croup. It occurs in infants and children and is marked by drooling, noisy and difficult mouth breathing, dysphagia, retraction of the head, and enlargement of the cervical lymph nodes. The diagnosis is established by a lateral roentgenogram of the neck and by finger palpation of a fluctuant mass on the posterior pharyngeal wall. Prompt institution of antibiotic therapy and controlled surgical drainage are the cornerstones of treatment.

Angioneurotic edema. Angioneurotic edema, seldom encountered in infants or young children, is characterized by supraglottic swelling in response to a specific food or some other allergen. The diagnosis is confirmed by finding pale red, rounded masses on either side of the superior isthmus of the larynx on direct laryngoscopic examination. Urticaria is an external sign pointing to the likely diagnosis. The rapid

response to epinephrine is a good therapeutic test.

Complications. A serious event in the course of laryngotracheobronchitis is the formation of *crusted exudate* in the tracheobronchial tree. Two factors are believed to promote this condition: (1) breathing of air that is not saturated with moisture and (2) temporary alterations of function of the mucus-secreting glands of the respiratory tract. In any event, crusting of the exudate may lead to further obstruction of the airway and collapse of a segment of the lung. The cough reflex is likely to be diminished in these patients. Cyanosis develops or increases. Signs of consolidation may be mistaken for pneumonia.

Mediastinal emphysema and *pneumothorax* are common complications. Extra-alveolar thoracic air may be produced through (1) the intrinsic route, in which minute perivascular ruptures occur in the alveoli, leading to pulmonary interstitial emphysema, mediastinal emphysema, pneumothorax, pneumoperitoneum, and subcutaneous emphysema, and (2) the extrinsic route, in which air enters the superior mediastinum behind the pretracheal fascia as a result of tracheostomy. From the superior mediastinum, air can penetrate adjacent areas. Both of these mechanisms may operate to produce mediastinal emphysema and pneumothorax. Tracheostomy is not the only factor nor even necessarily the most important factor, since instances of extra-alveolar thoracic air have been observed prior to or in the absence of tracheostomy.

The presence of *pneumothorax* may be suspected in a patient with absence of breath sounds and a hyperresonant percussion note on one side of the thorax and displacement of the heart and mediastinum to the opposite side. Roentgenographic examination will show the extent of the pneumothorax and is usually the means of detecting mediastinal emphysema. Subcutaneous emphysema produces a distinctive crackling or crepitus on palpation.

Interstitial bronchopneumonia in all likelihood enters the picture in every case of severe croup as the disease process extends to the terminal bronchioles, peribronchial tissues, and alveoli. It is often impossible even by roentgenographic examination to distinguish between patchy areas of atelectasis and interstitial pneumonia. The combination of infection and atelectasis if persistent is conducive to *bronchiectasis*, which may be seen as an end result. Travis et al. (1977) have pointed out the occurrence of pulmonary edema in several patients with laryngotracheitis and epiglottitis.

Although metastatic foci of infection are not common in *H. influenzae* type b epiglottitis, the experience in Denver as well as a review of the literature revealed that pneumonia, cervical lymphadenitis, and otitis media were the complications noted occasionally, while meningitis and pyarthrosis were quite rare (Molteni, 1976).

Prognosis. The prognosis of infectious croup is related to the character and extent of infection and to the amount of obstruction. As the disease progresses downward from simple laryngitis to laryngotracheobronchitis, the mortality increases from about 1% to 16% (Rabe, 1948). Only one death occurred among 262 nontracheostomized patients with viral croup. Of 35 patients with fatal cases, six had severe obstruction caused by crusted exudate in the trachea and bronchi.

In Rabe's series of 28 patients with epiglottitis caused by *H. influenzae* type b, there were five deaths. The fulminating character of this infection is indicated by the fact that four of the five deaths occurred from 9 to 20 hours after the onset of obstructive symptoms. The fifth patient, who received no specific treatment, died 48 hours after the onset of epiglottitis. All five patients had *H. influenzae* bacteremia.

In general, deaths from *H. influenzae* type b epiglottitis are attributable to bacteremia, toxemia, and rapid obstruction of the airway. This fact serves to highlight the importance of prompt specific chemotherapy and early nasotracheal intubation or tracheostomy.

Treatment. The keynote of treatment is to maintain the airway and to combat infection. It is important to place the patient promptly in an atmosphere with a high humidity level. In the home this can sometimes be achieved by turning on the hot water taps in a closed bathroom. In the hospital the patient should be placed in a room or tent in which the air is supersaturated with moisture, preferably by means of a mechanical humidifier with 30% to 40% oxygen. The temperature should be 21.1° to 23.9° C (70°

to 75° F). Higher temperatures, as generated in steam tents, are oppressive and not necessary. The patient should have plenty to drink. If fluids cannot be given by mouth, they must be administered parenterally. Rest is of paramount importance. The patient should be spared all needless medical examinations, details of nursing care, and especially, a succession of diagnostic or therapeutic venipunctures, taking of blood for blood counts, taking of nose and throat cultures, and other tests. Every effort should be made not to disturb a sleeping child. Expectorants have been tried and found wanting. Opiates and atropine are contraindicated.

In many cases, especially those in which infection is limited to the upper respiratory tract, a period of breathing supersaturated air, combined with rest, will be followed by no increase in the obstructive symptoms. Hoarseness, dyspnea, and inspiratory retraction or pulling are still present but are no worse. The child is not restless and sleeps from time to time. The color is good and there is no cyanosis. Little by little the signs and symptoms disappear, and in a few days the patient progresses to complete recovery. Severe cases with a similar onset are likely not to pursue such a favorable course. The obstructive phenomena are aggravated until it is obvious that the child will suffocate unless an airway is established.

Indications for tracheostomy or intubation. The decision to perform a tracheostomy or intubation for a patient with croup and *when* to do it calls for a nicety of clinical judgment. If this procedure is indicated, it is best done before the patient becomes exhausted and before it has to be done as an emergency, or last-ditch, procedure. If despite high humidity and oxygen levels, the patient shows increasing duskiness, dyspnea, inspiratory retraction, diminished air entry, and especially restlessness, it means there is increasing obstruction to the airway, and it is a clear indication for tracheostomy or intubation. Blood gas studies may show a falling Po_2 with a normal Pco_2. The establishment of an airway is usually followed by immediate and dramatic relief, and the child falls asleep as the tube is being installed.

The teamwork of pediatrician, bronchoscopist, respiratory therapist, and nurse is vitally important for the proper care of the patient. The bronchoscopist should see the patient, if possible, when he is admitted to the hospital, even though there may be no indication for an artificial airway at the moment. Someone with experience should be in attendance at all times. Special nursing care is essential because the tube may become plugged at any time. Frequent aspiration of tracheobronchial secretions is usually necessary. A bronchoscopist should be quickly available to deal with sticky exudates or crusts that cannot be aspirated by a catheter and that give rise to obstruction and pulmonary collapse.

Specific chemotherapy. Since most cases of infectious croup are viral in origin, the indications for administering antimicrobial agents are specific only in patients with *H. influenzae* and *C. diphtheriae* infections.

Corticosteroid therapy. The advocates of corticosteroid therapy postulate that its anti-inflammatory effect will reduce edema and improve the airway. The opponents of this therapy point to the equivocal clinical trials and the extensive studies on laboratory animals supported by clinical experience indicating that cortisone enhances susceptibility to infection. Although there is no evidence of harmful effects after the use of these drugs for a period limited to 2 or 3 days, the value of corticosteroids in the treatment of croup remains controversial (Eden et al., 1967; Cherry, 1979; Leipzig, et al., 1979). In an attempt to resolve the controversy over the use of high-dose corticosteroids in the treatment of croup, Koren et al. (1983) described a beneficial steroid effect in spasmodic croup with a prompt lowering of elevated respiratory rates. In contrast, there was no improvement when steroids were given to children with laryngotracheitis. At present the routine use of corticosteroids for acute laryngotracheitis is not recommended.

Other therapy. Nebulized racemic epinephrine administered by intermittent positive-pressure breathing (IPPB) apparatus has been helpful in the experience of some clinicians (Taussig et al., 1975; Westley et al., 1978). Treatments given at 2- to 4-hour intervals may produce acute beneficial results, but patients must continue under close observation because there may be a "rebound phenomenon," with relapse within several hours of the initial improvement.

A preparation of 2.25% racemic epinephrine is used for 10 to 15 minutes via a face mask attached to an IPPB machine driven by 40% oxygen. Considerable patient cooperation is required to complete this form of therapy.

Acute bronchiolitis

Acute bronchiolitis is seen mainly in the first 18 months of life with a peak at 6 months of age. One reason for this is that the small lumen of the infant's bronchioles is particularly vulnerable to obstruction by edema, cellular mucoid exudate, and muscular constriction. Partial obstruction results in trapping of air in the alveoli, which leads to hyperinflation. Expiration is prolonged and difficult. When the trapped air is absorbed, atelectasis follows. This sequence of events may lead to rapidly changing physical signs.

Bronchiolitis usually begins as an ordinary upper respiratory tract infection with nasal discharge, cough, slight fever, fretfulness, and loss of appetite. In a day or so, the infant gets rapidly worse and presents an alarming picture of rapid labored breathing, with retraction of the intercostal spaces, use of accessory respiratory muscles, cyanosis, and prostration. Increasing obstruction leads to progressive hypoxemia, which if unrelieved, may be followed by exhaustion and death. Respirations are rapid, shallow, difficult, and often wheezy, with a rate of 60 to 80 or more per minute. Inspiratory retraction is seen in the suprasternal notch and the intercostal and subcostal spaces. The cough is frequent, distressing, and often paroxysmal. Cyanosis appears or is intensified during coughing or crying and is likely to be continuous if the obstruction is severe. The patient is prostrate and takes little interest in his surroundings.

Physical findings, often changeable, are those of overinflated lungs; that is, the percussion note is hyperresonant, the diaphragm is depressed, and expiration is prolonged. Early, the breath sounds are diminished, and often no rales are heard. Later, fine, dry, or sibilant rales are audible. Fluoroscopic or roentgenographic examination of the chest shows the lung fields to be abnormally transparent, with increased bronchovascular markings. The diaphragm is depressed and the intercostal spaces are widened. Atelectatic areas are usually small and difficult to recognize in the roentgenogram. Occasionally, one or more segments are collapsed. Arterial blood gas determinations can be very helpful in assessing the patient's respiratory exchange, the need for further support, and the response to treatment. The anticipated findings are an initial hypoxemia, which may be followed by respiratory acidosis and hypercapnia as deterioration occurs.

The nonbacterial cause of bronchiolitis, long suspected on clinical grounds, became more clearly defined as a result of the studies of Parrott et al. (1962). RSV is the most important single agent causing bronchiolitis, followed by parainfluenza virus types 1 and 3, adenoviruses, rhinoviruses, and influenza virus. Measles virus may occasionally give rise to bronchiolitis. RSV infections occur annually in the temperate zone, with peaks in winter and early spring coinciding regularly with outbreaks of bronchiolitis in the population under 2 years of age. In school-age children, similar illnesses, wheezing-associated respiratory infections, are more often due to *Mycoplasma pneumoniae* (Henderson et al., 1979). RSV bronchiolitis and bronchopneumonia may be found as nosocomial infections among infants and children in nurseries and pediatric wards and may occur also among day-care center residents (Wenzel et al., 1977).

The treatment of acute bronchiolitis should aim at (1) relieving bronchiolar obstruction, (2) correcting hypoxemia and acidosis, (3) controlling potential cardiac complications, (4) providing supportive measures, and (5) combating any rare secondary bacterial infection.

The patient should breathe air well saturated with water vapor and high in oxygen content. The high humidity level is designed to render the exudates less sticky. Oxygen tends to dry bronchial secretions and must therefore be used only in conjunction with water vapor. Sometimes epinephrine (0.1 ml of 1:1000 solution given subcutaneously) or aminophylline seem to temporarily relieve bronchiolar spasm. Some groups have reported remarkable improvement following the administration of racemic epinephrine by IPPB apparatus. Cardiovascular support and drugs may be required in the presence of manifestations of developing heart failure, such as enlargement of the liver, gallop rhythm, change in quality of heart sounds,

tachycardia, and pulmonary edema. If the patient has very severe bronchiolitis that progresses in spite of these measures, it may be necessary to provide assisted ventilation and all the support available in an intensive care unit. Outwater and Crone (1984) described a logical program for the management of 15 small infants who in the course of acute bronchiolitis required ventilatory assistance. Fourteen of their 15 patients had positive immunofluorescence of tracheal secretions for RSV. They were all admitted to an intensive care unit, intubated, sedated, ventilated, diuresed, fluid restricted, given bronchiodilators, and fed by nasogastric tube.

As might be expected from the viral etiology of bronchiolitis, antimicrobial therapy is of no benefit. The routine prophylactic or therapeutic use of antimicrobial agents is contraindicated.

Ribavirin, a synthetic nucleoside with antiviral properties, has beneficial effects when administered by aerosol to infants with RSV bronchiolitis and pneumonia (Hall et al., 1983). It has also shown therapeutic efficacy in the treatment of young adults with influenza A and B illness (McClung et al., 1983; Wilson et al., 1984). There was a more rapid improvement in overall clinical signs, a decrease in virus shedding and an increase in arterial oxygen saturation. All three studies utilized placebo controls. The influenza patients also had a more rapid defervescence and resolution of rhinitis. Ribavirin is currently (1985) available only as an investigational drug.

Pneumonia

The term *pneumonia* is used to describe a variety of reactions of the lung to various agents, infectious and noninfectious. This discussion is limited to infectious pneumonia, bacterial and nonbacterial, that affects chiefly infants and children. The clinical manifestations vary greatly, depending on the causative agent, the age of the patient, his systemic reaction to the infection, the presence of any underlying host defense compromise, the extent of the lesions, and the degree of bronchial and bronchiolar obstruction.

Bacterial pneumonia. In the last three decades the incidence of pneumococcal and Group A streptococcal pneumonia has decreased sharply, in part due to the widespread use of antimicrobial agents. *H. influenzae* and other bacteria are also responsible for pneumonia in normal children. On the the other hand, staphylococcal pneumonia is a more common type of bacterial pneumonia in infancy and poses a formidable problem. The clinical manifestations, complications, and treatment of staphylococcal pneumonia are discussed in Chapter 27.

The unavailability of sputum or other materials for culture from the lower respiratory tract makes the etiologic diagnosis of bacterial pneumonia very difficult to establish with certainty in infants and young children. In most patients the diagnosis is based on clinical assessment and judgment. Occasionally, however, the following findings may be helpful: positive blood culture, empyema fluid available for sampling, or characteristic chest film, such as pneumatoceles in staphylococcal pneumonia. Leukocytosis with shift to the left, toxicity, grunting respirations, or splinting caused by pleural irritation may be clues to a bacterial etiology. Lung aspiration for culture may be necessary in patients who fail to respond to appropriate therapy and in those who are immunocompromised.

Pneumococcal pneumonia. The onset of pneumococcal pneumonia is typically sudden in a child who has been well or who has had an upper respiratory tract infection. In infants, vomiting or a convulsion may be the first manifestation. An older child may complain of a headache, abdominal pain, or chest pain. Examination reveals a temperature of 38.9° to 40° C (102° to 104° F), rapid pulse, rapid shallow respirations, a hot dry skin, and little else. In infants, the possibility of CNS involvement is suggested by high fever, convulsions, restlessness, stupor, stiff neck,

bulging anterior fontanelle, or Brudzinski's sign; examination of the CSF is often required to differentiate meningismus from meningitis. The course of pneumococcal pneumonia in a 9-year-old child is shown in Fig. 22-5.

By about the second day of illness, cough, expiratory grunt, dilation of the nostrils, suppression of breath sounds, and inconstant rales over the involved portion of the lungs point to the true nature of the disease. A pleural friction rub may be heard. Later, dullness and bronchial breathing indicate the area of consolidation, which may be confirmed by roentgenography. Resolution begins about 24 hours after appropriate antimicrobial treatment is started. Complications such as empyema, pericarditis, meningitis, arthritis, and peritonitis are seldom seen today. Otitis media is common but should be easily controlled. The etiologic diagnosis may be confirmed by culturing pneumococci from sputum, blood, or empyema fluid (Table 22-7). CIE of pleural fluids has been positive for pneumococcal antigens even when blood cultures have been negative (Siegel et al., 1978).

In evaluating children with pneumococcal pneumonia it is important to remember that as many as 25% of them may have a predisposing underlying condition (Burman et al., 1985). These include sickle cell disease, splenectomy, congenital heart disease, leukemia, immunoglobulin deficiency, asthma, galactosemia, and other metabolic disorders, especially those with hepatic damage. The peak incidence of pneumococcal disease is in the first 2 years of life, so some of these disorders may not yet have been detected.

Table 22-7. Some characteristics of pleural effusions

	Transudate	*Exudate*
Appearance	Light straw serum ultrafiltrate	Cloudy, opaque, cellular
Specific gravity	<1.016	>1.016
pH	≥7.3	<7.2 (6-7)
RBCs	up to 5000	>100,000 (malignancy)
WBCs	<1000	>1000 (usually >10000)
Protein concentrate	<3 gm	>3 gm (>0.5 serum level)
Glucose	70-95 mg	<60 mg
LDH	<200	>300
Gram stain	Negative	Positive
Culture	Negative	Positive
Antigen detection	Negative	Positive
Cytology	Negative	Especially with malignancy

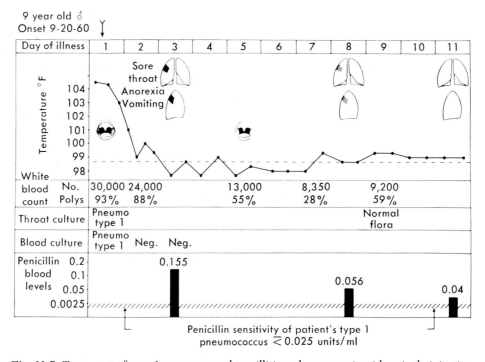

Fig. 22-5. Treatment of type 1 pneumococcal tonsillitis and pneumonia with a single injection of a penicillin preparation containing 600,000 units of aqueous procaine penicillin and 600,000 units of benzathine penicillin G. Note the dramatic subsidence of fever, the clearing of the exudative tonsillitis and pulmonary consolidation, and the rapid elimination of the type 1 pneumococci from the throat and blood. The penicillin blood level at 11 days (0.04 unit per milliliter) still exceeded the sensitivity of the patient's type 1 pneumococcus (less than 0.025 unit of penicillin per milliliter). (From Krugman S. Pediatr Clin North Am. 1961; 8:1199.)

Treatment. Pneumococcal pneumonia usually can be treated adequately by any one of a variety of antimicrobial agents, including penicillin, ampicillin, chloramphenicol, erythromycin, and the sulfonamides. Penicillin is the preferred drug (see p. 270). The response to therapy is usually observed within 1 to 2 days. The treatment should be continued for at least 5 days or more if the clinical findings warrant it. Only one drug is necessary.

Nonbacterial pneumonia. The clinical manifestations of nonbacterial pneumonia (atypical pneumonia or viral pneumonia) are diverse. The onset is usually gradual but may be sudden. Systemic signs, especially fever, may be striking or inconspicuous. A mild upper respiratory tract illness usually precedes the more acute episode. Cough, fever, chilliness, headache, malaise, anorexia, listlessness, and irritability are common manifestations. Anorexia may be prominent.

Cough appears early, is often severe and relentless, and interferes with sleep. Sputum, if obtainable, is mucoid or mucopurulent but may be blood streaked. Physical signs are variable; the child appears listless but only mildly or moderately ill. The temperature may be normal or elevated; respirations are usually normal. Chest findings are minimal, often limited to medium sticky rales and slight impairment of percussion note and breath sounds. The pneumonia is frequently discovered only on roentgenographic examination. The latter reveals a picture that also is not distinctive and varies from enlarged hilar shadows to patchy consolidation. Shifting areas of consolidation may be seen.

The clinical course is irregular but usually benign, complete recovery normally occurring in 1 to 3 weeks. Laboratory findings include a normal or slightly increased white blood cell count. Bacteriologic cultures are noncontributory. Cold agglutinins develop in the course of illness in about half of the patients with pneumonia caused by *M. pneumoniae*.

The performance of a quick qualitative cold agglutination test may help in the assessment of a patient suspected of mycoplasmal infection. To a standard citrated test tube add 5 drops of blood from the patient's fingertip, place the tube in a cup of ice water for 30 seconds, and then remove. When the tube is tilted, gross agglutination will be visible if the patient's serum titer is 1:64 or higher. Although a number of viral infections may induce cold agglutinins in infants and preschool children, their presence in high titer (greater than or equal to 1:64) in school-age children and adolescents correlates best with infection due to *M. pneumoniae*.

The etiologic agents associated with pneumonia are listed in Table 22-6. In the studies caried out by Parrott et al. (1962), RS virus, parainfluenza viruses, and adenoviruses appeared to be the major nonbacterial causes of pneumonia in children.

Immunocompromised patients may develop pneumonias of unusual etiology such as pneumocystis, cytomegalovirus (see Chapter 2), toxoplasmosis (see Chapter 31), or tuberculosis (see Chapter 3). Fungal pneumonias may also be associated with impaired host defenses or with exposure in endemic geographic areas. Blastomycosis has been reported in the valleys of the St. Lawrence, Ohio, and Mississippi rivers as well as in the southeastern United States. Histoplasmosis is endemic in certain parts of the United States, particularly the Ohio River valley. Coccidioidomycosis is endemic in the southwestern United States and in Argentina.

The wide spectrum of agents that may cause pneumonia in immunocompromised patients presents a serious diagnostic challenge. Viral (cytomegalovirus, herpes simplex, parainfluenza), protozoal *(Pneumocystis)*, fungal *(Candida, Asperigillus, Cryptococcus, Zygomycetes)*, and unusual bacterial (*Nocardia*, gram-negative bacilli, *Staphylococcus*) agents may be the etiologic culprits. Every case must be considered on its own individual features, but a precise diagnosis is often essential to successful intervention. Therefore, invasive techniques ranging from fiberoptic bronchoscopy to open lung biopsy may be necessary if antigen detection and cultures of blood, sputum, or other sources are

not helpful. Empiric therapy with amphotericin B, acyclovir, trimethoprim-sulfamethoxazole, and/or other drugs may be initiated on the basis of clinical clues while one is awaiting results.

Treatment. Most nonbacterial pneumonias are viral in origin and are not influenced by antimicrobial therapy. Chlamydial pneumonias are an exception, and patients should receive tetracycline for *Chlamydia psittaci* and erythromycin for *C. trachomatis* pneumonias. Erythromycin is recommended for *M. pneumoniae* pneumonia.

General therapeutic measures include bed rest and maintenance of fluid intake. Oxygen is indicated for patients who are cyanotic and dyspneic, and a moist atmosphere is helpful for those with obstructive bronchitis or bronchiolitis. Because of the lack of correlation between the results of upper respiratory tract cultures and the infecting flora of the lower respiratory tract, the etiology of pneumonia and other lower respiratory infections of infancy and childhood is often uncertain. The severity of illness, especially in infants, is often marked and the clinician is pressed to intervene with less than satisfying documentation of cause. For this reason antibiotics are often prescribed with a half-hearted zeal, "in case there is secondary bacterial invasion" superimposed on a likely viral infection. The small infant has a number of liabilities that predispose him to respiratory failure with an infection that in an older child might be relatively benign (Pagtakhan and Chernick, 1982):

1. Obligatory nasal breathing
2. Immature musculature of the chest wall
3. Tiny diameters and collapsibility of airways
4. Limited collateral ventilatory pathways
5. Increased tendency for parenchymal collapse
6. Fragility of metabolic and energy balances
7. Easy fatigability

The survival of infants with bronchopulmonary dysplasia has augmented the population of infants for whom a "minor" respiratory infection may become life-threatening and require a temporary period of mechanical ventilatory support. Similarly at high risk are infants with congenital heart disease (MacDonald et al., 1982) and with severe asthma.

Unusual pneumonias, such as those of fungal or protozoal origin, require the use of drugs with special problems of toxicity. Amphotericin B, which is effective for many of the fungi, should be used only with careful attention to its potential for nephrotoxicity, febrile reactions, anemia, hypokalemia, cardiac arrhythmias, and other adverse effects. Pentamidine isothionate, another agent with considerable toxicity, has been virtually replaced in the therapy of *Pneumocystis carinii* pneumonia by the combination trimethoprim-sulfamethoxazole, a far less toxic treatment (Siegel et al., 1984).

Influenza-like illness

The syndrome that is termed influenza-like illness is characterized by sudden onset, chills or chilliness, fever, headache, marked prostration, muscular pains in the back and extremities, respiratory symptoms, and lack of any clear-cut abnormal physical findings outside the upper respiratory tract.

It is now recognized that this syndrome may be caused by several viruses in addition to the influenza viruses A and B. The other agents include parainfluenza virus types 1, 2, and 3; adenoviruses; Coxsackie viruses Group A and Group B; and lymphocytic choriomeningitis virus.

The incubation period is short, usually 24 to 72 hours. The onset of illness is sudden, with chills or feelings of chilliness, fever, headache, aches and pains in the back and legs, malaise, anorexia, and prostration. Nausea and vomiting may occur. Pain or a burning sensation in the eyes may be present. Constitutional symptoms are more prominent, as a rule, than are respiratory symptoms. There is commonly a hacking cough accompanied by substernal soreness, which suggests tracheobronchitis. Dryness or scratchiness of the throat may occur together with hoarseness. Rhinitis, sneezing, and nasal discharge usually appear later.

The physical findings are characteristically scanty and ill defined. The patient often seems knocked out. In those patients who have fever, the temperature may go as high as 39.4° to 40° C (103° to 104° F). The temperature is likely to be higher in children than in adults. The pulse rate is usually in proportion to the degree of fever. The face may appear flushed, and the conjunctivae may seem injected. The throat may look normal, or it may be reddened and show glistening hypertrophied lymphoid nodules on the posterior pharyngeal wall. The lungs are usually clear. Signs of consolidation are not present in uncomplicated influenza-like illness.

The clinical laboratory findings are usually normal. The white blood cell count occasionally shows moderate leukopenia. The sedimentation rate is increased. Blood cultures are sterile. Results of roentgenographic examination of the chest are usually normal.

The course of the disease is usually one of rapid and progressive improvement. After severe infections, some patients tend to show persistent prostration and sweating and are easily tired for several days after the temperature comes down to normal. Complications are rarely seen outside a pandemic. Prompt and complete recovery is the rule in ordinary epidemics.

Like most other virus diseases, influenza-like illness is a self-limited infection. Treatment is symptomatic. Bedrest is recommended. There is no evidence that any antimicrobial agent affects the course. Complications are rarely encountered and are best dealt with as they arise. The routine prophylactic use of antimicrobial agents is discouraged. Antipyretics and codeine are usually effective in alleviating symptoms. Fluids should be given freely. The diet is best governed by the patient's appetite.

Prevention. Influenza virus vaccines may be somewhat reactogenic, especially in infants and children. The frequent antigenic drifts and occasional shifts of virus antigens make it difficult to keep up with the currently circulating strains of influenza A. Recommendations for vaccine use in children at high risk are found in Chapter 35. Amantadine hydrochloride has been used successfully in the prophylaxis of type A influenza strains in epidemic settings. Monto et al. (1979) reported a favorable result among University of Michigan students during the 1978 outbreak of H1N1 influenza. The drug was given orally, once daily (200-mg dose) for at least 6 weeks. Their results showed a 70% efficacy in prevention of illness and infection in contrast to a placebo control group. The available data on amantadine's effects and toxicity in the pediatric age group are limited (p. 503).

REFERENCES

Adair JC, Ring WH. Management of epiglottitis in children. Anesth Analg 1975; 54:622.

Adair JC, et al. Ten year experience with IPPB in the treatment of acute laryngotracheobronchitis. Anesth Analg 1971; 50:649.

Adams JM, Imagawa DT, Zike K. Epidemic bronchiolitis and pneumonitis related to respiratory syncytial virus. JAMA 1961; 176:1037.

Almeida JD, Tyrrell DAJ. The morphology of three previously uncharacterized human respiratory viruses that grow in organ culture. J Gen Virol 1967; 1:175.

Amman AJ, et al. Polyvalent pneumococcal-polysaccharide immunization of patients with sickle-cell anemia and patients with splenectomy. N Engl J Med 1977; 297:897.

Anas N, Boettrich C, Hall CB, et al. The association of apnea and respiratory syncytial virus infection. J Pediatr 1982; 101:65.

Anderson KC, Maurer MJ, Dajani AS. Pneumococci relatively resistant to penicillin: a prevalence survey in children. J Pediatr 1980; 97:939.

Andiman WA, McCarthy P, Markowitz RL, et al. Clinical, virologic, and serologic evidence of Epstein-Barr virus infection in association with childhood pneumonia. J Pediatr 1981; 99:880.

Andrewes CH. The taxonomic position of common cold viruses and some others. Yale J Biol Med 1961-1962; 34:200.

Andrewes CH, Bang FB, Chanock, RM, Zhdanov VM. Parainfluenza virus 1, 2, 3: suggested names for recently isolated myxoviruses. Virology 1959; 8:129.

Arth C, Von Schmidt BV, Grossman M, Schachter J. Chlamydial pneumonitis. J Pediatr 1978; 93:447.

Austrian R. Pneumococcal infection and pneumococcal vaccine. N Engl J Med 1977; 297:938.

Austrian R, et al. Prevention of pneumococcal pneumonia by vaccination. Trans Assoc Am Phys 1976; 89:184.

Beale AJ, McLeod DL, Stackiw W, Roads AJ. Isolation of cytopathic agents from respiratory tract in acute laryngotracheobronchitis. Br Med J 1958; 1:302.

Beare AS, Craig JW. Virulence for man of a human influenza A virus antigenically similar to "classical" swine viruses. Lancet 1960; 2:4.

Beaty HN, et al. Legionnaires' diseases in Vermont, May to October 1977. JAMA 1978; 240:127.

Beem M, et al. Association of the chimpanzee coryza agent with acute respiratory disease in children. N Engl J Med 1960; 263:523.

Beem MP, Saxon EM. Respiratory tract colonization and a distinctive pneumonia syndrome in infants infected with Chlamydia trachomatis. N Engl J Med 1977; 296:306.

Benfield GFA. Recent trends in empyema thoracis. Br J Dis Chest 1981; 75:358.

Beschamps GJ, Lynn HB, Wenzl JE. Empyema in children: review of Mayo Clinic experience. Mayo Clin Proc 1970; 45:43.

Bloom HH, Forsyth BR, Johnson KM, Chanock RM. Relationship of rhinovirus infection to mild upper respiratory disease. I. Results of a survey in young adults and children. JAMA 1963; 186:38.

Bloom HH, Johnson KM, Jacobsen R, Chanock RM: Recovery of parainfluenza viruses from adults with upper respiratory illnesses. Am J Hyg 1961; 74:50.

Bock BV, et al. Legionnaires' disease in renal-transplant recipients. Lancet 1978; 1:410.

Bradburne AS, Tyrrell DA. Coronaviruses of man. In Melnick JL, (ed). Progress in medical virology, vol. 12. New York: S Karger, 1970.

Brandt CD, et al. Infections in 18,000 infants and children in controlled study of respiratory tract disease. I. Adenovirus pathogenicity in relation to serologic type and illness syndromes. Am J Epidemiol 1969; 90:484.

Burman, LA, Norrby R, Trollfors B. Invasive pneumococcal infections; incidence, predisposing factors, and prognosis. Rev Inf Dis 1985; 7:133.

Burrows B, Knudson RG, Lebowitz MD. The relationship of childhood respiratory illness to adult obstructive airway disease. Am Rev Respir Dis 1977; 115:751.

Carson JL, Collier AM, Clyde WA Jr. Ciliary membrane alterations occurring in experimental *Mycoplasma pneumoniae* infection. Science 1979; 206:349.

Carson JL, Collier AM, Hu SS. Acquired ciliary defects in nasal epithelium of children with acute viral upper respiratory infections. N Engl J Med 1985; 312:463.

Cates KL, et al. A penicillin-resistant pneumococcus. J Pediatr 1978; 93:624.

Cattaneo SM, Kolman JW. Surgical therapy of empyema in children. Arch Surg 1973; 106:564.

Centers for Disease Control. Multiple-antibiotic resistance of pneumococci- South Africa. Morbid Mortal Weekly Rep 1977; 26:285.

Chandler FW, Hicklin MD, Blackmon JA. Demonstration of the agent of Legionnaires' disease in tissue. N Engl J Med 1977; 297:1218.

Chanock RM. Mycoplasma infections of man. N Engl J Med 1965; 273:1199.

Chanock RM, Bell JA, Parrott RH. Natural history of parainfluenza infection. In Pollard M (ed). Perspectives in virology, vol 2. Minneapolis: Burgess Publishing Co. 1961, p. 126.

Chanock RM, Finberg L. Recovery from infants with respiratory illness of a virus related to chimpanzee coryza agent (CCA). II. Epidemiologic aspects of infection in infants and young children. Am J Hyg 1957; 66:291.

Chanock RM, Hayflick L, Barile MD. Growth on artificial medium of an agent associated with atypical pneumonia and its identification as a PPLO. Proc Natl Acad Sci USA 1962; 48:41.

Chanock RM, et al. Respiratory syncytial virus. I. Virus recovery and other observations during 1960 outbreak of bronchiolitis, pneumonia, and minor respiratory diseases in children. JAMA 1961; 176:647.

Chanock RM, et al. Biology and ecology of two major lower respiratory tract pathogens—RS virus and Eaton PPLO. In Pollard M (ed). Perspectives in virology, vol 3. New York: Harper & Row, 1963, p. 257.

Chanock RM, et al. Possible role of immunologic factors in pathogenesis of RS virus lower respiratory tract disease. In Pollard M (ed). Perspectives in virology, vol 4. New York: Academic Press, Inc., 1969, pp. 125-139.

Chanock RM, et al. Influence of immunological factors in respiratory syncytial virus disease. Arch Environ Health 1970; 21:347.

Chany C, et al. Severe and fatal pneumonia in infants and young children associated with adenovirus. Am J Hyg 1958; 67:3967.

Chaudhary S, Bilinsky SA, Hennessy JL, et al. Penicillin V and rifampin for the treatment of group A streptococcal pharyngitis. J Pediatr 1985; 106:481.

Cherry JD. The treatment of croup: continued controversy due to failure of recognition of historic, ecologic, etiologic and clinical perspectives. J Pediatr 1979; 94:352.

Cowan MH, et al. Pneumococcal polysaccharide immunization in infants and children. Pediatrics 1978; 62:721.

Cradock-Watson JE, McQuillin J, Gardner PS. Rapid diagnosis of respiratory syncytial virus infection in children by the immunofluorescent technique. J Clin Pathol 1971; 24:347.

Cramblett HG. Croup—present day concept. Pediatrics 1960; 25:1071.

Dees SC. Asthma. In Kendig E (ed). Disorders of the respiratory tract in children. Philadelphia: W.B. Saunders Co. 1977, p. 820.

Denny FW, Clyde WA Jr, Glezon WP. *Mycoplasma pneumoniae* disease: clinical spectrum pathophysiology, epidemiology, and control. J Infect Dis 1971; 123:74.

Eaton MD, Meiklejohn G, van Herrick WJ. Studies on etiology of primary atypical pneumonia: filtrable agent transmissible to cotton rats, hamsters, and chick embryos. J Exp Med 1944; 79:649.

Eden AN, Kaufman A, Yu R. Corticosteroids and croup: controlled double blind study. JAMA 1967; 200:133.

Eliasson R, Mossberg B, Camner R, Afzelius BA. The immotile cilia syndrome. N Engl J Med 1977; 297:1.

Escobar JA, et al. Etiology of respiratory tract infections in children in Cali, Columbia. Pediatrics 1976; 57:123.

Evans AS, Brobst M. Bronchiolitis, pneumonitis, and pneumonia in University of Wisconsin students. N Engl J Med, 1961; 265:401.

Faden HS. Treatment of *Haemophilus influenza* type b epiglottitis. Pediatrics 1979; 63:402.

Fernald GW, Collier AM, Clyde WA Jr. Respiratory infections due to *Mycoplasma pneumoniae* in infants and children. Pediatrics 1975; 55:327.

Finland M. Pneumonia and pneumococcal infections, with special reference to pneumococcal pneumonia. Am Rev Respir Dis 1979; 120:481.

Forbes JA. Croup and its management. Br Med J 1961; 1389.

Forfar JO. Demography, vital statistics, and the pattern of disease in childhood. In Forfar JO, Arneil GC (eds). Textbook of paediatrics, London: Churchill Livingstone, 1984, pp. 9-16.

Fox JP, Cooney, MK, Hall CE. The Seattle virus watch. V. Epidemiologic observations of rhinovirus infections in families with young children. Am J Epidemiol 1975; 101:122.

Fox JP, et al. The virus watch program: a continuing surveillance of viral infections in metropolitan New York families. VI. Observations of adenovirus infections: virus excretion patterns, antibody response, efficiency of surveillance, patterns of infection and relation to illness. Am J Epidemiol 1969; 89:25.

Francis T Jr. Factors conditioning resistance to epidemic influenza. Harvey Lect 1942; 37:39.

Fraser DW, et al. Legionnaires' disease. Description of an epidemic of pneumonia. N Engl J Med 1977; 296:1150.

Freij BJ, Kusmiesz H, Nelson JD, et al. Parapneumonic effusions and empyema in hospitalized children: a retrospective review of 227 cases. Pediatr Inf Dis 1984; 3:578.

Friis B, Andersen P, Brenoe E, et al. Antibiotic treatment of pneumonia and bronchiolitis a perspective randomized study. Arch Dis Child 1984; 59:1038.

Frommell G, Bruhn FW, Schwartzman JD. Isolation of Chlamydia trachomatis from infant lung tissue. N Engl J Med 1977; 296:1150.

Gardner PS. How etiologic, pathologic and clinical diagnoses can be made in a correlated fashion. Pediatr Res 1977; 11:254.

Gardner PS, McQuillin J, Court SDM. Speculation on pathogenesis in death from respiratory syncytial virus infection. Br Med J 1970; 1:327.

Gardner PS, et al. Death associated with respiratory tract infections in children. Br Med J 1967; 4:316.

Ginsberg CM, Howard JB, Nelson JD. Report of 65 cases of *Hemophilus influenzae* b pneumonia. Pediatrics 1979; 64:283.

Glezen WP. Pathogenesis of bronchiolitis-epidemiologic considerations. Pediatr Res 1977; 11:234.

Glezen WP, Denny FW. Epidemiology of acute lower respiratory disease in children. N Engl J Med 1973; 228:498.

Glezen WP, Paredes A, Allison JE, et al. Risk of respiratory syncytial virus infection for infants from low-income families in relationship to age, sex, ethnic group, and maternal antibody level. J Pediatr 1981; 98:708.

Glezen WP, et al. Epidemiologic patterns of acute lower respiratory disease in children in a pediatric group practice. J Pediatr 1971; 78:397.

Glicklich M, Cohen RD, Jona JZ. Steroids and bag and mask ventilation in the treatment of acute epiglottitis. J Pediatr Surg 1979; 14:247.

Goldman AS, Schochet SS Jr, Howell JT: The discovery of defects in respiratory cilia in the immotile cilia syndrome. J Pediatr 1980; 96:244.

Gray BM, Converse GM III, Dillon HC Jr. Serotypes of Streptococcus pneumoniae causing disease. J Infect Dis 1980; 140:979.

Hall CB, Hall WJ, Gala CL, et al. Long term prospective study in children after respiratory syncytial virus infection. J Pediatr 1984; 105:358.

Hall CB, McBride JT, Walsh EE, et al. Aerosolized ribavirin treatment of infants with respiratory syncytial virus infection. N Engl J Med 1983; 308:1443.

Hall CB, et al. Neonatal respiratory syncytial virus infection. N Engl J Med 1979; 300:393.

Hall WJ, Hall CB, Speers DM. Respiratory syncytial virus infection in adults. Clinical, virologic and serial pulmonary function studies. Ann Intern Med 1978; 88:203.

Hammerschlag MR, et al. Prospective study of maternal and infantile infection with Chlamydia trachomatis. Pediatrics 1979; 64:142.

Harlap S, Davies AM. Infant admissions to hospital and maternal smoking. Lancet 1974; 1:529.

Harrison HR, English NG, Lee CK, Alexander ER. Chlamydia trachomatis infant pneumonitis: comparison with matched controls and other infant pneumonitis. N Engl J Med 1978; 298:702.

Henderson FW, Collier AM, Clyde WA Jr, Denny FW. Respiratory syncytial virus infections, reinfections and immunity. A prospective longitudinal study in young children. N Engl J Med 1979; 300:530.

Henderson FW, et al. The etiologic and epidemiologic spectrum of bronchiolitis in pediatric practice. J Pediatr 1979; 95:183.

Hendley JO, Wenzel RP, Gwaltney JM Jr. Transmission of rhinovirus colds by self-inoculation. N Engl J Med 1973; 288:1361.

Hierholzer JC, Hirsch MS. Croup and pneumonia in human infants associated with a new strain of respiratory syncytial virus. J Infect Dis 1979; 140:926.

Hilleman MR, et al. Appraisal of occurrence of adenovirus-caused respiratory illness in military populations. Am J Hyg 1957; 66:29.

Hilleman MR, et al. Polyvalent pneumococcal polysaccharide vaccines. J Infect 1979; 1 (suppl. 2):73.

Hirst GK. Studies of antigenic differences among strains of influenza A by means of red cell agglutination. J Exp Med 1943; 78:407.

Hoffman E. Empyema in childhood. Thorax 1961; 16:128.

Jackson GG. Sensitivity of influenza A virus to amantadine. J Infect Dis 1977; 136:301.

Jacobs JW, et al. Respiratory syncytial and other viruses associated with respiratory disease in infants. Lancet 1971; 1:871.

Jacobs MR, et al. Emergence of multiply resistant pneumococci. N Engl J Med 1978; 299:735.

Johnson KM, Bloom HH, Mufson MA, Chanock RM. Natural reinfection of adults by respiratory syncytial virus. N Engl J Med 1962; 267:68.

Johnson KM, et al. Acute respiratory disease associated with coxsackie A21 virus infection. I. Incidence in military personnel: observations in a recruit population. JAMA 1962; 179:112.

Joncas J, Berthiaume L, Pavilanis V. The structure of the respiratory syncytial virus. Virology 1969; 38:493.

Kapikian AZ, et al. An epidemiologic study of altered clinical reactivity to respiratory syncytial (RS) virus infection in children previously vaccinated with an inactivated RS virus vaccine. Am J Epidemiol 1969; 89:405.

Kaye HS, Marsh HB, Dowdle WR. Seroepidemiologic survey of coronavirus (strain OC 43) related infections in a children's population. Am J Epidemiol 1971; 94:43.

Kevy SV. Current concepts: croup. N Engl J Med 1964; 270:464.

Kim HW, et al. Respiratory syncytial virus neutralizing activity in nasal secretions following natural infection. Proc Soc Exp Biol Med 1969; 131:658.

Koraroff AL, Aronson MD, Pass TM, et al. Serologic evidence of chlamydial and mycoplasmal pharyngitis in adults. Science 1983; 222:927-929.

Koren G, Frand M, Barzilay Z, et al. Corticosteroid treatment of laryngotracheitis v spasmodic croup in children. Am J Dis Child 1983; 137:941.

Kosloske AM, Cushing AH, Shuck JM. Early decortication for anaerobic empyema in children. J Pediatr Surg 1980; 15:422.

Kovatch AL, Jardin DS, Dowling JN, et al. Legionellosis in children with leukemia in relapse. Pediatrics 1984; 73:811.

Lang WR, et al. Bronchopneumonia with severe sequelae in children with evidence of adenoviruses in the etiology of acute hemorrhagic cystitis. J Urol 1969; 1:73.

Lattimer GL, McCrone C, Galgon J. Diagnosis of Legionnaires' disease from transtracheal aspirate by direct fluorescent antibody staining and isolation of the bacterium. N Engl J Med 1978; 299:1172.

Leipzig B, et al. A prospective randomized study to determine the efficacy of steroids in treatment of croup. J Pediatr 1979; 94:194.

Li KI, Kiernan S, Wald ER, et al. Isolated uvulitis due to *Haemophilus influenzae* type b. Pediatrics 1984; 74:1054.

Light RW, Girard WM, Jenkinson SG, et al. Parapneumonic effusions. Am J Med 1980; 69:507.

Lin J-SL. Human mycoplasmal infections: serologic observations. Rev Infect Dis 1985; 7:216.

Lindsay MI Jr, et al. Hong Kong influenza: clinical, microbiologic and pathologic features in 127 cases. JAMA 1970; 214:1825.

Lionakis B, Gray SW, Skandalakis JE, et al. Empyema in children; a 25 year study. J Pediatr 1958; 53:719.

Liu C. Studies on primary atypical pneumonia. J Exp Med 1957; 106:455.

Loda FA, Glezen WP, Clyde WA Jr. Respiratory disease in group day care. Pediatrics 1972; 49:428.

Loda FA, et al. Studies on the role of viruses, bacteria and *M. pneumoniae* as causes of lower respiratory tract infections in children. J Pediatr 1968; 72:161.

MacDonald NE, Hall CB, Suffin SC, et al. Respiratory syncytial virus infection in infants with congenital heart disease. N Engl J Med 1982; 307:397.

Marmion BP, Goodburn GM. Effect of an organic gold salt on Eaton's primary atypical pneumonia agent and other observations. Nature 1961; 189:247.

Martin AJ, Gardner PS, McQuillin J. Epidemiology of respiratory viral infection among paediatric inpatients over a six-year period in northeast England. Lancet 1978; 2:1035.

McClung HW, Knight V, Gilbert BE, et al. Ribavirin aerosol treatment of influenza B virus infection. JAMA 1983; 249:2671.

McConnochie KM, Roghmann KJ. Bronchiolitis as a possible cause of wheezing in childhood: new evidence. Pediatrics 1984; 74:1.

McIntosh K, et al. The immunologic response to infection with respiratory syncytial virus in infants. J Infect Dis 1978; 138:24.

McLaughlin FJ, Goldman DA, Rosenbaum DM, et al. Empyema in children: clinical course and long term follow-up. Pediatrics 1984; 73:587.

Melnick JL, et al. Picornaviruses: classification of nine new types. Science 1963; 141:153.

Mills JL, et al. The usefulness of lateral neck roentgenograms in laryngotracheobronchitis. Am J Dis Child 1979; 133:1140.

Mintz L, et al. Nosocomial respiratory syncytial virus infections in an intensive care nursery: rapid diagnosis by direct immunofluorescence. Pediatrics 1979; 64:149.

Molteni RA. Epiglottitis: incidence of extraepiglottic infection: report of 72 cases and review of the literature. Pediatrics 1976; 58:526.

Monto AS, Cavallaro JJ: The Tecumseh study of respiratory illness. II. Patterns of occurrence of infection with respiratory pathogens, 1965-1969. Am J Epidemiol 1971; 94:280.

Monto AS, et al. Prevention of Russian influenza by amantadine. JAMA 1979; 241:1003.

Mufson MA. Pneumococcal infections. JAMA 1981; 246: 1942.

Mufson MA, Belshe RB: A review of adenoviruses in the etiology of acute hemorrhagic cystitis. J Urol 1976; 115:191.

Mufson MA, et al. Eaton agent pneumonia—clinical features. JAMA 1961; 178:369.

Murphy D, Lockhart CH, Todd JK. Pneumococcal empyema. Am J Dis Child 1980; 134:659.

Murphy TF, Henderson FW, Clyde WA, et al. Pneumonia: an 11 year study in a pediatric practice. Am J Epidemiol 1981; 113:12.

Neligan GA, et al. Respiratory syncytial virus infection of the newborn. Br Med J 1970; 3:146.

Nelson WE. Bacterial croup: a historical perspective. J Pediatr 1984; 105:52.

Ort S, Ryan JL, Barden G, et al. Pneumococcal pneumonia in hospitalized patients. JAMA 1983; 249:214.

Outwater KM, Crone RK. Management of respiratory failure in infants with acute viral bronchiolitis. Am J Dis Child 1984; 138:1071.

Pagtakhan RD, Chernick V. Respiratory failure in the pediatric patient. Pediatr Rev 1982; 3:247.

Parrott RH, et al. Respiratory diseases of viral etiology. III. Myxoviruses: parainfluenza. Am J Public Health 1962; 52:907.

Parrott RH, et al. Epidemiology of respiratory syncitial virus infection in Washington, D.C. Am J Epidemiol 1973; 52:907.

Pedreira FA, Guandolo VL, Feroli EJ, et al. Involuntary smoking and incidence of respiratory illness during the first year of life. Pediatrics 1985; 75:594.

Pullan CR, Hey EN. Wheezing, asthma, and pulmonary dysfunction 10 years after infection with respiratory syncytial virus in infancy. Br Med J 1982; 248:1665.

Rabe EF. Infectious croup. I. Etiology. II. "Virus" croup. III. Hemophilus influenza type b croup. Pediatrics 1948; 2:255, 415, 559.

Rooney JC, Williams HE. The relationship between proven viral bronchiolitis and subsequent wheezing. J Pediatr 1971; 79:744.

Rowe, WP, et al. Isolation of a cytopathogenic agent from human adenoids undergoing spontaneous degeneration in tissue culture. Proc Soc Exp Biol Med 1953; 84:570.

Ryan ME, Feldman S, Pruitt B, Fraser DW. Legionnaires' disease in a child with cancer. Pediatrics 1979; 64:951.

Sanford JP. Legionnaires' disease—the first thousand days. N Engl J Med 1979; 300:654.

Santosham M, Yolken RH, Zuiroz E, et al. Detection of rotavirus in respiratory secretions of children with pneumonia. J Pediatr 1983; 103:583.

Sanyal SK, Mariencheck WC, Hughes WT, et al: Course of pulmonary dysfunction in children surviving Pneumocystis carinii pneumonitis: a prospective study. Am Rev Respir Dis 1981; 124:161.

Schachter J. Chlamydial infections. N Engl J Med 1978; 298:428, 490, 540.

Schachter J, Sugg N, Sung M. Psittacosis—the reservoir persists. J Infect Dis 1978; 137:44.

Schachter J, et al. Pneumonitis following inclusion blennorrhea. J Pediatr 1975; 87:779.

Schachter J, et al. Prospective study of chlamydial infections in neonates. Lancet 1979; 2:377.

Schaefer C, Harrison R, Boyce WT, et al. Illnesses in infants born to women with Chlamydia trachomatis infection. Am J Dis Child 1985; 139:127.

Shands KN, Ho JL, Meyer RD, et al. Potable water as a source of legionnaires' disease. JAMA 1985; 253:1412.

Shope RE. The influenza of swine and man. Harvey Lect 1935-1936; 31:183.

Siegel JD, Gartner JC, Michaels RH. Pneumococcal empyema in childhood. Am J Dis Child 1978; 132:1094.

Siegel ST, Wolff LJ, Baehner RL, et al. Treatment of Pneumocystis carinii pneumonitis. Am J Dis Child 1984; 138:1051.

Smit P, et al. Protective efficacy of pneumococcal polysaccharide vaccines. JAMA 1977; 238:2613.

Smith CB, Purcell RH, Bellanti JA, Chanock RM. Protective effect of antibody to parainfluenza type 1 virus. N Engl J Med 1966; 275:1145.

Smith W, Andrewes CH, Laidlaw PO. A virus obtained from influenza patients. Lancet 1933; 2:66.

Stagno S, Brasfield DM, Brown MB, et al. Infant pneumonitis associated with cytomegalovirus, chlamydia, Pneumocystis, and Ureaplasma: a prospective study. Pediatrics 1981; 68:322.

Stagno S, Pifer LL, Hughes WT, et al. Pneumocystis carinii pneumonitis in young immunocompetent infants. Pediatrics 1980; 66:56-62.

Steen-Johnsen J, Orstavik I, Attramadal A. Severe illnesses due to adenovirus type 7 in children. Acta Paediatr Scand 1969; 58:157.

Steigman AJ, Lipton MM, Brapennicke H. Acute lymphonodular pharyngitis: a newly described condition due to coxsackie A virus. Am J Dis Child 1962; 102:713.

Stiles QR, Lindesmith GG, Tucker BL, et al. Pleural empyema in children. Ann Thorac Surg 1970; 10:37.

Strum R, Staneck JL, Myers JP, et al. Pediatric legionnaires' disease diagnosis by direct immunofluorescent staining of sputum. Pediatrics 1981; 68:539.

Stuart-Harris C. Swine influenza virus in man. Lancet 1976; 2:31.

Sussman SJ, Magoffin RL, Lennette EH, Schieble J. Cold agglutinins, Eaton agent, and respiratory infections of children. Pediatrics 1966; 38:571.

Taussig LM, et al. Treatment of laryngotracheobronchitis (croup). Am J Dis Child 1977; 238:2613.

Taylor-Robinson D, Tyrrell DA. Serotypes of viruses (rhinoviruses) isolated from common colds. Lancet 1962; 1:452.

Terranova W, Cohen MI, Fraser DW. 1974 outbreak of Legionnaires' disease diagnosed in 1977, clinical and epidemiological features. Lancet 1978; 2:122.

Travis KW, Todrez ID, Shannon DC. Pulmonary edema associated with croup and epiglottitis. Pediatrics 1977; 59:695.

Turner JAP, Corkey CWB, Lee JYC, et al. Clinical expressions of immotile cilia syndrome. Pediatrics 1981; 67:805.

Turner RB, Hayden FG, Hendley JO. Counterimmunoelectrophoresis of urine for diagnosis of bacterial pneumonia in pediatric outpatients. Pediatrics 1983; 71:780.

Unger A, Tapia L, Mimnich LL, et al. Atypical neonatal respiratory syncytial virus infection. J Pediatr 1982; 100:762.

Valenti WM, Clarke TA, Hall CB, et al. Concurrent outbreaks of rhinovirus and respiratory syncytial virus in an intensive care nursery: epidemiology and associated risk factors. J Pediatr 1982; 100:722.

Wang EL, Prober CG, Manson B, et al. Association of respiratory viral infections with pulmonary deterioration in patients with cystic fibrosis. N Engl J Med 1984; 311:1653.

Weber ML, et al. Acute epiglottitis in children—treatment with nasotracheal intubation. Pediatrics 1976; 57:152.

Welliver RC, Kaul A, Ogra PL. Cell-mediated immune response to respiratory syncytial virus infection: relationship to the development of reactive airway disease. J Pediatr 1979; 94:370.

Wenzel RP, et al. Hospital-acquired viral respiratory illness on a pediatric ward. Pediatrics 1977; 60:367.

Westley CR, Cotton EK, Brooks JG. Nebulized racemic epinephrine by IPPB for the treatment of croup. Am J Dis Child 1978; 132:484.

Wilson SZ, Gilbert BE, Quarles JM, et al. Treatment of influenza A (H1N1) virus infection with ribavirin aerosol. Antimicrob Agents Chemother 1984; 26:200.

Winterbauer RH, Dreis DF. Thoracic empyema: handling a dangerous infection wisely. J Respir Dis 1983; 116.

Wolfe WG, Spock A, Bradford WD. Pleural fluid in infants and children. Am Rev Respir Dis 1968; 98:1027.

Yunis EJ, et al. Adenovirus and ileocecal intussusception. Lab Invest 1975; 33:347.

Zollar LM, Krause HE, Mufson MA. Microbiologic studies on young infants and lower respiratory tract disease. Am J Dis Child 1973; 126:56.

Zuravleff JJ, Yu VC, Shonnard JW, et al. Diagnosis of legionnaires' disease. JAMA 1983; 250:1981.

23

RICKETTSIAL INFECTIONS

Rickettsiae are obligate intracellular gram-negative bacteria that multiply in arthropod vectors; the blood eating habits of these vectors involve their vertebrate hosts in the complex life cycle of these microorganisms. The geographic distribution of rickettsiae reflects that of the vector and except for epidemic typhus, man is an incidental host for most rickettsial infections. Although diseases such as typhus had been recognized for many years, it was only in the early twentieth century that rickettsiae were identified by Dr. Howard T. Ricketts. He injected blood from a patient with Rocky Mountain spotted fever (RMSF) into a guinea pig and produced disease.

Taxonomists have assigned the names Rickettsiales to the order, Rickettsiaceae to the family, Rickettsieae to the tribe, and created three genera: (1) *Rickettsia*, (2) *Rochalimaea*, and (3) *Coxiella*. The *Rickettsia* genus is further divided into groups, that is, typhus, spotted fever, and scrub typhus (Fig. 23-1). *R. quintana*, the etiologic agent of trench fever, grows extracellularly in the lumen of its host, the body louse, and on enriched medium. *Coxiella burnetti*, although similar to *Rickettsia* in morphology and intracellular growth, differs in major ways, for example, endospore production, DNA base composition, and transmission by aerosol to humans.

The diverse clinical illnesses produced by the three genera of the Rickettsieae tribe include vasculitis (RMSF), pneumonia (Q fever), febrile illness with vesicular rash (trench fever), recrudescent febrile infection (Brill-Zinsser disease), and endocarditis (Q fever). Endothelial damage and secondary inflammation is the hallmark of these rickettsiae infections. Rickettsial diseases include the following:

Rickettsia prowazekii—epidemic typhus, Brill-Zinsser disease

Rickettsia typhi—endemic typhus or murine typhus

Rickettsia canada—possibly disease like RMSF

Rickettsia rickettsii—Rocky Mountain spotted fever

Rickettsia akari—rickettsialpox

Rickettsia siberica—North Asian tick typhus

Rickettsia australis—Queensland tick typhus

Rickettsia conorii—boutonneuse fever

Rickettsia parkeri, R. rhipicephali, R. montana, R. belli—none known

Rickettsia tsutsugamushi—scrub typhus (chigger-borne typhus, mite-borne typhus, Japanese River fever, rural fever, tropical typhus)

Rochalimaea quintana—trench fever

Coxiella burnetti—Q fever

ETIOLOGY

Rickettsiales are pleomorphic coccobacillary organisms ranging from 0.3 to 0.6 μm in width to 0.8 to 2.0 μm in length. They are gram negative but poorly stained, and visualization is best accomplished using a Gimenez modification of the Macchiavello method, which stains organisms red. These bacteria have a three-layered

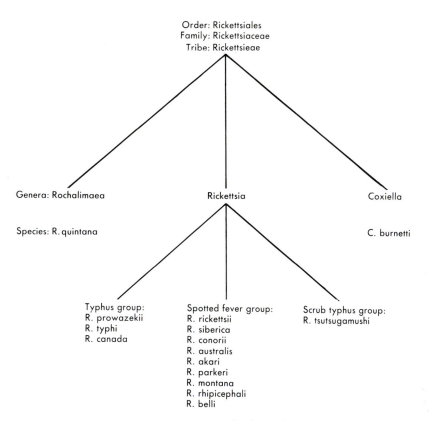

Order: Rickettsiales
Family: Rickettsiaceae
Tribe: Rickettsieae

Genera: Rochalimaea   Rickettsia   Coxiella

Species: R. quintana   C. burnetti

Typhus group:
R. prowazekii
R. typhi
R. canada

Spotted fever group:
R. rickettsii
R. siberica
R. conorii
R. australis
R. akari
R. parkeri
R. montana
R. rhipicephali
R. belli

Scrub typhus group:
R. tsutsugamushi

Fig. 23-1. Taxonomy of rickettsiales.

cell wall, trilaminar plasma membrane, ribosome-like particles, and intracellular organelles. They possess both RNA and DNA, and they divide by binary fission. The genome is large, varying from 1.0 to 1.5 × 10⁹ daltons. There seems to be a single chromosome as in other bacteria and plasmids. They have respiratory and synthetic capabilities independent of the cell. For example, they have mechanisms for production of adenosine triphosphate (ATP), carbohydrate breakdown, and protein and lipid synthesis. The genome size, DNA-DNA hybridization, and guanosine plus cytosine content is similar within species of a group, but significant differences exist between groups, for example, between *Coxiella* and *R. prowazeki*.

All members of the genus *Rickettsia* can obtain access to cytoplasm by traversing the host cell membrane and are unstable extracellularly, whereas *C. burnetti* is very resistant to heat and dryness. Only *R. quintana* can multiply extracellularly. All rickettsiae can be propagated in various tissue culture systems, embryonated eggs, laboratory animals, and certain arthropods. Generally, typhus-group organisms (ex-

cept *R. canada*), *C. burnetti*, and *R. tsutsugamushi* grow in cytoplasm. Spotted fever–group organisms grow in the cytoplasm and nucleus. Differences in virulence between strains have been noted but are not understood.

The antigenic differences help to classify these microorganisms. There is no common group antigen for all members of the Rickettsiaceae family or of the tribe Rickettsieae. Group-specific antigens are ether soluble and are thought to represent capsular material. Cell wall antigens are thought to be type specific.

THE SPOTTED FEVER GROUP

The RMSF rickettsiae cause a diffuse infectious vasculitis involving skin and produce a rash typically petechial and/or purpuric in character. Any of the viscera may be involved with the clinical disease, which encompasses a spectrum from unrecognized infection to fatal illness.

Rocky Mountain spotted fever (tick-borne typhus)

Rocky Mountain spotted fever, an acute infectious disease, is limited to the Western hemisphere. The disease is most prevalent in the Piedmont region of the southeastern United States and in Oklahoma. Small numbers of cases have been recognized over the years in almost every state (Fig. 23-2). Over 1100 cases of disease were reported to the Centers for Disease Control in 1983. This disease is responsible for 95% of all reported rickettsial infections in the United States. Exposure to the vectors determines the epidemiologic features of the disease. Thus, the incidence is seasonal, with most cases occurring between April and September, when exposure to ticks occurs. Rural and suburban dwellers are more likely to acquire disease than urban residents. Similarly, very young infants (less than 2 years old) are rarely exposed, and illness in this age group is unusual. Persons who are out of doors in the typical oak/hickory/pine forests that are the tick habitat are more likely to be exposed and acquire disease.

Four species of *Ixodes* (hard) ticks indigenous in the United States harbor *R. rickettsii*. The wood tick, *Dermacentor andersoni*, is the west-ern vector of *R. rickettsii*, and *D. variabilis*, or the dog tick, is the culprit in the southeast. Estimates vary, stating that less than 1% to 5% of tick vectors may harbor *R. rickettsii*. The Lone Star tick *(Amblyomma americanum)* and the rabbit tick *(Haemaphysalis leporispalustris)* only occasionally transmit disease to humans, but they may be important in maintenance of infection in animals. The infected tick must ingest a blood meal to "activate" the rickettsia. This phenomenon is probably related to increasing the temperature of the organism and microscopically correlates with presence of a microcapsular slime layer. Infection is transmitted to human beings by a tick bite or by handling an infected tick that has had a blood meal. Infection is transmitted within the laboratory by aerosol, but aerosol transmission is not known to occur in nature. Very rarely transmission from human to human has occurred by blood transfusion from a patient incubating disease or by an accidental needle stick contaminated with infected blood.

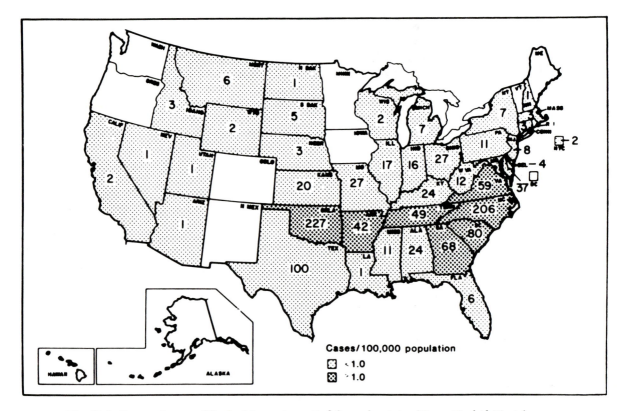

Fig. 23-2. Reported cases of Rocky Mountain spotted fever, by state. (From Morbid Mortal Weekly Rep 1984;33:188.)

Etiology and ecology. *R. rickettsii* is morphologically similar to other rickettsiae. *R. rickettsii* and *R. prowazekii* have a slime layer, probably composed of polysaccharide, external to the cell wall that could be antigenically important and/or relate to cell attachment. *R. rickettsii* is labile and killed by drying at room temperature or by moist heat (50° C) and by formalin or phenol. *R. rickettsii* organisms multiply in the nucleus and cytoplasm and produce demonstrable cytopathic effects. In vitro, in chick embryo fibroblasts and human endothelial cells the outer nuclear envelope and rough endoplasmic reticulum are dilated. The cisternal membranes envelope the organisms, which are released either as free forms or as enveloped forms. As cytopathic effects progress, a larger proportion of organisms are released in host cell membranes but shed these envelopes in supernatant fluid. Scanning electron microscopy (EM) studies have shown *R. rickettsii* exiting from cells on long cytoplasmic projections without cell lysis. Large numbers of cells become infected relatively quickly. These microorganisms live within ticks, causing no disease, and are transovarially transmitted to tick progeny. The ticks pass through four stages in their life cycle and they can acquire infection at any stage by feeding on a rickettsemic animal. The infection is passed by the vector through its sequential stages of development (egg to larvae to nymph to adult). These arthropods are both reservoirs and vectors of infection. *R. rickettsii* shares antigens with *R. montana* and in animals immunization with *R. montana* can protect against fatal *R. rickettsii* infection. It is theoretically possible that interrelationships of rickettsiae in nature may affect the clinical expression of human disease.

Pathogenesis and pathology. In mammals organisms multiply in the vascular endothelium and in smooth muscle, producing endothelial damage and small vessel occlusion, with extravasation of blood, fluid, and attendant serum electrolyte changes. Activation of the kallikrein-kinin system has been documented in humans as has disseminated intravascular coagulation. The vasculitis is apparent in many tissues (Fig. 23-3), especially skin, central nervous system, heart, lungs, liver, and kidney. Severe disease may cause occlusion of larger vessels and gangrene. In animal models, the rickettsiae themselves cause cellular damage. Cell-mediated immunity has been demonstrated in vitro to *R. rickettsii* antigens and may contribute to eradication of organisms in tissues, but the host immune response is not necessary or responsible for the tissue damage.

Clinical manifestations. The incubation period is usually 5 to 7 days with a range of 3 to 12 days. Recognized illness is characterized by a short prodromal period of headache, malaise, and myalgias. The abrupt onset of fever may be accompanied by chills, and the severity of myalgias and headache may increase. Usually the rash is noted from 2 to 4 days after onset of illness. It begins as a maculopapular eruption that has a peripheral distribution. The skin lesions appear first on the thenar eminence and flexural surfaces of the wrist and ankle. The rash then spreads to involve the arms, legs, chest and, last, the abdomen. The palms and soles are nearly always affected. The lesions are at first discrete, macular, and maculopapular, blanching on pressure. Within 1 to 3 days, the rash becomes hemorrhagic and lesions may become confluent with areas of necrosis at sites of maximal involvement. Gangrene of fingers, toes, genitalia, or nose may develop. During the period of convalescence, the rash becomes pigmented, and evidence of branny desquamation appears over the more severely affected areas.

The illness varies in severity even in the absence of specific antimicrobial therapy. Mortality rates are between 5% and 10%, and factors associated with increased fatality include increased age and an increased length of time from onset of illness to initiation of therapy. The diffuse nature of this infection results in protean manifestations. Myalgia and associated elevations of muscle enzymes are common. Hepatic involvement is frequent and may produce mild to severe hepatocellular dysfunction and jaundice. The gastrointestinal tract manifestations include abdominal pain, vomiting, and diarrhea. Myocardial involvement is common, and pathologically the vasculitis and inflammation are apparent (Fig. 23-3). The patient may have an altered sensorium or be comatose and the cerebrospinal fluid (CSF) frequently contains an increased cell count but usually fewer than 100 to 200 white blood cells per cubic millimeter. The peripheral white blood cell count is often normal but with a shift to the left with prominent vacuolization of polymorphonuclear cells. Hy-

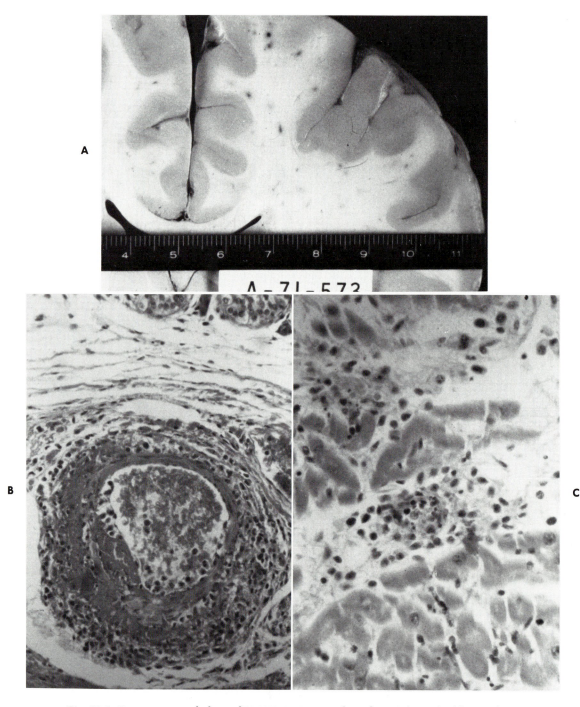

Fig. 23-3. Postmortem pathology of RMSF. **A,** Brain with evidence of petechial hemorrhages. **B,** Tunica testes showing prominent vasculitis with endothelial thickening and fibrin deposition. **C,** Vasculitis of myocardium.

ponatremia with mild peripheral edema are frequent consequences of the vasculitis, and corrective supportive measures may include transfusion of a colloid to increase intravascular volume. Increased antidiuretic hormone (ADH) levels have also been observed in this disease.

Hospitalized patients represent the more severely ill, and the course of illness may range from days to weeks. Prolonged fever of 10 days to several weeks or relapse upon cessation of therapy has been observed.

Diagnosis. Clinical suspicion of Rocky Mountain spotted fever is all important in endemic areas, especially during the months of seasonal prevalence of disease. A febrile illness, particularly with rash, often constitutes enough evidence for initiation of therapy. Additional features such as a known tick bite or attachment, myalgias, headache, and hyponatremia constitute a compelling clinical constellation. Laboratory diagnosis is dependent on the demonstration of antibodies, which are rarely present during the first 3 to 5 days of illness. Thus, specific therapy should not await confirmation of the diagnosis by serologic tests.

Laboratory diagnosis. Isolation of *R. rickettsii* from the blood is expensive and time consuming because it requires cell culture or animal inoculation and is done in only a few research lab-

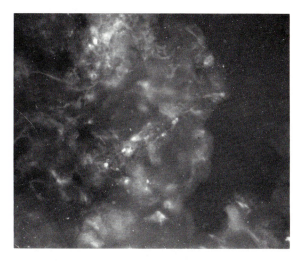

Fig. 23-4. Photomicrograph of a skin biopsy obtained from a 5-year-old child on the sixth day of illness. *Rickettsia rickettsii* are demonstrated by immunofluorescence. (×235.) (Courtesy Dr. David H. Walker, University of North Carolina at Chapel Hill.)

oratories. Recognition of positive cultures requires several days and therefore is not practical for early diagnosis.

Detection of intracellular *R. rickettsii* by fluorescein-conjugated antibody in skin biopsies obtained from an area of rash has yielded the earliest diagnosis (Fig. 23-4). Areas of normal skin do not demonstrate the presence of *R. rickettsii*. Preceding antibiotic therapy for longer than 24 hours may result in negative immunofluorescent stains of tissue from patients with known disease. If specific antisera are available it is possible to demonstrate the presence of intracellular organisms in autopsy tissues.

Confirmation of disease is generally accomplished by serologic demonstration of antibodies, which appear during convalescence. Nonspecific testing has traditionally been accomplished with the Weil-Felix reaction. Because of their polysaccharide O antigens several strains of *Proteus* (OX-19, OX-2, and OX-K) were found to be agglutinated by antibodies formed in response to rickettsial infections. Antibodies are detected after the first week of illness. The test is easy and inexpensive but lacks specificity and sensitivity.

Specific antibody to rickettsiae can be measured by indirect hemagglutination (IHA), microimmunofluorescence (MIF), latex agglutination, enzyme-linked immunosorbent assay (ELISA), and complement fixation (CF) tests. The last has been widely available but lacks sensitivity. Antibodies as detected by CF may be delayed in appearance, and their development has been aborted by specific antibiotic therapy. Neither the latex agglutination nor the ELISA are commercially available. The sensitivity and specificity of IHA, MIF, and latex agglutination are comparable (Philip et al., 1977). An antibody rise of fourfold or greater in two sera is diagnostic of acute infection.

Demonstration of specific IgM antibody by immunofluorescence or ELISA suggests recent infection. A comparison of antibody measurements on several patients is depicted in Fig. 23-5.

Host defenses. It seems probable that a single infection with *R. rickettsii* confers immunity. This is substantiated by volunteer studies. Persons who have been sequentially challenged twice with *R. rickettsii* have disease only after the first exposure (Dupont et al., 1973). A spec-

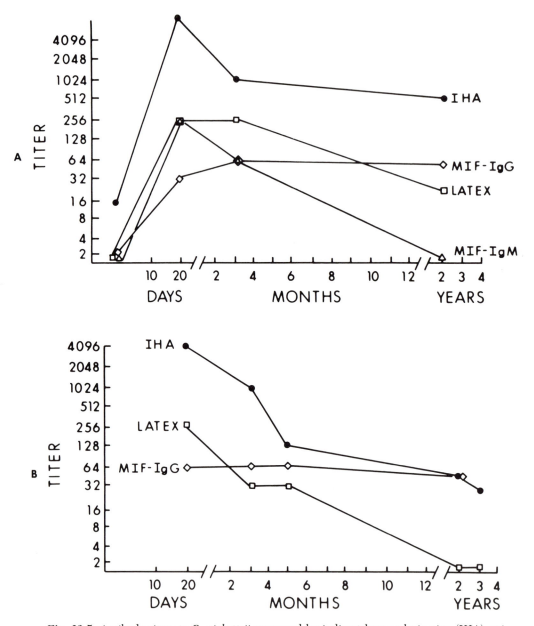

Fig. 23-5. Antibody titers to *R. rickettsii* measured by indirect hemagglutination (IHA), microimmunofluorescence (MIF) for IgG and IgM, and latex agglutination. Titers are plotted by the time they were obtained in relation to onset of symptomatic illness. **A,** Titers obtained from serum of 62-year-old man with rash and fever hospitalized for 5 days and treated with tetracycline. **B,** Titers obtained from serum of 3-year-old boy who had a rash and fever; he was not hospitalized and received only penicillin.

trum of antibodies can be demonstrated in response to *R. rickettsii* (Anacker et al., 1983). Crossed immunoelectrophoresis demonstrates antibody responses to different antigens of the organism. It is currently unknown which antibody or antibodies confers protection against *R. rickettsii*. Lymphocyte sensitization to *R. rickettsii* has been demonstrated in vitro with cells obtained from patients with prior infection. Antibody coating of *R. rickettsii* is necessary for phagocytosis and killing of the organism by guinea pig peritoneal macrophages in cell culture systems. The relative roles of antibody and cell-mediated immunity in recovery from infection or protection against subsequent infection in human beings is unknown.

Differential diagnosis. In the absence of rash, for example, in the early days of illness, or in the unusual patient in whom no rash develops during the illness, it is difficult to make a specific diagnosis. The disease must be suspected in endemic areas. The differential diagnosis includes other rash diseases. Meningococcemia is difficult to distinguish from Rocky Mountain spotted fever. Atypical measles, which occurs in individuals previously vaccinated with inactivated (killed) measles virus vaccine, may also resemble Rocky Mountain spotted fever. Other species of rickettsiae that cause tick-borne disease and resemble RMSF are found on several continents other than North America. Epidemic typhus is no longer present in the United States, but the clinical illness is similar to that of RMSF. The skin rash classically appears as a patchy cutaneous erythema and then progresses to the petechial form but usually spares the palms, soles, and face. Occasionally recrudescent typhus, Brill-Zinsser disease, occurs in the United States, but primarily it occurs in immigrants from previously endemic areas. Murine typhus is usually a mild illness and the rash tends to appear first on the trunk and spread to the extremities. Generally the rash is macular or maculopapular and does not become petechial. It is this rickettsial infection that is most likely to be confused with that of Rocky Mountain spotted fever within the United States.

Complications. Complications of RMSF are more likely to occur in untreated patients or patients whose specific therapy is initiated after more than 4 days of clinical illness. Central nervous system sequelae have been observed fol-

lowing infection, but generally the prognosis is excellent for recovery. Occasionally amputation of fingers and toes or other tissues may be necessitated by gangrene. Arrhythmias have been observed as a manifestation of the myocardial involvement.

Treatment. The only appropriate therapy is tetracycline or chloramphenicol, which alters the course of infection most significantly when instituted early in the course of illness. RMSF is not transmitted from human to human except for the unusual circumstance of blood transfusion or needle puncture. Therefore, patients do not need to be isolated.

Prevention. Nonspecific measures to diminish exposure to ticks should be taken but are not optimally successful. Individuals who are exposed to ticks and tick-infested environments should inspect themselves for ticks and carefully remove any ticks. A period of time is necessary for activation of rickettsiae in infected ticks, and therefore early removal of ticks could in theory prevent infection. Handling of attached ticks should preferably be accomplished by forceps and gentle traction. Tick tissues and tick feces are highly infectious if the vector contains *R. rickettsii*.

There is no available vaccine for prevention of RMSF. An early product made from egg-grown rickettsiae was used until it was shown conclusively that it failed to prevent infection. An experimental vaccine grown in cell culture systems was subjected to experimental trials in animals and humans. Although humoral antibodies and lymphocyte sensitization could be demonstrated, people were not protected against challenge with *R. rickettsii*, and therefore studies on this vaccine have been discontinued. Thus, therapy of disease is much more effective than available preventive measures.

Rickettsialpox

Rickettsialpox is caused by *Rickettsia akari*, an organism of the spotted fever group that cross-reacts serologically with *R. rickettsii*. The disease is usually a mild febrile illness heralded by the development of a local eschar. Subsequently a papulovesicular rash appears.

Etiology and ecology. The common house mouse is infested with a mite (formerly *Allodermanyssus*, now *Lipryssoides sanguineus*) that can be infected with *R. akari*. This rickettsial infection may also be transmitted transovarially to the progeny of an infected mite. Humans enter the cycle of infection accidentally; often this results from displacement of a rodent population by construction or during reduction of the rodent population by control programs. The mite attacks humans when its normal murine host is scarce. This rickettsia is infective for mice and guinea pigs but not for monkeys.

Epidemiology. All ages and both sexes are equally susceptible. The majority of cases of rickettsialpox have been reported in New York City, where the disease was originally described in the Kew area of the borough of Queens in 1946. It has also been identified in West Hartford, Boston, Philadelphia, Arkansas, Delaware, and Russia.

Clinical manifestations and pathology. The incubation period has been estimated to be between 10 and 24 days. A triad of symptoms occur in sequence. These are the initial eschar, a febrile illness, and a generalized papulovesicular eruption.

The primary lesion at the site of the original mite bite is a local erythematous papule that evolves into a vesicle over 2 days and then an eschar. The patient is usually not aware of either the bite or the lesion. The eschar resolves over 3 to 4 weeks, and this lesion is usually associated with enlarged regional lymph nodes.

Approximately 3 to 7 days after the appearance of the eschar, fever with chills may begin abruptly. Often there is headache, malaise, and myalgia. Within 72 hours of the onset of fever the generalized rash develops. These lesions are initially maculopapular and discrete, but small vesicles form on the summit of the papules. The lesions dry and may have tiny scabs that fall off without leaving scars. There is no characterisitc distribution of this rash. It may occur on any part of the body, but it only rarely involves the palms or soles. The entire course of illness is approximately 2 weeks. The WBC usually shows leukopenia (2400 to 4000) with relative lymphocytosis.

As there have been no reported deaths from this disease, the available pathology consists of examination of the cutaneous manifestations. The initial lesion is a firm nodule approximately 1 cm in diameter. It consists of a vesicle or pustule covered with dry epithelium or crust. Histologically the vesicle is situated subepidermally

and may arise from vacuolar changes of the basal layer. Mononuclear infiltration of the epidermis is seen with a mixed polymorphonuclear mononuclear cell infiltrate in the dermis. The capillaries of the corium are dilated and surrounded by mononuclear cells. There is endothelial swelling in blood vessels.

Diagnosis. The diagnosis may be made clinically and confirmed by antibody determinations. Weil-Felix antibodies do not appear after infection with *R. akari*. However, more specific testing including complement fixation can demonstrate an antibody response 1 to 2 months after the onset of illness. Shared antigens of *R. rickettsii* and *R. akari* may result in detectable antibodies for RMSF in patients with rickettsialpox.

R. akari has been isolated from both the blood and the vesicular fluid of infected persons. A research laboratory or one specifically interested in the diagnosis of this infection is necessary for diagnosis by culture, as animals and embryonated eggs are used.

Differential diagnosis. Rickettsialpox has been confused with chickenpox and is the only rickettsial disease characterized by the appearance of vesicular lesions. The presence of a primary eschar, however, should rule out varicella infection. The vesicular lesions in rickettsialpox are smaller than those in varicella, and those of rickettsialpox are usually situated on top of a papule. Rickettsialpox may affect all ages, but varicella is more likely to occur in children. The typical crusting of varicella lesions may not be observed in many of the rickettsialpox lesions. The diffuse nature of the vesicular lesions are in contrast to the characteristic distribution of chickenpox vesicles and should also help to distinguish this illness from primary herpes simplex infection. The demonstration of multinuclear giant cells and/or isolation of either of these viruses will easily distinguish these infections.

Hand-foot-and-mouth disease does not have a primary eschar and the scattered sparse lesions tend to be tender and painful.

Prognosis. Untreated rickettsialpox is a benign, self-limited, nonfatal disease. No complications have been described.

Treatment and control measures. Tetracycline and chloramphenicol have been reported to modify the course of illness. Prevention is directed at control of the rodent host of the vector. There are no vaccines available, and there is little stimulus to develop additional preventive measures because of the mild nature of this disease.

Additional tick-borne disease caused by members of the spotted fever group

An illness similar to RMSF but generally milder has been ascribed to several tick-borne rickettsiae. North Asian tick typhus is caused by *Rickettsia siberica* and occurs in Central Asia, the Siberian region of the USSR, and Mongolia. Queensland tick typhus is caused by *Rickettisa australis* and is found only in Australia. South African tick bite fever, boutonneuse fever occurring in the Mediterranean region, and Indian tick typhus are caused by *Rickettsia conorii* and are all very similar illnesses. All three of these rickettsiae infect species of *Ixodes* ticks and subsequently their wild animal host. As stated previously, humans are only incidentally infected and are not important as reservoirs or for transmission of these illnesses. In contrast to RMSF these rickettsial illnesses are characterized by a local skin lesion at the site of tick attachment with the formation of an eschar as described for rickettsialpox. Group-reactive complement-fixing antibodies have been demonstrated in response to infection with any of these three rickettsiae, but the Weil-Felix test is only inconsistently positive. These rickettsiae are also sensitive to chloramphenicol and tetracycline.

Rickettsiae not yet associated with human disease

R. rhipicephali, R. montana, R. parkeri, and *R. belli* are organisms in the spotted fever group. These organisms can be distinguished serologically but they also share antigens. They currently have no demonstrated relationship to human disease. In laboratory animals *R. rhipicephali* has the ability to lower immunity to challenge with virulent *R. rickettsii*. Antiserum raised to *R. montana* has modified illness in guinea pigs challenged with *R. rickettsii*. Thus, interactions of these other rickettsiae, their vectors, and human hosts should be delineated.

THE TYPHUS GROUP

The typhus group of rickettsiae causes epidemic typhus (including recrudescent disease) and murine typhus. These organisms share a common group-specific antigen and are characterized by intracytoplasmic growth.

Epidemic typhus (louse-borne typhus)

Epidemic typhus is an acute, potentially fatal infectious disease caused by *R. prowazekii* that has played an important role in history. It has been estimated, for example, that in World War I over 3 million Russians died as a result of this infection.

Etiology and ecology. *R. prowazekii* is similar to the previously described rickettsial species. The organisms multiply in cytoplasm much as do classic bacteria in liquid medium, and there are few cytopathic effects in the cells in which they grow. The organism is infectious for mice, guinea pigs, and embryonated eggs. Infectivity is preserved by lyophilization or storage at $-70°$ C. This organism can infect both the human body louse (*Pediculus humanus corporis*) and the head louse (*Pediculus humanus capitis*). *Pediculus corporis* feeds only on humans, and all three stages of the life cycle of the louse (egg, nymph, and adult) can occur on the same host. The louse becomes infected by taking a blood meal from a person with rickettsemia. *R. prowazekii* multiplies in the epithelial cells of the intestine of the louse. After 3 to 7 days, large numbers of rickettsiae are excreted in the feces. Fortunately, lice do not transmit the rickettsiae to their progeny, and infected lice die within several weeks. An infected louse transmits disease by moving to another person and excreting feces during the blood meal. The abrasions induced by scratching provide a portal of entry for the rickettsiae deposited on the skin. Rarely, infections may have been acquired by inhalation of dry infective feces of the louse. For practical purposes, man seems to be the only reservoir of infection; however, the flying squirrel (*Glaucomys volans*) has been reported to be an occasional reservoir responsible for disease in Virginia, North Carolina, and West Virginia (Sonenshine et al., 1978).

Clinical manifestations and pathology. After an incubation period of 7 to 14 days, the illness begins abruptly with fever, chills, headache, malaise, and generalized aches and pains. The fever and constitutional symptoms increase in severity and are followed by an eruption that appears between the fourth and sixth days of illness. The maculopapular rash appears first on the trunk near the axillae and subsequently spreads to involve the extremities. The face, palms, and soles are usually not involved. Initially the lesions are discrete pleomorphic macules that blanch on pressure. During the second week of illness, the skin lesions become petechial and purpuric and are subsequently followed by brownish pigmentation.

In the untreated patient fever lasts for 2 weeks and then falls by lysis over a period of 2 to 3 days. Severe illness is characterized by stupor, delirium, hallucinations, or excitability, mental dullness, marked weakness, prostration, and temporary deafness. Between the second and third weeks the patient either recovers or progresses to coma and death. The disease is also characterized by manifestations referable to the cardiovascular system. Early in the course of infection there may be relative bradycardia; later tachycardia and gallop rhythm may reflect the myocardial damage. Splenomegaly, albuminuria, and an elevation of BUN usually develop. The CBC may be characterized by leukopenia and anemia.

The typical pathologic lesion involves the endothelial cells of the small blood vessels. Multiplication of the rickettsiae causes edema, fibrin and platelet deposition, and obstruction of the vessels. This may be followed by thrombosis, hemorrhage, and perivascular accumulations of neutrophils, macrophages, and lymphocytes. The vascular lesions are widely disseminated but they are most numerous in the skin, myocardium, skeletal muscle, kidneys, and central nervous system.

Diagnosis. A compatible clinical picture should suggest the diagnosis, and appropriate therapy should not await laboratory confirmation of disease. Isolation of R. prowazekii can substantiate the clinical diagnosis but is potentially dangerous, difficult, and involves specifically trained personnel and special equipment. Primary isolations of R. prowazekii may be made by inoculating blood into guinea pigs and adult white mice or into the yolk sac of embryonated eggs.

Infection with R. prowazekii also induces the formation of antibodies that agglutinate Proteus vulgaris OX polysaccharide antigens. These agglutinins appear in the second week after onset of illness and agglutination is usually maximal with OX-19 strains. A fourfold rise in aggluti-

nation titers is suggestive of recent infection; serial specimens are often necessary to document the antibody increment. Complement-fixing antibodies are demonstrable in the third week after onset of illness and, as with RMSF, immunofluorescence tests as well as microagglutination procedures are more sensitive and available in specialized laboratories.

Differential diagnosis
Endemic typhus. Endemic typhus is clinically similar but usually much milder. The rash is less likely to be hemorrhagic. If the agent is isolated or injected into guinea pigs scrotal edema is produced, and this is not found after injection with R. prowazekii. Specific antibody measurements will establish the correct diagnosis.

Rocky Mountain spotted fever. The distribution of the rash should differ with concentration on the face and extremities. A specific antibody test will help distinguish these two illnesses.

Scrub typhus. A primary lesion is usually present with this infection, which consists of a papule progressing to a vesicle and then to a scab with an ulcer. This severe febrile illness and rash could be confused with typhus. Antibody determinations allow distinction of epidemic typhus and scrub typhus.

Meningococcemia. Meningococcemia usually progresses more rapidly than typhus, which may be helpful in making a clinical diagnosis. Isolation of the organism from the blood is diagnostic. This infection is commonly associated with meningitis.

Measles. The respiratory tract symptoms of coryza, conjunctivitis, and fever that precede the maculopapular eruption often provide a useful clinical distinction from typhus. The distribution of the rash with its initiation on the face and neck is different from that of typhus. Hemorrhagic lesions are uncommon in measles and usually fever subsides after the first week of illness.

Complications. Otitis media, parotitis, and bronchopneumonia may complicate epidemic typhus. Gangrene of portions of the extremities may also result from the vasculitis and thrombosis.

Prognosis. Untreated epidemic typhus fever is a severe and potentially fatal infection. The mortality ranges between 10% and 40%. The severe myocardial and CNS involvement are not usually followed by sequelae. The prognosis is considerably improved by specific antimicrobial therapy early in the course of disease. Case fatality rates have been shown to increase with increasing age.

Epidemiology. Epidemic typhus is worldwide in distribution. It occurs chiefly in Asia, Africa, Europe, Central America, and South America. During World War II the disease was epidemic in Russia, Poland, Germany, Spain, and North Africa. Conditions that promote louse infestation help to propagate the disease. These include crowding of destitute persons, lack of bathing, and conditions under which the same clothing is worn for prolonged periods. The conditions that are favorable for propagation of lice and disease have been seen in association with war, poverty, and famine. Lice apparently seek locations where the temperature is approximately 20° C and will abandon the host when the body temperature rises to 40° C. All ages and both sexes are equally susceptible.

A few sporadic cases of epidemic typhus in the United States have been associated with the flying squirrel and have raised questions as to whether this animal is a reservoir for this agent. The means of transmission of disease between these animals and man is not understood.

Brill-Zinsser disease. Recrudescent infection has occurred many years after an individual has had epidemic typhus. It was first suggested in 1934 that this recurrence was a relapse of a prior epidemic typhus infection. Thus, the disease may occur in an individual living in a louse-free environment and in the United States. It is most frequently observed in immigrants from endemic areas. An additional aspect of recrudescent disease is that lice feeding on such a patient can become infected and subsequently initiate another cycle of transmission. Thus, latent human infection represents an interepidemic reservoir. It is of interest that Weil-Felix antibodies usually do not develop in patients with Brill-Zinsser disease. However, as might be expected with an amnestic response, the demonstration of specific antibodies may occur earlier. These antibodies have been demonstrated to be IgG in immunoglobulin class. The IgG and IgM determinations are usually performed using microimmunofluorescence.

Management and therapy. Patients with epidemic typhus need to be deloused, which can be accomplished by bathing with soap and water

and weekly dusting with 10% DDT, 1% Lindane, or other effective agents lethal to the lice.

Tetracycline or chloramphenicol is appropriate specific antimicrobial therapy. A therapeutic response is ordinarily apparent within 48 hours, and the earlier therapy is initiated, the more likely the response is to be prompt.

After the patient and his or her clothing have been freed of lice no isolation is necessary, as the patient will not transmit disease to other persons. A susceptible contact who is known to have lice should be freed of his infestation. After that, quarantine is not necessary.

Prevention. In the 1940s a vaccine prepared by ether extraction of killed whole organisms grown in the yolk sac of embryonated eggs was developed. Although effective, it contained yolk sac and endotoxin and produced substantial local and systemic reactions.

Current studies have refined and purified species-specific protein antigens of *R. prowazekii* and *R. typhi* that are essential for protection. These purified large polypeptides do not have significant endotoxin content. Both humoral and cellular immunity to these antigens develops in man after natural infection and these "subunit vaccines" have been tested successfully for immunogenicity and efficacy in guinea pigs.

Murine typhus (endemic typhus, flea-borne typhus, rat typhus)

Endemic typhus fever is an acute, relatively mild infection caused by *R. typhi*. It is characterized clinically by headache, fever, malaise, and a maculopapular eruption with a centripetal distribution. Essentially, it is a modified version of epidemic typhus fever.

Etiology and ecology. *R. typhi* is a natural infection of rodents that is spread to man by the rat flea ((*Xenopsylla cheopis*) and the rat louse (*Polyplax spinulosa*). The vector, most frequently the rat flea, acquires *R. typhi* infection by feeding on a rickettsemic mouse or rat. The rickettsiae multiply in cells of the gut of the flea and in malpighian tubules. Thus infected, the flea may infect other susceptible rodents. Rickettsiae can be demonstrated in rodent brains for a period of up to several months. Fleas do not transmit *R. typhi* transovarially so that the murine hosts constitute the reservoir for the microorganisms. The occasional transmission of *R. typhi* to humans occurs when the infected flea that is taking a blood meal incites scratching; the host then inoculates the infected feces into the excoriation. Infection is not transmitted by the flea bite. The flea feces are also infective if accidentally transmitted through a mucosal surface such as the conjuctiva.

R. typhi is very similar to *R. prowazekii*. This organism is also infective for rats, mice, and guinea pigs as well as the yolk sac of embryonated eggs.

Clinical manifestations. The incubation period ranges from 1 to 2 weeks. The clinical picture of endemic typhus is indistinguishable from that of a mild case of epidemic typhus fever. The onset of fever, headache, malaise, myalgias, and a maculopapular nonpruritic skin rash that becomes apparent on the third to fifth day of disease are typical features of illness. The rash is typically sparse, discrete, and rarely hemorrhagic. In the untreated patient the febrile course seldom persists for more than 2 weeks. Reported mortality is less than 2%. Cardiac, central nervous system, and renal manifestations occur less frequently than in epidemic typhus.

Diagnosis. Weil-Felix agglutinins to *Proteus* OX-19 usually appear in the second week of infection. More sensitive and specific serologic assessment include antibodies measured by micro-IF. Complement fixation is a standard method, generally available but less sensitive.

Epidemiology. Murine typhus fever has a worldwide distribution and is endemic in many countries including the United States. In the United States the largest concentration of cases has occurred in the southern states along the Gulf of Mexico and the Atlantic Seaboard. Clearly, disease is related to areas that are rat or mice infested, and these animals tend to accumulate in large numbers where grains and feeds are stored. Over the past 10 years approximately half of the reported cases in the United States have occurred in Texas. The disease occurs most often during the summer months, and all ages and both sexes are equally susceptible.

Immunity. Endemic typhus is usually followed by lasting immunity. There is cross-protection between this disease and epidemic typhus fever, although they are caused by different organisms.

Treatment. Treatment is the same as that for epidemic typhus. This disease does not spread from human to human but is dependent totally on an infected vector.

Diagnosis. The serologic cross-reactions among members of the typhus group are common, but usually the response to the homologous antigen is the greatest. Inoculation of organisms or blood containing organisms into the peritoneal cavity of a guinea pig produces severe vesicular lesions and scrotal swelling. This is a much more severe disease for this animal than that induced by the inoculation of *R. prowazekii*.

Rickettsia canada infection

In 1967 a new species of rickettsia was isolated from rabbit ticks (*Haemaphysalis leporispalustris*) in Ontario, Canada. *R. canada* has been placed in the typhus group on the basis of guanosine plus cytosine content, DNA-DNA hybridization, and genome size, but it grows in both the cytoplasm and nuclei of infected cells, which is characteristic of the spotted fever group, and it has serologic cross-reactivity with the spotted fever–group organisms. The role of this organism in human disease is largely unknown, and it has not yet been isolated from a human source. Interestingly, there is serologic evidence that several patients with an RMSF-type illness had infection with this rickettsia.

THE SCRUB TYPHUS GROUP

There is an additional group of rickettsiae capable of producing a single clinical illness in humans. Demonstrably different surface antigens of these organisms do not seem to influence the manifestations of infection but allow persons to become infected and sustain clinical illness more than once by these rickettsiae.

Etiology. *R. tsutsugamushi* (or *Rickettsia orientalis*) is the etiologic agent. These rickettsiae have been studied in cell culture systems and observed to form blebs from their outer membranes just as some other gram-negative organisms do. These vesicles are intracellular in the cell cytoplasm. The organism infects several species of trombiculid mites. The mites have a four-stage life cycle, that is, egg, larva, nymph, and adult. The larva or chigger is the only stage that feeds on vertebrates. After a blood meal the chigger detaches and matures into a nymph and then into an adult. The nymphs and adults are free-living arthropods in the soil. *R. tsutsugamushi* can be transmitted transstadially, that is, from larva to nymph to adult, and transovarily from adult to egg. Therefore, trombiculid mites are the vectors and the reservoirs of the rickettsial infections that they transmit.

The natural cycle of infection involves chiggers in small mammals or ground-feeding birds. Humans accidentally enter the natural cycle of infection in areas of secondary or scrub vegetation. The disease is endemic in a triangular geographic area of about 5 million square miles, which includes Australia, Japan, Korea, India, and Vietnam. Appreciable morbidity was sustained during World War II by both American and Japanese soldiers. Disease usually occurs sporadically unless a group of people is brought into an endemic mite-infested area, when an outbreak may occur.

Clinical manifestations. The incubation period ranges from 1 to 3 weeks and the illness is very similar to other rickettsial infections, with abrupt onset of fever, headache, vomiting, myalgia, and abdominal pain. There is a local cutaneous lesion that evolves from a small indurated or vesicular lesion into an ulcerated area which is present at the time of onset of symptoms. An eschar is usually present as is local lymphadenopathy. Approximately 1 week after the onset of fever a rash appears that is characterized as macular or maculopapular and is apparent first on the trunk. Fatality ratios in epidemics have varied from 0% to 50%. Appropriate therapy alters the disease and prevents fatal illness.

Variation in surface antigenicity of the causative organism allows reinfection and clinically apparent disease in a single individual. Thus, infection with one strain of *R. tsutsugamushi* does not confer protection against another strain.

Diagnosis. The serologic diagnosis is somewhat complex because of the different antigens that do not cross-react. This means that a series of antigens, usually three, must be employed in a test such as the complement fixation assay. The strains represented are the Karp, Gilleam, and Kato. A Weil-Felix reaction may be postive with agglutinins to *Proteus* OX-K. The time course is similar to that of other rickettsial infections, with antibodies becoming detectable in the second week of illness.

Treatment. Tetracycline and chloramphenicol are effective agents that inhibit the growth of rickettsiae and usually produce prompt clin-

ical improvement. Relapse or recrudescence of self-limited fever has been observed in patients who have therapy initiated before 5 days of illness. If antibiotics are discontinued too early, relapse has also been observed.

TRENCH FEVER

Brief note of the illness caused by *Rochalimaea quintana* should be made as another rickettsial illness. It was originally recognized during World War I, disappeared, and then was recognized in epidemic form during World War II. The illness has been reported primarily in Europe, although *R. quintana* has been isolated from lice in Mexico. This is an interesting illness since the cycle is like that of epidemic typhus, that is, a louse-human-louse cycle, with no known animal reservoirs. *R. quintana* multiplies in an extracellular environment in the arthropod host, that is, in the lumen of the gut. Surprisingly the DNA of this organism hybridizes with that of the typhus group of organisms to the extent of 25% to 33%, suggesting more homology than would have been expected between genera. Transovarial transmission of infection does not occur. Once a louse is infected, it excretes rickettsiae in its feces for the duration of its life.

The incubation period in volunteers has been noted to be 8 to 18 days, and the clinical manifestations are variable. A mild, afebrile disease may occur with other symptoms, including headache, malaise, fever, myalgias, and bone pain. Rash is not prominent, but a macular eruption resembling rose spots of typhoid fever may occur. This rickettsial species can be isolated on enriched blood agar media or grown in the yolk sacs of embryonated eggs. Indirect immunofluorescence, complement fixation, and passive hemagglutination assays have been used to assess antibody status. *R. quintana* has been isolated from apparently healthy patients years after their original attack of disease.

In vitro sensitivity testing suggests that chloramphenicol and tetracycline would be effective therapy, although there are no data to substantiate their efficacy in people.

Q FEVER

Coxiella burnetti was simultaneously isolated from infected persons in Australia and from wood ticks in Montana and identified as a rickettsia in 1939. The name of the disease, Q fever, is derived from the first letter in *query*, which was the clinical description of this unusual febrile illness.

Etiology. *C. burnetti* grows intracellularly in membrane-bound vesicles, primarily in monocyte-macrophages. As an obligate intracellular organism it parasitizes eukaryotic cells and goes through its developmental cycle in the phagolysosome. These organisms actively metabolize at a pH of 4.5, which is the intravacuolar pH, and not at a pH of 7.0. Thus this organism thrives in the usually hostile environment of the phagolysosome. Surface antigenic differences define phase I and phase II organisms, which are morphologically the same. Phase I organisms exist in nature and phase II emerge with passage in embryonated eggs. Reversion occurs after animal passage. The ecology of this rickettsia is more complex than those previously described. One cycle involves arthropods, especially ticks, and a variety of vertebrates. Another cycle is maintained among domestic animals. These animals may have inapparent infections and shed large quantities of infectious organisms in urine, milk, feces, and placental products. *C. burnetti* resists desiccation and exposure to light or temperature after it is shed by the infected animal and therefore aerosolization of infectious material occurs. Humans and animals may be infected by inhalation of such material. An alternative mode of acquisition of infection has been documented to be ingestion of infected milk or handling of contaminated wool or hides. *C. burnetti* has also been shown to be able to penetrate through the skin, for example, with a minor abrasion, and through mucous membranes. Q fever has been an occupational risk in abatoir workers, dairy and other farm workers, persons employed in tanneries, wool, and felt plants, and in the laboratory setting. Four outbreaks have occurred recently in major university teaching hospitals involving as many as 100 persons. Thus this occupational hazard is receiving increased attention.

Clinical manifestations. The incubation period is 2 to 3 weeks, and illness usually begins abruptly with fever, chills, headache, malaise, and weakness. After 5 or 6 days of symptoms, cough and chest pain occur and rales may be audible. X ray films reveal pneumonia that is usually apparent by the third day of illness. The

consolidation clears over a period of 1 to 2 weeks. The reported pathology in the lungs consists of a peribronchial and perivascular lymphocytic and plasma cell infiltration. Fibrinous exudate fills the alveoli and bronchioles. The infiltrate is primarily mononuclear with lymphocytes, plasma cells, and monocytes. Skin rash is not a part of the clinical syndrome, and its absence is unique among the rickettsial diseases. There is a spectrum of illness, and people have been shown to be infected without any obvious symptoms. Asymptomatic recrudescence of infection has occurred during pregnancy. Prolonged fever, endocarditis, and hepatitis complete the clinical spectrum. Unfortunately Q fever endocarditis may occur months or years after the acute attack and should be thought of when a previous history of such illness in someone of the appropriate occupation or exposure history is ill with culture-negative disease.

Diagnosis. The compatible clinical picture and isolation of *C. burnetti* from the blood or sputum as well as serologic tests establish the diagnosis. Unfortunately, isolation of the organism requires inoculation of blood or sputum into an animal such as a guinea pig, mouse, or hamster, embryonated eggs, or cell cultures. Because of the possibility of transmission in the laboratory setting this is available only in research laboratories accustomed to dealing with the organism. Consequently, it is more reasonable to rely on serologic confirmation of the diagnosis.

Purified antigens are employed by several state health departments to perform the complement fixation test. *C. burnetti* exists in two phases and therefore reagents have been prepared using phase I and phase II antigens, which have been useful in distinguishing acute from chronic or past infection. Nevertheless, assessment by CF antibodies underestimates the prevalence of infection, and an intradermal skin test is more reliable. A microagglutination test has been a useful epidemiologic tool. An ELISA assay for specific IgM antibody to *C. burnetti* may prove to be helpful in diagnosis of acute infection. There are no Weil-Felix agglutinins in response to infection with *C. burnetti*.

Differential diagnosis. The differential diagnosis includes illness that relates to the particular system that is most prominently affected. Thus with respiratory complaints, influenza or

Mycoplasma pneumoniae might be considered, or with central nervous system complaints, meningitis. Abnormal liver function studies lead to a differential diagnosis including hepatitis, and with gastrointestinal manifestations, typhoid fever is sometimes considered.

Prognosis. The mortality before antimicrobial therapy was available was approximately 1%. With specific therapy fatalities are extraordinarily rare. The only exception to this is the unfortunate patient with endocarditis, where the mortality rate is higher.

Treatment. Tetracycline or chloramphenicol is indicated and should be administered for several days after the patient has become afebrile. Good clinical response is not as dramatic as that observed with some other rickettsial infections. Studies have suggested that replacement of an involved heart valve with a prosthetic valve as well as long-term therapy may improve the prognosis for patients with endocarditis due to *C. burnetti*.

Preventive measures. Preventive measures include sterilization by pasteurization of milk but otherwise it is difficult to interrupt the transmission of infection. Specific suggestions to protect laboratory personnel working with sheep or their tissues include research in a setting distinct from other hospital research and patient care. Seronegative flocks who have had negative testing by bioassay of amniotic fluid and placental tissues may be considered as an alternative to containment procedures, and a skin test is the best assessment of status of at-risk personnel. Lymphocyte transformation studies and skin testing are better predictors of immunity than antibody because antibody-negative persons may be immune. Human beings do not transmit disease to one another, so that isolation of the infected patient is not indicated. An early vaccine from phase II organisms had been used effectively in Public Health Service and Army laboratories, but adverse reactions limited any general applicability of the vaccine. Recently a formalin-inactivated phase I *C. burnetti* vaccine has undergone study. Phase I antigens increase the protective efficacy, and such a vaccine has provided protection in challenge studies. Thus a practical vaccine may become a reality in the foreseeable future.

REFERENCES
Rickettsia rickettsii

Anacker RL, Philip RN, Casper E, et al. Biological properties of rabbit antibodies to a surface antigen of *Rickettsia rickettsii*. Infect Immun 1983;40:292.

Ascher MS, et al. Initial clinical evaluation of a new Rocky Mountain spotted fever vaccine of tissue culture origin. J Infect Dis 1978;138:217.

Bradford WD, Croker BP, Tisher CC. Kidney lesions in Rocky Mountain spotted fever. Am J Pathol 1979;97:383.

Bradford WD, Hawkins HK. Rocky Mountain spotted fever in childhood. Am J Dis Child 1977;131:1228.

Centers for Disease Control: Rocky Mountain spotted fever—United States, 1983, Morbid Mortal Weekly Rep 1984;33:188.

Clements ML, Dumler JS, Fiset P, et al. Serodiagnosis of Rocky Mountain spotted fever: comparison of IgM and IgG enzyme-linked immunosorbent assays and indirect fluorescent antibody test. J Infect Dis 1983;148:876.

D'Angelo LJ, Winkler WG, Bergman DJ. Rocky Mountain spotted fever in the United States, 1975-1977. J Infect Dis 1978;138:273.

DuPont HL, Hornick RB, Dawkins AT, et al. Rocky Mountain spotted fever: a comparative study of the active immunity induced by inactivated and viable pathogenic *R. rickettsii*. J Infect Dis 1973;128:340.

Feng WC, Waner JL. Serological cross-reaction and cross-protection in guinea pigs infected with *Rickettsia rickettsii* and *Rickettsia montana*. Infect Immun 1980;28:627.

Hattwick MAW, O'Brien RJ, Hanson BF. Rocky Mountain spotted fever: epidemiology of an increasing problem. Ann Intern Med 1976;84:732.

Hattwick MAW, et al. Fatal Rocky Mountain spotted fever. JAMA 1978;249:1499.

Hayes SF, Burgdorfer W. Reactivation of *Rickettsia rickettsii* in *Dermacentor andersoni* Ticks: an ultrastructural analysis. Infect Immun 1982;37:779.

Hechemy KE, Michaelson EE, Anacker RL, et al. Evaluation of latex *Rickettsia rickettsii* test for Rocky Mountain spotted fever in 11 laboratories. J Clin Microbiol 1983;18:938.

King WV. Experimental transmission of Rocky Mountain spotted fever by means of the tick. Public Health Rep 1906;21:863.

Oster CN, et al. Laboratory-acquired Rocky Mountain spotted fever: the hazard of aerosol administration. N Engl J Med 1977;297:859.

Philip RN. et al. A comparison of serologic methods for diagnosis of Rocky Mountain spotted fever. Am J Epidemiol 1977;105:45.

Silverman DJ. *Rickettsia ricketsii*-induced cellular injury of human vascular endothelium in vitro. Infect Immun 1984;44:545.

Silverman DJ, Bond SB. Infection of human vascular endothelial cells by *Rickettsia rickettsii*. J Infect Dis 1984;149:201.

Silverman DJ, Wisseman CL. In vitro studies of rickettsia-host cell interactions: ultrastructural changes induced by *Rickettsia rickettsii* infection of chicken embryo fibroblasts. Infect Immun 1984;149:201.

Silverman DJ, Wisseman CL Jr, Waddell AD, Jones M. External layers of *Rickettsia prowazekii* and *Rickettsia rickettsii*: occurrence of a slime layer. Infect Immun 1978;22:233.

Todd WJ, Burgdorfer W, Wray GP. Detection of fibrils associated with *Rickettsia rickettsii*. Infect Immun 1983; 41:1252.

Walker DH, Firth WT, Edgell CJS. Human endothelial cell culture plagues induced by *Rickettsia rickettsii*. Infect Immun 1982;37:301.

Walker DH, Henderson FW. Effect of immunosuppression on *Rickettsia rickettsii* infection in guinea pigs. Infect Immun 1978;20:221.

Walker TS. Rickettsial interactions with human endothelial cells in vitro: adherence and entry. Infect Immun 1984;44:205.

Wells GM, Woodward TE, Fiset P, Hornick RB. Rocky Mountain spotted fever caused by blood transfusion. JAMA 1978;239:2763.

Wilfert CM, MacCormack JN, Kleeman K, et al. Epidemiology of Rocky Mountain spotted fever as determined by active surveillance. J Infect Dis 1984;150:469.

Woodward TE, et al. Prompt confirmation of Rocky Mountain spotted fever: indentification of rickettsiae in skin tissues. J Infect Dis 1976;134:297.

Spotted fever group

Burgdorfer A, Sexton DJ, Gerloff RK, et al. *Rhipicephalus sanguineus*: vector of a new spotted fever group rickettsia in the United States. Infect Immun 1975;12:205.

Hayes SF, Burgdorfer W. Ultrastructure of *Rickettsia rhipicephali*, a new member of the spotted fever group rickettsiae in tissues of the host vector *Rhipicephalus sanguineus*. J Bacteriol 1979;137:605.

Rickettsialpox

Brettman LR, Lewin S, Holzman RS, et al. Rickettsialpox: report of an outbreak and a contemporary review. Medicine 1981;60:363.

Dolgopol VB. Histologic changes in rickettsialpox. Am J Pathol 1948;24:119.

Greenberg M. Rickettsialpox in New York City. Am J Med 1948;4:866.

Huebner RJ, Jellison WL, Pomerantz C. Rickettsialpox—a newly recognized disease. IV. Isolation of a rickettsia apparently identical with the causative agent of rickettsialpox from *Allodermanyssus sanguineus*, a rodent mite. Public Health Rep 1946;61:1677.

Sussman LN. Kew Gardens' spotted fever. NY Med 1946;2:27.

Wong B, Singer C, Armstrong D, Millian SJ. Rickettsialpox: case report and epidemiologic review. JAMA 1979;242: 1998.

Typhus group

Bergman SJ, Kundin WD. Scrub typhus in South Vietnam, a study of 87 cases. Ann Intern Med 1973;79:26.

Brown GW, et al. Scrub typhus: a common cause of illness in indigenous populations. Trans R Soc Trop Med Hyg 1976;70:444.

Dasch GA, Samms JR, Weiss E. Biochemical characteristics of typhus group rickettsiae with special attention to the *Rickettsia prowazekii* strains isolated from flying squirrels. Infec Immun 1978;19:676.

Duma RJ, Sonenshine DE, Bozeman FM, et al. Epidemic typhus in the United States associated with flying squirrels. JAMA 1981;245:2318.

Older JJ. The epidemiology of murine typhus in Texas, 1969. JAMA 1970;214:2011.

Ormsbee RA, et al. Serologic diagnosis of epidemic typhus fever. Am J Epidemiol. 1977;105:261.

Osterman JV, Eisemann CS. Surface proteins of typhus and spotted fever group rickettsiae. Infect Immun 1978; 21:866.

Sonenshine DE, et al. Epizootiology of epidemic typhus (*R. prowazekii*) in flying squirrels. Am J Trop Med Hyg 1978;27:339.

Traub R, Wisseman CL. The ecology of chigger-borne rickettsiosis (scrub typhus). J Med Entomol 1974;11:237.

Q fever

Ascher MS, Berman MA, Ruppanner R. Initial clinical and immunologic evaluation of a new phase I Q fever vaccine and skin test in humans. J Infect Dis 1983;148:214.

Baca OG, Paretsky D. Q fever and *Coxiella burnetii*: a model for host-parasite interactions. Microbiol Rev 1983;47:127.

Burnet FM, Freeman M. A comparative study of rickettsial strains from an infection of ticks in Montana (United States of America) and from "Q" fever. Med J Aust 1939;2:887.

Derrick EH. The course of infection with *Coxiella burnetii*. Med J Aust 1973;1:1051.

Field PR, Hunt JG, Murphy AM. Detection and persistence of specific IgM antibody to *Coxiella burnetii* by enzyme-linked immunosorbent assay: a comparison with immunofluorescence and complement fixation tests. J Infect Dis 1983;148:477.

Hart RJC. The epidemiology of Q fever. Postgrad Med J 1973;49:535.

Williams JC, Peacock MG, McCaul TF. Immunological and biological characterization of *coxiella burnetii*, phases I and II, separated from host components. Infect Immun 1981;32:840.

24

RUBELLA (GERMAN MEASLES)

Rubella is an acute infectious disease characterized by minimal or absent prodromal symptoms, a 3-day rash, and generalized lymph node enlargement, particularly of the postauricular, suboccipital, and cervical lymph nodes. Prior to 1941, rubella was important chiefly because it was responsible for epidemics in schools and military installations and because it was frequently confused with measles and scarlet fever. Since 1941, a great deal of interest has been focused on this disease because of the association of rubella during pregnancy with an increased incidence of congenital malformations.

ETIOLOGY

Rubella is caused by a specific virus that has been shown to be present in the blood and nasopharyngeal secretions of patients with the disease. In 1914 Hess postulated, because of his transmission studies with rhesus monkeys, that rubella was caused by a virus. This observation was not confirmed until 1938 when Hiro and Tasaka produced the disease in children by inoculating them with filtered nasal washings obtained from patients during the acute phase of rubella. Habel in 1942 also successfully transmitted rubella to the rhesus monkey, using nasal washings and blood. Reports by Anderson in 1949 and by Krugman et al. in 1953 confirmed Hiro and Tasaka's findings. Krugman et al. also demonstrated that virus was present in the blood 2 days before and on the first day of rash and proved conclusively that rubella can occur without a rash (Krugman et al., 1953; Krugman and

Ward, 1954). The cultivation of rubella virus in tissue culture was reported independently and simultaneously by two groups. Weller and Neva in 1962 observed a cytopathic effect in human amnion cells. At the same time, Parkman et al. (1962) isolated the virus in cultures of African green monkey kidney tissue. Cells infected with rubella virus remained normal in appearance in spite of challenge with ECHO virus type 11, which characteristically causes a cytopathic effect.

Rubella virus is a moderately large virus. Its genome consists of single-stranded RNA. Its nucleocapsid is 30 nm in diameter and it is surrounded by a lipid envelope 60 to 70 nm in diameter containing glycoproteins. The nucleocapsid protein consists of four polypeptides. The envelope glycoprotein consists of E1 and E2 glycopeptides. Hemagglutination inhibition and neutralizing antibodies react with the E1 peptides (Dorsett et al., 1985).

Rubella virus is highly sensitive to heat, to extremes of pH, and to a variety of chemical agents. It is rapidly inactivated at 56° C and at 37° C. However, at 4° C the virus titer is relatively stable for 24 hours. For long-term preservation of the virus, a temperature of $-60°$ C is much better than the usual deep-freeze temperature of $-20°$ C. It is inactivated by a pH below 6.8 or above 8.1, ultraviolet irradiation, ether, chloroform, formalin, β-propiolactone, and other chemicals. It is resistant to thimerosal (Merthiolate) (1:10,000 solution) and antibiotics. Virus replication is not inhibited by 5-iodo-2′-

deoxyuridine (IDU) but is inhibited by amantadine hydrochloride. On the basis of its biochemical, biophysical, and ultrastructural properties, rubella virus is classified in the togavirus group, which includes most of the arboviruses. Its clinical and laboratory behavior, however, is more like that of the paramyxoviruses.

Rubella virus has been cultivated in a variety of tissue cultures. In general, the virus produces interference without a cytopathic effect in the following primary tissue culture cells: African green monkey kidney, bovine embryo kidney, guinea pig kidney, rabbit kidney, human amnion, and human embryonic kidney. Interference without a cytopathic effect has also been observed in rhesus monkey and human diploid cell lines. Cytopathic effect has been observed in a variety of continuous cell lines, including rabbit kidney (RK_{13}), rabbit cornea, and hamster (BHK-21). Rubella virus strains belong to one serologic type. Hemagglutination and complement-fixing antigens have been prepared in several tissue culture systems. The inhibition of these antigens by specific rubella antisera has formed the basis for practical serologic tests.

POSTNATALLY ACQUIRED RUBELLA
Clinical manifestations

The first symptoms of rubella occur after an incubation period of approximately 16 to 18 days, with a range of 14 to 21 days. The typical clinical course is illustrated in Fig. 24-1. In the child, the first apparent sign of illness is the appearance of the rash. In adolescents and adults, however, the eruption is preceded by a 1- to 5-day prodromal period characterized by low-grade fever, headache, malaise, anorexia, mild conjunctivitis, coryza, sore throat, cough, and lymphadenopathy. These symptoms rapidly subside after the first day of rash. The enanthem of rubella, described by Forchheimer in 1898, may be observed in many patients during the prodromal period or on the first day of rash. It consists of reddish spots, pinpoint or larger in size, located on the soft palate. In scarlet fever the soft palate may be covered with punctate lesions, and in measles it may have a red, blotchy appearance; these lesions are indistinguishable from the enanthem of rubella. Obviously, the so-called Forchheimer spots are not pathogno-

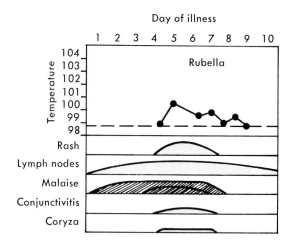

Fig. 24-1. Schematic diagram illustrating typical course of rubella in children and adults. Lymph nodes begin to enlarge 3 to 4 days before rash. Prodromal symptoms (malaise) are minimal in children (shaded area). In adults there may be a 3- to 4-day prodrome (hatched area). Conjunctivitis and coryza, if present, are usually minimal and accompany the rash.

monic for rubella and do not have the same diagnostic significance as Koplik's spots in measles.

Lymph node involvement. Observations made of patients with experimentally induced rubella or during epidemics indicate that lymph node enlargement may begin as early as 7 days before onset of rash (Fig. 24-2). There is generalized lymphadenopathy, but the nodes most commonly involved are the suboccipital, postauricular, and cervical nodes. The swelling and tenderness are most apparent and severe on the first day of rash. Subsequently, the tenderness subsides within a day or two, but the palpable enlargement of the nodes may persist for several weeks or more. As indicated in Table 24-1, the extent of the lymphadenopathy may be extremely variable, and occasionally it may even be absent. At times, splenomegaly also may be noted during the acute stage of the disease.

It is important to emphasize that involvement of the suboccipital, postauricular, and cervical lymph nodes is not pathognomonic for rubella. Lymphadenopathy is associated with diseases such as measles, chickenpox, adenovirus infections, and infectious mononucleosis as well as with many others.

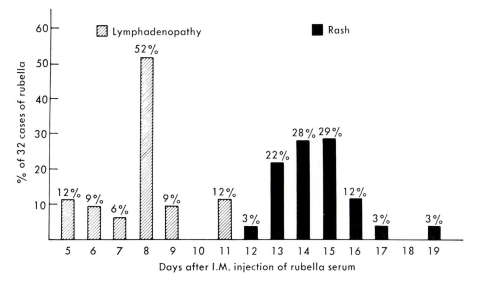

Fig. 24-2. Time of onset of lymphadenopathy and rash in 32 cases of experimentally transmitted rubella. Note appearance of lymphadenopathy 5 to 7 days before onset of rash. (From Green RH, et al.: Am J Dis Child 1965;110:348.)

Table 24-1. Clinical aspects of experimental rubella in children*

Patient	Maximum temperature (F°)	Rash	Lymph node enlargement	Leukopenia
C. R.	100.4	+	+ +	0
J. G.	101.6	0	+	0
P. K.	100.8	0	+ +	+ +
N. K.	99.6	+ +	+	+ +
E. T.	101.6	+ + +	+ + +	0
K. L.	100.4	+ +	+	+
J. S.	99.0	+ +	+	0
S. E.	99.4	+ +	0	0
G. O.	99.8	+ +	+ +	0
C. N.	99.4	+ + +	+ + +	—
P. A.	99.6	+ + +	+ +	—
T. B.	99.2	+	+	—
M. I.	99.4	+ +	+ + +	—

*From Krugman S, and Ward R: J Pediatr 1954;44:489.
Key: +, mild; + +, moderate; + + +, marked; 0, none; —, not done.

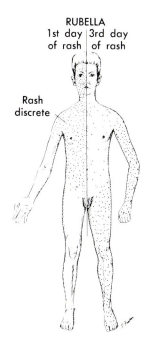

Fig. 24-3. Schematic drawing illustrating development and distribution of rubella rash.

Exanthem. The rash, particularly in children, may be the first obvious indication of illness. It appears first on the face and then spreads downward rapidly to the neck, arms, trunk, and extremities. The eruption appears, spreads, and disappears more quickly than does the rash of measles (Fig. 24-3). By the end of the first day, the entire body may be covered with the discrete pink-red maculopapules. On the second day, the rash begins to disappear from the face, and the lesions on the trunk may coalesce to form a uniform red blush that may resemble the rash of mild scarlet fever. The lesions on the extremities, however, remain discrete and generally do not coalesce. By the end of the third day in the typical case, the rash has disappeared. If the eruption has been intensive, there may be some fine branny desquamation; usually there is none.

The characteristic pink-red lesions of rubella differ from the purple-red lesions of measles and the yellow-red lesions of scarlet fever. In rubella the lesions are generally discrete and may or may not coalesce; if they do, a diffuse erythematous blush results. In contrast, the lesions of measles, particularly around the head and neck, tend to coalesce and form irregular blotches with crescentic margins. The similarities and differences between the eruptions of rubella and those of scarlet fever have been referred to previously. The circumoral area also differs in these two diseases; in rubella the rash involves this area, and in scarlet fever there is circumoral pallor.

The duration and extent of the rash may be variable. The eruption, which as a rule lasts for 3 days, may persist for 5 days or may be so evanescent that it disappears in less than a day. In an unknown number of instances, rubella may even occur without a rash. The existence of rubella without rash has been established. In 13 cases of experimentally induced rubella that we studied in 1954 (Table 24-1) the rash was extensive in three, moderate in six, mild in two, and absent in two. In 1965 Green et al. studied 24 children who were intimately exposed to rubella. A rise in rubella virus–neutralizing antibody titer was observed in 22 of the children. Rubella without rash occurred in eight of the 22 infected children. These two studies suggest that the incidence of subclinical rubella infections may be about 25%.

Fever. In children the temperature may be either normal or slightly elevated. Fever, if present, rarely persists beyond the first day of rash and is usually low grade. A typical temperature course is illustrated in Fig. 24-1. During epidemics, one occasionally sees patients with rubella whose temperatures are as high as 40° C (104° F). In adolescents and adults there may be low-grade fever during both the prodromal period and the first day of rash. The maximum temperature in a group of 13 children with experimentally induced rubella is listed in Table 24-1; in eight it was normal, and in five it ranged between 38° and 38.7° C (100.4° and 101.6° F).

Blood picture. Generally, the white blood cell count tends to be low. As indicated in Table 24-1, however, the white blood cell count may be normal. An increased number of plasma cells and Türk cells also have been described in rubella. Ocasionally there may be an increased percentage of abnormal lymphocytes or a decrease in platelets.

Diagnosis

Confirmatory clinical factors. A diagnosis of rubella is suggested by the appearance of a maculopapular eruption beginning on the face, progressing rapidly downward to the trunk and extremities, and subsiding within 3 days. Prodromal symptoms are minimal or absent, fever is low grade or absent, and lymphadenopathy precedes the appearance of the rash. A history of exposure, if available, is helpful.

Detection of causative agent. As indicated in Fig. 24-4, rubella virus may be recovered from the pharynx as early as 7 days before the onset of rash and as late as 14 days after onset of rash. The availability of virus isolation procedures has provided an important laboratory tool for the percise diagnosis of rubella. As indicated in Fig. 24-4, virus may be recovered from the pharynx with regularity within 5 days after the onset of rash; in contrast, viremia that is present before the onset of rash is rarely observed after the onset of rash.

Serologic tests. The pattern of appearance and persistence of rubella virus-neutralizing, complement-fixing (CF), and hemagglutination-inhibition (HI) antibody is shown in Fig. 24-4. Antibody is usually detectable by the third day of rash, and peak levels are reached about 1 month later. Complement-fixing antibody may

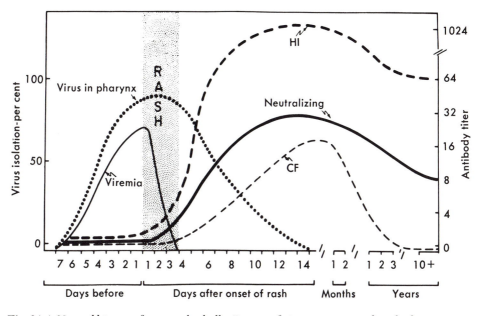

Fig. 24-4. Natural history of postnatal rubella. Pattern of virus excretion and antibody response. (Modified from Cooper LZ, and Krugman S: Arch Ophthalmol 1967;77:434.)

be short lived, declining to nondetectable levels within a year or more after infection. Neutralizing and HI antibodies usually persist for life. The HI antibody test has the advantages of high sensitivity and speed with which results are obtained. A serologic diagnosis is possible if acute- and convalescent-phase serum specimens are obtained. The acute-phase serum should be obtained as early as possible after onset of rash; convalescent-phase serum should be collected 2 to 4 weeks later. Evidence of a fourfold or greater rise in rubella antibody titer is indicative of a recent infection.

Differential diagnosis is discussed in Chapter 35.

Complications

Rubella in childhood is rarely followed by complications. Secondary bacterial infections, which are so common in measles, are not encountered in rubella. The following complications have been observed, especially during epidemics.

Arthritis. Joint involvement in adolescents and adults with rubella is much more common than is generally appreciated. It usually develops just as the rash is fading on the second to third day of illness. Either one or more of the larger and smaller joints may be involved. The

arthritis may be manifested by a return of fever and either transient joint pain without swelling or massive effusion into one or more joint spaces. These manifestations usually clear spontaneously within 5 to 10 days. Rubella arthritis, with involvement of the knees, ankles, or elbows, may simulate the polyarthritis of rheumatic fever. When there is fusiform swelling of the fingers, it may resemble rheumatoid arthritis. In 1958 Johnson and Hall studied 10 female patients with rubella arthritis of the small- and medium-sized joints that lasted 1 week. Positive latex fixation tests for rheumatoid factor were demonstrated in 9 of the 10 patients with arthritis as compared with only 2 of 7 patients who had rubella without arthritis. On the other hand, the euglobulin-sensitized sheep cell agglutination test was negative in 14 women with rubella arthritis observed by Kantor and Tanner (1962). None showed any clinical manifestations suggesting rheumatoid disease over a 2- to 5-year follow-up period. During an epidemic of rubella in a London suburb, Fry et al. (1962) observed arthritis in 15% of 74 adults who acquired the disease; they detected arthritis in 33% of 40 females and in 6% of 34 males. During an epidemic of rubella in Bermuda in 1971, joint manifestations were observed in 25% of children under the age of 11 years and in 52% of patients

11 years of age or older (Judelsohn and Wyll, 1973).

Encephalitis. Complications of rubella in the central nervous system (CNS) are extremely rare. Encephalitis is less commonly encountered after this disease than after measles or varicella. The incidence usually cited is 1 in 6000 cases of rubella. The clinical manifestations are similar to those observed in other types of postinfectious encephalitis. Complete recovery is generally the rule, but fatalities have been reported. Observations by Kenny et al. in 1965 indicated that demyelinization is apparently not a feature of rubella encephalopathy. Neurologic abnormalities are minor and occur infrequently, and intellectual function is generally unaffected if the patient survives. Electroencephalographic abnormalities, however, are relatively common and persistent.

Purpura. Thrombocytopenic as well as nonthrombocytopenic purpura may, in rare instances, complicate rubella. In addition to a reduction in platelet count, when present, there is usually prolonged bleeding time and increased capillary fragility. In some reported cases the clinical manifestations have included one or more of the following disorders: cutaneous hemorrhages, epistaxis, bleeding gums, hematuria, bleeding from the intestinal tract, and, rarely, cerebral hemorrhage. Most patients become symptom free within 2 weeks, and the platelet count returns to normal values.

Prognosis

The prognosis is almost uniformly excellent. Rubella is one of the most benign of all infectious diseases in children. The extremely rare complications of encephalitis and thrombocytopenic purpura may alter the prognosis. Many reported deaths attributed to rubella infection usually reflect errors in diagnosis.

Immunity

Active immunity. One attack of rubella is generally followed by permanent immunity. Many of the so-called second attacks represent errors in diagnosis. Active immunity is induced by infection after natural or artificial exposure. As indicated in Fig. 24-4, rubella-neutralizing antibody may persist for many years after infection.

Passive immunity. Neutralizing antibodies for rubella are present in gamma globulin and in convalescent-phase serum. Rubella, like measles and mumps, is rarely observed in the early months of life because of transplacentally acquired immunity.

Epidemiologic factors

Rubella is worldwide in distribution. It is endemic in most large cities. Localized epidemics occur at irregular intervals in contrast to the fairly consistent periodicity of measles. During the prevaccine era, major epidemics occurred at 6- to 9-year intervals. Rubella outbreaks usually occur during the spring months in the temperate zones.

The use of more than 125 million doses of live attenuated rubella vaccine since licensure in 1969 has had a major impact on the epidemiology of the disease. The last epidemic occurred in 1964. During the subsequent 20 years there was a progressive decrease in the number of reported cases of rubella. Major epidemics of the disease have been eliminated in the United States.

The age distribution of rubella during the prevaccine era was striking. It was rare in infancy and uncommon in preschool-age children. There was an unusually high incidence of the disease in older children, adolescents, and young adults. Rubella was a constant problem in boarding schools, colleges, and military installations. There was a significant number of man-days lost as a result of outbreaks among military personnel.

Rubella is probably spread via the respiratory route. Studies of human volunteers have confirmed this impression. The disease has been transmitted with nasopharyngeal secretions obtained from patients with rubella on the first day of the rash. The period of infectivity probably extends from the latter part of the incubation period to the end of the third day of the rash.

Isolation and quarantine

Isolation and quarantine precautions are generally not warranted. However, outbreaks of rubella have proved to be a problem in hospital and medical personnel in several states, including New York (McLaughlin and Gold, 1979), California, and Colorado (Edell et al., 1979). During the New York experience a male physician with rubella exposed 170 persons, including susceptible pregnant patients. These episodes create a difficult problem for institutions and staff—a problem that can be prevented by routine screening of male as well as female medical personnel caring for patients who may be pregnant and by immunization of those with no detectable rubella antibody.

Treatment

Symptomatic treatment. Rubella in many instances is asymptomatic, and no treatment at all is required. Even if the child has a low-grade fever, it may be unnecessary to keep him in bed. Headache, malaise, and pain in the lymph nodes can be easily controlled with aspirin.

Treatment of complications. Arthritis is usually well controlled by aspirin. Bed rest is advised if there is fever or involvement of the weight-bearing joints. A patient with encephalitis should be treated in the same way as a patient with measles encephalitis (p. 164). Corticosteroid therapy and platelet transfusions may be indicated in severe cases of thrombocytopenic purpura.

CONGENITAL RUBELLA

Congenital rubella was identified as a clinical entity more than a century after the disease was first recognized. In 1941 Gregg reported the occurrence of congenital cataracts among 78 infants born after maternal rubella infection acquired during the 1940 epidemic in Australia. More than half of these infants had congenital heart disease. Since 1941, Gregg's report of the rubella syndrome has been amply confirmed. The occurrence of rubella during the first trimester of pregnancy has been associated with a significantly increased incidence of congenital malformations, stillbirths, and abortions. The epidemic of rubella in the United States in 1964 was followed by the birth of many thousands of infants with the congenital rubella syndrome.

Pathogenesis

Studies by many investigators have provided evidence to support the following concept of the natural history of congenital rubella. As indicated in Fig. 24-4, viremia is present for several days before onset of rash. Maternal viremia may be followed by a placental infection and subsequent fetal viremia leading to a disseminated infection involving many fetal organs. Timing is the crucial element in the pathogenesis of con-

genital rubella. It is clear that a fetal infection is likely to be chronic and persistent if it is acquired during the early weeks and months of pregnancy. However, after the fourth month of gestation, the fetus no longer seems to be susceptible to the chronic infection that is characteristic of intrauterine rubella during the first 8 to 12 weeks.

The pathogenesis of rubella embryopathy is not entirely clear. Studies in human embryonic tissue culture cells indicated that rubella infection was associated with inhibition of mitosis and an increased number of chromosomal breaks (Plotkin et al., 1965). Autopsies of infants with congenital rubella revealed hypoplastic organs with a subnormal number of cells (Naeye and Blanc, 1965). Consequently, it is likely that rubella embryopathy may be caused by (1) inhibition of cellular multiplication; (2) chronic, persistent infection during the crucial period of organogenesis; or (3) a combination of both factors.

Clinical manifestations

The classic rubella syndrome described by Gregg and others in the 1940s was characterized by intrauterine growth retardation, cataracts, microcephaly, deafness, congenital heart disease, and mental retardation. Extensive studies of this syndrome during the 1964 rubella epidemic in the United States shed new light on this problem. The availability of specific virus isolation and serologic techniques provided information that revealed a broader spectrum of this disease. Intrauterine rubella infection may be followed by spontaneous abortion of the infected fetus, a stillbirth, a live birth of an infant with single or multiple malformations, or a normal infant. The various manifestations of congenital rubella are listed in Table 24-2. It is clear that the consequences of rubella infection during pregnancy are varied and unpredictable. Virtually every organ may be involved, singly, multiply, transiently, or progressively and permanently.

Neonatal manifestations. A variety of clinical manifestations may be present during the first weeks of life. Low birth weight in relation to period of gestation is common. Thrombocytopenic purpura characterized by a petechial and purpuric eruption may occur in association with other transient lesions such as hepatosplenomegaly, hepatitis, hemolytic anemia, bone le-

Table 24-2. Manifestations of congenital rubella

Growth retardation (low birth weight)
Eye defects
  Cataracts
  Glaucoma
  Retinopathy
  Microphthalmia
Deafness
Cardiac defects
  Patent ductus arteriosus
  Ventricular septal defect
  Pulmonary stenosis
  Myocardial necrosis
CNS defects
  Psychomotor retardation
  Microcephaly
  Encephalitis
  Spastic quadriparesis
  Cerebrospinal fluid pleocytosis
  Mental retardation
  Progressive panencephalitis
Hepatomegaly
Hepatitis
Thrombocytopenic purpura
Splenomegaly
Bone lesions
Interstitial pneumonitis
Diabetes mellitus
Psychiatric disorders
Thyroid disorders
Precocious puberty

sions (metaphyseal rarefaction), and bulging anterior fontanelle with or without pleocytosis in the CSF. These transient manifestations may occur in association with the classic cardiac, eye, hearing, and CNS defects. An infant with neonatal thrombocytopenic purpura characterized by the typical "blueberry muffin" skin lesions is shown in Plate 4.

Cardiac defects. Patent ductus arteriosus, with or without pulmonary artery stenosis, and atrial and ventricular septal defects are the most common cardiac lesions. Clinical evidence of congenital heart disease may be present at birth or delayed for several days. Other cardiac manifestations include myocardial involvement as indicated by electrocardiographic findings and necropsy evidence of extensive necrosis of the myocardium. Many infants have tolerated the cardiac lesions with little difficulty; others have developed congestive heart failure in the first months of life.

Eye defects. Cataracts, unilateral or bilateral, are common consequences of congenital rubella. They appear as pearly white nuclear lesions, frequently associated with microphthalmia. The cataracts may be too small at birth to be visible on casual examination. A careful ophthalmoscopic examination with a +8 lens held 15 to 20 cm from the eye may reveal an early cataract.

Rubella glaucoma is a less common eye lesion, and it may be clinically indistinguishable from hereditary infantile glaucoma. It may be present at birth, or it may appear after the neonatal period. The cornea is enlarged and hazy, the anterior chamber is deep, and ocular tension is increased. Glaucoma that requires prompt surgical therapy must be differentiated from transient corneal clouding.

Retinopathy is the most common eye manifestation of congenital rubella. It is characterized by discrete, patchy, black pigmentation that is variable in size and location. Retinopathy does not affect visual acuity if the lesions do not involve the macular area. The presence of this lesion is a valuable aid in the clinical diagnosis of congenital rubella.

Hearing loss. Deafness may be the only manifestation of congenital rubella. It may be unilateral but is usually bilateral. It is probably caused by maldevelopment and possibly by degenerative changes in the cochlea and organ of Corti. Hearing loss may be severe or so mild that it is overlooked unless detected by an audiometric examination. Severe bilateral hearing loss is responsible for speech defects.

Central nervous system involvement. Psychomotor retardation is a common manifestation of congenital rubella. In severe cases the brain is the site of a chronic, persistent infection, as indicated by the presence of pleocytosis, increased concentration of protein, and rubella virus in the CSF for as long as 1 year after birth. Microcephaly is a well-known manifestation of the rubella syndrome (Desmond et al., 1967). The most common consequence of CNS involvement is mental retardation that may be mild or profound. Behavioral disturbances and manifestations of minimal cerebral dysfunction also are common. Less common are severe spastic diplegia and autism.

Progressive rubella panencephalitis has been described in four patients with congenital rubella (Townsend et al., 1975; Weil et al., 1975). Severe, progressive neurologic deterioration was noted during the second decade of life. In two patients there was progression of spasticity, ataxia, intellectual deterioration, seizures, and subsequent fatality. Other findings included high levels of rubella antibody in serum and CSF, increased CSF protein and gamma globulin levels, histopathologic changes in the brain, and isolation of rubella virus from a brain biopsy of one of the patients. This syndrome in some ways resembled subacute sclerosing panencephalitis, a rare complication of measles.

Diagnosis

The presence of congenital rubella should be suspected under the following circumstances: (1) a history of possible rubella or exposure to rubella during the first trimester of pregnancy and (2) the presence of one or more of the various manifestations of congenital rubella listed on p. 314. However, final confirmation of the diagnosis is dependent on virus isolation and/or immunologic procedures.

Virus isolation. Rubella virus has been cultured from pharyngeal secretions, urine, CSF, and virtually every tissue and organ in the body. Infants with congenital rubella may remain chronically infected for many weeks or months. As indicated in Fig. 24-5, the incidence of virus shedding decreases with advancing age. Most infants with congenital rubella are no longer shedding virus and have a normal pattern of serum immunoglobulins by 1 year of age. However, infants with severe dysgammaglobulinemia may shed virus for a more prolonged period. Isolation of virus from the blood is very rare. Viremia has been observed chiefly in infants with immunologic disorders.

Immunologic response. The response to an intrauterine infection is shown in Fig. 24-6. It differs significantly from the response to rubella acquired postnatally. The chief difference lies in the pattern of virus excretion and antibody response. In rubella acquired after birth, virus excretion is transient, rarely persisting for more

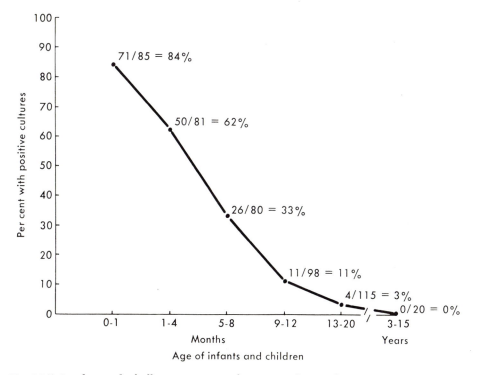

Fig. 24-5. Incidence of rubella virus excretion by age in infants with congenital rubella. (From Cooper LZ, Krugman S. Arch Ophthalmol 1967;77:434.)

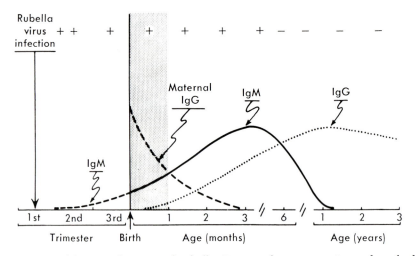

Fig. 24-6. Natural history of congenital rubella. Pattern of virus excretion and antibody response.

than 2 or 3 weeks (Fig. 24-4); in contrast, virus shedding may persist for many months after birth in congenital rubella.

As indicated in Fig. 24-6, the serum of an infant with congenital rubella contains actively acquired IgM-specific antibody and passively acquired maternal IgG antibody. Several months later, transplacentally acquired IgG is no longer detectable, and high levels of IgM may be present. By the end of 1 year, actively acquired IgG appears to be the dominant rubella antibody. Consequently, the presence and persistence of rubella antibody in the serum of an infant 5 to 6 months of age or older and the identification of the antibody in early infancy as IgM are indicative of congenital rubella infection.

The pattern of persistence of HI antibody following congenital rubella is different from that following naturally acquired infection. Detectable levels of antibody persist for many years in most children after a natural rubella infection. However, approximately 20% of children with congenital rubella by age 5 years may no longer have detectable rubella HI antibody (Cooper et al., 1971).

Differential diagnosis

Cytomegalovirus infection, congenital toxoplasmosis, and congenital syphilis also may be characterized by the following manifestations of congenital rubella: thrombocytopenic purpura, jaundice, hepatosplenomegaly, and bone le-

sions. Herpes simplex virus infection shows the same manifestations with the exception of bone lesions. The diagnosis may be clarified by the presence of other findings more compatible with congenital rubella, such as congenital cataract, glaucoma, patent ductus arteriosus, or maternal history of rubella. The precise diagnosis should be confirmed by specific laboratory tests.

Prognosis

Neonatal thrombocytopenic purpura carries a bad prognosis. The mortality exceeded 35% after the first-year follow-up of a large group of infants (Cooper and Krugman, 1967). The usual causes of death were sepsis, congestive heart failure, and general debility. In the absence of purpura, the mortality was approximately 10%. Deaths usually occurred during the first 6 months of life. The prognosis is excellent for children with minor defects.

Epidemiologic factors

The incidence of congenital rubella is dependent on the immune status of women of childbearing age and the occurrence of significant epidemics. In the United States approximately 15% of young women have no detectable rubella antibody. During the 1964 epidemic, 3.6% of pregnant women had rubella; in contrast, the infection rate was 0.1% to 0.2% during interepidemic years (Sever, 1967).

Congenital rubella is a contagious disease.

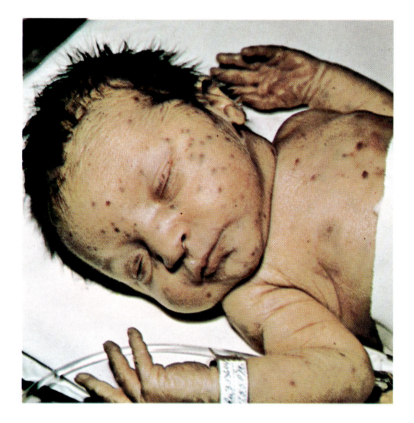

Plate 4
A 3-day-old infant with generalized macular lesions characteristic of neonatal purpura resulting from congenital rubella. His jaundice is caused by rubella hepatitis. (Courtesy Dr. Kenneth Schiffer, Albert Einstein College of Medicine, New York, NY; from Cooper LZ et al.: Am J Dis Child 1965;110:416.)

The infected newborn infant may disseminate the virus to close contacts for many months. This reservoir may provide a source for maintaining the virus in nature from year to year.

The risk associated with maternal rubella infection has been variously estimated. An evaluation of several prospective studies indicates that the risk of congenital malformations after maternal rubella may be as follows: (1) 30% to 50% during the first 4 weeks of gestation, (2) 25% during the first fifth to eighth weeks of gestation, and (3) 8% during the ninth to twelfth weeks of gestation. The overall risk of malformations from rubella during the first trimester is approximately 20%. There is a slight risk of deafness when rubella occurs during the thirteenth to sixteenth weeks.

Preventive measures

The major goal of preventive measures is the prevention of fetal infection that may cause congenital rubella. Active and passive immunization procedures have been used to achieve this objective.

Active immunization. The development of a live attenuated rubella virus vaccine by Meyer et al. (1966) was followed by field trials that culminated in the licensure of rubella vaccine in the United States in June 1969. The 1984 recommendations for the use of live attenuated rubella vaccine for prevention of rubella and congenital rubella are described in detail in Chapter 35, p. 539.

Passive immunization. The use of standard immune globulin (IG) for the prevention of rubella has been a controversial subject for many years. The available evidence indicates that human IG may modify or suppress the clinical manifestations of rubella without preventing viremia.

Since the use of standard IG has obvious limitations, it is difficult to justify its *routine* use for prophylaxis of rubella in early pregnancy. In a pregnancy in which a therapeutic abortion would not be considered because of religious or other contraindications, the use of IG may be justified; the suggested dose is 20 ml given intramuscularly.

If reliable laboratory facilities are available, use of the rubella HI antibody test will help in the management of the rubella problem in pregnancy. The following procedure is suggested:

1. Obtain a blood sample as soon as possible after exposure and test for presence or absence of antibody. The laboratory could complete this test within 24 hours.
2. If antibody is present, there is no risk of infection and the patient can be reassured.
3. If antibody is not detectable, IG may be given, and a second blood specimen should be obtained 4 weeks later. The HI antibody test should be repeated on the paired serum specimens. The detection of a fourfold or greater rise in antibody titer in the second serum specimen might be indicative of rubella infection in the mother. Failure to develop antibody would indicate absence of infection.

Isolation and quarantine

Isolation of infants with congenital rubella. The primary aim of isolation procedures is to prevent rubella infection in susceptible pregnant women. Infants with congenital rubella may shed virus for many weeks or months after birth. Intimate contact is generally required for the transmission of rubella. The risk of infection by the airborne route is probably inconsequential. Accordingly, potentially susceptible pregnant women should avoid close exposure to these infants.

Isolation in the hospital. Infants suspected of having congenital rubella should be admitted to a separate room designated as the isolation unit. Personnel assigned to this area should be selected on the basis of their childbearing potential and immune status. If appropriate laboratory facilities are available, it would be wise to screen all staff members for presence of rubella antibody. Isolation should be continued until the infant is ready to go home.

Isolation in the home. No special precautions are necessary for the parents and young sibling contacts. Potentially susceptible female visitors to the home should avoid physical contact with the infant during the contagious period. If laboratory facilities are available for identification of rubella virus, infants should be considered contagious until negative cultures have been obtained. As indicated in Fig. 24-5, evidence of virus shedding may disappear by 1 month of age in some infants; on the other hand, it may persist for a year or more in a small number of infants. If laboratory facilities are not available, the data shown in Fig. 24-5 may be used as a guide for the estimation of period of contagion. In general there appears to be some correlation between the severity of the infection and the duration of virus shedding. Infants with severe involvement will usually shed virus much longer than infants with minimal involvement.

REFERENCES

Anderson SG. Experimental rubella in human volunteers. J Immunol 1949;62:29.

Best JM, Banatvala JE, Bowen JM. New Japanese rubella vaccine: comparative trials. Br Med J 1974;3:221.

Boué A, Nicolas A, Montagnon B. Reinfection with rubella in pregnant women. Lancet 1971;1:1251.

Brody JA, et al. Rubella epidemic on St. Paul Island in the Pribilofs, 1963. JAMA 1965;191:619.

Burke JP, Hinman AR, Krugman S (eds). International symposium on prevention of congenital rubella infection. Rev Infect Dis 1985;7(Suppl 1):1.

Buser F, Nocolas A. Vaccination with RA 27/3 rubella vaccine. Am J Dis Child 1971;122:53.

Center for Disease Control. Rubella—Bermuda. Morbid Mortal Weekly Rep 1971;20:207.

Cooper LZ, Florman AL, Ziring PR, Krugman S. Loss of rubella hemagglutination inhibition antibody in congenital rubella. Am J Dis Child 1971;122:397.

Cooper LZ, Krugman S. Clinical manifestations of postnatal and congenital rubella. Arch Ophthalmol 1967;77:434.

Cooper LZ, et al. Neonatal thrombocytopenic purpura and other manifestations of rubella contracted in utero. Am J Dis Child 1965;110:416.

Cooper LZ, et al. Transient arthritis after rubella vaccination. Am J Dis Child 1969;118:218.

Davis WJ, et al. A study of rubella immunity and resistance to reinfection. JAMA 1971;215:600.

Desmond MM, et al. Congenital rubella encephalitis. J Pediatr 1967;71:311.

Dorsett PH, Miller DC, Green KY, et al. Structure and function of rubella virus proteins. Rev Infect Dis 1985; 7:S150.

Edell TA, et al. Rubella in hospital personnel and patients, Colorado. Morbid Mortal Weekly Rep 1979;28:325.

Enders JF. Rubella vaccination. N Engl J Med 1970;283:161.

Fleet WF Jr, et al. Exposure of susceptible teachers to rubella vaccines. Am J Dis Child 1972;123:28.

Fleet WF Jr, et al. Fetal consequences of maternal rubella immunization. JAMA 1974;227:621.

Forchheimer F. Enanthem of German measles. Philadelphia Med 1898;2:15.

Fry J, Dillane JB, Fry L. Rubella, 1962. Br Med J 1962;2:833.

Grayston JT, Watten RH. Epidemic rubella in Taiwan, 1957-1958. III. Gamma globulin in the prevention of rubella. N Engl J Med 1959;261:1145.

Green RH, et al. Studies on the natural history and prevention of rubella. Am J Dis Child 1965;110:348.

Greenberg M, Pelliteri O, Barton J. Frequency of defects in infants whose mothers had rubella during pregnancy. JAMA 1957;165:675.

Gregg NM. Congenital cataract following German measles in the mother. Trans Ophthalmol Soc Aust 1941;3:35.

Gregg NM, et al. Occurrence of congenital defects in children following maternal rubella during pregnancy. Med J Aust 1945;2:122.

Guyer B, et al. The Memphis State University rubella outbreak. JAMA 1974;227:1298.

Habel K, et al. Transmission of rubella to *Macacus mulatta* monkeys. Public Health Rep 1942;57:1126.

Halstead S, Diwan AR. Failure to transmit rubella virus vaccine—a close contact study in adults. JAMA 1971; 215:634.

Hermann KL, et al. Rubella immunization: persistence of antibody four years after a large-scale field trial. JAMA 1976;235:2201.

Hess AF. German measles (rubella): an experimental study. Arch Intern Med 1914;13:913.

Hill AB, Doll R, Galloway T McL, Hughes JPW. Virus diseases in pregnancy and congenital defects. Br J Prev Soc Med 1958;12:1.

Hiro Y, Tasaka S. Die Röteln sind eine Virus-krankheit. Monatsschr Kinderheilkd 1938;76:328.

Horstmann DM, et al. Rubella: reinfection of vaccinated and naturally immune persons exposed in an epidemic. N Engl J Med 1970;283:771.

Houser HG, Schalet N. Prevention of rubella with gamma globulin. Clin Res 1958;6:281.

Ingalls TH. Progress in pediatrics: German measles and German measles in pregnancy. Am J Dis Child 1957;93:555.

Jackson ADM, Fisch L. Deafness following maternal rubella, results of a prospective investigation. Lancet 1958;2:1241.

Johnson RE, Hall AP. Rubella arthritis; report of cases studied by latex tests. N Engl J Med 1958;258:743.

Judelsohn RG, Wyll SA. Rubella in Bermuda: termination of an epidemic by mass vaccination. JAMA 1973;223:401.

Kantor TG, Tanner M. Rubella arthritis and rheumatoid arthritis. Arthritis Rheum 1962;5:378.

Kenny FM, Michaels RH, Davis KS. Rubella encephalopathy: later psychometric, neurologic and encephalographic evaluation of seven survivors. Am J Dis Child 1965;110:374.

Kilroy AW, et al. Two syndromes following rubella immunization: clinical observations and epidemiological studies. JAMA 1970;214:2287.

Klock LE, et al. A clinical and serological study of women exposed to rubella vaccinees. Am J Dis Child 1972;123:465.

Korns RF. Prophylaxis of German measles with human serum globulin. J Infect Dis 1952;90:183.

Korones SB, et al. Congenital rubella syndrome: study of 22 infants. Am J Dis Child 1965;110:434.

Krugman S, ed. Proceedings of the International Conference on Rubella Immunization. Am J Dis Child 1969; 118:1.

Krugman S. Present status of measles and rubella immunization in the United States: a medical progress report. J Pediatr 1971;78:1; J Pediatr 1977;90:1.

Krugman S, Ward R. The rubella problem. J Pediatr 1954;44:489.

Krugman S, Ward R. Rubella: demonstration of neutralizing antibody in gamma globulin and reevaluation of the rubella problem. N Engl J Med 1958;259:16.

Krugman S, Ward R, Jacobs KG, Lazar M. Studies on rubella immunization. I. Demonstration of rubella without rash. JAMA 1953;151:285.

Landrigan PJ, Stoffels MA, Anderson E, Witte JJ. Epidemic rubella in adolescent boys. JAMA 1974;227:1283.

Levin MJ, et al. Diagnosis of congenital rubella in utero. N Engl J Med 1974;290:1187.

Lock FR, Gatling HB, Mauzy CH, Wells HB. Incidence of anomalous development following maternal rubella. Am J Obstet Gynecol 1961;81:451.

Lündström R. Rubella during pregnancy. A follow-up study of children born after an epidemic of rubella in Sweden, 1951, with additional investigations on prophylaxis and treatment of maternal rubella. Acta Paediatr 1962;51 (Suppl 133):1-110.

MacFarlane DW, Boyd RD, Dodrill CB, Tufts E. Intrauterine rubella, head size, and intellect. Pediatrics 1975; 55:797.

McLaughlin MD, Gold LH. The New York rubella incident: a case for changing hospital policy regarding rubella testing and immunization. Am J Pub Health 1979;69:287.

Menser MA, Forrest JM, Bransby RD. Rubella infection and diabetes. Lancet 1978;1:57.

Meyer HM, Parkman PD. Rubella vaccination—a review of practical experience. JAMA 1971;215:613.

Meyer HM Jr, Parkman PD, Panos TC. Attenuated rubella virus. II. Production of an experimental live-virus vaccine and clinical trial. N Engl J Med 1966;275:575.

Michaels RH, Mellin GW. Prospective experience with maternal rubella and the associated congenital malformations. Pediatrics 1960;26:200.

Modlin JF. Surveillance of the congenital rubella syndrome, 1969-73. J Infect Dis 1974;130:316.

Modlin JF, et al. A review of five years experience with rubella vaccine in the United States. Pediatrics 1975; 55:20.

Naeye RL, Blanc W. Pathogenesis of congenital rubella. JAMA 1965;194:1277.

Neff JM, Carver DH. Rubella immunization: reconsideration of our present policy. Am J Epidemiol 1970;92:162.

Parkman PD, Buescher EL, Artenstein MS. Recovery of rubella virus from army recruits. Proc Soc Exp Biol Med 1962;111:225.

Parkman PD, Meyer HM Jr, Kirschstein RL, Hopps HE. attenuated rubella virus. I. Development and laboratory characterization. N Engl J Med 1966;275:569.

Pitt DB. Congenital malformations and maternal rubella. Med J Aust 1957;1:233.

Plotkin SA, Boué A, Boué JG. The in vitro growth of rubella virus in human embryonic cells. Am J Epidemiol 1965;81:71.

Schiff GM, Donath R, Rotte T. Experimental rubella studies. I. Clinical and laboratory features of infection caused by the Brown strain rubella virus. II. Artificial challenge studies of adult rubella vaccinees. Am J Dis Child 1969;118:269.

Schiff GM, et al. Rubella vaccines in a public school system. Am J Dis Child 1974;128:180.

Shaffner W, et al. Polyneuropathy following rubella immunization. Am J Dis Child 1974;127:684.

Scott HD, Byrne EB. Exposure of susceptible pregnant women to rubella vaccinees; serologic findings during the Rhode Island immunization campaign. JAMA 1971; 215:609.

Sennett RA, Copeman WSC. Notes on rubella, with special reference to certain rheumatic sequelae. Br Med J 1940;1:924.

Seppala M, Vaheri A. Natural rubella infection of the female genital tract. Lancet 1974;1:46.

Siegel M. Unresolved issues in the first five years of the rubella immunization program. Am J Obstet Gynecol 1976;124:327.

Sever JL. Epidemiology of rubella. Washington DC: Pan American Health Organization, World Health Organization, May 1967, Scientific Publication No 147, p 366.

Stewart GL, et al. Rubella virus hemagglutination-inhibition test. N Engl J Med 1967;276:554.

Townsend JJ, et al. Progressive rubella panencephalitis: late onset after congenital rubella. N Engl J Med 1975; 292:990.

Vesikari T, Buimovici-Klein E. Lymphocyte responses to rubella antigen and phytohemagglutinin after administration of the RA 27/3 strain of live attenuated rubella vaccine. Infect Immun 1975;11:748.

Warkany J, Kalter H. Congenital malformations. N Engl J Med 1961;265:1046.

Weil ML, et al. Chronic progressive panencephalitis due to rubella virus stimulating SSPE. N Engl J Med 1975; 292:994.

Weller TH, Neva FA. Propagation in tissue culture of cytopathic agents from patients with rubella-like illness. Proc Soc Exp Biol Med 1962;111:215.

Wesselhoeft C. Rubella (German measles). N Engl J Med 1947;236:943,978.

Wilkins J, Leedon JM, Portnoy B, Salvatore MA. Reinfection with rubella virus despite live vaccine-induced immunity. Am J Dis Child 1969;118:275.

Ziring PR, Florman AF, Cooper LZ. The diagnosis of rubella. Pediatr Clin North Am 1971;18:87.

25

SEXUALLY TRANSMITTABLE DISEASES IN CHILDREN

The term *venereal diseases* has given way in recent years to the designation "sexually transmittable diseases" (STDs). Among the infections included in this category are gonorrhea, syphilis, lymphogranuloma venereum, *Chlamydia trachomatis*, herpes simplex virus, cytomegalovirus, *Trichomonas vaginalis*, venereal warts, and *Mycoplasma hominis*. The term *STD* includes acquisition of gonococcal ophthalmia or herpes simplex infection by newborns who encounter the organism in the maternal genital tract. All pediatric age groups may be infected with these diseases and gonorrhea is but one example. The patient with one diagnosed STD may have other simultaneous STDs so that the diagnosis of one is an indication to examine the child for others. Most investigators today would agree that STD in young children should be assumed to be sexually transmitted unless proven otherwise, which brings the infected child into the realm of suspected sexual child abuse.

SEXUAL ABUSE OF CHILDREN

Sexual abuse of children has been defined as the involvement of dependent, developmentally immature children and adolescents in sexual activities that they do not fully comprehend, to which they are unable to give informed consent, or that violate the social taboos of family roles. Sexual abuse includes all forms of adult involvement in sexual relations with children, including rape and incest. Pedophilia is the condition in which adults prefer sexual relations with chil-

dren, and it may take the forms of nonviolent fondling, viewing, and orogenital contact.

The incidence of sexual abuse is unknown, but many medical facilities find that increased efforts at recognition lead to identification of very significant numbers of involved children. Reported cases of sexual abuse comprise approximately 10% of all cases of abuse and neglect in some areas. Reluctance on the part of the perpetrator, family, medical community, and legal system to acknowledge the possibility of sexual abuse of children has undoubtedly hindered the understanding of this problem. Recent developments, including skilled interviewing techniques and the use of anatomically correct dolls, is allowing a fuller assessment of suspected cases. The statements from young children are gaining credibility; ". . .molestation may leave no evidence, except the child's story. This must be believed! Children do not fabricate stories of detailed sexual activities unless they have witnessed them, and they have indeed been witness to their abuse" (Kempe, 1978). There is a rapidly developing appreciation of the association between sexual abuse, other forms of child abuse, and other forms of behavioral disturbances in children including truancy, running away, depression, low self-esteem, weight disturbances, fears, and many other somatic complaints.

Although the minority of children who have experienced sexual abuse contract sexually transmittable diseases as a consequence, the diagnosis of a sexually transmittable disease is a

320

very important indication that the child has been in an abusive setting, and STD may be the sole finding on physical examination. For this reason, the examination should be thorough, all mucous membranes should be appropriately cultured, and the cultures should be handled in such a way as to ensure legal acceptability if that should become needed.

Although the list of infections that are known to be transmittable by a sexual route is very long for adults, in whom many of the infections are transmitted primarily during male homosexual activity, the main infections for which a child who is suspected of having an STD (see Table 25-1) should routinely be examined are syphilis, gonorrhea, condyloma acuminata (genital warts), herpes simplex of the genital area, *Chlamydia trachomatis*, and *Trichomonas vaginalis*. The following general cautions should be noted:

1. Many institutions have a medical service that is particularly skilled in the interview and examination of children suspected of having experienced sexual abuse. This may be a child protection team within the pediatric department or a person or group in obstetrics. This group, if available, should be involved in the work-up from the first contact.
2. If the child is symptomatic, all available and appropriate cultures and examinations should be done before the child is begun on therapy. For example, if the child has conjunctivitis, cultures of other mucosal areas should be taken before therapy is started.
3. All culture and examination samples must be thoroughly and clearly labeled, and delivery to the appropriate laboratory must be ensured by personal delivery if necessary.
4. If sexual abuse is documented by the presence of spermatozoa, presence of one of the listed STDs, or social history, the child should be hospitalized pending investigation and social/legal disposition.
5. The Child Abuse Reporting Law applies to sexual abuse or assault. Therefore reporting of confirmed cases is mandatory.
6. The majority of children who have been the victims of sexual abuse will not have specific physical findings to confirm the di-

agnosis. Subtle findings, such as bruising, may be present, but the physical examination is likely to be normal; a normal physical examination does not make a diagnosis of sexual abuse unlikely. Oral sexual contact is a common form of abuse, as is fondling and external genital contact.

7. If the child has gonorrhea, other members of the family usually also are infected. In particular, other female children are especially likely to be infected and should be examined. Admission to the hospital of the index child patient will facilitate a successful investigation.

Cultures that should be taken from children suspected of having been victims of sexual abuse are as follows:

1. Rectal, throat, urethral, and vaginal or endocervical cultures for *Neisseria gonorrhoeae* should be plated on Thayer-Martin media. Vaginal cultures are satisfactory for prepubertal females. Blood cultures should be taken if there is reason to consider disseminated disease. Other sites (conjunctivae, joint fluid) should be cultured if clinically indicated.
2. Vulvovaginal or pharyngeal cultures for *Chlamydia trachomatis*, if available, are indicated.
3. Serum for a VDRL should be collected at the first examination and repeated in 6 to 8 weeks.
4. Wet smears of vaginal secretions (saline lavage or aspirate may be used) for spermatozoa and saline lavage with aspiration of pharyngeal or vaginal secretions for quantitative acid phosphatase assay should be performed if there has been reason to think that a sexual contact occurred within the past day.
5. Presence of venereal warts should be sought and noted if present.
6. Urinalysis with attention to the presence of *Trichomonas* should be performed.
7. Pregnancy should be determined if indicated.

The subject of child abuse and sexual abuse of children is one of the most rapidly advancing fields of pediatric interest and requires the physician to give attention to changes in concepts concerning diagnosis and management as they emerge.

Table 25-1. Sexually transmittable diseases in prepubertal children who are evaluated for suspected sexual abuse

References	Number of children evaluated	Number (%) who had diagnosis of				
		Gonorrhea	Chlamydia	Syphilis	Trichomonas	Condyloma acuminata
Rimsza and Niggemann (1982)	285	21 (7.4)	—	0	—	—
White et al. (1983)	409	46 (10)	—	6 (1.5)	4 (1)	3 (1)
Ingram et al. (1984)	50	10 (20)	3 (6)	—	2 (4)	—

GONORRHEA

Gonorrhea is the most frequently reported infectious disease in the United States. The World Health Organization estimates that there are about 100 million gonorrheal infections each year throughout the world. The reported number of cases of gonorrhea in the United States exceeds 1 million annually, and it is estimated that more than 2.5 million cases occur. An unknown number of cases escape detection and contribute to the silent reservoir of infection in males and females. The reported age-specific rate for gonococcal disease in children up to 14 years was 10.6 per 100,000 for males and 30.6 per 100,000 for females in 1982.

Gonorrhea is an inflammatory disease of the mucous membranes of the genitourinary tract that only occurs in humans. It is caused by the gonococcus, *Neisseria gonorrhoeae*, which was first described by Neisser in 1879. The most common portal of entry is the genitourinary tract, and the organism may then cause various inflammatory diseases of adjacent tissues such as cervicitis, salpingitis, and vulvovaginitis in children. The newborn may acquire the organism during delivery when direct contact with contaminated vaginal secretions leads to conjunctivitis. Bacteremia may occur and most often causes cutaneous lesions and arthritis, rarely endocarditis and meningitis. Children may present with gonococcal proctitis and pharyngitis as well as asymptomatic carriage of gonococci in the rectum, pharynx, and genitourinary tract.

In stained smears of urethral pus, gonococci appear as gram-negative, biscuit-shaped intracellular diplococci. Gram stains of synovial fluid, urethral discharge, or urine sediment in the male may reveal the characteristic organism. The female adult cervix may be colonized with other organisms, including *Neisseria* species, rendering the Gram stain less reliable. The genitourinary tract of the prepubertal girl with nonestrogenized mucosa supports the growth of the gonococcus, so the vaginal smears are useful in the diagnosis of vulvovaginitis in that age range.

Cultivation of the gonococcus on artificial media is difficult because of its fastidious growth requirements, but heated, blood-enriched media are satisfactory. The lysed red blood cells provide a source of iron required by the organism. Gonococci grow best aerobically, at a temperature of 35° to 36° C, in an atmosphere with 2% to 10% carbon dioxide, and humidity. The only sugar fermented by the gonococcus is glucose, with production of acid but no gas.

The use of Thayer-Martin selective medium, which contains vancomycin, colistimethate, and nystatin, inhibits growth of many competing saprophytes of the genitourinary tract, allowing the detection of gonococci. Specimens of areas that are normally sterile, such as joint fluid, should be plated on chocolate agar. Specimens for gonococci should be plated quickly and not allowed to stand at room temperature. The availability of commercial, prepackaged media with a 4-week "shelf life" in the refrigerator greatly facilitates office cultures by the practitioner. Identification of gonococci is dependent on oxidase-positive, catalase-positive colonies and sugar fermentations.

Virulence factors

There are several developing systems for typing strains of *N. gonorrhoeae*. Typing systems include (1) auxotyping, which determines nutritional requirements; (2) coagglutination and microimmunofluorescence, which relates to components of the outer membrane of the organism; (3) enzyme-linked immunosorbent assay (ELISA) for the principal outer membrane protein; and (4) typing of the pilus composition. The ability to type strains of *N. gonorrhoeae* has enabled the identification of bacterial factors that contribute to virulence. The following is a brief summary of some of the principal components of virulence, as they are currently understood.

There are five major colony types, designated T1 through T5, which reflect differences in the surface antigens of the orgnaisms in the colony. Differences in colony form may be distinguished by indirect microscopic examination. Colony types 1 and 2 are pilated and are virulent for humans, and colony types 3, 4, and 5 are nonpilated and are relatively avirulent. Pili confer to cell walls an enhanced ability to adhere to host cells and to each other.

Organisms from the pilated colony types are relatively resistant to phagocytosis. Although gonococci of all colony types are readily destroyed following phagocytosis, ingestion of pilated gonococci by macrophages is very inefficient compared with that of nonpilated strains. Pilated gonococci adhere to polymorphonuclear leukocytes. The polymorphonuclear leukocyte that is in contact with an adherent gonococcus discharges the contents of the phagocytic granules against the adherent organism. The attack on the gonococcus is usually unsuccessful. The polymorphonuclear leukocyte may then be parasitized by the viable gonococcus, leading to multiple intracellular organisms characteristic of the Gram stain of the discharge from a patient with gonorrhea.

All gonococci produce IgA_1 protease, an enzyme that cleaves IgA_1 at the hinge region of the antibody molecule. This enzyme presumably allows gonococci to adhere to mucosal surfaces even in the presence of a secretory antibody response.

Increased clinical virulence of some strains is suggested by the observation of microepidemics of gonorrhea involving an unusually high rate of severe disease. Characterization of strains of *N. gonorrhoeae* obtained from patients with disseminated disease has revealed the following properties.

1. Isolates of *N. gonorrhoeae* from patients with disseminated gonococcal infection are not susceptible to the bactericidal activity of sera from patients with uncomplicated gonorrhea, even though sera from those patients are usually bactericidal for other strains. This resistance to serum bactericidal activity may be due to a change in the outer membrane of the organism.

2. The isolates are auxotrophic for arginine, uracil, and hypoxanthine, nutrients not usually required for growth of strains from patients with asymptomatic or genitourinary disease.

3. A high degree of sensitivity to penicillin is characteristic of strains from patients with disseminated disease. Penicillin sensitivity and serum resistance appear to be independent variables.

4. The cell wall also contains several types of outer membrane proteins. The predominant type, as defined by polyacrylamide gel electrophoresis, is protein I (PI), or principal outer membrane protein (POMP). In general, strains with higher molecular weight PI are more resistant to serum bactericidal effects.

Protein II (PII), which occurs in lesser amounts than PI, is heat sensitive and occurs in the outer leaflet of the outer membrane. Its presence in strains is associated with adherence to mucosal cells, opaque colony formation on agar media, and sensitivity to serum bactericidal activity. Loss of PII occurs at a high frequency and is associated with increased invasive potential. Such organisms are recovered from the fallopian tubes of women with salpingitis and from the blood and joints of persons with disseminated gonococcal infection. Strains lacking PII are less sticky, are transparent on agar media, and are more resistant to serum bactericidal activity.

5. Patients with deficiency of one of the terminal components of the complement system (especially factors 5, 6, 7, or 8) are at considerable risk of disseminated, chronic, or recurrent gonococcal disease.

Pathology and pathogenesis

Stratified squamous epithelium has the capacity to resist invasion by the gonococcus, whereas columnar epithelium is susceptible. This difference accounts for the absence of lesions in the adult vagina and on the external genitalia of both sexes. The susceptibility of columnar epithelium leads to infection of urethra, prostate gland, seminal vesicles, and epididymis in males. In females infection occurs primarily in the urethra, Skene's and Bartholin's glands, cervix, and fallopian tubes. Gonorrhea may occur in males or females without signs or symptoms. Primary infection may take place in the rectal or pharyngeal mucosa of either sex. The alkaline pH of secreted mucus and the lack of estrogenization permit vaginal infections with overt vulvovaginitis in the prepubertal girl.

Gonococci penetrate the surface cell layers through the intracellular spaces and reach the subepithelial connective tissue by the third or fourth day of infection. An inflammatory exudate quickly forms beneath the epithelium. In the acute phase of infection, numerous leukocytes, many with phagocytosed gonococci, are present in the lumen of the urethra, causing a characteristic profuse yellow-white discharge in males. In the absence of specific treatment, the inflammatory exudate in the subepithelial connective tissue is replaced by fibroblasts and eventually by fibrous tissue around the urethra with ensuing stricture of the urethra.

Direct extension occurs via the lymphatic vessels and less often via the blood vessels. Infection spreads to the posterior urethra, Cowper's glands, seminal vesicles, prostate, and epididymis, which leads to perineal, perianal, ischiorectal, or periprostatic abscesses. In teenage adult males, acute prostatitis may result in prostatic abscess or chronic prostatitis, and epididymitis is the most frequent complication. After healing has taken place, scar formation may destroy the lumen of the epididymis, and azospermia may result from bilateral involvement. Antimicrobial treatment usually prevents these complications. As many as 50% of untreated teenage and adult males become asymptomatic but remain infectious for periods up to 6 months.

In females, primary infection most frequently affects the columnar epithelium of the postpubertal cervix, and the histopathologic appearance resembles that of the male urethra. Spread of infection to the fallopian tubes may be acute or subacute, without signs and symptoms, and sometimes it is extremely difficult to diagnose. Acute stages may result in peritonitis. As a rule, the infection is confined to the pelvis. The end result of untreated or inadequately treated salpingitis is complete or partial obstruction of the tubes, which often leads to tubal pregnancy or sterility. Pelvic inflammatory disease (PID) is an especially common complication of gonorrhea in female adolescents, and when it occurs in this age range it is especially likely to result in infertility (see Pelvic inflammatory disease and salpingitis).

Clinical manifestations

In pregnancy. The effects of gonococcal disease on the infant may begin before delivery, since there is evidence that gonococcal disease in pregnant women may have an adverse effect on both the mother and the infant. Edwards et al. (1978) compared 19 women who had intrapartum gonorrhea with 41 case controls. The women with gonorrhea had a significantly greater occurrence of premature rupture of membranes, prolonged rupture of membranes, chorioamnionitis, and premature delivery. Other studies have shown an alarming incidence of perinatal deaths and abortions (see Table 25-2). In addition to the effect on the fetus, postpartum complications in the mother are common. Therefore the diagnosis of gonococcal disease should be sought and controlled during pregnancy. Control should consider several issues:

1. Recurrent infection following an initial episode during pregnancy is very common. Therefore, the woman who had been infected in early pregnancy should be recultured in later pregnancy. This is also true in any other high-risk situation.

2. Many mothers conceive their first child while they are teenagers, an age range in which gonococcal disease has a particularly high prevalence and at an age in which they may look to their pediatrician for medical care.

3. Gonococcal disease in this age range is especially dangerous to women, because PID is a relatively frequent complication (see Pelvic inflammatory disease and salpingitis).

In infancy

Ophthalmia neonatorum. Gonococcal ophthalmia is the most common form of gonorrhea in infants and results from perinatal contamination of infants by their infected mothers. After an initially nonspecific conjunctivitis, serosanguinous discharge is rapidly replaced by a thick, purulent exudate. Corneal ulceration and iridocyclitis appear unilaterally or in both eyes. Unless therapy is initiated promptly, destruction of the involved eye(s) may supervene, leading to blindness.

Table 25-2. Outcome of pregnancy in mothers who were infected with *N. gonorrhoeae* at delivery

References	Number studied	Normal or term infants	Aborted infants	Perinatal death	Premature infants
Sarrel and Pruett (1968)	37	13 (35%)	13 (35%)	3	6 (17%)
Israel et al. (1978)	39	30 (77%)	1	1	5 (13%)
Amstey and Steadman (1976)	222	142 (64%)	24 (11%)	15 (7%)	49 (22%)
Edwards et al. (1978)	19	7 (37%)		2 (11%)	8 (42%)

Ophthalmia neonatorum, formerly a leading cause of blindness, has been controlled by prophylaxis with silver nitrate (Credé's method) or with other antimicrobial agents such as erythromycin. Bacitracin and sulfonamides are known to be ineffective in prophylaxis. Gonococcal ophthalmia occurs in children who have had prophylaxis, although rarely, and probably as a result of fetal infection before delivery. Gonococcal ophthalmia, for example, has been observed after delivery by cesarean section, in which case the infant had no direct contact with the maternal cervix or lower genital tract.

Scalp abscess. Gonococcal infections of scalp wounds that occur during fetal monitoring have been observed quite frequently. The lesions may produce extensive local inflammatory disease and necrosis and be a focus for disseminated infection. A scalp wound in a neonate should be cultured for gonococci as well as other likely pathogens, which include *Staphylococcus* species, group B streptococci, and gram-negative enteric flora. Herpes simplex may also be present in areas of injury to the scalp of newborns. Overall, approximately 1 of every 200 births that are monitored with fetal scalp electrodes have been complicated by infections at the monitoring site.

In young children. Prepubertal gonorrhea occurs most often in females. Gonococcal vulvovaginitis accounts for about 75% of gonococcal disease in children. It must be distinguished bacteriologically from vulvovaginitis caused by other agents. This is done by isolation of *N. gonorrhoeae* from a vaginal swab; an endocervical culture is not necessary. In preadolescent females, the vaginal exudate may be minimal and may be confused with a benign discharge. Gonococci on Gram stain or cultures may be very

sparse. Symptoms referable to the urinary tract may predominate. Asymptomatic disease is well reported and is usually recognized because the child is cultured during an investigation of suspected sexual abuse.

Ascending pelvic infection may occur in prepubertal females and may occur in the absence of significant vaginal discharge. The main signs of early disease are dysuria and vaginal discharge. When gonococcal infection spreads from the cervix into the fallopian tubes, it is characterized by lower abdominal pain. The onset of acute salpingitis, or pelvic inflammatory disease (PID), may be abrupt and must be distinguished from those of acute appendicitis, cystitis, pyelonephritis, cholecystitis, and ectopic pregnancy (see pelvic inflammatory disease and salpingitis).

Children who have experienced sexual abuse, homosexual men, and women with primary genitourinary infection often have anorectal gonorrhea, which, in general, produces only a minor inflammatory reaction. In most patients anorectal infection is asymptomatic but may cause local burning and discharge. Rectal cultures for *N. gonorrhoeae* are essential in the work-up of a child for gonococcal disease.

In teenage males, the onset of gonococcal urethritis is marked by sudden burning on urination occurring 2 days to 2 weeks after sexual exposure, similar to the presentation in adult males. This is followed by a mucopurulent discharge from the urethra. Involvement of the prostate gland is manifested by retention of urine, pain, and fever. Epididymitis is characterized by severe pain, tenderness, and swelling.

Asymptomatic infection may also occur in about 50% of teenage and adult females.

Extragenital manifestations

Arthritis. Arthritis is the most common extragenital complication of asymptomatic gonorrhea and may occur in any age, including the newborn. In the prepenicillin days, arthritis occurred in 3% to 5% of patients with gonorrhea; today the incidence is much lower, probably less than 1%. Females are affected twice as often as males, and the genitourinary infection is usually asymptomatic. The onset is usually sudden, with chills, fever, and acute migratory polyarthritis occurring from 1 to 4 weeks after the initial infection. Any joint may be involved, but the knees, wrists, and ankles are most commonly affected.

Tenosynovitis. Tenosynovitis occurs more frequently in gonococcal arthritis than in any other type of infectious arthritis, thus providing a valuable clue to the cause. It usually involves the hands, wrists, and feet. The diagnosis may be difficult since gonococci are cultivated from joint fluid in only about one fourth of the cases. The probable diagnosis is based on recovery of the gonococcus from a genitourinary site, the clinical manifestations, and the response to antimicrobial therapy.

Rash. Gonococcal bacteremia may produce, in addition to arthritis and tenosynovitis, a characteristic rash. The lesions are sparse, rarely more than 20 in all, and are distributed over the dorsal aspects of distal extremities. They are painful, vesiculopustular, sometimes hemorrhagic lesions with an erythematous base. Immunofluorescent preparations of skin biopsies may be positive for gonococcal antigens.

Proctitis. Proctitis may be a primary form of infection or in the female may result from spread of adjacent infection. In males, proctitis is almost always the result of sodomy and frequently occurs in homosexuals. Rectal involvement may be asymptomatic or characterized by tenesmus, bloody mucoid diarrhea, burning, and discharge.

Perihepatitis. Gonococcal perihepatitis (Fitz-Hugh–Curtis syndrome) results from extension of infection from salpingitis to the capsule and outer surface of the liver. It should be considered in females with right upper quadrant pain, palpable liver, abnormal liver function tests, and adnexal and uterine cervical tenderness. A positive endocervical culture for gonococcus supports the diagnosis.

Conjunctivitis. Conjunctivitis beyond the newborn period follows direct spread, usually via fingers contaminated with genital secretions, or rarely results from gonococcemia.

Oropharyngitis. Gonococcal oropharyngitis is common among homosexuals and in children who are the victims of sexual abuse. Infection follows orogenital contact and may simulate streptococcal pharyngitis with swollen tonsils, exudate, and enlarged cervical lymph nodes, or it may be asymptomatic. Temporomandibular arthritis has been reported recently as a complication of gonococcal pharyngitis.

PELVIC INFLAMMATORY DISEASE AND SALPINGITIS

Vaginal infection of females who are adolescent or younger may progress to involve the fallopian tubes or may disseminate to the pelvis, leading to pelvic inflammatory disease (PID). This is the most serious complication of sexually transmitted diseases. Salpingitis appears to be a disease of multiple microbiologic causes, the end results of which are purulent infection of the fallopian tubes, which causes scarring during healing. Because of the fibrosis, patency is compromised and fertility jeopardized. PID in adolescents is particularly likely to result in infertility, and PID is the single most common cause of infertility in young women.

The identification of the etiology of cases of PID is complicated by the difficulty of obtaining fallopian tube specimens before therapy. Studies of women with acute PID have recovered *N. gonorrhoeae* from the endocervix from approximately 35% to 80% of cases and from a smaller proportion of samples of fallopian tube aspirates. Most investigators believe that gonococcal infections are a very common cause of acute PID but not necessarily the only one. Other etiologies include *Chlamydia trachomatis* and *Ureaplasma urealyticum*. Following the acute event, chronic polymicrobial disease develops in the scarred areas of distortion. Mixed aerobic and anaerobic flora, especially including *Peptostreptococcus* and *Peptococcus* species, are often recovered.

Risk factors for PID and acute salpingitis have been shown to include young age at acquisition of gonococcal disease, a history of previous PID, multiple sexual partners, and use of an intrauterine device (IUD) for contraception. Approximately 15% of teenagers who develop gonorrhea will progress to PID.

Diagnosis of PID may be difficult and the differential diagnosis includes numerous other conditions of the lower abdomen, including appendicitis, ectopic pregnancy, cholecystitis, mesenteric adenitis, pyelonephritis, and septic abortion. Misdiagnosis of PID is common and is one of the more common causes of medically nonindicated laparotomy. Laparoscopy may assist in establishing a diagnosis. Recommendations by Shafer et al. (1982) suggest that a clinical diagnosis of PID be supported by the presence of lower abdominal pain and tenderness, cervical motion tenderness, and adnexal tenderness. Fever, leukocytosis, elevated sedimentation rate, and adnexal mass on abdominal ultrasound support the diagnosis. Culdocentesis, if performed, may reveal evidence of purulent reaction in the peritoneal cavity. It is probable that the outcome for fertility is improved with prompt and vigorous therapy. Indications for hospitalization for therapy of PID include young age of patients and are listed as follows:

1. All adolescents
2. Diagnostic uncertainty
3. Failure to respond to prior regimen
4. Pregnancy
5. Fever, peritoneal signs
6. Adnexal mass
7. IUD use
8. Noncompliance

Other complications, such as meningitis, endocarditis, pericarditis, and, in adults, uveitis and liver abscesses, are rare.

TREATMENT

During the 20 years prior to 1976, all *N. gonorrhoeae* were sensitive to penicillin, but a gradual increase had been noted in the mean minimal inhibitory concentration (MIC). In March 1976 reports appeared of the first clinical isolations of penicillinase-producing *N. gonorrhoeae* (PPNG) arising in the Far East. These resistant strains carried a plasmid coding for production of betalactamase, the same R factor responsible for penicillinase elaboration by *Haemophilus influenzae*. PPNG now cause approximately 0.5% of all gonococcal disease in the United States. They are rare in children but have been reported. These resistant strains cause the same disease spectrum as penicillin-sensitive organisms.

In 1983 an outbreak of chromosomally mediated penicillin resistant gonococci was reported from North Carolina and has subsequently occurred in other areas of the country. They are also rare in children. They do not produce penicillinase.

Therapy of gonococcal disease

Prevention of neonatal infection. All pregnant women should have endocervical culture examinations for gonococci as an integral part of prenatal care at the first prenatal visit. A second culture late in pregnancy should be obtained from women who are at high risk of gonococcal infection.

Routine prevention of gonococcal ophthalmia. Routine preventive treatment includes (1) 1% silver nitrate (do not irrigate with saline, as this may reduce efficacy) or (2) ophthalmic ointments containing tetracycline, erythromycin, or neomycin. Bacitracin ointment (not effective) and penicillin drops (sensitizing) are not recommended.

Management of infants born to mothers with untreated gonococcal infection. The infant born to a mother with untreated gonorrhea should have orogastric and rectal cultures taken routinely and blood cultures taken if symptomatic. A term infant should receive aqueous crystalline penicillin G, 100,000 units IM or IV in a single dose. The preterm infant may receive 20,000 units aqueous crystalline penicillin G.

Neonatal disease

Gonococcal ophthalmia. Patients should be hospitalized. Antimicrobial agents include aqueous crystalline penicillin G, 100,000 units per kilogram of body weight every 24 hours in two doses intravenously for 7 days plus frequent saline irrigations until the discharge ceases. Topical antimicrobial therapy is optional.

Complicated infection. Arthritis, abscess, and septicemia should be treated by hospitalization and administration of aqueous crystalline penicillin G, 75,000 to 100,000 U per kilogram of body weight per 24 hours in four doses for a minimum of 7 days. Meningitis should be treated with aqueous crystalline penicillin G, 100,000 U per kilogram of body weight per 24 hours divided into three or four intravenous doses a day and continued for at least 10 days.

Childhood disease beyond infancy. Gonococcal ophthalmia should be treated with hospitalization and by the administration of aqueous crystalline penicillin G, intravenously, 75,000 to 100,000 U per kilogram of body weight per 24 hours in four doses, or procaine penicillin G, intramuscularly 75,000 to 100,000 U per kilogram of body weight per 24 hours in two doses for 7 days plus saline irrigations. Topical antibiotics alone are not adequate therapy of gonococcal ophthalmitis. The source of the infection must be identified.

Uncomplicated vulvovaginitis and urethritis may not require hospitalization. Both may be treated at one visit by amoxicillin, 50 mg/kg plus probenecid, 25 mg/kg both given orally. Alternative single dose parenteral therapy is aqueous penicillin G, 100,000 U/kg IM, and probenecid, 25 mg/kg by mouth. Topical and systemic estrogen therapy are of no benefit in vulvovaginitis. All patients should have follow-up cultures, and the source of infection should be identified, examined, and treated.

Anorectal or pharyngeal gonococcal infection. Treatment of anorectal and pharyngeal gonococcal disease in adults with oral amoxicillin has been less effective than with intramuscular penicillin. If the oral regimen is used for a child with this form of infection, repeat examinations with culture must be made at 3 days and 2 weeks to ensure cure of the infection. This is true also of all other forms of gonococcal disease in children.

Treatment and prevention of salpingitis and pelvic inflammatory disease. Coinfection with both chlamydiae and gonococci is common in children as well as adults. In female adolescents treatment of gonorrhea with drug regimens that are effective against gonococci but not chlamydiae has led to a high incidence of residual salpingitis and, in males, of urethritis, both associated with continued disease due to chlamydia. Optimal therapy for known or possible coinfection with both diseases is not certain in adults and has also not been explored in children. The following regimen may be employed pending further data. The reader is advised to look for recommendations in the *Morbidity and Mortality Weekly Report* from the CDC.

Penicillin, amoxicillin, cefuroxime, and spectinomycin alone will fail to eradicate chlamydia. Trimethoprim-sulfamethoxazole (TMP-SMX), tetracycline, and erythromycin are effective in vitro and in many clinical forms of chlamydial disease. The pediatrician may elect to treat the child with a combination of one of the first five agents and to add a 7-day course of TMP-SMX, erythromycin, or tetracycline orally.

Treatment of children who are allergic to penicillin or who are infected with penicillinase-producing N. gonorrhoeae or chromosomally mediated penicillin-resistant strains. Spectinomycin, 40 mg/kg IM as a single injection is the treatment of choice for these circumstances. Cefotaxime, 100 to 200 mg/kg/day in four doses IV represents the alternative drug of choice. However, both spectinomycin and cefotaxime may fail to eradicate pharyngeal disease due to penicillinase-producing strains.

Children who are 8 years of age or older may receive tetracycline, 40 mg/kg/day orally in four divided doses for 7 days if they are allergic to penicillin. Tetracycline is not effective in treating penicillinase-producing *N. gonorrhoeae*.

Follow-up

Follow-up urethral specimens should be obtained from males 7 days after treatment is completed. Cervical and rectal specimens should be obtained from females 7 to 14 days after treatment is completed. If the infection is related to possible PPNG from the Far East, follow-up should be done after 3 to 7 days.

• • •

Test for syphilis

All patients with gonorrhea should have a serologic test for syphilis done at the time of diagnosis. Patients receiving the recommended amount of penicillin parenterally need not have follow-up serologic tests. Patients treated with ampicillin, spectinomycin, or tetracycline should have follow-up serologic tests done for syphilis each month for 4 months to detect syphilis that may have been missed by treatment of gonorrhea.

Patients with gonorrhea who also have syphilis should be given additional treatment appropriate to the stage of syphilis.

Although long-acting forms of penicillin, such as benzathine penicillin G, are effective in therapy of some forms of syphilis, they are not efficacious in the treatment of gonorrhea.

CHLAMYDIA TRACHOMATIS

Chlamydiae are bacteria that are obligate intracellular parasites. There are two species, *Chlamydia trachomatis* and *Chlamydia psittaci*. Both species require tissue-culture methods for recovery from clinical specimens. *C. trachomatis* has become the source of a great deal of medical interest in the past decade because it is one of the most common of the STDs. It resembles gonorrhea epidemiologically in that it causes ophthalmia in newborns born to mothers with infected birth canals and causes vaginitis, PID, and urethritis in infected children, adolescents, and adults. It is also an important cause of newborn pneumonitis. The major syndromes associated with *C. trachomatis* infection are as follows:

1. Nongonococcal urethritis
2. Cervicitis
3. Salpingitis
4. Pelvic inflammatory disease
5. Inclusion conjunctivitis
6. Pneumonia in newborns
7. Lymphogranuloma venereum
8. Endemic trachoma

C. psittaci causes pulmonary psittacosis in humans, birds, and other animals and will not be discussed any further in this section.

The diagnosis of disease caused by *C. trachomatis* may be made through inoculation of a specimen from the infected site onto one of several tissue culture systems and subsequent identification of the development of the intracellular, cytoplasmic microcolonies that result. Fig. 25-1 shows a tissue-culture monolayer with a microcolony that has been stained with iodine.

Tissue culture systems are expensive, require technical skills not present in many laboratories, and require several days to develop a positive result. Alternative diagnostic methods include the following.

1. Direct stain is used to detect inclusions in infected material. This method is most appropriate when examining conjunctival scrapings for endemic trachoma or neonatal ophthalmia. A smear may be made of epithelial cells (not the polymorphonuclear leukocytes of the exudate) and stained using iodine, Giemsa, or fluorescent antibody stain. In neonates, the Giemsa and fluorescent stains provide very satisfactory results if the sample is appropriately collected. Recently studies of urethral and cervical smears have been examined with fluorescein-conjugated monoclonal antibody, indicating that culture-independent diagnosis of genital tract disease may become possible.

2. Serologic methods are used for identification of persons with chlamydial infections; these methods are improving. Chlamydial organisms share a common group antigen, and the complement-fixation test measures antibody to that antigen. This test will yield a titer of 1:16 or greater in most patients with psittacosis or lymphogranuloma venereum but is unreliable for

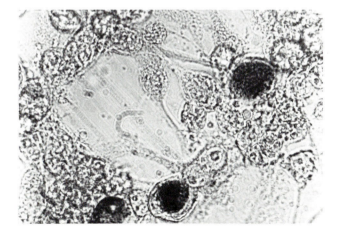

Fig. 25-1. Tissue culture inoculation of *C. trachomatis*, stained with iodine, showing cytoplasmic microcolonies of organisms.

Table 25-3. Microimmunofluorescent types of *Chlamydia trachomatis* in clinical disease

Microimmunofluorescent type	Usual disease	Geographic distribution
A, B, C	Classic ocular trachoma	Primarily endemic in Asia and Africa
D, E, F, G, H, I, J, K, L, M	Inclusion conjunctivitis Salpingitis Nongonococcal urethritis Infant pneumonitis	Worldwide, sporadic
Lymphogranuloma venereum I, II, and III	Lymphogranuloma venereum Genital trachoma	Worldwide, sporadic

other forms of infection, including those of the newborn.

Microimmunofluorescent tests were initially introduced as a method of serotyping strains. Table 25-3 lists the serotypes of strains causing the major forms of human chlamydial disease. This method has subsequently been adapted to diagnostic purposes by assay of serotype-specific antibody. It is a difficult test to perform and not widely available. Infants with chlamydial pneumonia have elevated titers compared with other chlamydial syndromes.

Inclusion conjunctivitis (IC)

IC occurs in infants who are born to mothers with cervical chlamydial infection. The mother's infection may be asymptomatic during pregnancy, but there is a high incidence of postpartum fever and pelvic disease following parturition. Numerous studies of the incidence of cervical chlamydial infection have been performed in cities in the United States, and rates of infection in pregnancy range in most series from about 7% to 12%, with women in lower socioeconomic classes tending to have a higher incidence. Subsequently, studies concerning transmission of chlamydia from an infected mother to the newborn have shown that at least 25% of such infants develop clinically apparent conjunctivitis. Chlamydial infections account for about one third of all conjunctivitis in the first few months of life, most of the remaining cases being due to pneumococci, staphylococci, gonococci, chemical irritants, and viral infections.

Chlamydial conjunctivitis resembles endemic trachoma initially and is characterized by a mucopurulent discharge that may be unilateral. Systemic signs are usually minimal, although otitis media is common. Edema of the lids and prominence of small blood vessels occurs. Superinfection with other bacteria is very common. Untreated cases recover without any residua in about 35% of cases, and the remainder have only mild residual abnormalities, including micropannus and pannus formation, scars, focal neovascularization, and limbal pocks. All of these are also characteristic of early endemic ocular trachoma. Treatment within 2 weeks of onset will almost always avert all sequelae.

Neonatal pneumonitis

It has been recognized for decades that there was a constellation of disease within families in which the adult males had urethritis, the women had PID and fever following delivery, and the infant had conjunctivitis, sometimes associated with pulmonary disease. Not until recently, however, was the pulmonary disease carefully described and related to infection with *C. trachomatis*.

Of infants born to cervically infected women, the most common site of infection in the infant is the conjunctiva (about 20%), and the nasopharynx or rectum are both infected in about 20% of instances. Nasopharyngeal infection may lead to pneumonia, probably occurring in about one half of the infants with positive nasopharyngeal cultures. Chlamydial pneumonia appears to account for about one half of the cases of newborn pneumonia in children aged 3 weeks to 3 months.

The clinical characteristics of the pneumonia have been well described. The onset occurs at anytime from 3 weeks to 3 months of life and is accompanied by a prominent cough, wheezing, and congestion. Systemic signs of disease such

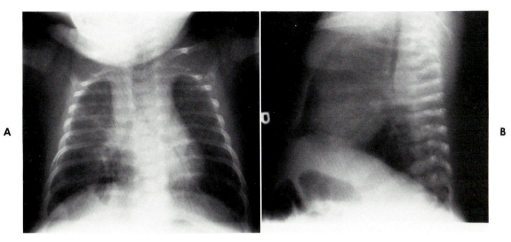

Fig. 25-2. Roentgenographic findings of a child with chlamydial pneumonia demonstrating hyperinflation and atelectasis.

as fever and acidosis are rare. Roentgenographic examination shows hyperinflation with occasional areas of atelectasis (Fig. 25-2). The child may also have otitis media or conjunctivitis. Laboratory findings that may be helpful include eosinophilia from a tracheal aspirate or peripheral blood, hyperglobulinemia of both IgG and IgM, and a pronounced antibody response to the infecting serotype by microimmunofluorescence. Apnea, gastrointestinal disturbances, lethargy, and "bronchiolitis" may accompany the illness.

Although children usually recover, there are fatalities with this condition. Chronic pulmonary disease may result. More severely affected infants may also be infected with another agent, especially cytomegalovirus.

Treatment

The responses to treatment are not dramatic, and placebo-controlled trials are lacking, but therapy is believed by most clinicians to help the child. Both ocular and pulmonary infections should be treated systemically. Chlamydial infections often relapse if therapy is short. Recommended therapy is erythromycin 50 mg per kilogram of body weight per day for 3 weeks. If the child is old enough to receive a sulfonamide, that may provide an alternative regimen.

Genitourinary tract disease. As in the adult, children may acquire genitourinary tract infections with *C. trachomatis*. In male children or adolescents, that will usually lead to urethritis

or, occasionally, proctitis or epididymitis. Females will usually experience urethritis, proctitis, or cervicitis that may progress to salpingitis or endometritis. Table 25-4 lists several recent studies of the prevalence of chlamydial and gonococcal disease in various groups of children, including those with known sexual abuse and those who are sexually active. The route of infection outside infancy should be assumed to be sexual, and the child should be evaluated for the possibility of sexual abuse. All children who are being evaluated for sexual abuse should have cultures for chlamydiae taken from pharynx, rectum, urethra, and vagina if methods are available. Conjunctivitis may be evaluated by Giemsa stain as with the newborn. Recommended treatment of genitourinary *Chlamydia* outside the newborn period is erythromycin for 2 weeks, tetracycline if the child is of an appropriate age, or, finally, sulfonamide.

Lymphogranuloma venereum (LGV). LGV is caused by any one of three strains of *C. trachomatis*, which exhibit particular virulence. These strains kill infected egg embryos rapidly and have enhanced pathogenicity in mice. Similarly, human genitourinary tract disease with these strains is likely to result in deep infections, a relatively severe exudative response, and sequelae due to fibrosis at the sites of chronic infection. Pediatric disease caused by LGV strains is seldom recognized, but approximately 20 cases have been reported, often because an adult

Table 25-4. Studies on prevalence of STD in various groups of children

Date	Infection	Age, sex	Infected (%)	Population group	Special risks
Chacko and Louchik (1984)	*Chlamydia*	Adolescent, M	7/20 (35)	Adolescent clinic, Baltimore	Adolescent clinic
		Adolescent, F	19/70 (27)	Adolescent clinic, Baltimore	Pregnant F
		Adolescent, F	47/190 (23)	Adolescent clinic, Baltimore	Nonpregnant F
Ingram et al. (1984)	*Chlamydia*	1 to 12 years, F	3/50 (6)	North Carolina	Known sexual contact or abuse
Hammerschlag et al. (1984)	*Chlamydia*	2 to 14 years, F	2/48 (4)	Brooklyn, NY	Known sexual abuse
Golden et al. (1984)	*Chlamydia*	12 to 17 years, F	19/186 (10.2)	Adolescent Ob-Gyn Center (AOGC), New York	Sexually active
	Gonorrhea	12 to 17 years, F	18/186 (10)	AOGC, New York	
	Syphilis	12 to 17 years, F	6/186 (3)	AOGC, New York	
Hein et al. (1977)	Gonorrhea	Adolescent, M	40/2098 (1.9)	Youth detention center	Asymptomatic, sexually active
		Adolescent, F	26/574 (7)	Youth detention center	Sexually active
Ingram et al. (1984)	Gonorrhea	1 to 12 years, F	10/50 (20)	North Carolina	Known sexual contact

member of the family was also diseased. Rectal disease, inguinal adenopathy, and cervicitis were the usual presentations. Patients with LGV usually have very high titers to chlamydial group antigen, and therefore the complement-fixation (CF) test to either lygranum or psittacosis is very high. These serologic tests are available in most State Health Department laboratories and should be ordered for children of either sex with proctitis and inquinal adenopathy of unknown etiology.

SYPHILIS

The reported rate of primary and secondary syphilis had declined to four per 100,000 in the 1950s with the widespread use of penicillin. However, during the two decades from 1960 to 1980 there occurred an increase in incidence to the current plateau of 10 reported cases of syphilis per 100,000 population. Approximately 34,000 cases of early syphilis (primary, secondary, and early latent) and 76,000 cases of all stages of syphilis occurred in the calendar year

1982 in the United States. The disease continues to occur, posing problems of accurate detection and appropriate management because physicians have become less familiar with the multiple manifestations of this infection.

In 1982 there were 159 reported cases of congenital syphilis in infants less than 1 year of age, whereas 107 cases were reported in 1978. The incidence of congenital syphilis reflects the occurrence of infectious syphilis among women of childbearing age. There are about 1.5 cases of congenital disease for 100 cases of primary and secondary disease in women of childbearing age.

Most public health authorities believe that the reported number of cases of syphilis underestimates the actual incidence of disease. Failure to report recognized disease may lead to inadequate tracing of sexual contacts. The reservoir of unreported, untreated cases serves to increase the number of persons with undiagnosed syphilis. Primary and secondary disease occurs most frequently in urban centers. Young adults have the disease most often, with almost 5000 cases reported in individuals from birth to 19 years of age in 1982. Physicians caring for children and adolescents must therefore be prepared to diagnose and treat this infection.

Bacteriology

The causative agent of syphilis is *Treponema pallidum*, a thin, delicate organism with tapering ends. It varies in length from 5 to 20 μm and has a uniform cylindrical thickness of approximately 0.25 μm. *T. pallidum* usually has 6 to 14 flat waves per cell with the appearance of a helical coil. It exhibits a sluggish motility with flexuous movement, usually without rotation in a wet preparation; this may help to identify it when seen through a dark-field microscope. Although several mammals (rabbits and monkeys) can be experimentally infected by *T. pallidum*, man is the only natural host. Outside the host, *T. pallidum* is very fragile and easily destroyed by various physical and chemical agents including heat of 42° C, drying, and soap and water.

Pathogenesis

The central problem in understanding the pathogenesis of syphilis is that although there is a vigorous host response to infection, prior disease has a minimal effect on resistance to reinfection, and the infection may persist for life. Some of the information concerning host and bacterial interaction that may pertain to these questions are as follows.

Treponemal virulence-associated factors. Virulent *T. pallidum* attach to host cells during parasitism and are oriented by the proximal hook to the host cell surface. There appears to be a ligand-receptor adherence mechanism involving the treponemal outer membrane proteins. Virulent strains attach to metabolically active mammalian cells and treponemes are capable of multiplication only during attachment. Fetal and infant cells appear to support treponemal growth maximally, and capillary cells are the prime target of parasitism. Virulent treponeme strains produce hyaluronidase, which may facilitate the perivascular infiltration that is apparent by histopathology. These strains may also invade the ground substance that joins capillary endothelial cells.

Virulent *T. pallidum* attracts an avidly adherent coating by fibronectin, a protein of host origin. This coating appears to protect the organism from antibody-mediated phagocytosis, allows the organism to adhere to the surface of host phagocytes with only limited ingestion of the organisms, may block complement-mediated lysis by the coated treponeme, and, finally, may allow the treponeme to acquire physiologically active host proteins, such as ceruloplasmin and transferrin, on which they are dependent.

Host response. Treponema appear to persist in extracellular loci with little or no inflammatory response elicited. It is known that polymorphonuclear leukocytes ingest virulent treponema, incorporate them into phagocytic vacuoles, degranulate, and digest *T. pallidum*. However, relatively large numbers of treponema are needed in order to elicit this response and small numbers may escape recognition by host phagocytes.

Alterations in host cell–mediated immunity occur during primary and secondary stages of syphilis. During early stages of disease all aspects of cell–mediated immunity are suppressed, including responses to nonspecific T-cell mitogens. Blastogenesis to treponemal antigens is not demonstrable until late in secondary disease. Natural killer cell activity is increased in early primary syphilis and depressed in secondary and latent syphilis. There is some evidence to support the idea that lymphocytes from recovered infected animals confer moderate protection for nonimmune animals. However, the extent to which these alterations in cellular function during infection affect the outcome or progression of disease remains uncertain.

The lesions of syphilis that are most infectious occur on mucous membranes in the anogenital region or the mouth, and transmission occurs during close physical or sexual contact. The exception to this is congenital syphilis, which is transmitted from the infected mother to the fetus in utero. The infection may, rarely, be transmitted through a break in the skin.

Acquired syphilis

Acquired syphilis in childhood appears to follow a course similar to that of adults. Although most recognized syphilitic disease of children is congenital, it appears that approximately one third is acquired, and almost always it represents the result of sexual abuse or assault. The natural course of acquired (not congenital) syphilis can be summarized as follows:

1. An incubation period of approximately 3 weeks (10 to 90 days) is followed by the primary stage, characterized by a hard, indurated, nontender chancre at the original site of infection that persists from 1 to 5 weeks.

2. The secondary stage is manifested by cutaneous and systemic symptoms resulting from the earlier spirochetemia. This secondary stage appears approximately 6 weeks after the primary stage (2 weeks to 6 months) and heals in 2 to 6 weeks.

3. The subclinical latent state follows and is diagnosed by the presence of a reactive serologic test and lasts from 1 to 40+ years. Approximately one third of infected individuals develop late syphilis, characterized by cardiovascular, CNS, cutaneous, or visceral lesions.

4. Approximately two thirds of untreated, infected individuals will go through life with little or no physical abnormality, although more than half of these will remain serologically positive. However, the life expectancy of persons with latent syphilis is also shorter than normal.

Primary syphilis. Primary syphilis is characterized by a painless chancre that appears at the site of contact 10 to 90 days after exposure, the average being 21 days. The lesion is usually single and is most often found on the glans penis of the male and on the cervix or external genitalia of the female. It has a variety of forms, the most distinctive form being an indurated chancre. Since primary lesions in the female may be located within the vagina and/or cervix, all females should have a complete pelvic examination if primary disease is to be ruled out. Chancres are frequently accompanied by hard, nonfluctuant, painless, enlarged inguinal lymph nodes called *satellite buboes*. Primary lesions may also appear on the labia or scrotum, in the anus or rectum, and on the lips, tongue, tonsil, nipple, and fingers.

Often a definite diagnosis of primary syphilis can be established only by a positive dark-field examination since serology may be nonreactive at this stage. A presumptive diagnosis can be based on the following evidence: exposure to an infected person within 3 months; presence of

indolent lesions, active or healing; lymphadenitis; and, most importantly, a rising serologic titer. In the course of making a presumptive diagnosis, the physician should consider other venereal and nonvenereal genital infections. Since serologic tests for syphilis (STSs) may be nonreactive, a single negative STS does not by itself exclude infection. Repeated testing may establish the diagnosis. Primary symptoms usually disappear without treatment within 3 to 5 weeks. In the course of untreated syphilis, the chancre frequently disappears spontaneously before the appearance of the secondary lesions, although it may still be evident at the onset of the secondary stage.

Secondary syphilis outside of the neonatal period. Secondary manifestations generally appear 6 weeks to several months after infection and last for a few days to 1 year. These manifestations usually appear about the time involution of the primary chancre occurs, but there may be an asymptomatic period between the two stages. Signs and symptoms include a local or generalized cutaneous rash, condylomata lata of the anogenital region, malaise, fever, sore throat, generalized adenopathy, alopecia, mucous patches of the mouth, and positive serology. It is not unusual to find pleocytosis or increased protein in the cerebrospinal fluid (CSF) of patients with secondary syphilis. However, it is not routine practice to examine the CSF at this stage of the disease. Skin lesions may be macular, papular, papulosquamous, or bullous in adults as they are sometimes in early congenital syphilis in infants. The lesions are bilateral and symmetrical; they are seldom pruritic. As a rule, *T. pallidum* may be demonstrated in any mucous or cutaneous secondary lesion but most easily in a moist one. Failure to demonstrate the spirochete in suspicious lesions does not rule out a diagnosis of secondary syphilis. Alopecia and condylomata lata are less common than cutaneous lesions.

Latent syphilis. Latency is arbitrarily divided into early latency and late latency. Early latency is 2 to 4 years (depending on classification used) after the last evidence of secondary disease has ended. Late latency occurs thereafter and is the time period during which tertiary manifestations usually emerge.

Latent syphilis is by definition clinically inapparent. A diagnosis is usually established on the basis of positive serology after the possibility of the presence of other stages of syphilis has been ruled out by physical and CSF examinations. All untreated cases of syphilis are latent at some time during the course of the disease, and in some instances the disease may be latent for the duration of the infection or the life of the patient. Patients with latent syphilis may progress to develop gummatous lesions, cardiovascular syphilis, or neurosyphilis, which represent tertiary syphilis. After an infection has persisted for more than 4 years, it is rarely communicable, except in the case of the pregnant woman (see congenital syphilis).

Late syphilis. All late manifestations of syphilis are those of a vascular disease, except for the gumma, which is probably a hypersensitivity phenomenon; the other lesions of late syphilis are a consequence of obliterative endarteritis of terminal arterioles and small arteries and the resulting inflammatory and necrotic changes. Children may develop late forms of syphilis.

Untreated late syphilis may have a broad range of signs and symptoms, varying from none apparent to those indicating severe damage to one or more systems of the body. A list of the most common types and their incidence follows:

Type of late syphilis	Frequency (%)
Latent syphilis	70
Neurosyphilis (symptomatic)	8
Late benign syphilis	17
Cardiovascular syphilis	10

These diagnostic categories are not mutually exclusive. For example, (1) of patients with neurosyphilis, about 15% also have cardiovascular syphilis; (2) of patients with cardiovascular syphilis, about 12% also have neurosyphilis; and (3) of patients with late benign syphilis, about 13% have cardiovascular involvement, and another 10% have neurosyphilis.

Neurosyphilis. The essential pathologic process of all types of neurosyphilis is obliterative endarteritis, usually of terminal vessels, with associated parenchymatous degeneration. Neurosyphilis may be arbitrarily divided into the following groups, depending on the type and degree of CNS pathologic condition: asymptomatic; meningovascular; and parenchymatous, consisting of paresis and tabes dorsalis.

Optic atrophy is a serious complication of neu-

rosyphilis. Examination of the peripheral visual fields is imperative in every patient suspected of having neurosyphilis. Pupillary changes may be seen in late neurosyphilis; the classic change is the Argyll Robertson pupil, which is small and irregular and fails to react to light but responds normally to accommodation.

Asymptomatic neurosyphilis. The patient with asymptomatic neurosyphilis is usually seen because of a positive serology and without signs or symptoms of CNS involvement. However, CSF shows an increase in number of cells and total amount of protein and a reactive serology.

Meningovascular neurosyphilis. In meningovascular neurosyphilis, definite signs and symptoms of CNS damage are present, indicating cerebrovascular occlusion, infarction, and encephalomalacia with focal neurologic signs, depending on the size and location of the lesion. The CSF is always abnormal, with pleocytosis, increase in amount of protein, and a reactive serology.

Parenchymatous neurosyphilis. This form of neurosyphilis appears as paresis or tabes dorsalis. The manifestations of paresis may be myriad and are always indicative of widespread damage to the parenchyma. Personality changes range from minor ones to obvious psychosis. Focal neurologic signs are common. The CSF is invariably abnormal; the number of cells and the concentration of cells and protein are increased, and CSF serology is positive.

Cardiovascular syphilis. The damage in cardiovascular syphilis is usually caused by medial necrosis of the aorta, with aortic dilation often extending into the valve commissures. The essential signs are those of aortic insufficiency or saccular aneurysm of the thoracic aorta. In the differential diagnosis, other possibilities such as arteriosclerosis, hypertension, and rheumatic heart disease deserve careful evaluation. Saccular aneurysm of the thoracic aorta is pathognomonic of cardiovascular syphilis. Aortic insufficiency with no other valvular lesions in a middle-aged person with reactive serology should be considered cardiovascular syphilis until proved otherwise.

Other conditions that may resemble a chancre or secondary syphilis include carcinoma, scabies, lichen planus, psoriasis, drug reactions, Behçet's syndrome, Reiter's syndrome, pityriasis, and tinea vesicolor.

Congenital syphilis

Congenital syphilis usually results from transplacental infection of the developing fetus. An untreated syphilitic pregnant woman may transmit infection to the fetus at any clinical stage of her disease. Transmission to the fetus occurs in almost all pregnant women with untreated primary syphilis, 90% of women with secondary syphilis, and approximately 30% of women with early latent disease. Evidence of fetal damage, such as abortion, is rare before the eighteenth week of gestation. However, pathologic examination of tissues obtained from therapeutic abortions prior to 12 weeks of gestation have shown treponemal organisms to be present in fetuses from mothers who had untreated syphilis. No inflammatory response was present unless gestation was 15 weeks or more in duration. It is possible that the fetal immune system cannot recognize the spirochete until at least 15 weeks of gestation. Sequential acquisition by the fetus of the ability to respond to a number of antigens has been demonstrated.

A woman who has been adequately treated with penicillin and followed with quantitative serology and has no evidence of reinfection does not need to be retreated with each subsequent pregnancy. However, if any doubt exists about the adequacy of previous treatment or the presence of active infection, a course of treatment should be given to prevent congenital syphilis. Women who have been treated for syphilis in the past may become reinfected, and their babies may develop congenital syphilis.

The signs and symptoms of congenital syphilis are arbitrarily divided into early manifestations, which appear in the first 2 years of life, and late manifestations, which emerge anytime thereafter. The outcome of untreated fetal infection is variable. Intrauterine death occurs in an estimated 25% of infections, with abortion usually occurring after the first trimester. Perinatal death may occur in another 25% to 30% of untreated infected babies. Those infants who survive have a broad spectrum of manifestations.

Early congenital syphilis. The abnormal physical and laboratory findings in early congenital syphilis are varied and unpredictable. The onset is between birth and about 3 months of life, with most cases occurring within the first 5 weeks of age. The baby with congenital syphilis may appear perfectly normal at birth only to appear later in the newborn period with "septic" syphilis, characterized by multiorgan system involvement. The neonate in the immediate newborn period may have only hepatosplenomegaly with or without jaundice.

Skeletal system. Because of their frequency and early appearance, the roentgenographic changes in the bones are of diagnostic value. The changes are usually present at birth but may appear in the first few weeks of life. The bony changes, osteochondritis and periostitis, are self-limited and are usually healed in the first 6 months, even in the absence of specific therapy. These are painful lesions, and pain on motion often leads an affected infant to appear to have a limb paralysis.

The femur and humerus are most often involved. Roentgenographically, accumulating calcified matrix is seen at the epiphyseal margin, which may be smooth or serrated. The serrated appearance is known as Wegner's sign; this represents points of calcified cartilage aimed at the nutrient cartilage canal. A zone of rarefaction at the epiphyseal line, which represents syphilitic granulation tissue containing a few scattered calcified remnants and a mass of connective tissue containing areas of perivascular infiltration of small round cells, may also be found. Irregular areas of increased density and rarefaction produce the moth-eaten appearance of the roentgenogram. Epiphyseal separation may occur due to a fracture of the brittle layer of calcified cartilage. Roentgenographic findings in congenital syphilis are shown in Figs. 25-3 to 25-5. Irregular periosteal thickening is also common.

Rhinitis. Rhinitis (coryza or snuffles) is likely to mark the onset of congenital syphilis. Usually it appears in the first week of life and seldom later than third month. The snuffles is more severe and persists longer than the common cold, is often bloody, and is frequently associated with laryngitis.

Rash. The syphilitic rash usually appears 1 or 2 weeks after the rhinitis. The typical eruption is maculopapular and consists of small dark-red-copper–colored spots. If the rash is present at birth, it is often bullous. The rash is most severe on the hands and feet. The rash comes out slowly, taking 1 to 3 weeks, and is followed by desquamation. As the rash fades, the lesions become coppery or dusky red, and pigmentation may persist.

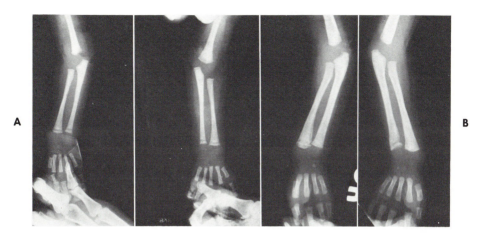

Fig. 25-3. Congenital syphilis. **A,** Typical wide horizontal metaphyseal radiolucent bands. **B,** Destructive syphilitic metaphysitis of the radius and ulna in a 6-week-old infant. Note subperiosteal reaction.

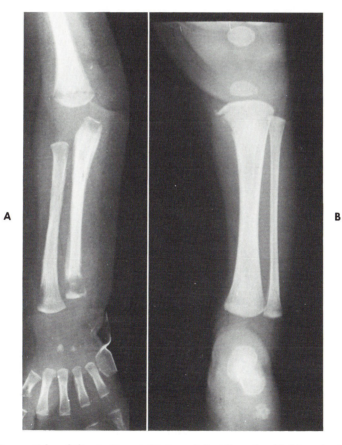

Fig. 25-4. Congenital syphilis. **A,** Panosteitis in an infant 9 weeks old. Metaphysitis is present and subperiosteal bone is appearing. **B,** Radiolucent area of the medial aspect of the proximal tibial metaphyses. This is called Wimberger's sign.

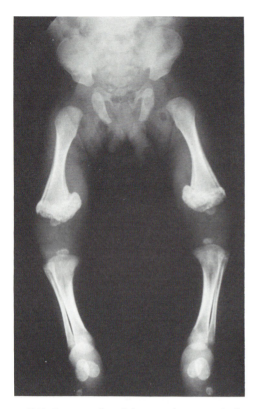

Fig. 25-5. Congenital syphilis. Diaphysitis with abundant callus formation secondary to pathologic fractures through the metaphyseal lesions. The lesions healed, and there were no sequelae.

Fissures and mucous patches. Fissures and mucous patches are not seen often but are highly characteristic features of congenital syphilis. The fissures develop about the lips, nares, and anus. They bleed readily and heal with scarring. A cluster of scars radiating around the mouth is named "rhagades." Mucous patches may be found on any of the mucous membranes, especially in the mouth and genitalia. Condylomata are raised, moist lesions appearing on areas of the skin where there is moisture or friction. They are highly infectious.

Constitutional manifestations. Infants with congenital syphilis may have fever. The white blood cell count may reveal a leukemoid reaction, and the differential may show many myelocytes and metamyelocytes. Although the infant may not have evidence of CNS involvement, examination of the CSF may show increased protein, pleocytosis, and, in some infants, a positive VDRL test. Involvement of the kidneys with either nephritis or nephrosis can

be present. Generalized adenitis may occur. Hepatosplenomegaly is usually a major finding, as in Coombs'-negative hemolytic anemia.

Ectodermal changes. Ectodermal changes in syphilitic infants include suppuration and exfoliation of the nails, loss of hair and eyebrows, choroiditis, and iritis.

Neonates and infants with congenital syphilis may resemble babies with other illnesses peculiar to newborns, including toxoplasmosis, rubella, cytomegalovirus, herpes simplex virus, "sepsis" of the newborn, blood group incompatibilities, battered child syndrome, "periostitis" of prematurity, neonatal hepatitis, and osteomyelitis.

Late congenital syphilis

Late manifestations of congenital syphilis are the result of scarring from the early systemic disease and include involvement of the teeth, bones, eyes, and eighth nerve; gummas in the viscera, skin, or mucous membranes; and neurosyphilis.

Teeth. Characteristic changes are found in the permanent upper central incisors, which present a notched appearance of the biting edges; roentgenographic study leads to diagnosis even while deciduous teeth are in place (Fig. 25-6). These are "Hutchinson's teeth." If first molars show maldevelopment of the cusps (Fig. 25-7), the finding is called mulberry or Moon's molars.

Interstitial keratitis. Interstitial keratitis is the most common late lesion. It may appear at any age between 4 and 30 years or later but characteristically it appears when the patient is close to puberty. A ground-glass appearance may develop in the cornea accompanied by vascularization of the adjacent sclera. These changes become bilateral and lead to blindness.

Neurosyphilis. The same manifestations of neurosyphilis seen in acquired syphilis may occur in congenital syphilis. Paresis is seen more frequently and tabes dorsalis less frequently in the congenital form than in the acquired form of the disease.

Eighth nerve deafness. Hearing loss is usually sudden and appears around 8 to 10 years of age. It often accompanies interstitial keratitis.

Bone changes. Bone changes include the sclerosing lesions, saber shin and frontal bossing, and the gummatous or destructive lesion of sad-

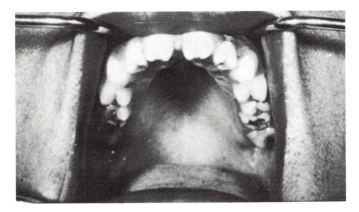

Fig. 25-6. Hutchinson's teeth. Note the notched edges and screwdriver shape of the central incisors.

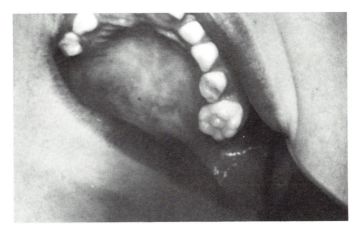

Fig. 25-7. Mulberry or Moon's molar.

dle nose. Perforation of the hard palate is almost pathognomonic of congenital syphilis.

Clutton's joint. Clutton's joint is painless arthritis of the knees and, rarely, other joints.

Cutaneous lesions. Rhagades represent scars resulting from persistent rhinitis during infancy and are rarely seen today.

Laboratory procedures in the diagnosis of syphilis

Dark-field examination. The diagnosis of syphilis can be made by a positive dark-field examination of appropriate specimens. This test requires a compound microscope equipped with a dark-field condenser with which the specimen is illuminated by reflected light against a dark background. A positive diagnosis can be made

by an experienced worker on the basis of characteristic morphologic aspects and motility.

Dark-field examination is most productive during primary, secondary, early congenital, or infectious relapsing syphilis in which fresh lesions may be sampled. Specimens should consist of serous fluid and should be free of red blood cells, cellular debris, and other organisms. Physiologic saline with no additives should be used to cleanse suspected lesions for dark-field examination. Aspirated material from involved regional lymph nodes can also be examined for *T. pallidum*. Gloves should be worn by the physician in examining any lesion suspected of being syphilis and in obtaining any material for dark-field examination.

Failure to demonstrate *T. pallidum* in the exudate from the lesion suspected of being syphilitic in repeated examinations may mean that (1) the lesion is not syphilitic, (2) the patient has received systemic or local treatment, (3) too much time has elapsed since the appearance of the lesion, or (4) the lesion is one of late syphilis. If the results continue to be negative, the patient should return the following day for further tests. Only after extensive study has failed to reveal *T. pallidum* should a report of negative results be made. It is common practice in adults to make a dark-field examination daily for 3 consecutive days after which the patient's case is followed with serologic tests. When serology and dark-field are negative but typical lesions are present, prophylactic treatment may be advisable on the basis of clinical judgment of the appearance of the lesion, the history, and the epidemiologic aspects. When all examinations over a period of time are negative, the decision to treat or not to treat must be made by the physician after consideration of all the available evidence.

Serologic tests. The serologic diagnosis of syphilis employs the use of two general types of tests: reaginic and treponemal (see Table 25-5).

The reaginic tests employ cardiolipid lecithin as antigen. The antibody measured has been termed *reagin*, which has no relationship to the reaginic IgE in allergic patients. Antibody appears in the blood 1 to 3 weeks after the chancre appears or approximately 4 to 6 weeks after infection, which in the newborn may be at 4 to 6 weeks of life.

The reaginic tests are basically of two types, depending primarily on whether the antibody is detected by flocculation or by complement fixation. Flocculation tests include the VDRL, Kline, Kahn, Hinton, and Mazzini tests. Rapid reagin tests employing a modified VDRL antigen are currently in use and include the automated reagin test (ART) and the rapid plasma reagin (RPR) circle card test. These two tests are very useful when large numbers of sera are screened and speed is essential. These tests are inexpensive, can be well controlled, and are quantitated. However, these tests are not specific for syphilis and may also be reactive in patients with liver disease, collagen-vascular diseases, and other conditions.

A positive serology will be found in approximately 75% of sera from patients with primary syphilis, in 100% from patients with secondary syphilis, in 95% from those with early latent syphilis, but in only 70% of patients with late latent or late (tertiary) syphilis. Thus false-negative serology using the reaginic tests is a problem in very early and again in late stages of untreated syphilis.

With adequate treatment, the reaginic tests should become nonreactive in 6 to 12 months after primary syphilis and in 12 to 18 months after secondary syphilis. Patients with primary syphilis or secondary syphilis who have had adequate treatment will occasionally maintain a lower titer (so-called Serofast) 2 years after their therapy.

The fluorescent treponemal antibody absorption (FTA-ABS) test is quite sensitive and specific. It is technically more difficult and used for confirmation of positive nontreponemal tests and in later stages of syphilis. The antigen used

Table 25-5. Serologic tests for syphilis

Antigen	Antigen source	Tests	Percent reactivity during		
			Primary stage	Secondary stage	Tertiary stage
Nontreponemal reagin	Extracts of tissue (cardiolipin-lecithin-cholesterol)	Complement fixation (Wassermann, Kolmer)			
		Flocculation (VDRL, Hinton, Kahn)	78	97	77
Treponemal	*T. pallidum* Reiter strain	Reiter protein CF	61	85	72
	T. pallidum	TPI	56	94	92
		FTA-ABS	85	99	95
		IgM-FTA-ABS			

in this test is whole dead *T. pallidum*. The results of this test are usually reported as non-reactive, borderline, and reactive. Borderline results with this test do not negate the presence or absence of syphilis and should be repeated. The FTA-ABS is the most sensitive serologic test in all stages of syphilis. It becomes reactive earlier in primary syphilis than do treponemal tests and remains positive longer in latent or late syphilis.

Another treponemal test, the *Treponema pallidum* immobilization (TPI) test, has been used in the past but is presently available only for research purposes. When serum containing specific antibody combines with *T. pallidum* and complement, *T. pallidum* is immobilized.

Use of fluorescein-conjugated antihuman IgM treponemal antibodies (IgM-FTA-ABS) is helpful for diagnosis. IgM antibodies in serum from an infant indicate congenital infection. Although the validity of this test has been questioned, the presence of IgM-FTA-ABS in an infant is strongly suggestive of congenital infection. A negative determination does not rule out congenital syphilis, since syphilis may infect the infant at the time of delivery. Infants with congenital syphilis may have a negative IgM-FTA-ABS assay at delivery.

Criteria for diagnosis of early congenital syphilis. The diagnosis of early congenital syphilis is based on clinical, serologic, and epidemiologic considerations. Indications for the diagnosis, which have been modified from Rathbun (1983a), are found in Table 25-6. It should

Table 25-6. Indications for the diagnosis of early congenital syphilis (patient younger than 2 years)*

Clinical indications

Absolute
1. Specimen from lesions showing *Treponema pallidum* on dark-field or histologic examination

Major
2. Positive reagin test of cerebrospinal fluid
3. Condyloma lata
4. Osteochondritis, periostitis
5. Snuffles, hemorrhagic rhinitis
6. Bullous lesions, palmar/plantar rash

Minor
7. Mucous patches
8. Hepatomegaly, splenomegaly
9. Generalized lymphadenopathy
10. Central nervous system signs
11. Hemolytic anemia, diffuse intravascular coagulation
12. Elevated cell count or protein in cerebrospinal fluid
13. Pneumonitis
14. Edema, ascites
15. Placental villitis or vasculitis
16. Intrauterine growth retardation

Serologic indications

Major
1. Fourfold rise in reagin titer and positive treponemal antibody test
2. Development of a positive treponemal antibody test after birth
3. Positive reagin test or treponemal antibody test after 4 months of age

Epidemiologic indications

Major
1. Untreated early syphilis in the mother within 4 weeks of delivery
2. Contact of pregnant woman with person with untreated primary or secondary syphilis

Minor
3. Untreated late latent syphilis in the mother
4. Early syphilis in the mother within 3 months after child's birth
5. Mother treated for syphilis during pregnancy with a drug other than penicillin
6. Mother treated for syphilis during pregnancy and not followed serologically to delivery

---

*Modified from Rathbun KC. Sex Transm Dis 1983a;10:102.

be noted that patients with early congenital syphilis have a significant incidence of other infections, including CMV, toxoplasmosis, other STDs, and bacteremia. The diagnosis for congenital syphilis may be particularly difficult when another infection is present. Both VDRL and FTA-ABS measure IgG antibody and therefore do not distinguish disease of the infant from maternally derived antibody. Many infants are born to women who have had syphilis in the past, have received therapy, and have remained seroreactive. Their infants will also be seroreactive. Assuring that the infant does not have congenital disease in the immediate newborn period may not be possible.

In Fig. 25-8 are depicted the four major patterns of serologic results from infants who were initially clinically well and were not treated in the perinatal period. Pattern (a) describes children who receive passive transfer of maternal antibody, do not have disease, have progressive decrease of titer of antibody to a nondetectible level, and have a nondetectible reaction at 2 to 3 months of age. These children need not receive therapy.

Pattern (b) depicts infants to whom disease is transmitted at delivery and who are clinically well at delivery. In this group the mothers are seroreactive and the infant receives maternal antibody, which is catabolized and decreases for a few weeks. However, the infant begins to produce antibody at about 3 to 4 weeks of age and, if untreated, will present with congenital syphilis at about 3 to 6 weeks of age.

Pattern (c) is difficult to interpret. These children often have a relatively low titer of antibody at birth but the antibody does not decrease to nonreactive, and at 6 weeks to 3 months the children are still seroreactive. Though these children may or may not have active disease, we would recommend that they receive a full course of therapy.

Pattern (d) depicts infants whose mothers have acquired syphilis very near to the time of delivery, and the infant therefore is clinically well, receives no maternal antibody, and is seronegative. In these instances the infection is transmitted to the infant at delivery, and if left untreated the child will usually present with disease at about 3 to 6 weeks of life. These children will be recognized prior to development of symptomatic illness only if the mother's illness is recognized (a chancre or early secondary eruption) or she is identified as a contact.

Children who have a reactive serology at birth who may be observed with repeated serologic assessment and clinical examination, and not receive treatment at the time of birth, should meet the following criteria:

1. The child must be clinically well and remain so.

2. The child must be available for follow-up examinations. Children of families who are known to avoid medical care may require therapy before discharge. Sera should be examined appropriately during alternate weeks until nonreactive or until the diagnosis is proved or disproved.

3. Before the child is proved to be free of congenital disease, he or she must have (a) a serologic test for syphilis that decreases to nonreactive and (b) if the titer decreased to nonreactive within a few weeks of birth, he or she must have a serologic test that has been taken at about 2 to 3 months that is also nonreactive.

4. If the mother had primary or secondary disease during pregnancy, she must be documented to have received adequate therapy with penicillin. Other forms of therapy and poorly documented therapy may not be adequate for the treatment of the fetus.

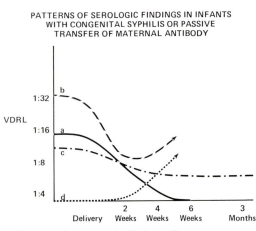

PATTERNS OF SEROLOGIC FINDINGS IN INFANTS WITH CONGENITAL SYPHILIS OR PASSIVE TRANSFER OF MATERNAL ANTIBODY

a. Passive transfer of maternal antibody: no disease.
b. Passive transfer of maternal antibody: later onset of disease.
c. Passive transfer of maternal antibody: indeterminate status for infant.
d. Perinatal infection of mother and infant: later onset of disease.

Fig. 25-8. Schematic presentation of major serologic results during first months of life of infants who are being evaluated for possible congenital syphilis.

Infants who should receive therapy for presumed congenital syphilis at the time of birth include the following:

1. The newborn who has signs of illness compatible with congenital syphilis and has a reactive serology
2. The newborn who has signs of illness compatible with congenital syphilis and is born to a mother who was known to have been exposed during pregnancy to a person with primary or secondary syphilis
3. The newborn who is clinically well but was born to a mother who had primary or secondary syphilis during pregnancy and was not treated or inadequately treated, including infants who have a reactive serology as well as infants who have a nonreactive serology
4. The newborn who is clinically well but was born to a mother who had contact within 90 days before delivery with a person with primary or secondary syphilis and who had not been treated or had been inadequately treated, including infants with a reactive serology and infants who have a nonreactive serology.

Note that although most recommendations for therapy assume that adequate therapy of a mother with primary or secondary syphilis during pregnancy will prevent congenital syphilis with a high degree of reliability, there is reason to doubt this premise (see, for example, Woolf et al. [1980] and Mascola et al. [1984]). Therefore, physicians who wish to treat all infants of mothers who had primary or secondary syphilis during pregnancy before the infant is discharged from the hospital may elect to do so.

Cerebrospinal fluid examination. The indications for a CSF examination are discussed under Treatment. Studies obtained on the CSF should include a VDRL, total cell count with differential, and total protein. Dark-field examination of the CSF may be useful but is rarely performed.

Treatment

T. pallidum is exquisitely sensitive to penicillin, with a minimal inhibitory concentration of 0.004 unit of 0.0025 μg/ml having been defined by animal experimentation. Effective therapy of acquired syphilis must maintain a minimal concentration of 0.3 U/ml in the serum or CSF

for 7 to 10 days. Thus therapy is designed to achieve and to maintain several times the necessary inhibitory levels. Penicillin has minimal toxicity and remains the drug of choice because of established efficacy and no evidence that the organism has increasing resistance to this drug.

Congenital syphilis. The decision that an apparently well or ill infant does or does not have congenital syphilis must rest on the physical examination, history of disease and treatment of the mother, results of a lumbar puncture (LP), and serology. If the child is thought to have congenital syphilis on any of these bases, even if asymptomatic, the child should receive a complete course of therapy similar to that which a symptomatic infant would receive. Although many treatment schedules differentiate between a course for infants with CNS involvement and those without, clinical experience has shown that CNS involvement may be inapparent if the LP is performed early. Furthermore, asymptomatic infants treated with benzathine penicillin G in a single dose may progress to florid systemic disease. For these reasons it is our recommendation that the infant with presumed or established diagnosis of congenital syphilis should be treated with aqueous crystalline penicillin G, 50,000 U per kilogram of body weight per day in two divided doses IM or IV for 10 days. Alternately, aqueous procaine penicillin G, 50,000 U per kilogram of body weight per day IM for 10 days may be prescribed.

Primary and early secondary acquired syphilis. Benzathine penicillin G, 2.4 million units (approximately 50,000 U per kilogram) at a single session in two injection sites, is the preferred regimen. The alternative regimens are tetracycline, 40 mg per kilogram of body weight per day for 15 days, or erythromycin, 40 mg per kilogram of body weight per day for 15 days.

Late syphilis (more than 2 years in duration). The recommended therapy is benzathine penicillin G (50,000 U per kilogram) in two injection sites weekly for three doses. Alternately, tetracycline, 40 mg per kilogram of body weight per day for 30 days or erythromycin, 40 mg per kilogram of body weight per day for 30 days, may be employed.

All forms of neurosyphilis in persons older than 1 year. Aqueous crystalline penicillin, 50,000 U per kilogram of body weight per day IV divided into six doses for 10 days, is followed by benzathine penicillin G, 50,000 U per kilogram of body weight per day weekly for 3 weeks.

Follow-up

The list below summarizes recommendations concerning follow-up of infants after treatment or prophylaxis for congenital syphilis. The patient should be thoroughly evaluated for the extent of disease if there is serologic evidence of failure of treatment or of recurrent disease.

1. For patients diagnosed as having congenital syphilis
   a. Reagin testing every 3 months for the first 15 months, then every 6 months until negative or stable at low titer
   b. Treponemal antibody test after 15 months of age
   c. Repeat cerebrospinal fluid evaluation 2 years after treatment if the patient was treated for syphilis or showed any signs of central nervous system disease
   d. Careful developmental evaluation, vision testing, and hearing testing before 3 years of age or at the time of diagnosis
2. For patients treated in utero or at birth because of maternal syphilis*
   a. Reagin testing at birth and then every 3 months until at least 6 months of age and test is negative
   b. Treponemal antibody test after 15 months of age
3. For women treated for syphilis during pregnancy
   a. Reagin testing monthly until delivery, then every 3 months until negative
   b. Retreatment anytime there is a fourfold rise in reagin titer

---

*Any time the patient meets the criteria for diagnosis of congenital syphilis, follow-up should be that indicated for a diagnosed case.

REFERENCES
Child abuse and sexual abuse

DeJong AR, Weiss JC, Brent RL. Condyloma accuminata in children. Am J Dis Child 1982;136:704-706.

Farrell MK, Billimire ME, Shamroy JA, Hammond JG. Prepubertal gonorrhea: a multidisciplinary approach. Pediatrics 1981;67:151-153.

Gardner M, Jones JG. Genital herpes acquired by sexual abuse of children. J Pediatr 1984;104:243-244.

Hammerschlag MR, Doraiswamy B, Alexander ER, et al. Are rectogenital chlamydial infections a marker of sexual abuse of children? Pediatr Infect Dis 1984;3:100-101.

Ingram DL, Runyan DK, Collins AD, et al. Vaginal *Chlamydia trachomatis* infection in children with sexual contact. Pediatr Infect Dis 1984;3:97-99.

Ingram DL, White ST, Durfee MF, Pearson AW. Sexual contact in children with gonorrhea. Am J Dis Child 1982;136:994-996.

Kempe CH. Sexual abuse, another hidden pediatric problem. Pediatrics 1978;62:382-389.

Neinstein LS, Goldenring J, Carpenter S. Non-sexual transmission of sexually transmitted diseases: an infrequent occurence. Pediatrics 1984;74:67-76.

Orr DP, Prietto SV. Emergency management of sexually abused children: the role of the pediatric resident. Am J Dis Child 1979;133:628-631.

Rimsza ME, Niggemann EH. Medical evaluation of sexually abused children: a review of 311 cases. Pediatrics 1982;69:8-14.

Summit RC. The child sexual abuse accommodation syndrome. Child Abuse Neglect 1983;7:177-193.

Tilelli JA, Turek D, Jaffe AC. Sexual abuse of children. Clinical findings and implications for management. N Engl J Med 1980;302:319-323.

White ST, Loda FA, Ingram DL, Pearson A. Sexually transmitted diseases in sexually abused children. Pediatrics 1983;72:16-21.

Gonococcal diseases

Amstey MS, Steadman KT. Asymptomatic gonorrhea and pregnancy. J Am Vener Dis Assoc 1976;3:14.

Apicella MA. Serogrouping the *Neisseria gonorrhoeae*: identification of four immunologically distinct acidic polysaccharides. J Infect Dis 1976;134:377.

Baker C. Sexually-transmitted diseases and child abuse. Am J Vener Dis Assoc 1978;5:169.

Brown RC. The prevalence of infectious syphilis in patients with acute gonorrhea. South Med J 1978;61:98.

Cooperman MB. Gonococcal arthritis in infancy: a clinical study of forty-four cases. Am J Dis Child 1927;33:932.

Crawford G, Knapp JS, Hale J, Holmes KK. Asymptomatic gonorrhea in men: caused by gonococci with unique nutritional requirements. Science 1977;196:1352.

Crede CSF. Reports from the obstetrical clinic in Leipzig. Prevention of eye inflammation of the newborn. Am J Dis Child 1971;121:3.

Edwards LE, et al. Gonorrhea in pregnancy. Am J Obstet Gynecol 1978;132:637.

Eisenstein BI, Lee TJ, Sparling SF. Penicillin sensitivity and serum resistance are independent attributes of strains of *Neisseria gonorrhoeae* causing disseminated gonococcal infection. Infect Immun 1977;15:834.

Handsfield HH, Hodson EA, Holmes KK. Neonatal gonococcal infection. JAMA 1973;225:697.

Hein K, Marks A, Cohen MI. Asymptomatic gonorrhea: prevalence in a population of urban adolescents. J Pediatr 1977;90:634-635.

Holmes KK, Counts GW, Beaty HN. Disseminated gonococcal infection. Ann Intern Med 1971;74:979.

Holt LE. Gonococcus infections in children, with special reference to their prevalence in institutions and means of prevention. NY Med J, Phil Med J 1905;81:521,589.

Israel KS, Rissing KB, Brooks GF. Neonatal and childhood gonococcal infections. Clin Obstet Gynecol 1975;18:143.

Karney WW, et al. Spectinomycin versus tetracycline for the treatment of gonorrhea. N Engl J Med 1977;296:889.

Knapp JS, Holmes KK. Disseminated gonococcal infections caused by *Neisseria gonorrhoeae* with unique nutritional requirements. J Infect Dis 1975;132:204.

Kohen DP. Neonatal gonococcal arthritis: three cases and review of the literature. Pediatrics 1974;53:436.

Litt IF, Cohen MI. Perihepatitis associated with salpingitis in adolescents. JAMA 1978;240:1253.

Litt IF, Edberg SC, Finberg L. Gonorrhea in children and adolescents; a current review. J Pediatr 1974;85:595.

Nelson JD, Mohs E, Dajani AS, Plotkin SA. Gonorrhea in preschool and school aged children. A report of the prepubertal gonorrhea cooperative study group. JAMA 1976;236:1359.

O'Reilly RJ, Lee L, Welch BG. Secretory IgA antibody responses in *Neisseria gonorrhoeae* in the genital secretions of infected females. J Infect Dis 1976;133:113.

Patamasucon P, Rettig PJ, Nelson JD. Cefuroxide therapy of gonorrhea and co-infection with *Chlamydia trachomatis* in children. Pediatrics 1981;68:534-538.

Plavidal FJ, Werch A. Fetal scalp abscess secondary to intrauterine monitoring. Am J Obstet Gynecol 1976;125:65.

Sarrel PM, Pruett KA. Symptomatic gonorrhea during pregnancy. Obstet Gynecol 1968;32:670.

Sgroi SM. Pediatric gonorrhea beyond infancy. Pediatr Ann 1979;8:326.

Snowe RJ, Wilfert CM. Epidemic reappearance of gonococcal ophthalmia neonatorum. Pediatrics 1973;57:110.

Stamm WE, Guinan ME, Johnson C, et al. Effect of treatment regimens for *Neisseria gonorrhoeae* on simultaneous infection with *Chlamydia trachomatis*. N Engl J Med 1984;310:545-549.

Wald ER. Gonorrhea diagnosis by Gram stain in the female adolescent. Am J Dis Child 1977;131:1044.

Wiesner PJ, et al. Clinical spectrum of pharyngeal gonococcal infection. N Engl J Med 1973;288:181.

Pelvic inflammatory disease

Cates W. Sexually transmitted organisms and infertility: the proof of the pudding. Sex Transm Dis 1984;II:113-116.

Eschenbach DA, Buchanan TM, Pollock HM, et al. Polymicrobial etiology of acute pelvic inflammatory disease. N Engl J Med 1975;293:166-171.

Shafer M-AB, Irwin CE, Sweet RL. Acute salpingitis in the adolescent female. J Pediatr 1982;100:339-350.

Chlamydia

Alexander ER, Harrison HR. Role of *Chlamydia trachomatis* in perinatal infection. Rev Infect Dis 1983;5:713-719.

Chacko MR, Louchik JC. *Chlamydia trachomatis* infection in sexually active adolescents: prevalence and risk factors. Pediatrics 1984;73:836-840.

Friedman AD, Harrison HR, Alexander ER. Coinfection with cytomegalovirus and *Chlamydia trachomatis*: seroepidemiologic data. J Infect Dis 1983;148:332.

Golden N, Hammerschlag M, Newhoff S, et al. Prevalence of *Chlamydia trachomatis* cervical infections in female adolescents. Am J Dis Child 1984;138:562-564.

Hammerschlag MR, Anderson M, Semine DZ, et al. Prospective study of maternal and infantile infection with *Chlamydia trachomatis*. Pediatrics 1979;64:142-148.

Harrison HR, English MG, Lee CK, Alexander ER. *Chlamydia trachomatis* infant pneumonia. N Engl J Med 1978;298:702-708.

Martin DH, Koutsky L, Eschenbach DA, et al. Prematurity and perinatal mortality in pregnancies complicated by maternal *Chlamydial trachomatis* infections. JAMA 1982;247:1585-1588.

Podgore JK, Holmes KK, Alexander ER. Asymptomatic urethral infections due to *Chlamydial trachomatis* in male U.S. military personnel. J Infect Dis 1982;146:828.

Potter ME, Kaufmann AK, Plikaytis BD. Psittacosis in the United States, 1979. Morbid Mortal Weekly Rep 1980;32:27ss-31ss.

Rettig PJ, Nelson JD. Genital tract infection with *Chlamydia trachomatis* in prepubertal children. J Pediatr 1981;99:206-210.

Schachter J. Chlamydial infections. N Engl J Med 1978;298:428-435, 490-495, 540-549.

Sweet RL, Schachter J, Robbie MO. Failure of beta-lactam antibiotics to eradicate *Chlamydia trachomatis* in the endometrium despite apparent clinical care of acyte salpingitis. JAMA 1983;250:2641-2645.

Tam MR, Stamm WE, Handsfield HH, et al. Culture-independent diagnosis of *Chlamydia trachomatis* using monoclonal antibodies. N Engl J Med 1984;310:1146-1150.

Tipple MA, Beem MO, Saxon EM. Clinical characteristics of the febrile pneumonia associated with *Chlamydia trachomatis* infection in infants less than 6 months of age. Pediatrics 1979;63:192-197.

Syphilis

Deacon WE, Lucas JB, Price EV. Fluorescent treponemal antibody-absorption (FTA-ABS) test for syphilis. JAMA 1966;198:624.

Drew FL, Sarandria JL. False-positive FTA-ABS in pregnancy. J Am Vener Dis Assoc 1975;1:165.

Dunlop EMC, Al-Egaily MB, Houang ET. Penicillin levels in blood and CSF achieved by treatment of syphilis. JAMA 1979;241:2538.

Frenz G, Hideon PB, Espersen F, et al. Penicillin concentrations in blood and spinal fluid after a single intramuscular injection of penicillin G benzathine. Eur J Clin Microbiol 1984;3:147.

Handsfield HH, Lukehart SA, Sell S, et al. Demonstration of *Treponema pallidum* in a cutaneous gumma by indirect immunofluorescence. Arch Dermatol 1983;119:677.

Harter CA, Benirschke K. Fetal syphilis in the first trimester. Am J Obstet Gynecol 1976;124:705.

Jaffe HW. The laboratory diagnosis of syphilis. Am Intern Med 1975;83:846.

Jenson JR, Thestrup-Pederson K, From E. Fluctuations in natural killer cell activity in early syphilis. Br J Vener Dis 1983;59:30-32.

Lee TJ, Sparling PF. Syphilis, an algorithm. JAMA 1979;242:1187.

Luxon L, Lees AJ, Greenwood RJ. Neurosyphilis today. Lancet 1979;1:90.

Mascola L, Pelosi R, Blount JH, et al. Congenital syphilis: why is it still occurring? JAMA 1984;252:1719-1722.

McCracken GH Jr, Kaplan JM. Penicillin treatment for congenital syphilis. JAMA 1974;228:855.

Musher DM, Hague-Park M, Gyorkey F, et al. The inter-action between *Treponema pallidum* and human poly-morphonuclear leukocytes. J Infect Dis 1983;147:74-86.

Peterson KM, Baseman JB, Alderete JF. *Treponema palli-dum* receptor binding proteins interact with fibronectin. J Exp Med 1983;157:1958-1970.

Rathbun KC. Congenital syphilis: a proposal for improved surveillance, diagnosis and treatment. Sex Transm Dis 1983;10:102.

Rathbun KC. Congenital syphilis. Sex Transm Dis 1983; 10:93.

Rosen EW, Richardson NJ. A reappraisal of the value of the IgM fluorescent treponemal antibody absorption test in the diagnosis of congenital syphilis. J Pediatr 1975;87:38.

Sparling PF. Diagnosis and treatment of syphilis. N Engl J Med 1971;284:642.

Speer ME, Taber LH, Clark DB, Rudolph AJ. Cerebro-spinal fluid levels of benzathine penicillin G in the neo-nate. J Pediatr 1977;9:996.

Taber LH, Feigin RD. Spirochetal infections. Pediatr Clin North Am 1979;26:377.

Taber LH, Huber TW. Congenital syphilis. Prog Clin Biol Res 1975;3:183.

Woolf A, Wilfert CM, Kelsey DB, Gutman LT. Childhood syphilis in North Carolina. NC Med J 1980;41:443.

Wong GHW, Steiner B, Faine S, et al. Factors affecting the attachment of *Treponema pallidum* to mammalian cells in vitro. Br J Vener Dis 1983;59:21-29.

26

SMALLPOX AND VACCINIA

A full discussion of smallpox and vaccinia was included in Chapter 28 of the seventh (1981) edition of this book. Because the disease has been successfully eradicated and the requirement, with a solitary exception, for vaccination has been abolished, we have chosen to restrict this chapter to brief general sections, comments on contemporary issues, remarks on related viruses and illnesses, and a list of significant references for those readers who choose to explore further this fascinating example of man's conquest of a disease.

For more than 3000 years smallpox was a widespread illness with serious morbidity and mortality. Nations in Africa and the Asian subcontinent reported millions of cases annually as recently as 1967. In that year the World Health Organization (WHO) began its 10-year program of smallpox eradication. On October 26, 1977 Ali Maow Maalin, a cook in the district hospital at Merka, Somalia, had the onset of his smallpox rash. He may well go down in history as the last known patient with endemic smallpox. In the years after Maalin's recovery, the only known smallpox victims acquired their infection as the result of a laboratory contamination in Birmingham, England.

Nearly 200 episodes of suspected endemic smallpox have been reported to the WHO since the case of Ali Maow Maalin, but none has been verified. Instead, they have proved to be chickenpox, herpes simplex, monkeypox, drug erup-

tions, or other skin disorders. Of special note is monkeypox, which has been reported with regularity from West and Central Africa. Originally recovered from monkeys who became ill in captivity, the virus has been responsible for more than 80 cases of human illness closely resembling smallpox, usually in children with no history of previous smallpox vaccination. Secondary spread among humans is quite unusual, but several cases have been documented. Serologic assays can differentiate variola, vaccinia, and monkeypox infections (Walls et al., 1981).

The WHO Assembly in 1980 received the documentation of the final global eradication of smallpox. This is an achievement unique in the history of man's interaction with the microorganisms of his environment. Smallpox virus exists today only in the deep freezers of two selected laboratories.

The two laboratories that maintain stocks of variola virus are at the Centers for Disease Control in Atlanta, Georgia, and the Research Institute for Viral Preparations in Moscow, USSR. They participate in the smallpox eradication surveillance and research program of the World Health Organization (WHO, 1983). In addition, WHO has stockpiled 300 million doses of vaccine in Geneva, Switzerland, Toronto, Canada, and New Delhi, India, as an insurance in case of the unexpected reemergence of smallpox. Several nations have independently set aside their own vaccinia reserves.

SMALLPOX (VARIOLA MAJOR; VARIOLA MINOR OR ALASTRIM; VARIOLOID)

Smallpox was an acute, highly contagious, preventable disease caused by poxvirus variola, a specific virus immunologically related to vaccinia virus. It was characterized by a 3- to 4-day prodromal period of chills, high fever, headache, backache, vomiting, and prostration. The temperature began to subside as the eruptive stage commenced on the third or fourth day. The eruption progressed from macular to papular to vesicular to pustular and finally to crusting during an 8- to 14-day period. The temperature rose again and the constitutional symptoms intensified during the pustular stage. The rash had a characteristic peripheral or centrifugal distribution, with lesions at the same stage in any one regional area.

Variola major, variola minor or alastrim, and varioloid were the three chief forms of the disease. *Variola major* was classic smallpox. It had a high mortality that varied with the type of lesions as follows: ordinary-discrete, <10%; ordinary-semiconfluent, 25% to 50%; ordinary-confluent, 50% to 75%; flat, >90%; hemorrhagic, nearly 100% (Koplan and Foster, 1979). In general infants, pregnant women, and elderly patients had higher fatality rates. *Variola minor*, or alastrim, was a mild type of smallpox occurring in nonvaccinated persons. It was caused by a less virulent strain of the virus that bred true. The mortality was usually under 1% except in rare instances when the rash became confluent or hemorrhagic. *Varioloid* was a mild form of smallpox occurring in previously vaccinated persons who had partial immunity. This mild disease was caused by a virulent strain of the virus capable of causing variola major in a nonimmunized contact.

Etiology

The poxviruses are a group of large, ellipsoid, complex DNA viruses. They include more than 20 mammalian viruses as well as groups of bird (avipox) and insect (entomopox) viruses. A number of the group can initiate human infection but only variola (smallpox) has been of worldwide significance. The other agents are of importance in various species, which include monkeys, elephants, camels, sheep, rabbits, swine, buffalo, goats, cows, mice, turkeys, canaries, pigeons, and other birds. Variola and vaccinia are members of the genus *Orthopoxvirus;* others in that genus are cowpox, monkeypox, and whitepox viruses.

Smallpox and vaccinia viruses are morphologically indistinguishable and closely related immunologically. The elementary bodies can be identified in smears of vesicular fluid stained by the Paschen, Giemsa, or Gutstein method. Under the electron microscope they are brick shaped or ovoid and approximately 230 × 400 nm in size. Aggregates of these bodies in infected host cells form the so-called Guarnieri bodies. These are intracytoplasmic inclusions measuring approximately 10 μm in diameter. The viral genome is a single molecule of double-stranded DNA contained within a central core that in turn is enclosed by an external coat of lipid and protein surrounding two lateral bodies as well. Research continues on the classification and genetic relatedness of the many poxviruses and their interrelationships. All poxviruses apparently share a common inner core nucleoprotein antigen.

Infection with smallpox and vaccinia viruses stimulates the production of at least four types of antibody: antihemagglutinin, complement-fixing antibodies, neutralizing antibodies, and antibodies that inhibit agar gel precipitation. Levels of antihemagglutinin and complement-fixing antibodies rise significantly by the end of the second week of illness or vaccination; they persist for several months. Neutralizing antibodies develop later but persist for years.

Pathogenesis, pathology, clinical manifestations, diagnosis, differential diagnosis, complications, prognosis, immunity, epidemiologic factors, treatment, preventive measures, isolation, quarantine, and control are discussed in Chapter 28 of the seventh edition as well as in many of the references listed at the end of this chapter.

VACCINIA

Vaccinia is an acute infectious disease caused by deliberate smallpox vaccination or by the accidental contact of abraded skin with infective material. It is characterized by the development of a localized lesion that progresses in sequence from papule to vesicle to pustule to crust. Fever and regional lymphadenitis may develop during the vesicular or pustular stage. The infection

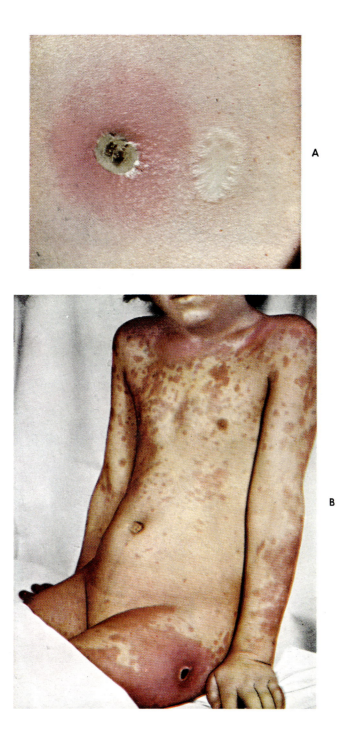

Plate 5
A, Primary take in a previously vaccinated person. **B,** Toxic eruption complicating vaccinia.
(From Top FH, Wehrle PF, eds. Communicable and infectious diseases, ed 8. St. Louis. The
CV Mosby Co., 1976.)

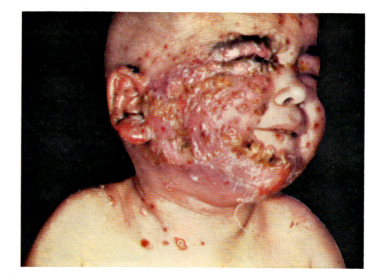

Plate 6
Eczema vaccinatum. (Courtesy Dr. Otto E. Billo; from Stimson PM, Hodes HLA. Manual of the common contagious diseases. Philadelphia. Lea & Febiger, 1956.)

stimulates the production of antibodies that are protective against smallpox.

Clinical manifestations

The clinical manifestations of vaccinia are dependent for the most part on the immune status of the individual. Two types of reactions may result from a successful vaccination: a "major" response (pustular lesion or an area of definite induration or congestion surrounding a central lesion, scab, or ulcer 6 to 8 days after vaccination) or an "equivocal" response.

Major response. Three days after vaccination, the inoculated site becomes reddened and pruritic. It becomes papular on the fourth day and vesicular by the fifth or sixth day. A red areola surrounds the vesicle, which becomes umbilicated and then pustular by the eighth to the eleventh day. By this time the red areola has enlarged markedly. The pustule begins to dry, the redness subsides, and the lesion becomes crusted between the second and third week. By the end of the third week, the scab falls off, leaving a permanent scar that at first is pink in color but eventually becomes white.

At the end of the first week, between the vesicular and pustular phases, there may be a variable amount of fever, malaise, and regional lymphadenitis. These symptoms usually subside within 1 to 2 days and are more likely to occur in older children and adults than in infants.

Accelerated, modified, or vaccinoid reaction. Revaccination of a partially immune person is followed by an attenuated form of vaccinia with the following characteristics: (1) usually there is no fever or constitutional symptoms; (2) a papule appears by the third day, becomes vesicular by the fifth to seventh day, and dries shortly thereafter; (3) the vesicle and its red areola are relatively small; and (4) the scar, if present, is usually insignificant and disappears within a year or two.

Accelerated reactions may also result from scratching and autoinoculation with the vesicular fluid of a primary vaccinia pox. The accelerated lesions mature simultaneously with the initial primary lesion and heal without scarring as a rule.

• • •

The absence of a reaction does *not* mean that the person is immune. In most instances, either the vaccine is not potent or the technique is at fault. Occasionally a papule may result from needle trauma. Consequently, when there is doubt, it is wise to repeat the vaccination.

In order to evaluate a vaccination, it would be ideal to inspect the lesion daily. When this is not practical, the optimum times of inspection are the third, seventh, and fourteenth days.

Vaccination procedures

Methods. The most commonly employed methods of vaccination are the multiple pressure method, multiple puncture method with bifurcated needles, and jet injection method when large numbers of individuals are to be vaccinated at one place in a short time.

Precautions. Since vaccination is generally an elective procedure, it should be postponed in instances of intercurrent infection. Primary vaccination of individuals with eczema or other types of exfoliative dermatitis may be complicated by eczema vaccinatum, a severe and potentially fatal disease. Vaccination should be deferred until the skin lesions clear.

It is recommended that vaccination, in those few instances when indicated, be given as *one* inoculation over the *deltoid area*, with the *multiple pressure* or *multiple puncture* technique and a fully potent vaccine.

Immunity

Immunity develops between the eighth and eleventh days after vaccination. Antihemagglutinin, complement-fixing, and virus-neutralizing antibodies are demonstrable between the tenth and thirteenth days.

Duration of immunity is extremely variable; it may range between 2 and 10 years. During the mass vaccination program in New York City in 1947, a random sampling of 25,000 of the 5 million vaccinated persons indicated that 74% had successful takes, indicating probable susceptibility to smallpox. Revaccination at 3-year intervals is generally adequate to maintain optimum immunity.

Complications

Until May 1983 when it was withdrawn by Wyeth Laboratories (the sole U.S. producer) from general availability, smallpox vaccine was occasionally administered to patients with recurrent herpes simplex or papillomas in the mistaken expectation that it would interfere with development of new lesions or accelerate the resolution of older ones. Because some of these patients suffered from underlying immunodeficiency disorders they acquired life-threatening progressive vaccinia due to unarrested local replication of vaccinia virus.

Currently smallpox vaccine is available and recommended only for laboratory workers who may be engaged in surveillance or research involving variola or other closely related orthopoxviruses. The largest use of vaccine, however, is by the armed forces, who continue to administer vaccinia to active duty personnel, recruits, reserves, and national guardsmen—nearly 1 million doses annually. Therefore it seems appropriate and prudent to retain the following paragraphs on the possible complications of vaccination.

Secondary bacterial infection. The local lesion may become secondarily infected with staphylococci or streptococci, causing cellulitis.

Accidental infection. Autoinoculation by means of scratching an active lesion may produce secondary pocks over various parts of the body. The severity of this complication is governed by the site of inoculation. For example, a lesion of the eye with corneal involvement may result in ulceration, scarring, and blindness.

Toxic eruptions. An erythema multiforme type of eruption occasionally occurs between the seventh and tenth days at the height of the vaccinia reaction. The rash may be generalized or localized to a particular area. It usually clears within 3 to 5 days. It is thought to be due to a sensitivity reaction (Plate 5). This rash was most often seen in infants vaccinated before their first birthday.

Generalized vaccinia. This potentially serious complication arose between the seventh and fourteenth days after vaccination. A generalized eruption develops, with crops of lesions simulating a primary vaccination. Healing without scars takes place rapidly, being completed at the same time as the healing of the primary vaccinia lesion.

Eczema vaccinatum. This potentially fatal complication of vaccinia develops in patients with eczema or other forms of exfoliative dermatitis who have been either vaccinated or exposed to an active case of vaccinia. The disease is characterized by high fever, severe toxicity, and an extensive vesicular and pustular eruption

chiefly confined to the area of dermatitis (Plate 6 and Fig. 26-1). Healthy areas of skin also may become involved. The mortality may be significant.

Progressive vaccinia (vaccinia necrosum; prolonged vaccinia; vaccinia gangrenosa). Progressive vaccinia, a highly fatal complication, is fortunately rare. The initial vaccinal lesion fails to heal and progresses to involve more and more areas of adjacent skin. The necrosis of the tissues continues to extend, often over a period of months. Metastatic lesions may develop in other parts of the skin, bones, and viscera. This complication has been observed in patients with immunologic disorders. The common denominator has been depression of T-lymphocyte function, either congenital or acquired. Progressive vaccinia is also likely to occur in patients with immunologic deficits caused by malignant disease of the lymphatic system (leukemia or lymphomas) and/or their therapy. Treatment has been attempted with vaccinia-immune globulin (VIG), N-methylisatin-B-thiosemicarbazone (methisazone, marboran), interferon, transfer factor, acyclovir, and rifampin. Cases have been too infrequent to evaluate therapy in an acceptable fashion.

Postvaccinal encephalitis. Postvaccinal encephalitis is a serious but rare complication. The incidence of postvaccinal encephalitis in Sweden from 1947 to 1954 was 1.9 per 100,000. Surveillance of complications of smallpox vaccination in the United States in 1968 revealed 2.9 cases of encephalitis per 1 million primary vaccinations; the highest incidence, 6.5 per 1 million, was observed in infants less than 12 months old.

The clinical picture is the same as that in other postinfectious encephalitides. The usual manifestations include fever, headache, vomiting, meningeal signs, paralysis, drowsiness, coma, and convulsions. The spinal fluid contains an increase in number of mononuclear cells and amount of protein. Pathologically, the brain shows the same type of perivascular infiltration and demyelination as occurs in encephalitis-complicating measles and chickenpox. The mortality may be as high 30% to 40%.

Treatment

Primary vaccinia requires no treatment. Dressings are unnecessary. Fever and pain in

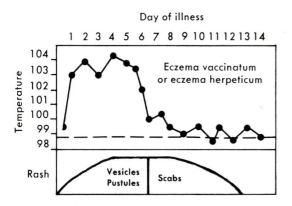

Day of illness

Fig. 26-1. Schematic diagram of the clinical course of eczema herpeticum or eczema vaccinatum.

the arm may be treated with appropriate doses of aspirin. Superimposed pyogenic infections may require hot compresses and antimicrobial therapy. Patients with eczema vaccinatum need intensive supportive therapy; they should receive VIG, 0.6 ml per kilogram of body weight intramuscularly. The same dose would be indicated for patients with vaccinia necrosum. In general, the treatment of encephalitis is the same as that of any infectious or postinfectious encephalitis.

Preventive measures

Most complications of vaccinia are preventable. Vaccination is contraindicated under the following circumstances: evidence of eczema or other chronic forms of dermatitis in the vaccinated person or a close contact; or altered immune status from disease or immunosuppressive therapy.

An experimental attenuated vaccinia virus vaccine was used by Kempe (1967) for the primary vaccination of more than 1000 patients suffering from eczema. The vaccination was well tolerated; local and systemic reactions were not significant, and there was no evidence of virus dissemination. The success of the WHO smallpox eradication program obviated the need for this product.

In 1971 the United States Public Health Service accepted the recommendation of its Advisory Committee on Immunization Practices that *routine* smallpox vaccination in the United States be discontinued. In 1976 the former recommendation of routine smallpox vaccination for hospital employees was also rescinded. Since

that time the sole civilian group for whom vaccine has been indicated is laboratory workers directly involved with smallpox or related orthopoxviruses. As mentioned previously, however, nearly 1 million armed forces personnel annually receive the vaccine.

It is worth noting a potential renaissance of interest in widespread vaccinia administration. Smith et al. (1983) have reported the successful incorporation into the vaccinia virus genome of coding sequences for the hepatitis B surface antigen. Gene portions from other human viral pathogens have similarly been exploited to provide a vaccinia "carrier virus" that could serve to induce immunity to a number of viral infections. It is premature to debate here the advisability of utilizing vaccinia virus in this way.

REFERENCES
Smallpox

American Public Health Association. Smallpox. In Control of communicable diseases in man, ed 12. New York. The Association, 1975.

Bauer DJ, St Vincent L, Kempe CH, Downie AW. Prophylactic treatment of smallpox contacts with N-methylisatin-β-thiosemicarbazone (compound 33T57). Lancet 1963; 2:494.

Bauer DJ, et al. Prophylaxis of smallpox with methisazone. Am J Epidemiol 1970;90:130.

Baxby D. Identification and interrelationships of the variola/vaccinia subgroup of poxviruses. Prog Med Virol 1975; 19:216.

Baxby D. The origins of vaccinia virus. J Infect Dis 1977;136:453.

Behbehani AB. The smallpox story: life and death of an old disease. Microbiol Rev 1983;47:455-509.

Breman JG, Arita I. The confirmation and maintenance of smallpox eradication. N Engl J Med 1980;303:1263-1273.

Center for Disease Control. Smallpox certification—East Africa. Morbid Mortal Weekly Rep 1979;28:497.

Cho CT, Wenner HA. Monkeypox virus. Bacteriol Rev 1973;37:1.

Esposito JJ, Obijeski JF, Nakano JH. Orthopoxvirus DNA: strain differentiation by electrophoresis of restriction endonuclease fragmented virion DNA. Virology 1978;89:53.

Fenner F. The eradication of smallpox. Prog Med Virol 1977;23:1.

Fenner F. Global eradication of smallpox. Rev Infect Dis 1982;4:916-922.

Guarnieri G. Ricerche sulla patogenesi et etiologia dell' infezione vaccinica e variolosa. Arch Sci Med 1982;16:403.

Henderson DA. The eradication of smallpox. Sci Am 1976;235:25.

Koplan JP, Foster SO. Smallpox: clinical types, causes of death, and treatment. J Infect Dis 1979;140:440.

Mazumder DNG, De S, Mitra AC, Mukherjee MK. Clinical observations on smallpox: a study of 1233 patients admitted to the Infectious Diseases Hospital, Calcutta, during 1973. Bull WHO 1975;52:301.

Moss B. Reproduction of poxviruses. In Fraenkel-Conrat H, and Wagner RR, eds. Comprehensive virology, vol 3. New York. Plenum Press, 1974, pp 405-474.

Ricketts TF, Byles JB. The diagnosis of smallpox, vols I and II. Reprinted from the 1908 London edition. U.S. Department of Health, Education, and Welfare, Bureau of Disease, Prevention and Environmental control, Division of Foreign Quarantine, 1966.

Walls HH, Ziegler DW, Nakano JM. Characterization of antibodies to orthopoxviruses in human sera by radioimmunoassay. Bull WHO 1981;59:253-262.

Vaccinia

Goldstein JA, Neff JM, Lane JM, Koplan JP. Smallpox vaccination reactions, prophylaxis, and therapy of complications. Pediatrics 1975;55:342.

Jenner E. An inquiry into the causes and effects of the variolae vaccinae, a disease discovered in some of the western counties of England, particularly Gloucestershire, and known by the name of cowpox. Reprinted by Cassell and Co, Ltd, 1896. Available in Pamphlet vol 4232, Army Medical Library, Washington, DC.

Kempe CH. Studies on smallpox and complications of smallpox vaccination. Pediatrics 1960;26:176.

Kempe CH. Attenuated vaccinia in the elective primary vaccination of eczema patients. Abstracts, American Pediatric Society, 77th Annual Meeting, April 26-29, 1967.

Kempe CH. Smallpox: recent developments in selective vaccination and eradication. Am J Trop Med Hyg 1974;23:775.

Lane JM, Ruben FL, Neff JM, Millar JD. Complications of smallpox vaccination, 1968. N Engl J Med 1969;281:1201.

Neff JM, et al. Complications of smallpox vaccination. I. National survey in the United States, 1963. N Engl J Med 1967;276:125.

Stimson PM, Hodes HL. A manual of the common contagious diseases. Philadelphia. Lea & Febiger, 1956.

Top FA, Wehrle PF, eds. Communicable and infectious diseases, ed 8. St Louis. The CV Mosby Co., 1976.

Smith GL, Mackett M, Moss B. Infectious vaccinia virus recombinants that express hepatitis B virus surface antigens. Nature 1983;302:490-495.

Tyzzer EE. The etiology and pathology of vaccinia. J Med Res 1904;11:180.

27

STAPHYLOCOCCAL INFECTIONS

Staphylococcal infections continue to pose serious problems for infants and children, particularly those under 1 year of age and those who are hospitalized. Staphylococcal infections of the skin, such as impetigo, boils, and wound infections, may lead to septicemia and serious complications, such as osteomyelitis and other metastatic foci in the heart, lungs, brain, and kidney. Staphylococcal septicemia and pneumonia with various complications, such as lung abscess, pneumatoceles (emphysematous blebs), empyema, and pyothorax, give rise to clinical manifestations of major importance. A rare meningococcemia-like disease caused by staphylococcal bacteremia has been recognized. Staphylococci also are major contributors to bacterial food poisoning.

There is considerable evidence indicating that there is a high incidence of severe staphylococcal infections resistant to antimicrobial therapy. It appears, furthermore, that staphylococci differ from other gram-positive cocci in basic biologic relationships within the host. Staphylococci possess a remarkable capacity to adapt to changes in the environment, to mutate rapidly, and, so far, to survive all the weapons devised by man. *Staphylococcus aureus* is remarkably adaptable, being able to change by direct mutation, harboring plasmids that can be passed, and transferring genetic material by transduction.

ETIOLOGY

Staphylococci, from the Greek word meaning "a bunch of grapes," are gram-positive, rounded microorganisms occurring in characteristic grapelike clusters. They flourish on artificial media. Three species, *S. aureus*, *S. epidermidis*, and *S. saprophyticus*, are currently identified. *S. aureus* is responsible for various human illnesses but may also be found as a normal inhabitant of the skin or mucous membranes. *S. epidermidis* is less pathogenic for man than *S. aureus* but may produce minor skin lesions and, with increasing frequency, is the cause of more serious diseases such as bacteremia and endocarditis in debilitated patients and in those with prosthetic heart valves and other devices. It is a major cause of meningitis in children with spina bifida, meningomyelocele, hydrocephalus, and shunts draining cerebrospinal fluid from the cerebral ventricles to other body spaces. An atypical *S. epidermidis*, presumed to be the cause of some urinary tract infections occurring in young women, has been reclassified as *S. saprophyticus*.

The cell wall of staphylococci contains peptidoglycan, teichoic acid, and protein A. Protein A has a high affinity for the Fc fragment of immunoglobulins, and thus it binds to and agglutinates IgG and fixes complement. Some strains of staphylococci also possess a capsule that acts to inhibit phagocytosis by host cells and thus plays the role of a spreading factor. Demonstration of antibodies to teichoic acid is useful in managing patients with severe staphylococcal diseases (Sheagren, 1984).

Coagulase

Most strains of *S. aureus* pathogenic for man have the capacity to grow in human blood, to ferment mannitol, and to form several enzymes, toxins, and hemolysins. The formation of the enzyme coagulase is the most important distinguishing feature that characterizes most strains of *S. aureus*; it is absent from *S. epidermidis*.

Coagulase has the ability to clot plasma. Formation of the clot is induced by the combination of the following factors: (1) coagulase, which is formed by staphylococci, and (2) a substance called coagulase-reacting factor, which is normally present in human plasma and the plasma of certain animals. The interaction of plasma coagulase-reacting factor and coagulase produces a thrombinlike substance that converts fibrinogen to fibrin. Human and rabbit plasmas contain the factor and are readily clotted.

The injection of coagulase-positive strains of staphylococci seldom results in abscess formation in certain species of animals lacking the plasma coagulase-reacting factor. Localized abscesses are induced in these animals, however, when a coagulable plasma is introduced simultaneously. In 1956 Rammelkamp and Lebovitz observed that, in general, the serum titers of coagulase-reacting factor are appreciably lower in infants under 2 years of age than in adults (Fig. 27-1). In this respect it may be significant that infants infected by staphylococci are more likely to develop septicemia and diffuse inflammatory processes in contrast to focal lesions typical of infection in the adult.

Although it is generally agreed that there is a high correlation between coagulase formation and virulence of staphylococci for man, the part played by coagulase in the pathogenesis of human infections is not clear.

Toxins

Staphylococci produce a variety of exotoxins. Some also have a substance (teichoic acid–pep-

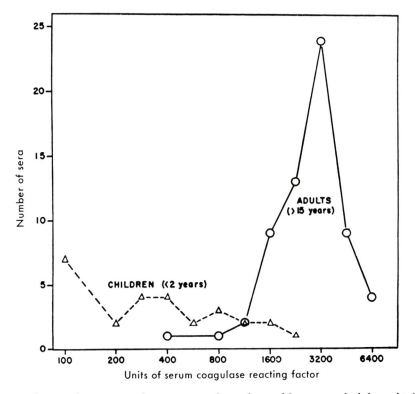

Fig. 27-1. The coagulase-reacting factor content of sera obtained from normal adults and infants. (From Rogers DE. Ann. Intern Med 1956;45:748; data from Rammelkamp CH, Jr, Lebovitz JL. Ann NY Acad Sci 1956;65:144.)

tidoglycan complex) in the cell wall that mimics the effects of endotoxin and has clinical importance (Wilkinson et al., 1981). Six enterotoxins (A through F) have been described; when inadvertently injested in spoiled food, these cause acute gastroenteritis. Enterotoxin F is also thought to cause the toxic shock syndrome.

An exotoxin capable of producing exfoliation in newborn mice was identified and characterized in 1972 by Melish et al. This exfoliative toxin has been particularly associated with coagulase-positive staphylococci of phage group II. The toxin has been shown to be the cause of the so-called staphylococcal scalded skin syndrome, which includes the following conditions: (1) generalized exfoliative disease (Ritter's disease) in infants, (2) toxic epidermal necrolysis (Lyell's disease) in older individuals, (3) localized bullous impetigo, and (4) staphylococcal scarlatiniform eruption. The toxin has a selective effect on the cells of the stratum granulosum epidermis, whereas other cells of the skin remain unaffected.

Other enzymes

Staphylococci form several other extracellular enzymes in vitro. *Leukocidin* is produced by most pathogenic tissue-invading staphylococci and has the capacity to destroy leukocytes in vitro. *Staphylokinase* (fibrinolysin) is formed by most pathogenic coagulase-positive strains. It lyses the coagulase-induced clots by activating plasma plasminogen to the fibrinolytic enzyme plasmin. Four *hemolysins*—alpha, beta, gamma, and delta—are produced by various strains of staphylococci. The most important hemolysin with respect to human infection is alpha hemolysin, which appears to be identical to the lethal necrotizing exotoxin *hyaluronidase*. This spreading factor is formed by more than 90% of strains of staphylococci. The well-known resistance of many strains of staphylococci to penicillin is caused by an enzyme, *penicillinase*, a beta-lactamase that inactivates penicillin by hydrolysis.

Bacteriophage typing

The problem of identifying staphylococci has been aided and clarified by bacteriophage typing. The method consists of determining the patterns of susceptibility of cultures of staphylococci to a series of bacteriophages. Staphylococci to be typed are seeded on the surface of an agar plate. Small amounts of the phages are dropped on the agar surface in an orderly sequence. Incubation is followed by the appearance of distinctive patterns of lysis of the staphylococci at the sites of the phages. These patterns serve to identify related strains and to differentiate types that are unrelated. The 19 basic phages recommended for typing are divided into four groups—groups I, II, III, and IV—each of which possesses considerable specificity. For example, cultures of staphylococci that are lysed by the phages in group II are not lysed by phages in the other groups. Only coagulase-positive staphylococci are susceptible to the typing phages. The method has proved useful in epidemiologic investigations of staphylococcal infections.

Attempts continue to be made to classify staphylococci by serotyping. As yet, however, no clinically useful system has been developed.

PATHOGENESIS AND PATHOLOGY

Staphylococci are ubiquitous organisms. They are part of the normal flora of the human skin and the respiratory and gastrointestinal tracts. About 15% of normal persons are nasal carriers of staphylococci (Tuazon and Sheagren, 1974). The pathogenicity of a particular strain is dependent on the combined effects of the various enzymes and toxins as well as the invasive properties of the strain, which were described previously.

The formation of an abscess is characteristic of staphylococcal infection in man, and the site of invasion is usually the skin. Staphylococci multiply locally and produce hyaluronidase, which increases the permeability of connective tissue and probably serves to promote the spread of these organisms. There is exudation of plasma and migration of granulocytes in large numbers to the scene of action. Rapid necrosis and destruction of tissue usually follow invasion of staphylococci. Thrombosis of the blood vessels and formation of fibrin occur. If the organisms are not consumed and killed during the first inflammatory response, more plasma and phagocytes collect at the site. The fully developed local lesion consists of a central necrotic core filled with dead and dying leukocytes and organisms, surrounded and sharply demarcated by a fibroblastic wall within which lie viable leukocytes and bacteria. Without treatment, the abscess may rupture spontaneously, drain, and eventually heal.

Usually the fibroblastic barrier serves to prevent extension of the infection. Any trauma that breaks this barrier, such as squeezing of a pimple or premature incision of a furuncle, may give rise to a spreading infection, often with bacteremia.

Rogers and Tompsett (1952) showed that coagulase-positive staphylococci may survive for long periods within the cytoplasm of human and rabbit leukocytes and monocytes after phagocytosis. This phenomenon may be an important factor in the mechanism of resistance of antimicrobial agents, or it may interfere with host factors concerned with the destruction of staphylococci.

It has been suggested that the typical walled-off avascular lesion containing the staphylococci accounts for (1) the lack of antibody formation, (2) the persistence of infection, and (3) the failure of antimicrobial agents with high in vitro activity to destroy staphylococci in vivo.

It seems likely that antimicrobial agents along with tissue fluids penetrate the barrier and reach the staphylococci. It does not necessarily follow that effective antistaphylococcal action ensues. Serum proteins and other tissue substances may exert a powerful effect on the antimicrobial agent, the metabolism of the staphylococcus, or both. It has been shown that there is vigorous glycolytic activity with accumulation of large quantities of lactic acid in local inflammatory areas. Glucose levels drop sharply, oxygen is consumed, the carbon dioxide level rises, and the pH falls. It appears possible that such drastic physiologic changes taking place in the lesion may be associated with drug-parasite relationships quite different from those found in vitro. Antimicrobial agents may be inactivated or the staphylococci may be rendered resistant to antimicrobial action in the abscess.

Bacteria in an abscess may also no longer be in the phase of growth, due to the high local concentration of organisms and other metabolic factors. Antimicrobials such as methicillin and oxacillin, which exert their antibacterial effect by interfering with cell wall synthesis, are poorly effective in this setting in which the bacteria are barely multiplying.

Staphylococci tolerant to penicillins and their related antimicrobials may also play a role in the pathology induced by these organisms. Such organisms, originally described by Sabath et al. (1977), have minimal bacterial concentrations (MBCs) that exceed their minimal inhibitory concentrations (MICs) by a factor of at least 32. Growth of these organisms is easily inhibited by drugs such as oxacillin, but the organisms are extremely difficult to kill. This property of resistance of certain staphylococci is entirely separate from beta-lactamase production. There have been several reports of staphylococcal infections that have responded inadequately to proper antibiotic therapy caused by penicillin-tolerant staphylococci (Rajashekaraiah et al., 1980). Therefore, laboratories should be prepared to measure MICs and MBCs of staphylococci from patients whose response to antimicrobials has been poor in the event that the cause of treatment failure is a tolerant organism.

HOST FACTORS

Certain changes in the host may interfere with native resistance and lead to increased incidence of staphylococcal infections. It has been known for a long time that diabetes and staphylococcal infections go hand in hand. Dubos (1953) demonstrated experimentally that in the presence of ketone bodies, the antibacterial action of lactic acid on staphylococci is diminished. There also is evidence that the leukocytes of diabetic patients form less lactic acid from glucose than do leukocytes of normal persons.

Severe nutritional deficiencies and poor skin defenses are known to promote staphylococcal infections. Indwelling catheters, intravascular foreign bodies, and instrumentation may cause a predisposition in the host to staphylococcal bacteremia. Staphylococcal pneumonia may be secondary to a preceding viral infection such as varicella or influenza. The use of corticosteroids may predispose to serious staphylococcal infections.

Patients with chronic granulomatous disease and other functional defects of leukocytes are especially susceptible to staphylococcal infections.

IMMUNITY

Although the sera of most normal adults contain antibodies to the various antigenic components of *S. aureus* and to toxins and enzymes produced by *S. aureus*, evidence is lacking for correlation between the level of any of these antibodies and immunity or susceptibility to disease.

Antibodies seem to play little if any role in host defense against staphylococci. These organisms are mainly controlled by nonspecific complement-mediated phagocytosis by polymorphonuclear leukocytes (Verhoef and Verbrugh, 1981). Patients with defective intracellular killing of bacteria, such as those with chronic granulomatous disease, are therefore at high risk to develop severe staphylococcal infections.

The acquisition of immunity by adult persons, however, is suggested by the changing patterns of disease in relation to age. For example, local abscesses develop in adults more commonly than in infants. Serious forms of infection, such as staphylococcal pneumonia, empyema, septicemia, and osteomyelitis, occur more frequently in infants and children than in older persons. In the preantibiotic era, staphylococcal pneumonia was seldom seen in adults, and then usually as a complication of epidemic influenza. It is true that the incidence of staphylococcal pneumonia in adults has been rising since the advent of antimicrobial agents, but this may be related to factors extraneous to the present argument, such as (1) the intensified use of hospitals for people with major illnesses, particularly elderly persons with debilitating or malignant conditions associated with lowered resistance in general, and (2) exposure of this particular population in hospital to increasing numbers of staphylococci resistant to antimicrobial agents.

CLINICAL MANIFESTATIONS

The clinical manifestations of staphylococcal infections vary with the site of involvement. Thus the same microorganism may cause either a simple benign furuncle, debilitating osteomyelitis, or fulminating septicemia. This discussion of clinical manifestations will be devoted chiefly to staphylococcal pneumonia, osteomyelitis, enterocolitis, scalded skin syndrome, and toxic shock syndrome.

The various infections of the skin and subcutaneous tissue include impetigo, paronychia, furunculosis, and cellulitis. Mastitis and omphalitis are occasionally seen in newborn infants. These minor infections may be followed by serious consequences. During the late 1950s and

early 1960s, many newborn infants developed severe staphylococcal infections as a result of being colonized with virulent organisms in the hospital nursery. For reasons that have never been clear, this form of staphylococcal disease began to disappear in the mid-1960s and has not been a significant problem since that time period.

Staphylococcal meningitis has been referred to in Chapter 15. It is usually seen in newborn infants with hydrocephalus and cerebrospinal fluid (CSF) shunts, or following other neurosurgical procedures. Endocarditis may occur in children with congenital heart disease and after cardiac surgery.

STAPHYLOCOCCAL PNEUMONIA
Clinical manifestations

Staphylococcal pneumonia usually occurs as a primary infection of the respiratory tract. It may also occur as a complication of measles, chickenpox, influenza, or cystic fibrosis of the pancreas. The highest incidence occurs among infants. In older individuals it may occur as a complication of a preceding viral infection, acute bacterial endocarditis, or septic thrombophlebitis; septic emboli may involve the lungs.

The illness usually begins as an upper respiratory tract infection with fever, nasal obstruction or discharge, and cough associated with irritability and anorexia. The symptoms may progress rapidly or gradually to increasing cough, tachypnea, dyspnea, and subcostal retractions. Severe infections in young infants may be manifested by increasing respiratory distress, abdominal distention, pallor, cyanosis, prostration, and possibly death.

The physical findings vary with the type of pulmonary involvement. Staphylococcal infection of the lung may be followed by consolidation, abscess formation, pneumatoceles, empyema, pneumothorax, or pyopneumothorax, either singly or in combination. In children the roentgenographic lesion is apt to appear as multiple cysts because of the characteristic pneumatocele formation. In adults the pulmonary lesions appear as confluent areas of consolidation with rapid progression to abscess formation and cavitation.

Pneumatocele formation is a hallmark of staphylococcal pneumonia. A pneumatocele is thought to be an emphysematous bleb within the pulmonary interstitial tissue, presumably produced as follows: The staphylococci invade the bronchial wall and peribronchiolar tissues, producing inflammation and abscess formation. The perforation of the bronchial wall by the abscess enables air to pass into the interstitial space. A ball-valve effect traps the air, thereby producing a cyst, or pneumatocele. Thus the bleb is a secondary manifestation of the bronchial and peribronchial infection. Pneumatoceles usually clear spontaneously within a variable period of 4 weeks to 4 months.

Pneumothorax results from the rupture of a pneumatocele. Sudden onset of severe dyspnea, cyanosis, prostration, and shock may indicate tension pneumothorax. Empyema occurs as the result of rupture of an abscess into the pleural cavity. Pyopneumothorax develops if the abscess connects with a bronchus. Pneumatoceles,

pneumothorax, empyema, and pyopneumothorax may occur singly or in combination in more than 50% of cases.

The blood picture characteristically reveals an increase in number of polymorphonuclear leukocytes. Occasionally, however, the white blood cell count is normal or low. The roentgenographic findings may reveal rapidly changing infiltrations, pneumatoceles, pneumothorax, empyema, or pyopneumothorax (Fig. 27-2).

Complications

The following conditions may complicate staphylococcal pneumonia.

Congestive heart failure. Severe infections with extensive pulmonary involvement may be complicated by tachycardia, enlarging liver, and increasing rales, all indicative of cardiac decompensation.

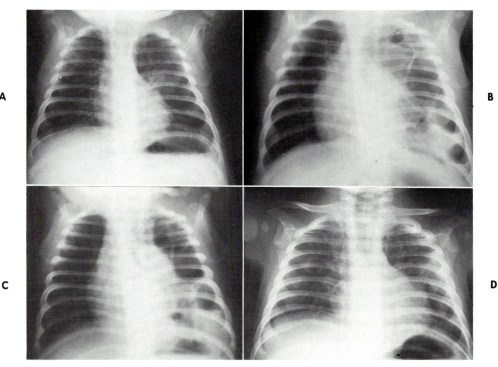

Fig. 27-2. Roentgenograms of E. R., a 3-month-old infant with acute staphylococcal pneumonia, showing the typical progression from consolidation to pneumatocele formation and pyopneumothorax to final resolution. **A,** Roentgenogram taken at admission, Feb. 6, 1958 (third day of illness), showing an area of consolidation in the left midlung field. **B,** Roentgenogram taken Feb. 10, 1958 (seventh day of illness), showing pneumatocele formation and pyopneumothorax. The heart and mediastinum are displaced to the opposite side. **C,** Roentgenogram taken Feb. 28, 1958 (twenty-fifth day of illness), showing pneumatoceles, pyopneumothorax, and shift of mediastinum still present. **D,** Roentgenogram taken March 28, 1958 (fifty-third day of illness), showing considerable clearing.

Fibrothorax. Inadequate drainage of empyema may very rarely be complicated by a fibrothorax.

Diagnosis

A diagnosis of staphylococcal pneumonia is suggested by two or more of the following factors: (1) acute respiratory distress in a young infant, (2) history of recent pyoderma, omphalitis, or mastitis, and (3) roentgenographic evidence of pneumatocele, empyema, or pyopneumothorax.

The staphylococcal etiology is confirmed by the demonstration of a positive blood or empyema fluid culture. A positive throat culture may not be significant because approximately 60% of all newborn infants are carriers of the microorganisms in the nasopharynx. The nasopharyngeal culture would be strongly suggestive, however, if it yields 100% growth of hemolytic S. aureus that is coagulase positive.

Differential diagnosis

The following conditions may simulate staphylococcal pneumonia.

Pneumococcal pneumonia. The pulmonary consolidation in the early stages of staphylococcal pneumonia may resemble pneumococcal infection. The lack of a prompt response to antimicrobial drugs and subsequent roentgenographic evidence of pneumatocele, empyema, or pyopneumothorax favor staphylococcal cause (Fig. 27-2).

Coliform bacillus pneumonia. Pneumonia caused by *Escherichia coli*, *Enterobacter aerogenes*, *Klebsiella pneumoniae*, or *Pseudomonas aeruginosa* may be clinically indistinguishable from staphylococcal infection. A premature infant in Bellevue Hospital acquired pneumonia with roentgenographic evidence of pneumatoceles; this suggested a staphylococcal etiology. Blood and throat cultures, however, were positive for *E. coli*.

Acute bronchiolitis. Acute respiratory disease in an infant, associated with wheezing, tachypnea, and roentgenologic evidence of obstructive emphysema, is more typical of bronchiolitis than of staphylococcal pneumonia.

Cystic fibrosis. Staphylococcal pneumonia may complicate underlying cystic fibrosis. The demonstration of abnormally high levels of sodium and chloride in the sweat would suggest this diagnosis.

Aspiration of foreign body. Pulmonary disease secondary to a nonopaque foreign body may be confused with staphylococcal pneumonia.

Prognosis

Staphylococcal pneumonia in infants was a highly fatal disease before antibacterial drugs were available. The availability and use of effective antistaphylococcal antibiotics have reduced the number of fatalities significantly. In general the younger the infant, the smaller the chance for survival. On the other hand, the prognosis is favorable for older infants and children who have had the benefit of early optimum antimicrobial therapy. The prognosis in complicated patients with underlying problems depends on the prognosis of the associated disease.

In spite of extensive pulmonary involvement, infants who recover usually show no apparent residual pulmonary damage. Pneumatoceles subside completely, and chronic lung abscess is an uncommon sequela. In view of the local pulmonary lesions, however, subsequent bronchiectasis is a possibility.

Treatment

Staphylococcal pneumonia in an infant is an acute medical emergency. *Early*, *optimum*, and *intensive* antimicrobial therapy will considerably improve the chances for survival. Early treatment is particularly important because of the rapidity with which staphylococci produce focal necrosis of tissues. Delay in therapy may be followed by an irreversible chronic suppurative process. Optimum therapy includes the proper dose of the appropriate antibiotic and surgical drainage of an abscess cavity, that is, empyema, if present. Intensive prolonged therapy is necessary because staphylococci tend to persist in tissues, thereby providing a potential focus for relapse.

Antimicrobial therapy. A physician responsible for the care of an infant with staphylococcal pneumonia is faced with a dilemma. Many antistaphylococcal agents are available for the treatment of the disease. The selection of drugs for initial therapy will have a profound effect on the course of the disease. The various antistaphylococcal drugs and recommended doses for the treatment of severe staphylococcal infections are listed on p. 562.

A severe staphylococcal infection should be assumed to be caused by penicillin-resistant, coagulase-positive microorganisms until proved otherwise. Accordingly, initial therapy should be with a penicillinase-resistant penicillin such as oxacillin or methicillin. There appear to be increasing numbers of methicillin-resistant staphylococci, however, particularly among hospital-acquired organisms. Therefore, consideration should be given to the use of vancomycin as initial therapy for patients who are very ill and in certain clinical situations such as hospital-acquired infection. Even if a staphylococcus appears to be sensitive to cephalosporins in vitro, these drugs may be poorly effective against staphylococci if they are methicillin resistant (Sheagren, 1984). Methicillin-resistant staphylococci are also resistant to clindamycin. Rifampin, which enters phagocytic cells, is effective against many staphylococci. It may therefore be particularly useful for patients with chronic granulomatous disease. Patients infected with tolerant organisms (an equal to or greater than 32-fold difference between MIC and MBC) may require treatment with two bactericidal antibiotics, particularly if the initial response to therapy is poor.

The duration of antimicrobial therapy must be individualized for each patient. It may vary between 2 weeks and 2 months and will depend on the sensitivity of the organism, the extent and character of the pulmonary involvement, and the presence or absence of complications. A relapse is likely to occur if therapy is discontinued too soon. Measurement of antibodies to teichoic acid may be helpful in deciding whether to stop or to continue antibiotics; ideally these antibodies should be measured early in the course of the infection, somewhat later, and when discontinuation of therapy is being considered. The presence of these antibodies after a course of therapy suggests continuing disease and the likelihood of occult metastatic abscesses. Measurement of these antibodies is also useful in patients with staphylococcal bacteremia, endocarditis with negative blood cultures, and those with deep tissue infections that are not accessible to culturing such as osteomyelitis (Sheagren, 1984).

Supportive therapy. Infants with severe staphylococcal pneumonia should be placed in a Croupette in an atmosphere of high humidity level and, if necessary, high oxygen content. Some patients will require mechanical ventilation. Hydration must often be maintained by

parenteral routes. Anemia that may develop during the course of the infection should be corrected by blood transfusion.

Treatment of complications. The complications of staphylococcal pneumonia may be treated as follows.

Pneumatocele. Pneumatocele usually clears up spontaneously. As a rule, there is no need for needle aspiration or surgical intervention. The blebs usually disappear over a period of weeks or months (Fig. 27-2). If the bullae cause mechanical compression of the trachea or main bronchi, however, aspiration or excision may be necessary.

Empyema and pyopneumothorax. The preferred treatment of empyema and pyopneumothorax is *early* closed suction drainage, which is best accomplished by the intercostal insertion of a catheter with the patient under local anesthesia. This procedure is much more satisfactory than repeated aspirations. It relieves respiratory distress due to either tension pneumothorax or massive empyema. Evacuation of the pleural space promotes reexpansion of the compressed lung.

Fibrothorax. Surgical intervention (decortication) for a fibrothorax is rarely necessary. It usually subsides spontaneously after a variable period of time. When there is doubt, it is best to defer decortication until it has been shown to be definitely indicated.

• • •

In summary, infants with acute staphylococcal pneumonia may either be a medical or surgical emergency. Optimum antimicrobial therapy instituted early, and suction drainage instituted promptly in the event of a tension pneumothorax, may be lifesaving procedures.

ACUTE STAPHYLOCOCCAL OSTEOMYELITIS

The incidence of osteomyelitis in infants and children has decreased considerably in recent years. The clinical manifestations may be preceded by trauma, pyoderma, varicella, or other antecedent infections. Physical findings will depend on the site and degree of involvement; localized tenderness and swelling are important signs. Although any bone may be affected, the femur, tibia, and humerus are the most frequent sites. In infants under 1 year of age osteomyelitis is commonly accompanied by pyogenic arthritis.

Treatment includes antimicrobial therapy and surgical drainage. After a period of parenteral antibiotics, it is possible to continue therapy with oral medication in certain patients. Further discussion on osteomyelitis may be found in Chapter 18.

STAPHYLOCOCCAL ENTEROCOLITIS

Staphylococcal enterocolitis (pseudomembranous enterocolitis; postantibiotic diarrhea) was a well-known entity prior to the antibiotic era; however, the intensive use of broad-spectrum antibacterial drugs has undoubtedly increased the incidence of this disease. It is now recognized that this illness may not only be caused by staphylococci but also (and possibly more frequently) by *Clostridium difficile*.

Staphylococci are normal inhabitants of the gastrointestinal tract, but they are present in small numbers. Antimicrobial agents that inhibit the normal intestinal flora create fertile soil for the multiplication of resistant strains of staphylococci. The enteritis is thought to be caused by two factors: (1) presence of an antimicrobial-resistant enterotoxigenic strain of hemolytic *S. aureus* and (2) suppression of the normal bacterial flora in the feces. Enteritis need not occur, however, despite the presence of both factors.

Clinical manifestations

The severe illness is characterized by copious watery diarrhea associated with high fever, weakness, nausea, vomiting, abdominal distention, mental confusion, shock, and, occasionally, death. On the other hand, the symptoms may be mild, subsiding spontaneously within a short period of time.

Complications

Shock and dehydration resulting from excessive fluid loss are the complications that are probably responsible for most of the deaths.

Diagnosis

The diagnosis is confirmed by demonstration of a predominance of staphylococci on smear and culture of stool.

Differential diagnosis

Postantibiotic diarrhea may also be caused by *C. difficile*, which is diagnosed by isolation of this organism from the stool and/or detection of

clostridial toxin in feces. Staphylococcal food poisoning, which is a separate entity, can easily be differentiated because of its epidemic nature; in this condition, the formation of staphylococcal enterotoxin has taken place in the contaminated food before ingestion. Detailed aspects of other forms of gastroenteritis are discussed in Chapter 9.

Prognosis

Early diagnosis and prompt therapy will improve the prognosis considerably. In severe cases there may be a rapid progression from dehydration to shock to death.

Treatment

As soon as staphylococcal enterocolitis is recognized, use of the offending broad-spectrum antibiotic should be discontinued. In mild cases the normal bacterial flora will return and the symptoms will subside rapidly. In severe cases, however, the dehydration should be rapidly corrected, and specific antimicrobial therapy should be instituted. Antistaphylococcal drugs such as oral vancomycin as indicated on p. 562 are frequently used to treat enterocolitis caused by staphylococci or clostridia. Eradication of *Staphylococcus* organisms is generally followed by improvement.

STAPHYLOCOCCAL FOOD POISONING

Food poisoning caused by *S. aureus* follows the ingestion of preformed enterotoxin. The toxin itself is not produced by *S. aureus* within the gastrointestinal tract. Staphylococci are common causes of food poisoning in the United States. Certain foods, particularly custard-filled pastries, when left at room temperature for several hours, provide fertile soil for the growth of staphylococci and the formation of enterotoxin.

Clinical manifestations

The illness has an explosive onset approximately 1 to 6 hours after the contaminated food has been ingested. Severe cases are characterized by nausea, vomiting, severe abdominal cramps, profuse diarrhea, prostration, and even shock. Occasionally the symptoms are milder. Generally the temperature is normal or subnormal. The patient improves within 8 to 24 hours, but weakness may persist for several days.

Diagnosis

The short incubation period and multiple cases are highly suggestive of this disease. No practical laboratory test is available to confirm the diagnosis. The epidemiologic circumstances, however, usually provide adequate confirmatory evidence.

Prognosis

Rapid uncomplicated recovery is the rule. Fatalities are rare.

Treatment

Patients with severe cases require parenteral administration of fluids, treatment for shock, and analgesics for pain.

STAPHYLOCOCCAL SCALDED SKIN SYNDROME

Staphylococcal scalded skin syndrome, described by Melish and Glasgow in 1970 and 1971, includes a spectrum of diseases of the skin caused by phage types I and II coagulase-positive staphylococci that elaborate an exfoliative toxin.

The following description of the syndrome by Melish and Glasgow (1970) stems from their experience with at least 28 patients.

The newborn infants with generalized disease followed a similar clinical course [Fig. 27-3]. They had the abrupt onset of generalized erythema with "sandpaper" texture of the involved skin, increased erythema in skin creases similar to Pastia's lines and marked tenderness of the skin surface. Within 2 days, and often within a few hours, the upper layer of the epidermis remained wrinkled after light stroking, resulting in the characteristic Nikolsky sign. Shortly thereafter, large, flaccid bullae filled with clear fluid appeared. The epidermis separated in large sheets, revealing a moist, red, glistening surface. Within 48 hours the exfoliated areas dried, and large, thick seborrheic flakes appeared over these areas and around the mouth [Fig. 27-4]. The secondary desquamation continued for 3 to 5 days. Phage Group II staphylococci were cultured from the skin surface and from distant sites in all these patients.

The patients with staphylococcal scarlatiniform disease had generalized erythema, sandpaper skin texture and diffuse tenderness. The early course was indistinguishable from that of the patients in the previous group, but in none of these patients did exfoliation develop. After 1 or 2 days of erythema, cracks appeared in skin creases and about the eyes and

mouth. This was followed by the appearance of the large, thick seborrhea-like flakes over nearly the entire skin surface. This flaky desquamation continued for 3 to 5 days. Although in the early course of the disease the skin changes were identical with those in streptococcal scarlet fever, there were important clinical differences. There was no strawberry tongue or palatal enanthem, and the throat cultures were negative for streptococci. The patterns of desquamation were also markedly different, desquamation in scarlet fever occurring later with fine, branny flakes or thin sheets of skin. Phage Group 2 staphylococci were cultured from all these patients. Two patients had purulent staphylococcal conjunctivitis immediately before the rash appeared.*

STAPHYLOCOCCAL TOXIC SHOCK SYNDROME

Toxic shock syndrome (TSS) has been described in detail by Todd et al. (1978), who observed seven children, 8 to 17 years of age, with this severe disease. The illness was characterized by an acute onset of high fever, headache, confusion, and a scarletiniform rash. Other manifestations included sore throat, vomiting, watery diarrhea, decreased urine output, hepatic abnormalities, evidence of disseminated intravascular coagulation (DIC), and shock. These findings were associated with the isolation of a toxin-producing strain of phage group I S. aureus from various mucosal surfaces and abscess sites. The toxin produced by this organism was shown to be biochemically and immunologically distinct from phage group II staphylococcal exfoliative toxin, which is responsible for the scalded skin syndrome. It is now recognized to be enterotoxin F (formerly also termed pyrogenic exotoxin C). It is not known whether the toxin acts directly on host tissues or enhances endotoxin effects on these tissues. The staphylococcal infection itself is often minor and may go unnoticed (Sheagren, 1984).

Skin biopsy demonstrates the different histologic effects of staphylococcal toxins in TSS and the scalded skin syndrome. In TSS, epidermal cleavage occurs in the basilar layers. In the scalded skin syndrome, cleavage occurs in the middle layers of the epidermis. In toxic epidermal necrolysis (TEN), an exfoliative syndrome often due to drug therapy or a viral infection,

---

*Melish ME, Glasgow LA: N Engl J Med 1970;282:1114.

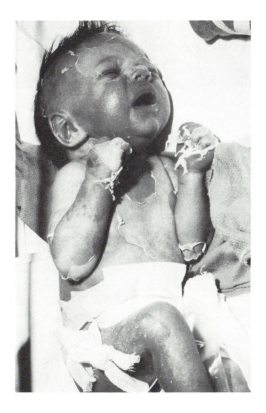

Fig. 27-3. Newborn infant with scalded-skin syndrome in exfoliative stage. (From Melish ME, Glasgow LA. Reprinted by permission of New England Journal of Medicine 1970;282:1114.)

Fig. 27-4. Two-year-old girl in the resolving phase of the scalded-skin syndrome undergoing secondary desquamation. There are large, thick flakes of dried skin concentrated particularly about the mouth. (From Melish ME, Glasgow LA. Reprinted by permission of the New England Journal of Medicine 1970;282:1114.)

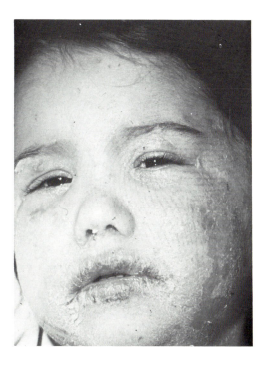

cleavage is beneath the basilar layer of the epidermis. For very ill patients in whom the clinical picture is unclear, a skin biopsy may be helpful for diagnosis.

The following case report by Todd et al. (1978) highlights the extraordinary clinical manifestations of TSS.

CASE 1. Patient 5 was a white girl, aged 15 years 9 months, who entered the Children's Hospital, Denver, on September 25, 1977, delirious and in shock after a 2-day history of worsening pharyngitis and vaginitis, associated with vomiting and watery diarrhea. On admission her temperature was 40.9° C [105.6° F] and her blood pressure was 66/0 mm Hg. She had very injected conjunctivae, a diffuse erythroderma covering her entire body, facial and limb edema, abdominal guarding, and a purulent vaginal discharge. She was confused and aggressive; there were no localizing or meningeal signs.

The initial white cell count was 18,800/µl (32% segmented neutrophils, 59% nonsegmented neutrophils); the initial platelet count of 270,000/µl later fell to 18,000/µl. Her urine contained protein (3+ proteinuria), pus cells (7-10 cells/high power field), and occasional red blood cells. Her blood urea was 41 mg/dl, and her serum creatinine was 2.5 mg/dl. The bilirubin and SGOT concentrations were slightly raised. The arterial Po_2 in room air was 44 mm Hg, the Pco_2 was 24 mm Hg, and the pH was 7.25. The chest x-ray showed bilateral interstitial and early alveolar infiltrates suggestive of "shock lung." Multiple specimens were taken for bacterial and viral cultures, and the patient was given intravenous fluids, antibiotics, parenteral steroids, heparin, isoproterenol, digitalis, and controlled ventilation with increased end expiratory pressure.

Her illness was marked by persistent hypotension and acidosis, oliguria, and disseminated intravascular coagulation with severe thrombocytopenia. A skin biopsy showed no abnormalities. With intensive care she gradually improved; her blood pressure stabilized, the fever and rash subsided, and by the sixth hospital day she was alert and awake and extubated. She had fully recovered by the eighth day except for necrosis of parts of the distal phalanges of her left foot and the skin of her left forearm. Fine desquamation of the face, trunk, and extremities had started on the third hospital day and progressed to marked peeling of the palms and soles by the fourteenth hospital day.

A throat culture taken at admission gave a heavy growth of *Staph. aureus* (phage type 29/52/80), as did her vaginal culture. All other cultures, including those of blood, cerebrospinal fluid, and urine, were sterile. Antistaphylococcal therapy was given for 21 days. The patient was discharged on the seventeenth hospital day. Parts of the third and fifth toe on the left foot had to be amputated because of gangrene.*

Special susceptibility to TSS has been reported in a group of young women using tampons during their menstrual periods. Since the original description of the syndrome, it has been appreciated that menstruating women are the predominant population at risk, probably related to staphylococcal colonization of the genitourinary tract and tampon usage.

Antibiotics do not influence the course of the illness. There is some evidence that patients who develop the syndrome lack antibodies to enterotoxin F. Thus vaccine development and treatment with specific antiserum are theoretically possible (Sheagren, 1984).

ENDOCARDITIS

Acute bacterial endocarditis is a fulminant highly fatal disease, seen mainly in adults, in which valves on the left side of the heart are involved. Physicians who care for children and adolescents are more likely to encounter patients with staphylococcal endocarditis involving valves of the right side of the heart. This illness is much less fulminant; it is almost always seen in parenteral drug abusers. Complications include septic emboli to the lungs as well as to the meninges, joints, and kidneys.

MENINGOCOCCEMIA-LIKE DISEASE

Certain staphylococci have the ability to activate the complement and coagulation systems; bacteremia with one of these strains can result in an illness that resembles meningococcemia. Therefore it has been recommended that patients presenting with signs and symptoms of septic shock and disseminated intravascular coagulation in whom the causative organism cannot immediately be identified have included in their therapy a penicillinase-resistant antimicrobial pending definitive culture results (Sheagren, 1984).

TRACHEITIS

Tracheitis caused by staphylococci was described in 1979 by Jones et al. This illness causes

---

*From Todd J, Fishaut M, Karpel F, Welch T. Lancet 1978;2:1116.

obstruction of the upper airway and may be mistaken for croup or epiglottitis. Subglottic edema is present along with purulent tracheal secretions and high fever. The most important aspect of therapy is maintenance of a clear airway. The role of antibiotics in treatment of this disease has not yet been established, but usually antistaphylococcal drugs are employed.

DIAGNOSIS

Standard microbiologic techniques such as culture and Gram stain are satisfactory for diagnosis of most staphylococcal infections. Gram stains of exudates from staphylococcal infections characteristically reveal organisms in grapelike clusters along with inflammatory cells.

As has been mentioned, assay for antibodies to teichoic acid has proved useful for further evaluation of patients with staphylococcal bacteremia and other deep-seated staphylococcal infections, especially with regard to decisions concerning termination of therapy. This may be accomplished by gel diffusion or more rapidly by enzyme immunosorbent assay (Thisyakorn et al., 1984). Another useful diagnostic tool is the lysostaphin-sensitivity test, which permits rapid differentiation between coagulase-positive and coagulase-negative staphylococci in blood cultures (Sheagren, 1984). This test may be particularly helpful in differentiating between staphylococcal infection and a contaminated blood culture.

EPIDEMIOLOGIC FACTORS

Human carriers of staphylococci are common, but staphylococcal disease is rare. Most healthy adults carry coagulase-positive staphylococci in the nose or on the skin. The nasal carrier state varies, according to Miles et al. (1944), "not with the environment of the person, but with the person himself. There is a marked tendency for persons to be either persistent carriers or persistently free from nasal *Staphylococcus aureus*."* Staphylococci discharged into the air remain viable on sheets and blankets, are disseminated in dust, and can be recovered from the air of hospital wards and operating rooms when people are present. As a rule, such carrier strains are epidemiologically dangerous only for patients with open wounds or persons with lowered resistance. On the other hand, there is suggestive evidence that a person with acute illness caused by staphylococci is a more dangerous source of infection than a healthy carrier. Barber and Burston (1955) observed that, although most of the nurses in a maternity unit carried a single phage type of staphylococcus in the nose, few infections occurred. The development of a facial boil in a nurse working in the unit was promptly followed by two severe infections in infants in the nursery. The phage type of staphylococci recovered from the furuncle and from the infected infants was the same as that which had been carried by the nurses and infants for months.

Direct transmission of staphylococcal infection from carrier to recipient probably seldom takes place by means of droplets expelled from the nose. Indirect routes appear more likely, the first step being contamination of the skin and clothing of the carrier. Staphylococci may then reach a recipient who touches the carrier, contaminated bedding, or towels. The microorganisms may also reach a recipient through airborne particles released from the carrier's skin or clothing by friction, movement, or washing.

The present-day hospital is a major source of serious staphylococcal infections. The increasing incidence of infections in hospitals caused by staphylococci resistant to antimicrobial agents has been widely observed. Since the early 1940s the incidence of penicillin-resistant strains detected in hospital patients has steadily risen from between 0% and 12% to 100%. Nonhospitalized persons also rarely yield penicillin-sensitive strains of staphylococci.

Staphylococci are endowed with a striking ability to adapt to changes in their environment produced by antimicrobial agents. The selective emergence of strains resistant to antimicrobial agents in general has followed the use of each antistaphylococcal drug. Strains of *S. aureus* and *S. epidermidis* resistant to methicillin and oxacillin are becoming problems in some hospitals, especially in intensive care units. At this time such organisms are almost invariably sensitive to vancomycin, but it is obvious that newer drugs for control of staphylococci will have to be developed in the future.

---

*From Miles AA, Williams REO, Clayton-Cooper B. J Pathol Bacteriol 1944;56:513.

Staphylococcal food poisoning

Staphylococci can multiply in a variety of foods, and refrigeration is essential to prevent elaboration of toxin. Contamination of food is usually not suspected until after illness occurs. Presumably contamination may occur from multiple potential sources, including persons harboring organisms.

PREVENTIVE MEASURES

The ubiquity of staphylococci, their ready adaptability, and the nature of the parasite-host relationship make it difficult to control human staphylococcal infections.

Measures in hospitals

Since there is little eivdence that healthy persons carrying staphylococci in the nose are primarily responsible for transmitting infection even to premature and newly born infants (potentially the most susceptible recipients), masks are not recommended. Washing the hands with a detergent before and after handling patients and putting on a clean gown before entering the ward are recommended for all persons.

It is most important to exclude from hospitals all persons with acute staphylococcal infections of the skin or mucous membranes, who may be shedding particularly virulent staphylococci. The topical application of antistaphylococcal creams and ointments for the control of organisms carried in the nose or skin is not advisable.

In view of the possibility of airborne infection in the newborn and premature infant nurseries, the following preventive measures are suggested:

1. All infant beds and bassinets should be thoroughly decontaminated after being occupied by newborn infants. Soiled nursery linen should be autoclaved.
2. No *dry* sweeping, dusting, or cleaning should be permitted.
3. Prophylactic use of antimicrobial agents is not recommended.
4. Guidelines for care and maintenance of respiratory equipment should be made and strictly adhered to.

Bacterial interference

A bacterial interference measure proved useful for control of staphylococcal infections in newborn infants in the late 1950s and early 1960s. A penicillin-sensitive, relatively nonpathogenic strain of *S. aureus* (502A) was implanted on the nasal mucosa and umbilical stumps of newborn infants. This artificial colonization served to prevent natural colonization with epidemic pathologic strains, thereby interrupting the chain of transmission from infant to infant (Shinefield et al., 1963a-d). A similar strategy also proved useful in interrupting transmission of staphylococcal infections in families (Fine et al., 1967).

This measure is rarely used today. It is not without hazard, since occasional infants implanted with 502A have been reported to develop fatal sepsis (Houck et al., 1972). Nevertheless, it is a measure that might potentially be useful in the future, should outbreaks of staphylococcal disease due to resistant organisms again become a problem in newborn nurseries.

Prevention of food poisoning

Persons with obvious staphylococcal infections of the skin, especially of the hands, should be excluded temporarily from the preparation or handling of food. Sliced and chopped meats, custards, and cream fillings should be refrigerated promptly to avoid multiplication of staphylococci accidentally introduced. Pastries should be filled with custard immediately before sale, or there should be adequate heating of the finished product. All leftover foods should be refrigerated promptly.

Antimicrobial prophylaxis

One or two doses of vancomycin or a second generation cephalosporin such as cefazolin are at times administered to patients just prior to surgery of the abdomen, pelvis, or head and neck and in patients with prosthetic heart valves or patches to prevent wound infection and/or endocarditis. While the frequency of prosthetic valve endocarditis has decreased since the introduction of antistaphylococcal prophylaxis, controlled studies have not indicated that these measures are effective (Van Scoy and Wilkowske, 1983). The potential risks of allergic reactions, emergence of resistant bacterial strains, and superinfection must be weighed against potential benefits to the patient (Hirschmann and Inui, 1980).

REFERENCES

Barber M, Burston J. Antibody resistant staphylococcal infection: a study of antibiotic sensitivity in relation to phage types. Lancet 1955;2:578.

Barton LL, Feigin RD. Childhood cervical lymphadenitis. J Pediatr 1974;84:846.

Beaven DW. Staphylococcal pneumonia in the newborn: an epidemic of 8 fatal cases. Lancet 1956;2:211.

Blair JE. The staphylococci. In Dubos R, ed. Bacterial and mycotic infections of man, ed 3. Philadelphia: JB Lippincott Co., 1958, 310.

Boris M, Shinefield HR, Ribble JC, Eichenwald HF. Bacterial interference: its effect on nursery-acquired infection with *Staphylococcus aureus*. IV. Louisiana epidemic. Am J Dis Child 1963;105:674.

Brigg JN. Staphylococcic pneumonia in infants and young children. Can Med Assoc J 1957;76:269.

Campbell JA, Gastineau DC, Velios F. Roentgen studies in suppurative pneumonia of infants and children. JAMA 1954;154:468.

Dearing WH. Micrococcic enteritis and pseudomembranous enterocolitis as complications of antibiotic therapy. Ann NY Acad Sci 1956;65:235.

Disney ME, Wolff J, Wood BSB. Staphylococcal pneumonia in infants. Lancet 1956;1:767.

Drutz AJ, Van Way MH, Schaffner W, Koenig MG. Bacterial interference in the therapy of recurrent staphylococcal infections. Multiple abscesses due to the implanation of the 502A strain of staphylococcus. N Engl J Med 1966;275:1161.

Dubos RJ. Effect of ketone bodies and other metabolites on the survival and multiplication of staphylococci and tubercle bacilli. J Exp Med 1953;98:145.

Dutton AAC, Elines PC. Vancomycin: report on treatment of patients with severe staphylococcal infections. Br Med J 1959;1:1144.

Faden HS, Burke JP, Glasgow LA, Everett JR. Nursery outbreak of scalded-skin syndrome. Am J Dis Child 1976;130:265.

Fine RN, Onslow JM, Erwin ML, Cohen JO. Bacterial interference in the treatment of recurrent staphylococcal infections in a family. J Pediatr 1967;70:548.

Fisher JH, Swenson O. Surgical complications of staphylococcic pneumonia. Pediatrics 1957;20:835.

Forbes GB, Emerson GL. Staphylococcal pneumonia and empyema. Pediatr Clin North Am 1957;4:215.

Green M, Nyhan WL Jr, Fousek MD. Acute hematogenous osteomyelitis. Pediatrics 1956;16:368.

Hirschmann JV, Inui TS. Antimicrobial prophylaxis: a critique of recent trials. Rev Infect Dis 1980;2:1-23.

Hieber JP, Davis AT. Staphylococcal cervical adenitis in young infants. Pediatrics 1976;57:424.

Houck PW, Nelson JD, Kay JL. Fatal septicemia due to *Staphylococcus aureus* 502A: report of a case and review of the infectious complications of bacterial interference programs. Am J Dis Child 1972;123:45-48.

Jeljaszewicz J, ed. Proceedings of the Third International Symposium on Staphylococci and Staphylococcal infections. New York: Springer-Verlag, 1976.

Johnson AD, Metzger JF, Spero L. Production, purification and chemical characterization of *Staphylococcus aureus* exfoliative toxin. Infect Immun 1975;12:1206.

Jones R, Santos JI, Overall JC. Bacterial tracheitis, JAMA 1979;242:721-726.

Kayser FH. Methicillin-resistant staphylococci. Lancet 1975;2:650.

Klein JO, Finland M. The new penicillins. N Engl J Med 1963;269:1019, 1074, 1129.

Knight V, Holzer AR. Studies on staphylococci from hospital patients. I. Predominance of strains of group III phage patterns which are resistant to multiple antibodies. J Clin Invest 1954;33:1190.

Krugman S, Ward R. Air sterilization in an infant's ward. Effect of triethylene glycol vapor and dust-suppressive measures on the respiratory cross infection rate. JAMA 1951;145:775.

Le CT, Lewin EB. Teichoic acid serology in staphylococcal infections of infants and children. J Pediatr 1978;93:572.

Light IJ, Sutherland JM, Schott JE. Control of staphylococcal outbreak in nursery: use of bacterial interference. JAMA 1965;193:699.

Lindskog GE. Present-day management of pleural empyema in infants and adults. N Engl J Med 1956;225:320.

Lyell AA. A review of toxic epidermal necrolysis in Britain. Br J Dermatol 1967;79:662.

Melish ME, Glasgow LA. The staphylococcal scalded-skin syndrome: development of an experimental model. N Engl J Med 1970;282:1114.

Melish ME, Glasgow LA. The staphylococcal scalded skin syndrome: the expanded clinical syndrome. J Pediatr 1971;78:958.

Melish ME, Glasgow LA, Turner MD. The staphylococcal scalded-skin syndrome: isolation and partial characterization of the exfoliative toxin. J Infect Dis 1972;125:129.

Miles AA, Williams REO, Clayton-Cooper B. Carriage of *Staphylococcus aureus (pyogenes)* in man and its relation to wound infections. J Pathol Bacteriol 1944;56:513.

Pildes RS, Ramamurthy RS, Vidyasagar D. Effect of triple dye on staphylococcal colonization in the newborn infant. J Pediatr 1973;82:978.

Prober CG. Oral antibiotic therapy for bone and joint infections. Pediatr Infect Dis 1982;1:8-10.

Pryles CV. Staphylococcal pneumonia in infancy and childhood: an analysis of 24 cases. Pediatrics 1958;21:609.

Rajashekaraiah KR, Rice T, Rao VS, et al. Clinical significance of tolerant strains of *S. aureus* in patients with endocarditis. Ann Intern Med 1980;93:796-801.

Rammelkamp CH Jr, Lebovitz JL. The role of coagulase in staphylococcal infections. Ann NY Acad Sci 1956;65:144.

Rebhan AW, Edwards HE. Staphylococcal pneumonia: a review of 329 cases. Can Med Assoc J 1960;82:513.

Rogers DE, Tompsett R. The survival of staphylococci within human leukocytes. J Exp Med 1952;95:209.

Sabath LD, Wheeler N, Laverdiere M. A new type of penicillin resistance of *Staphylococcus aureus*. Lancet 1977;1:443-447.

Shaffer TE, Baldwin JN, Rheins MS, Sylvester RF. Staphylococcal infections in newborn infants. I. Study of an epidemic among infants and nursing mothers. Pediatrics 1956;18:750.

Sheagren JN. *Staphylococcus aureus:* the presistent pathogen. N Engl J Med 1984;310:1368-1373, 1439-1442.

Shinefield HR, Ribble JC, Boris M, Eichenwald HF. Bacterial interference: its effect on nursery-acquired infection with *Staphylococcus aureus*. I. Preliminary observations on artificial colonization of newborns. Am J Dis Child 1963a;105:646.

Shinefield HR, Sutherland JM, Ribble JC, Eichenwald HF. Bacterial interference: its effect on nursery-acquired infections with *Staphylococcus aureus*. II. Ohio epidemic. Am J Dis Child 1963b;105:655.

Shinefield HR, et al. Bacterial interference: its effect on nursery-acquired infection with *Staphylococcus aureus*. V. Analysis and interpretation. Am J Dis Child 1963c; 105:683.

Shinefield HR, et al. Bacterial interference: its effect on nursery-acquired infection with *Staphylococcus aureus*. III. Georgia epidemic. Am J Dis Child 1963d;105:663.

Shinefield HR, et al. Interactions of staphylococcal colonization: influence of normal nasal flora and antimicrobials on inoculated *Staphylococcus aureus* strain 502A. Am J Dis Child 1965;111:11.

Simon JH, Rantz LA. The newer penicillins. I. Bacteriological and clinical pharmacological investigations with methicillin and oxacillin. Ann Intern Med 1962;57:335. II. Clinical experiences with methicillin and oxacillin. Ann Intern Med 1962;57:344.

Clinical experiences with methicillin and oxacillin. Ann Intern Med 1962;57:344.

Thisyakorn U, Shelton S, Tzou-yien, et al. Detection of teichoic antibodies in children with staphylococcal infection. Pediatr Infect Dis 1984;3:222-225.

Todd J, Fishaut M, Kapral F, Welch T. Toxic shock syndrome associated with phage-group-1 staphylococci. Lancet 1978;2:116.

Tuazon CU, Sheagren JN. Increased staphylococcal carrier rate among narcotic addicts. J Infect Dis 1974;129:725-727.

Van Scoy RE, Wilkowske CJ. Prophylactic use of antimicrobial agents. Mayo Clin Proc 1983;58:241-245.

Verhoef J, Verbrugh HA. Host determinants in staphylococcal disease. Annu Rev Med 1981;32:107-122.

Wallman IS, Godfrey RC, Watson JRH. Staphylococcal pneumonia in infancy. Br Med J 1955;2:1423.

Wilkinson BJ, Kim Y, Peterson PK. Factors affecting complement activation by *S. aureus* cell walls, their components, and mutants altered in teichoic acid. Infect Immun 1981;32:216-224

28

STREPTOCOCCAL INFECTIONS, GROUP A, INCLUDING SCARLET FEVER

Group A hemolytic streptococci are responsible for a large variety of infections in childhood, including streptococcal tonsillitis or pharyngitis, scarlet fever, and erysipelas. The type of infection induced depends on a variety of factors, including (1) the properties of the particular type of streptococcus, (2) the portal of entry, and (3) host factors, such as age and immune status. The infections are characterized by fever, constitutional symptoms, inflammatory or purulent lesions at the portal of entry, leukocytosis, and sequelae such as rheumatic fever and acute glomerulonephritis.

ETIOLOGY

Streptococci pathogenic for humans are for the most part members of group A. These microorganisms are characterized by their tendency to grow in chains. The capsules are composed largely of hyaluronic acid. Loss of the capsule by desiccation is thought to account for lability of these organisms, explaining why transmission by fomites is rare. The optimal temperature for growth of the streptococcus is 37° C; it is inhibited at temperatures above 40° C.

The serologic grouping of hemolytic streptococci is based on the presence of group-specific antigens, designated as C carbohydrates. Lancefield (1933) identified 12 groups, A through L. Although group A streptococci are responsible for most human infections, occasionally other groups may be associated with disease in man. Grouping is achieved by means of the precipitin technique (Lancefield, 1933) or by a fluorescent antibody (FA) method. Group A streptococci may also be differentiated from other groups by a nonserologic procedure described in 1953 by Maxted, who used bacitracin in a simple antibiotic plate method. The principle of this test is that group A strains are more sensitive to bacitracin than other groups of streptococci. Growth of most group A strains is inhibited by a 0.01 unit bacitracin disk. In an analysis of 12,560 strains, the bacitracin test agreed with the precipitin test in 95.8% of cases (Moody, 1972). Grouping by immunofluorescence tests provides similar agreement with precipitin assays.

The major component of the bacterial cell wall is group A carbohydrate, which has antigenic components that cross react with glycoprotein from human cardiac valves (Goldstein et al., 1968).

The most important surface protein is the M protein; it determines the type specificity of group A streptococci. More than 60 types have been identified. In addition, M proteins play an important role in virulence. They inhibit the phagocytosis of streptococci by host leukocytes by obscuring the C_3b receptor. This antiphagocytic effect can be neutralized by specific antibody. Cross protection between different types does not occur, and M proteins are also poorly antigenic in man. Two additional protein antigens, T and R, have no role in virulence or protection.

The inner layer of the cell wall is composed of mucopeptide or peptidoglycan; injection of this material intravenously into rabbits induces carditis, suggesting that this substance too may be involved in the pathogenesis of acute rheumatic fever (Rotta and Bednat, 1969).

Group A hemolytic streptococci secrete a number of toxins and enzymes such as streptokinase, deoxyribonuclease, streptolysin S and O, hyaluronidase, and erythrogenic toxin. Streptolysins cause beta hemolysis observed on blood agar cultures. Infection with streptococci that elaborate any of these substances is also followed by the production of specific antibodies for the substance, such as antistreptokinase, antideoxyribonuclease, and antistreptolysins S and O, hyaluronidase, and erythrogenic antitoxin. The measurement of these antibodies may be used as an aid to diagnosis. Antistreptolysin O, for example, is present in high titer in the serum of most patients recovering from a recent streptococcal infection. The streptozyme test measures antibodies not only to streptolysin O but also to nicotinamide dinucleotidase, streptokinase, and other unspecified streptococcal antigens using a single reagent, sheep erythrocytes coated with extracellular products from cultured streptococci (Janeff et al., 1971).

The erythrogenic toxin is responsible for the rash of scarlet fever. The identification of three immunologically distinct rash-producing toxins explains the occasional occurrence of several episodes of scarlet fever in the same person (Zabriskie, 1964; Watson and Kim, 1970). Production of erythrogenic toxin is mediated by lysogeny (Zabriskie, 1964).

PATHOLOGY

The local lesions caused by the hemolytic streptococcus show the characteristic inflammatory reaction of hyperemia, edema, and polymorphonuclear cell infiltration. In scarlet fever the pathogenic changes are due to both the toxin and the microorganism. There is generalized lymphoid hyperplasia. Some cases reveal the characteristic findings of acute glomerulonephritis. The skin during the height of the rash shows signs of hyperemia, edema, and polymorphonuclear cell infiltrates in the corium.

EPIDEMIOLOGIC FACTORS

People of all ages, sexes, and races are susceptible to streptococcal infections. The incidence varies with age according to the clinical type of infection. In general, however, it is low-est in infancy, begins to rise gradually thereafter, and reaches a peak just before adolescence. In the pediatric age group, streptococcal infections of the throat are most common in children between 6 and 12 years of age; the incidence is lower among preschool-age children. In contrast, streptococcal infections of the skin are more common in preschool-age children.

Geographic distribution appears to be related to climate. The incidence of streptococcal pharyngitis and tonsillitis is higher in temperate areas than in tropical or warmer areas. In the United States the highest incidence of streptococcal infections occurs in the north, particularly in the Rocky Mountain states. The geographic distribution of skin infections is different. In general, streptococcal impetigo is more common in warmer or tropical climates than in cooler ones.

The seasonal distribution varies with the particular geographic area. In the United States streptococcal pharyngitis occurs most often during late winter and early spring. Skin infections, however, are more common during the late summer or early fall.

The chief sources of pathogenic streptococci are discharges from the nose, throat, ears, and skin of patients or carriers. People who carry streptococci in the nose have been shown to be a particularly rich source. The transmission of infection is effected chiefly by indirect contact with either a patient or a carrier. The streptococci can also be transmitted indirectly by contaminated objects or by unwashed hands. The air can be easily contaminated by streptococci after sneezing or coughing, since the organisms are spread chiefly by large airborne droplets. Contaminated milk, ice cream, and eggs have been responsible for food-borne epidemics on rare occasions.

Streptococcal throat infections are endemic in most large cities in the temperate zone. In smaller, more isolated communities, the disease may be absent for a period of time, after which an epidemic may occur.

IMMUNITY

As indicated earlier, group A hemolytic streptococci are composed of various antigenic constituents and elaborate extracellular antigenic material. Two of these antigens, type-specific M protein and erythrogenic toxin, stimulate the production of antibodies that provide a person with at least two types of resistance—antibacterial immunity and antitoxic immunity.

It has been postulated that the development of immunity and hypersensitivity may play a role in the changing pattern of streptococcal disease with advancing age. The nonspecific, nonlocalizing character of streptococcal disease in infants may represent the initial type of response to the microorganism. The more localized manifestations of disease, such as streptococcal tonsillitis, may be manifestations of hypersensitivity as well as bacterial infection.

Antibacterial immunity

Antibacterial immunity is related to the type-specific M component of group A hemolytic streptococci. A person who is infected with a given type of streptococcus develops antibodies against strains of the same type only. For example, infection with type 4 streptococcus is followed by development of antibodies against type 4 but not against type 19 or other types. These bacteriostatic antibodies have been demonstrated in patients' sera for several years after infection.

The current hypothesis of type-specific antibacterial immunity is supported by data obtained from many immunologic and epidemiologic studies. Theoretically, during a lifetime a person may develop at least 40 or more streptococcal infections, some apparent and others inapparent. Each infection in turn would in all probability be caused by a different type of streptococcus. It has been demonstrated that the serum of infants and young children has a limited number of these type-specific bacteriostatic antibodies. As the person's age increases, a larger number of these type-specific antibodies develops as a result of repeated infections. However, second attacks of streptococcal infection with the same type have occurred. The capacity of early penicillin therapy to decrease the response to various streptococcal antigens may explain some of these second attacks.

Antitoxic immunity

Antitoxic immunity is acquired either passively or actively. The antitoxic immunity of infancy is transplacental in origin and disappears before the end of the first year. Actively acquired antitoxin resulting from infection probably persists for life. Antitoxic immunity for the most part has group rather than type specificity, which is characteristic of antibacterial immunity.

• • •

In summary, the immune status of a person may affect the type of infection acquired after exposure to a particular pathogenic strain of streptococcus. The hypothetical example in Fig. 28-1, which assumes exposure to toxic group A

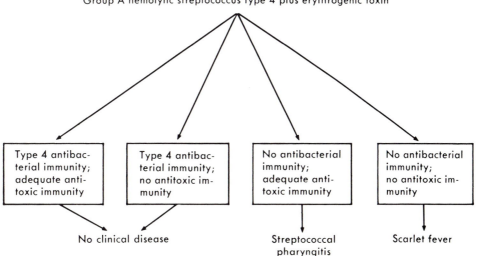

Group A hemolytic streptococcus type 4 plus erythrogenic toxin

| Type 4 antibacterial immunity; adequate antitoxic immunity | Type 4 antibacterial immunity; no antitoxic immunity | No antibacterial immunity; adequate antitoxic immunity | No antibacterial immunity; no antitoxic immunity |

No clinical disease   Streptococcal pharyngitis   Scarlet fever

Fig. 28-1. Effect of immune status on streptococcal infections (see text).

hemolytic streptococcus type 4, illustrates this graphically. It may be noted that (1) type 4 antibacterial immunity prevents clinical disease regardless of the antitoxic status; (2) when type 4 antibacterial immunity is absent but antitoxic immunity is present, streptococcal pharyngitis or tonsillitis may develop, but scarlet fever will not occur; and (3) when neither type 4 antibacterial nor antitoxic immunity is present, scarlet fever may develop.

CLINICAL MANIFESTATIONS

The clinical manifestations of streptococcal disease are governed by many factors, the most important being the portal of entry, the variety of infecting streptococci, the patient's age, and the immune status of the host. The effect of type-specific immunity has been discussed. Powers and Boisvert (1944) emphasized the importance of the age factor in relation to the type of clinical response. They described the manifestations of streptococcal infections, or streptococcosis, for three pediatric age groups: under 6 months, 6 months to 3 years, and 3 to 12 years.

Streptococcosis in infants under 6 months of age

Streptococcosis in infants under 6 months of age is characterized by nasopharyngitis associated with a thin mucopurulent nasal discharge and irregular rises in temperature. Frequently, there are excoriations around the nares. The acute symptoms last for approximately 1 week, but persistent nasal discharge and irritability may continue for 6 weeks. The disease is clinically indistinguishable from the common cold. It can be identified only by means of a culture of the nasal discharge.

Streptococcosis in children 6 months to 3 years of age

In streptococcosis in children 6 months to 3 years of age there is an insidious onset of low-grade fever, mild constitutional symptoms, and mild nasopharyngitis. The nasal discharge is purulent, and the anterior cervical lymph nodes are usually enlarged and tender. Sinusitis and otitis media are frequent complications. The low-grade fever and symptoms may persist for as long as 4 to 8 weeks. This type of infection is clinically similar to various nonspecific respiratory tract infections. Diagnosis can best be established by nasopharyngeal culture.

Streptococcal infection in children 3 to 12 years of age

In children 3 to 12 years of age, streptococcosis is manifested as acute follicular tonsillitis, pharyngitis, or scarlet fever. Streptococcal tonsillitis is essentially scarlet fever without a rash. The clinical picture, complications, prognosis, and treatment are identical to those of scarlet fever; consequently they are considered in the discussion of scarlet fever.

Scarlet fever

The incubation period of scarlet fever is 2 to 4 days, with a range of 1 to 7 days. The disease is ushered in abruptly by fever, vomiting, sore throat, and constitutional symptoms such as headache, chills, and malaise. Within 12 to 48 hours after onset, the typical rash appears. In some cases abdominal pain is an early and prominent symptom. The association of this manifestation with vomiting may suggest the possibility of a surgical abdomen. The combination of vomiting and abdominal pain in streptococcal tonsillitis without rash is also frequently seen.

The significant findings are fever, enanthem, and exanthem.

Fever. In the typical case (Fig. 28-2), the temperature rises abruptly to 39.4° C (103° F) and reaches its peak by around the second day. It then gradually falls to normal by lysis within 5 or 6 days. A severe case has a higher and more protracted temperature course. Occasionally in mild scarlet fever the temperature may be low (under 38.3° C; 101° F) or normal. The pulse rate is frequently increased out of proportion to

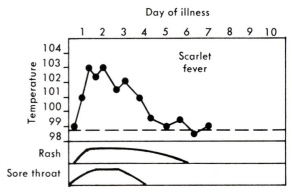

Fig. 28-2. Schematic diagram of a typical case of untreated uncomplicated scarlet fever. The rash usually appears within 24 hours of onset of fever and sore throat.

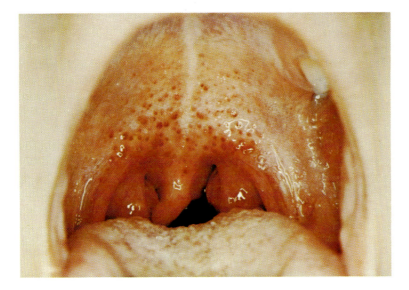

Plate 7
Marked petechial stippling of the soft palate in scarlet fever. (From Stillerman M, Bernstein SH. Am J Dis Child 1961;101:476.

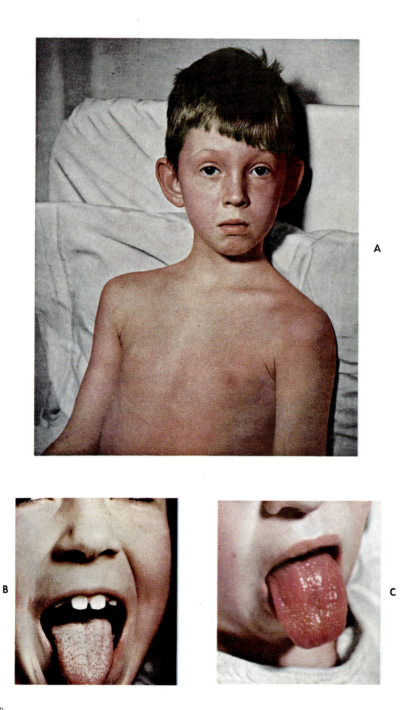

Plate 8
Scarlet fever, **A,** Punctate, erythematous rash (second day). **B,** White strawberry tongue (first day). **C,** Red strawberry tongue (third day). (Courtesy Dr. Franklin H. Top, Professor and Head of the Department of Hygiene and Preventive Medicine, State University of Iowa, College of Medicine, Iowa City, Iowa; and Parke, Davis & Company's *Therapeutic Notes*.)

the fever. Today, one rarely observes a typical temperature course; it usually drops precipitously to normal within 24 hours after penicillin therapy is begun.

Enanthem. The enanthem includes lesions of the tonsils, pharynx, tongue, and palate. The tonsils are enlarged, edematous, reddened, and covered with patches of exudate. The pharynx also is edematous and beefy red in appearance. In mild cases the tonsils and pharynx show moderate erythema and little or no exudate. Severe cases may be characterized by membranous ulcerative tonsillitis clinically indistinguishable from diphtheria (Plate 7). The tongue changes in appearance as the disease progresses. During the first 1 or 2 days, the dorsum has a white fur coat, and the tip and edges are reddened. As the papillae become reddened and edematous, they project through the coat, producing the so-called white strawberry tongue. By the fourth or fifth day the white coat has peeled off. The red glistening tongue studded with prominent papillae presents the appearance of a red strawberry (Plate 8). The palate is usually covered with erythematous punctiform lesions and occasionally with scattered petechiae. The uvula

and the free margin of the soft palate are reddened and edematous (Plate 7).

Exanthem. The rash usually appears within 12 hours after onset of the illness; occasionally it may be delayed for 2 days. The rash is an erythematous punctiform eruption that blanches on pressure. The punctate lesions, pinhead in size, give the skin a rough sandpaperlike texture. The rash of scarlet fever resembles a "sunburn with goose pimples" (Plate 8).

The exanthem (Fig. 28-3) has the following distinctive features:

1. It becomes generalized very rapidly, usually within 24 hours.
2. The punctiform lesions are usually not present on the face. The forehead and cheeks are red, smooth, and flushed, and the area around the mouth is pale (circumoral pallor).
3. It is more intense in skin folds such as the axillae and the groin and at sites of pressure such as the buttocks.
4. It has areas of hyperpigmentation, occasionally with tiny petechiae in the creases of the folds of the joints, particularly in the antecubital fossae. These lesions form transverse lines (Pastia's sign) that persist for a day or so after the rash has faded.
5. If the eruption is severe, minute vesicular lesions (miliary sudamina) may be scattered over the abdomen, hands, and feet.
6. It desquamates.

The rash, fever, sore throat, and other clinical manifestations clear up by the end of the first week. The period of desquamation follows shortly thereafter.

Desquamation. Desquamation is one of the most characteristic features of scarlet fever. The extent and duration of the desquamation are directly proportional to the intensity of the rash. It becomes apparent first on the face at the end of the first week as fine branny flakes. Then it spreads to the trunk and finally to the extremities, becoming generalized by the third week (Fig. 28-4). The desquamating skin of the trunk comes off in larger, thicker flakes. Frequently, circular areas of epidermis of variable size peel off, giving the skin a punched-out or pinhole appearance. The hands and feet usually are the last to desquamate, becoming involved between the second and third weeks. The tips of the fin-

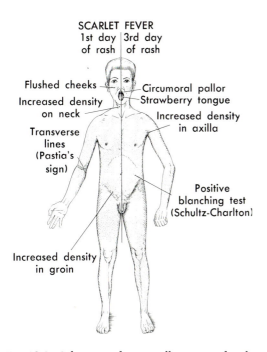

Fig. 28-3. Schematic drawing illustrating development and distribution of scarlet fever rash.

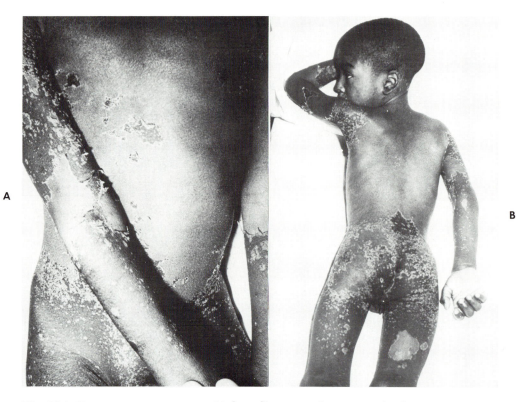

Fig. 28-4. Desquamation in a patient 16 days after onset of severe scarlet fever. **A,** Typical circular punched-out areas in groin and upper thighs. **B,** Sequence of spread from face to trunk and finally to extremities.

gers characteristically show a splitting of the skin at the free margins of the nails. In severe cases an epidermal cast of the fingers, hands, or feet may be shed. In mild cases of scarlet fever, the process of desquamation may be complete in 3 weeks; in severe cases it may persist for as long as 8 weeks. Sometimes a retrospective diagnosis may be made on the basis of peeling skin and a history of a sore throat associated with a rash several weeks previously. Occasionally, the eruption may be missed entirely.

Surgical scarlet fever

The portal of entry in classic scarlet fever is the nasopharynx. Occasionally, however, hemolytic streptococci may infect the site of a wound, a burn, or other type of skin lesion. Under these circumstances, so-called surgical scarlet fever may develop. The clinical manifestations are identical to those described earlier, except that the pharyngeal and tonsillar involvement are absent. However, there may be local inflammatory signs at the wound or operative site.

Streptococcal sepsis

Although today group A streptococci are most often considered in the context of surface infections of the respiratory tract or skin, it is important to remember that they may cause serious invasive disease in normal children, newborns, and compromised hosts. These are usually fulminant bacteremic or septicemic infections with pneumonia, empyema, osteomyelitis, endometritis, meningitis, or soft tissue abscesses (Burech et al., 1976).

Streptococcal infections of the skin

Eczema streptococcum. Infants with weeping eczematoid lesions are prone to develop secondary infections, particularly with hemolytic streptococci. The resulting lesion shows extensive erythema, serosanguineous exudate, crusting, weeping, and regional adenopathy.

Impetigo. The characteristic superficial purulent crusting lesions may be caused by either hemolytic streptococci or staphylococci. The vesicular stage of streptococcal impetigo may be transient, and vesicles are small (1 to 2 mm in diameter). The typical lesion is a thick, adherent amber-colored crust on an erythematous base; there is often an associated local lymphadenopathy. Bullous impetigo is usually caused by staphylococci. These vesicular lesions are large (1 to 2 cm in diameter); they rupture and form thin crusts without accompanying lymphadenopathy.

Erysipelas. Erysipelas, formerly very common, is rarely seen today. It is characterized by a red, indurated thickening of the skin. It begins as a small lesion that spreads marginally for approximately 4 to 6 days. The margins have a raised, firm, tender, palpable border. On the face the rash may assume a butterfly distribution. The skin lesion is usually associated with fever and constitutional symptoms that subside when the rash stops progressing.

Histologically, there is evidence of an inflammatory reaction involving the superficial lymph vessels. The lymph channels are crammed with fibrin, leukocytes, and streptococci. The progressively diffuse lymphatic involvement accounts for the peculiar spread and evolution of the lesion.

DIAGNOSIS

The diagnosis of streptococcal infections, including scarlet fever, can be established by (1) characteristic clinical features, (2) isolation of the causative agent, (3) serologic tests, and (4) other confirmatory tests.

Characteristic clinical features

The triad of fever, vomiting, and sore throat associated with an exudative tonsillitis and an erythematous punctiform eruption suggests scarlet fever. The same symptoms and signs without a rash point to streptococcal tonsillitis.

Stillerman and Bernstein (1961) observed that groups of symptoms and signs are better indicators of streptococcal pharyngitis than single symptoms and signs. The following four syndromes were found to be associated with positive cultures in more than 70% of the cases:

1. Moderate redness of the oropharynx, exudate over the tonsils, and cervical adenitis (75%)
2. Marked redness of the oropharynx with or without tonsillar exudate, and cervical adenitis (74%)
3. Moderate or marked redness of the oropharynx, no tonsillar exudate, and petechiae on the palate, with or without cervical adenitis (95%)
4. Moderate or marked redness of the oropharynx, tonsillar exudate, and petechiae on the palate, with or without cervical adenitis (100%)

Isolation of causative agent

The throat culture is the most useful and most important confirmatory test. Group A hemolytic streptococci may be isolated from the throat, the nasopharynx, or an infected wound. A positive throat culture is usually indicative of an acute streptococcal infection; it may also indicate the presence of a carrier state. A quantitative throat swab culture usually reveals a correlation between the isolation of large numbers of streptococci and the presence of a streptococcal pharyngitis (Breese et al., 1972). Studies by Bell and Smith (1976) revealed a heavy growth of *Streptococcus pyogenes* in 71% of throat swabs taken from 1054 children with pharyngitis, as compared with 1.7% of 462 normal children who were carriers.

Diagnosis of streptococcal impetigo is made by isolation of the organism from a skin lesion. Staphylococci may also be isolated simultaneously.

Serologic tests

Rapid tests for diagnosis of group A streptococcal infections from throat swabs are now commercially available (Slifkin and Gil., 1984). These tests appear to be sensitive and specific, and they may become standard in physicians' offices in the future since results are usually available within 15 minutes. Additional experience will be necessary, however, before such rapid tests can be recommended for routine testing.

A significant rise in antistreptolysin O titer during convalescence is indicative of a streptococcal infection. This test is especially helpful if the throat culture is negative as a result of previous antimicrobial therapy. Increases in titers of serum antibodies to other streptococcal enzymes may be helpful as sensitive indicators of recent infection (antihyaluronidase, antistreptokinase, antideoxyribonucleases, and others). Early eradication of hemolytic streptococci by

Table 28-1. General features of streptococcal infections at different sites*

	Streptococcal pharyngitis and tonsillitis	Streptococcal impetigo and pyoderma
Clinical features		
Erythema	Usually present and generalized	Often minimal and localized to immediate area around lesion
Vesicular stage	Absent	Typical of early lesion but transient
Pustular stage	Patchy exudate; pustules sometimes confluent	Pustules usually discrete; flora often mixed
Crusted stage	Absent	Frequent and characteristic
Local pain	Common; may be intense	Usually absent
Systemic reaction	Fever, headache, and malaise common	Unusual
Regional adenitis	Common	Less common, but adenopathy frequently seen
Deep-seated cellulitis	May occur	Perhaps less common
Bacteremia	Rare	May be relatively more frequent
Scarlatiniform rash	Sometimes present	Rare
Course	Typically acute, except in infants	Often chronic; lesions may become ecthymatous
Laboratory findings		
Leukocytosis	Usually present	Often absent
Bacterial agent	Group A streptococci	Group A streptococci; often also large numbers of staphylococci
Serologic types of group A streptococci	Many different types	Few types predominate
Antistreptolysin O response	Common	Uncommon
Epidemiologic factors		
Seasonal occurrence	Winter and spring	Late summer and early fall
Common-source epidemics	May occur	Not described
Geographic distribution	More common in temperate or cold climates	Common in hot or tropical climates
Age	Young school-age children	Children of preschool age
Sex	Equal incidence	Equal incidence
Transmission	Direct spread from human reservoirs, particularly nasal carriers	Unknown; insects may be mechanical vectors
Carrier state	Common in pharynx of many populations	Unusual on skin, except in certain situations
Preceding trauma	Not present	May predispose to natural or experimental infection
Preceding viral infection	Uncommon	Uncommon
Complications		
Acute nephritis	Occurs; partially preventable (50%)	Occurs; preventability unknown
Acute rheumatic fever	Occurs; preventable	Does not occur
Treatment		
Local	Not important	Removal of crusts and scrubbing with hexachlorophene soap
Systemic	Single intramuscular injection of benzathine penicillin or oral administration of penicillin for 10 days	May not be necessary; extensive lesions may require intramuscular injection of benzathine penicillin

*From Wannamaker LW. N Engl J Med 1970;282:23.

antimicrobial therapy may suppress the development of antibodies.

Following impetigo, it is rare for antibodies to antistreptolysin O to rise. While all group A streptococci produce streptolysin O, cholesterol in the skin binds to the toxin and prevents development of the immune response after impetigo (Kaplan and Wannamaker, 1976).

Other confirmatory tests

The typical blood picture shows leukocytosis with a predominance of polymorphonuclear leukocytes. An increase in number of eosinophils to between 5% and 10% of the total white blood cell count is a common finding in scarlet fever.

DIFFERENTIAL DIAGNOSIS

The differential diagnosis of scarlet fever is discussed in detail in Chapter 34. Some of the conditions that may be confused with this disease are rubella, measles, exanthem subitum, erythema infectiosum, infectious mononucleosis, staphylococcal scalded skin syndrome, Kawasaki's syndrome, and toxic shock syndrome. Sunburn in a child with nonspecific pharyngitis may be confused with scarlet fever; the absence of eruption in the bathing suit area clarifies the diagnosis. Heat rash (miliaria) also may simulate a scarlatiniform eruption.

The differential diagnosis of exudative and membranous tonsillitis has been covered in the chapters on diphtheria (p. 26) and infectious mononucleosis (p. 67).

Wannamaker in 1970 and Peter and Smith in 1977 described the comparative features of streptococcal infections of the throat and skin. The organisms causing disease in these two organ systems appear to be different. For example, nephritogenic types that cause pharyngitis are rarely isolated from the skin (Anthony et al., 1969). The various features of these infections are listed in Table 28-1.

COMPLICATIONS

Complications following streptococcal infections may occur early or late in the course of the disease.

Early complications

Early complications are generally the result of an extension of the streptococcal infection; they usually occur during the first week of illness. Thus a spread of the infection to the regional lymph nodes results in cervical adenitis. A progression of the infection into the middle ear is followed by otitis media. Sinusitis also may be produced by invading hemolytic streptococci. Bronchopneumonia is a rare early complication of streptococcal involvement of the upper respiratory tract. Early bacterial complications rarely occur in adequately treated patients. Other less common complications include mastoiditis, septicemia, and osteomyelitis.

Late complications

Late complications or sequelae are rheumatic fever and acute glomerulonephritis. Their pathogenesis is uncertain, but they are thought to be due to a hypersensitivity reaction to group A hemolytic streptococci or some of their by-products. These complications usually develop after a latent period of approximately 1 to 3 weeks, and their incidence is not related to the severity of the initial infection. They may follow mild or inapparent infections as well as severe ones.

Rheumatic fever. Rheumatic fever is a relatively uncommon but serious complication of streptococcal infections; its incidence is approximately 3% after exudative pharyngitis. Rheumatic fever has not been associated with streptococcal impetigo. With optimum penicillin therapy for the preceeding streptococcal infection, the incidence may be reduced to less than 1%. Recurrent attacks of rheumatic fever, on the other hand, are a frequent complication of streptococcal infection, but most of these can be prevented by prophylactic penicillin. The disease is rare in children under 3 years of age; it occurs most often in older children. The clinical manifestations of fever, polyarthritis, and carditis occur 7 or more days after the onset of the streptococcal infection.

Nephritis. Nephritis is a more common complication than rheumatic fever, but its incidence is variable. Certain strains of group A hemolytic streptococci, particularly types 12, 4, and 49, are nephritogenic, and infections with these microorganisms may be followed by a high incidence of nephritis. Nephritis, unlike rheumatic fever, may complicate streptococcal infections of the skin as well as those of the throat. Nephritis is usually manifested by fever, bloody urine, moderate edema, and, occasionally, hypertension and azotemia. In contrast to rheumatic fever, only one attack usually occurs; recurrences are unlikely. The rarity of recurrences may be due to the limited number of nephritogenic types of streptococci. The prognosis for complete recovery is usually excellent, although longitudinal studies on patients followed for many years after their attack indicate that hypertension and uremia may be late sequelae of nephritis (Schacht et al., 1976).

PROGNOSIS

The prognosis for adequately treated streptococcal infections is excellent. Serious septic complications can be easily prevented and treated. Adequate therapy will also reduce the incidence of rheumatic fever, thereby improving the prognosis. Deaths caused by scarlet fever and other streptococcal infections, very common several decades ago, are rare today.

TREATMENT
Antimicrobial therapy

The treatment of streptococcal infections, including scarlet fever, has been revolutionized by antimicrobial therapy. Penicillin is without question the preferred drug. Strains of group A hemolytic streptococci are uniformly susceptible to penicillin. Penicillin therapy is consistently followed by a dramatic subsidence of fever and constitutional symptoms. While at one time it was believed that penicillin had little effect on the acute symptoms of streptococcal sore throat, it is now apparent that this belief is erroneous. For years some investigators (Breese et al., 1972; Hall and Breese, 1984) have maintained that penicillin reduces the symptoms of streptococcal sore throat more rapidly than no treatment. Nelson (1984), in a double blind study, demonstrated this phenomenon. Thus not only does prompt penicillin therapy prevent the sequelae of streptococcal infection of the throat, but also it rapidly alleviates symptoms. Optimum treatment eradicates the streptococci from the site of infection, prevents septic complications, and reduces the incidence of rheumatic fever. Early institution of therapy interferes with the development of antistreptolysin O antibodies. It is uncertain whether the incidence of nephritis is affected by early penicillin therapy.

Optimum penicillin therapy can be achieved by a variety of regimens. The goal in treating streptococcal pharyngitis is to maintain an adequate blood level against group A hemolytic streptococci for at least 10 days. The 10-day period of penicillinemia may be achieved by oral or intramuscular therapy. Oral therapy is usually not reliable because it requires the patient's compliance for 10 days. Optimum therapy is achieved by use of benzathine penicillin G, a long-acting preparation. Benzathine penicillin G, 600,000 units, in combination with aqueous procaine penicillin, 600,000 units, is well tolerated, and, as indicated in Fig. 28-5, it provides an effective blood level for at least 10 days after a single intramuscular injection in children up to 10 years of age. For older children, adolescents, and adults a larger dose is recommended (benzathine penicillin G, 900,000 units, in combination with 300,000 units of aqueous procaine penicillin).

Impetigo is best treated with penicillin given parenterally as well as bacitracin given topically. While it is unclear whether antibiotic therapy can prevent nephritis, therapy will decrease the spread of the organism to others.

Patients who are allergic to penicillin may be treated with erythromycin estolate (Ginsberg et al., 1984) or a cephalosporin. Sulfonamides are not effective for the treatment of an established streptococcal infection. Tetracyclines are not recommended because of the high incidence of strains resistant to this antibiotic.

Supportive therapy

Although bed rest is recommended during the febrile period of streptococcal pharyngitis, it is virtually impossible to keep most children in bed when they feel well. Aspirin or acetaminophen are indicated for sore throat and malaise. An adequate fluid intake should be encouraged during the febrile period. A regular diet should be offered when tolerated.

PREVENTIVE MEASURES

Administration of penicillin will effectively prevent most cases of streptococcal infection if the drug is administered *prior to exposure*. The indications for prophylactic therapy are not clear-cut and are difficult to define because (1) the susceptibility of the contact is unknown, (2) the contact may have acquired a subclinical infection, and (3) the antibiotic may cause a toxic reaction. Ideally, the results of a throat culture should resolve the question of whether or not

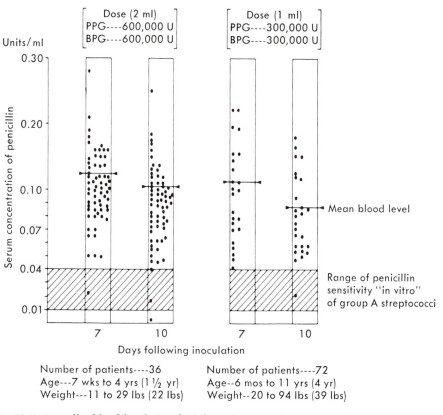

Fig. 28-5. Penicillin blood levels 7 and 10 days after a single injection of a mixture of aqueous procaine penicillin G (PPG) and benzathine penicillin G (BPG). Each black dot represents one blood level determination. (From Drescher AN, Krugman S. Unpublished studies.)

to treat a person. If facilities for culture are not available, the following circumstances may warrant the use of prophylaxis for children who are contacts: (1) intimate household exposure, (2) obvious epidemic in a school or institutional group, (3) previous history of rheumatic fever in any member of a family, (4) intercurrent illness in the exposed person, and (5) evidence that the particular strain of hemolytic streptococcus is a nephritogenic strain. For the isolated school type of exposure (a single case in a class), we would be inclined to withhold prophylactic therapy and observe the child very carefully. In general, penicillin prophylaxis is employed more often in children than in adults, since children are more susceptible to streptococcal infections and they are less likely to develop drug reactions.

If prophylactic therapy is indicated because of specific exposure, penicillin should be ad-

ministered orally or as a single injection of benzathine penicillin G as recommended in the discussion on treatment. This recommendation is based on the assumption that the contact has acquired a subclinical infection.

If penicillin is contraindicated because of hypersensitivity, erythromycin may be given.

For long-term streptococcal prophylaxis of patients with rheumatic fever, monthly injections of benzathine penicillin have been most effective, although breakthrough cases of rheumatic fever have been reported (Nordin, 1984). Sulfonamides are recommended for penicillin-sensitive patients.

ISOLATION AND QUARANTINE

Specific penicillin therapy that rapidly eradicates hemolytic streptococci has reduced the need for periods of isolation.

Quarantine measures are not indicated.

REFERENCES

Anthony BF, Kaplan EL, Wannamaker LW, et al. Attack rates of acute nephritis after type 49 streptococcal infection of the skin and of the respiratory tract. J Clin Invest 1969;48:1697-1704.

Bass JW, Crast FW, Knowles CR, Onafer CN. Streptococcal pharyngitis in children. A comparison of prior treatment schedules with intramuscular penicillin G benzathine. JAMA 1976;235:1112.

Bell SM, Smith DD. Quantitative throat swab culture in the diagnosis of streptococcal pharyngitis in children. Lancet 1976;2:61.

Breese BB, et al. Beta-hemolytic streptococcal infection: the clinical and epidemiologic importance of the number of organisms found in culture. Am J Dis Child 1972;124:352.

Burech DL, Koranyi KI, Haynes RE. Serious group A streptococcal diseases in children. J Pediatr 1976;88:972.

Coffey JM. Further observations on the toxigenic properties of hemolytic streptococci. J Immunol 1938;35:121.

Denny FW, et al. Prevention of rheumatic fever. JAMA 1950;143:151.

Derrick CW, Dillon HC. Erythromycin therapy for streptococcal pharyngitis. Am J Dis Child 1976;130:175.

Durack DT, Kaplan EL, Bisno A. Apparent failures of endocarditis prophylaxis of 52 cases submitted to a national registry. JAMA 1983;250:2318-2322.

Ferrieri P, Dajani AS, Wannamaker LW. Benzathine penicillin in the prophylaxis of streptococcal skin infections: a pilot study. J Pediatr 1973;83:572.

Ginsberg CM, McCracken GH, Steinberg JB, et al. Treatment of group A streptococcal pharyngitis in children. Clin Pediatr 1984;21:83-88.

Ginsberg CM, McCracken GH, Crow SD, et al. Erythromycin therapy for group A streptococcal pharyngitis. Results of a comparative study of the estolate and ethylsuccinate formulations. Am J Dis Child 1984;138:536-539.

Goldstein I, Rebeyotte P, Parlebas J, et al. Isolation from heart valves of glycopeptides which share immunological properties with *Streptococcus hemolyticus* group A polysaccharides. Nature 1968;219:866-868.

Hall CB, Breese BB. Does penicillin make Johnny's strep throat better? Pediatr Infect Dis 1984;3:7-9.

Hamburger MH, Jr, Green MJ, Hamburger VG. The problem of the "dangerous carrier" of hemolytic streptococci. I. Number of hemolytic streptococci expelled by carriers with positive and negative nose cultures. J Infect Dis 1945;77:68.

Janeff J, Janeff D, Taranta A, et al. A screening test for streptococcal antibodies. Lab Med 1971;2(7):38-40.

Kaplan EL. The group A streptococcal upper respiratory tract carrier state: an enigma. J Pediatr 1980;97:337-345.

Kaplan EL, Wannamaker LW. Suppression of the antistreptolysin O response by cholesterol and by lipid extracts of the rabbit skin. J Exp Med 1976;144:754-767.

Kaplan JM, McCracken GH, Jr, Culbertson MC. Penicillin and erythromycin concentration in tonsils. Am J Dis Child 1974;127:206.

Krugman S, Ebin EV. Improved local tolerance to penicillin. Pediatrics 1958;21:243.

Lancefield RC. A serological differentiation of human and other groups of hemolytic streptococci. J Exp Med 1933;57:571.

Maxted WR. The use of bacitracin for identifying group A haemolytic streptococci. J Clin Pathol 1953;6:224.

Maxted WR, Fraser CAM, Parker MT. Streptococcus pyogens type 49. A nephritogenic streptococcus with a wide geographical distribution. Lancet 1967;1:644.

Moody MD. Old and new techniques for rapid identification of group A streptococci. In Wannamaker LW, Matsen JM, eds. Streptococci and streptococcal diseases: recognition, understanding, management. New York: Academic Press, 1972;177-188.

Nelson JD. The effect of penicillin therapy on the symptoms and signs of streptococcal pharyngitis. Pediatr Infect Dis 1984;3:10-13.

Nordin JD. Recurrence of rheumatic fever during prophylaxis with monthly benzathine penicillin G. Pediatrics 1984;73:530-531.

Peter G, Smith AL. Group A streptococcal infections of the skin and pharynx. N Engl J Med 1977;297:311.

Powers GF, Boisvert PL. Age as a factor in streptococcosis. J Pediatr 1944;25:481.

Rotta J, Bednat B. Biological properties of streptococcal cell wall particles III. J Exp Med 1969;130:31-45.

Schacht RG, Gluck MC, Gallo GR, et al. Progression to uremia after remission of acute poststreptococcal glomerulonephritis. N Engl J Med 1976;295:977-981.

Schwentker FF, Janney JH, Gordon JE. The epidemiology of scarlet fever. Am J Hyg 1943;38:27.

Siegel AC, Johnson EE, Stollerman GH. Controlled studies of streptococcal pharyngitis in a pediatric population. I. Factors related to the attack rate of rheumatic fever. II. Behavior of the type-specific immune response. N Engl J Med 1961;265:559.

Silverman BK, et al. Comparative serological changes following treated group A streptococcal pharyngitis. Am J Dis Child 1974;127:498.

Slifkin M, Gil GM. Evaluation of the culturette bound ten-minute group A strep 10 technique. J Clin Microbiol 1984;20:12-14.

Stillerman M, Bernstein SH. Streptococcal pharyngitis; evaluation of clinical syndromes in diagnosis. Am J Dis Child 1961;101:476.

Swift HF. The relationship of streptococcal infections to rheumatic fever. Am J Med 1947;2:168.

Wannamaker LW. Differences between streptococcal infections of the throat and of the skin. N Engl J Med 1970;282:23, 78.

Wannamaker LW, et al. Effect of penicillin prophylaxis on streptococcal disease rates and the carrier state. N Engl J Med 1953;249:1.

Watson DW, Kim YB. Erythrogenic toxins. In Montie TC, Kadia S, Ajl SJ, ed. Microbial toxins. New York:Academic Press, Inc., 1970;173-186.

Zabriskie JB. The role of temperate bacteriophage in the production of erythogenic toxin by group A streptococci. J Exp Med 1964;119:761.

29

TETANUS (LOCKJAW)

Clostridium tetani produces a potent soluble exotoxin that is responsible for the clinical manifestations of tetanus. The disease is an acute toxemia characterized by tonic spasms of voluntary muscles with a high fatality rate. *C. tetani* infection usually occurs at a break in the skin that may be trivial or unrecognized, but it may also complicate burns, puerperal infections, infections of the umbilical stump (tetanus neonatorum), and certain surgical operations in which the source of infection may be contaminated sutures, dressings, or plaster. The illness begins with tonic spasms of the skeletal muscles and is followed by paroxysmal contractions. The muscle stiffness involves the jaw (lockjaw) and neck first and later becomes generalized.

ETIOLOGY

The tetanus bacillus is a long, thin (2 to 5 μm × 3 to 8 μm), motile, gram-positive anaerobic rod. Older cultures of these organisms and smears from wounds frequently stain as gram-negative microbes, and this may be confusing to the uninitiated. These organisms may develop a terminal spore that does not take the Gram stain and gives the bacterium a drum-stick appearance. The spores are very resistant to heat and the usual antiseptics. They may persist in tissues for many months in a viable although dormant state. Under anaerobic conditions, the organisms are easily isolated on blood agar or in cooked meat broth. The organism does not ferment carbohydrates, does not usually liquefy gelatin, and produces little change in litmus milk.

The bacilli are widely distributed in soil, street dust, and feces of some horses, sheep, cattle, dogs, cats, rats, guinea pigs, and chickens. Consequently, manure-containing soil may be highly infectious. In agricultural areas a significant number of normal human adults may harbor the organisms, and agricultural workers have a higher incidence of infection. The spores have also been found in contaminated heroin.

Tetanus bacilli produce a potent neurotoxin (tetanospasmin) that may be plasmid encoded. Despite demonstrable strain differences in *C. tetani* there is only a single tetanus toxin produced. Tetanus toxin is synthesized intracellularly as a single polypeptide chain with a molecular weight of 160,000. This toxin is released from the cell, is nicked by a clostridial protease, and then consists of two components that are held together by at least one disulfide bond as well as noncovalent bonds. Experimentally, reduction will separate the toxin's components into a heavy, or beta, chain (molecular weight 105,000) and a light, or alpha, chain (molecular weight 55,000). The receptor of the toxin is present in the heavy chain, and the molecular weight of this portion of the heavy chain is about 47,000. The toxin binds to two sialidase-sensitive gangliosides (GDlb and GTlb) of neurons. The light, or alpha, chain is probably the toxic portion of the molecule, but it requires the receptor, or beta, portion to gain access to cells.

PATHOGENESIS

The portal of entry is usually a site of minor puncture wounds or scratches and the organism can proliferate only if the oxidation-reduction (Eh) potential is lower than that of normal living tissues. Deep puncture wounds, burns, crush, and other injuries that promote favorable conditions for the growth of anaerobic organisms may be followed by tetanus. Occasionally, no apparent portal of entry can be found. Under these circumstances, it is conceivable that the site of infection may have been the alimentary tract. When conditions are favorable the bacilli multiply at the site of primary inoculation and produce toxin.

Toxin then travels centripetally in the axoplasm of the alpha motor fibers and accumulates in the motor neurons in the membrane-bound endoplasmic reticulum. Marie and Morax proposed this route of access of toxin to the central nervous system in 1902 as did Meyer and Ransome in 1903. Experimentally, it was shown that toxin was not lethal if the local motor nerves were severed. Toxin is neutralizable when it is free and is only partially neutralizable when it is on the cell surface. Pinocytosis of toxin renders it nonneutralizable as it is internalized in the cell. Thus, fixation of toxin to nerves and its internalization results in irreversible effects. The toxin acts presynaptically, presumably at the inhibitory terminals where glycine is the mediator. Internuncial neurons are affected, and presynaptic inhibition is blocked. This results in the uncontrolled spread of impulses, hyperreflexia, and constant muscle contraction. The strongest muscles, usually extensors, exert the greatest effects. The toxin also affects the sympathetic nervous system.

PATHOLOGY

There are no specific pathologic lesions caused by the infectious agent. Secondary effects of the muscle contractions may include vertebral fractures, pneumonia, and hemorrhages into the muscles.

CLINICAL MANIFESTATIONS

The incubation period is extremely variable. The usual range is 5 to 14 days; however, it may be as short as 1 day or as long as 3 weeks or more.

The appearance of the site of infection, if obvious, provides no clue to the impending toxemia. The disease begins insidiously with progressively increasing stiffness of the voluntary muscles; generally the muscles of the jaw and neck are the first to be involved. Within 24 to 48 hours after the onset of the disease, rigidity may be fully developed and may spread rapidly to involve the trunk and extremities. With spasm of the jaw muscles, trismus (lockjaw) develops. The wrinkling of the forehead and the distortion of the eyebrows and the angles of the mouth produce a peculiar facial appearance called *risus sardonicus* (sardonic grin). The neck and back become stiff and arched (opisthotonos). The abdominal wall is boardlike. The extremities are usually stiff and extended.

A variety of excitants may initiate painful paroxysmal spasms that may persist for a few seconds or several minutes. These seizures may be provoked by the most trivial kind of visual, auditory, or cutaneous stimuli, such as bright lights, sudden noises, and movement of the patient. The sardonicus and opisthotonos are most marked during these spasms.

Initially the spasms may occur at infrequent intervals, with complete relaxation between attacks. Later the spasms occur more often and are more prolonged and more painful. Involvement of the muscles of respiration, laryngeal obstruction due to laryngospasm, or accumulation of secretions in the tracheobronchial tree may be followed by respiratory distress, asphyxia, coma, and death. Involvement of the bladder sphincter leads to urinary retention.

The manifestations of sympathetic nervous system involvement may include labile hypertension, tachycardia, peripheral vasoconstriction, cardiac arrhythmias, profuse sweating, hypercapnia, increased urinary excretion of catecholamines, and late-appearing hypotension.

During the illness, the patient's sensorium is usually clear. The fever is generally low grade or absent. Patients who recover are usually afebrile. After a period of weeks, the paroxysms decrease in frequency and severity and gradually disappear. Generally the trismus is the last symptom to subside. Patients with fatal disease are usually febrile; in most instances, death occurs before the tenth day of illness.

The spinal fluid in tetanus is normal. The peripheral white blood cell count may be normal or slightly elevated. Most patients with tetanus show the generalized manifestations described. Occasionally, however, generalized tetanus may be preceded by cephalic tetanus. In this case, the incubation period is only 1 to 2 days; it follows a head injury or otitis media and has a poor prognosis (Bagratuni, 1952). Cephalic tetanus is characterized by involvement of various cranial nerves, especially the seventh, but the third, fourth, ninth, tenth, and twelfth may be affected also. Cephalic tetanus can occur without subsequent generalized disease.

Tetanus neonatorum

The onset of tetanus usually begins when the newborn infant is between 3 and 10 days old and is manifested by difficulty in sucking and by excessive crying. Soon the infant's jaw becomes too stiff to suck, and there is also difficulty in swallowing. Shortly thereafter, stiffness of the body appears, and intermittent jerking spasms may begin. Variable degrees of trismus, sustained, tonic, or rigid states of muscle contraction, and spasms or convulsions occur. The spasms may occur frequently or rarely, spontaneously or in response to stimuli. Deep tendon reflex activity may be increased, or the deep tendons may show no response on testing because of constant generalized stiffness. Opisthotonos may be absent or so extreme that the head almost touches the heels. The cry varies from a repeated, short, mildly hoarse cry to a strangled-sounding voiceless noise. Color varies from normal to slate-blue cyanosis, due to poor aeration and impending shock. Severe spasms may be followed by gray color and flaccidity, anoxia, and exhaustion.

CASE 1. F.F., a 13-day-old male infant, was brought to Children's Hospital of Los Angeles with respiratory arrest. The infant was born at another hospital to a gravida 5, para 5 mother. On the second day of life, the patient left the other hospital. On the tenth day, the umbilical stump fell off, and purulent drainage was observed at the site. On the thirteenth day of life, the infant had trismus, was irritable, and refused feedings. On the morning of the fourteenth day, the day of admission, the infant was febrile, his body was rigid, his respirations were noisy, and he was drooling. The infant had frequent spasms of the extremities and the body triggered by external stimuli. The mouth was locked in an open position. Respirations were shallow, and an inspiratory rattle was heard that was suggestive of laryngospasm.

Gram-positive rods and spores were present in pus from the umbilicus. Treatment included the use of tetanus antitoxin (human), surgical debridement of the umbilical stump, tracheostomy, reduction of environmental stimuli, and the use of diazepam (Valium), meprobamate, phenobarbital, thorazine, penicillin, and kanamycin. The infant received feedings by gavage, and the bladder was emptied by Crede's method.

The patient's condition improved steadily. Spasms decreased in frequency and stopped altogether after 4 weeks. The use of medications was also discontinued then, without return of spasms, and the patient was discharged well after 48 days in the hospital.

DIAGNOSIS

The development of trismus, risus sardonicus, generalized tonic rigidity, and spasms in a patient with a clear sensorium and a recent history of trauma is highly suggestive of a diagnosis of tetanus. The recovery of *C. tetani* from the wound would confirm the diagnosis; however, in most instances the organism is not detected.

DIFFERENTIAL DIAGNOSIS
Acute bacterial meningitis

Trismus is rarely present in acute bacterial meningitis. The patient is usually acutely ill, febrile, and has an altered sensorium. The positive spinal fluid examination identifies the disease as meningitis.

Encephalitis

Patients with viral and postinfectious encephalitides rarely have trismus, do not have clear minds as a rule, and usually have abnormal spinal fluid findings.

Rabies

Continuous tonic seizures are not present in rabies; they are usually intermittent and clonic. Trismus is rarely observed.

Strychnine poisoning

There is usually complete relaxation between convulsions in strychnine poisoning. When trismus occurs, it occurs late.

Reaction to phenothiazines

Among the extrapyramidal neurologic syndromes that may accompany the use of some phenothiazine drugs are acute dystonic reactions with facial grimacing, torticollis, and muscle rigidity. These disappear with discontinuation of the drug.

Tetany

In tetany, trismus is usually absent, but carpopedal spasms and laryngospasm may be present. A low blood calcium content confirms the diagnosis.

Peritonsillar abscess

Peritonsillar abscess, a febrile painful condition, is usually accompanied by trismus. However, there are no generalized muscular spasms.

COMPLICATIONS

The interference with pulmonary ventilation by laryngospasm, respiratory muscle spasm, or accumulation of secretions may be followed by pneumonia and atelectasis. Vertebral compression fractures and lacerations of the tongue may follow a seizure.

PROGNOSIS

Tetanus continues to be a very serious disease. Despite new methods of treatment, a person with tetanus today has a high probability of dying. The declines in incidence and mortality of tetanus over the past two decades have been parallel, resulting in minor changes in the case fatality rate. The incidence and death rates are shown in Fig. 29-1. In patients who survive, recovery is complete—without sequelae if supportive measures have provided adequate ventilation. The prognosis is significantly affected by the following factors.

Age

The highest mortality is found among patients in the extremes of life. For neonates the case fatality rate is 66%, and for persons 50 years of age or older it is 70%. By contrast, for patients 10 to 19 years old, the case fatality rate lies between 10% and 20%.

Incubation period

The median incubation period of fatal and nonfatal tetanus cases with known wounds was 6.2 and 7.6 days, respectively, in 1968 to 1969, and similar observations were made during 1963, 1966, and 1967. Consistently lower case fatality rates have been observed in those below the age of 50 years as compared to those above 50 years, irrespective of the length of incubation period.

Christie (1969) believes that a more reliable guide to the prognosis is the length of the period of onset, defined as the interval between the first evidence of trismus and the first general convulsion. If this period is shorter than 48 hours, the attack is likely to be severe; if the interval is longer, the illness will be milder. Nevertheless, the course of tetanus cannot be predicted until the severity and frequency of the

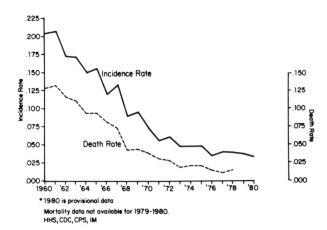

Fig. 29-1. Tetanus incidence rate per 100,000 population and death rate per 100,000 population, United States, 1960-1980*

convulsions have been made clear. It is easy to be misled in the first day or two.

Fever

In mild or moderately severe cases of tetanus, fever is not a common finding. In patients with involvement of the brain stem, fever or hyperpyrexia is often present. Afebrile patients have a better chance of recovery.

Extent of involvement

In local tetanus, the symptoms are confined to the wound area, and the prognosis is usually good. Generalized involvement, however, is followed by a more serious outcome. Convulsions occurring in patients less than 20 years of age correlate with a poorer prognosis.

Antitoxin therapy

In general, antitoxin therapy does not significantly affect the prognosis. Toxin has usually been fixed and is not available for neutralization. However, antitoxin may modify the disease if it is given during the incubation period or very early in the course of the illness.

EPIDEMIOLOGIC FACTORS

Tetanus is worldwide in distribution. The spores are widely disseminated in soil and in animal feces. Tetanus spores or toxin may contaminate a variety of biologic and surgical products such as vaccines, sera, and catgut. Persons of all ages and both sexes are equally susceptible. In spite of the ubiquity of *C. tetani*, tetanus is relatively rare but tetanus neonatorum is still a serious problem in developing countries. The disease can be prevented in newborns by proper handling of the umbilical cord and by immunization of pregnant women. In fact, with available tools of modern aseptic technique and active immunization, this is a disease that could be eliminated.

IMMUNITY

It is estimated that 0.01 unit of antibody is protective in humans. Maternal IgG antibodies, if present, are transmitted through the placenta. This passively acquired immunity, however, is of short duration, as maternal globulins are metabolized by the infant. The administration of tetanus toxoid to infants, children, and adults will stimulate the production of antibodies that provide protection against the effects of toxin. This can be maintained at a protective level by periodic injections. Patients recovering from tetanus should be actively immunized because the extremely potent toxin may not stimulate an antibody response in the patient.

TREATMENT
Control of muscular spasms

The patient should be admitted to a quiet, darkened room where all possible auditory, visual, tactile, or other stimuli are reduced to a minimum. The first priority in the management should be the administration of appropriate drugs to reduce the number and severity of the spasms.

Diazepam (Valium) has proved to be a very valuable drug, because it effectively controls spasms and hypertonicity without depressing the cortical centers. The recommended dose for infants under 2 years of age is 8 mg per kilogram of body weight per day given in doses of 2 to 3 mg every 3 hours. The dosage should be increased to 10 to 40 mg per kilogram of body weight per day for children 2 to 5 years of age and older. The intramuscular dose should be decreased as indicated, and the drug should be given orally when tolerated.

Antitoxin therapy

It is recommended that after adequate sedation has been achieved, human tetanus immunoglobulin be given in a single dose, 3000 to 6000 units, intramuscularly. If human immune serum globulin is unavailable, bovine tetanus antitoxin should be given if the sensitivity reactions to horse serum (p. 29) are negative. The antitoxin is given intravenously and intramuscularly, with half the dose given via each route.

Antimicrobial therapy

It is recommended that aqueous penicillin G be given in a dose of 1 million units intravenously every 6 hours of 1.2 million units of procaine penicillin once daily. Tetracycline, 2 gm daily (adult dose), may be used if the patient is sensitive to penicillin. Penicillin is effective against the vegetative form of the tetanus bacillus and kills growing bacteria, thus stopping toxin production. Penicillin does not alter the effects of existing toxin.

Surgical treatment

After the patient has been sedated and has received antitoxin, any wound should be thoroughly cleansed and debrided. Extensive surgical excision is usually not indicated.

Supportive treatment

Good medical and nursing care must be concerned with minimizing stimuli that may precipitate a convulsion. Procedures such as catheterization or placement of indwelling lines should be carried out at a time when any sedative is exerting its maximum effect. Such procedures are best accomplished early in the course of clinical illness. In addition, care should be taken to anticipate and prevent such complications as aspiration pneumonia, lower bowel obstruction due to fecal impaction, urinary retention, and decubitus ulcers. Adequate sedation may prevent a compression fracture of the vertebra. Respiratory support is essential, and this may require intubation or tracheostomy with respirator ventilation.

Tracheostomy

The combination of heavy sedation, difficulty in swallowing, laryngospasm, and accumulation of secretions leads to obstruction of the airway. A tracheostomy or intubation can be lifesaving if it is performed when there is an appropriate indication. The following problems may be considered specific indications for this procedure: (1) prolonged spasm of the respiratory muscles, (2) inability to cough or swallow, (3) laryngeal obstruction due to spasm or secretions, and (4) coma.

A relatively low mortality of 10% was reported by Edmondson and Flowers (1979), who treated 100 patients with tetanus on an intensive care unit. They attributed this favorable mortality rate to early resort to tracheostomy and paralysis in the severe cases.

PREVENTIVE MEASURES
Active immunization

Since many cases of tetanus follow minor abrasions and lacerations that are ignored, control of the disease can be best achieved by active immunization with toxoid before exposure. All infants should be routinely immunized with tetanus toxoid that is incorporated with diphtheria toxoid and pertussis vaccine. The usual basic series of the triple antigen is given at 8-week intervals for three doses beginning at 2 to 4 months of age. Booster doses are given at approximately 1 and 4 years later and at 10-year intervals thereafter.

In the event of an injury, an additional booster dose of tetanus toxoid may be indicated; a protective antitoxin level is usually achieved within 1 week (see p. 483). It has been shown that a booster dose can provoke an adequate response after a 10-year lapse since the last injection. In severe, crushing, and heavily contaminated wounds, particularly compound skull fractures, human tetanus immunoglobulin, 250 units, should be given intramuscularly in conjunction with the toxoid. This procedure should prevent a potential short-incubation–period disease. It is important to emphasize that patients recovering from tetanus may not be immune; therefore, they should be actively immunized with tetanus toxoid.

Passive immunization

Persons who have not been actively immunized should be protected with human tetanus immunoglobulin in the event of an injury. The usual dose is 250 units given intramuscularly; in severe wounds 500 units may be indicated.

Care of a wound

A wound should be cleansed thoroughly, foreign bodies and necrotic tissue should be removed, and the area should be debrided when indicated.

REFERENCES

Abel JJ, et al. Researches on tetanus. Bull Johns Hopkins Hosp 1935;56:84, 317; 1936;59:307; 1938;62:91, 522, 610; 1938;63:373.

Adams JM, Kenny JD, Rudolph AJ. Modern management of tetanus neonatorum. Pediatrics 1979;64:472.

Armitage P, Clifford R: Prognosis in tetanus: use of data from therapeutic trials. J Infect Dis 1978;138:1-8.

Bagratuni L. Cephalic tetanus: with report of a case. Br Med J 1952;1:461.

Bizzini B. Tetanus toxin. Microbiol Rev 1979;43:224-240.

Brand DA, Acampora D, Gottlieb ZD, et al. Adequacy of antitetanus prophylaxis in six hospital emergency rooms. N Engl J Med 1983;309:636-40.

Brooks VB, Asanuma H. Action of tetanus toxin in the cerebral cortex. Science 1962;137:674.

Brooks VB, Curtis DR, Eccles JC. Mode of action of tetanus toxin. Nature 1955;175:120.

Center for Disease Control. Tetanus surveillance. United States Department of Health, Education, and Welfare,

Public Health Service, Health Services and Mental Health Administration report no. 4, March 31, 1974.

Christie AB. Infectious diseases: epidemiology and clinical practice. Baltimore: The Williams & Wilkins Co., 1969.

Cole L, Youngman H. Treatment of tetanus. Lancet 1969;1:1017.

Edmondson RS, Flowers MW. Intensive care in tetanus: management, complications and mortality in 100 cases. Br Med J 1979;1:1401.

Edsall G. Specific prophylaxis of tetanus. JAMA 1959; 171:417.

Edsall G. Passive immunization. Pediatrics 1963;32:599.

Eidels L, Proia RL, Hart DA. Membrane receptors for bacterial toxins. Micro Rev 1983;47:596-620.

Goyal RK, Neogy CN, Mathur GP. A controlled trial of antiserum in the treatment of tetanus. Lancet 1966; 2:1371.

Kaeser HE, Sauer A. Tetanus toxin: a neuromuscular blocking agent. Nature 1969;223:842.

Kessimer JG, Habig WH, Hardegree MC. Monoclonal antibodies as probes of tetanus toxin structure and function. Infect Immun 1983;42:942-948.

Kerr JH, et al. Involvement of the sympathetic nervous system in tetanus: studies on 82 cases. Lancet 1968;2:236.

Kryzhanovsky G. Tetanus: a polysystemic disease. In Comptesrendus de la patrieme Congerence Internationale sur la tetanos (Proceedings of the Fourth International Conference on Tetanus). Lyon, France: Lips, 1975;189.

Laird WJ, Aronson W, Silver RP, et al. Plasmid associated toxigenicity in Clostridium tetani. J Infect Dis 1980; 142:623.

Levine L, Edsall G. Tetanus toxoid: what determines reaction proneness? J Infect Dis 1981;144:376.

Long AP. Tetanus toxoid, its use in the United States Army. Am J Public Health 1943;33:53.

Looney JM, Edsall G, Ispen J, Jr, Chasen WH. Persistence of antitoxin levels after tetanus toxoid inoculation in adults and effects of a booster dose after intervals. N Engl J Med 1956;254:6.

Marie A, Morax V. Recherches sur l'absorption de la toxine tetanique. Ann Inst Pasteur 1902;16:818.

McCracken GH, Jr, Dowell DL, Marshall FN. Double-blind trial of equine antitoxin and human immune globulin in tetanus neonatorum. Lancet 1971;1:1146.

Meyer H, Ransome F. Untersuchungen uber den Tetanus. Arch Exp Pathol Pharmakol 1903;49:369.

Millard AH. Local tetanus. Lancet 1954;2:844.

Pratt EL. Clinical tetanus: a study of 56 cases, with special reference to methods of prevention and a plan for evaluating treatment. JAMA 1945;129:1243.

Rubbo SD, Suri JC. Passive immunization against tetanus with human immune globulin. Br Med J 1962;2:79.

Rubinstein HM. Studies on human tetanus antitoxin. Am J Hyg 1962;76:276.

Sanders RKM, Martyn B, Joseph R, Peacock ML. Intrathecal antitetanus serum (horse) in the treatment of tetanus. Lancet 1977;1:974.

Smolens J, Vogt A, Crawford MN, Stokes J, Jr. The persistence in the human circulation of horse and human tetanus antitoxins. J Pediatr 1961;59:899.

Spaeth R. A clinical study of tetanus. Am J Dis Child 1940;59:693.

Stanfield JP, Gall D, Braden PM. Single dose-antenatal tetanus immunization. Lancet 1973;1:215.

Veronesi R. Clinical observations on 712 cases of tetanus subject to four different methods of treatment: 18.2 per cent mortality rate under a new method of treatment. Am J Med Sci 1956;232:629.

30

TOXOPLASMOSIS

Toxoplasmosis is a widespread, usually asymptomatic zoonotic infection caused by the ubiquitous obligate intracellular protozoon parasite *Toxoplasma gondii*. It may be congenital or acquired. Both forms are characterized by a wide variety of clinical patterns ranging from an asymptomatic course to a severe generalized infection with a fatal outcome. The chief clinical manifestations of congenital infection include chorioretinitis, abnormal spinal fluid, convulsions, intracranial calcifications, anemia, jaundice, splenomegaly, hepatomegaly, fever, and lymphadenopathy. Acquired toxoplasmosis, when it is apparent, may be mild (resembling infectious mononucleosis), or severe, manifested by any of the following: fever, encephalitis, maculopapular rash, pneumonia, hepatitis, polymyositis, pericarditis, and myocarditis.

ETIOLOGY

T. gondii was first isolated from a North African rodent, *Ctenodactylus gondi*, and was described as a new protozooan species in 1909. Thirty years later its role in the causation of human disease was established.

Toxoplasmas exist in three forms: the tachyzoite (the proliferative form), the tissue cyst, and the oocyst (which produces sporozoites). The parasite exists in two cycles. The complete cycle with gametogeny and formation of oocysts occurs only in members of the cat family. Cats are the definitive host for this parasite. Infected cats shed millions of noninfectious oocysts in the feces; after excretion sporulation must occur to render the oocysts infectious.

In other animal hosts, only an incomplete cycle of the organism occurs, and no oocysts develop. Tachyzoites and tissue cysts are formed. Tachyzoites are crescent shaped, ranging in size from 4 to 7 μm long and 2 to 4 μm wide. They may be demonstrated with both Giemsa and Wright's stain. This form of the organism is used in serologic tests. It is also the form seen in acute infections, during which it invades every kind of mammalian cell.

Within the recovering host, tachyzoites, some of which remain viable, are incorporated into cysts. Each cyst may contain hundreds to thousands of toxoplasmas. Cysts are most commonly found in brain and in skeletal and heart muscle; they may be demonstrated in tissue sections with periodic acid–Schiff stain. They persist for years and may be one source of latent infection with this organism. Presumably, immunity to the parasite prevents reactivation of symptomatic infection. Remington (1983) also speculates that the immune system is responsible for controlling the primary infection at least in part by causing cyst formation. Some toxoplasmas may also, after primary infection, remain viable in monocytes; these too may be a source for reactivation of latent infection, especially in immunocompromised hosts.

Humans may be infected by inadvertent ingestion of sporulated oocysts or tissue cysts in meat, by iatrogenic inoculation of cysts or tachyzoites, by organ transplantation or blood transfusion, respectively, or by transplacental transmission of tachyzoites from mother to fetus when the mother has a primary infection during pregnancy. Human-to-human transmission, with the exception of transplacental passage, has not been demonstrated.

Natural toxoplasmic infection is found throughout the world in a wide variety of species of mammals, birds, and reptiles. Infections with *T. gondii* occur among domestic animals and birds, including dogs, cats, sheep, goats, swine, cattle, rabbits, rats, guinea pigs, chickens, and pigeons.

Various studies indicate that *T. gondii* probably originated as an intestinal coccidian in cats, with fecal-to-oral spread. Congenital transmission in humans is ecologically unimportant but medically very important. In pregnant women consumption of raw and undercooked meat laden with cysts, and contact with contaminated cat feces seem to be important methods of transmission. The carnivorous nature of cats not only provides an effective means of spread but also can lead to widespread contamination of the environment with a profusion of oocysts.

T. gondii oocysts require at least 24 hours for sporulation to occur at 25° C. Sporulation and the development of infectivity are temperature dependent. Higher temperatures arrest infectivity; 24 hours at 37° C or 30 minutes at 50° C prevent sporulation (Frenkel et al., 1970).

Infection of humans with toxoplasma is followed by the formation of antibodies detectable by a variety of methods and by the development of cellular immunity. In 1948 Sabin and Feldman discovered a new immune phenomenon in which the affinity of *T. gondii* for certain dyes serves as an indicator of the presence or absence of antibody. This so-called dye test depends on the fact that toxoplasmas incubated with normal nonimmune serum are stained with methylene blue. When they are incubated with specific immune serum (together with a heat-labile accessory factor present in fresh normal human serum), they lose their staining affinity for the dye. The dye test provides the most effective and quantitative method of measuring toxoplasma-neutralizing antibodies.

PATHOLOGY

The pathologic changes observed in toxoplasmic infections in humans vary with the age of the person. In the fetus and young infant the principal lesion is a marked destruction of nervous tissue. Toxoplasmas are often widely disseminated in other tissues, including the heart, lungs, adrenal glands, and striated muscles. In these tissues, necrotizing and focal inflammatory lesions may or may not be present. The central nervous system (CNS) shows a severe meningoencephalitis characterized by large inflammatory lesions, necrosis, calcification, and cyst formation. The areas involved are the cortex, subcortical white matter, caudate and lenticular nuclei, midbrain, pons and medulla, and spinal cord. Severe lesions are likely to occur around the ventricles, the walls of which may be covered with exudate or ependymal granulomas. Obstruction of the foramina of Monro or aqueduct of Sylvius may give rise to internal hydrocephalus. Miliary granulomas, often associated with focal necrotic and inflammatory lesions, are numerous in the brain and spinal cord.

Chorioretinitis is characterized by edema and necrosis of the retina, necrosis and disruption of the pigmented layer and the layer of rods and cones, and infiltration of the retina and choroid with inflammatory cells. In the later stages, an increase in glial tissue is seen in the affected areas of the retina. Granulation tissue is formed and may invade the vitreous.

The main pathologic findings in acquired cases appear to be interstitial pneumonitis, focal necrosis in the liver and spleen, foci of necrosis and cellular infiltration in the myocardium, and focal lesions in the brain.

CLINICAL MANIFESTATIONS
Congenital toxoplasmosis

The congenital form of toxoplasmic infection has a varied assortment of clinical manifestations ranging from a generalized infection dominated by signs of irreversible CNS damage to a mild or asymptomatic infection. These clinical manifestations of congenital toxoplasmosis are similar to those observed in infants with congenital cytomegalovirus and rubella virus infections and neonatal herpes simplex infections.

The classic combination of chorioretinitis, cerebral calcification, and hydrocephalus (or microcephalus) was observed by Eichenwald in 1957 in only about 60% of 150 confirmed cases of congenital toxoplasmosis. Chorioretinitis was the most common single feature, occurring in

86% of the cases. It may not be apparent at birth but can develop within a few weeks after birth. Bilateral as a rule, the lesions are found in the macula and on the periphery of the retina. In some instances, the observation of peripheral lesions may require examination with the patient under anesthesia, after full dilation of the pupils.

Abnormal cerebrospinal fluid (CSF) was the second most common finding. It was present in 63% of cases (Eichenwald, 1957). In congenital toxoplasmosis the CSF is often xanthochromic. There are increased levels of both red blood cells and white blood cells, predominantly mononuclear elements. The protein content is elevated. In the ventricular fluid, protein levels have been reported to be as high as 2000 mg/100 ml CSF. Toxoplasmas may be seen in smears of the sediment stained with Wright's stain or in cell blocks of the sediment embedded and stained with hematoxylin and eosin. Toxoplasmas may also be detected in the CSF by inoculation of animals.

Other common features include convulsions, intracranial calcifications, anemia, jaundice, hepatomegaly, and splenomegaly. In addition, such diverse manifestations as lymphadenopathy, pneumonitis, vomiting, diarrhea, and maculopapular rash are not uncommon.

The various forms and the severity of congenital toxoplasmosis are related in part to the time of gestation when intrauterine infection takes place. When infection occurs in the first or second trimester of pregnancy, the infant may be born dead or may show generalized severe disease. When the infection occurs in the third trimester the infant is likely to be normal or less severely affected.

Desmonts and Couvreur (1974, 1975) found that only a minority of infants born to mothers who acquired acute toxoplasmosis during pregnancy showed signs of clinical infection. Sixty percent of the infants were not infected. Of those who were infected, the majority had subclinical infection; only 11% of the total were overtly affected. Although the rate of intrauterine infections increases throughout the 9 months of pregnancy, first trimester infections are most often associated with severe disease of the infant.

The following case report illustrates generalized disease in a low birth weight infant.

CASE 1. A Puerto Rican female infant (birth weight 2410 gm) was jaundiced from birth. The skin showed numerous petechiae and ecchymoses with large confluent areas (Fig. 30-1). Both the liver and spleen were enormous. Bilateral chorioretinitis was observed. The infant died on the seventh day after birth. Postmortem examination showed generalized toxoplasmosis.

Acquired toxoplasmosis

Infection acquired after birth also is characterized by a variety of clinical patterns. They include the following syndromes: (1) benign lymphadenitis and fever, resembling infectious mononucleosis; (2) severe illness with some or all of the following manifestations: fever, maculopapular rash, pneumonia, hepatitis, polymyositis, pericarditis, and myocarditis; and (3) chorioretinitis. The three clinical syndromes

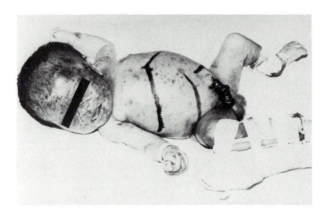

Fig. 30-1. Infant with congenital toxoplasmosis. Note rash and hepatosplenomegaly.

may occur singly or in combination in the same patient (case 2). Most acquired infections, however, are without obvious symptoms. For example, most women who give birth to an infant with congenital infection can recall no illness during pregnancy.

Benign lymphadenitis. Benign lymphadenitis is characterized by fatigue, fever, coryza, and generalized lymphadenopathy. The clinical picture resembles infectious mononucleosis. Lymphocytosis with atypical lymphocytes is commonly observed, but the heterophil antibody test is negative. Fatigue is the main symptom. The lymph nodes are enlarged to the size of hazelnuts or walnuts. They may be tender during the acute stage, but later they are usually painless. They are firm, discrete, and smooth and not attached to underlying tissues. The overlying skin is not affected. The lymphadenitis is often generalized, but one superficial area only may be affected. Enlarged hilar shadows may be seen in the roentgenogram of the chest. The infection runs a benign course, sometimes with persistent fatigue for months but ending in complete recovery.

Severe disease. The onset may be insidious, with weakness and malaise that persist for 6 to 10 days, often followed by fever, rash, and signs of pneumonia. The temperature may be as high as 41.1° C (106° F). The rash is maculopapular, generalized, and similar to that of Rocky Mountain spotted fever except that the scalp, the palms of the hands, and the soles of the feet are spared. The skin lesions are bright red to pale pink, and some may blanch on pressure.

Signs of pneumonia may appear simultaneously with the rash, or they may emerge later. Coarse rales and dullness over both lung bases may be accompanied by cough, dyspnea, and cyanosis. Roentgenographic examination of the chest may show irregular areas of increased density in the lower lobes or only accentuation of the hilar and lower lobe markings. The prognosis is often unfavorable.

Severe infections have also been reported in which the clinical picture has included hepatitis, polymyositis, pericarditis, myocarditis, and encephalitis. Acute encephalitis is characterized by headache. vomiting, generalized convulsions, unsteady gait, or transitory confusion. The temperature may not be elevated at the onset. En-

larged lymph nodes and spleen may be present. The results of neurologic examination are usually normal. The CSF shows an increase in number of white blood cells, predominantly mononuclear cells, from 30 to 2000/mm³ of CSF. Protein and glucose concentrations are usually normal. The patient's condition may steadily deteriorate, ending in death or survival with residual brain injury manifested by recurrent convulsions and personality changes. Patients who recover completely with no residual damage have also been described.

Immunocompromised patients such as those with an underlying malignancy or acquired immunodeficiency syndrome (AIDS) are at greater risk to develop severe toxoplasmosis than immunologically normal persons. In many cases in immunocompromised persons, the infection is believed to be the result of reactivation of latent toxoplasmosis rather than a primary infection with this organism.

Chorioretinitis. Although chorioretinitis is a common manifestation of congenital infection, it is rare in acquired toxoplasmosis. It has been observed to occur in about 1% of patients with confirmed toxoplasmosis of the acquired type (Perkins, 1973). In most patients who present with it beyond the newborn age it is believed to have resulted from reactivation of latent infection acquired congenitally. There is considerable evidence that it represents an allergic inflammatory response to ruptured pseudocysts.

CASE 2. A 2.5-year-old boy was admitted to Bellevue Hospital on May 15, 1959, because of fever of unknown origin. He was born in Puerto Rico but had lived in New York City for 9 months before onset of this illness. The clinical course of the disease is illustrated in Fig. 30-2. The clinical manifestations included fever, maculopapular rash, pneumonitis, lymphadenopathy (Fig. 30-3), and chorioretinitis. There was no evidence of encephalitis. Other manifestations included periorbital edema, hepatosplenomegaly, leg pain, leg tenderness, and edema of both feet. During the first 3 weeks of his illness, he was subjected to a battery of laboratory tests that shed no light on the diagnosis.

A *Toxoplasma* dye test performed during the fifth week was positive in a titer of 1:4096. The titer increased to 1:16,384 in the tenth week. Toxoplasmas were isolated from a postauricular lymph node in the ninth week. Small areas of chorioretinitis were noted in both eyes during the seventeenth week. *Toxo-*

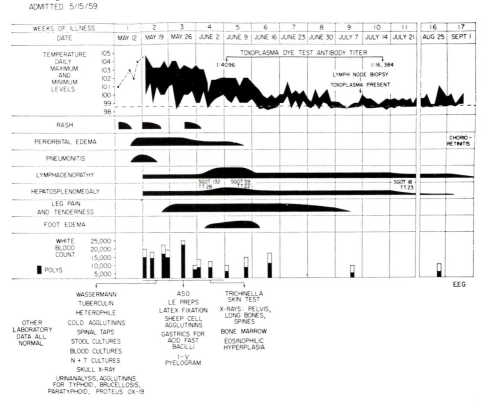

R.A. 2½ YEAR ♂
ADMITTED 5/15/59

Fig. 30-2. Schematic diagram of clinical course of acquired toxoplasmosis in a child. (From Neumann CG, Hilton C, Barreda A. Am J Dis Child 1960;100:117.)

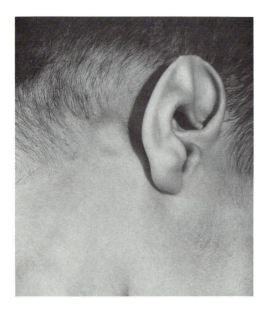

Fig. 30-3. Enlarged postauricular lymph node of patient with acquired toxoplasmosis.

plasma dye tests performed on sera obtained from the mother and father were negative.

Clinical manifestations of the following syndromes associated with acquired toxoplasmosis were observed in this patient: (1) lymphadenitis; (2) fever, pneumonitis, and rash; and (3) chorioretinitis. The source of his *Toxoplasma* infection was unknown.

DIAGNOSIS

Congenital toxoplasmosis

A diagnosis of congenital toxoplasmosis should be considered in the presence of the following clinical manifestations in a newborn or young infant: chorioretinitis, abnormal spinal fluid, anemia, convulsions, intracranial calcifications, splenomegaly, jaundice, hepatomegaly, rash, lymphadenopathy, fever, vomiting, and hydrocephalus or microcephalus. These diverse signs occur in various combinations. The classic triad of chorioretinitis, cerebral calcification, and hydrocephalus or microcephalus is seen in only about 60% of the patients. Neither the CNS signs, which occur most frequently, nor the visceral manifestations, such as jaundice and enlargement of the liver and spleen, are sufficiently characteristic to warrant a diagnosis on clinical grounds alone. It is important to emphasize that chorioretinitis, intracranial calcifications, hepatosplenomegaly, and jaundice may also be associated with congenital infection with cytomegalovirus.

A *specific* diagnosis is established by the demonstration of *T. gondii* and by serologic methods. The organism may be isolated in cell cultures or demonstrated by inoculation of laboratory animals. When isolation of the organism is to be attempted, tissues should be inoculated as quickly as is possible. The best method of storage, if it is required, is refrigeration at 4° C.

Serodiagnosis is more widely used and more practical than isolation of the parasite. A primary infection with *T. gondii* is followed by the rapid formation of antibodies, as measured by the dye test, or by complement fixation (CF), indirect immunofluorescence (IFA), or enzyme-linked immunosorbent assay (ELISA). In most laboratories one of the latter tests has replaced the dye test, which requires the use of viable infectious *T. gondii*. An indirect hemagglutination assay (IHA) has been developed, but it is not sensitive enough for diagnosis of congenital toxoplasmosis, although it has been used successfully for seroepidemiologic studies. Within 1 or 2 weeks after infection, the dye test antibody and IFA levels rise to not less than 1:256 and occasionally as high as 1:32,000 or more. CF antibody is usually absent during the early weeks of infection, but then its level rises and ranges from 1:16 to 1:256. All types of toxoplasma antibodies may persist at high levels for several years. CF antibody often disappears completely, but the other types fall more slowly and tend to persist indefinitely. Even the lowest titers are indicative of past infection with *T. gondii*. For serodiagnosis of acute primary toxoplasmosis in a pregnant woman, a significant rise in antibody titer in *two* serum samples run in one test is required; even high antibody titers may not be indicative of *acute* infection.

Specific IgM antibody measured by immunofluorescence has been detected in neonatal and cord sera. This method may be useful for diagnosis of congenital infection in some laboratories, but it is technically difficult and may not always be reliable because false-positive and false-negative results can occur. IgM antibody in adults and older children can develop after both primary and recurrent toxoplasmosis.

Antibodies to *T. gondii* cross the placenta from mother to infant. If the child is not infected, these passively acquired antibodies disappear from the infant's blood with time. The diagnosis of congenital toxoplasmosis is untenable in the absence of specific antibody in the serum of the child, regardless of how high the titer may be in the mother's serum. When congenital toxoplasmosis is suspected in an asymptomatic infant, antibody titers should be obtained during the first weeks of life, and the test should be repeated after several months. If the infant's antibody titer is high because of infection with *T. gondii*, it will still be elevated in the second test. If the second test is negative or the titer is low, it indicates disappearing antibody passively acquired from the mother, and the diagnosis of congenital toxoplasmosis cannot be made. Varying patterns of antibody synthesis in infected infants have been observed, however, so that if the second titer is *low*, a third titer should be performed after several more months, and the infant should continue to be observed closely, especially for chorioretinitis.

In older children, particularly those over the age of 6 years, when the IFA or dye test antibody titers may be less than 1:256 in the mother or child or in both, the diagnosis is still possible if the child shows clinical manifestations compatible with congenital toxoplasmosis. Ocular disease in children and adults is often associated with *low* specific antibody titers. If only the mother's serum is available for examination because the child died before toxoplasmosis was suspected of being present, an antibody titer of 1:256 or more *does not* prove that the child had toxoplasmosis.

In 1965 Glasser and Delta described a prospective diagnosis of congenital toxoplasmosis achieved by chance observation of cysts in the placenta of monozygotic twins. Although they were observed closely, the twins showed no evidence of disease until 7 months of age, when alternating strabismus was observed in both infants. At 10 months of age they both had bilateral strabismus, bilateral chorioretinitis, and calcifications in the region of the basal ganglia; CF antibody titers were 1:64 in both infants. When congenital toxoplasmosis is suspected, if possible, placental tissue should be examined histologically and/or cultured for the presence of cysts or tachyzoites.

Acquired toxoplasmosis

The acquired forms of toxoplasmosis may be suspected of being present in patients showing a variety of clinical manifestations, including (1) fever, fatigue, and lymphadenopathy resembling infectious mononucleosis but with negative heterophil antibody tests and negative serologic tests for Epstein-Barr virus; (2) fever, maculopapular rash resembling rickettsial disease, encephalitis, pneumonia, myocarditis, and a variety of other severe manifestations; and (3) ocular signs such as chorioretinitis and granulomatous uveititis. Disseminated infections with toxoplasma have been reported with increasing frequency in immunocompromised patients. A specific diagnosis is established similar to the ways already described for congenital toxoplasmosis. Toxoplasmas must be demonstrated in tissues or fluids from the patient, or antibody formation, or an increase in antibody titer must be demonstrated in the course of the illness to make the diagnosis. Demonstration of tachyzoites indicates acute infection. The presence of cysts in tissue specimens does not differentiate between acute and chronic (latent) infection.

Although the *skin test* may be a useful epidemiologic tool for estimating the incidence of subclinical infection, it is of no diagnostic value in the individual case. This is because a considerable proportion of persons with congenital toxoplasmosis who possess circulating antibody fail to give a positive skin test. A positive test also fails to differentiate between persons with low dye test titers of dubious significance and those with highly significant titers.

PROGNOSIS
Congenital toxoplasmosis

The mortality rate may range between 3% and 12% irrespective of the clinical manifestations. Death is not the only end result of toxoplasmosis. Serious sequelae pertaining to the CNS have been observed in a high proportion of survivors. Mental retardation has occurred in about 85% of those with manifest illness who were observed for 4 years or more. Convulsions have occurred in about 80%, spasticity and palsies in 58% to 75%, severely impaired sight in 42% to 68%, and hydrocephalus or microcephalus in 44% of those with neurologic disease but in only 6% of those with generalized disease. Deafness has occurred in a small fraction. Only 8% to 16% of the patients were normal after the 4-year follow-up period (Eichenwald, 1957). No matter what the early manifestations are, the eventual outcome may be severe, irreversible damage to the CNS. Subclinical toxoplasmosis in the newborn may also result in progressive CNS abnormalities, according to the studies of Alford et al. (1975), which has implications for treatment.

A *good prognosis* can be given for subsequent children of a mother who has given birth to a child with congenital toxoplasmosis. Many mothers who gave birth to children with proved congenital toxoplasmosis have had children subsequently. None of the children from subsequent pregnancies has had toxoplasmosis.

Acquired toxoplasmosis

The prognosis depends on the clinical form of the illness and the immune status of the host. The outlook is serious for patients with the syndrome of fever, rash, pneumonia, encephalitis, and other evidence of disseminated infection. A fatal course may result, although recoveries have been reported. The syndrome of fever, fatigue, and lymphadenitis resembling infectious mononucleosis is usually benign. Complete recovery is the rule, although it may be delayed for weeks.

EPIDEMIOLOGIC FACTORS

The exact source of infection and mode of transmission are not fully known. *T. gondii* is a ubiquitous parasite. Cats, dogs, rodents, swine, cattle, sheep, goats, and other mammals as well as pigeons, chickens, and other birds serve as reservoirs of infection. Evidence of excretion of *Toxoplasma* oocysts in cat feces indicates that this is a likely source of human infection (Teutsch et al., 1979).

Another source of infection is raw or undercooked meat. One outbreak of acute lymphadenitic toxoplasmosis involved five medical students. Fever, headache, myalgia, lymphadenopathy, and splenomegaly characterized the illness. Extremely high Sabin-Feldman dye test titers and rising CF antibody titers confirmed the diagnosis. All five students ate rare hamburgers at the same place on the same night, and circumstantial evidence indicated that this was the source of infection (Kean et al., 1969).

The incidence of subclinical or unrecognized *Toxoplasma* infection varies greatly among different age groups and in different parts of the world. Antibody surveys of different population groups have shown infection rates ranging from 20% to 80%. Infection appears to be rare in the far north and most common in the tropics. In a longitudinal study of 40 families from an upper socioeconomic group in Cleveland, Ohio, antibodies were found in 4.9% of 123 children and in 35% of adults. In these families, toxoplasmosis appeared to be distributed at random, it did not appear to be highly contagious, no common source was found, and inapparent infection or mild febrile episodes without lymphadenopathy were associated with acquisition of antibody (Warren and Dingle, 1966). The incidence of positive skin tests in normal persons in Cincinnati was shown by Feldman and Sabin in 1949 to rise progressively from 5% in persons 5 to 9 years of age to 65% in those 40 years of age and older. The same rising incidence with age was found by Thalhammer in Vienna in 1954, except

that there the 60% level was reached as early as 21 years of age. Feldman (1958) observed a similar rapid rise in patients in Syracuse. He also found great variation in incidence in different parts of the world, ranging from zero among Eskimos in Alaska to 70% for all age groups in Tahiti. Antibodies occur with equal frequency in males and females. There seems to be no seasonal concentration of cases of congenital toxoplasmosis.

TREATMENT

The most effective treatment for acute toxoplasmosis is the combination of sulfadiazine (or triple sulfonamides) with pyrimethamine. Spiramycin has been used to treat pregnant women in France with apparent success (Desmonts and Couvreur, 1974, 1975). It is not licensed in the United States, although it is available from the Centers for Disease Control (CDC) in Atlanta, Georgia, for use in some cases of toxoplasmosis such as congenital infection and that involving the CNS.

Immunologically normal persons with acute toxoplasmosis characterized by lymphadenopathy do not require specific treatment. However, sulfonamide and pyrimethamine therapy is indicated for persons with severe, disseminated disease, for those with vital organ involvement, such as chorioretinitis, and for those who are immunocompromised (Ruskin, 1976). In newborn infants chemotherapy is also indicated for the treatment of early active infection, which may be identified only by serologic means. The combined therapy is not recommended for pregnant women because of the teratogenicity of pyrimethamine. Under these circumstances, sulfonamides should be used alone if the pregnancy will not be terminated by abortion. It may be possible to obtain spiramycin from the CDC.

The dose of pyrimethamine is 0.5 mg per kilogram of body weight every 12 hours; the maximum daily dose should not exceed 25 mg. Sulfadiazine, 150 mg per kilogram of body weight per day is given every 6 hours. These drugs should be given by mouth for 4 weeks. Because pyrimethamine is a folic acid antagonist that can induce leukopenia and thrombocytopenia, patients receiving this drug should have white blood cell and platelet counts at least once weekly. The effects can be reversed by adding folinic acid (1 mg per kilogram of body weight per 24 hours in one dose) to the patient's therapy. The use of corticosteroids is contraindicated.

PREVENTION

Immunosuppressed persons and presumably susceptible pregnant women should be protected against exposure. Hands should be washed after touching uncooked meat. Cysts in meat can be killed by heating to 60° C or by freezing to −20° C (Swartzberg and Remington, 1975). Fruits and vegetables should be washed because of potential contamination with oocysts. Cat feces should be avoided. It is reasonable to screen women of childbearing years before they become pregnant to determine whether they have already experienced toxoplasmosis and thus are at no risk during pregnancy.

REFERENCES

Alford CA, Stagno S, Reynolds DW. Toxoplasmosis: silent congenital infection. In Krugman S, Gershon AA, ed. Infections of the fetus and the newborn infant. Proceedings of an NYU–National Foundation Symposium, March 1975. New York:Alan R Liss, 1975;133.

Desmonts G, Couvreur J. Congenital toxoplasmosis: a prospective study of 378 pregnancies. N Engl J Med 1974;290:1110.

Desmonts G, Couvreur J. Toxoplasmosis: epidemiologic and serologic aspects of perinatal infection. In Krugman S, Gershon AA, ed.s. Infections of the fetus and the newborn infant. Proceedings of an NYU–National Foundation Symposium, March 1975. New York:Alan R Liss, 1975;115.

Dorfman RF, Remington JS Value of lymph node biopsy in the diagnosis of acute acquired toxoplasmosis. N Engl J Med 1973;289:878.

Dubey JP, Miller NL, Frenkel JK. The *Toxoplasma gondii* oocyst from cat feces. J Exp Med 1970;132:636.

Dubey JP, Miller NL, Frenkel JK. Isolation of parasites in congenital toxoplasmosis. Arch Fr Pediatr 1974;31:157.

Dubey JP, Miller NL, Frenkel JK. Toxoplasmosis: epidemiologic and serologic aspects of perinatal infection. In Krugman S, Gershon AA, eds. Infections of the fetus and the newborn infant. Proceedings of an NYU–National Foundation Symposium, March 1975. New York:Alan R Liss, 1975;115.

Eichenwald HF. The laboratory diagnosis of toxoplasmosis. Ann NY Acad Sci 1956;64:207.

Eichenwald HF. Congenital toxoplasmosis. A study of 150 cases. Am J Dis Child 1957;94:411-412.

Eichenwald HF. A study of congenital toxoplasmosis with particular emphasis on clinical manifestations, sequelae and therapy. In Siim JC, ed. Human toxoplasmosis. Copenhagen:Munksgaard, International Booksellers and Publishers Ltd, 1960.

Eyles DE, Coleman N. Evaluation of curative effects of pyramethamine and sulfadiazine, alone and in combination, on experimental mouse toxoplasmosis. Antibiotics Chemother 1955;5:529.

Feldman HA. Toxoplasmosis (review article). Pediatrics 1958;22:559.

Feldman HA. Nationwide serum survey of United States military recruits, 1962. IV. Toxoplasma antibodies. Am J Epidemiol 1965;81:385.

Feldman HA. Congenital toxoplasmosis, at long last. (editorial), N Engl J Med 1974;290:1138.

Feldman HA, Sabin AB. Skin reactions to toxoplasmic antigen in people of different ages without known history of infection. Pediatrics 1949;4:798.

Frenkel JK. Toxoplasma in and around us. Bio-Science 1973a;23:343.

Frenkel JK. Toxoplasmosis: parasite life cycle, pathology, and immunology. In Hammond DM, Long PL, eds. The coccidia. Baltimore:University Park Press, 1973b;343-410.

Frenkel JK, Dubey JP. Toxoplasmosis and its prevention in cats and man. J Infect Dis 1972;126:664.

Frenkel JK, Dubey JP, Miller NL. *Toxoplasma gondii* in cats: fecal stages identified as coccidian oocysts. Science 1970;167:893.

Glasser L, Delta BG. Congenital toxoplasmosis with placental infection in monozygotic twins. Pediatrics 1965;35:276.

Gleason TH, Hamlin WB. Disseminated toxoplasmosis in the compromised host. Arch Intern Med 1974;134:1059.

Grantz CG, Hilton C, Barreda A. A case of acquired toxoplasmosis presenting as an interesting diagnostic problem. Am J Dis Child 1960;100:141.

Hutchison WM. Coccidian-like nature of *Toxoplasma gondii*. Br Med J 1970;1:142.

Jacobs L. New knowledge of toxoplasma and toxoplasmosis. Adv Parasitol 1973;11:631.

Jones TC, Len L, Hirsch JG. Assessment in vitro of immunity against *Toxoplasma gondii*. J Exp Med 1975;141:466.

Kean BH, Kimball AC. The complement-fixation test in the diagnosis of congenital toxoplasmosis. Am J Dis Child 1977;131:21.

Kean BH, Kimball AC, Christenson WN. An epidemic of toxoplasmosis. JAMA 1969;208:1002.

Krick JA, Remington JS. Toxoplasmosis in the adult—an overview. N Engl J Med 1978;298:550.

Perkins ES. Ocular toxoplasmosis. Br J Ophthalmol 1973;57:1-17.

Pinkerton H, Henderson RG. Adult toxoplasmosis: a previously unrecognized disease entity simulating typhus-spotted fever group. JAMA 1941;116:807.

Quinn EL, Fischer EJ, Cox F, Jr, Madhaven T. The clinical spectrum of toxoplasmosis in the adult. Cleve Clin Q 1975;42:71.

Remington JS. Toxoplasmosis. In Charles D, Finland M, eds. Obstetric and perinatal infections. Philadelphia:Lea & Febiger, 1973;27.

Remington JS, Dalrymple W, Jacobs L, Finland M. Toxplasma antibodies among college students N Engl J Med 1963;269:1394.

Remington JS, Desmonts G. Congenital toxoplasmosis: variability in the IgM-fluorescent antibody response and some pitfalls in diagnosis. J Pediatr 1973;83:27.

Remington JS, Desmonts G. Toxoplasmosis. In Remington J, Klein JO, eds. Infectious diseases of the fetus and newborn infant. Philadelphia:WB Saunders Co., 1983;144-263.

Ruskin J. Toxoplasmosis in the compromised host. Ann Intern Med 976;84:193.

Sabin AB. Toxoplasmic encephalitis in children. JAMA 1941;116:801.

Sabin AB. Toxoplasmosis: a recently recognized disease of human beings. In DeSanctis AG, ed. Advances in pediatrics, vol 1. New York:Interscience Publishers, Inc., 1942.

Sabin AB, Eichenwald HF, Feldman HA, Jacobs L. Present status of clinical manifestations of toxoplasmosis in man. Indications and provisions for routine serologic diagnosis. JAMA 1952;150:1063.

Sabin AB, Feldman HA. Dyes as microchemical indicators of a new immunity phenomenon affecting a protozoon parasite *(Toxoplasma)*. Science 1948;108:660.

Siim JC. Clinical and diagnosic aspects of acquired toxoplasmosis. Abstracts of Conference on Toxoplasmosis. Eighth International Congress of Pediatrics, Copenhagen, July 22-27, 1956.

Stagno S. Congenital toxoplasmosis. Am J Dis Child 1980;134:635.

Stray-Pedersen B. A prospective study of acquired toxoplasmosis in 8,043 pregnant women in the Oslo area. Am J Obstet Gynecol 1980;136:399.

Swartzberg JE, Remington JS. Transmission of toxoplasma. Am J Dis Child 1975;129:777.

Teutsch SM. Epidemic toxoplasmosis associated with infected cats. N Engl J Med 1979;300:695.

Thalhammer O. Zwei bemerkenswerte Fälle frischer Toxoplasmainfektion Osterr, Z Kinderh 1954;10:316.

Thalhammer O. Congenital toxoplasmosis. Lancet 1962;1:23.

Wallace GD. Isolation of *Toxoplasma gondii* from the feces of naturally infected cats. J Infect Dis 1971;124:227.

Warren KS, Dingle JH. A study of illness in a group of Cleveland families. XXII. Antibodies to Toxoplasma gondii in 40 families observed for ten years. N Engl J Med 1966;274:993.

Werner H, Janitschke K. Fases evolutivas, ciclo evolutivo y posecion sistematica de *Toxoplasma gondii*. Bol Chil Parasitol 1970;25:57.

Whiteside JD, Regent RHJ. Toxoplasma encephalitis complicating Hodgkin's disease. J Clin Pathol 1975;28:443.

Wolf A, Cowan D, Paige BH. Toxoplasmic encephalomyelitis. IV. Experimental transmission of the infection to animals from a human infant. J Exp Med 1940;71:187.

Work K, Hutchison WM. The new cyst of *Toxoplasma gondii*. Acta Pathol Microbiol Scand 1969;77:414.

31

TUBERCULOSIS

Tuberculosis is an ancient disease that is known to have existed in prehistoric times. It is worldwide in distribution, affecting not only human beings but also many species of wild and domestic animals. In the early nineteenth century tuberculosis was the cause of death in more than one third of the autopsies performed in Paris. Tuberculosis was not considered an infectious disease until 1882, when Koch reported the discovery of the tubercle bacillus (Tb). The spread of tuberculosis became a concern of public health authorities, and measures directed toward its control were established. In the 1830s the death rate due to tuberculosis in large cities in the United States was about 400 per 100,000 of the population. By 1900 the death rate had already fallen to 200 per 100,000. The downward trend accelerated after antimicrobial therapy became available, and in 1983 there were only about 2000 deaths in the United States due to tuberculosis. However, although there is almost universal evidence of a declining death rate, tuberculosis continues to be a serious cause of illness. The reported number of new active cases of tuberculosis, both in children and in adults, has not decreased as rapidly as the death rate. In 1980 the new active case rate for all ages in the United States varied from 2.4 per 100,000 in New Hampshire to 53.5 per 100,000 in the District of Columbia. There were 23,000 cases of clinically apparent new disease due to Tb in 1983.

Surveys using the tuberculin test have provided additional information about the prevalence of infection. In 1907, infection was almost universal in large cities. Surveys in St. Louis and Philadelphia in the following years showed that more than 50% of the general population reacted to tuberculin. By 1937 the rate of reactivity to purified protein derivative of tuberculin (PPD) of United States naval recruits 15 to 19 years old was 31.9%. Thirty years later, in the period from 1965 to 1969, 3% of naval recruits 17 to 21 years old showed reactions measuring 10 mm or more to tuberculin, and in 1973 only 2% reacted. In the United States in 1973 only 0.2% of children entering school at age 6 years reacted to tuberculin.

ETIOLOGY

Mycobacterium tuberculosis organisms are usually referred to as acid-fast bacilli. They do not stain with Gram stain but when heated they do absorb a carbol-fuchsin stain, and once stained, they resist decolorization by strong acids and alcohol. They also absorb auramine-rhodamine dye, which is a fluorescent dye. This technique differs from many fluorescent studies in that it is not a fluorescent antibody. The stain is not specific for *M. tuberculosis* and is also reactive with other Mycobacteriaceae. Tubercle bacilli grow best in the presence of oxygen and at body temperature. They can survive in a dried state for a long time, but they can be killed rapidly by exposure to direct sunlight or to ultraviolet rays.

Both *M. tuberculosis* and *M. bovis* are pathogenic for man. Children are equally susceptible to infection with either, but in the United States the campaign for the eradication of tuberculosis in cattle has made infection with *M. bovis* very rare. In addition, asymptomatic infection with atypical bacilli is found in all parts of the world. Such infections may result in skin sensitivity to tuberculin and occasionally in disease, especially cervical adenitis.

PATHOGENESIS
Initial infection

The lung is the most common portal of entry of tubercle bacilli. If the bacilli are ingested, tuberculosis at the portal of entry in the upper respiratory or intestinal tract may result. The initial infection produces a complex consisting of the local disease at the portal of entry of tubercle bacilli and in the regional lymph nodes that drain that area, the Ghon complex. The term *primary tuberculosis* includes the primary complex and the local progression of disease. *Primary tuberculosis* is no longer used under the modern classification of tuberculosis developed by the American Thoracic Society, but the concept of a special response of the body to the first infection with tubercle bacilli is still valid and is basic to an understanding of tuberculosis in children.

At the site of entry, the bacilli multiply and create an area of inflammatory exudate. Almost as soon as infection occurs, bacilli are carried through the lymphatic system to the nearest group of lymph nodes that drain the area in which the focus is situated. When the portal of entry is in the lung, the bronchopulmonary nodes usually form the complex. Until delayed hypersensitivity develops, the area of infection may expand and remains unencapsulated. With the onset of delayed hypersensitivity the perifocal infiltration generally increases very rapidly, regional lymph nodes enlarge and the initial lesion may become caseous and may become walled off. Caseous lesions may eventually calcify. Living tubercle bacilli may persist within these foci for years.

Progression of tuberculous disease usually involves the bronchi, the blood vessels, and the lymphatic channels supplying and draining the lung, all of which converge in the hilar area. Enlargement of hilar nodes may encroach upon any of these structures. The ones most commonly affected are the bronchi, especially in in-

fants who often develop tuberculous endobronchitis. The infection may erode the bronchial wall to cause a fistula between the node and the bronchial lumen with dissemination of the infection through the bronchi. The swelling of the bronchial mucosa may interfere with aeration and drainage of segments or of an entire lobe of the lung. Sequelae in the involved portion of lung are fibrosis, bronchiectasis, distortion of the bronchi, and pneumonia. Tuberculous lymph nodes sometimes compress or invade other adjacent structures, such as the pericardium, esophagus, or blood vessels. During resolution of infection, the nodal component of the primary complex resolves less rapidly than does the parenchymal focus.

Hematogenous tuberculosis

During the early stage of disease small numbers of tubercle bacilli reach the bloodstream either directly from the initial focus or by way of the regional nodes and the thoracic duct. This sporadic dissemination (occult hematogenous tuberculosis) ceases after delayed hypersensitivity develops. Some disseminated tubercle bacilli progress at varying rates into foci of active disease. Such lesions may regress and heal completely, may progress immediately, or may remain quiescent but contain viable tubercle bacilli. These latent foci may become active again years after the initial infection.

Most complications resulting from hematogenous dissemination are caused by the invasion of an adjoining viscus or space by a tubercle or group of tubercles. For example, caseous tubercles in the cerebral cortex or on the meninges cause meningitis by the discharge of tubercle bacilli into the subarachnoid space. Acute generalized miliary tuberculosis usually results from the invasion of a blood vessel by a caseating focus of tuberculosis or by dissemination from a tubercle within the lumen of a blood vessel originally seeded during the early lymphohematogenous spread.

Although most complications result from hematogenous dissemination, a few do not. The frequent association of spondylitis with pleurisy or with renal tuberculosis is often due to involvement of adjacent paravertebral nodes. Most complications of primary tuberculosis develop during the first year after onset of the disease. In the Bellevue Hospital experience with untreated children, only about 5% of the survivors developed complications more than 1 year after the first infection. Chronic pulmonary tuberculosis of the type usually seen in adults rarely developed in children before adolescence; it occurred twice as often in girls as boys. Twenty percent of the cases in girls were diagnosed within 2 years of the date of menarche.

IMMUNITY
Host defense

Virulent strains of *M. tuberculosis* are remarkable for the ability to persist within the human host for years in spite of a vigorous response to the infection on the part of the infected person. Recent evidence suggests that one mechanism by which strains evade destruction is by preventing the fusion between macrophage phagosomes, in which they are encased after being ingested, and macrophage lysosomes. Lysosomal enzymes do not, therefore, have access to the area around the organisms. Whether this is a sufficient explanation of bacterial intramacrocytic survival and multiplication remains uncertain.

The host response to mycobacterial infection is complex and incompletely understood. Delayed hypersensitivity, measured clinically by cutaneous reactivity to PPD, accompanies the response. During this response, circulating monocytes demonstrate increased bactericidal function for a variety of organisms, an increase in the density of surface Fc receptors, an in-

crease in hexose monophosphate shunt activity, and enhanced adherence. Some of these alterations appear to reflect a plasma factor that is present in patients with tuberculosis. These aspects of the immunologic response to tuberculosis are the subject of current research.

Sex

In the children studied in Bellevue Hospital, before chemotherapy there were equal numbers of boys and girls. The mortality and incidence of meningitis were equal in both sexes. However, among tuberculin-reactive teenagers, active disease occurred more frequently in adolescent girls than in adolescent boys. Before chemotherapy was available, there was a higher death rate from tuberculosis in girls 15 to 18 years old than in boys of the same age group. At the present time the case rate and the death rate in most countries are highest among elderly men.

Genetic factors

Genetically determined susceptibility to tuberculosis has been demonstrated by inbreeding rabbits, and in humans there is evidence that the degree of resistance to tuberculosis may vary in different ethnic groups.

Age

Infants who are exposed to *M. tuberculosis* have a very high incidence of active and disseminated disease, which has been estimated to be

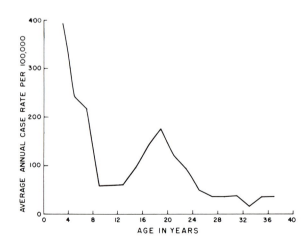

Fig. 31-1. Incidence of tuberculosis among children who were initially PPD reactive by age when tuberculous disease was first diagnosed. Reprinted with kind permission of G W Comstock. (From Comstock GW, et al. Am J Epidemiol 1974;99:141.)

at least 35% of infected cases. It is probable that the infective dose for infants is less than 10 organisms. The majority of untreated infants who develop disease die. This extreme susceptibility of the very young decreases during early childhood until adolescence, when there again occurs an enhanced susceptibility to disease. Following the early twenties, humans are relatively resistant, and probably about 1% of untreated and otherwise healthy young adults who are exposed to *M. tuberculosis* develop clinically apparent disease (Fig. 31-1).

Nutrition

It is difficult to separate the effects of poor nutrition on resistance to tuberculosis from those of other socioeconomic factors. Active disease, however, is inversely proportional to the degree of nutrition, and excellent nutrition is essential to the recovery of young children with tuberculosis.

Intercurrent infections

Measles has the closest association with activation of latent disease, but other infectious diseases, especially pertussis, have also been incriminated. The skin reactivity to tuberculin disappears in the preeruptive stage of measles and does not reappear for 2 or 3 weeks, and disease may worsen during this time. There is abundant evidence that corticosteroid therapy without concurrent antituberculous therapy may precipitate disease.

EPIDEMIOLOGIC FACTORS
Mode of spread

The source of infection in children is usually an adult or occasionally an adolescent who is usually a member of the household. When a person with contagious pulmonary tuberculosis coughs or sneezes, droplets of varying sizes containing tubercle bacilli are dispersed into the air. The particle must be of a particular size to gain access to an alveolus where infection begins. The number of tubercle bacilli discharged into the atmosphere by a patient depends on the number of organisms in the sputum, the amount and character of the sputum, and the type and frequency of cough. Almost all initial infections occur in the lungs. Occasionally, ingested bacilli find a portal of entry in the intestinal tract and, more rarely, in a tonsil or in the mucous membranes of the mouth. Other extrapulmonary sites of infection such as those in the skin or conjunctiva are due to local contact with tubercle bacilli.

Although the index case for children is most often a member of the family, it may also be a nurse, a babysitter, a domestic worker, or a frequent visitor. An infant may be subjected to a small but appreciable risk of infection when exposed to an adult with apparently quiescent tuberculosis. The source of tuberculosis in a child may be an elderly person with a cough caused by unrecognized chronic tuberculosis.

Epidemic spread is possible whenever a large proportion of a population has never been exposed to tubercle bacilli, a situation that now exists in most schools. Epidemics are characterized by the finding of a number of newly infected children within a short period of time. The index case is often a teacher, other school personnel, or another student with active pulmonary disease.

Contagion of childhood tuberculosis

In general, primary pulmonary tuberculosis in young children is noninfectious for older children or adults. Bacilli are rarely recovered by culture, even from children with recent infections, unless gastric lavage is performed early in the morning. The number of colonies is usually very small, rarely over 10 and often only one or two. The contagiousness of chronic pulmonary tuberculosis in older children and adolescents is comparable to that of similar pulmonary disease in adults. Cavitation at the site of the initial focus is also an especially contagious form of tuberculosis. Fortunately, these forms of disease are uncommon in children, and when they occur, drug therapy usually causes a rapid decrease in the number of bacilli. Probably of greater concern in the prevention of spread of disease is the possibility that other infected members of a child's family will visit the hospital. For that reason, the child and all visitors may need to be restricted to the child's room pending investigation of the family.

DIAGNOSTIC CRITERIA
Tuberculin tests

The tuberculin skin test is the primary method of identifying persons who have been infected with tubercle bacilli. PPD, used for intradermal testing in the United States, is prepared by heating tubercle bacilli; it was developed by Seibert and designated by the World Health Organization as the international PPD-tuberculin, usually called PPD-S. The potency of tuberculin is expressed in terms of international tuberculin units (TU): 1 TU is equivalent to about 0.00002 mg of PPD; five TU is the standard dose for intradermal testing. PPD is available commercially in a buffered diluent. Tuberculin is adsorbed to glass or plastic. To avoid reduction in potency by such adsorption, manufacturers add Tween 80 to the diluent. This stabilized PPD will expire in 1 year. Transfer of tuberculin from one container to another should be avoided, and skin tests should be administered within 24 hours after the syringe has been filled.

The Mantoux test (intradermal test) is the most accurate and reliable method of testing if it is done properly. A tuberculin syringe should be used. The best site for testing is the central part of the volar surface of the forearm. The skin should be washed with alcohol and allowed to dry. The needle is inserted transversely into, but not beneath, the skin, and exactly 0.1 ml of test material is injected. A wheal at least 5 mm in diameter should be formed. The operator must ensure that the needle is within the dermal layers, since a false-negative result may be obtained if the tuberculin is injected subcutaneously. For mass tuberculin surveys the Mantoux test may be administered with a jet injector using a specially adapted head for intracutaneous injection.

Tests should be read between 48 and 72 hours after the injection. If there is erythema without induration, the reaction should be considered negative. When there is an area of induration, it should be carefully palpated, and its maximum transverse diameter should be measured with a millimeter rule. Induration of less than 5 mm is considered a negative reaction. The test should be considered doubtful if the induration is more than 5 mm but less than 10 mm in diameter. The test should be repeated at a different site; a second test may give a decisive result. A test with 5 TU that results in 10 mm or more of induration is positive. Local reactions that may occur at the site of injection include marked swelling, erythema, vesiculation, and ulceration. In the case of such reactions, there may be lymphangitis and swelling of the regional lymph nodes. Application of topical steroids will help to control a severe local reaction.

The use of greater concentrations of PPD, such as 250 TU, is valuable only in excluding the diagnosis of generalized anergy. In testing as part of a physical examination or in surveys, it is not necessary to start with 1 TU.

Testing for skin reaction to tuberculin may also be done with multiple puncture devices. These introduce concentrated tuberculin into the skin. The exact amount introduced in a test cannot be measured. Several types of multiple puncture tests are available including the Tine test, which is a plastic device to which are attached four metal prongs carrying dried tuberculin, the Applitest, the Monovacc, which utilizes many plastic points that are pressed through a concentrated solution of tuberculin, and the Heaf test, which may be administered using a spring-activated apparatus that pushes a circle of six metals points through a concentrated solution of PPD. All these tests should be considered screening tests rather than diagnostic tests. Reactions of 2 mm or less at each prong should be considered negative. Reactions larger than 2 mm are considered doubtful unless vesiculation has occurred. Doubtful screening reactions should be confirmed by means of a diagnostic Mantoux test with 5 TU of PPD. A Mantoux test should always be used if the physician suspects tuberculosis in an ill child.

When potent testing material is properly administered, a tuberculin skin test should produce positive results in the majority of tuberculous persons. Among the exceptions are severely dehydrated or moribund patients and those receiving treatment with corticosteroids. In addition, anergy to tuberculin is often present for 2 or 3 weeks after the onset of measles and during the incubation period of primary tuberculous infection. If the physician suspects tuberculosis and the PPD is nonreactive, the test may be repeated weekly until the problem is resolved. In addition, an intradermal application of *Candida* 1:1000 will help to determine whether the patient is experiencing generalized anergy.

History of exposure

One of the most helpful, and sometimes the most crucial, aspect of the diagnosis of tuberculosis in children is the elicitation of a history of exposure to a patient with active pulmonary disease. If tuberculosis is suspected, members of the family should be asked on more than one occasion if persons within the extended household have had compatible pulmonary disease, weight loss, or sweating. Visitors to the home in the prior 3 months should be discussed, since a transient exposure to an alcoholic relative is a fairly common contact. In extended households, close friends of older household members should be included in the discussion of the health of persons to whom the child has been exposed. Many extended families live in several adjacent homes, and all members of these homes should be considered as potential contacts. If the diagnosis remains uncertain, tuberculin testing of all household members will help to determine if the child is living in an environment in which there has been tuberculous exposure.

Roentgenologic examination

Roentgenographic examination of the chest should be done if tuberculosis is suspected and should include a lateral view.

Recovery of tubercle bacilli

The proof of the tuberculous origin of a lesion is the identification of tubercle bacilli. The finding of acid-fast bacilli on direct examination does not identify them as *M. tuberculosis*, since mycobacteria cannot be speciated by their morphologic aspects; however, it is helpful in suggesting a diagnosis. Mycobacteria are impervious to Gram stain and usually do not show on a specimen stained with Gram's method alone. Auramine-rhodamine allows a more sensitive and rapid identification of the presence of acid-fast organisms in a clinical sample than do the traditional acid-fast stains such as the Kinyoun stain. Direct stains are of great value in the examination of cerebrospinal fluid (CSF), since meningitis due to acid-fast bacilli other than tubercle bacilli is rare. Diagnostic specimens from suspected cases should be cultured for identification of *M. tuberculosis* and other mycobacteria and for determination of susceptibility of the organisms to antituberculous drugs. Cultures of tubercle bacilli usually display some growth in 3 to 4 weeks; however, they should be observed for at least 2 months.

In adults, expectorated sputum is the most common source of pulmonary secretions for cul-

ture or animal inoculation. In children, sputum is usually swallowed, and gastric lavage is a method of attempting recovery of tubercle bacilli that will yield organisms in about 35% of children with pulmonary tuberculosis. The number of bacilli recovered from the gastric lavage is usually very small in children, and the yield is increased when washings obtained on 3 successive days are pooled. Cultures obtained during the early phase of primary pulmonary tuberculosis are most likely to yield tubercle bacilli. Bronchoscopy provides a better yield. For adults and children old enough to cooperate, an effective method of inducing sputum is the inhalation of nebulized, warmed, hypertonic saline solution. This method is more acceptable to patients than gastric lavage, and the yield of positive cultures from it has been reported to be good. Guinea pig inoculation of CSF or pleural fluid was an important method of diagnosis in the past, but it is now seldom used.

Histopathologic examinations

Biopsies from diseased areas of the skeletal system, pleura, superficial lymph nodes, and liver may yield a diagnosis. Histopathologic findings include noncaseating granulomas, caseating granulomas, and presence or absence of mycobacteria or acid-fast stains of the tissue.

Hematologic examinations

Hematologic examinations usually offer little help in making a diagnosis or prognosis. Mild secondary anemia is often present. The total white blood cell count is often within normal limits. During some active phases of tuberculosis, there may be an elevation in the total count with an increase in number of polymorphonuclear leukocytes. The erythrocyte sedimentation rate is moderately elevated in most patients and decreases as the disease becomes inactive. No serologic tests have as yet been devised that are of significant help in making a diagnosis or prognosis.

TREATMENT

The general care and supervision of a child with tuberculosis require careful planning. Close liaison should be maintained between the physicians caring for adults and those caring for children in the same family. The pediatrician should work closely with members of the local department of health, including the public health nurses and social workers. To function properly, social investigation should be organized on a family basis.

Most children with asymptomatic or early initial infection do not require hospital or sanatorium care. They may lead an essentially unrestricted life. Asymptomatic children remaining at home should be shielded against the anxiety of parents. The usual immunizations are indicated, including measles vaccine after therapy has begun.

Antituberculous drugs

In the child whose contact is known, it is almost certain that the sensitivity pattern of the contact's isolate will be the same as that of the child. Therefore determining the sensitivity of the contact's isolate may guide therapy for the child.

A combination of drugs for initial therapy is usually employed to prevent treatment failures and to prevent the emergence of resistant *M. tuberculosis*. The possibility that resistant organisms may be included in the population increases with the size of the population of infecting organisms. The number of bacilli present in a cavity is vastly greater than the number in a nodular lesion, and numbers of organisms in asymptomatic persons who are PPD reactive are fewer still. When the estimated number of organisms is very large, the use of three drugs may be advisable. For other forms of symptomatic disease, two are usually sufficient, unless there

is reason to expect an increased chance that the child has acquired a drug-resistant infection (primary resistance).

Chemotherapy for childhood tuberculosis

The therapy for childhood tuberculosis has included a number of standard regimens that appear to have had a high degree of success. Many of these regimens reflect adult experience and have been only moderately well studied in children. There are drug regimens that are highly recommended for adults for which there have been virtually no reported trials involving children. The following comments and suggested regimens are based on a number of years of successful experience in children. Improved understanding of the use of newer drugs in children will undoubtedly lead to changes in accepted courses of therapy (Table 31-1).

The three antituberculous drugs that are used in children and are considered to be *first line* are isoniazid, rifampin, and streptomycin. Most courses of childhood tuberculosis, in which drug resistance is not proven or highly likely, are well managed by a combination of these drugs.

Isoniazid. Isoniazid remains the single most valued form of therapy and has been available for 32 years. It is mycobactericidal and may be given orally, intravenously, or intramuscularly. It is inexpensive and may be administered as a single daily dose. It is distributed to all areas of the body. There are genetically determined racial differences in the rate of acetylation of INH that may influence rates of adverse reaction to

Table 31-1. Preferred therapy of tuberculosis in children

Drug	Daily dose	Route of administration	Notes on adverse reactions
Isoniazid	10 to 20 mg/kg, 300 mg total maximum may be given in one dose	PO IM IV	Peripheral neuritis, prevented by pyridoxine; hepatotoxicity; use caution when combined with rifampin
Streptomycin	20 to 30 mg/kg, 1 gm maximum	IM	Eighth nerve damage; assay serum concentration, if renal impairment present
Rifampin	15 to 20 mg/kg, 600 mg maximum	PO	Hepatotoxicity; orange staining of secretions; use with caution with INH; gastric irritation
Ethambutol	15 to 20 mg/kg	PO	Optic neuritis; for this reason, avoid in children less than 12 years old
Ethionamide	15 to 20 mg/kg	PO	Hepatotoxicity; gastric irritation

some extent but do not appear to influence the efficacy of therapy.

There is competitive inhibition by INH of pyridoxine utilization, which leads to peripheral neuritis. Although this is most common in older adults, it may also occur in children. Supplementation of the diet with pyridoxine will prevent the reaction, and the usual dose is approximately 1 mg pyridoxine for every 10 mg INH prescribed.

The other major adverse reaction to INH is hepatotoxicity. It is very rarely of clinical significance in children but is a source of concern to everyone. Conditions that appear to enhance the hepatotoxicity of INH include concomitant use of phenytoin and rifampin. The great majority of hepatotoxic INH reactions are asymptomatic, involve minor degrees of hepatic enzyme elevations, and resolve with continued therapy. Rare but serious reactions, which may be life-threatening, are associated with continued use of INH (and/or rifampin) after the onset of symptomatic disease. For this reason, it is good practice to warn the parents of signs and symptoms of early INH hepatotoxicity and instruct them to discontinue the use of INH if these signs occur and to return to clinic for evaluation. During the course of 1 year of therapy for tuberculosis, most patients will have an episode in which the drug is discontinued for symptoms compatible with INH toxicity.

Signs of INH toxicity that are recognizable to a layman include:
1. Right upper abdominal aching or pain
2. Dark urine
3. Poor appetite or vomiting
4. Yellow sclera
5. Fever of 38.3° C (101° F) for 2 days or more

One of the purposes of monthly follow-up visits during therapy is to ensure that the parent understands the indications for discontinuing therapy as well as for ensuring compliance with medication. Routine monitoring of liver function is not recommended.

If INH is prescribed alone, doses of 10 to 20 mg per kilogram of body weight per day are usual. Tablets of 100 and 300 mg are readily available; the tablet may be crushed and mixed with a tasty food. If INH is given in a regimen also containing rifampin, the INH dose should not exceed 10 mg per kilogram of body weight per day.

Rifampin. Rifampin is relatively newly available for treatment of tuberculosis and has only recently become a first-line drug for use in children. It is orally absorbed, widely distributed throughout the body, and highly efficacious in treatment of tuberculosis. It has been particularly helpful in the treatment of difficult forms of tuberculosis such as extrapulmonary disease, advanced pulmonary disease, and tuberculosis due to strains resistant to other drugs. Nevertheless, there are several difficulties with the use of rifampin. They are as follows:
1. The drug is relatively expensive.
2. It is not licensed for use by the FDA in children younger than 5 years.
3. There is no liquid preparation commercially available, although pharmacies may prepare one.
4. A metabolite may cause orange coloration of urine and secretions that may stain contact lenses and clothing, harmless but potentially alarming.
5. Hypersensitivity reactions may occur with intermittent use.
6. Gastrointestinal irritation may occur and be severe.

Rifampin should be administered with another antituberculous drug for persons with clinically apparent disease. Particular alertness to hepatic toxicity when it is combined with INH is important, and the dose of each when used in combination should not exceed 10 mg/kg/day INH and 15 mg/kg/day rifampin.

Streptomycin. Streptomycin remains a first-line drug in the treatment of advanced cases of tuberculosis in children. It is bactericidal. It must be administered parenterally, which the manufacturer recommends be intramuscularly. It is frequently used for 3 to 12 weeks to initiate therapy and is discontinued after the disease is fully controlled. The main adverse reaction is eighth nerve deafness. Monitoring of serum concentrations of streptomycin probably assists in preventing this complication. Peak serum concentrations of 20 to 30 µg/ml are the goal.

Other agents. Other antituberculous agents are far less frequently used. Para-aminosalicylic acid (PAS) is administered orally, is inexpensive, and is well tolerated by children. However, it is marginally effective, large doses are required, and therefore, it is often bypassed. Ethambutol is a mainstay of adult regimens. However, the main complication, optic neuritis, is difficult to diagnose in children in early stages; thus many pediatricians refrain from its use unless the patient is a teenager or an older adolescent. Pyrazinamide is also coming into increased use in adults, but pediatric experience with the drug is almost nonexistent. Finally, ethionamide is an INH congener and, like INH, is bactericidal and widely distributed throughout the body. INH-resistant strains are usually ethionamide sensitive. It is well tolerated by children; the main form of adverse reaction is hepatotoxicity. It is a very important drug when INH resistance is known or suspected.

The remaining antituberculous agents that are available are used almost entirely for retreatment or in patients whose tubercle bacilli are resistant to one or more major drugs. Kanamycin sulfate and viomycin sulfate are both effective antituberculous agents that are administered intramuscularly. Pyrazinamide, which is given orally, exerts good antituberculous effects but produces severe hepatotoxicity in some patients. Cycloserine is a moderately effective drug, given orally; it is toxic for the central nervous system (CNS), and it may cause convulsions.

Corticosteroids. The use of steroid hormones in persons with tuberculosis is contraindicated unless antituberculous drugs are given at the same time. Steroid therapy may diminish the inflammatory changes in the tuberculous lesions and eliminate systemic manifestations such as fever and malaise. In most forms of tuberculosis in which steroid therapy has been used, proof of its effectiveness has not been obtained. Possible indications for its use include (1) tuberculous meningitis with actual or impending block and (2) severe respiratory distress in a child with tuberculous endobronchitis.

PREVENTION

Tuberculosis occurs more frequently in urban than in rural populations. The new active case rate in the District of Columbia is 11 times that in Iowa. Within cities the death rate and the rate of newly reported cases continues to be highest in persons at the low end of the socioeconomic scale. Philadelphia had an overall new case rate of 49 per 100,000 population in 1973; in the extreme northeastern portion of the city,

a middle-class area, the rate was 14 per 100,000, whereas West Philadelphia had a rate of 131 per 100,000.

Case finding surveys are most fruitful in groups with a high probability of tuberculous infection, such as contacts of newly diagnosed cases of tuberculosis, residents of economically depressed areas of large cities, and indigent patients suffering from diseases such as silicosis and alcoholism that predispose them to tuberculosis. As the rate of infection has decreased, the use of tuberculin surveys with roentgenographic examination of the reactors has become the method of case finding. The object of discovering persons with active tuberculosis is not only to cure the patient by specific therapy but also to prevent spread to other individuals, especially children. Studies have shown that treated patients rarely infect their contacts, even in the home. The major risk of infection occurs before the index case is diagnosed.

Schedules for routine screening with tuberculin have changed over the past few decades. Currently, most children receive a PPD at 1 year of age. Thereafter, some children continue to receive yearly examinations while others will not receive another unless they are being examined as part of a diagnostic work-up. It is prudent to plan a schedule that takes account of the extent of tuberculous disease in the patient's environment. If the disease is rare, a PPD at 1 year, at entrance to school, and during high school would be a satisfactory schedule. However, for many populations, it should remain a part of the yearly examination during early childhood.

Any plan for prevention of tuberculosis should be concerned particularly with children. In areas with a low rate of infection, much of the active tuberculosis found in adults is due to reactivation of disease originally acquired in early life. The identification of children who are PPD reactive may furnish clues to previously unknown cases of active tuberculosis in adults.

Preventive therapy

Soon after isoniazid was introduced, it was noticed that meningitis did not develop in infected children who were receiving this therapy, even when they had miliary tuberculosis. In 1955, 2750 children with positive tuberculin tests were randomly assigned to receive either isoniazid or placebo for 1 year. During a follow-up period of 10 years, the rate of complications in the group that received placebo was 30.2 per 1000 children as compared with 3.6 per 1000 children who received isoniazid. Thirty-one of the 41 complications in the placebo group occurred within the first year, including six cases of meningitis and one of miliary tuberculosis. There were no instances of meningitis or miliary tuberculosis in the group that received isoniazid.

Since that time the concept of *preventive therapy* has developed. Preventive therapy is applied to the prevention of tuberculosis in two primary settings.

The first primary setting involves the patient who has been exposed within a household or other close setting to a person with active pulmonary tuberculosis but is nonreactive to PPD. In this circumstance, the physician cannot determine if the patient has not acquired the infection or if the patient is infected but has not yet manifested delayed hypersensitivity to tuberculin. Since some patients, especially children, may progress rapidly during the first weeks after infection, it is not safe merely to observe such a patient. Therefore, persons at significant risk of having recently been infected but who are PPD nonreactive should receive preventive therapy. The usual course of therapy is INH, and the duration is 2 to 3 months. At the end of that time the patient may be retested with PPD. If he has remained PPD nonreactive and is no longer exposed to an active case, therapy may cease. If he has become PPD reactive, he should complete a full course of preventive therapy, which is 1 year in duration.

It should be noted that preventive therapy with INH is not efficacious if the strain is resistant to INH. If that is the case, rifampin is usually used in a similar regimen, but clinical studies concerning the efficacy of rifampin for prophylaxis have not been accomplished.

Some health departments exclude children from their protocols for administration of preventive therapy. However, the precepts of preventive therapy apply with particular urgency to children, who are at increased risk of progressive tuberculosis compared to adults. The pediatrician should ensure that the children who are in contact with an infected adult receive adequate prophylaxis.

Other settings in which preventive therapy of PPD-nonreactive persons may be indicated include institutional outbreaks of tuberculosis and any closed setting in which it has been found that the development of disease or delayed hypersensitivity is occurring in several persons.

The other common setting in which preventive therapy is indicated is for the patient who is clinically well, has normal or minimal changes in the chest roentgenogram, and is PPD reactive. In this instance, if the patient is a child, a full course of preventive therapy should be planned, which would usually be INH, 10 mg per kilogram of body weight per day, for 1 year. Persons who are particularly likely to progress to active disease include those who are very young, who have become infected within the past year, and who become immunosuppressed due to malignant disease, use of adrenocorticosteroids, or other illnesses such as measles.

When a positive tuberculin test is associated with tuberculous disease, delayed hypersensitivity ordinarily persists for many years, even if the disease has responded well to specific therapy. In contrast are those children whose only evidence of tuberculosis is delayed hypersensitivity to tuberculin. When they are retested a few years after the original reaction, it is not uncommon to find reversion of the tuberculin test to negative.

Bacille Calmette-Guérin vaccination

Bacille Calmette-Guérin (BCG), live attenuated strains of a related mycobacteria, has been used as a vaccine for over 50 years. It produces a varying degree of immunity to infection with virulent tubercle bacilli. Although the immunity is not complete and superinfections with human *M. tuberculosis* can occur, the illness is moderated and rarely progressive. The most important benefit of BCG vaccination is that the risk of disseminated disease is markedly diminished; both miliary tuberculosis and meningitis usually can be prevented by vaccination.

In the United States, Rosenthal et al. reported a 74% reduction of morbidity in BCG-vaccinated children. Palmer et al. (1958) of the Public Health Service, after controlled-community trials in Puerto Rico and in Georgia, concluded that BCG was only about 30% effective in these populations. A study very similar in design and execution, conducted by the British Medical Research Council among adolescents, reported that the vaccine was more than 80% effective. The discrepancies in results may be due to variations in the vaccine strains but are probably also related to prior subclinical infections with atypical acid-fast bacilli. In experimental animals, atypical mycobacteria have the capacity to modify the course of subsequent infection with tubercle bacilli.

In the United States there are families in which tuberculosis is uncontrolled and active, and BCG vaccination may provide the wisest form of protection for some children. It should be noted that the majority of PPD reactions within 1 year or more after BCG vaccination are less than 10 mm in diameter. Reactions larger than that are likely to represent infection with *M. tuberculosis*, and the child should be assessed accordingly. A very small number of deaths due to BCG vaccination have been reported. These have mainly occurred in patients with immunodeficiency disorders. Since millions of children have been vaccinated, the procedure may be regarded as relatively safe.

Two strains of BCG are available in the United States. Glaxo Laboratories distributes BCG through Eli Lilly Co. This strain is applied intradermally. The second strain is the *Tice* strain and is available from the Research Foundation of Chicago. This vaccine is applied percutaneously. Some pediatricians believe that the rate of conversion following use of the Tice strain is superior to that of the Glaxo strain.

CLINICAL SPECTRUM OF TUBERCULOSIS
Classification

The classification of tuberculous disease has undergone many revisions, and the literature is burdened with terms that have changed meaning with changing understanding of the disease process. In the late 1970s the American Thoracic Society proposed the most recent classification, which is compatible with the disease in both children and adults. This classification is based on the patient's history of exposure, tuberculin reaction, symptomatic state, location of apparent disease, and treatment, and is as follows:

0. No tuberculosis exposure, not infected (no history of exposure, negative tuberculin skin test)

I. Tuberculosis exposure, no evidence of infection (history of exposure, negative tuberculin skin test)

II. Tuberculous infection, without disease (positive tuberculin skin test, negative bacteriologic studies if done, no roentgenographic findings compatible with tuberculosis, no symptom due to tuberculosis)
Chemotherapy status (preventive therapy)
   A. None
   B. On chemotherapy since (date)
   C. Chemotherapy terminated (date)
      1. Complete (prescribed course of therapy)
      2. Incomplete

III. Tuberculosis: infected, with disease
The current status of the patient's tuberculosis shall be described by the following characteristics:
   A. Location of disease
      1. Pulmonary
      2. Pleural
      3. Lymphatic
      4. Bone or joint
      5. Genitourinary
      6. Miliary
      7. Meningeal
      8. Peritoneal
      9. Other
   The predominant site shall be listed for each patient. Other sites may also be listed if significant. More precise anatomic sites may be specified.
   B. Bacteriologic status
      1. Positive by
         a. Microscopy only (date)
         b. Culture only (date)
         c. Microscopy and culture (date)
      2. Negative (date)
      3. Pending
      4. Not done
   C. Chemotherapy status
      1. None
      2. On chemotherapy since (date)
      3. Chemotherapy terminated (date)
         a. Complete (prescribed course of therapy)
         b. Incomplete
   D. Roentgenogram findings
      1. Normal

2. Abnormal
   a. Cavitary or noncavitary
   b. Stable or worsening or improving
E. Tuberculin skin test
   1. Positive reaction
   2. Doubtful reaction
   3. Negative reaction
   4. Not done

Tuberculosis suspect: Patients may be so classified until diagnostic procedures are complete. This classification should not be used for more than 3 months.

Tuberculous infection without disease

Asymptomatic primary infection is tuberculous infection in which the child is tuberculin reactive but has no apparent clinical illness and normal or minimally abnormal roentgenogram of the chest. This condition may occur very early in an illness in which the child will progress to active disease or may remain quiescent and heal. Infants are most likely to have progressive disease, but over 80% of children who are over 4 years of age and have not reached puberty will not progress. Adolescence is another period in which progression of primary disease is likely to occur. In any event, preventive therapy should be instituted.

Tuberculous infection with disease

Almost all cases of tuberculous disease in children are first (primary) infections. The incubation period of primary tuberculosis varies from 2 to 8 weeks. During this period the skin test does not react. Tubercle bacilli may be cultured from material obtained by gastric lavage during the prereactive period before any changes appear on a chest roentgenogram. The usual mode of onset of the initial tuberculous infection is insidious. The patient, especially an infant, often has signs or symptoms of an infection of the upper respiratory tract that appear at the same time as the fever. Except for the anorexia and lassitude that can accompany any fever, there are not other symptoms associated with the onset of primary tuberculosis. Erythema nodosum can appear concomitantly with the fever of onset, but today this finding is infrequent. Abnormal physical findings from the pulmonary examination are rarely found even when an extensive lesion is seen on the roentgenogram.

Occasionally the onset of the initial pulmonary infection may be pneumonic, resembling lobar pneumonia, with fever, rapid respiratory rate, and signs of dullness, bronchial breath sounds, and moist rales. These signs and symptoms often subside in a few days to 2 weeks. The white blood cell count, if it has been elevated, returns to a normal range, the abnormal physical signs disappear, and the child seems to have recovered from the acute illness. The roentgenogram, however, continues to show parenchymal infiltrates and enlargement of mediastinal nodes (Fig. 31-2). This type of onset may be due to an associated nontuberculous pneumonia and would respond initially to antimicrobial therapy.

Course. There is nothing diagnostic about the appearance of a child with initial tuberculous infection. If the pulmonary lesion progresses locally or if there is marked progression by the lymphohematogenous route, the child will experience a period of illness that usually resolves. In a few weeks, if treatment has not begun, afternoon fevers ensue. In a large percentage of older children with primary pulmonary tuberculosis, the initial lesion remains localized and causes no major symptoms or signs, and even without specific therapy the fever is unlikely to continue more than 2 to 3 months. Alternately, the pulmonary component of the primary complex may progress locally, in which case extension into the bronchi produces disseminated areas of tuberculous pneumonia.

In the early stage of bronchial involvement infants often have a harsh expiratory cough. Older children usually have no cough even when extensive disease is present. Small infants may have respiratory distress, especially during an intercurrent infection. Occasionally the clinical picture may be indistinguishable from nonspecific laryngotracheobronchitis. Transient wheezes or rhonchi are often heard, especially in infants. Bronchoscopic studies have shown that tuberculous bronchitis may persist for months or years, even in patients receiving specific therapy, and bronchiectasis has been a sequel of tuberculous bronchitis in many patients.

Roentgenographic appearance. The initial complex may appear on the roentgenogram at the time of onset or it may be inapparent. Parenchymal infiltrates that appear weeks or months after onset usually represent segmental obstruction or nontuberculous infection. In the

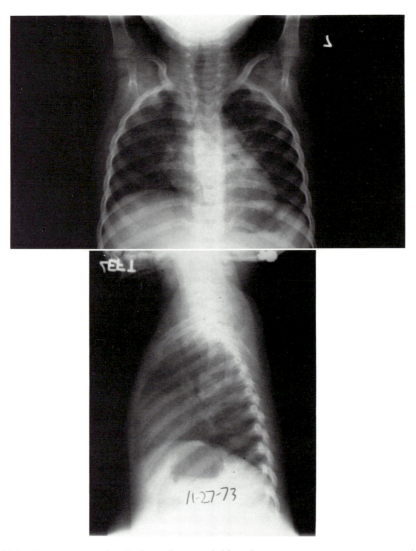

Fig. 31-2. Roentgenographic findings from a child with asymptomatic recent onset of pulmonary tuberculosis, demonstrating hilar and paratracheal adenopathy.

adolescent or adult, new infiltrates may be due to chronic pulmonary tuberculosis. The appearance of the initial focus may vary from a round area less than 2 cm in diameter to one that occupies an entire lobe. Regardless of its size at onset there is usually little change for at least 3 months, when the area of involvement may begin to diminish gradually. Infiltrates persisting for 2 years or longer are not rare.

A primary focus without enlarged regional lymph nodes is rare, but enlarged lymph nodes without apparent parenchymal infiltrates are common. Hilar adenopathy may be the only roentgenographic evidence of tuberculosis and

is best identified in a lateral view, where the nodes may form a rounded mass obscuring the bifurcation. Enlarged carinal nodes, often associated with foci in the lower lobes, are seen most easily in an oblique or in a lateral view. The mass of nodes around the bifurcation may be so large that it displaces the heart and mediastinum.

In patients who have received antimicrobial therapy, calcification rarely is seen in the area of the parenchymal focus unless treatment was begun after the occurrence of extensive caseation necrosis. Calcification occurs more often in lymph nodes than in pulmonary foci. The usual

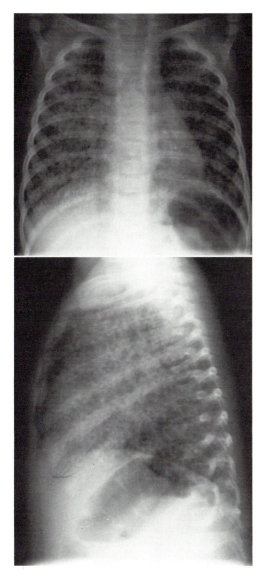

Fig. 31-3. Roentgenographic findings from a 6-month-old child with miliary tuberculosis. Note the nodular appearance and uniform size of the lesions. (Courtesy Drs. G. Gaisie and W. Clyde, University of North Carolina, Chapel Hill, NC.)

minimal interval in an older child is 1 year, and calcification may not be found for 5 or more years in an adolescent or young adult.

Differential diagnosis. The differential diagnosis of tuberculosis includes mycotic infections such as histoplasmosis and blastomycosis. Local epidemiologic patterns may be helpful. The clinical and roentgenographic picture of locally progressive pulmonary tuberculosis may be con-

fused with that of staphylococcal pneumonia in the infant or lung abscess in the older child. Biopsy or bronchoscopic examination may be required. The results of a tuberculin test also help to distinguish between enlargement of the hilar nodes due to tuberculosis and similar findings in sarcoidosis, Hodgkin's disease, or chronic pneumonia.

Hematogenous tuberculosis

Generalized tuberculosis in children may be caused by three types of hematogenous spread: (1) an occult dissemination in which clinical manifestations may or may not occur, (2) a single generalized dissemination that usually causes acute disease, and (3) repeated or protracted dissemination.

Occult hematogenous tuberculosis. The dissemination of a small number of tubercle bacilli through the blood early in the course of the first infection with tuberculosis has been termed *occult hematogenous tuberculosis*. Most of the dissemination takes place during the incubation period and for a short time after onset of disease, and it is unlikely to continue after hypersensitivity to tuberculin has been established. The bacilli are most commonly seeded to the apices of the lungs, the liver and spleen, and the superficial lymph nodes. Clinical manifestations during this episode usually last only a few days and are mild.

Acute miliary tuberculosis. Miliary tuberculosis is a complication of tuberculous infection that usually occurs within the first 6 months after onset of infection. All tubercles resulting from an acute generalized hematogenous spread are of approximately the same size and are often the size of millet seed. The pulmonary infiltrates seen on the roentgenogram may be so small that they are barely visible.

An abrupt rise in temperature usually heralds the onset of miliary tuberculosis. Infiltrates become visible on the roentgenogram about 1 to 3 weeks after onset of fever. At this time there are usually no respiratory symptoms and no abnormal physical signs in the lungs. If diagnosis and treatment are delayed, fine rales may be heard, and dyspnea and cyanosis may develop. Enlargement of the liver, spleen, and superficial lymph nodes has occurred in about half of the children at the time of diagnosis. Choroid tubercles may occur but, in spite of an intensive search, are found in only about 13% of tuberculous children. Specific therapy for miliary tuberculosis may prevent meningitis, but many patients present with both conditions.

Roentgenographic appearance. The even distribution of infiltrates throughout both lung fields is the most characteristic feature of the roentgenogram. Segmental obstruction, if present, produces the appearance of discrete areas of pneumonia. Examination of lateral views will usually reveal an equal distribution of tubercles over the entire lung fields. The lesions may resemble multiple nodules (Fig. 31-3).

Diagnosis. The PPD is nonreactive in many children who have miliary tuberculosis. If the tuberculin test is positive and if there is no roentgenographic evidence of miliary tuberculosis, the roentgenogram should be repeated weekly. Choroidal tubercles, if present, may be of great diagnostic importance. When they occur, however, they often do not appear until several weeks after the onset of miliary tuberculosis.

Culture of blood, bone marrow, or other tissue may confirm the diagnosis eventually, but these positive findings are obtained too late to be of help in establishing the initial diagnosis. Biopsy of the liver or bone marrow may be of greater value in achieving a rapid diagnosis.

Prognosis. In the preantibiotic era, miliary tuberculosis was usually fatal within 3 months; most untreated children developed meningitis. The use of antituberculous therapy has improved the prognosis so that most treated patients recover if they are not moribund when first diagnosed and if they survive meningitis, if present.

COMPLICATIONS
Chronic pulmonary tuberculosis

Chronic tuberculosis is very uncommon in children; less than 5% of patients younger than 15 years old develop this form of pulmonary tuberculosis. Most cases of pulmonary tuberculosis of the adult type (chronic pulmonary tuberculosis) are caused by endogenous pulmonary reinfection or extension from a focus that was established during the initial bacteremic phase of primary disease and differs markedly from primary tuberculosis. Chronic pulmonary tuberculosis usually remains a pulmonary disease; unlike the initial infection, it does not represent the onset of a systemic disease.

The risk of developing chronic pulmonary tuberculosis increases during adolescence and usually develops within 1 or 2 years after the initial infection. When the date of conversion of the tuberculin test is known, the relatively short interval between initial infection and chronic pulmonary tuberculosis that can often be demonstrated suggests that many instances of chronic pulmonary tuberculosis, especially in young adults, represent local progression of initial disease. Evidence of early chronic pulmonary tuberculosis is most commonly seen roentgenographically above or below the clavicle in one or both lungs. Most small lesions in children and adolescents are unstable and tend to progress. Oblique and lordotic views may be valuable, and films made in expiration may help to uncover an apical focus. Frank hemoptysis is practically never seen in children and adolescents.

Pleural effusion

Pleural effusion is diagnosed in about 8% of children with initial pulmonary tuberculosis; two thirds of the cases of pleural effusion develop within 6 months of the onset of the primary disease. The complication occurs twice as frequently in boys as in girls and more often in children of school age than in younger children. Pleural effusion in children may occur as an extension from a subpleural primary focus, or the pleural lesion may result from hematogenous seeding to the pleura (Fig. 31-4). The onset of disease is occasionally insidious but more often is accompanied by fever and chest pain that is increased by deep breathing. The patient remains febrile for 1 to 2 weeks, followed by a gradual defervescence. By the end of the third week the temperature is usually normal, and most of the fluid has been absorbed.

The diagnosis of tuberculous pleural effusion is suggested by a positive tuberculin test, examination of the pleural fluid, or history. The diagnosis is confirmed by recovery of tubercle bacilli on culture from pleural fluid or from material obtained by pleural biopsy or by histologic examination of biopsy material. Most often the fluid is clear, but occasionally it is slightly cloudy, and rarely it is frankly hemorrhagic. The albumin content is increased, and the white blood cell count is highly variable with a predominance of lymphocytes. Tubercle bacilli are recovered by culture in about 50% of cases. Nee-

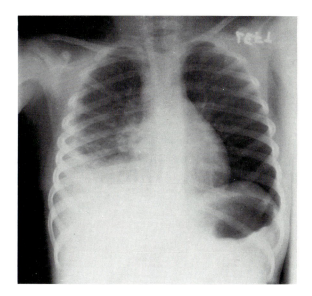

Fig. 31-4. Roentgenographic findings from a child with recent onset of pulmonary tuberculosis complicated by pleural effusion.

dle biopsies of the parietal pleura show typical tubercles in about 60% of cases, and cultures of tissues obtained by this method also yield tubercle bacilli in most cases.

The immediate and long-term outlook of children with tuberculous pleural effusion has always been good. In untreated children the incidence of chronic pulmonary tuberculosis in later life was no greater than in those who never had this complication. Moderate to severe scoliosis developed in 5% of children with untreated tuberculous pleurisy, but few instances have been seen since the advent of chemotherapy. Thoracenteses that remove large amounts of fluid at one time or repeated thoracenteses for drainage of pleural fluid are not advised, as the fluid will resolve during therapy. Arm and shoulder exercises designed to prevent scoliosis should be started.

Tuberculous meningitis

Meningitis is the most serious complication of tuberculosis; it is the most common cause of death from tuberculosis in childhood. Tuberculous meningitis was almost always fatal before effective therapy was available. Today it can be cured in at least 9 out of 10 patients, but complete neurologic recovery in children depends to a large extent on early diagnosis followed by prompt and prolonged therapy, and it is not always attained. During the preantibiotic era the

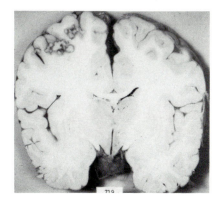

Fig. 31-5. Cerebral granulomas found at autopsy in a patient with tuberculous meningitis. Extension of the intracerebral focus to the CSF probably preceded and developed into meningeal disease.

average course of meningitis from first symptom to death was only 19 days. Knowledge of the pathogenesis of meningitis helps in diagnosis and in interpretation of the early physical signs and early changes in the CSF.

Pathogenesis. Tubercle bacilli that lodge in the cerebral cortex behave as metastatic foci elsewhere; a caseous lesion forms, increases in size until it reaches the overlying meninges, and infects the subarachnoid space (Fig. 31-5). Sometimes the tuberculous focus may discharge caseous material and bacilli into the ventricular fluid, causing fulminating meningitis. Usually the infection of the meninges is gradual. Even in this early stage of meningeal involvement, examination of the CSF usually shows some deviations from normal.

A caseous focus may form, become encapsulated, and form a tuberculoma to produce symptoms simulating a brain tumor. A quiescent lesion may be activated by trauma or by an intercurrent systemic infection such as measles. The caseous focus that drains into the subarachnoid space may originate not only in the cortex, meninges, or choroid plexus but also in the bones enclosing the CNS. Thus tuberculous meningitis may also be due to direct extension from tuberculous mastoiditis or spondylitis.

Meningitis is an early complication of primary and of miliary tuberculosis, usually developing within 6 months of the onset of infection. The first symptoms appear within 4 months of the estimated date of onset of tuberculosis in 40% of the cases. Fig. 31-6 demonstrates a tuber-

culous focus in a patient with miliary tuberculosis, shown by contrast-enhanced computer-assisted tomographic scan.

The greatest involvement of the meninges surrounds the brain stem. The exudate at the base of the brain may cause obstruction of the basal cisterns, leading to hydrocephalus. Involvement of cerebral arteries and veins is common, and acute tuberculous arteritis may cause occlusion of the vessels with resulting severe neurologic sequelae such as hemiparesis and seizure disorders.

The signs and symptoms of tuberculous meningitis often can be related to pathologic changes in the CNS. The involvement of the cranial nerves is due to the exudate at the base of the brain (Fig. 31-7). Exudate or edema around the optic nerve causes visual disturbances in which changes in the optic disks are usually found. Impairment of extraocular muscles is common. Hemipareses usually result from cerebral in-

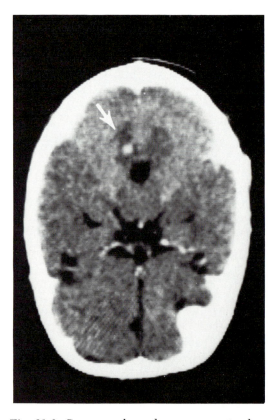

Fig. 31-6. Contrast-enhanced computer-assisted tomographic identification of focal cerebral granuloma in a child with miliary tuberculosis and minimal abnormalities in cerebrospinal fluid examination.

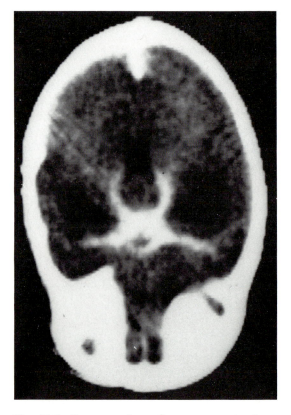

Fig. 31-7. Contrast-enhanced computer-assisted tomographic visualization of the basilar view of the head, recording the extent of inflammatory activity in a child with advanced tuberculous meningitis.

volvement secondary to vascular changes. Neurologic signs may be transient if they are due to cerebral edema or if the vascular lesion causing them can be reversed by therapy. If the area of infarction is large, the deficits may be permanent.

The onset of tuberculous meningitis is usually insidious. Fever, vomiting, and apathy are the most striking symptoms, and about 20% have infections of the upper respiratory tract at the time of onset of the meningitis, many with evidence of otitis media. Children over 4 years of age often complain of headache and abdominal pain.

The course of meningitis is classically divided into three stages. The initial stage of general symptoms lasts about a week. The second stage of neurologic involvement may start abruptly with drowsiness, some resistance to neck flexion, sluggish pupillary reactions, strabismus, ptosis, positive Kernig's or Brudzinski's signs, absent abdominal reflexes, or increased deep tendon reflexes. In spite of drowsiness, patients usually respond to stimuli. Occasionally, patients in the second stage have no evidence of meningeal irritation, but they develop signs or symptoms of encephalitis such as confusion, disorientation, slurred speech, grimacing, chewing, athetoid movements of the extremities, or peripheral tremors. Funduscopic examination is usually normal. Patients in the third stage of meningitis are usually unresponsive and exhibit neurologic signs such as opisthotonos, decerebrate rigidity, marked irregular respirations, hemipareses, and cranial nerve palsies. Obstructive hydrocephalus may develop even during optimal therapy. The fluid is frequently xanthochromic, and the protein content is usually greater than 300 mg/100 ml of spinal fluid.

Diagnosis. Tuberculous meningitis usually is seen in children who have not previously been diagnosed as having tuberculosis. Diagnosis during the first stage will depend largely on the family or social history indicating the possibility of tuberculosis, appreciation of the importance of a history of marked apathy or drowsiness, and administration of a tuberculin test. Many children with tuberculous meningitis react to tuberculin, and many children who develop meningitis have evidence of tuberculosis on chest roentgenogram. However, both of these findings may be absent (Table 31-2).

The characteristic findings from the CSF are clear fluid and white blood cell counts ranging from 10 to 350 cells/mm^3, with a predominance of lymphocytes or monocytes. Occasionally the initial count may be as high as 1000 cells/mm^3, with a predominance of polymorphonuclear leukocytes, and the glucose concentration may be decreased (less than 40 mg/100 ml), particularly in disease of longer duration. The protein content of the spinal fluid is usually above normal and increases on successive examinations. The chloride content of the fluid is frequently below normal in the second or third stage of meningitis but may be normal in the first stage. Tubercle bacilli often can be found on direct smear of CSF sediment but usually only after a meticulous search. In most patients tubercle bacilli can be recovered on culture. Confirmation of the diagnosis by this means is always desirable, but treatment should never be deferred pending the results of culture if there is reason to suspect this diagnosis.

Early in the second stage of tuberculous meningitis, differentiation from other infections by means of the CSF may be difficult, but the decreasing glucose and increasing protein content may help distinguish tuberculous meningitis from viral encephalomyelitis or lead encephalopathy. However, herpes simplex encephalitis may resemble that due to tuberculosis, as may tumors. Treatment may occasionally be begun while the diagnosis is being pursued,

Table 31-2. Diagnostic findings in recent studies of tuberculous meningitis in children

Finding	Cases
History of exposure to case with active tuberculosis	40% to 69%
Abnormal roentgenogram of chest	44% to 88%
Intermediate PPD < 10 mm	6% to 48%
CSF cell predominance of polymorphonuclear leukocytes	14% to 27%
Papilledema	9% to 33%
Cranial nerve palsies	12% to 13%
Normal CSF glucose	13% to 22%

since there is a close correlation between the prognosis and the stage of the disease in which treatment is begun. Children treated during the first stage of meningitis almost invariably survive, often without significant sequelae, while children first treated after severe neurologic changes have occurred are at great risk of a poor or fatal outcome.

Serous tuberculous meningitis

Serous meningitis is a clinical entity that resolves spontaneously; it occurs in tuberculous children who develop signs or symptoms that suggest tuberculous meningitis. This diagnosis was of great importance before specific therapy was available, because the favorable prognosis was in marked contrast to that of true tuberculous meningitis. The differential diagnosis is less important today, because all forms of active tuberculosis receive specific therapy.

Tuberculoma

Tuberculomas of the brain or spinal cord are isolated foci of active tuberculosis. Like other foci they may produce symptoms within a short period after initial infection, or they may remain silent for a time and later cause caseous meningitis or serous meningitis. Many tuberculomas are diagnosed as intracranial neoplasms.

Tuberculosis of the skeletal system

In most instances complications in the bones or joints appear early in infection and afflict about 4% of children with tuberculosis. In children who receive antituberculous therapy the risk of late skeletal complications has all but vanished. As with other complications, tuberculosis of the skeletal system usually results from early hematogenous dissemination of tubercle bacilli. Spondylitis may be due to lymphatic drainage from another area of tuberculosis, such as pleura or kidney. Spondylitis is rare in infants, and dactylitis occurs almost exclusively in infants.

The skeletal disease usually begins in the metaphyseal portions of the epiphyses, and the necrotic process may invade the surrounding tissue to form cold abscesses that often appear at points far from their sources. The destruction may involve only the bone, but often it extends through the epiphysis into the capsule of the joint. The spine is the most common site of tuberculous bone involvement, with the hip and then the knee next in order of frequency. Dactylitis of the

hands and feet is now uncommon. Multiple bony lesions are seen in disseminated forms of tuberculosis, especially in protracted hematogenous tuberculosis. Occasionally, biopsy for culture or pathologic examination may be indicated to confirm the diagnosis.

In tuberculosis of the spine (Pott's disease) the infection usually begins in the vertebral body. Destruction of the vertebral bodies may result in collapse producing a kyphotic deformity (gibbus), and narrowing of the intervertebral space may occur. Rigidity of the spine is due to muscular spasm from the resulting pain. Pain is a more prominent symptom of tuberculosis of the joints. It is usually localized to the involved joint and is increased by motion.

Local disability and referred pain often respond rapidly to therapy. Until pain on motion in the affected area is no longer present, some degree of rest is indicated, which may be secured by a splint or by bed rest to avoid the trauma of weight-bearing bones. When treatment is given early, relatively little destruction of bone occurs. The need for surgical fusion in spondylitis has almost been eliminated by antituberculous drug therapy.

Tuberculosis of the superficial lymph nodes

Lymphadenitis of the superficial lymph nodes was formerly the most common complication of tuberculosis in children. Cervical adenitis was believed to represent the regional adenopathy of tuberculosis of the tonsils, but this portal of entry is now very rare. In most instances generalized adenitis is an early hematogenous complication of tuberculosis. Excluding the patients with extrapulmonary primary tuberculosis, most persons with superficial adenitis of tuberculous origin also have pulmonary roentgenographic evidence of tuberculosis. If the diagnosis is otherwise in doubt, a biopsy may be done.

At the present time in the United States, adenitis of the superficial cervical nodes is far more likely to be due to atypical acid-fast bacilli than to *M. tuberculosis*. The main findings differentiating those with atypical infection from those with tuberculosis of the lymph nodes are the tuberculin test, the lack of history of contact with tuberculous persons, the normal chest roentgenogram, the response to antituberculous therapy, and the results of cultures. In atypical mycobacteriosis, the tuberculin test is usually indeterminate (5 to 9 mm) or positive but weakly so (10 to 12 mm). This is especially true in the southeastern portion of the United States, where atypical mycobacterial colonization and disease are very prevalent. The chest roentgenogram is normal whereas most children with tuberculous adenitis show evidence of the pulmonary infection. In cervical adenitis due to atypical bacilli, the nodes that are most often involved are those at the angle of the jaw, the submental group, and those in the preauricular area; response to therapy with antituberculous drugs is poor. The recovery of bacilli by culture from a needle biopsy or from material obtained from surgical resection is desirable to confirm the differential diagnosis. Pathologic examination of biopsy material from both conditions show findings which are identical. Atypical mycobacteria seldom are sensitive to INH.

Antibiotic therapy directed toward possible pyogenic infection may initiate the treatment of cervical adenitis. A favorable response within 1 to 2 weeks is consistent with the diagnosis of a nontuberculous infection. If the lymph nodes remain unchanged or increase in size, an aspirate or excision may be obtained. If nodal excision is done before the overlying skin has become involved there should be no difficulty with wound healing. The biopsy provides material for pathologic examination and culture.

Tuberculosis of the tonsils and adenoids, larynx, middle ear, and mastoids. Tuberculosis of a tonsil can result from infection caused by contact with material containing tubercle bacilli. This route of infection was important when the incidence of bovine tuberculosis was high and milk was not pasteurized, but it is now extremely rare in the United States. Tuberculous infection of the larynx is usually caused by infectious sputum in adolescents and adults who have chronic pulmonary tuberculosis. The onset of the middle ear and mastoid disease is without pain or fever. Discharge from the ear canal and deafness are early symptoms. Facial paralysis develops more often in tuberculous otitis media than in other chronic infections of the middle ear. Infection of the labyrinth is also more common than in purulent infections, but it develops so gradually that symptoms are uncommon, even when function is destroyed.

Tuberculosis of the abdomen. Peritonitis may be localized, in which case it is called *plastic peritonitis*. This most often results from direct extension of infection from lymph nodes or may originate from tuberculous salpingitis. In early cases there may be a small amount of loculated fluid. If the disease process is unchecked, the omentum becomes attached by adhesions and forms a mass in the epigastrium. The onset of peritonitis may be insidious, with low-grade fever as the only symptom. Occasionally the first symptoms are those of partial intestinal obstruction, vomiting, and pain. The lymph nodes and the surrounding exudate can often be palpated as irregular tender masses with a characteristic doughy feeling. Efforts to confirm the diagnosis by paracentesis incur the risk of perforating the intestine if it has become adherent to the abdominal wall.

Generalized peritonitis with effusion may be due to direct extension from an initial infection in the gastrointestinal tract, but such instances are rare in the United States. The ascites also may result from hematogenous spread of the bacilli. The fluid increases rapidly, and a patient with a scaphoid abdomen may develop a tense, rounded abdomen within 48 hours. In children, ascites appears to be an early complication of tuberculosis.

Tuberculous enteritis was formerly a sequela of advanced pulmonary tuberculous disease in adults and adolescents. Its usual location is the lower half of the jejunum, the ileum, and the cecum. It is caused by superinfection of the mucosa with tubercle bacilli from swallowed sputum. Shallow ulcers produce pain and diarrhea alternating with constipation. Fistulas from the GI tract may develop if therapy is neglected.

Tuberculosis of the skin

Extensive tuberculous disease of the skin, such as progressive lupus vulgaris, has always been rare in the United States. Cutaneous manifestations fall into two groups. The disease may be localized and the infection is caused by direct contact with tubercle bacilli, or scattered lesions may be conveyed to the skin by the bloodstream or lymphatics. In addition to tuberculous infection of the skin, other nonspecific skin conditions such as erythema nodosum are manifestations of tuberculosis as well as of other diseases.

Tuberculosis of the eye

The conjunctiva and cornea are the usual sites of disease in children. Most often the organisms reach the eye by bacteremic spread. However, inoculation of *M. tuberculosis* into the conjunctiva can be caused by a cough or sneeze from a tuberculous individual or by inoculation of the bacilli by contaminated hands. A few yellowish gray nodules may be found on the palpebral conjunctiva that resemble the early nodular lesions of trachoma. When the nodules coalesce a small ulcer is formed.

The lesions of phlyctenular conjunctivitis are small, grayish, jellylike nodules usually seen on the limbus and accompanied by injection of the blood vessels of the adjacent conjunctiva. They do not contain tubercle bacilli and are thought to be phenomena of hypersensitivity to tuberculin that occur in the initial stage of tuberculosis.

Tuberculosis of the endocrine and exocrine glands

Isolated instances of tuberculosis of the thyroid, parotid, pineal, and pituitary glands as well as the thymus, pancreas, ovary, and testis have been observed. The adrenal gland is the gland in which tuberculosis has been diagnosed most frequently premortem. About 100 proved cases have been reported in children and many more in adults. The peak age incidence of Addison's disease is at about 30 years. Formerly it usually was caused by tuberculosis, but at present tuberculosis of the adrenal glands is rarely encountered.

Tuberculosis of the genital tract

The genital tract may be the portal of entry of tuberculous infection, but seeding through the blood or from a contiguous focus of active disease may also occur. The most common evidence of genital tuberculosis in boys is epididymitis. The nodular and painless or slightly painful enlargement is usually discovered in the course of a physical examination. Tuberculosis of the fallopian tubes is the most common form of genital involvement in females and is often associated with some degree of endometritis, especially in women.

Tuberculosis of the urinary tract

Renal tuberculosis can occur at any age but is mainly a disease of young adults. Tuberculous disease of the kidney usually stems from hematogenous dissemination of bacilli to the cortex of the kidney, very often during the initial in-

fection. Tubercle bacilli have been recovered from the urine of children during occult hematogenous dissemination and from the urine of persons with miliary tuberculosis. Bacilluria indicates a focus of active disease, although it may originate in a single caseous tubercle. When renal tuberculosis progresses, the necrosis usually results in fistulous tracts leading into the pelvis of the kidney, when the infection may spread through the ureter into the bladder. In males the prostate and epididymis may be involved.

In children who are not known to be tuberculous, renal disease is usually first suggested by persistent pyuria from which no organisms can be cultured by routine methods. A common additional finding is albuminuria and hematuria.

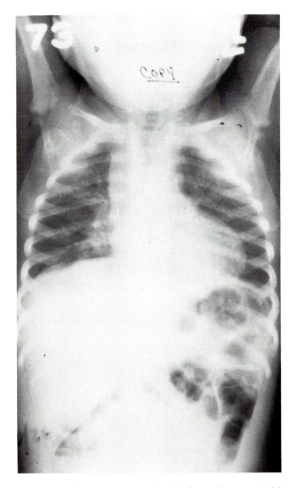

Fig. 31-8. Roentgenographic findings from a child with pulmonary tuberculosis complicated by pericardial effusion. Pericardiocentesis revealed serosanguineous fluid from which *M. tuberculosis* was not isolated.

A urologic examination is necessary to define the site and extent of renal and ureteral involvement. The earliest changes are usually in the upper or lower calyces, where there may be an irregularity due to the erosion of the parenchyma. Cavities may be seen in more advanced disease.

Tuberculous pericarditis

This complication is also usually the result of hematogenous dissemination to the pericardium, is most common in older children, and, if advanced, may lead to restrictive compromise of cardiac function (Fig. 31-8).

REFERENCES

Abernathy RS, Dutt AK, Stead WW, et al. Short-course chemotherapy for tuberculosis in children. Pediatrics 1983;72:801.

American Academy Pediatrics, Section on Diseases of the Chest. The tuberculin test. Pediatrics 1974;54:650.

American Lung Association. Diagnostic standards and classification of tuberculosis and other mycobacterial diseases. New York: The Association, 1974.

American Thoracic Society. Preventive therapy of tuberculous infection. Am Rev Respir Dis 1974;110:371.

Armstrong JA, D'Arcy Hart P. Phagosome-lysosome interactions in cultured macrophages infected with virulent tubercle bacilli. Reversal of the usual nonfusion pattern and observations on bacterial survival. J Exp Med 1975;142:1.

Barksdale L, Kimm KS. Mycobacterium. Bacteriol Rev 1977;41:217.

Brickman HF, Beaudry PH, Marks MI. The timing of tuberculin tests in relation to immunization with live viral vaccines. Pediatrics 1975;55:392.

Brooks SM, Lassiter NL, Young EC. A pilot study concerning the infection risk of sputum positive tuberculous patients on chemotherapy. Am Rev Respir Dis 1973;108:799.

Brown RC, Atuk NO. A second reversion of the tuberculin reaction after isoniazid prevention therapy. A case report. Am Rev Respir Dis 1973;107:658.

Campbell PB. Defective leukotaxis in monocytes from patients with pulmonary tuberculosis. J Infect Dis 1979;139:409.

Centers for Disease Control. BCG vaccines. Morbid Mortal Weekly Rep 1979;28:241.

Christensen WI. Genitourinary tuberculosis: review of 102 cases. Medicine 1974;53:377.

Comstock GW. Frost revisited: the modern epidemiology of tuberculosis. Am J Epidemiol 1975;101:363.

Comstock GW, Livesay VT, Woolpert SF. The prognosis of a positive tuberculin reaction in childhood and adolescence. Am J Epidemiol 1974;99:141.

Dahlstrom G, Sjogren I. Side-effects of BCG vaccination. J Biol Stand 1977;5:147.

Edwards LB, Livesay VT, Acquaviva FA, Palmer CE. Height, weight, tuberculous infection and tuberculous disease. Arch Environ Health 1971;22:106.

Edwards PQ. Screening for tuberculosis. Chest 1975;68:451.

Ellard GA. Variations between individuals and populations in the acetylation of isoniazid and its significance for the treatment of pulmonary tuberculosis. Clin Pharmacol Ther 1976;19:610.

Farer LS, Lowell AM, Meador MP. Extrapulmonary tuberculosis in the United States. Am J Epidemiol 1979;109:205.

Ferebee SH. Controlled chemoprophylaxis trials in tuberculosis. A general review. Adv Tuberc Res 1970;17:28.

Furey WW, Stefancic MF. Tuberculosis in a community hospital. JAMA 1976;235:168.

Harding GE, Smith DW: Host-parasite relationships in experimental airborne tuberculosis. VI. Influence of vaccination with Bacille Calmette-Guerin on the onset and/or extent of hematogenous dissemination on virulent *Mycobacterium tuberculosis* to the lungs. J Infect Dis 1977;136:439.

Hendin AS, Margolis MT, Glickman MG. Occlusion of the basilar artery in tuberculous meningitis. Neuroradiology 1973;6:193.

Ho RS, Fok JS, Harding GE, Smith DW. Host-parasite relationships in experimental airborne tuberculosis. VII. Fate of *Mycobacterium tuberculosis* in primary lung lesions and in primary lesion-free lung tissue infected as a result of bacillemia. J Infect Dis 1978;138:237.

Hsu KHK. Thirty years after isoniazid. Its impact on tuberculosis in children and adolescents. JAMA 1984;251:1283.

Kalish SB, Radin RC, Phair JP, et al. Use of an enzyme-linked immunosorbent assay technique in the differential diagnosis of active pulmonary tuberculosis in humans. J Infect Dis 1983;147:523.

Katz P, Goldstein RA, Fauci AS. Immunoregulation to infection caused by *Mycobacterium tuberculosis:* the presence of suppressor myocytes and the alteration of subpopulations of T lymphocytes. J Infect Dis 1979;140:12.

Kendig EL, Jr. The place of BCG vaccine in the management of infants born of tuberculous mothers. N Engl J Med 1969;281:520.

Kopanoff DE, et al. A continuing survey of tuberculosis primary drug resistance in the United States: March 1975 to November 1977. A U.S. Public Health Service cooperative study. Am Rev Respir Dis 1978;118:835.

Lifschitz M. The value of the tuberculin skin test as a screening test for tuberculosis among BCG-vaccinated children. Pediatrics 1965;36:624.

Light IJ, Saidleman M, Sutherland JM. Management of newborns after nursery exposure to tuberculosis. Am Rev Respir Dis 1974;109:415.

Lincoln EM. Course and prognosis of tuberculosis in children. Am J Med 1950;9:623.

Lincoln EM. Epidemics of tuberculosis. Arch Environ Health 1967;14:473.

Lincoln EM, Sewell EM. Tuberculosis in children. New York: McGraw-Hill Co., 1963.

Lincoln EM, Sordillo SVR, Davies PA. Tuberculosis meningitis in children: a review of 167 untreated and 74 treated patients with special reference to early diagnosis. J Pediatr 1960;57:807.

Litt IF, Cohen MI, McNamara H. Isoniazid hepatitis in adolescents. J Pediatr 1976;89:133.

Lunn JA, Johnson AJ. Comparison of the Tine and Mantoux tuberculin tests. Report of the Tuberculin Subcommittee of the Research Committee of the British Thoracic Association. Br Med J 1978;1:1451.

Mintz AA. Tuberculous meningitis in children before and since isoniazid. South Med J 1976;69:1061.

Mitchell JR, et al. Increased incidence of isoniazid hepatitis in rapid acetylators: possible relation in hydrazine metabolites. Clin Pharmacol Ther 1975;18:70.

Moulding T. Chemoprophylaxis of tuberculosis: when is the benefit worth the risk and cost? Ann Intern Med 1971;74:761.

Olazabal F, Jr. Chloidal tubercles. JAMA 1967;200:374.

Palmer CE, Edwards LB, Hopwood L, Edwards PQ. Experimental and epidemiologic basis for the interpretation of tuberculin sensitivity. J Pediatr 1959;55:413.

Palmer CE, Shaw LW, Comstock GW. Community trials of BCG vaccination. Am Rev Tuberc 1958;77:877.

Pessayre D, et al. Isoniazid-rifampin fulminant hepatitis. A possible consequence of the enhancement of isoniazid hepatotoxicity by enzyme induction. Gastroenterology 1977;72:284.

Porter JM, Snowe RJ, Silver D. Tuberculous enteritis with perforation and abscess formation in childhood. Surgery 1972;71:254.

Powell KE, Meador MP, Farer LS. Recent trends in tuberculosis in children. JAMA 1984;251:1289.

Rideout VK, Hiltz JE. An epidemic of tuberculosis in a rural high school in 1967. Can J Public Health 1969;60:22.

Rose CE, Jr, Zerbe GO, Lantz SO, Bailey WC. Establishing priority during investigation of tuberculosis contacts. Am Rev Respir Dis 1979;119:603.

Sifontes JE. Rifampin in tuberculosis meningitis. J Pediatr 1975;87:1015.

Smith AM, Lattimer JK. Genitourinary tract involvement in children with tuberculosis. Overview of subtle and surprisingly frequent involvement. NY State J Med 1973;73:2325.

Spyridis P, et al. Isoniazid liver injury during chemoprophylaxis in children. Arch Dis Child 1973;54:65.

Stead WW, Bates JH. Evidence of a "silent" bacillemia in primary tuberculosis. Ann Intern Med 1971;74:559.

Steiner M. Newer and second-line drugs in the treatment of drug-resistant tuberculosis in children. Med Clin North Am 1967;51:1153.

Steiner P, Portugaleza C. Tuberculous meningitis in children. A review of 25 cases observed between the years of 1965 and 1970 at the Kings County Medical Center of Brooklyn with special reference to the problem of infection with primary drug-resistant strains of *M. tuberculosis*. Am Rev Respir Dis 1973;107:22.

Steiner P, Rao M, Goldberg R, Steiner M. Primary drug resistance in children. Drug susceptibility of strains of *M. tuberculosis* isolated from children during the years of 1969 to 1972 at the Kings County Hospital Medical Center of Brooklyn. Am Rev Respir Dis 1974;110:98.

Steiner P, Rao M, Victoria M, Steiner M. Primary isoniazid-resistant tuberculosis in children. Clinical features, strain, resistance, treatment and outcome in 26 children treated at Kings County Medical Center at Brooklyn between the years 1961 and 1972. Am Rev Respir Dis 1974;110:306.

Steiner P, et al. Miliary tuberculosis in two infants after nursery exposure: epidemiologic, clinical and laboratory findings. Am Rev Resp Dis 1976;113:267.

Stottmeier KD. Emergence of rifampin-resistant *Mycobacterium tuberculosis* in Massachusetts. J Infect Dis 1976;133:88.

Sumaya CV, et. Tuberculosis in children during the isoniazid era. J Pediatr 1975;87:43.

Thompson NH, Glassroth JL, Snider DE, Jr, Farer LS. The booster phenomenon in serial tuberculin testing. Am Rev Respir Dis 1979;119:587.

Vestal AL. Procedures for the isolation and identification of mycobacteria. Atlanta: Department of Health, Education, and Welfare, 1975.

Visudiphan P, Chiemchanya S. Evaluation of rifampin in the treatment of tuberculous meningitis in children. J Pediatr 1975;87:893.

Wallgren A. Pulmonary tuberculosis: relation of childhood infection to the disease in adults. Lancet 1938;1:417.

Wallgren A. The time-table of tuberculosis. Tubercle 1945;29:245.

Zarabi M, Sane S, Girdany BR. The chest roentgenogram in the early diagnosis of tuberculous meningitis in children. Am J Dis Child 1971;121:389.

32

URINARY TRACT INFECTIONS

The term *urinary tract infection* (UTI) refers to a clinical entity that may involve the urethra, bladder (lower urinary tract), and/or the ureters, renal pelvis, calyces, and renal parenchyma (upper urinary tract). It is a convenient designation because it is often impossible to localize the infection to either the lower tract or the upper tract. Most bacterial urinary tract infections are characterized by the presence of significant numbers of bacteria in the urine.

The designation *significant bacteriuria* refers to the number of bacteria in excess of the usual bacterial contamination of the anterior urethra. The presence of more than 100,000 bacteria per milliliter of urine in a clean voided specimen is likely to be the result of infection, not contamination at the time of voiding. *Asymptomatic bacteriuria* is defined as significant bacteriuria in a patient who has no clinical evidence of active infection.

Lower UTI is usually characterized by dysuria, frequency, urgency, and possibly suprapubic tenderness. The clinical manifestations of acute pyelonephritis may include fever, lumbar pain and tenderness, dysuria, urgency, and frequency associated with significant bacteriuria.

Recurrence of a UTI may be caused by a relapse or a reinfection. A relapse is a recurrence of the infection with the *same* infecting microorganism, perhaps indicating inadequate therapy. A reinfection is a new infection caused by a bacterium that is different from the one responsible for the previous episode. Specific identification may require serotyping of the bacterium, for

example, *Escherichia coli*, a procedure that is not uniformly available to the clinician. Persistence of the UTI, associated with the same organism, for many months or years indicates the presence of a chronic infection.

ETIOLOGY

The microorganisms that cause UTIs include:
Gram-negative bacteria
  E. coli
  Klebsiella pneumoniae
  Proteus mirabilis
  Enterobacter aerogenes
  Pseudomonas aeruginosa
  Serratia marcescens
  Salmonella
Gram-positive bacteria
  Staphylococcus epidermidis
  Enterococcus
  Staphylococcus aureus
  Staphylococcus saprophyticus
Other agents
  Adenovirus types 11 and 21
  Candida albicans
The most common pathogens are the gram-negative bacilli. Of this group, *E. coli* is responsible for most acute infections. The other gram-negative bacteria, such as *Proteus*, *Pseudomonas*, and *Klebsiella-Enterobacter* species, are more likely to be associated with chronic or recurrent infections. Salmonella bacteriuria is usually associated with salmonella sepsis.

Gram-positive bacteria, such as *S. epidermidis*, *S. saprophyticus*, and *S. aureus*, have been identified as causes of UTIs. Coagulase-negative staphylococci have been detected as urinary tract pathogens in sexually active young women (Bailey, 1973; Vosti, 1975) and newborns (Khan et al., 1975). Coagulase-positive staphylococci may invade the urinary tract via the hematogenous route.

Adenovirus types 11 and 21 have been reported as causes of acute hemorrhagic cystitis (Mufson and Belshe, 1976). Fungi, such as *C. albicans*, may be responsible for UTIs in patients with indwelling catheters during the course of their treatment with antibiotics, in immunocompromised patients, and as a result of renal seeding during fungemia.

PATHOGENESIS

Bacterial invasion of the urinary tract may occur by direct extension, ascending via the urethra, or by the hematogenous route. Lymphatic spread has been suggested, but it has not been proved (Murphy et al., 1960).

The ascending route is the most common pathway of infection. Bacteria that colonize the distal urethra may eventually spread to the bladder. Massage of the urethra and sexual intercourse have been shown to force bacteria into the bladder (Bran et al., 1972; Buckley et al., 1978). Hematogenous spread may occur during the course of neonatal sepsis. In older children and adolescents with staphylococcal sepsis and/or endocarditis, the kidney may be the site of abscesses.

The pathogenesis of a UTI is dependent in great part on factors associated with both the microorganism and the host. The following virulence factors of microorganisms are associated with UTIs:

1. Size of inoculum
2. Pili (mucosal cell adherence)
   a. Mannose sensitive type 1, common
   b. P pili
   c. X pili
3. Motility
4. Urease production

Microorganism

Experimental studies in mice have revealed that the greater the number of organisms delivered to the kidney, the greater the chance of inducing pyelonephritis (Gorrill and De Navas-

quez, 1964). Thus the size of the inoculum is an important factor. Evidence accumulated during the course of studies by Gruneberg et al. (1968) and Kaijser (1973) indicates that certain organisms appear to be particularly virulent for the urinary tract. Of the 150 or more *E. coli* O serogroups, only a few (01, 02, 04, 06, 07, 075) have been responsible for most UTIs, and these especially include those that possess large quantities of K1 antigen.

A primary pathogenic factor is the presence of pili. Pili have been shown to be important for the attachment of *E. coli* and *P. mirabilis* to the urinary tract epithelium (Silverblatt, 1974). Almost all *E. coli* contain type 1 common pili that bind to mannose (Ofek et al., 1977). Attachment to mannose-containing receptors on epithelial cells of the urethra and vagina is thought to be of primary importance in colonizing the lower urinary tract (Iwahi et al., 1983; Svanborg-Eden et al., 1983). *E. coli* isolates from patients with cystitis have a greater avidity and adhere in higher numbers to uroepithelial cells than do *E. coli* fecal isolates (Svanborg-Eden et al., 1976, 1981). Uropathogenic *E. coli* and *P. mirabilis* are capable of altering their surface composition (phase variation) and tend to lose their type 1 pili on arrival in the kidney (Silverblatt, 1974; Ofek et al., 1981). This ability to vary phase characteristics constitutes a selective advantage by promoting renal cell attachment and, more so, because mannose receptors of type 1 pili facilitate phagocytosis by polymorphonuclear leukocytes (Perry et al., 1983).

P pili cause mannose-resistant hemagglutination and bind to specific glycolipid receptor sites on human epithelial cells (Kallenius et al., 1981; Leffler et al., 1981; Svanborg-Eden et al., 1981, 1983). *E. coli* with P pili have their favored site of attachment on the uroepithelium of the kidneys where receptors are distributed with greatest density (Svanborg-Eden et al., 1976, 1983). UTIs are more likely to occur in persons who express the P blood group antigen (Lomberg et al., 1983).

A third type of pili, X pili, are also capable of binding to uroepithelium. Their receptor sites have not been identified; however, they also have an affinity for the upper urinary tract.

Motility is also likely to be an important pathogenic factor. Weyrauch and Bassett (1951) have shown that motile bacteria can ascend in the ureter against the flow of the urine. Moreover, the ascent of these bacteria may be facilitated by the decreased ureteral peristalsis attributed to the endotoxin of gram-negative bacilli.

It has been shown that the production of urease by the infecting bacteria may affect their capacity to cause pyelonephritis. When urinary tract infection was induced in experimental animals by the retrograde administration of *P. mirabilis*, a urease-producing organism, there was a high degree of correlation between the number of bacteria in the kidney and the extent of renal damage. However, treatment with a urease inhibitor reduced the extent of renal damage and the number of bacteria in the kidney without a significant decrease in the number of bacteria in the urine (Musher et al., 1975).

Host

The known host defense mechanisms of the urinary tract are:
Antibacterial activity of urine
Prostatic secretions of postpubescent males
Flushing mechanisms of the bladder
Low vaginal pH
Antiadherence effect of uromucoid
Antiadherence effect of mucopolysaccharide
Humoral immunity
Local secretory immunity
Lack of P blood group antigen
Normal flora
Antibacterial activity of urine against certain bacteria has been described. Kaye (1968) has reported that extremes of osmolality, high urea concentration, low pH, and high concentration of organic acids may inhibit the growth of some bacteria that cause UTIs. However, with the usual range of pH (5.5 to 7.0) and osmolality (300 to 1200), the rate of growth of *E. coli* has been reported to be unaffected (Asscher et al., 1966). Prostatic fluid may inhibit bacterial growth (Stamey et al., 1968). In contrast, glucose makes urine a better culture medium, and it has been shown to inhibit the migrating, adhering, aggregating, and killing functions of polymorphonuclear leukocytes.

The flushing mechanism of the bladder enhances the spontaneous clearance of bacteria. Voiding and dilution probably play an important role. In addition the intact mucosal surfaces of

animal bladders have been shown to be resistant to bacterial invasion (Cobbs and Kaye, 1967).

Low vaginal pH appears to be an important factor responsible for lack of colonization (Stamey and Timothy, 1975). For example, serogroups of *E. coli* that usually cause UTIs are more resistant to low pH than serogroups that are less common causes of infection (Stamey and Kaufman, 1975). In contrast, low pH has been shown to have an inhibitory effect on *P. mirabilis* and *P. aeruginosa* (Stamey and Mihara, 1976). This phenomenon may possibly account for the high incidence of *E. coli* infection.

Tamm-Horsfall protein is secreted by renal tubular cells and is present in the urine as uromucoid (Orskov et al., 1980). Since uromucoid is rich in mannose residues it may bind, prevent attachment, and allow adequate flushing out of bacteria. This hypothesis is substantiated in an animal model by prevention of colonization with mannose blocking (Aronson et al, 1979). Parsons et al. (1975) have demonstrated that an antiadherence mechanism of the bladder (in rabbits) exists by pretreatment of the bladder with dilute hydrochloric acid. Acid-treated bladders had 20- to 50-fold increases of bacterial adherence than controls. Adherence was enhanced by ablation of mucopolysaccharide and glycosaminoglycan from the surface of bladder epithelium (Parsons et al, 1978, 1979). Increased adherence appears to be species specific (Sobel and Vardi, 1982).

It is possible that antibacterial mechanisms are responsible for the rapid disappearance of bacteria applied to bladder mucosa in an experimental model (Vivaldi et al., 1965; Cobbs and Kaye, 1967; Norden et al., 1968); however, the nature of these mechanisms has yet to be established. Secretory IgA does decrease adherence and colonization of perineal cells by *E. coli* (Stamey et al., 1978) and is increased in children with UTIs (Uehling and Stiehm, 1971).

The role of humoral immunity as a mechanism of the host's defense against UTI has not been satisfactorily clarified. Hanson et al. (1977) reported that *E. coli* acute pyelonephritis induced serum antibodies to O antigens but rarely to K antigens. In contrast, increased levels of O antibodies were not detected in sera from patients with cystitis or asymptomatic bacteriuria. Using the sensitive enzyme-linked immunosorbent assay (ELISA), Hanson et al. (1977) found high levels of *E. coli* O antibody in the urine of most patients with acute pyelonephritis, lower levels in those with asymptomatic bacteriuria and cystitis, and minimal or no detectable levels in the urine of healthy children. Serum antibody to O antigen, K antigen, and type 1 pili have been found in patients with pyelonephritis (Hanson et al., 1977, 1981; Mattsby-Baltzer et al., 1982; Rene and Silverblatt, 1982), and IgM is the predominant species detected during acute infections. IgG antibody to the lipid A component of gram-negative rods is also detectable and may be a measure of the severity of renal disease and tissue destruction (Mattsby-Baltzer et al., 1981).

Animal studies suggest that humoral antibody is protective against ascending infection due to organisms with P pili and O and K antigens (Mattsby-Baltzer et al., 1982; Kaijser et al., 1983; O'Hanley et al., 1983). The protective effect appears to be mediated by blocking of attachment to the uroepithelium of the upper urinary tract (Svanborg-Eden and Svennerholm, 1978). The role of the host's normal perineal flora—lactobacilli, *Staphylococcus epidermidis*, corynebacteria, streptococci, and anaerobes—in preventing colonization with uropathogens is not understood.

A number of factors intrinsic and extrinsic to the host combine to predispose to UTI. They include:

Intrinsic
  Obstruction
  Stasis
  Reflux
  Pregnancy
  Sexual intercourse (in females)
  Hyperosmolality of renal medulla
  Host cell receptor sites for attachment
  Immunologic crossreactivity of bacterial antigen and human protein
  Chronic prostatitis
  B or AB blood type
  Genetic predisposition (?)
Extrinsic
  Instrumentation (catheters)
  Antimicrobial agents

Probably the single most important host factor affecting the occurrence of UTIs is urinary stasis resulting from obstruction of urine flow or bladder dysfunction. This predisposing host condition is more frequently observed in the younger patient and should prompt a more rapid roentgenographic investigation of the urinary system. The most common causes are:
  Congenital anomalies of ureter or urethra
    Valves
    Stenosis
    Bands
  Calculi
  Dysfunctional voiding
  Extrinsic ureteral or bladder compression
  Neurogenic bladder (functional obstruction)
The stasis resulting from these factors is associated with increased susceptibility to infection.

There is a striking correlation between vesicoureteral reflux and the occurrence of UTIs. Reflux, the retrograde flow of urine into the ureter and kidney, is caused by the incompetence of the normal valvular action of the ureterovesicular junction. It may occur when this area is affected by congenital anatomic defects, disease, or distal obstruction. Reflux tends to perpetuate infection by maintaining a residual pool of infected urine in the bladder after voiding. Children with reflux may develop upper UTIs and renal scarring. Smellie and Normand (1975) have reported that reflux may be detected in 30% to 50% of children with symptomatic or asymptomatic bacteriuria and that the scarred kidney associated with reflux is more susceptible to reinfection.

Physiologic alterations of the urinary tract that increase the likelihood of UTI occur as a result of pregnancy. These changes include decreased bladder and ureteral tone, decreased ureteral peristalsis, hydroureter, and increased residual bladder urine, all of which serve to cause or aggravate obstruction, stasis, and reflux.

Sexual intercourse in females produces transient bacteriuria and is associated with an increased risk of UTI. This is substantiated by the studies of Nocolle et al. (1982) and Pfau et al. (1983), showing that 80% of UTIs begin within 24 hours of intercourse in sexually active women.

Hyperosmolality of the renal medulla inhibits the migration of polymorphonuclear leukocytes to damaged medullary tissue and decreases phagocytosis of bacteria (Rocha and Fekety, 1964).

There are several facts that suggest a genetic predisposition to UTI, including the association of blood group P antigen (Lomberg et al., 1983) with blood groups B and AB, that is, those lacking anti-B isohemagglutinin (Kinane et al., 1982). Studies on the occurrence of periurethral or vaginal defects in host defenses have been inconclusive. The finding of Stamey (1973) that persons subject to recurrences have a propensity to more frequent and prolonged colonization has not been supported by the work of others (Parsons et al., 1979; Kunin et al., 1980).

Adult males with chronic prostatitis are at risk for recurrent urinary tract infections due to intermittent seeding of their urinary bladders.

Finally, there is evidence that chronic interactions of the host's immune system with retained bacterial antigens or mimicking host antigens is responsible for chronic progressive renal damage. Bacterial antigen may not be eradicated and may trigger formation of antigen-antibody complexes (Hanson et al., 1977). Tamm-Horsfall protein antigen can permeate the renal interstitial spaces and evoke an aggressive humoral and cellular immune response (Work and Andriole, 1980; Mayrer et al., 1983). The most aggressive response occurs in persons with vesicoureteral reflux independent of bacteriuria. Furthermore, Tamm-Horsfall protein cross reacts with gram-negative bacilli (Fasth et al., 1980).

Two important extrinsic host factors, instrumentation and antimicrobial agents, predispose to UTI. This is particularly true in hospitalized patients with short-term indwelling catheters and patients with chronic bladder dysfunction. Catheters produce their damage by eroding the slime layer of the urethra and bladder and by serving as a nidus for intraluminal concretions and bacterial colonization (Rubin, 1980). The pericanular space is not subject to mechanical washing out of bacteria as is the uncatheterized urethra. Suction ulcers of the bladder mucosa develop at the site of the bladder portal when urine drainage systems are not properly vented (Monson et al., 1977). Antimicrobial agents apparently have the effect of altering the host's normal perineal flora, allowing easier colonization with uropathogens. In patients with urinary catheters antibiotics have the effect of shifting colonization to antibiotic-resistant strains (Britt et al., 1977; Butler and Kunin, 1968; Warren et al., 1982, 1983).

PATHOLOGY

Mucosal and submucosal edema and infiltration of the tissue with leukocytes are the prominent histopathologic changes of cystitis.

In acute pyelonephritis and upper UTIs, the kidney is usually enlarged; its capsular surface is smooth, and the pelvic mucosa may also be involved. The microscopic findings include edema, congestion, polymorphonuclear infiltration of the interstitium, and abscess formation. Tubules may be distended by exudate consisting of leukocytes, bacteria, and debris, occasionally causing necrosis. The medulla is involved to a greater degree than the cortex.

In chronic pyelonephritis the kidney is usually contracted; its surface is scarred, and its capsule is thickened. The calyces and pelvis are fibrotic, and the thickness of the parenchyma is decreased. The glomeruli show evidence of proliferation, crescents, and hyalinization, and they are surrounded by pericapsular fibrosis. The renal architecture is disrupted by fibrotic bands and collections of lymphocytes, eosinophils, and plasma cells. Tubules are atrophied and dilated.

CLINICAL MANIFESTATIONS

The clinical manifestations of UTIs are dependent on the age of the patient. The following symptoms in newborn infants and in those under 2 years of age are characteristically nonspecific, and they appear to be related to the gastrointestinal tract rather than the urinary tract: failure to thrive, feeding problems, vomiting, diarrhea, abdominal distention, and jaundice. Infants may have signs of balanitis, prostatitis, and orchitis or manifestations of overt sepsis.

The infection in children over 2 years of age may be characterized by fever, frequency, dysuria, abdominal pain, flank pain, and hematuria. The occurrence of enuresis in a child who has been toilet trained could be a manifestation of a UTI. Young infants and boys may have an obstructive uropathy characterized by dribbling of urine, straining with urination, or a decrease in the force and size of the urinary stream. These findings of obstruction can be aggravated by infection.

The manifestations of UTIs in adolescents and adults are fairly specific. Lower urinary tract symptoms include frequency and painful urination of a small amount of turbid urine that occasionally may be grossly bloody. Fever is usually absent. In contrast, upper UTI may be characterized by fever, chills, flank pain, and such lower tract symptoms such as frequency, urgency, and dysuria. Occasionally, the lower tract symptoms may appear 1 to 2 days before the upper tract symptoms. The clinical manifestations in some patients may be so atypical that they resemble gallbladder disease, because of epigastric pain, and acute appendicitis, because of right lower abdominal pain.

Given the appropriate clinical setting, the diagnosis is suggested by the detection of white blood cells and bacteria in the urine. The diagnosis of UTI requires confirmation by quantitative culture of urine and localization of the site of infection.

Presumptive tests

Pyuria. Pyuria is usually defined as the presence of more than five to eight white blood cells (WBCs) per cubic millimeter of *uncentrifuged* urine. This usually represents more than one WBC per high-power field; it would be 50 to 100 WBCs/mm³, that is, more than five WBCs per high-power field in *centrifuged* urine.

Pyuria does not necessarily indicate the presence of a UTI. Patients with or without pyuria may or may not have an infection. False-positive results on the order of about 30% have been reported (Brumfitt, 1965). Nevertheless, it is likely that most patients with symptomatic UTIs will have pyuria.

Microscopic examination of urine for bacteria. A Gram stain of uncentrifuged urine is a useful test for the presumptive diagnosis of UTI. Infection is suggested by the presence of at least one bacterium per oil-immersion field in a midstream, clean-catch urine specimen, equivalent to about 100,000 bacteria per milliliter.

Bioluminescence. The quantitative detection of bacterial production of ATP is another sensitive and specific screening test for UTI and detects both gram-positive and gram-negative organisms (Hanna et al., 1983).

Specific tests

Quantitative culture of urine. Urine for culture may be obtained as a midstream clean-catch specimen, by catheterization, or by suprapubic aspiration. A negative culture of a clean-catch specimen would obviate the need for catheterization or suprapubic aspiration.

Organisms, in any number, are considered significant when obtained by suprapubic aspiration. If the quantitative culture from a midstream sample reveals 100,000 bacteria or more per milliliter of urine, it indicates the presence of significant bacteriuria. A count of less than 10,000 bacteria per milliliter suggests probable contamination. A false-positive test may be due to contamination or prolonged incubation of urine before culture. False-negative results may reflect prior antimicrobial therapy, the presence of a fastidious organism that is difficult to culture, rapid flow of urine, or inactivation of bacteria by a break in technique such as spilling soap or other cleansing agents into the urine. Therefore, there are clinical situations where colony counts of less than 100,000 may indicate significant bacteriuria.

Convenient, accurate, inexpensive culture techniques have become available for clinic or office practice. These include the filter-strip, dip-slide, and dip-strip techniques. The filter-strip technique does not differentiate gram-negative and gram-positive bacteria. The dip-slide and dip-strip techniques do use discriminating agars that allow differentiation of gram-negative and gram-positive organisms.

The specific bacterium recovered by culture should be identified and tested for antimicrobial susceptibility as a guide to appropriate therapy.

Localization of site of infection. It is important to determine if the infection involves the lower tract (probably cystitis) or the upper tract (probably pyelonephritis). Although pyelonephritis is classically associated with fever, flank pain or tenderness, decreased renal concentrating ability, and an elevated erythrocyte sedimentation rate (ESR), the absence of these findings does not reliably exclude upper tract disease. Collection of urine by ureteral catheterization for quantitative culture is the most reliable method of localizing the site of infection; however, it is an invasive test and may require general anesthesia. Stamey et al. (1965) evaluated 95 females and 26 males by this method. Their observation that the site of infection was limited to the bladder in 50% of this group could not be predicted by history and physical examination. Localization by bladder washout (Fairley technique) is less invasive and does not require anesthesia; however, this is a cumbersome test and is not routinely performed.

The detection of antibody coating of bacteria has been reported to be a sensitive, reliable, *noninvasive* indicator of renal bacteriuria in women (Jones et al., 1974; Thomas et al., 1974). After addition of fluorescein-conjugated anti-human globulin to urine, the demonstration of fluorescence of the antibody-coated bacteria indicates upper tract involvement. This immunofluorescence technique has been applied to children with bacteriuria; however, its usefulness in children appears to be limited (Hellerstein et al., 1978; McCracken et al., 1981). Urinary lactic dehydrogenase (LDH) isoenzyme 5 has been shown to be more accurate for localizing the site of infection in infants and children. Lorentz and Resnick (1979) have reported that urinary LDH is a good indicator of acute pyelonephritis.

C-reactive protein (CRP) is another useful method for distinguishing upper from lower UTI and has a sensitivity and specificity of approximately 90% when compared to bladder washout (McCracken et al., 1981). A CRP value greater than 30 μg/ml suggests upper tract disease.

Finally, response to therapy is a clinical indication of the site of infection in adults. Studies in women indicate that more than 90% of patients with lower UTI but less than 50% of those with upper UTI are cured by a single dose of antibiotic if the organism is susceptible (Ronald et al., 1976; Fang et al., 1978). In children, however, recurrences of infection after short duration therapy occur in approximately 30% of those treated (McCracken, 1982). This does not differ from the frequency of recurrences following conventional therapy.

DIFFERENTIAL DIAGNOSIS

The differential diagnosis of UTIs is dependent in great part on the age of the patients. The clinical manifestations in newborn infants and in infants under 2 years of age are nonspecific. The findings of irritability, failure to thrive, vomiting, diarrhea, and jaundice suggest the possibility of *bacterial sepsis*, *acute gastroenteritis*, or *hepatitis*. The appropriate blood, stool,

and urine cultures should provide a clue to the correct diagnosis.

In older children and adults the various conditions that may simulate cystitis or pyelonephritis should be considered. For example, the symptoms of gonorrheal or chlamydial urethritis may suggest a lower UTI. A right-sided pyelonephritis could be confused with acute appendicitis, gallbladder disease, or hepatitis. Again, the appropriate cultures and serologic tests should help identify the true diagnosis.

COMPLICATIONS

Failure to recognize and to treat acute UTIs may result in recurrent infections and progression to chronic pyelonephritis. Children with chronic pyelonephritis associated with ureteral reflux and obstructive uropathy may develop such consequences of chronic renal failure as anemia, hypertension, growth failure, and metabolic abnormalities. Nephrolithiasis and stricture formation may also develop and further complicate management. A rare complication is that of renal abscess, which may rupture into the perirenal space.

PROGNOSIS

The prognosis depends on the site of involvement, the presence or absence of obstructive uropathy, and vesicoureteral reflux and therefore is related to the age of the patient. Young patients with obstructive uropathy and infection are much more likely to have serious long-term sequelae. Most single, uncomplicated episodes of infection respond to specific antimicrobial therapy. However, about one third of these patients may relapse within 1 year. Relapses decrease in frequency beyond this time; however, 1% of patients may relapse up to 6 years after initial infection. The prognosis is less favorable for patients with obstructive lesions and for those with chronic pyelonephritis. In spite of specific antimicrobial therapy, most of these patients have repeated recurrences, and those with bilateral renal involvement may progress to chronic renal insufficiency.

EPIDEMIOLOGY

Urinary tract infections involve all age groups from neonatal to geriatric. A study involving routine suprapubic puncture in over 1000 infants revealed bacteriuria in 1%; it was more common in boys. Premature infants have two to three times this rate of UTI. During preschool years, UTI is more common in girls (4.5%) than in boys (0.5%).

Long-term surveillance studies by Kunin et al. (1962) and Kunin (1970, 1976) of school-children revealed persistent bacteriuria in 1.2% of girls and in 0.4% of boys. Each year an additional 0.4% of girls developed bacteriuria. Thus the overall prevalence in school girls was 5%. These studies indicated that the peak incidence of UTI in children occurred between 2 and 6 years of age. White girls tended to have more frequent reinfections than black girls. The incidence of UTI in females of high school and college age is approximately 2%.

TREATMENT

The objectives of treatment of children with UTIs are fourfold: (1) to eliminate the infection, (2) to detect and correct functional or anatomic abnormalities, (3) to prevent recurrences, and (4) to preserve renal function. The achievement of these goals will require successful identification of the causative microorganism, selection of optimum antimicrobial drugs and patient compliance in their use, roentgenographic evaluation of the urinary tract, screening for recurrent infections with periodic urine cultures, and use of general hygienic measures to prevent reinfections. Surgery may be required to correct se-vere reflux in children with UTIs and especially to correct obstructive lesions.

Antimicrobial therapy

Newborn infants with UTIs and children suspected of having pyelonephritis should be treated empirically at the time of diagnosis because of the frequency of associated bacteremia. Empiric therapy for newborn infants should include ampicillin (100 to 200 mg/kg/day) and gentamicin (5 mg/kg/day for infants less than 1 week of age and 7.5 mg/kg/day for infants more than 1 week of age, or another aminoglycoside). Table 32-1 provides recommendations for initial therapy of newborn infants without sepsis or meningitis when a specific organism can be predicted or when an organism has been isolated and susceptibilities are not yet available.

Older children with suspected pyelonephritis should be treated empirically with gentamicin (5 to 7.5 mg per kilogram of body weight per day) possibly with the addition of ampicillin. Table 32-2 contains recommendations for initial therapy of older children when a specific organism can be predicted or when an organism has been isolated and susceptibilities are not yet available. Children with mild symptoms and those with lower UTIs may not require antimicrobial therapy until the results of urine culture are available. If therapy is indicated before the results of culture become available, oral sulfisoxazole or triple sulfonamides are sug-

Table 32-1. Initial therapy for predicted cause of acute urinary tract infections in newborn infants while awaiting susceptibility results

Gram stain	Etiology	Initial therapy
Gram-negative rods	Coliforms (*Escherichia coli, Klebsiella pneumoniae, Enterobacter aerogenes*)	Gentamicin 3 mg/kg/day or amikacin 10 mg/kg/day
	Proteus mirabilis	Ampicillin 50 to 75 mg/kg/day
	Pseudomonas aeruginosa	Mezlocillin 75 to 100 mg/kg/day
Gram-positive cocci in chains	*Streptococcus fecalis*	Ampicillin 30 mg/kg/day IM or 50 mg/kg/day PO; add an aminoglycoside if synergy is needed
Gram-positive cocci in clusters	*Staphylococcus aureus*	Methicillin or oxacillin 50 to 75 mg/kg/day
	Staphylococcus aureus, methicillin resistant (MRSA)	Vancomycin 30 mg/kg/day
	Staphylococcus epidermidis	As for *S. aureus*

gested because *E. coli* and other gram-negative bacilli are the most common pathogens. Ampicillin or amoxicillin (30 mg per kilogram of body weight per day in three doses) may be used as an alternative to sulfonamides. When the results of urine culture and antibiotic sensitivities are known, the antimicrobial therapy can be changed if necessary. If a repeat urine culture 48 hours after initiation of therapy is negative, the treatment should be continued, regardless of the results of in vitro sensitivity studies. If the repeat culture is still positive and the colony count has not decreased, the results of the sensitivity tests should be used as a basis for changing the antimicrobial therapy.

For children in whom clinical and laboratory parameters indicate lower tract infection, the use of single-dose or short-term regimens should be restricted to those beyond the newborn period with their first UTI. Reexamination of the patient and reculture of the urine after short-term therapy is mandatory. Amoxicillin, cefadroxil, nitrofurantoin, and trimethoprim-sulfamethoxazole have all been used as short-term regimens.

McCracken and Eichenwald (1978) recommend that treatment be continued for 10 to 14 days. A "cure" is determined by the demonstration of several negative cultures after cessation of therapy. Therapeutic failures after short

Table 32-2. Initial therapy for predicted cause of urinary tract infection in older children while awaiting susceptibility results

Clinical condition	Etiology	Initial therapy*
Acute nonobstructive		
Gram-negative rods	Coliforms	Trisulfapyrimidines 120 to 150 mg/kg/day or sulfisoxazole 120 to 150 mg/kg/day or amoxicillin 30 mg/kg/day
	Pseudomonas	Carbenicillin 30 to 50 mg/kg/day PO or parenteral carbenicillin or mezlocillin 100 mg/kg/day
Gram-positive cocci in chains	*Streptococcus fecalis*	Ampicillin 50 to 100 mg/kg/day; add aminoglycoside if necessary for synergy
Gram-positive cocci in clusters	*Staphylococcus aureus, Staphylococcus epidermidis*	Nafcillin 100 mg/kg/day or vancomycin 40 mg/kg/day
	Staphylococcus aureus, methicillin resistant (MRSA)	Vancomycin 40 mg/kg/day
Acute nonobstructive with suspected sepsis	Coliforms	Kanamycin 15 mg/kg/day or gentamicin 6 to 7.5 mg/day
Acute obstructive	Coliforms	Trimethoprim (TMP) 6 mg with sulfamethoxazole (SMX) 30 mg/kg/day or nitrofurantoin 5 to 7 mg/kg/day × 3 weeks or gentamicin 3 mg/kg/day
Chronic, recurrent, or hospital acquired (acute therapy)	Coliforms	Amikacin 15 to 22 mg/kg/day or carbenicillin indanyl 10 to 30 mg/kg/day or TMP 30 mg with SMX, 6 mg/kg/day
Chronic, recurrent, or hospital acquired with sepsis	Coliforms	Amikacin 15 to 22 mg/kg/day or cefuroxime 75 to 150 mg/kg/day or moxalactam 150 to 200 mg/kg/day or mezlocillin 200 to 300 mg/kg/day or piperacillin 200 to 300 mg/kg/day
Prophylaxis for chronic or recurrent infection		TMP with 2 mg SMX 10 mg/kg/day or nitrofurantoin 1 to 2 mg/kg/day

*Alterations and subsequent therapy should be based on culture and sensitivity reports. The usual duration of therapy for acute infection is 10 days (Nelson, 1985).

course or conventional antibiotic treatment of susceptible organisms suggest upper tract disease. Consideration should be given to a 6-week regimen in patients who do not respond to conventional therapy. Follow-up should continue for at least 2 years with monthly urine culture for the first 3 months followed by three cultures 3 months apart and two semiannual cultures. If reinfection occurs, the susceptibility of the organism should be determined, and the appropriate therapy should be instituted. Reinfection is differentiated from recurrence by typing the causative agent.

After initial infection in infants under 2 years of age, in boys of any age, and, possibly, girls beyond 2 years, an intravenous pyelogram and voiding cystourethrogram should be performed. Information developed by these radiographic studies affects management. Children with no reflux or grade 1 reflux require only follow-up examination. Children with grade II or III reflux are candidates for suppressive therapy. Children with grade IV reflux are also candidates for suppressive therapy, and urologic consultation should be obtained.

If radiographic studies are not performed in older girls following primary infection, they are indicated if there is a recurrence. Radiographic studies are usually performed 6 weeks or longer after acute infection to avoid detection of grade I or II reflux caused by irritation of the vesicoureteral junction. Children with clinical signs of upper tract disease who fail to respond promptly to antibiotic therapy probably warrant intravenous pyelography during their acute infection to investigate the role of obstruction. If grade III or IV reflux is detected it is likely to be persistent and not the result of acute infection.

PROPHYLAXIS

Patients with frequent recurrences and those with chronic infections may require suppressive therapy for many years. As indicated in Table 32-2, the use of nitrofurantoin or trimethoprim-sulfamethoxazole should be considered.

Several regimens are available when breakthrough infections occur. The finding that low-dose ampicillin interferes with adherence of *E. coli* may have dramatic impact on the prophylaxis of UTIs in the future (Redjeb et al., 1982),

but further studies must be carried out before this form of prophylaxis can be recommended.

Various nonspecific general measures may be helpful in preventing recurrences of UTIs. These include adequate fluid intake; frequent voiding, especially before bedtime; proper perineal hygiene, particularly after defecation; and avoidance of chronic constipation, which could produce rectal distention that might distort the bladder. Persons with functional abnormalities of the bladder benefit from intermittent catheterization programs.

REFERENCES

Aronson M, Medalia O, Schori L, et al. Prevention of colonization of the urinary tract of mice with *Escherichia coli* by blocking of bacterial adherence with methyl-a-D-mannopyanoside. J Infect Dis 1979;139:329-332.

Asscher AW, et al. Urine as a medium for bacterial growth. Lancet 1966;2:1037.

Bailey RR. Significance of coagulase-negative *Staphylococcus* in urine. J Infect Dis 1973;127:179.

Bran JL, Levison ME, Kaye D. Entrance of bacteria into the female urinary bladder. N Engl J Med 1972;286:626.

Britt MR, Garibaldi RA, Miller WA, et al. Antimicrobial prophylaxis for catheter-associated bacteriuria. Antimicrob Agents Chemother 1977;11:240-243.

Brumfitt W. Urinary cell counts and their value. J Clin Pathol 1965;18:550.

Buckley RM, McGuckin M, MacGregor RR. Urine bacterial counts following sexual intercourse. N Engl J Med 1978;298:321.

Butler HK, Kunin CM. Evaluation of specific systemic antimicrobial therapy in patients while on closed catheter drainage. J Urol 1968;100:567-572.

Cobbs CG, Kaye D. Antibacterial mechanisms in the urinary bladder. Yale J Biol Med 1967;40:93.

Fang LST, Tolkoff-Rubin NE, Rubin R. Efficacy of single-dose and conventional amoxicillin therapy in urinary tract infection localized by the antibody-coated bacteria technique. N Engl J Med 1978;298:413-416.

Fasth A, Ahlstedt S, Hanson LA, et al. Cross-reaction between Tamm-Horsfall glycoprotein and *Escherichia coli*. Int Arch Allergy Appl Immunol 1980;63:303-311.

Gorrill RH, De Navasquez SJ. Experimental pyelonephritis in the mouse produced by *Escherichia coli, Pseudomonas aeruginosa* and *Proteus mirabilis*. J Pathol Bacteriol 1964;87:79.

Gruneberg RN, Leigh DA, Brumfitt W. *Escherichia coli* serotypes in urinary tract infection: studies in domiciliary, antenatal and hospital practice. In O'Grady F, Brumfitt W, ed. Urinary tract infection. Oxford: Oxford University Press, 1968;68-70.

Hanna B, Larrier L, Fam C, et al. Bacteriuria screening by bioluminescence. Interscience Conference on Antimicrobial Agents and Chemotherapy, Abstract 737, Las Vegas, Nevada, October 1983.

Hanson LA, Fasth A, Jodal U, et al. Biology and pathology of urinary tract infection. J Clin Pathol 1981;34:695-700.

Hanson LA, et al. Antigens of *Escherichia coli*, human immune response, and the pathogenesis of urinary tract infections. J Infect Dis 1977;136:S144.

Hellerstein S, Kennedy E, Nussbaum L, et al. Localization of the site of urinary tract infections by means of antibody-coated bacteria in the urinary sediments. J Pediatr 1978;92:188-193.

Iwahi T, Abe Y, Nakao M, et al. Role of type I fimbriae in the pathogenesis of ascending urinary tract infection induced by *Escherichia coli* in mice. Infect Immun 1983; 39:1307-1315.

Jones SR, Smith JW, Sanford JP. Localization of urinary tract infections by detection of antibody-coated bacteria in urine sediment. N Engl J Med 1974;290:591.

Kaijser B. Immunology of *Escherichia coli:* K. antigen and its relation to urinary-tract infection. J Infect Dis 1973; 127:670.

Kaijser B, Larsson P, Olling S, et al. Protection against acute ascending pyelonephritis caused by *Escherichia coli* in rats, using isolated capsular antigen conjugated to bovine serum albumin. Infect Immun 1983;39:142-146.

Kaijser B, Olling S. Experimental hematogenous pyelonephritis due to *Escherichia coli* in rabbits: the antibody response and its protective capacity. J Infect Dis 1973; 128:41.

Kallenius G, Mollby R, Svensson SB, et al. Occurrence of P-fimbriated *Escherichia coli* in urinary tract infection. Lancet 1981;2:1369-1372.

Kaye D. Antibacterial activity of human urine. J Clin Invest 1968;47:2374.

Khan AJ, Evans HE, Bombeck E, et al. Coagulase negative-staphylococcal bacteriuria—a rarity in infants and children. J Pediatr 1975;86:309-313.

Kinane DF, Blackwell CC, Brettle RP, et al. ABO blood group, secretor state and susceptibility to recurrent urinary tract infection in women. Br Med J 1982;285:7–9.

Kunin CM. The natural history of recurrent bacteriuria in school girls. N Engl J Med 1970;282:1443.

Kunin CM. Urinary tract infections in children. Hosp Pract 1976;113:91.

Kunin CM, Polyak R, Postel E. Periurethral bacterial flora in women. Prolonged intermittent colonization with *Escherichia coli*. JAMA 1980;243:134-139.

Kunin CM, Zacha E, Paquin AJ. Urinary tract infections in school children. I. Prevalence of bacteriuria and associated urologic findings. N Engl J Med 1962;206:1287.

Leffler H, Svanborg-Eden C. Glycolipid receptors for uropathogenic *Escherichia coli* on human erythrocytes and uroepithelial cells. Infect Immun 1981;34:920-929.

Lomberg H, Hanson LA, Jacobsson B, et al. Correlation of P blood group, vesicoureteral reflux, and bacterial attachment in patients with recurrent pyelonephritis. N Engl J Med 1983;308:1189-1192.

Lorentz WB, Resnick MI. Comparison of urinary lactic dehydrogenase with antibody-coated bacteria in the urine sediment as a means of localizing the site of urinary tract infection, Pediatrics 1979;64:672.

Mattsby-Baltzer I, Claesson I, Hanson LA, et al. Antibodies to lipid A during urinary tract infection. J Infect Dis 1981;144:319-328.

Mattsby-Baltzer I, Hanson LA, Kaijser B, et al. Experimental *Escherichia coli* ascending pyelonephritis in rats: changes in bacterial properties and the immune response to surface antigens. Infect Immun 1982;35:639-646.

Maybeck CE. Significance of coagulase negative staphylococcal bacteriuria. Lancet 1969;2:1150-1152.

Mayrer AR, Miniter P, Andriole VT. Immunopathogenesis of chronic pyelonephritis. Am J Med 1983;75:59-70.

McCracken GH, Jr. Management of urinary tract infections in children. Pediatr Infect Dis 1982;1(suppl):52-56.

McCracken G, Eichenwald H. Antimicrobial therapy: therapeutic recommendations and a review of new drugs. J Pediatr 1978;93:366.

McCracken GH, Jr, Ginsburg CM, Namasanthi V, et al. Evaluation of short-term antibiotic therapy in children with uncomplicated urinary tract infections. Pediatrics 1981;67:796-801.

Miller TE, North JD. Host response in urinary tract infections. Kidney Int 1974;5:179.

Monson TP, Macalalad FV, Hamman JW, et al. Evaluation of a vented drainage system in prevention of bacteriuria. J Urol 1977;177:216-219.

Mufson MA, Belshe RB. A review of adenoviruses in the etiology of acute hemorrhagic cystitis. J Urol 1976; 115:191.

Murphy JJ et al. The role of the lymphatic system in pyelonephritis. Surg Forum 1960;10:880.

Musher DM, et al. Role of urease in pyelonephritis resulting from urinary tract infection with *Proteus*. J Infect Dis 1975;131:177.

Nelson JD. Pocketbook of pediatric antimicrobial therapy. 6th ed. Dallas: Jodone Publishing Co, 1985.

Nicolle L, Harding GKM, Preiksaitis J, et al. The association of urinary tract infection with sexual intercourse. J Infect Dis 1982;278:635-642.

Norden CW, Green GM, Kass EH. Antibacterial mechanisms of the urinary bladder. J Clin Invest 1968;47:2689-2700.

Ofek I, Mirelman D, Sharon N. Adherence of *Escherichia coli* to human mucosal cells mediated by mannose receptors. Nature 1977;265:623-625.

Ofek I, Mosek A, Sharon N. Mannose-specific adherence of *Escherichia coli* freshly extracted in the urine of patients with urinary tract infections and of isolates subcultured from the infected urine. Infect Immun 1981;34:708-711.

O'Hanley PD, Lark D, Falkow S, et al. A globaside binding *Escherichia coli* pilus vaccine prevents pyelonephritis (Abstract). Clin Res 1983;31:372A.

Orskov I, Ferencz A, Orskov F. Tamm-Horsfall protein or uromucoid is the normal urinary slime that traps type I fimbriated *Escherichia coli*. Lancet 1980;1:887.

Parsons CL, Anwar H, Stauffer C, et al. *In vitro* adherence of radioactively labelled *Escherichia coli* in normal and cystitis prone women. Infect Immun 1979;26:453-457.

Parsons CL, Greenspan C, Mulholland SG. The primary antibacterial defense mechanism of the bladder. Invest Urol 1975;13:72-76.

Parsons CL, Schrom SH, Hanno P, et al. Bladder surface mucin: examination of possible mechanisms for its antibacterial effect. Invest Urol 1978;6:196-200.

Perry A, Ofek I, Silverblatt FJ. Enhancement of mannose-mediated stimulation of human granulocytes by type I fimbriae aggregated with antibodies on *Escherichia coli* surfaces. Infect Immun 1983;39:1334-1335.

Pfau A, Sacks T, Engtestein D. Recurrent urinary tract infections in premenopausal women: prophylaxis based on an understanding of the pathogenesis. J Urol 1983; 129:1152-1157.

Redjeb SB, Slim A, Horchani A, et al. Effects of ten milligrams of ampicillin per day on urinary tract infections. Antimicrob Agents Chemother 1982;22:1084-1086.

Rene P, Silverblatt FJ. Serological response to *Escherichia coli* pili in pyelonephritis. Infect Immun 1982;37:749-754.

Rocha H, Fekety FR. Acute inflammation in the renal cortex and medulla following thermal injury. J Exp Med 1964;119:131-138.

Ronald AR, Boutros P, Mourtada H. Bacteriuria localization and response to single-dose therapy in women. JAMA 1976;235:1854-1856.

Rubin M. Effect of catheter replacement on bacterial counts in urine aspirated from indwelling catheters. J Infect Dis 1980;142:291.

Silverblatt FS. Host-parasite interaction in the rat renal pelvis: a possible role of pili in the pathogenesis of pyelonephritis, J Exp Med 1974;140:1696-1711.

Smellie JM, Normand ICS. Bacteriuria, reflux and renal scarring. Arch Dis Child 1975;50:581.

Sobel JD, Vardi Y. Scanning electron microscopy study of *Pseudomonas aeruginosa in vivo* adherence to rat bladder epithelium. J Urol 1982;128:414-417.

Stamey TA. The role of introital enterobacteria in recurrent urinary infections. J Urol 1973;109:467-472.

Stamey TA, Govan DE, Palmer JM. The localization and treatment of urinary tract infections: the role of bactericidal urine levels as opposed to serum levels. Medicine 1965;44:1.

Stamey TA, Kaufman MF. Studies of introital colonization in women with recurrent urinary infections. II. A comparison of growth in normal vaginal fluid of common versus uncommon serogroups of *E. coli*. J Urol 1975;114:264.

Stamey TA, Mihara G. Studies of introital colonization in women with recurrent urinary infections. V. The inhibitory activity of normal vaginal fluid on *Proteus mirabilis* and *Pseudomonas aeruginosa*. J Urol 1976;115:416.

Stamey TA, Timothy MM. Studies of introital colonization in women with recurrent urinary infections. I. The role of vaginal pH. J Urol 1975;114:261.

Stamey TA, Wehner N, Mihara G, et al. The immunologic basis of recurrent bacteriuria: role of cervicovaginal antibody in enterobacterial colonization of the introital mucosa. Medicine 1978;57:47-56.

Stamey TA, et al. Antibacterial nature of prostatic fluid. Nature 1968;218:444.

Svanborg-Eden C, Gotschlich EC, Korhonan TK, et al. Aspects of structure and function of pili of uropathogenic *E. coli*. Prog Allergy 1983;33:189-202.

Svanborg-Eden C, Hagberg L, Hanson LA, et al. Adhesion of *Escherichia coli* in urinary tract infection. CIBA Found Symp 1981;80:161-187.

Svanborg-Eden C, Hanson LA, Jodol U, et al. Variable adherence to normal human urinary tract epithelial cells of *Escherichia coli* strains associated with various forms of urinary tract infection. Lancet 1976;2:490-492.

Svanborg-Eden C, Svennerholm AM. Secretory immunoglobulin A and G antibodies prevent adhesion of *Escherichia coli* to human urinary tract epithelial cells. Infect Immun 1978;22:790-797.

Thomas V, Shelokov A, Forland M. Antibody-coated bacteria in the urine and the site of urinary tract infection. N Engl J Med 1974;290:588.

Uehling DT, Stiehm ER. Elevated urinary secretory IgA in children with urinary tract infection. Pediatrics 1971; 47:40-46.

Vivaldi E, Munoz J, Cotran R, et al. Factors affecting the clearance of bacteria within the urinary tract. In Kass EH, ed. Progress in pyelonephritis. Philadelphia: FA Davis, 1965;531-535.

Vosti CL. Recurrent urinary tract infections. Prevention by prophylactic antibiotics after sexual intercourse. JAMA 1975;231:934.

Warren JW, Anthony WC, Hoopes JM, et al. Cephalexin for susceptible bacteriuria in afebrile, long-term catheterized patients. JAMA 1982;248:454-458.

Warren JW, Hoopes JM, Muncie HL, et al. Ineffectiveness of cephalexin in treatment of cephalexin-resistant bacteriuria in patients with chronic indwelling urethral catheters. J Urol 1983;129:71-73.

Weyrauch HM, Bassett JB. Ascending infection in an artificial urinary tract. An experimental study. Stanford Med Bull 1951;9:25.

Work J, Andriole VT. Tamm-Horsfall protein antibody in patients with end-stage kidney disease. Yale J Biol Med 1980;53:133-148.

33

VARICELLA-ZOSTER INFECTIONS

Varicella (chickenpox)
Zoster (shingles)

Varicella is a common, contagious disease of childhood that is caused by primary infection with varicella-zoster (V-Z) virus. It is characterized clinically by a short or absent prodromal period and by a pruritic rash consisting of crops of papules, vesicles, and scabs, with eventual crusting of nearly all the lesions. In normal children the systemic symptoms are usually mild, and serious complications are unusual. In adults and in children with deficiencies in cell-mediated immunity the disease is more likely to be characterized by an extensive eruption, severe constitutional symptoms, and, occasionally, complicating varicella pneumonia with a potentially fatal outcome.

Zoster, which is caused by reactivation of latent V-Z virus, is characterized by localized crops of varicella-like lesions along the course of the sensory nerve distribution of dorsal root ganglia or extramedullary ganglia of cranial nerves. It is most common in immunocompromised individuals and more common and more painful in adults than in children.

ETIOLOGY

Varicella-zoster virus, a member of the herpesvirus group, consists of a core, containing protein and DNA, surrounded by protein layers, termed the *capsid*. The capsid has an icosahedral shape. These structures are surrounded by two additional membranes, the tegument and the envelope. The V-Z particles range in size between 150 and 200 nm (Fig. 33-1). The agent

does not cause clinical disease in common laboratory animals, although simian forms of varicella have been described. Weller first propagated the virus in tissue cultures of human embryonic cells, using infectious vesicular fluid as source material. He demonstrated the presence of eosinophilic inclusion bodies and multinucleated cells typical of varicella and successfully passed the agent in series, using the cellular components of the tissue culture. With the use of tissue culture fluid as antigen, a rise in complement-fixing antibody was demonstrated in convalescent-phase serum.

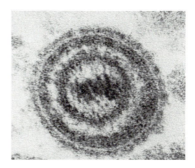

Fig. 33-1. Electron micrograph of varicella-zoster (V-Z) virus. This specimen was obtained from vesicular fluid of a child 1 day after the onset of varicella. The structural elements of the virion are the central DNA core, the protein capsid, the tegument, and the envelope. The last structure is required for infectivity of the virion. ($\times 175,000$.) (Courtesy Michael D. Gershon, M.D.)

433

The following impressive body of evidence indicates that the viruses that cause varicella and zoster are identical:

1. Electron microscopic study of vesicular fluids reveals the presence of morphologically identical particles in both varicella and zoster.
2. The cytopathic effect of varicella virus in tissue cultures is neutralized not only by varicella immune serum but also by zoster immune serum. Both of these sera also neutralize herpes zoster virus. The two viruses are indistinguishable by immunofluorescence assays.
3. Biopsies of lesions produced by both viruses reveal the same type of eosinophilic inclusion body.
4. Smears of varicella and zoster lesions show the same type of multinucleated giant cells.
5. Varicella has been transmitted to susceptible children by inoculating them with zoster vesicular fluid. The experimental disease was contagious and it did produce chickenpox in other susceptible children.
6. They have the same DNA structure.

PATHOLOGY

The following sequence of events is believed to occur when a varicella-susceptible person is infected. The virus gains entry at the conjunctivae and/or mucosa of the upper respiratory tract. The virus then multiplies in regional lymph nodes, and a primary viremia occurs about 4 to 6 days after infection. The virus then reaches and replicates in the liver, spleen, and possibly, other organs as well, resulting in a secondary viremia, at which time virus is delivered to the skin; rash results on the average 14 days after infection (Grose, 1982). Viremia has been demonstrated during the first few days of varicella. It is more difficult to document in normal than in immunocompromised persons (Feldman and Epp, 1976; Myers, 1979; Ozaki et al., 1984). Viremia has also been reported in some patients with zoster (Gershon et al., 1978; Pichini et al., 1983).

The initial skin lesion of varicella begins as a macule, which in the majority of instances progresses to be a papule, vesicle, and scab in rapid sequence. Rarely, lesions regress after the macular and papular stages. The vesicle is located chiefly in the prickle cell layer of the skin, the roof being formed by the stratum corneum and lucidum and the floor by the deeper prickle cell layer. The vesicular fluid has been attributed to fluid filling intercellular spaces produced by degeneration of cells in the prickle cell layer of the epidermis. Ballooning degeneration of the cells is followed by the formation of multinucleated giant cells, many of which contain the typical type A intranuclear inclusion bodies.

As the lesion progresses, polymorphonuclear leukocytes invade the corium and the vesicular fluid, which changes from a clear to a cloudy appearance. The absorption of the fluid is followed by the formation of a scab, which is at first adherent but later becomes detached. Mucous membrane lesions develop in the same way but do not progress to scab formation. The vesicles usually rupture and form shallow ulcers, which heal rapidly.

Ordinarily the target organ for the virus is the skin, although children with benign cases of varicella and transiently elevated AST levels (greater than 50 IU/liter) have been described (Pitel et al., 1980). However, postmortem examination of infants and adults who died of varicella reveals evidence of involvement of many organs. Areas of focal necrosis and acidophilic inclusion bodies may be present in the esophagus, liver, pancreas, kidney, ureter, bladder, uterus, and adrenal glands. The lungs show evidence of widely disseminated interstitial pneumonia with numerous hemorrhagic areas of nodular consolidation. Histologically, the exudate consists chiefly of red cells, fibrin, and many mononuclear cells, some containing intranuclear inclusion bodies (Fig. 33-2). Encephalitis complicating varicella is pathologically similar to measles and other types of postinfection encephalitis showing perivascular demyelination in the white matter.

The pathology of skin lesions associated with zoster and varicella is the same. Zoster, however, also causes an inflammatory lesion in the posterior nerve roots and ganglia. Spread of the inflammation to the anterior horn cells may cause temporary or permanent paralysis. The lesion in the posterior root is characterized by infiltration of small round cells and red blood cells, necrosis of nerve cells and fibers, and an inflammatory reaction of the ganglion sheath.

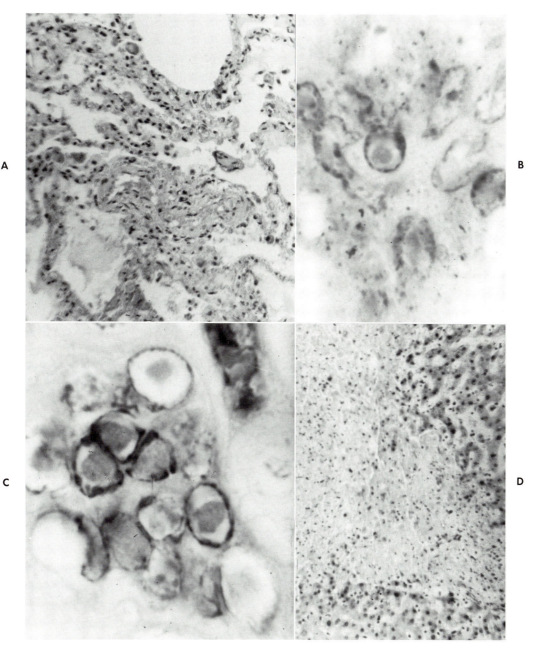

Fig. 33-2. Microscopic sections from E.W., a 44-year-old man who died of pulmonary edema after 5 days of hemorrhagic varicella associated with severe right upper quadrant abdominal pain, cough, dyspnea, tachypnea, cyanosis, and hemoptysis. **A,** Interstitial mononuclear cell infiltration and fibrinous exudate in the alveoli of the lung. **B,** Intranuclear inclusion bodies in the lung. **C,** Multinucleated cell with intranuclear inclusions in the skin. **D,** Typical focus of necrosis in the liver. (From Krugman S, Goodrich CH, Ward R. N Engl J Med 1957;257:843.)

Using in situ hybridization techniques, V-Z DNA and RNA have been demonstrated in human sensory ganglia obtained from autopsy material (Gilden et al., 1983; Hyman et al., 1983). This indicates that the site of V-Z latency is sensory ganglia, although efforts to culture infectious virus from such ganglia have been unsuccessful.

CLINICAL MANIFESTATIONS OF VARICELLA

Following an incubation period of 14 to 16 days, with outside limits of 10 to 21 days, the disease begins with low-grade fever, malaise, and the appearance of a rash. In children the exanthem and constitutional symptoms usually occur simultaneously. In adolescents and adults the rash may be preceded by a 1- to 2-day prodromal period of fever, headache, malaise, and anorexia. The typical clinical course of varicella is illustrated in Fig. 33-3.

Rash

The most striking manifestation of the lesion of chickenpox is the rapidity of its progression from macule to papule to vesicle to beginning crusting (Fig. 33-3). This transition may take place within 6 to 8 hours. The typical vesicle of chickenpox is superficially located in the skin. It has thin, fragile walls that rupture easily. In appearance it resembles a dewdrop, usually elliptical in shape, 2 to 3 mm in diameter, and surrounded by an erythematous area. This red areola is most distinct when the vesicle is fully formed, and it fades as the lesion begins to dry. The drying process, which begins in the center of the vesicle, produces an umbilicated appearance first and then a crust. After a variable interval of 5 to 20 days, depending on the depth of skin involvement, the scab falls off, leaving a shallow pink depression. The site of the lesion eventually becomes white, with no evidence of scar formation. Secondarily infected lesions and prematurely removed scabs may be followed by scarring.

The lesions appear in crops that generally involve the trunk, scalp, face, and extremities. The distribution is typically central, with the greatest concentration of lesions on the trunk (Fig. 33-4). The rash is more profuse on the proximal parts of the extremities (upper arms and thighs) than on the distal parts (forearms and legs). A distinctive manifestation of the eruption is the presence of lesions in all stages in any one general anatomic area; macules, papules, vesicles, and crusts are usually located in proximity (Fig. 33-5).

In the typical case of chickenpox, three successive crops of lesions appear over a 3-day period in the characteristic central distribution just

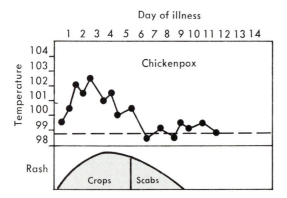

Fig. 33-3. Schematic diagram illustrating clinical course of typical case of chickenpox. Crops of lesions appear with rapid progression from macules to papules to vesicles to scabs.

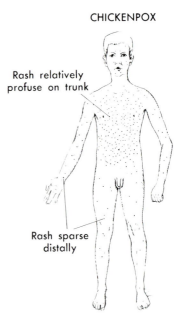

Fig. 33-4. Schematic drawing illustrating typical distribution of rash of chickenpox.

described. The extremes of this picture may range from (1) a single crop of a few scattered lesions to (2) a series of five or more crops developing over a week with an uncountable number of lesions covering the entire skin surface of the body. In a study of almost 1000 cases of chickenpox in normal children, the average number of vesicles was 250 to 500 (Ross et al., 1962).

Vesicles develop on the mucous membranes of the mouth as well as on the skin. They occur most commonly over the palate and usually rupture so rapidly that the vesicular stage may be missed. In appearance, they resemble the shallow white 2- to 3-mm ulcers of herpetic stomatitis. The palpebral conjunctiva, pharynx, larynx, trachea, and rectal and vaginal mucosa may also be involved.

In areas of local inflammation, such as ammoniacal dermatitis in the diaper area or sunburned skin, there may be a significant increase in the number of lesions. These vesicles are generally smaller than usual, tend to be in the same stage of development, and may become confluent.

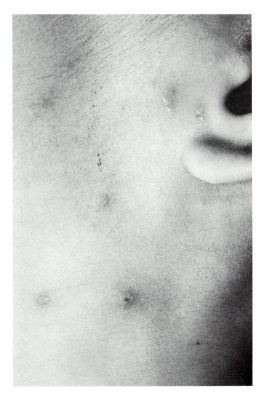

Fig. 33-5. Chickenpox lesions in various stages.

In summary, the rash of chickenpox is characterized by (1) a rapid evolution of macule to papule to vesicle to crust, (2) a central distribution of lesions that appear in crops, (3) the presence of lesions in all stages in any one anatomic area, and (4) an eventual crusting of nearly all the lesions.

Fever

The temperature curve of a typical case of chickenpox is illustrated in Fig. 33-3. The height of the fever usually parallels the severity of the rash. When the eruption is sparse, the temperature is usually normal or slightly elevated; an extensive rash is more likely to be associated with high and more prolonged fevers. Temperatures up to 40.6° C (105° F) are not unusual in severe cases of chickenpox with involvement of almost the entire skin surface.

Other symptoms

Headache, malaise, and anorexia usually accompany the fever. In many cases the most distressing symptom is pruritus, which is present during the vesicular stage of the disease.

Unusual types of chickenpox

Various unusual types of varicella are observed occasionally.

Hemorrhagic, progressive, and disseminated varicella. Varicella in an immunocompromised host may be characterized by a hemorrhagic, progressive, and/or disseminated infection and a potentially fatal outcome. Feldman et al. (1975) observed 77 children with cancer who contracted varicella. Of this group, 17 were off therapy and 60 were receiving anticancer therapy at the time of varicella infection. No complications were observed among the 19 children who were not treated with corticosteroids or chemotherapeutic agents at the time of infection. In contrast, of the 60 treated children, 19 (32%) had evidence of visceral dissemination and four (7%) died. Deaths were associated with varicella pneumonia (all four patients) and encephalitis (two of the four patients). Disseminated varicella occurred more frequently in children with absolute lymphopenia, less than 500 lymphocytes/mm^3.

The characteristic course of progressive varicella was observed in four children at Bellevue Hospital after onset of the disease. All four children were treated for malignancies with chemotherapeutic agents and/or radiotherapy. In each child the varicella infection appeared to be mild initially, but new crops of vesicles continued to appear for up to 2 weeks after onset of rash. Two of these children developed hemorrhagic lesions and varicella pneumonia before death. The two survivors continued to get new lesions for a prolonged period of time.

Severe, progressive, fatal varicella infection has also been observed in children treated with high doses of corticosteroids for conditions other than cancer. Gershon et al. (1972) described the development of fulminating varicella in two boys treated with corticosteroids for rheumatic fever; deaths occurred 2 and 4 days after onset of rash. Feldman et al. (1977) and Feldman and Epp (1979) have detected V-Z viremia in immunocompromised patients. They observed a direct correlation between the duration of viremia and the severity of the disease.

Congenital varicella syndrome. Congenital varicella syndrome is extremely rare. Since the 1940s, when it was first recognized, 20 cases have been recorded in the world literature (Hanshaw and Dudgeon, 1978; Weller, 1983; Young and Gershon, 1983). The incidence of this syndrome following gestational varicella is unknown. In one prospective study of 135 pregnant women with varicella, no infants were born with the syndrome (Siegal, 1973). The incidence of congenital malformations in this cohort, 3%, was no different than that for the control group of 146 infants whose mothers had no known viral infection during pregnancy. The congenital varicella syndrome has occurred when maternal varicella has developed as late as 28 weeks of gestation; it has followed maternal zoster as well as chickenpox. Fortunately it is rare because there is no known way to diagnose it in utero or to prevent it. The major reported malformations are listed in Table 33-1, and an infant with the syndrome is shown in Fig. 33-6. The pathogenesis is not understood, but the rarity of the illness and the pattern of cicatricial skin lesions suggest that the fetus may have experienced both varicella and zoster.

Severe or fatal varicella in 5- to 10-day-old infants may occur when their mothers have varicella 5 days or less before delivery. It is believed that in infants who contract the illness between 5 to 10 days of age (an incubation period of about

Table 33-1. Clinical and laboratory data of 20 infants with the congenital varicella syndrome*

Number following maternal varicella	15
Number following maternal zoster	5
Time (weeks) of maternal infection	
Mean	13
Range	8 to 28
Major malformations described	
Ocular abnormalities (chorioretinitis/ microphthalmia/cataract)	14
Cortical atrophy or other CNS involvement	11
Cicatricial skin lesions	11
Hypotrophic limb	10
Low birth weight	10
Laboratory data	
Immunologic confirmation of varicella in mother	6
Immunologic confirmation of varicella in infant	8
Number of infants from whom virus was isolated	0

*Modified from Young NA, Gershon AA. Chickenpox, measles and mumps. In Remington JS, Klein JO, eds. Infections of the fetus and newborn infant. 2nd ed. Philadelphia: W.B. Saunders Co., 1983, pp 375-427; and Hanshaw JB, Dudgeon JA. Viral diseases of the fetus and newborn. In Major Problems of Pediatrics. Philadelphia: W.B. Saunders Co., 1978;17:192-208.

10 days), the cellular immune response to V-Z virus has not yet matured. Therefore the infection may become disseminated, as in a leukemic child with varicella. Maternally transmitted antibody may act as a form of passive immunization for the infant, but when the mother has had varicella for less than 5 days she has not yet made or transferred this antibody to her baby. The attack rate of varicella in newborn infants under these conditions is about 20%. However, in infants who contract the disease, the mortality is about 35% (Meyers, 1974).

The disseminated varicella infection is characterized by hemorrhagic lesions and involvement of the lungs and the liver. The effect on the fetus when maternal varicella occurred near term is shown in Table 33-2.

Bullous varicella. Bullous varicella is an unusual type of varicella characterized by the si-

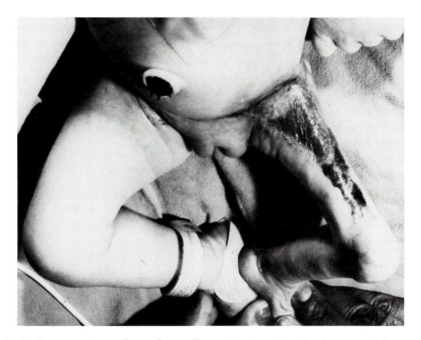

Fig. 33-6. Congenital varicella syndrome illustrating cicatricial skin lesions and hypotrophic left lower limb. (From Srabstein JC, et al. J Pediatr 1974;84:239.)

Table 33-2. Maternal varicella near term: effect on the fetus (50 cases)*

Onset	Effect
Maternal varicella, 5 or more days before delivery; baby's varicella, age 0-4 days	27 of 27 survived
Maternal varicella, 4 days or less before delivery, baby's varicella, age 5-10 days	16 of 23 survived (7 died of disseminated varicella, 2 had severe disease with survival)

*From Gershon, AA. Prog Clin Biol Res 1975a;3:79.

multaneous occurrence of typical varicelliform lesions and bullae. The reports by Melish (1973) and by Wald et al. (1973) indicated that the bullous lesions were caused by phage group II staphylococci. These staphylococci produce epidermolytic toxin, the cause of staphylococcal scalded skin syndrome. Thus it appears that in bullous varicella the lesions may be superinfected by an exfoliative toxigenic *Staphylococcus aureus*. Varicella-zoster virus has not been cultivated from the bullous fluid.

Varicella in the adult. Varicella, like many other virus infections, is likely to be more severe in adults than in children. In general, the fever is higher and more prolonged, the constitutional symptoms are more severe, the rash is more profuse, and complications are more frequent. Since 1956 we have observed more than 40 cases of primary varicella pneumonia in adults and only a few cases in children (see discussion of complications). This diagnosis was confirmed pathologically in four cases that came to necropsy. Postmortem studies of three adults who died of severe varicella showed evidence not only of extensive pneumonitis but also of hepatitis. Typical intranuclear inclusion bodies were demonstrated in the lung and liver lesions.

Although varicella pneumonia is less common than our experience with hospitalized patients might indicate, it is certainly a significant complication of varicella. Weber and Pellecchia (1965) have reported a prospective evaluation of 114 military personnel with varicella that revealed roentgenographic evidence of pulmonary involvement in 16%, but clinical signs were present in only 4%.

Second attacks of varicella. It was generally accepted at one time that varicella occurs only once in a lifetime. Second attacks of clinical illness are difficult to confirm by laboratory means because most first attacks are diagnosed only clinically. However, there is a growing body of evidence suggesting that second attacks of varicella may occur (Weller, 1983). Varicella has been observed in persons known to have specific antibodies before onset of illness (Zaia et al., 1983; Gershon et al., 1984a). Serologic evidence of subclinical infection of varicella-immune individuals closely exposed to V-Z virus has also been reported (Gershon et al., 1982; Arvin et al., 1983). Most second attacks have been mild. It is likely that second attacks may prove to be more common in immunocompromised persons.

CLINICAL MANIFESTATIONS OF ZOSTER

The incubation period of zoster is unknown because it is impossible to determine the time of activation of latent V-Z virus. The predilection of the virus for the posterior nerve root areas accounts for the severe pain and tenderness along the involved nerve roots and the corresponding areas of skin. Fever may or may not be present.

It is believed that zoster occurs when cellular immunity to varicella-zoster virus is depressed. This depression may be very transient, as when otherwise normal persons develop the illness, or it may be secondary to severe immunosuppression induced by diseases such as malignancy, anticancer chemotherapy or radiotherapy, or following immunosuppression for organ transplantation.

The classical case of zoster is characterized by a typical rash. The lesions begin as macules and papules and progress through the same stages as a varicella eruption. The regional lymph nodes may be enlarged and tender. The lesions may appear on the trunk (involvement of dorsal roots), on the shoulders, arms, and neck (involvement of second to fourth cervical ganglia), or on the perineal area and lower extremities. Cranial nerve involvement may affect the trigeminal nerve. Inflammation of the maxillary division of the nerve is associated with lesions of the uvula and tonsillar area. Mandibular division involvement is associated with lesions of the buccal mucosa, floor of the mouth, and anterior part of the tongue, and involvement of the ophthalmic division is followed by scleral and corneal lesions. Involvement of the geniculate ganglion of the facial nerve may be followed by pain, a vesicular eruption in the auditory canal, and facial paralysis, which usually subsides but may be permanent. The severe neuralgia, which may persist following convalescence, is more common in adults than in children.

Herpes zoster is chiefly a disease of the immunocompromised and of adults, but it is not unusual to observe it in infants and children. A previous clinical or subclinical episode of varicella is a prerequisite. Winklemann and Perry (1959) reported seven cases observed during a 3-year period in patients 7 months to 4 years of age. A previous attack of varicella occurred 2 months to 2 years before the zoster infection in five of the seven patients. Brunell et al. (1968) observed 15 infants and children with herpes zoster on the New York University–Bellevue Hospital Pediatric Service during the 2-year period 1964 to 1966. The youngest patient was a 3½ month-old infant whose mother had had varicella during the seventh month of pregnancy. The other children, 3 years to 14 years of age, had a history of varicella; the interval between onset of varicella and herpes zoster ranged between 1 and 9 years.

Brunell and Kotchmar (1981) have proposed that varicella acquired in utero predisposes to early postnatal development of zoster. They reported on five infants whose mothers had varicella between 3 and 7 months gestation. These infants had no evidence of varicella after birth. Presumably all had varicella in utero, since they developed zoster after an average latent period of only 21 months (range 3 to 41 months). The usual latent period between varicella and zoster is measured in decades.

Disseminated zoster

Within 1 or 2 weeks after appearance of the localized lesions the rash may become generalized, resembling varicella. Fever may be low grade or high, and it usually subsides within 1 week. Disseminated zoster is not common, but when it does occur, it usually is seen in children and adults with severe immunologic defects due to malignancy or immunosuppressive therapy. Fatalities may occur when there is extensive visceral involvement in patients with depressed cell-mediated immunity (Goffinet et al., 1972; Feldman et al., 1973).

DIAGNOSIS OF VARICELLA
Confirmatory clinical factors

The typical case of chickenpox can be recognized clinically with ease. The characteristic diagnostic features include (1) the development of a papulovesicular eruption concentrated on the face and trunk associated with fever and mild constitutional symptoms; (2) the rapid progression of macules to papules to vesicles to crusts; (3) the appearance of these lesions in crops, with a predominant central distribution including the scalp; (4) the presence of shallow white ulcers on the mucous membranes of the mouth; and (5) the eventual crusting of all the skin lesions. The knowledge of a definite exposure to the disease is always helpful when present.

Detection of causative agent

Varicella virus may be readily isolated from vesicular fluid obtained within the first 3 to 4 days of rash. Primary human amnion or human fetal fibroblast tissue cultures will support the growth of the virus. The isolation of virus is unnecessary for the routine diagnosis of chickenpox. V-Z antigen can be detected in vesicular fluid by countercurrent immunoelectrophoresis (CIE) or indirect immunofluorescence.

Serologic tests

Complement-fixing antibody has been detected in serum obtained as early as 7 days after onset of the disease. Consequently, a retrospective diagnosis is possible if acute and convalescent serum specimens are available. The first sample of blood should be collected as soon as possible after the onset of disease; the second specimen should be obtained 2 or more weeks later. Additional practical serologic tests, more sensitive than the complement-fixing assay, have been described: (1) the V-Z fluorescent antibody to membrane antigen (FAMA) test (Williams et al., 1974; Zaia and Oxman, 1977); (2) the immune adherence hemagglutination antibody (IAHA) test (Gershon et al., 1976); (3) enzyme-linked immunosorbent assay (ELISA) (Forghani et al., 1978; Gershon et al., 1981; Shehab and Brunell, 1983); and (4) radioimmunoassay (RIA) (Friedman et al., 1979; Arvin and Koropchak, 1980; and Richman et al., 1981).

Isolation of virus and serologic procedures may be indicated for the identification of atypical or unusual types of chickenpox.

Ancillary laboratory findings

The white blood cell count is not consistent. In most cases it is within the normal range. It is not unusual for adults with primary varicella pneumonia to have leukocytosis with a predominance of polymorphonuclear leukocytes.

DIAGNOSIS OF ZOSTER

Implication of V-Z virus is essential for a definitive diagnosis of zoster infection of the skin because classical zosterlike lesions have on occasion been observed in herpes simplex infections. A fourfold rise in complement-fixing (CF) FAMA, IAHA, ELISA, or RIA V-Z antibody titer 2 to 4 weeks after appearance of lesions provides additional confirmation of the diagnosis. Alternatively, the diagnosis may be made by demonstration of virus or viral antigens in vesicular fluid.

DIFFERENTIAL DIAGNOSIS OF VARICELLA

The differential diagnosis of varicella is also discussed in Chapter 34. Varicella may resemble the following conditions.

Impetigo

The lesions of impetigo are vesicular at first but rapidly progress to the pustular and crusting stage. They differ from chickenpox in appearance and distribution. They do not appear in crops, do not involve the mucous membranes of the mouth, and are not accompanied by constitutional symptoms. The lesions commonly involve the nasolabial area because of the tendency for a child to scratch this area with his contaminated fingers. Other areas that are easily scratched also become involved.

Insect bites, papular urticaria, and urticaria

Insect bites, papular urticaria, and urticaria are not accompanied by constitutional symptoms. They are papular and pruritic but do not have the typical vesicular appearance and distribution. Vesicles, if present, are pinpoint in size. The scalp and mouth are devoid of lesions.

Scabies

The differential points of scabies are the same as those for insect bites. In addition, the observation of burrows between the fingers and toes and the microscopic identification of *Sarcoptes scabiei* help to confirm the diagnosis.

Dermatitis herpetiformis

The lesions in dermatitis herpetiformis are usually symmetrical and consist of erythematous, papulovesicular, and urticarial lesions that are markedly pruritic, have a chronic course, and heal with residual pigmentation.

Rickettsialpox

Rickettsialpox has the classic triad of signs and symptoms in the following order: (1) the appearance of a primary lesion or eschar on some part of the body, (2) the development of an influenza-like syndrome, and (3) the occurrence of a generalized papulovesicular eruption. The rash of rickettsialpox differs from that of varicella in that the vesicles are much smaller and are superimposed on a firm papule. Crusts do not develop regularly; if they do, they are very small. The diagnosis is confirmed by a specific CF test.

Eczema herpeticum or vaccinatum

In eczema herpeticum or vaccinatum there may be a history of smallpox vaccination or contact with a person who either has a fever blister or has been vaccinated recently. The vesicular and pustular lesions are most profuse over the sites of eczema. The different type of distribution and the absence of mouth lesions are helpful differential points. Virus isolation and serologic studies can identify the agent as either herpes simplex or vaccinia.

Smallpox

The elimination of smallpox in the 1970s now makes this diagnosis extremely unlikely.

COMPLICATIONS OF VARICELLA

Complications of varicella are not common; uneventful recovery is the rule except in immunocompromised persons.

Secondary bacterial infection

The secondary infection of skin lesions is not common enough to warrant the use of prophylactic antimicrobials. Staphylococci or beta-hemolytic group A streptococci may gain entry into the lesions and produce impetigo, furuncles, cellulitis, and, possibly, erysipelas. These infections may become foci for possible septicemia, pneumonia, suppurative arthritis, osteomyelitis, or local gangrene. Even in the era before antibiotics were available, there was a low incidence of this type of complication. Bullous impetigo caused by exfoliative toxigenic *S. aureus*, stage II, may be considered a secondary bacterial infection.

Encephalitis

Encephalitis occurs in less than one of every 1000 cases of varicella and may complicate a mild as well as a severe infection. The clinical and pathologic picture is similar to that of measles and postvaccinal encephalitis. Cerebellar involvement with ataxia is more common in varicella than in measles encephalitis (Peters et al., 1978). If it occurs as an isolated phenomenon, the prognosis is excellent. The symptoms of central nervous system (CNS) involvement usually develop between the third and eighth days following onset of rash; at times they may precede the exanthem. The signs are those of meningoencephalomyelitis, with fever, headache, stiff neck, change in sensorium, and, occasionally, convulsions, stupor, coma, and paralysis. Cerebral involvement in contrast to cerebellar carries a more guarded prognosis.

In both cerebellar and cerebral types CSF changes include pleocytosis with a predominance of lymphocytes, an elevated protein value, and a normal glucose value. In a survey of 59 cases of varicella encephalitis, Applebaum et al. (1953) reported complete recovery in 80%, evidence of brain damage in 15%, and death in 5%. Of 302 cases of varicella encephalitis reported in the United States during 3 years (1963 to 1965), 82, or 27.1%, were fatal. Encephalitis was present in 90% of 254 cases of neurologic complications of varicella reviewed by Miller et al. (1956). Other rare nervous system complications included transverse myelitis, peripheral neuritis, and optic neuritis.

Specific antibody has been detected in the CSF of patients with encephalitis caused by V-Z virus (Gershon et al., 1980). Demonstration of V-Z antibody in CSF may therefore be used to confirm the clinical diagnosis. Encephalitis ranging from mild to severe following zoster with a facial distribution is not an uncommon occurrence. The use of antiviral therapy in patients with CNS complications of varicella or zoster is controversial because the underlying pathology is not well understood. Many physicians elect to treat immunocompromised patients with antiviral drugs but not those who are immunologically normal.

Varicella pneumonia

Varicella pneumonia has been recognized chiefly in normal adults and immunocompromised patients of all ages. It has rarely been observed in normal children. It is more apt to occur in immunocompromised patients and infants with neonatal varicella. One to 5 days after chickenpox begins, there is an onset of cough, chest pain, dyspnea, tachypnea, and, possibly, cyanosis and hemoptysis. Rales are usually heard over both lung fields. The roentgenogram shows characteristic nodular densities throughout both lung fields (Fig. 33-7). The nodular infiltrates vary in size and occasionally coalesce to form larger areas of consolidation. The leukocyte count may either be normal or be slightly elevated.

The course of the pneumonia is variable. It may be extremely mild with little or no cough and no respiratory distress, and roentgenographic evidence of the disease may subside within 1 week. On the other hand, there may be severe respiratory embarrassment, with chest pain, hemoptysis, cyanosis, a stormy course of 7 to 10 days, and roentgenographic findings that persist for as long as 4 to 6 weeks. Occasionally there is a fatal outcome. Varicella pneumonia may be further complicated by pleural effusion, subcutaneous emphysema, and pulmonary edema. Severe cases of varicella pneu-

monia may show evidence of other visceral involvement, such as varicella hepatitis. The development of right upper quadrant pain associated with icterus should suggest probable varicella hepatitis. A summary of the epidemiologic and clinical manifestations of primary varicella pneumonia is given in Table 33-3.

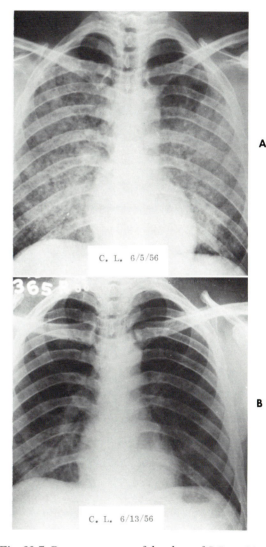

Fig. 33-7. Roentgenograms of the chest of C.L., a 24-year-old man with varicella, characterized on the third day by severe cough, dyspnea, tachypnea, cyanosis, and hemoptysis. **A,** Roentgenogram taken on the fourth day of pneumonia, showing extensive nodular infiltrates throughout both lung fields. **B,** Appearance 8 days later; there was considerable clearing. (From Krugman S, Goodrich CH, Ward, R. N Engl J Med 1957;257:843.).

Table 33-3. Summary of epidemiologic and clinical manifestations of 30 cases of primary varicella pneumonia

Age	Range: 4 to 82 yr			Mean average: 33years
	(only two children, 4 and 6 years of age, both with leukemia)			

Sex	Male: 22			Female: 8

Season	Jan. to March: 15	April to June: 14		Oct. to Dec.: 1

Day of onset of cough	First: 5	Second: 15	Third: 7	Fourth and fifth: 3

Clinical manifestations	*Severe*	*Moderate*	*Mild*	*None*
Cough	11	7	12	—
Dyspnea	10	6	3	11
Cyanosis	6	3	2	19
Hemoptysis	4	5	5	15
Rales	3	9	8	10
Roentgenographic findings	8	11	10	—

White blood count	Range: 4000 to 16,200			Mean average: 8600

Complications	Hepatitis (4)
	Pleural effusion (3)
	Pulmonary abscesses (2)
	Subcutaneous emphysema (1)
	Gastric ulcers (1)

Deaths	Pulmonary edema (1)
	Pulmonary abscesses and gastric ulcers (1)
	Hepatitis (3)
	Pulmonary abscesses and Hodgkin's disease (1)
	Leukemia (1)

CASE REPORT. C.B., a 26-year-old black woman, was admitted to the communicable disease unit of the Bellevue Hospital Center in 1956 in acute respiratory distress. Three days before admission she developed a fever and rash. Two days later she developed rapid labored respirations and a cough productive of bloody sputum. These symptoms became progressively more severe until the time of entry into the hosptial. Past history was negative for chickenpox. Family history was noncontributory.

Physical examination revealed an acutely ill patient in severe respiratory distress: temperature 40° C (104° F), pulse 124, respirations 46, and blood pressure 110/78 mm Hg. She was cyanotic, tachypneic, and dyspneic. There was a generalized eruption over her scalp, face, trunk, and extremities, with crops of papules, vesicles, and crusted lesions typical of chickenpox. Typical lesions of varicella were also present on the soft palate in the form of shallow white ulcers. There were coarse rales and rhonchi over the lower left chest posteriorly. The heart was not enlarged, the sounds were of good quality, and there were no murmurs. There was generalized lymphadenopathy.

Laboratory findings. Findings were hemoglobin, 16 gm per 100 ml; leukocytes, 12,800; polymorphonuclears, 83% (27% band cells); lymphocytes, 16%; monocytes, 1%. A smear showed normal red blood cells and platelets. Urinalysis was normal. The sputum culture revealed α-streptococci and *S. aureus*. Blood culture was negative. Roentgenogram of the chest revealed an extensive nodular infiltrate throughout both lung fields.

Course. The patient was placed in an oxygen tent, and treatment with tetracycline was begun. Dyspnea, tachypnea, and cyanosis persisted, and rales appeared over both lung fields. Her course was progressively downhill, and she died 24 hours after admission to the hospital.

Necropsy. Necropsy revealed evidence of varicella with involvement of the skin, lungs, trachea, bronchi, vaginal mucosa, and, probably, liver and uterus. Both pleural surfaces were studded with small hemorrhagic areas; some of these areas had white centers and others felt nodular. On the cut surface both lungs contained numerous hemorrhagic nodular areas of consolidation measuring 3 to 5 mm in diameter. These were widely distributed in all lobes. There was a severe degree of pulmonary edema bilaterally.

Microscopic examination of the lungs revealed lobular areas of consolidation with some tendency to confluence in zones of greatest involvement. The alveoli contained an exudate made up principally of red cells, fibrin, and mononuclear cells. Plasma cells and polymorphonuclear leukocytes were also present. In the intervening lesser involved zones of the lung, the alveoli contained edema fluid and mononuclear cells. Characteristic inclusion bodies were identified in the mononuclear cells of the pulmonary exudate.

Mackay and Cairney (1960) reported roentgenographic evidence of widespread, evenly distributed 1- to 3-mm nodules of calcific density in seven adults who had severe varicella after the age of 19 years. The roentgenograms were taken 3 to 32 years after the onset of varicella.

Reye syndrome

Epidemiologic surveys of the infections that have preceded Reye syndrome demonstrate a large variety of associated agents. In an epidemiologic study of Reye syndrome in Las Cruces, New Mexico, the incidence of Reye syndrome was estimated to be 2.5 per 1000 cases of varicella, four to nine times greater than its incidence after influenza B (Hurwitz and Goodman, 1982).

It has also been recognized that elevations of liver enzyme levels are not infrequent in otherwise normal children following varicella (Ey et al., 1981; Myers, 1982). In one study of 39 children with varicella, AST elevations were greater than normal in 77% (Pitel et al., 1980). Jaundice rarely develops in these patients. The condition is almost always self-limited and requires no specific therapy. Until these studies were reported, it was not realized that the liver can be involved in uncomplicated varicella. The relationship, if any, between this asymptomatic form of varicella hepatitis and Reye syndrome is not known, although some children have experienced severe vomiting episodes during the period of abnormal liver enzyme activity. Lichtenstein et al. (1983) obtained liver biopsies from 19 children who had marked elevation of ami-

notransferase activity with minimal neurologic symptoms (lethargy) following varicella (eight children) or an upper respiratory infection (11 children). Microscopic evidence of Reye syndrome was found in 14 children (74%). Therefore, they proposed that patients with vomiting, hepatic dysfunction, and minimal neurologic impairment after varicella have Reye syndrome.

Disseminated varicella

For a discussion of disseminated varicella, see p. 437.

Other rare complications

Uveitis and orchitis have also been reported as complications of varicella. Acute glomerulonephritis has been described as a complication of varicella in patients either with or without evidence of associated streptococcal infection (Yuceoglu et al., 1967).

Varicella arthritis is another rare complication. The association was reported by Ward and Bishop (1970) and by Mulhern et al. (1971), who described the occurrence of a monoarticular arthritis of the knee with effusion, tenderness, and pain, and no erythema. The synovial fluid contained 3000 to 4000 white blood cells per cubic millimeter, predominantly lymphocytes, and it was bacteria free. The effusion cleared spontaneously in 3 days. Priest et al. (1978) reported the isolation of V-Z virus from joint fluid obtained from a patient with varicella arthritis.

Purpura fulminans and gangrene of several toes were observed in a 7-year-old child admitted to the Bellevue Hospital Infectious Disease Unit. This rare complication has been described by Smith (1967) and by de Koning et al. (1972).

PROGNOSIS

Varicella is usually a benign disease of childhood. The typical case clears up spontaneously without sequelae and without scarring. Lesions that are secondarily infected are likely to be followed by permanent scars if the deep layers of the skin are involved. The rare case of sepsis, bacterial pneumonia, or osteomyelitis should respond to appropriate antibacterial therapy.

Varicella may be a very serious disease in newborn infants, adults, patients receiving high doses of corticosteroids for any reason, and patients treated with chemotherapy or radiotherapy for an underlying malignancy. Varicella pneumonia is potentially fatal.

IMMUNITY

An attack of chickenpox usually confers lasting immunity; second attacks are unusual (Weller, 1983). Varicella-zoster antibody has been shown to persist for many years after infection. Most immune adults have detectable FAMA, ELISA, RIA, or IAHA V-Z antibody. The complement-fixing test is not sensitive enough to be of use for determining immune status to varicella.

Transplacental immunity was studied by Gershon et al. (1976). They tested 200 mother-infant (cord) serum specimens for V-Z antibody by the FAMA test; 10% of this group were seronegative. The maternal and cord blood antibody titers were essentially the same. Women born in the United States were more likely to be immune than those who were born in Latin American countries. Only 5% of U.S. women were seronegative, as compared with 16% of the Latin American group. The disappearance of passively acquired antibody in the first year of life is shown in Fig. 33-8. By 6 months of age most infants no longer have detectable V-Z antibody. Transplacentally acquired V-Z antibody has been detected in the blood of low birth weight infants, even those of less than 1500 gm (Raker et al., 1978).

Development of mild varicella in young infants despite the presence of transplacental maternal antibody has been reported by Baba et al. (1982). They observed nine cases of mild to moderate varicella in young infants who had detectable V-Z antibody titers prior to illness.

During the course of vaccine trials with the live attenuated varicella vaccine (see p. 449) it was also recognized that the presence of specific serum antibody at the time of exposure to the virus does not necessarily guarantee protection from clinical varicella. Eight recipients of varicella vaccine who had underlying leukemia developed mild clinical varicella following an exposure several months after immunization despite serum V-Z antibody titers that were predicted to be protective (Gershon et al., 1984b). In addition, varicella has also been reported in persons having detectable V-Z antibody following natural infection (Zaia et al., 1983; Gershon et al., 1984a). These observations have led to a reexamination of the mechanism

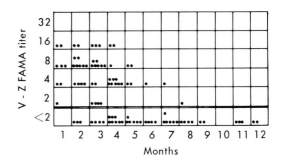

Fig. 33-8. Detection of varicella-zoster (V-Z) antibody in the first year of life in 67 infants. The sensitive fluorescent antibody against membrane antigen (FAMA) test was used for the assay. (From Gershon AA, et al. Pediatrics 1976;58:692.)

by which immunity to varicella is mediated. Serum antibody is not fully protective. Secretory antibody at the level of the respiratory tract may be important but it has thus far not been studied in detail.

Cellular immunity is also of undoubted importance, both in protection from reinfection with V-Z virus and in recovery from V-Z infection. It was recognized many years ago that the prognosis of varicella in children with isolated defects in humoral immunity was excellent. In contrast, children with congenital defects in cellular immunity were recognized to be at high risk to develop severe infections.

Specific cell-mediated immunity to V-Z virus develops following an attack of varicella. Failure to develop a positive cellular immune response correlates with death from varicella (Patel et al., 1979; Gershon and Steinberg, 1979). Various types of cell-mediated immune reactions to V-Z virus have been described, including T-cell and macrophage cytotoxicity, antibody-dependent cytotoxicity (ADCC), and natural killer (NK) cells (Weller, 1983). The role of these reactions in protection against V-Z infection is under current investigation. A diagram depicting the summary of the natural history of V-Z infections is shown in Fig. 33-9.

EPIDEMIOLOGIC FACTORS

Chickenpox is worldwide in distribution, being endemic in all large cities. Epidemics do not have the periodicity of measles; they occur at irregular intervals determined chiefly by the size and concentration of new groups of susceptible children. All races and both sexes are

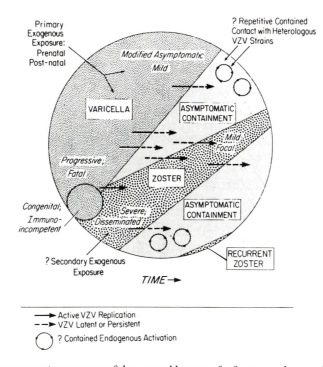

Fig. 33-9. Diagrammatic summary of the natural history of infection with varicella-zoster virus. Two variables are depicted: time and clinical severity. In the competent host the containment period is on the order of decades; however, in the immunocompromised person the two clinical processes may merge without an intervening asymptomatic interval. The containment period after congenital varicella is typically of short duration. During the asymptomatic containment period episodes of endogenous viral replication probably occur, and contact with heterologous exogenous strains may stimulate host defenses, usually in the absence of overt disease. (From Weller TH. N Engl J Med·1983;309:1362-1368, 1434-1440.)

equally susceptible. Seasonal distribution varies with the particular zone. In temperate areas the incidence rises during the late autumn, winter, and spring. The seasonal distribution of zoster is different from that of varicella; zoster occurs with equal frequency throughout the year.

Varicella is predominantly a disease of childhood, with the highest age incidence between 2 and 8 years. It is extremely rare in adults who have lived in heavily populated urban areas, but not uncommon in those who have come from isolated rural areas. Ross et al. (1962) observed a group of 641 adults and 501 children who had intimate household exposure to varicella. The overall attack rates were 1.4% for adults and 78% for children. Of 79 adults with a negative history of varicella, only 8% acquired the disease. In contrast, 87% of 441 presumably susceptible children acquired the disease.

Studies in our laboratory have indicated that of 92 consecutive adults with no history of var-

icella 23 (25%) were actually susceptible (La-Russa, et al., 1985). Steele et al. (1982) have noted a similar percentage of susceptibility in adults.

The age distribution of zoster is different from that of varicella. A study of 108 patients by Miller and Brunell (1970) revealed that 69% were 50 years of age or older and less than 10% were children.

Immunocompromised children, however, are at some risk to develop zoster; it is considerably higher than the risk in normal children. In a study of children with malignant disease the overall incidence of zoster was 9% (Feldman et al., 1973). This study involved 1132 patients over a 10-year period. The incidence of zoster in patients with Hodgkin's disease was 22%; it was 10% in children with acute lymphocytic leukemia and 5% in children with solid tumors. No specific chemotherapy was found to be associated with increased risk of infection.

Chickenpox is one of the most highly contagious diseases, comparable to measles and smallpox in this respect. The infection is spread chiefly by direct contact with a patient. Under hospital conditions indirect contact through the medium of a third person occurs within the limitations of time and distance. It would be unlikely, however, for a physician to carry the infection from one building to another; adequate hand washing and "airing" would probably eliminate the infective agent. There is evidence to suggest that varicella can be transmitted via the airborne route (Leclair et al., 1980; Gustafson et al., 1982).

A patient with chickenpox may transmit the disease to other susceptible persons from approximately 1 day before onset of rash until all of the vesicles have become dry. A mild case will show complete crusting within 5 days and a severe case within 10 days. In contrast with those of smallpox, the dry scabs of varicella do not contain active virus.

TREATMENT

Chickenpox is a self-limited disease for which the treatment is entirely symptomatic. Acetaminophen is indicated for high fever and severe constitutional symptoms. Aspirin should not be given until the relationship between this drug, if any, and Reye syndrome is clarified. Local applications of calamine lotion or antipruritic ointments may help to control the itching. Occasionally the pruritus is partially relieved by oral antihistamines. Fingernails should be kept short and clean in an attempt to minimize secondary skin infections caused by scratching.

Treatment of complications

The following measures are recommended for the treatment of complications of chickenpox.

Bacterial infections. Bacterial infections complicating chickenpox are most often caused by *S. aureus* or group A beta-hemolytic streptococci. Infection of a local lesion usually responds to simple measures such as warm compresses. Antimicrobial therapy is indicated for cellulitis, sepsis, or pneumonia. The treatment of severe staphylococcal infections is discussed in detail on p. 350.

Encephalitis. Patients in coma require careful observation and supportive treatment for the maintenance of hydration and adequate nutri-

tion. Parenteral fluids and tube feeding should be employed as indicated. Care should be exercised to prevent aspiration.

Corticosteroids have not been effective therapy for varicella encephalitis. Antiviral therapy may be used, although data concerning efficacy are not available.

Severe varicella. There are several useful antiviral drugs (acyclovir, vidarabine, and interferon) for treatment of severe or potentially severe varicella. Since acyclovir is well tolerated, it has been used to treat immunocompromised patients with varicella early in the course of disease. Such therapy is not usually necessary, however, for immunocompromised patients who have received active or passive immunization. One of our patients, a 17-year-old male with T-cell leukemia, developed varicella after no known exposure. He was immediately admitted to Bellevue Hospital and treated with intravenous acyclovir for 7 days. He developed a high fever and extensive maculopapular skin lesions but no pneumonia. He was discharged within 10 days. Previously, when only interferon and vidarabine were available, no treatment would have been given, unless the patient developed varicella pneumonia or extensive hemorrhagic skin lesions. By this time, however, it is often too late for an antiviral drug to be beneficial. Therefore, early treatment of varicella in high-risk patients is warranted.

In our opinion, acyclovir is currently the drug of choice for severe or potentially severe V-Z infection because it is effective and well tolerated. It does not prevent development of postherpetic pain, although it may shorten the duration. When given within 3 to 5 days after rash acyclovir is effective treatment for varicella in immunocompromised patients (Prober et al., 1982; Balfour et al., 1984). Acyclovir has also been used successfully to treat zoster in both normal and immunocompromised patients (Peterslund et al., 1981; Bean et al., 1982; Balfour et al., 1983a,b).

For treatment of immunocompromised patients with varicella or zoster, acyclovir should be administered intravenously at a dose of 750 mg to 1500 mg per square meter of body surface area per day in three divided doses for 7 to 10 days. Toxicity is unusual, although phlebitis has been reported.

Neither active nor passive immunization will

protect entirely against development of clinical varicella after an exposure. "Breakthrough" varicella, if it does occur, however, is almost always mild. Therefore, such patients will require antiviral therapy only if their illness seems to be becoming severe, for example, development of over 500 skin lesions, hemorrhagic vesicles, or pneumonia.

Acyclovir is relatively nontoxic because it interferes mainly with synthesis of viral rather than host DNA. Acyclovir itself is not an antiviral. It requires phosphorylation by a thymidine kinase present only in virus-infected cells in order to interfere with DNA synthesis. Therefore, its effect on uninfected host cells is minimal, accounting for its lack of significant toxicity.

Alternative drugs, vidarabine and interferon, are also effective in treatment of varicella and zoster (Whitley et al., 1976, 1982a,b; Merigan et al., 1978; Arvin et al., 1982). However, these drugs are more toxic than acyclovir and they are more difficult to administer. Nausea, vomiting, rash, and tremors have been reported with vidarabine therapy; fever, fatigue, myalgia, and weight loss have been associated with interferon therapy (Hirsch and Schooley, 1983). Both drugs require hospitalization of the patient, and both must be given intravenously.

In general all of the antiviral drugs have been most effective when administered within 3 days after the onset of illness. It is more compelling to treat immunosuppressed patients with varicella early, because the mortality rate approaches 15%, than to treat zoster patients, for whom mortality is only 1% to 2%. Among zoster patients, those with lymphoproliferative cancers who are over 38 years of age were at greatest risk (Whitley et al., 1982b). In this study of 121 patients, treatment with vidarabine within 72 hours of onset decreased the incidence of disseminated zoster.

PREVENTIVE MEASURES

Varicella is usually a benign and uncomplicated disease of childhood. Consequently, no preventive measures are recommended for a normal child who has been exposed. On the other hand, susceptible newborn infants, corticosteroid-treated children, and proven susceptible adults should be protected, if possible. Infants whose mothers have the rash of varicella within 5 days of delivery should be protected.

Successful passive immunization against varicella has been accomplished with zoster immune globulin (ZIG). ZIG was shown by Brunell et al. (1972) and Gershon et al. (1974) to modify the course of varicella in high-risk children. The spectrum of illness in 15 recipients of ZIG following a household exposure ranged from subclinical infections in five to modified varicella with no more than 44 skin lesions in nine, to severe varicella in one child who recovered. All 15 children had persistence of V-Z antibody by the FAMA test for a 2-year follow-up period. The dose of ZIG in this study was 5 ml intramuscularly given within 72 hours of exposure.

Judelsohn et al. (1974) of the Center for Disease Control gave ZIG to nonhousehold as well as household high-risk patients exposed to varicella. The clinical attack rate was not affected but the disease was significantly modified. Most of the ZIG recipients had fewer than ten lesions. The dose of ZIG was 5 ml given within 72 hours after exposure. Neither ZIG nor immune globulin (IG) nor zoster immune plasma (ZIP) has been effective for the prevention or modification of disseminated zoster (Groth et al., 1978; Merigan and Stevens, 1978).

Varicella-zoster immune globulin (VZIG) is as efficacious in modifying varicella in the immunocompromised as is ZIG, and it has replaced ZIG. VZIG is prepared from lots of outdated plasma that contain relatively high V-Z antibody titers. In a comparison study, 49 of 81 (60.4%) immunosuppressed children who received VZIG and 57 of 83 (68.6%) who received ZIG were protected from varicella after household exposure (Zaia et al., 1983). The dose of VZIG is 1.25 ml per 10 kg of body weight.

A live attenuated varicella vaccine was developed in Japan by Takahashi et al. (1974). Studies with this Oka strain of varicella virus have been conducted in normal, ambulatory children (Takahashi et al., 1975), in hospitalized children with chronic diseases such as nephrotic syndrome (Asano et al., 1975), and in children with leukemia (Izawa et al., 1977). The vaccine was immunogenic, well tolerated, and protective (Asano and Takahashi, 1977; Asano et al., 1977).

Studies in the United States have included immunization of normal children (Arbeter et al., 1982, 1984; Weibel et al., 1984). The vaccine was well tolerated and immunogenic. In one study (Weibel et al., 1984) it was 100% effective in prevention of clinical varicella in normal vaccinees. In contrast, children who received placebo experienced about a 50% attack rate of clinical varicella following household exposures to the virus.

Vaccine trials in leukemic children in the United States and Canada have demonstrated that about 80% of these vaccinees are protected against clinical varicella. "Breakthrough" cases have been described, but these are usually extremely mild illnesses (Brunell et al., 1982; Gershon et al., 1984b). Gershon et al. (1984b) have observed eight cases of mild varicella in vaccinees, on the average 8 months after vaccination. In this collaborative study, of 235 leukemic children, mild to moderate vaccine-associated rashes were noted in about 40% of leukemic children vaccinated while in remission but still receiving chemotherapy with a 1-week hiatus before and after vaccination. These children were at a slight risk to transmit vaccine virus to others, although these contact cases in normal children were extremely mild (Gershon et al., 1984b).

Because the vaccine is so well tolerated and because the incidence of zoster after immunization is not increased, it is likely that this vaccine may eventually be administered routinely to normal children if it is found to provide long-lasting protection. A 5-year follow up study by Asano et al. (1983) indicated that positive antibody titers were maintained in normal vaccinees for this period of time.

ISOLATION AND QUARANTINE

Isolation and quarantine procedures have been drastically modified in recent years for the following reasons: (1) they not only have proved to be ineffective in the past but also have contributed to unnecessary loss of time from school and other activities, (2) in most instances exposure has usually occurred before the diagnosis has become apparent, and (3) it makes little sense to prevent an inevitable disease that is generally mild in childhood and postpone it until adulthood when it is more likely to be severe and potentially fatal.

Unless there are specific local regulations, isolation and quarantine procedures should be individualized. Most authorities agree (1) that the patient with chickenpox should be kept at home until the vesicles have dried, (2) that contacts should not be quarantined but merely observed, and (3) that efforts to institute isolation precautions within the home to protect siblings are useless and should not be attempted.

On the other hand, rigid isolation precautions should be employed for the prevention of the infection of infants and high-risk children. Appropriate measures should be instituted to prevent contact with a definite or potential case of chickenpox. If exposure has occurred or is inevitable, the preventive measures already described would be indicated.

REFERENCES

Aimes CR. The elementary bodies of zoster and their serological relationship to those of varicella. Br J Exp Pathol 1934;15:314.

Applebaum E, Rachelson MH, Dolgopol VB. Varicella encephalitis. Am J Med 1953;15:523.

Arbeter AM, Starr SE, Preblud SA, et al. Varicella vaccine trials in health children: a summary of comparative and follow up studies. Am J Dis Child 1984;138:434-438.

Arbeter AM, Starr SE, Weibel RE, et al. Live attenuated varicella vaccine: immunization of healthy children with the OKA strain. J Pediatr 1982;100:886-893.

Arvin AM, Koropchak CM. Immunoglobulins M and G to varicella zoster virus measured by solid-phase radio immunoassay: antibody responses to varicella and herpes zoster infections. J Clin Microbiol 1980;12:367-374.

Arvin AM, Koropchak CM, Wittek AE. Immunologic evidence of reinfection with varicella-zoster virus. J Infect Dis 1983;148:200-205.

Arvin AM, Kushner JH, Feldman S, et al. Human leukocyte interferon for the treatment of varicella in children with cancer. N Engl J Med 1982;306:761-765.

Asano Y, Albrecht P, Vujcic LK, et al. Five-year follow-up study of recipients of live varicella vaccine using enhanced neutralization and fluorescent antibody membrane antigen assays. Pediatrics 1983;72:291-294.

Asano Y, Takahashi M. Clinical and serologic testing of a live varicella vaccine and two-year follow-up for immunity of the vaccinated children. Pediatrics 1977;60:810.

Asano Y, et al. Application of a live attenuated varicella vaccine to hospitalized children and its protective effect on spread of varicella infection. Biken J 1975;18:35.

Asano Y, et al. Protective efficacy of vaccination in children in four episodes of natural varicella and zoster in the ward. Pediatrics 1977;59:8.

Baba K, Yabuuchi H, Takabashi M, et al. Immunologic and epidemiologic aspects of varicella infection acquired during infancy and early childhood. J Pediatr 1982;100:881-885.

Balfour HH. Intravenous acyclovir therapy for varicella in immunocompromised children. J Pediatr 1984;104:134-136.

Balfour HH, Bean B, Laskin OL, et al. Acyclovir halts progression of herpes zoster in immunocompromised patients. N Engl J Med 1983a;308:1448-1453.

Balfour HH, McMonigal KA, Bean B. Acyclovir therapy of varicella-zoster virus infections in immunocompromised patients. J Antimicrob Chemother 1983b;12(Suppl B): 169-179.

Bean B, Braun C, Balfour HH. Acyclovir therapy for acute herpes zoster. Lancet 1982;2:118-121.

Brunell PA. Varicella-zoster infections in pregnancy. JAMA 1967;199:93.

Brunell PA, Casey HL. Crude tissue culture antigen for determination of varicella-zoster complement fixing antibody. Public Health Rep 1964;79:839.

Brunell PA, Cherry JD, Ector WL, et al. Expanded guidelines for use of varicella-zoster immune globulin. Pediatrics 1983;72:886-889.

Brunell P, Kotchmar GS. Zoster in infancy: failure to maintain virus latency following intrauterine infection. J Pediatr 1981;98:71-73.

Brunell PA, Miller L, Lovejoy F. Zoster in children. Am J Dis Child 1968;115:432.

Brunell PA, Ross A, Miller LH, Kuo B. Prevention of varicella by zoster immune globulin. N Engl J Med 1969; 280:1191.

Brunell PA, Shehab Z, Geiser C, et al. Administration of live varicella vaccine to children with leukaemia. Lancet 1982;2:1069-1072.

Brunell PA, et al. A gel precipitin test for the diagnosis of varicella. Bull WHO 1971;44:811.

Brunell PA, et al. Prevention of varicella in high risk children: a collaborative study. Pediatrics 1972;59:718.

Bullowa JGM, Wishik SM. Complications of varicella. I. Their occurrence among 2,534 patients. Am J Dis Child 1935;49:923.

Cheatham WJ, Weller TH, Dolan TF, Jr, Dower JC. Varicella: report of two fatal cases with necropsy, virus isolation, and serologic studies. Am J Pathol 1956;32:1015.

Davis CM, Van Dersarl JV, Coltman CA, Jr. Failure of cytarabine in varicella-zoster infections. JAMA 1973; 224:122.

de Koning J, Frederiks E, Kerkhoven P. Purpura fulminans following varicella: Helv Paediatr Acta 1972;27:177.

Ehrlich RM, Turner JAP, Clarke M. Neonatal varicella. J Pediatr 1958;53:139.

Eisenbud M. Chickenpox with visceral involvement. Am J Med 1952;12:740.

Ey JL, Smith SM, Fulginiti VA. Varicella hepatitis without neurologic symptoms or findings. Pediatrics 1981;67:285-287.

Feldman S, Chaudary S, Ossi M, Epp E. A viremic phase for herpes zoster in children with cancer. J Pediatr 1977; 91:597.

Feldman S, Epp E. Isolation of varicella zoster virus from blood. J Pediatr 1976;88:265-267.

Feldman S, Epp E. Detection of viremia during incubation of varicella. J Pediatr 1979;94:746.

Feldman S, Hughes WT, Daniel CB. Varicella in children with cancer: seventy-seven cases. Pediatrics 1975;56:388.

Feldman S, Hughes WT, Kim HY. Herpes zoster in children with cancer. Am J Dis Child 1973;126:178.

Finkel KC. Mortality from varicella in children receiving adrenocorticosteroids and adrenocorticotropin. Pediatrics 1961;28:436.

Forghani B, Schmidt NJ, Dennis J. Antibody assays for varicella-zoster virus: comparison of enzyme immunoassay with neutralization, immune adherence hemagglutination, and complement fixation. J Clin Microbiol 1978; 8:545.

Freund P. Congenital varicella. Am J Dis Child 1958;96:730.

Friedman MG, Leventon-Kriss S, Sarov I. Sensitive solid-phase radioimmunoassay for detection of human immunoglobulin G antibodies to varicella-zoster virus. J Clin Microbiol 1979;9:1.

Garland J. Varicella following exposure to herpes zoster. N Engl J Med 1943;228:336.

Gershon AA. Clinical trial of live attenuated varicella vaccine in high risk susceptibles—a preliminary report. Prog Clin Biol Res 1975a;3:79.

Gershon AA. Varicella in mother and infant: problems old and new. In Krugman J, Gershon AA, eds. Infections of the fetus and newborn infants. New York: Alan R. Liss, 1975b;79.

Gershon AA. Live attenuated varicella-zoster vaccine. Rev Infect Dis 1980;2:393-407.

Gershon AA, Brunell PA, Doyle EF, et al. Steroid therapy and varicella. J Pediatr 1972;81:1034.

Gershon AA, Frey HM, Steinberg SP, et al. Determination of immunity to varicella using an enzyme-linked-immunosorbent-assay. Arch Virol 1981;70:169-172.

Gershon AA, Kalter ZG, Steinberg S. Detection of antibody to varicella-zoster virus by immune adherence hemagglutination. Proc Soc Exp Biol Med 1976;151:762.

Gershon AA, Krugman S. Seroepidemiological survey of varicella: value of specific fluorescent antibody test. Pediatrics 1975;56:1005.

Gershon AA., Steinberg SP. Cellular and humoral immune responses to VZV in immunocompromised patients during and after VZV infections, Infect Immun 1979;25:828.

Gershon AA, Steinberg SP. Inactivation of varicella zoster virus *in vitro:* effect of leucocytes and specific antibody. Infect Immun 1981;33:507-511.

Gershon AA, Steinberg SP, Borkowsky W, et al. IgM to varicella-zoster virus: demonstration in patients with and without clinical zoster. Pediatr Infect Dis 1982;1:164.

Gershon AA, Steinberg S, Brunell PA. Zoster immune globulin: a further assessment. N Engl J Med 1974;290:243.

Gershon AA, Steinberg SP, Gelb L, et al. Clinical reinfection with varicella-zoster virus. J Infect Dis 1984a;149:137-142.

Gershon AA, Steinberg S, Gelb L, et al. Efficacy of live attenuated varicella vaccine in children with acute leukemia in remission. JAMA 1984b;252:355-362.

Gershon AA, Steinberg S, Greenberg S, et al. Varicella-zoster–associated encephalitis: detection of specific antibody in cerebrospinal fluid. J Clin Microsc 1980;12:764-767.

Gershon AA, Steinberg S, Silber R. Varicella-zoster viremia. J Pediatr 1978;92:1033-1034.

Gershon AA, et al. Antibody to varicella-zoster virus in parturient women and their offspring during the first year of life. Pediatrics 1976;58:692.

Gilden DH, Vafai A, Shtram Y, et al. Varicella zoster virus DNA in human sensory ganglia. Nature 1983;306:478-480.

Goffinet DR, Glatstein EJ, Merigan TC. Herpes zoster-varicella infections and lymphoma. Ann Intern Med 1972;76:235.

Gold E. Serologic and virus isolation sutdies of patients with varicella or herpes zoster. N Engl J Med 1966;274:181.

Goldson AS, Millichap JG, Miller RH. Cerebellar ataxia with pre-eruptive varicella. Am J Dis Child 1963;106:197.

Good RA, Vernier RL, Smith RE. Serious untoward reactions to therapy with cortisone and adrenocorticotropin in pediatric practice. Pediatrics 1957;19:272.

Grose C. Varicella-zoster virus infections: chickenpox (varicella) and shingles (zoster). In Glasser R, Gotleib-Stematsky T, eds. Human herpesvirus infections, clinical aspects. New York: Marcel Dekker, Inc,, 1982;85-150.

Grose C, Edmond BJ, Brunell PA. Complement-enhanced neutralizing antibody response to varicella-zoster virus. J Infect Dis 1979;139:432.

Groth KE, et al. Evaluation of zoster immune plasma: treatment of cutaneous disseminated zoster in immunocompromised patients. JAMA 1978;239:1877.

Gustafson TL, Lavely GB, Brawner ER, et al. An outbreak of airborne nosocomial varicella. Pediatrics 1982;70:550-556.

Haggerty RJ, Eley RC. Varicella and cortisone. Pediatrics 1956;18:160.

Hanshaw JB, Dudgeon JA. Viral diseases of the fetus and newborn. In Major problems in pediatrics. Philadelphia: W.B. Saunders Co., 1978;17:192-208.

Hirsch MS, Schooley RT. Treatment of herpesvirus infections. N Engl J Med 1983;309:963-970, 1034-1038.

Hurwitz ES, Goodman RA. A cluster of cases of Reye syndrome associated with chickenpox. Pediatrics 1982;70:901-906.

Hyman RW, Ecker JR, Tenser RB. Varicella-zoster virus RNA in human trigeminal ganglia. Lancet 1983;2:814-816.

Izawa T, et al. Application of a live varicella vaccine in children with acute leukemia or other malignant disease. Pediatrics 1977;60:805.

Jemsek J, Grenberg S, Taber L, et al. Herpes-zoster associated encephalitis: clinicopathologic report of 12 cases and review of the literature. Medicine 1983;62:81-94.

Jordan GW, Merigan TC. Cell-mediated immunity to varicella-zoster virus; in vitro lymphocyte responses. J Infect Dis 1974;130:495.

Judelsohn RG, Meyers JD, Ellis RJ, Thomas EK. Efficacy of zoster immune globulin. Pediatrics 1974;53:476.

Knyvett AF. The pulmonary lesions of chickenpox. Q J Med 1966;35:313.

Krugman S, Goodrich CH, Ward R. Primary varicella pneumonia. N Engl J Med 1957;257:843.

La Russa P, Steinberg S, Seeman M, et al. Determination of immunity to VZ virus by means of an intradermal skin test. J Infect Dis 1985;152.

Leclair JM, Zaia JA, Levin MJ, et al. Airborne transmission of chickenpox in a hospital. N Engl J Med 1980;302:450-453.

Lichtenstein PK, Heubi JE, Daugherty CC, et al. A frequent cause of vomiting and liver dysfunction after varicella and upper-respiratory tract infection. N Engl J Med 1983;309:133-139.

Luby JP, et al. Adenine arabinoside therapy of varicella-zoster virus infections. In Pavan-Langston D, Buchanan RA, Alford CA (eds). Adenine arabinoside: an antiviral agent. New York: Raven Press, 1975;237.

Mackay JB, Cairney P. Pulmonary calcification following varicella. N Z Med J 1960;59:453.

Melish ME. Bullous varicella: its association with the staphylococcal scalded skin syndrome. J Pediatr 1973;83:1019.

Merigan T, Rand K, Pollard R, et al. Human leukocyte interferon for the treatment of herpes zoster in patients with cancer. N Engl J Med 1978;298:981-987.

Merigan TC, Stevens DA. The use of zoster immune globulin in the prevention of varicella and the treatment of zoster. Fifteenth Congress of the International Blood Transfusion Society, Paris, July 23, 1978.

Merigan TC, et al. Human leukocyte interferon for the treatment of herpes zoster in patients with cancer. N Engl J Med 1978;298:981.

Merselis JG, Jr, Kaye D, Hook EW. Disseminated herpes zoster: a report of 17 cases. Arch Intern Med 1964;113:679.

Meyers JD. Congenital varicella in term infants: risk reconsidered. J Infect Dis 1974;129:215.

Miller HG, Stanton JB, Gibbons JL. Parainfectious encephalomyelitis and related syndromes: critical review of neurological complications of certain specific fevers. Q J Med 1956;25:427.

Miller LH, Brunell PA. Zoster, reinfection or activation of latent virus? Am J Med 1970;49:480.

Mortimer EA, Lepow ML. Varicella with hypoglycemia possibly due to salicylates. Am J Dis Child 1962;103:583.

Mulhern LM, Friday GA, Perri JA. Arthritis complicating varicella infection. Pediatrics 1971;48:827.

Myers MG. Viremia caused by varicella-zoster virus: association with malignant progressive varicella. J Infect Dis 1979;140:229-233.

Myers MG. Hepatic cellular injury during varicella. Arch Dis Child 1982;57:317-319.

O'Neil RR. Congenital varicella. Am J Dis Child 1962;104:39.

Oppenheimer EH. Congenital chickenpox with disseminated visceral lesions. Bull Johns Hopkins Hosp 1944;74:240.

Ozaki T, Ichikawa T, Matsui Y, et al. Viremia phase in nonimmunocompromised children with varicella. J Pediatr 1984;104:85-87.

Patel PA, Toonessi S, O'Malley J, et al. Cell-mediated immunity to varicella zoster virus in subjects with lymphoma or leukemia. J Pediatr 1979;94:223-230.

Peters ACB, Versteeg J, Lindenman J, et al. Varicella and acute cerebellar ataxia. Arch Neurol 1978;35:769.

Peterslund NA, Seyer-Hansen K, Ipsen J, et al. Acyclovir in herpes zoster. Lancet 1981;2:827-830.

Pichini B, Ecker JR, Grose C, et al. DNA mapping of paired varicella-zoster virus isolates from patients with shingles. Lancet 1983;2:1223-1225.

Pitel PA, McCormick KL, Fitzgerald E, et al. Subclinical hepatic changes in varicella infection. Pediatrics 1980;65:631-633.

Priest JR, Urick JJ, Groth KE, Balfour HH. Varicella arthritis documented by isolation of virus from joint fluid. J Pediatr 1978;93:990.

Prober CG, Kirk LE, Keeney RE. Acyclovir therapy of chickenpox in immunosuppressed children—a collaborative study. J Pediatr 1982;101:622-625.

Raker RK, Steinberg S, Drusin LM, Gershon A. Antibody to varicella-zoster virus in low-birth-weight newborn infants. J Pediatr 1978;93:505.

Rand KH, et al. Cellular immunity and herpes virus infections in cardiac-transplant patients. N Engl J Med 1976;296:1372.

Reye RDK, Morgan G, Baral J. Encephalopathy and fatty degeneration of viscera: disease entity in childhood. Lancet 1963;2:749.

Richman DD, Cleveland PH, Oxman MN, Zaia JA. A rapid radioimmunoassay using ^{125}I-labeled staphylococcal protein A for antibody to varicella zoster virus. J Infect Dis 1981;143:693-699.

Ross A, Lencher E, Reitman G. Modification of chickenpox in family contacts by administration of gamma globulin. N Engl J Med 1962; 267:369.

Sargent EN, Carson MJ, Reilly ED. Varicella pneumonia: a report of 20 cases with postmortem examination in 6. Calif Med 1967;107:141.

Serota FT, Starr SE, Bryan CK, et al. Acyclovir treatment of herpes zoster infections. JAMA 1982;247:2132-2135.

Shehab Z, Brunell PA. Enzyme-linked immunosorbent assay for susceptibility to varicella. J Infect Dis 1983;148:472-476.

Siegel M. Congenital malformations following chickenpox, measles, mumps, and hepatitis. Results of a cohort study. JAMA 1973;226:1521-1524.

Smith EWP, et al. Varicella gangrenosa due to group A β-hemolytic streptococcus. Pediatrics 1976;57:306.

Smith H. Purpura fulminans complicating varicella: recovery with low molecular weight dextran and steroids. Med J Aust 1967;2:685.

Srabstein, JC et al. Is there a congenital varicella syndrome? J Pediatr 1974;84:239.

Steele RW, Coleman MA, Fiser M, Bradsher RW. Varicella zoster in hospital personnel: skin test reactivity to monitor susceptibility. Pediatrics 1982;70:604-608.

Stevens CA, Jordon GW, Waddell TF, Merigan TC. Adverse effect of cytosine arabinoside on disseminated zoster in a controlled trial. N Engl J Med 1973;289:873.

Strachman J. Uveitis associated with chickenpox. J Pediatr 1955;46:327.

Straus S, Reinhold W, Smith H, et al. Endonuclease analysis of viral DNA from varicella and subsequent zoster infections in the same patient. N Engl J Med 1984;311:1362.

Takahashi M, et al. Live vaccine used to prevent the spread of varicella in children in hospital. Lancet 1974;2:1288.

Takahashi M, et al. Development of a live attenuated varicella vaccine. Biken J 1975;18:25.

Thompson CA, Cantrell FP. Chickenpox pneumonia treated with prednisone: a case report. Ann Intern Med 1958; 49:1239.

Uduman SA, Gershon AA, Brunell PA. Should patients with zoster receive zoster immune globulin? JAMA 1975; 234:1049.

Wald ER, Levine MM, Togo Y. Concomitant varicella and staphylococcal scalded skin syndrome. J Pediatr 1973; 83:1017.

Ward JR, Bishop B. Varicella arthritis. JAMA 1970;212:1954.

Weber DM, Pellecchia JA. Varicella pneumonia: study of prevalence in adult men. JAMA 1965;192:572.

Weibel RE, Neff BJ, Kuter BJ, et al. Live attenuated varicella virus vaccine. Efficacy trial in healthy children. N Engl J Med 1984;310:1409-1415.

Weller TH. Serial propagation in vitro of agents producing inclusion bodies derived from varicella and herpes zoster. Proc Soc Exp Biol Med 1953;83:340.

Weller TH. Varicella and herpes zoster. Changing concepts of the natural history, control, and importance of a not-so-benign virus. N Engl J Med 1983;309:1362-1368.

Weller TH, Coons AH. Fluorescent antibody studies with agents of varicella and herpes zoster propagated in vitro. Proc Soc Exp Biol Med 1954;86:789.

Wesselhoeft C, Pearson CM. Orchitis in the course of severe chickenpox with pneumonitis, followed by testicular atrophy. N Engl J Med 1950;242:651.

White HH. Varicella myelopathy. N Engl J Med 1962; 266:772.

Whitley R, Hilty M, Haynes R, et al. Vidarabine therapy of varicella in immunosuppressed patients. J Pediatr 1982a;101:125-131.

Whitley RJ, Soong SJ, Dolin R, et al. Early vidarabine therapy to control the complications of herpes zoster in immunosuppressed patients. N Engl J Med 1982b;307:971-975.

Whitley RJ, et al. Adenine arabinoside therapy of herpes zoster in the immunosuppressed. N Engl J Med 1976; 294:1193.

Williams DL, Gershon AA, Gelb L et al. Herpes zoster following varicella vaccine in a child with acute lymphocytic leukemia. J. Pediatr 1985;106:259.

Williams V, Gershon AA, Brunell PA. Serologic response to varicella-zoster membrane antigens measured by indirect immunofluorescence. J Infect Dis 1974;130:669.

Winkelmann RK, Perry HO. Herpes zoster in children. JAMA 1959;171:876.

Wright EM, Lipson MJ, Mortimer EA, Jr. Varicella and severe hypoglycemia: a previously undescribed syndrome. Am J Dis Child 1956;92:512.

Young NA, Gershon AA. Chickenpox, measles and mumps. In Remington JS, Klein JO, eds. Infections of the fetus and newborn infant. 2nd ed. Philadelphia: W.B. Saunders Co., 1983, pp 375-427.

Yuceoglu AM, Berkovich S, Minkowitz S. Acute glomerular nephritis as a complication of varicella. JAMA 1967; 202:113.

Zaia JA, Oxman MN. Antibody to varicella-zoster virus-induced membrane antigen: immunofluorescence assay using monodisperse glutaraldehyde-fixed target cells. J Infect Dis 1977;136:519.

Zaia JA, Levin MJ, Preblud SR, et al. Evaluation of varicella-zoster immune globulin: protection of immunosuppressed children after household exposure to varicella. J Infect Dis 1983;147:737-743.

34

DIAGNOSIS OF ACUTE EXANTHEMATOUS DISEASES

Under certain circumstances a physician who examines a patient with a rash is charged with a grave responsibility. An error in diagnosis may have a profound effect on the patient, the contacts, and the community. The following examples (effect on the patient, effect on contacts, and effect on the community) will serve as illustrations.

Effect on the patient

The disease of a patient with meningococcemia was mistakenly diagnosed as measles. Specific therapy was not started early; however, a potential fatality was averted when the disease was finally recognized and treated. Another patient with scarlet fever was said to have rubella. Complicating otitis media could have been prevented if the correct diagnosis had been made and appropriate treatment had been instituted.

Effect on contacts

A classical clinical picture of exanthem subitum in an infant was erroneously labeled as rubella. Under normal circumstances this mistake would have been of little consequence. In this instance, however, the patient's mother was 2 months pregnant and had never had rubella. The error in diagnosis created an unnecessary period of anxiety for the parents who had visions of the future birth of a congenitally malformed infant.

A child with mild measles was said to have rubella. A young sibling contact developed severe measles complicated by pneumonia. This situation could have been prevented by a correct diagnosis that would have dictated the use of gamma globulin to attenuate the sibling's disease.

Effect on the community

On March 5, 1947, a 47-year-old businessman was admitted to a general hospital in New York City because of fever and rash. The initial diagnosis was toxic eruption, and the patient was admitted to a dermatology ward. On March 8 he was transferred to a communicable disease hospital where he subsequently died. The cause of his death proved to be smallpox. A small outbreak of the disease was initiated in the general hospital, spreading out from these foci. In the end there were 12 cases of smallpox and two deaths. There were several additional deaths among the 5 million persons who were vaccinated in New York City. The cost in time, effort, and money was incalculable, and the affairs of the entire city and its inhabitants were seriously disrupted. It is unlikely that a similar situation will occur again because smallpox has been eradicated from the world. However, occasionally an adult with severe hemorrhagic varicella may be erroneously diagnosed as having smallpox.

DIFFERENTIAL DIAGNOSIS

The rashes of various exanthematous diseases are so similar in appearance that they may be clinically indistinguishable. On the other hand, each disease has its characteristic total clinical picture that is distinctive. The differential diagnosis of the acute exanthems is based on a number of factors, including (1) the past history of infectious disease and immunization, (2) type of prodromal period, (3) features of the rash, (4) presence of pathognomonic or other diagnostic signs, and (5) laboratory diagnostic tests.

An attack of many of the exanthematous diseases is followed by permanent immunity. Consequently, a past history of measles, for example, might preclude that diagnosis. However, the history is only as reliable as the memory of the patient or the parent or the accuracy of the original diagnosis.

The character and duration of the prodromal period are also important. Some diseases have a prolonged (4 or more days) prodromal period before the rash appears; in others it may be short or absent. In certain diseases the prodrome is characterized by respiratory tract symptoms; in others, influenza-like symptoms predominate.

The character, distribution, and duration of the rash require evaluation. An eruption may be discrete or confluent and central or peripheral in distribution, and it may persist for 1 to 2 weeks or disappear within 1 day.

Pathognomonic and other signs are always helpful diagnostic clues. Koplik's spots, for example, simplify the recognition of measles.

The final diagnosis in many instances cannot be made on clinical grounds alone. Laboratory diagnostic tests must be employed for identification of the causative agent or for demonstration of the development of specific antibodies.

CLASSIFICATION OF ACUTE EXANTHEMATOUS DISEASES

The acute exanthematous diseases may be conveniently separated into two categories: those characterized by an erythematous maculopapular or punctiform eruption and those characterized by a papulovesicular eruption. These two types of rash are associated with many conditions other than the acute exanthematous diseases. These diseases and other conditions are given in the accompanying lists.

The following diseases and conditions are characterized by a *maculopapular eruption:*

Measles
Atypical measles
Rubella
Scarlet fever

Staphylococcal scalded skin syndrome
Staphylococcal toxic shock syndrome
Meningococcemia
Typhus and tick fevers
Toxoplasmosis
Cytomegalovirus infection
Erythema infectiosum
Exanthem subitum
Enteroviral infections
Infectious mononucleosis
Toxic erythemas
Drug eruptions
Sunburn
Miliaria
Mucocutaneous lymph node syndrome (Kawasaki's disease)

The following diseases and conditions are characterized by a *papulovesicular eruption:*

Varicella-zoster infections
Smallpox
Eczema herpeticum
Eczema vaccinatum
Coxsackie virus infections
Atypical measles
Rickettsialpox
Impetigo
Insect bites
Papular urticaria
Drug eruptions
Molluscum contagiosum
Dermatitis herpetiformis

The preceding lists do not include all the conditions associated with a rash.

DIFFERENTIAL DIAGNOSIS OF MACULOPAPULAR ERUPTIONS

The acute exanthems and other conditions listed previously are frequently or occasionally characterized by a maculopapular eruption. These diseases may be differentiated by a complete evaluation of four of the categories described in this discussion of differential diagnosis: (1) prodromal period, (2) rash, (3) presence of pathognomonic or other diagnostic signs, and (4) laboratory diagnostic tests.

Prodromal period

Measles. As indicated in Fig. 34-1, the rash of measles is preceded by a 3- or 4-day prodromal period of fever, conjunctivitis, coryza, and cough.

Atypical measles. The prodromal period of atypical measles is usually characterized by fe-

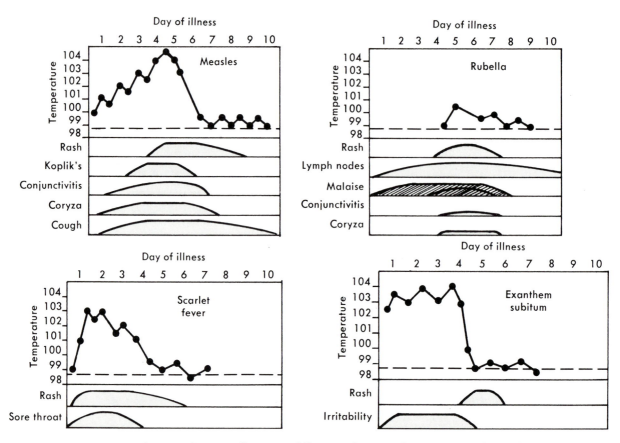

Fig. 34-1. Schematic diagrams illustrating differences between four acute exanthems characterized by maculopapular eruptions.

ver, cough, headache, myalgia, and occasionally pleuritic chest pain preceding the onset of rash by 2 to 4 days.

Rubella. In rubella in children there is usually no prodromal period (Fig. 34-1). The appearance of the rash may be the first obvious sign of illness. Lymphadenopathy that precedes the rash is usually asymptomatic in children. Adolescents and adults may have a variable 1- to 4-day period of malaise and low-grade fever before the rash appears. The temperature may be normal.

Scarlet fever. The rash of scarlet fever occurs within 12 hours of the onset of fever, sore throat, and vomiting. Occasionally the prodromal period may be prolonged to 2 days (Fig. 34-1).

Staphylococcal scalded skin syndrome. Fever and irritability occur at the time of onset of rash in staphylococcal scalded skin syndrome; there is no prodromal period.

Staphylococcal toxic shock syndrome. High fever, headache, confusion, sore throat, vomiting, diarrhea, and shock may precede or may be associated with the rash of staphylococcal toxic shock syndrome.

Meningococcemia with or without meningitis. The prodrome of meningococcemia with or without meningitis is variable. Usually the rash appears within 24 hours. The initial symptoms are fever, vomiting, malaise, irritability, and possibly a stiff neck.

Epidemic and murine typhus. A 4- to 6-day prodromal period precedes the appearance of the rash of epidemic and murine typhus. It is characterized by high fever, chills, headache, and generalized aches and pains.

Rocky Mountain spotted fever. In Rocky Mountain spotted fever the onset of rash is preceded by a 3- to 4-day period of fever, chills, headache, malaise, and anorexia.

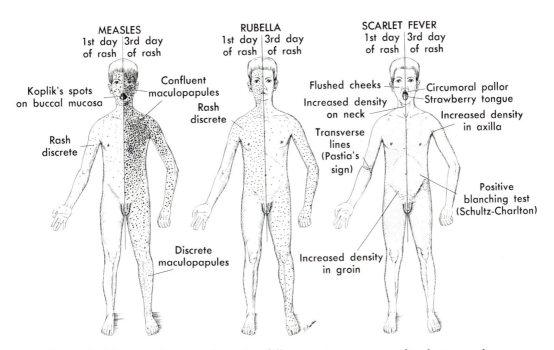

Fig. 34-2. Schematic drawings illustrating differences in appearance, distribution, and progression of rashes of measles, rubella, and scarlet fever.

Erythema infectiosum. In erythema infectiosum no prodromal period is typically present. Usually the first sign of the illness is the appearance of the rash.

Exanthem subitum. A 3- or 4-day prodromal period of high fever and irritability precedes the rash of exanthem subitum, which appears as the temperature falls to normal by crisis (Fig. 34-1).

Enteroviral infections. ECHO virus type 16 infection (Boston exanthem) may have a prodromal period resembling exanthem subitum, but the fever tends to be lower. Fever and constitutional symptoms in ECHO virus types 4, 6, and 9 and in Coxsackie virus infections may precede but usually coincide with the appearance of the rash.

Mucocutaneous lymph node syndrome (Kawasaki's disease). A nonspecific febrile illness with sore throat precedes the rash of mucocutaneous lymph node syndrome by 4 to 6 days.

Toxic erythemas, drug eruptions, sunburn, and miliaria. Toxic erythemas, drug eruptions, sunburn, miliaria, and other noninfectious conditions with a maculopapular eruption do not have prodromal periods.

Rash

Measles. The rash of measles is reddish brown in color, appears on the face and neck first, and progresses downward to involve the trunk and extremities in sequence. As indicated in Fig. 34-2, the eruption is generalized by the third day. The lesions on the face, neck, and upper trunk tend to be confluent; those on the lower trunk and extremities are usually discrete. The eruption fades by the fifth or sixth day, with brownish staining first followed by branny desquamation. The hands and feet do *not* desquamate.

Atypical measles. The rash of atypical measles associated with previous immunization with killed measles vaccine resembles Rocky Mountain spotted fever more than typical measles. The eruption is characterized by erythematous, urticarial, papular, petechial, and purpuric lesions with a predilection for the extremities, especially the hands, wrists, feet, and ankles; occasionally the lesions may be vesicular.

Rubella. The rash of rubella is pink in color, begins on the face and neck, and progresses downward to the trunk and extremities more rapidly than in measles; it becomes generalized within 24 to 48 hours. The lesions are usually discrete rather than confluent, and those that develop first are the earliest to fade. Consequently, on the third day the face is usually clear and only the extremities may be involved. The eruption usually disappears by the end of the third day, and as a rule it does not desquamate. The striking contrast between the distribution of measles and rubella rashes on the third day of eruption is illustrated in Fig. 34-2.

Scarlet fever. The rash of scarlet fever is an erythematous punctiform eruption that blanches on pressure. It appears first on the flexor surfaces and rapidly becomes generalized, usually within 24 hours. The forehead and cheeks are smooth, red, and flushed, but the area around the mouth is pale (circumoral pallor). The lesions are most intense and prominent in the neck, axillary, inguinal, and popliteal skin folds (Fig. 34-2). Desquamation is characteristic, and in contrast to measles, it involves the hands and feet.

Staphylococcal scalded skin syndrome. In staphylococcal scalded skin syndrome the rash is a generalized, erythematous, scarlatiniform eruption; it has a sandpaperlike texture. The erythema is accentuated in the skin folds, simulating Pastia's lines. The skin is tender. The course of the rash is different from that of scarlet fever. Within 1 to 2 days bullae may appear, and the epidermis may separate into large sheets revealing a moist, red, shiny surface beneath. In contrast, the pattern of desquamation is different in scarlet fever; it occurs 1 to 2 weeks later and is characterized by fine, branny flakes or thin sheets of skin.

Staphylococcal toxic shock syndrome. The rash of staphylococcal toxic shock syndrome is scarlatiniform in appearance; it occurs most prominently on the trunk and extremities and is associated with edema of the face and limbs and desquamation.

Meningococcemia. In meningococcemia an early, transient maculopapular eruption may precede the petechial, purpuric rash, which often is present when the patient seeks medical attention. In contrast to measles, this early exanthem has no regular, predictable distribution.

Epidemic and murine typhus. The characteristic rash of epidemic and murine typhus is a maculopapular and petechial eruption that has a *central* distribution. The face, palms, and soles are not involved as a rule.

Rocky Mountain spotted fever. The eruption of Rocky Mountain spotted fever is maculopapular and petechial, with a *peripheral* distribution. The palms and soles are usually involved, and occasionally the face also may be affected.

Erythema infectiosum. The afebrile patient with asymptomatic erythema infectiosum develops a characteristic rash that erupts in three stages in the following sequence: (1) red, flushed cheeks with circumoral pallor (slapped-cheek appearance); (2) maculopapular eruption over upper and lower extremities (the rash assumes a lacelike appearance as it fades); and (3) an evanescent stage characterized by subsidence of the eruption, followed by a recurrence precipitated by a variety of skin irritants.

Exanthem subitum. The lesions of exanthem subitum are typically discrete rose-red maculopapules that frequently appear on the chest and trunk first and then spread to involve the face and extremities. The eruption usually disappears within 2 days. Occasionally it fades within several hours.

Enteroviral infections. The rashes of ECHO virus and Coxsackie virus infections are often rubella-like in appearance. The lesions are usually maculopapular, discrete, nonpruritic, and generalized. Unlike measles, desquamation and staining do not occur. Petechial lesions suggesting meningococcemia may rarely be noted in ECHO virus type 9 and group A Coxsackie virus type 9 infections.

Mucocutaneous lymph node syndrome (Kawasaki's disease). In mucocutaneous lymph node syndrome there is a generalized erythematous rash with elements of macules and papules. The palms and soles are swollen and reddened, eventually peeling after several days or weeks. Dryness with erythema of the lips, mouth, and tongue accompanies bilateral conjunctival injection.

Drug eruptions and toxic erythemas. Drug eruptions and toxic erythemas may be characterized by maculopapular eruptions that may simulate any of the diseases listed previously.

Sunburn. Sunburn may be confused with the rash of scarlet fever, particularly if there is a coincident sore throat. The eruption is confined to the area not protected by a bathing suit.

Miliaria. The fine punctiform lesions of miliaria are chiefly confined to the flexor areas. The rash is usually not generalized, and it does not desquamate as a rule.

Presence of pathognomonic or other diagnostic signs

Measles. Koplik's spots are pathognomonic for measles.

Atypical measles. Atypical measles is frequently associated with roentgen evidence of pneumonia and occasionally with pleural effusion.

Rubella. In rubella, lymphadenopathy, particularly postauricular and occipital, is a common manifestation, but it also occurs in other diseases.

Scarlet fever. A strawberry tongue and exudative or membranous tonsillitis are typical of scarlet fever.

Staphylococcal scalded skin syndrome. An associated staphylococcal infection, such as impetigo or purulent conjunctivitis, may be present with staphylococcal scalded skin syndrome. Nikolsky's sign is present.

Staphylococcal toxic shock syndrome. The scarlatiniform eruption of staphylococcal toxic shock syndrome is associated with high fever, toxicity, and shocklike state.

Meningococcemia. A petechial purpuric eruption associated with meningeal signs would point to meningococcemia.

Epidemic and murine typhus. A maculopapular petechial eruption centrally distributed in a person living in an area where epidemic typhus is endemic is suggestive of the disease.

Rocky Mountain spotted fever. A history of a recent tick bite in a person with a maculopapular, petechial, peripherally distributed eruption is characteristic of Rocky Mountain spotted fever.

Toxoplasmosis. The acquired infection of toxoplasmosis may be characterized by one or more of the following syndromes: (1) fever, pneumonitis, and rash, (2) lymphadenopathy, (3) encephalitis, and (4) chorioretinitis.

Erythema infectiosum. Erythema infectiosum is suggested by the slapped-face appearance in a well child.

Enteroviral infections. The rash of enteroviral infections may be associated with aseptic meningitis. The infections occur most commonly during the summer and fall months.

Infectious mononucleosis. A triad of membranous tonsillitis, lymphadenopathy, and splenomegaly suggests infectious mononucleosis as a possibility.

Laboratory diagnostic tests

Measles. The measles hemagglutination-inhibition (HI) test is the most practical diagnostic test. The pattern of appearance of antibody is shown in Fig. 13-4. A fourfold or greater rise in measles HI antibody is detected during convalescence; the peak titer usually ranges between 1:256 and 1:1024. The blood picture typically shows leukopenia.

Atypical measles. Extraordinary rises in measles HI antibody have been detected within 2 weeks after onset of atypical measles. The titers may exceed 1:100,000.

Rubella. As indicated in Fig. 24-4, a positive throat culture for rubella virus and evidence of a rise in antibody level are helpful diagnostic aids. The blood picture shows either a normal or low white blood cell count.

Scarlet fever. Group A hemolytic streptococci may be cultured from the nasopharynx. There is usually a rise in antistreptolysin O titer.

Staphylococcal scalded skin syndrome. A culture of skin or other sites of infection is positive for phage group II staphylococci in staphylococcal scalded skin syndrome.

Staphylococcal toxic shock syndrome. Cultures of various mucosal surfaces or purulent lesions should be positive for phage group I *Staphylococcus aureus* in staphylococcal toxic shock syndrome.

Meningococcemia. The microorganism causing meningococcemia may be observed on Gram stain and recovered from the blood, spinal fluid, or petechiae.

Epidemic and murine typhus. The Weil-Felix agglutination reaction with *Proteus* OX-19 is positive. A specific complement fixation test is available for epidemic and murine typhus.

Rocky Mountain spotted fever. The Weil-Felix agglutination reaction with *Proteus* OX-19 and OX-2 is positive. Thrombocytopenia, hyponatremia, and hypoalbuminemia are common. A specific Rocky Mountain spotted fever complement fixation test is available.

Toxoplasmosis. A rise in *Toxoplasma* antibody titer during convalescence indicates acute toxoplasmosis.

Erythema infectiosum. No diagnostic test is available for erythema infectiosum.

Exanthem subitum. There is no diagnostic test for exanthem subitum. The blood picture shows leukopenia when the rash appears.

Enteroviral infections. ECHO viruses and Coxsackie viruses may be recovered from stools, throat, blood, or cerebrospinal fluid (CSF). The diagnosis is confirmed by demonstrating a rise in neutralizing antibody titer to the specific virus.

Infectious mononucleosis. In infectious mononucleosis the blood smear is positive for abnormal lymphocytes. The monospot test and heterophil agglutination test are positive. Results of liver function tests, such as aminotransferases, are abnormal. Epstein-Barr virus antibody appears during convalescence.

DIFFERENTIAL DIAGNOSIS OF PAPULOVESICULAR ERUPTIONS

The acute exanthems and other conditions listed on p. 455 are usually characterized by a papulovesicular eruption. The following differ-ential criteria are similar to those employed for the maculopapular eruptions.

Prodromal period

Varicella. As indicated in Fig. 34-3, a prodromal period is usually absent in chickenpox. The rash and constitutional symptoms, particularly in children, occur simultaneously. In adolescents and adults, however, there may be a 1- or 2-day prodromal period of fever, headache, malaise, and anorexia.

Smallpox. The smallpox rash is preceded by a 3-day period of chills, headache, backache, and severe malaise (Fig. 34-3). A transient rash with bathing-trunks distribution may occur during the prodrome.

Herpes simplex, herpes zoster, and vaccinia. Herpes simplex, herpes zoster, and vaccinia occur without any prodromal period (eczema vaccinatum and herpeticum, Fig. 34-3).

Rickettsialpox. In rickettsialpox a generalized papulovesicular eruption is preceded by the de-

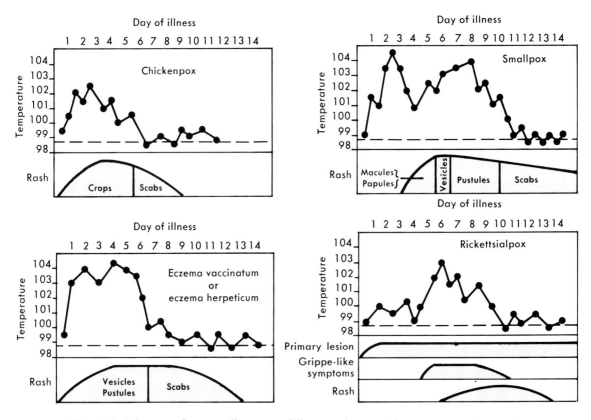

Fig. 34-3. Schematic diagrams illustrating differences between four acute exanthems characterized by papulovesicular eruptions.

velopment of (1) an initial lesion (an eschar) and (2) an influenzalike syndrome (Fig. 34-3).

Rash

Varicella. The rash of chickenpox is characterized by (1) *rapid* evolution of macules to papules to vesicles to crusts, (2) central distribution of lesions, which appear in crops (Fig. 34-4), (3) presence of lesions in all stages in any one anatomic area, (4) presence of scalp and mucous membrane lesions, and (5) eventual crusting of nearly all the skin lesions.

Smallpox. The rash of smallpox is characterized by (1) *slow* evolution of macules to papules to vesicles to pustules to crusts, (2) peripheral distribution of lesions, which are most prominent on the exposed skin surfaces (Fig. 34-4), (3) presence of lesions in the same stage in any one anatomic area, and (4) skin lesions that are more deep seated than those of varicella.

Eczema herpeticum and vaccinatum. In eczema herpeticum and vaccinatum the vesicular and pustular lesions are most profuse on the sites of eczema. Mouth and scalp lesions are generally absent. (See Plate 6.)

Herpes zoster. The lesions of herpes zoster are unilateral and distributed along the line of the affected nerves; vesicles are grouped together and tend to become confluent.

Atypical measles. The papulovesicular lesions of atypical measles may appear on the face and the trunk. During the crusting phase they resemble varicella. This eruption may or may not be associated with the characteristic maculopapular eruption that resembles Rocky Mountain spotted fever in its peripheral distribution.

Rickettsialpox. The primary lesion of rickettsialpox is an eschar that measures 1.5 cm or more in diameter. The generalized papulovesicular eruption is made up of tiny vesicles superimposed on a firm papule. The vesicles are much smaller than those of chickenpox. Many lesions do not crust.

Impetigo. The lesions of impetigo, at first vesicular, become confluent and rapidly progress to the pustular and crusting stage. They do not appear in crops, they commonly involve the nasolabial area and other sites available for scratching, and they do not involve the oral mucous membranes.

Insect bites and papular urticaria. Insect bites and papular urticaria do not have a typical vesicular appearance and do not involve the scalp or mucous membranes.

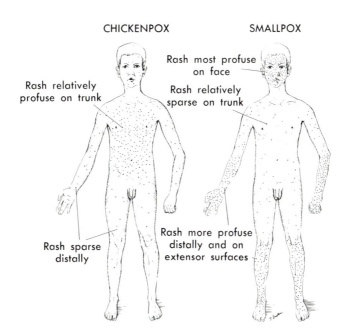

Fig. 34-4. Schematic drawings illustrating differences in distribution of rashes of chickenpox and smallpox.

Molluscum contagiosum. The lesions of molluscum contagiosum are scattered, discrete, firm, small nodular el_____ rounding red areolae.

Dermatitis herpetiforn_____
petiformis is characterized_____
papulovesicular lesions that a_____
distribution, by a chronic course, and by hea_____
with residual pigmentation.

Laboratory diagnostic tests

Varicella. The virus of varicella is isolated from vesicular fluid. Detection of specific varicella-zoster (V-Z) antibody during convalescence is accomplished by means of one of the following tests: complement fixation (CF), fluorescent antibody to membrane antigen (FAMA), immune adherence hemagglutination antibody (IAHA), or enzyme linked immunosorbent assay (ELISA).

Smallpox. The virus of smallpox may be identified by electron microscopy or gel diffusion.

Smallpox vesicular fluid may be used as antigen for a CF test. A rise in the level of CF or HI
_____
_____

1____
demo____

Eczen____
eczema vaccinatum a____
smallpox.

Herpes zoster. The laboratory tests for herpes zoster are the same as those for chickenpox.

Rickettsialpox. The isolation of *Rickettsia akari* from the blood may be achieved by inoculation of the yolk sac of embryonated eggs. The rise in the level of rickettsialpox and Rocky Mountain spotted fever CF antibodies occurs during convalescence.

35

ACTIVE IMMUNIZATION FOR THE PREVENTION OF INFECTIOUS DISEASES

Vaccines for prevention of the 18 infectious diseases listed below have been licensed by the Office of Biologics of the Food and Drug Administration (FDA).

BCG
Cholera
Diphtheria
H. influenzae, type b
Hepatitis B
Influenza
Measles
Meningococcus
Mumps
Pertussis
Plague
Poliomyelitis
Rabies
Rubella
Smallpox
Tetanus
Typhoid fever
Typhus fever
Yellow fever

Recommendations for the use of these vaccines are reviewed periodically by at least two committees: the Public Health Service on Immunization Practices Advisory Committee (ACIP) and the Committee on Infectious Diseases of the American Academy of Pediatrics (AAP). A close liaison exists between representatives of the FDA, ACIP, and AAP. The final recommendations for the use of various vaccines usually represent the consensus of the committees based on their evaluation of the available current data. The acquisition of new knowledge about vaccines and significant changes in the epidemiologic aspects of the various infectious diseases provide the basis for modifications of the recommendations.

The ACIP is sponsored by the Centers for Disease Control. The recommendations that are developed and revised are published in the Centers of Disease Control *Morbidity and Mortality Weekly Report*. The recommendations of the Committee on Infectious Diseases of the AAP are published by the Academy in the so-called Red Book. The 1982 report was the nineteenth edition since the first issue in 1938. Revisions of special sections are published periodically in AAP Newsletters.

This chapter includes the collected recommendations of the ACIP. The statement about each of the 19 diseases includes the dates of the revisions. In addition, a brief list of selected references is appended to each statement. In general, these recommendations are essentially the same as those proposed by the AAP Committee on Infectious Diseases. However, occasionally, minor differences may be noted because the ACIP is concerned chiefly with public health and the AAP Committee is concerned with pediatric and general practice as well.

GENERAL RECOMMENDATIONS ON IMMUNIZATION

This 1983 revision of the "General Recommenda-

ments by public health officials and specialists in clinical and preventive medicine. Benefits and risks are associated with the use of all products—no vaccine is completely safe or completely effective. The benefits range from partial to complete protection from the consequences of disease, and the risks range from common, trivial, and inconvenient side effects to rare, severe, and life-threatening conditions. Thus, recommendations on immunization practices balance scientific evidence of benefits, costs, and risks to achieve optimal levels of protection against infectious or communicable diseases.

These recommendations describe this balance and attempt to minimize the risk by providing specific advice regarding dose, route, and spacing of immunobiologics and by delineating situations warranting precautions or contraindicating their use. These recommendations may apply only in the United States, as epidemiological circumstances and vaccines may differ in other countries. The relative balance of benefits and risks may change as diseases are brought under control or eradicated. For example, because smallpox has been eradicated throughout the world, the very small risk from smallpox vaccine now exceeds the risk of smallpox; consequently, smallpox vaccination of civilians is now indicated only for laboratory workers directly involved with smallpox or closely related orthopox viruses (e.g., monkeypox, vaccinia, and others).

Definitions

A. Immunobiologic. Immunobiologics include vaccines, toxoids, and antibody containing preparations from human or animal donors, including globulins and antitoxins. These products are used for immunization.

1. *Vaccine:* A suspension of attenuated live or killed microorganisms (bacteria, viruses, or rick-

ettsiae), or fractions thereof administered to induce immunity and thereby prevent infectious disease.

Hepatitis B Immune Globulin (HBIG), Varicella Zoster Immune Globulin (VZIG), Rabies Immune Globulin (RIG), and Tetanus Immune Globulin (TIG).

5. *Antitoxin:* A solution of antibodies derived from the serum of animals immunized with specific antigens (diphtheria, tetanus) used to achieve passive immunity or to effect a treatment.

B. Vaccination and immunization. Today, these terms are often used interchangeably. The words *vaccination* and *vaccine* derive from vaccinia, the cowpox virus once used as smallpox vaccine. Thus, *vaccination* originally meant the inoculation of vaccinia virus to render individuals immune to smallpox. Some people still prefer that the term *vaccination* be restricted to this use, but many have come to use the term in a more general sense, to denote the administration of any vaccine or toxoid without regard to whether the recipient is successfully made immune.

Immunization is a more inclusive term denoting the process of inducing or providing immunity artificially by administering an immunobiologic. Immunization can be *active* or *passive*.

Active immunization denotes the production of antibody or antitoxin in response to the adminstration of a vaccine or toxoid. *Passive immunization* denotes the provision of temporary immunity by the administration of preformed antitoxin or antibodies (e.g., immunoglobulin, maternal antibodies). Three types of immunobiologics are used for passive immunization: (1) pooled human IG, (2) specific IG preparations, and (3) antitoxin.

Although there is lack of consensus that vaccination and immunization are completely synonymous, these words are used interchangeably in ACIP statements when referring to active immunization. Regardless of which term is used, it must be emphasized that administration of an immunobiologic cannot be automatically equated with the development of (or conferring of) adequate immunity because of a variety of specific factors, many of which are discussed in this statement.

---

*Replaces previous recommendations on this subject in MMWR 1980;29:76, 81-83.

C. Antigen(s). Substance(s) inducing the formation of antibodies. In some vaccines, the antigen is highly defined (e.g., pneumococcal polysaccharide, hepatitis B surface antigen, tetanus or diphtheria toxoids); in others, it is complex or incompletely defined (e.g., killed pertussis bacteria, live, attenuated viruses).

Immunobiologics

The specific nature and content of immunobiologics may differ. When immunobiologics against the same infectious agents are produced by different manufacturers, active and inert ingredients among the various products may differ. Practitioners are urged to become familiar with the constituents of the products they use. The constituents of immunobiologics include:

A. Suspending fluid. This frequently is as simple as sterile water or saline, but it may be a complex fluid containing small amounts of proteins or other constituents derived from the medium or biologic system in which the vaccine is produced (serum proteins, egg antigens, cell-culture-derived antigens).

B. Preservatives, stabilizers, antibiotics. These components of vaccines are used to inhibit or prevent bacterial growth in viral culture or the final product, or to stabilize the antigen. They include such materials as mercurials and specific antibiotics. Allergic reactions may occur if the recipient is sensitive to one of these additives.

C. Adjuvants. An aluminum compound is used in some vaccines to enhance the immune response to vaccines containing inactivated microorganisms or their products (e.g., toxoids and hepatitis B virus vaccine). Vaccines with such adjuvants must be injected deeply in muscle masses, since subcutaneous or intracutaneous administration may cause local irritation, inflammation, granuloma formation, or necrosis.

Route, site, and technique of immunization

A. Route. There is a recommended route of administration of each immunobiologic. To avoid unnecessary local or systemic effects and/or ensure optimal efficacy, the practitioner should not deviate from the recommended route of administration.

B. Site. Injectable immunobiologics should be administered in an area where there is minimal opportunity for local, neural, vascular, or tissue injury. Subcutaneous injections are usually administered into the thigh of infants and in the deltoid area of older children and adults. Intradermal injections are generally given on the volar surface of the forearms, except for human diploid cell rabies vaccine, with which reactions are less severe in the deltoid area.

In the past, the upper, outer quadrant of the buttocks was the usual site of intramuscular vaccination. The buttocks should not be routinely used as a vaccination site for infants and children; and, to avoid injury to the sciatic nerves, they are generally not used in adults. The central region of the buttocks should be avoided for all injections; the upper, outer quadrant should be used only for the largest volumes of injection or when multiple doses need to be given, such as when large doses of IG must be administered. The site selected should be well into the upper, outer mass of the gluteus maximus and away from the central region of the buttocks.

Currently, preferred sites for intramuscular injections are the anterolateral aspect of the upper thigh and the deltoid muscle of the upper arm. In most infants, the anterolateral aspect of the thigh provides the largest muscle mass and, therefore, is the preferred site. In older children, the deltoid mass is of sufficient size for intramuscular injection. An individual decision must be made for each child, based on the volume of the injected material and the size of the muscle into which it is to be injected. Many practitioners prefer to continue using the anterolateral thigh until age 3 years before switching to the deltoid area. In adults, the deltoid is generally used for routine intramuscular vaccine administration.

C. Techniques. Before giving the injection, the needle is inserted in the site, and the syringe plunger is pulled back to see if blood appears; if so, the needle should be withdrawn and a new site selected. The same procedure is followed until no blood appears. A separate needle and syringe should be used for each injection. Disposable needles and syringes should be discarded in labeled containers to prevent accidental inoculation or theft. If more than one vaccine preparation is administered, each should be given at a different site.

Dosage

The recommended doses of immunobiologics are derived from theoretical considerations, experimental trials, and clinical experience. Administration of dose volumes smaller than those recommended, such as split doses or intradermal administration (unless specifically recommended), may result in inadequate protection. Exceeding the recommended dose volumes might be hazardous because of excessive local or systemic concentrations of antigens.

Some practitioners use divided doses of vaccine (particularly diphtheria and tetanus toxoids and pertussis vaccine [DTP]) to reduce reaction rates. There has not been adequate study of the efficacy of such practices by serologic confirmation or clinical efficacy or of the effects on the subsequent frequency and severity of adverse reactions. The Committee does not recommend dividing doses of any vaccine.

Age at which immunobiologics are administered

Several factors influence recommendations concerning the age at which vaccine is administered (Tables 35-1 to 35-3). These include: age-specific risks of disease, age-specific risks of complications, ability

Table 35-1. Recommended schedule for active immunization of normal infants and children (See individual ACIP recommendations for details).

†For all products used, consult manufacturer's package enclosure for instructions for storage, handling, and administration; immunobiologics prepared by different manufacturers may vary, and those of the same manufacturer may change from time to time. The package insert should be followed for a specific product.

§DTP–Diphtheria and tetanus toxoids and pertussis vaccine.

¶OPV–Oral, attenuated poliovirus vaccine contains poliovirus types 1, 2, and 3;

**Simultaneous administration of MMR, DTP, and OPV is appropriate for patients whose compliance with medical care recommendations cannot be assured.

††MMR–Live measles, mumps, and rubella viruses in a combined vaccine (see text for discussion of single vaccines versus combination).

§§Up to the seventh birthday.

¶¶Td–Adult tetanus toxoid and diphtheria toxoid in combination, which contains the same dose of tetanus toxoid as DTP or DT and a reduced dose of diphtheria toxoid.

Table 35-2. Recommended immunization schedule for infants and children up to 7th birthday not immunized at the recommended time in early infancy* (See individual ACIP recommendations for details.)

Timing	Vaccine(s)	Comments
First visit	DTP-1† OPV-1 § (if child is ≥15 mo. of age, MMR¶)	DTP, OPV, and MMR can be administered simultaneously to children ≥ 15 mo. of age
2 mo. after first DTP, OPV	DTP-2, OPV-2	
2 mo. after second DTP	DTP-3	An additional dose of OPV at this time is optional for use in areas with a high risk of polio exposure
6-12 mo. after third DTP	DTP-4, OPV-3	
Preschool** (4-6 yr.)	DTP-5, OPV-4	Preferably at or before school entry
14-16 yr.	Td††	Repeat every 10 years throughout life

*If initiated in the first year of life, give DTP-1, 2, and 3, OPV-1 and 2 according to this schedule and give MMR when the child becomes 15 months old.

†DTP–Diphtheria and tetanus toxoids with pertussis. DTP may be used up to the seventh birthday.

§OPV–Oral, attenuated poliovirus vaccine contains poliovirus types 1, 2, and 3.

¶MMR–Live measles, mumps, and rubella viruses in a combined vaccine (see text for discussion of single vaccines versus combination).

**The preschool dose is not necessary if the fourth dose of DTP and third dose of OPV are administered after the fourth birthday.

††Td–Adult tetanus toxoid and diphtheria toxoid in combination, which contains the same dose of tetanus toxoid as DTP or DT and a reduced dose of diphtheria toxoid.

Table 35-3. Recommended immunization schedule for persons 7 years of age or older (See individual ACIP recommendations for details.)

Timing	Vaccine(s)	Comments
First visit	Td-1,* OPV-1† and MMR§	OPV not routinely administered to those ≥ 18 years of age
2 mo. after first Td, OPV	Td-2, OPV-2	
6-12 mo. after second Td, OPV	Td-3, OPV-3	OPV-3 may be given as soon as 6 weeks after OPV-2
10 years after Td-3	Td	Repeat every 10 years throughout life

*Td–Tetanus and diphtheria toxoids (adult type) are used after the seventh birthday. The DTP doses given to children under 6 who remain incompletely immunized at age 7 or older should be counted as prior exposure to tetanus and diphtheria toxoids (e.g. a child who previously received 2 doses of DTP, only needs 1 dose of Td to complete a primary series).
†OPV–Oral, attenuated poliovirus vaccine contains poliovirus types 1, 2, and 3. When polio vaccine is to be given to individuals 18 years or older, IPV is preferred. See ACIP statement on polio vaccine for immunization schedule for IPV.
§MMR–Live measles, mumps, and rubella viruses in a combined vaccine. Persons born before 1957 can generally be considered immune to measles and mumps and need not be immunized. Rubella vaccine may be given to persons of any age, particularly to women of childbearing age. MMR may be used since administration of vaccine to persons already immune is not deleterious. (See text for discussion of single vaccines versus combination.)

of individuals of a given age to respond to the vaccine(s), and potential interference with the immune response by passively transferred maternal antibody. In general, vaccines are recommended for the youngest age group at risk with an acceptable level of antibody response following vaccine administration. For example, while infants as young as 6 months of age may be at risk for measles, most are protected by maternal antibody, which may inhibit successful active immunization at this age. In the United States, measles vaccine is routinely administered at 15 months of age, by which time maternal antibody is no longer detectable.

In certain measles epidemics, public health officials may recommend measles vaccine for infants as young as 6 months of age. Although a smaller proportion of those given vaccine before the first birthday develop antibody to measles, compared with older infants, the higher risk of disease during an epidemic may justify earlier immunization. Such infants should be reimmunized at the recommended age for measles vaccination to achieve protection.

Spacing of immunobiologics

A. Multiple doses of same antigen. Some products require more than one dose for full protection. In addition, it is necessary to give periodic reinforcement (booster) doses of some preparations to maintain protection. In recommending the ages and/or intervals for multiple doses, the Committee takes into account current risks from disease and the objective of inducing satisfactory protection. Intervals between doses that are longer than those recommended do not lead to a reduction in final antibody levels. Therefore,

it is unnecessary to restart an interrupted series of an immunobiologic or to add extra doses. By contrast, giving doses of a vaccine or toxoid at less than recommended intervals may lessen the antibody response; doses given at less than recommended intervals should not be counted as part of a primary series.

B. Different antigens. Experimental evidence and extensive clinical experience have strengthened the scientific basis for giving certain vaccines at the same time. Most of the widely used antigens can safely and effectively be given simultaneously. This knowledge is particularly helpful in circumstances that include imminent exposure to several infectious diseases, preparation for foreign travel, or uncertainty that the patient will return for further doses of vaccine.

In general, inactivated vaccines can be administered simultaneously at separate sites. It should be noted, however, that when vaccines commonly associated with local or systemic side effects (such as cholera, typhoid, and plague vaccines) are given simultaneously, the side effects theoretically might be accentuated. When practical, these vaccines should be given on separate occasions.

Field observations indicate that simultaneous administration (on the same day) of the most widely used live-virus vaccines has not resulted in impaired antibody response or increased rates of adverse reactions. Observation of children indicates that antibody responses to trivalent oral polio vaccine (OPV) given simultaneously with licensed combination measles-mumps-rubella (MMR) vaccine are comparable to those obtained when the same vaccines are given at separate visits. It is reasonable to expect equivalent immunologic responses when other licensed combination or live, attenuated-virus vaccines or their component antigens are given simultaneously with OPV. While data are lacking on potential interference with

C. Immune globulin. Immune globulin (IG,) formerly called Immune Serum Globulin, [ISG] and various specific immune globulins contain antibodies

Data on the response to simultaneous administration of diphtheria and tetanus toxoids and pertussis vaccine (DTP), OPV, and MMR vaccine are lacking. However, field experience and antibody data regarding simultaneous administration of either DTP and measles vaccine or DTP and OPV indicate that the protective response is satisfactory and adverse reactions do not increase. Therefore, simultaneous administration of all these antigens is recommended when individuals require multiple antigens and there is doubt that the recipient will return to receive further doses of vaccine. Children 15 months of age or older who have received fewer than the recommended number of DTP and OPV doses fall into this category (Table 35-2). Simultaneous administration of pneumococcal polysaccharide vaccine and whole-virus influenza vaccine gives a satisfactory antibody response without increasing the occurrence of adverse reactions. Simultaneous administration of the pneumococcal vaccine and split-virus influenza vaccine may also be expected to yield satisfactory results. However, it should be kept in mind that influenza vaccine should be administered annually to the target population, whereas, under current recommendations, pneumococcal polysaccharide vaccine should only be administered in a single dose.

An inactivated vaccine and a live, attenuated-virus vaccine can be administered simultaneously at separate sites, with the precautions that apply to the individual vaccines. Some data suggest that the simultaneous administration of cholera and yellow fever vaccines may interfere with the immune response to each other. Decreased levels of antibodies have been observed when the vaccines are administered within 3 weeks of each other, compared with administration of the vaccines at longer intervals. However, there is no evidence that protection to either of these diseases diminishes when these vaccines are administered simultaneously. Therefore, the Committee believes that yellow fever and cholera vaccines can be administered simultaneously, if necessary.

least 6 weeks, but preferably 3 months after the administration of IG. Preliminary data indicate that IG does not interfere with the immune response either to OPV or yellow fever vaccine.

If IG administration becomes necessary after a live vaccine has been given, interference may occur. In general, vaccine virus replication and stimulation of immunity will occur within 7 to 10 days. Thus, if the interval between vaccine and IG is less than 14 days, vaccine should be repeated about 3 months after IG was given, unless serologic testing indicates that antibodies have been produced; if the interval was longer, vaccine need not be readministered. If administration of IG becomes necessary because of imminent exposure to disease, live virus vaccines may be administered simultaneously with IG, with the recognition that vaccine-induced immunity may be compromised. The vaccine should be administered in a site remote from that chosen for IG inoculation. Vaccination should be repeated about 3 months later, unless serologic testing indicates antibodies have been produced.

Hypersensitivity to vaccine components

Vaccine antigens produced in systems or with substrates containing allergenic substances, e.g., antigens derived from growing microorganisms in embryonated chicken eggs, may cause hypersensitivity reactions. These reactions may include anaphylaxis when the final vaccine contains a substantial amount of the allergen. Yellow fever vaccine is such an antigen. Vaccines with such characteristics should not be given to persons with known hypersensitivity to components of the substrates. Contrary to this generalization, influenza vaccine antigens (whole or split), although prepared from viruses grown in embryonated eggs, are highly purified during preparation and have only very rarely been reported to be associated with hypersensitivity reactions.

Live virus vaccines prepared by growing viruses in cell cultures are essentially devoid of potentially allergenic substances related to host tissue. On very rare occasions, hypersensitivity reactions to measles vaccine have been reported in persons with anaphylactic hypersensitivity to eggs. Measles vaccine, however, can be given safely to egg-allergic individuals provided the allergies are not manifested by anaphylactic symptoms. Since mumps vaccine is grown in similar cell cultures, the same precautions apply.

Screening persons by history of ability to eat eggs without adverse effects is a reasonable way to identify those possibly at risk from receiving measles, mumps and influenza vaccine. Individuals with anaphylactic hypersensitivity to eggs (hives, swelling of the mouth and throat, difficulty breathing, hypotension, or shock)* should not be given these vaccines.

Rubella vaccine is grown in human diploid cell culture and can be safely given, regardless of a history of allergy to eggs or egg proteins.

Bacterial vaccines, such as cholera, DTP, plague, and typhoid, are frequently associated with local or systemic adverse effects; these common reactions do not appear to be allergic.

Some vaccines contain preservatives (e.g., thimerosal, a mercurial) or trace amounts of antibiotics (e.g., neomycin) to which patients may be hypersensitive. Those administering vaccines should carefully review the information provided with the package insert before deciding whether the rare patients with known hypersensitivity to such preservatives or antibiotics should be given the vaccine(s). No currently recommended vaccine contains penicillin or its derivatives.

Some vaccines (e.g., MMR vaccine or its individual component vaccines) contain trace amounts of neomycin. This amount is less than would usually be used for the skin test to determine hypersensitivity. Persons who have experienced anaphylactic reactions to neomycin should not receive these vaccines. Most often, neomycin allergy is contact dermatitis, a manifestation of a delayed-type (cell-mediated) immune response rather than anaphylaxis. In such individuals, the adverse reaction, if any, to neomycin in the vaccines would be an erythematous, pruritic papule at 48-96 hours. A history of delayed-type reactions to neomycin is not a contraindication to receiving these vaccines.

Altered immunocompetence

Virus replication after administration of live, attenuated-virus vaccines may be enhanced in persons with immune deficiency diseases, and in those with suppressed capability for immune response, as occurs with leukemia, lymphoma, generalized malignancy, or therapy with corticosteroids, alkylating agents,

---

*Any of these signs or symptoms constitutes a systemic anaphylactic response.

antimetabolites, or radiation. Patients with such conditions should not be given live, attenuated-virus vaccines. Because of the possibility of familial immunodeficiency, live, attenuated-virus vaccines should not be given to a member of a household in which there is a family history of congenital or hereditary immunodeficiency until the immune competence of the potential recipient is known. OPV should not be given to a member of a household in which there is a family history of immunodeficiency or immunosuppression, regardless whether acquired or hereditary, until the immune status of the recipient and the other family members is known. Individuals residing in the household of an immunocompromised individual should not receive OPV, because vaccine viruses are excreted by the recipient of the vaccine and may be communicable to other persons.

Severe febrile illnesses

Minor illnesses, such as mild upper-respiratory infections, should not postpone vaccine administration. However, immunization of persons with severe febrile illnesses should generally be deferred until they have recovered. This precaution is to avoid superimposing adverse effects from the vaccine on the underlying illness or mistakenly identifying a manifestation of the underlying illness as a result of the vaccine. In persons whose compliance with medical care cannot be assured, it is particularly important to take every opportunity to provide appropriate vaccinations.

Vaccination during pregnancy

On the grounds of a theoretical risk to the developing fetus, live, attenuated-virus vaccines are not generally given to pregnant women or those likely to become pregnant within 3 months after receiving vaccine(s). With some of these vaccines—particularly rubella, measles, and mumps—pregnancy is a contraindication. Both yellow fever vaccine and OPV can be given to pregnant women at substantial risk of exposure to natural infection. When vaccine is to be given during pregnancy, waiting until the second or third trimester to minimize any concern over teratogenicity is a reasonable precaution. If a pregnant woman receives a live, attenuated-virus vaccine, there is not necessarily any real risk to the fetus. In particular, although there are theoretical risks in giving rubella vaccine during pregnancy, data on previously and currently available rubella vaccines indicate that the risk, if any, of teratogenicity from live rubella vaccine is quite small. There has been no evidence of congenital rubella syndrome in infants born to susceptible mothers who received rubella vaccine during pregnancy.

Since persons given measles, mumps, or rubella vaccine viruses do not transmit them, these vaccines may be administered with safety to children of pregnant women. Although live polio virus is shed by children recently immunized with OPV (particularly

less vaccine is otherwise contraindicated.

Official health agencies should take whatever steps are necessary, including development and enforce-

tion of pregnant women with IG (see below). For further information regarding immunization of pregnant women, refer to the American College of Obstetricians and Gynecologists (ACOG) Technical Bulletin Number 14, May 1982.

Adverse events following immunization*

Modern vaccines are extremely safe and effective, but not completely so. Adverse events following immunization have been reported with all vaccines. These range from frequent, minor, local reactions to extremely rare, severe, systemic illness such as paralysis associated with OPV. To improve knowledge about adverse reactions, all temporally associated events severe enough to require the recipient to seek medical attention should be evaluated and reported in detail to local or state health officials and to the vaccine manufacturer. It is frequently impossible to establish cause-and-effect relationships when untoward events occur after receiving vaccine(s) since temporal association alone does not necessarily indicate causation.

Disease control through continuing programs

The best means of reducing the occurrence of vaccine-preventable diseases of childhood (diphtheria, pertussis, tetanus, polio, measles, mumps, and rubella) is by having a highly immune population. Universal immunization is an important part of good health care and should be accomplished through routine and intensive programs carried out in physicians' offices and public health clinics. Programs aimed at ensuring that all children are immunized at the recommended age should be established and maintained in all communities. In addition, all other susceptible persons (regardless of age) should be immunized, un-

ness of the need for vaccines. The Committee recommends the use of these standard records by all health care providers.

A permanent, comprehensive immunization record should be established for each newborn infant and maintained by the parent. Physicians should encourage parents to use the record and should record all immunization data. Parents or guardians should be urged to bring the record every time the child sees a health care provider. Health care providers should review the immunization status of children at each visit. At a minumum, the type of immunobiologic administered and the date of administration should be entered into the patient's immunization record.

Maintenance of personal immunization records is very important, since persons in this country relocate frequently. This will facilitate accurate record-keeping for the patient, assist with physician encounters, and fulfill the need for documentation of immunization in schools and other institutions and organizations.

Every health care provider should maintain a permanent record of the immunization history of each patient so information can be updated when subsequent vaccine(s) are administered, and patients in need of immunization can easily be identified and recalled. These records should contain the type of vaccine or other immunobiologic administered, date of administration, manufacturer, and lot number.

Recall or tickler systems have been developed to identify children who are due for immunizations or behind schedule for immunizations so parents can be contacted to have them immunized. The Committee recommends the use of these systems by all health care providers.

Dates of immunization (at least month and year) should be required on institutional immunization records, such as those kept in schools and day-care centers, to assure that children have received vaccines at an acceptable age and according to an appropriate

---

*More complete information on adverse reactions to a specific vaccine may be found in the ACIP recommendations for specific vaccines.

schedule. This will facilitate assessment that a primary vaccine series has been completed and that any needed boosters have been obtained at the appropriate time. Measles, mumps, and rubella immunizations should be considered adequate only if they were administered on or after the first birthday (the currently recommended age for routine measles immunization is 15 months). Administration of MMR vaccine at 15 months is desirable for use in routine infant-child immunization programs.

Sources of vaccine information

Apart from these general recommendations, which are published at approximately 2-year intervals, the practitioner can draw on a variety of sources for specific data and updated information including:

A. Official package circular. Manufacturers provide product-specific information along with each vaccine; some of these are reproduced in their entirety in the *Physician's Desk Reference* (PDR) and dated.

B. Morbidity and Mortality Weekly Report (MMWR). This report is published weekly by CDC and contains vaccine recommendations, reports of specific disease activity, policy statements, and the regular and special recommendations of this Committee. The MMWR will contain any necessary updated information on the ACIP recommendations. Subscription price for domestic (United States, Canada, and Mexico) is $70.00 (third class) and $90.00 (first class), and the foreign price is $140 (airmail printed matter) and $155 (airmail letter). Write: MMWR, National Technical Information Services, 5282 Port Royal Road, Springfield, Virginia 22161.

C. Health Information for International Travel. This booklet is published annually by CDC as a guide to requirements and recommendations for specific immunizations and health practices for travel to various countries. It can be obtained for $5 from the Superintendent of Documents, U.S. Government Printing Office, Washington, D.C. 20402.

D. Advisory memoranda. Memoranda are published when necessary by CDC to advise international travelers or those who provide information to travelers about specific outbreaks of communicable diseases abroad. These memoranda include health information for prevention and specific recommendations for immunization and may be obtained at the present time at no cost by writing the Division of Quarantine, Centers for Disease Control, Atlanta, Georgia 30333, to request placement on the mailing list.

E. The Report of the Committee on Infectious Diseases of the American Academy of Pediatrics (Red Book). The full report containing recommendations on all licensed vaccines is usually updated every 4-5 years. The most recent Red Book was published in 1982. The cost is $15.00, plus mailing. It may be ordered from: American Academy of Pediatrics, P.O. Box 1034, Evanston, Illinois 60204.

F. Red Book Update. The Committee on Infectious Diseases of the American Academy of Pediatrics publishes its recent positions and specific recommendations in *Pediatrics* after each quarterly meeting. A yearly subscription costs $30.00. It may be ordered from the address listed in E above.

G. Control of Communicable Diseases in Man. This manual is published by the American Public Health Association at approximately 5-year intervals. The thirteenth edition (1980) is available now. The manual contains valuable information concerning infectious diseases, their occurrence worldwide, immunization, diagnostic and therapeutic information, and up-to-date recommendations on isolation and other control measures for each disease presented. It may be ordered at a cost of $7.50 from: The American Public Health Association, 1015 Fifteenth Street, N.W., Washington, D.C. 20005.

H. Technical Bulletins of the American College of Obstetricians and Gynecologists (ACOG). These bulletins, which are updated periodically, contain important information on immunization of pregnant women. A set may be ordered at a cost of $7.50 from: American College of Obstetricians and Gynecologists, Attention: Distribution Center, 600 Maryland Avenue, S.W., Suite 300 East, Washington, D.C. 20024.

I. Routine reports. Most state and many local health departments provide routine immunizations, immunization cards, and schedules to patients. They also send out routine reports of disease incidence.

J. Additional information. Additional information can also be obtained from city, county, or state health departments, medical schools, and large hospitals. Specific questions may be addressed to the Division of Immunization, Centers for Disease Control, Atlanta, Georgia 30333, telephone, (404) 329-3311.

Patient information

Parents and patients should be informed about the benefits and risks of vaccines. It is essential that the patient or responsible person be given information concerning the risks of vaccines as well as the major benefits from vaccines in preventing disease in both individuals and the community. Benefit and risk information should be presented in terminology that is as simple as possible. No formal and legally acceptable statement has been universally adopted for the private medical sector. CDC has developed "Important Information Statements" for use with federally purchased vaccines given in public health clinics. Practitioners may wish to consider these or similar materials for parents and patients. The Committee recommends that there be ample opportunity for questions before each immunization.

From MMWR 1983;32(1):1-17.

BCG VACCINES
Introduction

1955—of liquid vaccines prepared from different BCG strains showed protection ranging from 0 to 80%.

0.03%, based on the prevalence among 6-year olds.

The incidence of tuberculosis cases varies broadly among different segments of the population and in different localities. Cases occur twice as frequently in males as in females. Rates increase sharply with age in both sexes and all races. More than 80% of reported cases are in persons over 25 years of age, most of whom were infected several years previously. Reported cases are generally typical post-primary pulmonary disease. The risk of infection is greatest for those who have repeated exposure to persons with unrecognized or untreated sputum-positive pulmonary tuberculosis. Chemotherapy rapidly reduces the infectivity of cases.

Efforts to control tuberculosis in the United States are directed toward the early identification and treatment of cases and preventive therapy with isoniazid for infected persons at high risk of developing disease. In this country, vaccine prepared from the Bacillus of Calmette and Guérin (BCG) has been used mainly for selected groups of uninfected persons who live or work where they have an unavoidable risk of exposure to tuberculosis.

BCG vaccines

BCG was derived from a strain of *Mycobacterium bovis* attenuated through years of serial passage in culture by Calmette and Guérin at the Pasteur Institute, Lille, France. It was first administered to humans in 1921.

There are many BCG vaccines* available in the world today; all are derived from the original strain, but they vary in immunogenicity, efficacy, and reactogenicity. Variation probably has been the result of genetic changes in the bacterial strains; differences in techniques of production; methods and routes of vaccine administration; and characteristics of the populations and environments in which vaccine has been studied. Controlled trials—all conducted prior to

---

*Official name: BCG Vaccine.

capable of inducing tuberculin sensitivity in guinea pigs and humans. (The assumed relationship between sensitivity and immunity has not been proven.)

Freeze-dried vaccine should be reconstituted, protected from exposure to light, and used within 8 hours.

Vaccine usage

General recommendations. Modern methods of case detection, chemotherapy, and preventive treatment can be highly successful in controlling tuberculosis. Nevertheless, an effective BCG vaccine may be useful under certain circumstances. In particular, BCG may benefit uninfected persons with repeated exposure to infective cases who cannot or will not obtain or accept treatment.

Recommended vaccine recipients

1. BCG vaccination should be seriously considered for individuals, such as infants in a household, who are tuberculin skin-test negative (1) but who have repeated exposure to persistently untreated or ineffectively treated patients with sputum-positive pulmonary tuberculosis.

2. BCG vaccination should be considered for groups in which an excessive rate of new infections can be demonstrated and the usual surveillance and treatment programs have failed or are not feasible. Such groups might exist among those without a regular source of health care.

Adequate surveillance and control measures should be possible to protect groups such as health workers (2). However, some health workers may be at increased risk of repeated exposure, especially those working in institutions serving major urban population centers in which the endemic prevalence of tuberculosis is relatively high. BCG vaccine should be considered when the frequency of skin-test conversion representing new infections (3) exceeds 1% annually.

Schedule. BCG should be reserved for persons who are skin-test negative to 5 TU* of tuberculin, PPD.† Those who receive BCG should have a tuberculin skin test 2-3 months later. If that skin test is negative and the indications for BCG remain, a second dose of vaccine should be given. Dosage is indicated by the manufacturer in the package labeling; one-half of the usual dose should be given to persons under 28 days old. If the indications for immunization persist, these children should receive a full dose after attaining 1 year of age.

Administration technique. The World Health Organization recommends that BCG be given by the intradermal route in order to provide a uniform and reliable dose. In the United States, however, vaccines for intradermal and for percutaneous administration are licensed, and vaccination should be only by the route indicated in the package labeling.

Risks and side effects

BCG vaccine has been associated with adverse reactions including severe or prolonged ulceration at the vaccination site, lymphadenitis, and—very rarely—osteomyelitis, lupoid reactions, disseminated BCG infection, and death. Available data on adverse reactions do not necessarily pertain to the vaccines currently licensed in the United States, and the reported frequency of complications has varied greatly, depending in part on the extent of the surveillance effort. For example, the frequency of ulceration and lymphadenitis has been reported to range from 1% to 10%, depending on the vaccine, the dosage, and the age of vaccinees. Osteomyelitis has been reported to occur in 1 per 1,000,000 vaccinees, although limited information indicates that with newborns it may be higher. Disseminated BCG infection and death are very rare (1-10 per 10,000,000 vaccinees) and occur almost exclusively in children with impaired immune responses.

Precautions and contraindications

Altered immune states. BCG for prevention of tuberculosis should not be given to persons with impaired immune responses such as occur with congenital immunodeficiency, leukemia, lymphoma, or generalized malignancy, and when immunologic responses have been suppressed with steroids, alkylating agents, antimetabolites, or radiation.

Pregnancy. Although no harmful effects of BCG on the fetus have been observed, it is prudent to avoid vaccination during pregnancy unless there is an immediate excessive risk of unavoidable exposure to infective tuberculosis.

---

*Tuberculin unit.
†Purified protein derivative of tuberculin.

Interpretation of tuberculin test. After BCG vaccination, it is usually not possible to distinguish between a tuberculin reaction caused by virulent suprainfection and one resulting from persistent postvaccination sensitivity. Therefore, caution is advised in attributing a positive skin test to BCG (except in the immediate postvaccination period), especially if the vaccinee has recently been exposed to infective tuberculosis.

Tuberculosis in vaccinated persons. Since full, lasting protection from BCG vaccination cannot be assured, tuberculosis should be included in the differential diagnosis of any tuberculosis-like illness in a BCG vaccinee.

Surveillance

All suspected adverse reactions to BCG should be carefully investigated and reported to health authorities. These reactions occasionally occur as long as a year or more after vaccination.

REFERENCES

1. American Lung Association. Diagnostic standards and classification of tuberculosis and other mycobacterial diseases. New York, American Lung Association, 1974.
2. CDC. Guidelines for Prevention of TB Transmission in Hospitals (HEW Pub. No. [CDC] 79-8371). Atlanta, CDC, Jan 1979.
3. Thompson N, Glassroth JL, Snider D, Farer LS. The booster phenomenon in serial tuberculin testing. Am Rev Respir Dis 1979;119:587-597.

SELECTED BIBLIOGRAPHY

CDC. Tuberculosis in the United States 1977 (HEW Pub. No. [CDC] 79-8322). Atlanta, CDC, Mar 1979.

Eickhoff TC. The current status of BCG immunization against tuberculosis. Annu Rev Med 1977;28:411-423.

National Institutes of Health. Status of Immunization in Tuberculosis in 1971: Report of a Conference on Progress to Date, Future Trends, and Research Needs (HEW Pub. No. [NIH] 72-68). Washington, Government Printing Office, 1972.

Rouillon A, Waaler H. BCG vaccination and epidemiological situation: a decision making approach to the use of BCG. Adv Tuberc Res 1976;19:64-126.

World Health Organization. Ninth Report of the Expert Committee on Tuberculosis (WHO Tech Rep No. 552). Geneva, WHO, 1974.

From MMWR 1979;28:241-244.

CHOLERA VACCINE
Introduction

Historically, cholera has commonly occurred in endemic and epidemic form in parts of southern and southeastern Asia. Since 1961, cholera due to the El Tor biotype has been epidemic throughout much of Asia, the Middle East, and Africa, and in certain parts of Europe. Infection is acquired primarily from contaminated water or food; person-to-person transmission is not important except in rare instances. The risk of cholera for travelers who use the usual tourist

Vaccine is not recommended for infants under 6 months of age and is not required for travel by most countries.

Health Organization (WHO) no longer recommends cholera vaccination for travel to or from cholera-infected areas. Surveillance and treatment are sufficient to prevent spread of the disease if it were to be introduced into the United States.

Vaccine available in the United States is prepared from a combination of phenol-inactivated suspensions of classic Inaba and Ogawa strains of *Vibrio cholerae* grown on agar or in broth.

Vaccine usage

General recommendations. The only indications for cholera vaccine are travel to and residence in countries with cholera. Vaccine should not be used to manage contacts of imported cases or to control the spread of infection.

Repeated vaccination may sometimes be required of, or advised for, laboratory workers and airline and ship crews. Since groups such as these are unlikely to acquire or transmit cholera, and since there is limited information on the long-term safety of repeated vaccination, such practices should be continued only when resolutely demanded by some countries for international travel.

a single dose of vaccine is sufficient to satisfy International Health Regulations. With the threat or occurrence of epidemic cholera, health authorities of some countries may require evidence of a complete primary series of 2 doses or a booster dose within 6 months before arrival. The complete primary series is otherwise suggested only for special high-risk groups that work and live in highly endemic areas under less than sanitary conditions. (See Table 35-4 for appropriate dose.)

Vaccination requirements published by WHO are regularly updated and summarized for travelers by the Public Health Service and distributed to state and local health departments, airlines, travel agents, many physicians, and others. Physicians and travelers should seek information on requirements from these sources.

Physicians administering vaccine to travelers should emphasize that an International Certificate of Vaccination against cholera must be validated for it to be acceptable to quarantine authorities. Validation can be obtained at most city, county, and state health departments as well as many private clinics and physicians' offices. Failure to secure validation may cause travelers to be revaccinated or quarantined. A properly documented Certificate is valid for 6 months beginning 6 days after vaccination or beginning on the

---

*Official name: Cholera Vaccine.

Table 35-4. Recommended doses, by volume (ml), for immunization against cholera

Dose number	Route and age			
	Intradermal* 5 years and over	Subcutaneous or intramuscular		
		6 mos-4 years	5-10 years	Over 10 years
1 and 2	0.2 ml	0.2 ml	0.3 ml	0.5 ml
Boosters	0.2 ml	0.2 ml	0.3 ml	0.5 ml

*Higher levels of protection (antibody) may be achieved in children less than 5 years old by the subcutaneous or intramuscular routes.

date of revaccination, if this revaccination is within 6 months of a previous injection.

Primary immunization. Complete primary immunization consists of 2 doses of vaccine given 1 week to 1 month or more apart. (This is not required to satisfy International Health Regulations). Dose volume by age group and by route of administration is shown in the table below. The intradermal route is satisfactory for persons 5 years of age and older.

Booster doses. Booster doses may be given every 6 months if necessary for travel or for residence in highly endemic, unsanitary areas. In areas where cholera occurs in a 2-3 month "season", protection is best if the booster dose is given at the beginning of the season. The primary series does not ever need to be repeated for booster doses to be effective.

Summary. The recommended doses for primary and booster immunization are in Table 35-4.

Precautions and contraindications

Reactions. Vaccination often results in 1-2 days of pain, erythema, and induration at the site of injection. The local reaction may be accompanied by fever, malaise, and headache.

Serious reactions following cholera vaccination are extremely rare. If a person has experienced a serious reaction to the vaccine, revaccination is not advisable. Most governments will permit an unvaccinated traveler to proceed if he or she carries a physician's statement of medical contraindication. However, some countries may quarantine such unvaccinated persons or place them under surveillance if they come from areas with cholera.

Pregnancy. There is no specific information on the safety of cholera vaccine during pregnancy. Its use should be individualized to reflect actual need.

SELECTED BIBLIOGRAPHY

Bart KJ, Gangarosa EJ. Cholera, in Kelley VC (ed): Brennemann's Practice of Pediatrics, II(1) Chap 18 c. New York, Harper and Row, 1977, pp 1-12.

Barus D, Burrows W (eds). Cholera, Philadelphia, WB Saunders Co, 1974.

Gangarosa EJ, Barker WH. Cholera: implications for the United States. JAMA 1974;227:170-171.

McCormack WM, Chowdhury AM, Jahangir N, et al. Tetracycline prophylaxis in families of cholera patients. Bull WHO 1968;38:787-792.

Philippines Cholera Committee. A controlled field trial on the effectiveness of the intradermal and subcutaneous administration of cholera vaccine in the Philippines. Bull WHO 1973;49:389-394.

Sommer A, Khan M, Mosley WH. Efficacy of vaccination of family contacts of cholera cases. Lancer 1973;1:1230-1232.

Published in MMWR 1978;27:173.

DIPHTHERIA, TETANUS, AND PERTUSSIS: GUIDELINES FOR VACCINE PROPHYLAXIS AND OTHER PREVENTIVE MEASURES

This revision of the Immunization Practices Advisory Committee (ACIP) statement on diphtheria, tetanus, and pertussis updates the statement issued in 1981 (1) and incorporates the 1984 supplementary statement on the risks of pertussis disease and pertussis vaccine for infants and children with personal histories of convulsions. (2) It includes a review of the epidemiology of the three diseases, a description of the available immunobiologic preparations, and the appropriate immunization schedules. Also included are revisions in the schedule for combined diphtheria and tetanus toxoids (DT) when pertussis vaccine is contraindicated, and revisions in the recommendations on precautions and contraindications to vaccine use, on immunization for infants and children who have underlying neurologic disorders, and on tetanus prophylaxis in wound management.

Introduction

Simultaneous immunization against diphtheria, tetanus, and pertussis during infancy and childhood has been a routine practice in the United States since the late 1940s. This practice has played a major role in markedly reducing the incidence rates of cases and deaths from each of these diseases.

Diphtheria

At one time, diphtheria was common in the United States. More than 200,000 cases, primarily among children, were reported in 1921. Approximately 5%-10% of cases were fatal; the highest case-fatality ratios were in the very young and the elderly. Reported cases of diphtheria of all types declined from 306 in 1975 to 59 in 1979; most were cutaneous diphtheria reported from a single state. After 1979, cutaneous diphtheria was no longer reportable. From 1980 through 1983, only 15 cases of respiratory diphtheria were reported; 11 occurred among persons 20 years of age or older.

The current rarity of diphtheria in the United States is due primarily to the high level of appropriate immunization in children (96% of children entering school have received three or more doses of diptheria and tetanus toxoids and pertussis vaccine [DTP]) and to an apparent reduction of the circulation of toxigenic strains of *Corynebacterium diphtheriae*. Most cases occur in unimmunized or inadequately immunized persons. The age distribution of recent cases and the results of serosurveys indicate that many adults in the United States are not protected against diphtheria. Thus, it appears that more emphasis should be placed on adult immunization programs.

Both toxigenic and nontoxigenic strains of *C. diphtheriae* can cause disease, but only strains that produce toxin cause myocarditis and neuritis. Furthermore, toxigenic strains are more often associated with

series generally induces protective levels of serum antitoxin that persist for 10 or more years.

Complete immunization significantly reduces the risk of developing diphtheria, and immunized persons who develop disease have milder illnesses. Protection is thought to last at least 10 years. Immunization does not, however, eliminate carriage of *C. diphtheriae* in the pharynx or nose or on the skin.

Tetanus

The occurrence of tetanus in the United States has decreased dramatically as a result of the routine use of tetanus toxoid. Nonetheless, the number of reported cases has remained relatively constant in the last decade at an annual average of 90 cases. In 1983, 91 tetanus cases were reported from 29 states. In recent years, approximately two-thirds of patients have been 50 years of age or older. The age distribution of recent cases and the results of serosurveys indicate that many U.S. adults are not protected against tetanus. The disease has occurred almost exclusively among persons who are unimmunized or inadequately immunized or whose immunization histories are unknown or uncertain.

In 6% of tetanus cases reported during 1982 and 1983, no wound or other condition could be implicated. Nonacute skin lesions, such as ulcers, or medical conditions, such as abscesses, were reported in 17% of cases.

Neonatal tetanus occurs among infants born under unhygienic conditions to inadequately immunized mothers. Immune pregnant women confer protection to their infants through transplacental maternal antibody. From 1974 through 1983, 20 cases of neonatal tetanus were reported in the United States.

Spores of *Clostridium tetani* are ubiquitous. Serologic tests indicate that naturally acquired immunity to tetanus toxin does not occur in the United States. Thus, universal primary immunization, with subsequent maintenance of adequate antitoxin levels by means of appropriately timed boosters, is necessary to protect persons in all age groups. Tetanus toxoid is a highly effective antigen, and a completed primary

cases go unrecognized or unreported, and diagnostic tests for *Bordetella pertussis*—culture and direct-immunofluorescence assay (DFA)—may be unavailable, difficult to perform, or incorrectly interpreted.

For 1982 and 1983, 53% of reported illnesses from *B. pertussis* occurred among children under 1 year of age and 78% among children under 5 years of age; 13 of 15 deaths reported to the CDC occurred in children under 1 year old. Before widespread use of DTP, about 20% of cases and 50% of pertussis-related deaths occurred in children under 1 year old.

Pertussis is highly communicable (attack rates of over 90% have been reported in unimmunized household contacts) and can cause severe disease, particularly in very young children. Of cases under 1 year of age reported to CDC during 1982 and 1983, 75% were hospitalized; approximately 22% had pneumonia; 2.5% had one or more seizures; and 0.7% died. Because of the substantial risks of complications of the disease, completion of a primary series of DTP vaccine early in life is essential.

In older children and adults—including, in some instances, those previously immunized—infection may result in nonspecific symptoms of bronchitis or an upper respiratory tract infection, and pertussis may not be diagnosed because classic signs, especially the inspiratory whoop, may be absent. Older preschool-aged children and school-aged siblings who are not fully immunized and develop pertussis can be important sources of infection for young infants, the group at highest risk of disease and disease severity. The importance of the infected adult in overall transmission remains to be defined.

Controversy regarding use of pertussis vaccine led to a formal reevaluation of the benefits and risks of this vaccine. The analysis indicated that the benefits of the vaccine continue to outweigh its risks (3).

Because the incidence rate and severity of pertussis decrease with age, and because the vaccine may cause side effects and adverse reactions, pertussis immunization is not recommended for children after their seventh birthday, except under unusual circumstances (see VACCINE USAGE).

Preparations used for immunization

Diphtheria and tetanus toxoids are prepared by formaldehyde treatment of the respective toxins and are standardized for potency according to the regulations of the U.S. Food and Drug Administration (FDA). The Lf content of each toxoid (quantity of toxoid as assessed by flocculation) may vary among different products. Because adverse reactions to diphtheria toxoid are apparently directly related to the quantity of antigen and to the age of the recipient, the concentration of diphtheria toxoid in preparations intended for use in adults is reduced.

Pertussis vaccine is a suspension of inactivated *B. pertussis* cells. Potency is assayed by comparison with the U.S. Standard Pertussis Vaccine in the intracerebral mouse protection test. The protective efficacy of pertussis vaccines in humans has been shown to correlate with the potency of vaccines.

Diphtheria and tetanus toxoids and pertussis vaccine, as single antigens or various combinations, are available as aluminum salt adsorbed preparations. Only tetanus toxoid is available in nonadsorbed (fluid) form. Although the rate of seroconversion is essentially equivalent with either type of tetanus toxoid, the adsorbed toxoid induces a more persistent antitoxin titer.

The two toxoids and the pertussis vaccine are currently available in the United States as the following preparations:

1. Diphtheria and Tetanus Toxoids and Pertussis Vaccine Adsorbed (DTP) and Diphtheria and Tetanus Toxoids Adsorbed (For Pediatric Use) (DT) are combinations for use in infants and children under 7 years old.
2. Tetanus and Diphtheria Toxoids Adsorbed (For Adult Use) (Td) is a combined preparation for use in persons 7 years old and older.
3. Pertussis Vaccine Adsorbed (P)*, Tetanus Toxoid (Fluid), Tetanus Toxoid Adsorbed (T), and Diphtheria Toxoid Adsorbed (D)†, are single antigen products for use in instances when combined antigen preparations are not indicated.

Work is in progress to develop an effective acellular pertussis vaccine with a reduced reaction rate. Current research is directed toward development of a vaccine consisting principally of one or more of the bacterial components thought to provide protection.

---

*Distributed by the Biologics Products Program, Michigan Department of Public Health for use within that state; may be available for use outside Michigan under special circumstances, by consultation with that program.
†Distributed by Sclavo, Inc.

Prominent candidate antigens include filamentous hemagglutinin and lymphocytosis promoting factor (pertussis toxin). However, several years will be necessary to complete development, and to document the potency, safety, and efficacy of a new vaccine.

Vaccine usage

The standard, single-dose volume of DTP, DT, Td, single-antigen adsorbed preparations of pertussis vaccine, tetanus toxoid and diphtheria toxoid, and the nonadsorbed tetanus toxoid is 0.5 ml. Adsorbed preparations should be administered intramuscularly (IM). Vaccine administration by jet injection may be associated with more frequent local reactions. (See also ACIP: General recommendations on immunization. MMWR 1983;32:1-8, 13-17.)

Primary immunization

Children 6 weeks through 6 years old (up to the seventh birthday) (Table 35-5). One dose of DTP should be given IM on four occasions—the first three doses at 4- to 8-week intervals, beginning when the infant is approximately 6 weeks-2 months old. The fourth dose is given approximately 6-12 months after the third to maintain adequate immunity for the ensuing preschool years. This dose is an integral part of the primary immunizing course. If a contraindication to pertussis vaccination exists (see PRECAUTIONS AND CONTRAINDICATIONS), DT should be substituted for DTP as outlined under Special Considerations below.

Persons 7 years old and older and adults (Table 35-6). Pertussis-containing preparations are not recommended routinely in these age groups. A series of three doses of Td should be given IM; the second dose is given 4-8 weeks after the first; and the third dose, 6-12 months after the second. Td rather than DT is the agent of choice for immunization of all patients 7 years old and older, because side effects from higher doses of diphtheria toxoid are more common in older children and adults.

Interruption of primary immunization schedule. Interrupting the recommended schedule or delaying subsequent doses probably does not lead to a reduction in the level of immunity reached on completion of the primary series. Therefore, there is no need to restart a series regardless of the time elapsed between doses.

Booster immunization

Children 4-6 years old (up to the seventh birthday). Those who received all four primary immunizing doses before their fourth birthday should receive a single dose of DTP just before entering kindergarten or elementary school. This booster dose is not necessary if the fourth dose in the primary series was given after the fourth birthday.

Persons 7 years old and older. Tetanus toxoid

Table 35-5. Routine diphtheria, tetanus, and pertussis immunization schedule summary for children less than 7 years old—United States 1985*

¶DT, if pertussis vaccine is contraindicated. If the child is 1 year of age or older at the time that primary dose 3 would be due, a third dose 6-12 months after the second completes primary immunization with DT.

Table 35-6. Routine diphtheria and tetanus immunization schedule summary for persons 7 years old and older—United States, 1985*

Dose	Age/interval	Product
Primary 1	First visit	Td
Primary 2	4-8 weeks after first dose†	Td
Primary 3	6-12 months after second dose†	Td
Boosters	Every 10 years after last dose	Td

*Important details are in the text.
†Prolonging the interval does not require restarting series.

should be given with diphtheria toxoid as Td every 10 years. If a dose is given sooner as part of wound management, the next booster is not needed for 10 years thereafter (see TETANUS PROPHYLAXIS IN WOUND MANAGEMENT). More frequent boosters are not indicated and have been reported to result in an increased occurrence and severity of adverse reactions. One means of ensuring that persons receive boosters every 10 years is to vaccinate persons routinely at mid-decade ages, e.g. 15 years, 25 years, etc.

Special considerations

Children with a contraindication to pertussis vaccination (see PRECAUTIONS AND CONTRAINDICATIONS). For children under 7 years old with a contraindication to pertussis vaccine, DT should be used rather than DTP. To ensure that there will be no interference with the antigens from maternal antibodies, unimmunized children under 1 year of age

receiving their first DT dose should receive a total of four doses of DT as the primary series, the first three doses at 4- to 8-week intervals and the fourth dose 6-12 months later (similar to the recommended DTP schedule). If further doses of pertussis vaccine become contraindicated after beginning a DTP series in the first year of life, DT should be substituted for each of the remaining scheduled DTP doses.

Unimmunized children 1 year of age or older for whom DTP is contraindicated should receive two doses of DT 4-8 weeks apart, followed by a third dose 6-12 months later in order to complete the primary series. Children 1 year of age or older who have received one or two doses of DT or DTP and for whom further pertussis vaccine is contraindicated should receive a total of three doses of a preparation containing diphtheria and tetanus toxoids, with the third dose administered 6-12 months after the second dose.

Children who complete a primary series of DT before their fourth birthday should receive a single dose of DT just before entering kindergarten or elementary school. This dose is not necessary if the last dose of the primary series was given after the fourth birthday.

Pertussis immunization for persons 7 years old or older. Routine immunization against pertussis is not recommended for persons 7 years old and older. In exceptional cases, such as persons with chronic pulmonary disease exposed to children with pertussis or health-care personnel exposed during nosocomial or community outbreaks, a booster dose of adsorbed pertussis vaccine may be considered. A reduced dose is used for adults (4). Routine pertussis vaccination of hospital personnel is not recommended.

Persons recovering from tetanus or diphtheria. Tetanus or diphtheria infection may not confer immunity; therefore, active immunization should be initiated at the time of recovery from the illness and arrangements made to ensure that the remaining doses of a primary series are administered as early as possible.

Children recovering from pertussis. Children who have recovered from culture-confirmed pertussis need not receive further doses of pertussis vaccine. Lacking culture confirmation of the diagnosis, DTP immunization should be completed because pertussis syndrome may have been caused by other *Bordetella* species, chlamydia, or some viruses.

Neonatal tetanus prevention. There is no evidence that tetanus and diphtheria toxoids are teratogenic. A previously unimmunized pregnant woman who may deliver her child under unhygienic circumstances or surroundings should receive two properly spaced doses of Td before delivery, preferably during the last two trimesters. Incompletely immunized pregnant women should complete the three-dose series. Those immunized more than 10 years previously should have a booster dose.

Adult immunization with Td. Limited serosurveys done since 1977 indicate that the proportion of the population lacking protective levels of circulating antitoxin against diphtheria and tetanus increases with increasing age and that at least 40% of persons 60 years of age or older lack protective levels of antitoxins. Every visit of an adult to a health-care provider should be an opportunity to assess the patient's immunization status and, if indicated, to provide protection against tetanus and diphtheria using the combined toxoid, Td. Adults with uncertain histories of a complete primary series should receive a primary series. To ensure continued adequate protection in the individual, booster doses of Td could be given routinely at mid-decade ages, e.g., 15 years, 25 years, 35 years, etc.

Use of single-antigen preparations. Multiple antigen preparations should be used, unless there is a contraindication to one or more antigens in a preparation.

A single-antigen adsorbed pertussis vaccine preparation may be used to complete immunization against pertussis for children under 7 years of age who have received fewer than the recommended number of doses of pertussis vaccine but have received the recommended number of doses of diphtheria and tetanus toxoids for their age. Alternatively, doses of DTP can be given for protection against pertussis, although it is suggested that the total number of doses of diphtheria and tetanus toxoids not exceed six each before the seventh birthday.

Available data do not indicate substantially more reactions following receipt of Td than following receipt of single-antigen, adsorbed tetanus toxoid. Furthermore, adults, in general, are even less likely to have adequate circulating levels of diphtheria anti-

toxin than adequate circulating levels of tetanus antitoxin. The routine use of Td in all medical settings, e.g., private practice, clinics and emergency rooms, for all persons 7 years of age or older requiring primary immunization or booster doses will improve levels of protection against both tetanus and diphtheria, especially among adults.

Side effects and adverse reactions

Local reactions, generally erythema and induration with or without tenderness, are common after the administration of vaccines containing diphtheria, tetanus, or pertussis antigens. Occasionally, a nodule may be palpable at the injection site of adsorbed products for several weeks. Abscesses at the site of injection have been reported (6-10 per million doses). Mild systemic reactions, such as fever, drowsiness, fretfulness and anorexia, occur quite frequently. These reactions are significantly more common following DTP than following DT, are usually self-limited, and need no therapy other than, perhaps, symptomatic treatment (e.g., antipyretics).

Moderate to severe systemic events, such as fever of 40.5 C (105 F) or higher, unusual high-pitched crying, collapse, or convulsions, occur relatively infrequently. Other more severe neurologic complications, such as a prolonged convulsion or encephalopathy, occasionally fatal, have been reported to be associated with DTP administration, although rarely.

Approximate rates for adverse events following receipt of DTP vaccine (regardless of dose number in the series) are indicated in Table 35-7 (5, 6).

The frequency of local reactions and fever following DTP vaccination is significantly higher with increasing numbers of doses of DTP while other mild to moderate systemic reactions (e.g., fretfulness, vomiting) are significantly less frequent (5). If local redness of 2.5 cm or greater occurs, the likelihood of recurrence after another DTP dose increases significantly (7).

In the National Childhood Encephalopathy Study (NCES) a large, case-control study in England (6), children 2-35 months of age with serious, acute neurologic disorders, such as encephalopathy or complicated convulsion(s), were more likely to have received DTP in the 7 days preceding onset than their age-, sex-, and neighborhood-matched controls. Among children known to be neurologically normal before entering the study, the relative risk* of a neurologic illness occurring within the 7-day period following receipt of a dose of DTP, compared to children not receiving DTP vaccine in the 7-day period before onset of their illness, was 3.3 (p < 0.001). Within this 7-day period, the risk was significantly increased in

---

*Relative risk was estimated by odds ratio.

Table 35-7. Adverse events occurring within 48 hours of DTP immunizations

ized by severe local reactions (generally starting 2-8 hours after an injection), may follow receipt of tetanus toxoid, particularly in adults who have received fre-

More serious systemic	
Persistent, inconsolable crying (duration ≥3 hours)	1/100 doses
High-pitched, unusual cry	1/900 doses
Fever ≥40.5 C (≥105 F)	1/330 doses
Collapse (hypotonic-hypore-sponsive episode)	1/1,750 doses
Convulsions (with or without fever)	1/1,750 doses
Acute encephalopathy†	1/110,000 doses
Permanent neurologic deficit†	1/310,000 doses

*Number of adverse events per total number of doses regardless of dose number in DTP series.
†Occurring within 7 days of DTP immunization.

immunized children only within 3 days of vaccination (relative risk 4.2, p < 0.001). The relative risk for illness occurring from 4-7 days after vaccination was 2.1 (0.05 < p < 0.1). The attributable risk estimate for a serious acute neurologic disorder within 7 days after DTP vaccine (regardless of outcome) was one in 110,000 doses of DTP, and for a permanent neurologic deficit, one in 310,000 doses. No specific clinical syndrome was identified. Overall, DTP vaccine accounted for only a small proportion of cases of serious neurologic disorders reported in the population studied.

Although there are uncertainties in the reported studies, recent data suggest that infants and young children who have had previous convulsions (whether febrile or nonfebrile) are more likely to have seizures following DTP than those without such histories (8).

Rarely, an anaphylactic reaction (i.e., hives, swelling of the mouth, difficulty breathing, hypotension, or shock) has been reported after receiving preparations containing diphtheria, tetanus, and/or pertussis antigens. The ACIP finds no good evidence for a causal relationship between DTP and hemolytic anemia or thrombocytopenic purpura.

Arthus-type hypersensitivity reactions, character-

4 months of age. By chance alone some SIDS victims can be expected to have recently received vaccine.

Onset of infantile spasms has occurred in infants who have recently received DTP or DT. Analysis of data from the NCES on children with infantile spasms showed that receipt of DTP or DT was not causally related to infantile spasms (10). The incidence of onset of infantile spasms increases at 3-9 months of age, the time period when the second and third doses of DTP are generally given. Therefore, some cases of infantile spasms can be expected to be related by chance alone to recent receipt of DTP.

Reporting of adverse events

Reporting by parents and patients of all adverse events occurring within 4 weeks of antigen administration should be encouraged. Adverse events which require a visit to a health-care provider should be reported by health-care providers to manufacturers and local or state health departments. The information will be forwarded to an appropriate federal agency (the Bureau of Biologics Research and Review of the FDA, or CDC.

Comments on the use of reduced dosage schedules or multiple small doses

The ACIP recommends giving only the full dose of DTP vaccine; if a specific contraindication to DTP exists, none should be given. In the United States the full course of primary immunization is considered to be four 0.5 ml doses of DTP.

Concern about adverse events following pertussis vaccine has led some practitioners to reduce the volume of DTP vaccine administered to less than 0.5 ml per dose in an attempt to reduce side effects. There is no evidence that a reduction in dosage decreases the frequency of severe events, such as seizures, hypotonic-hyporesponsive episodes, and encephalopathy. The mechanisms for these reactions are not known. Some studies reported significantly lower rates of local reactions to one half of the recommended dose (0.25 ml) compared to those following a full dose *(7,11)*. A recent study also showed significantly lower pertussis serologic responses after the second and third half doses although the differences were small *(11)*. This investigation used pertussis agglutinins as a measure of clinical protection; however, agglutinins are not absolute measures of clinical protection against pertussis disease. Further, there is no evidence that the low screening titer used in this investigation (1 : 16) is indicative of protection. Currently, there are no reliable measures of efficacy other than clinical protection. Further evidence against the use of reduced doses comes from earlier studies of vaccine *(12,13)* with potency equivalent to that of half-doses of current vaccine. Attack rates of pertussis for exposed household members who received a lower potency vaccine (equivalent to a half dose of the current vaccine) were approximately twice as high as attack rates for exposed household members who had received vaccines of potency equivalent to full doses of current vaccine (29% compared to 14% or lower).

The use of an increased number of reduced volume doses of DTP in order to equal the total volume of the five recommended doses of DTP vaccine is not recommended. It is unknown whether such a practice reduces the likelihood of vaccine related events. In addition, by increasing the number of immunizations the likelihood of a temporally-associated but etiologically unrelated event may be enhanced.

Neither the use of reduced individual doses of DTP vaccine nor the use of multiple doses of reduced volume that, in total, equal a full immunizing dose has been adequately studied. Neither the efficacy of such practices in reducing the frequency of associated serious adverse events, nor the resulting protection against disease has been determined.

Simultaneous administration of vaccines

The simultaneous administration of DTP, oral polio virus vaccine (OPV), and/or measles-mumps-rubella vaccine (MMR) has resulted in seroconversion rates and rates of side effects similar to those observed when the vaccines are administered separately (12). Therefore, if there is any doubt that a vaccine recipient will return for further vaccine doses, the ACIP recommends the simultaneous administration of all vaccines appropriate to the age and previous vaccination status of the recipient. This would especially include the simultaneous administration of DTP, OPV and MMR to such persons at 15 months of age or older.

Precautions and contraindications

A febrile illness is reason to defer routine vaccination. Minor illness, such as mild upper respiratory infection, should not ordinarily be a reason for postponing vaccination. A history of prematurity generally is not a reason to defer vaccination *(13)*.

Immunosuppressive therapies including irradiation, antimetabolites, alkylating agents, cytotoxic drugs, and corticosteroids (used in greater than physiologic doses) may reduce the immune response to vaccines. Short-term (less than 2 weeks) corticosteroid therapy or intra-articular, bursal, or tendon injections with corticosteroids should not be immunosuppressive. Although no specific studies with pertussis vaccine are available, if immunosuppressive therapy will be discontinued shortly, it would be reasonable to defer immunization until the patient has been off therapy for 1 month *(16)*, otherwise vaccinate the patient while still on therapy.

When an infant or child returns for the next dose of DTP, the parent should be questioned about any reactions occurring after the previous dose.

Pertussis-containing preparations

Absolute contraindications. If any of the following adverse events occurs after DTP or single antigen pertussis vaccination, further vaccination with a vaccine containing pertussis antigen is contraindicated:

1. Allergic hypersensitivity.
2. Fever of 40.5 C (105 F) or greater within 48 hours.
3. Collapse or shock-like state (hypotonic-hyporesponsive episode) within 48 hours.
4. Persisting, inconsolable crying lasting 3 hours or more or an unusual, high-pitched cry occurring within 48 hours.
5. Convulsion(s) with or without fever occurring within 3 days. (All children with convulsions, especially those with convulsions occurring within 7 days of receipt of DTP, should be fully evaluated to clarify their medical and neurologic status before a decision is made on initiating or continuing vaccination with DTP (see next section, item 3).
6. Encephalopathy occurring within 7 days: this includes severe alterations in consciousness with generalized or focal neurologic signs. (A small but significantly increased risk of encephalopathy has been shown only within the 3 day period following DTP receipt. However, most authorities believe that an encephalopathy occurring within 7 days of DTP should be considered a contraindication to further doses of DTP.)

Immunization of infants and young children who have underlying neurologic disorders. The presence of a neurologic condition characterized by changing developmental or neurological findings, regardless of whether a definitive diagnosis has been made, is also considered a contraindication to receipt of pertussis vaccine as administration of DTP may coincide with or possibly even aggravate manifestations of the disease. Such disorders include uncontrolled epilepsy, infantile spasms, and progressive encephalopathy.

Stable conditions, such as cerebral palsy and developmental delay, are not considered contraindications to pertussis vaccination.

3. Incompletely immunized children with a neurologic event occurring between doses. Infants and children who have received one or more doses of DTP

duce permanent brain damage in those children.

Whether to administer DTP to children with proven or suspected underlying neurologic disorders, and when, must be decided on an individual basis. An important consideration is the current low frequency of pertussis reported in most areas of the United States, indicating a relatively low risk of exposure. Other considerations include the current near-absence of diphtheria in the United States and the low risk that an infant will acquire an infection with *C. tetani.* Based on these considerations and the nature of the child's disorder, the following approaches are recommended:

1. Infants as yet unimmunized who are suspected to have underlying neurologic disease. Possible latent central nervous system disorders that are suspected because of perinatal complications or other phenomena may become evident as they evolve over time. Because DTP administration may coincide with onset of overt manifestations of such disorders and result in confusion about causation, it is prudent to delay initiation of immunization with DTP or DT (but not OPV) until further observation and study have clarified the child's neurologic status. In addition, the effect of treatment, if any, can be assessed. The decision whether to commence immunization with DTP or DT should be made no later than the child's first birthday. In making this decision, it should be recognized that children with severe neurologic disorders may be at enhanced risk of exposure to pertussis from institutionalization or from attendance at clinics and special schools or in which many of the children may be unimmunized. In addition, because of neurologic handicaps, these children may be in greater jeopardy from complications of the disease.

2. Infants and children with neurologic events temporally-associated with DTP. Infants and children who experience a seizure within 3 days of receipt of DTP or an encephalopathy within 7 days should not receive further pertussis vaccine, even though cause and effect may not be established (see PRECAUTIONS AND CONTRAINDICATIONS).

disorder occurs after the first birthday, the child's neurologic status should be evaluated to ensure the disorder is stable before a subsequent dose of DTP is given (see next section).

4. Infants and children with stable neurologic conditions. Infants and children with stable neurologic conditions, including well-controlled seizures, may be vaccinated. The occurrence of single seizures (temporally unassociated with DTP) in infants and young children, while necessitating evaluation, need not contraindicate DTP immunization, particularly if the seizures can be satisfactorily explained. Anticonvulsant prophylaxis should be considered when giving DTP to such children. Parents of infants and children with histories of convulsions should be made aware of the slightly increased chance of postimmunization seizures.

5. Children with resolved or corrected neurologic disorders. DTP administration is recommended for infants with certain neurologic problems that have clearly subsided without residua or have been corrected, such as neonatal hypocalcemic tetany or hydrocephalus (following placement of a shunt and without seizures).

Immunization of infants and young children who have a family history of convulsion or other central nervous system disorders. The ACIP, after evaluating the evidence available concerning the risk of a neurologic illness following pertussis vaccination of a child with a family history of convulsion or other central nervous disorder, does not believe that such a history is a contraindication to pertussis vaccination.

Preparations containing diphtheria toxoid and tetanus toxoid. The only contraindication to tetanus and diphtheria toxoids is a history of a neurologic or severe hypersensitivity reaction following a previous dose. Immunization with tetanus and diphtheria toxoids is not known to be associated with an increased risk of convulsions. Local side effects alone do not preclude continued use. If an anaphylactic reaction to a previous dose of tetanus toxoid is suspected, intradermal skin testing with appropriately diluted tetanus toxoid may be useful before a decision is made to discontinue tetanus toxoid immunization (15). In one study, 94 of 95 persons giving histories of anaphylactic symptoms following a previous tetanus toxoid dose were non-reactive following intradermal testing and tolerated a further tetanus toxoid challenge without other reaction (15). One person had immediate erythema and induration following skin testing but tolerated a full intramuscular dose without adverse effects. Mild, nonspecific skin-test reactivity to tetanus toxoid, particularly if used undiluted, appear to be fairly common. Most vaccinees develop inconsequential cutaneous delayed hypersensitivity to the toxoid.

Persons who experienced Arthus-type hypersensitivity reactions or fever greater than 103 F (39.4 C) following a prior dose of tetanus toxoid usually have very high serum tetanus antitoxin levels and should not be given even emergency doses of Td more frequently than every 10 years, even if they have a wound that is neither clean nor minor.

If a contraindication to using tetanus toxoid-containing preparations exists in a person who has not completed a primary immunizing course of tetanus toxoid and other than a clean, minor wound is sustained, *only* passive immunization should be given using tetanus immune globulin (see TETANUS PROPHYLAXIS IN WOUND MANAGEMENT).

Although there is no evidence that tetanus and diphtheria toxoids are teratogenic, waiting until the second trimester of pregnancy to administer Td is a reasonable precaution to minimize any theoretical concern.

Diphtheria prophylaxis for case contacts

All household contacts with less than three doses of diphtheria toxoid should receive an immediate dose of a diphtheria toxoid-containing preparation and should complete the series according to schedule (see Tables 1 and 2). Household contacts with 3 or more doses who have not received a dose of a preparation containing diphtheria toxoid within the previous 5 years should receive a booster dose of a diphtheria toxoid-containing preparation appropriate for their age.

All close contacts should be examined daily for 7 days for evidence of disease. Asymptomatic unimmunized or inadequately immunized household contacts should receive prompt chemoprophylaxis with either an IM injection of benzathine penicillin (600,000 units for persons under 6 years old and 1,200,000 units for those 6 years old or older) or a 7-10 day course of oral erythromycin (children, 40 mg/kg/day; adults, 1 gm/day). Erythromycin may be slightly more effective, but IM benzathine penicillin may be preferred, since it avoids possible problems of noncompliance with a multi-day oral drug regimen.

Bacteriologic cultures before and after antibiotic prophylaxis may be useful in the follow-up and management of contacts. Identified untreated carriers of toxigenic *C. diphtheriae* should receive antibiotics as recommended above for unimmunized household contacts. Those who continue to harbor the organism after either penicillin or erythromycin should receive an additional 10-day course of oral erythromycin.

Even when close surveillance of unimmunized close contacts is impossible, the use of equine diphtheria antitoxin is not generally recommended because of the risks of allergic reaction to horse serum. Immediate hypersensitivity reactions occur in about 7% and serum sickness in 5% of adults receiving the recommended prophylactic dose of equine antitoxin. The risk of adverse reactions to equine antitoxin must be weighed against the small risk of diphtheria occurring in an unimmunized household contact who receives chemoprophylaxis. If antitoxin is to be used, the usually recommended dose is 5,000-10,000 units IM—after appropriate testing for sensitivity—at a site different from that of toxoid injection. The immune response to simultaneous diphtheria antitoxin and toxoid inoculation is unlikely to be impaired, but this has not been adequately studied.

Cases of cutaneous diphtheria generally are caused by infections with nontoxigenic strains of *C. diphtheriae*. However, a lesion suspected of being cutaneous diphtheria should be considered to be caused by a toxigenic strain until proven otherwise. Recommendations for prophylaxis of close case contacts are the same as for respiratory diphtheria, since cutaneous diphtheria may be more contagious for close contacts than is respiratory infection. If a cutaneous case is known to be due to a nontoxigenic strain, routine investigation or prophylaxis of contacts is not necessary.

Tetanus prophylaxis in wound management

Chemoprophylaxis against tetanus is neither practical nor useful in managing wounds; wound cleaning, debridement when indicated, and proper immunization are important. The need for tetanus toxoid (active immunization), with or without tetanus immune globulin (TIG) (passive immunization), depends on both the condition of the wound and the patient's immunization history (Table 35-8, see also PRECAUTIONS AND CONTRAINDICATIONS). Rarely have cases of tetanus occurred in persons with a documented primary series of toxoid injections.

A thorough attempt must be made to determine whether a patient has completed primary immunization. Patients with unknown or uncertain previous immunization histories should be considered to have had no previous tetanus toxoid doses. Persons who had military service since 1941 can be considered to have received at least one dose; although most may have completed a primary series of tetanus toxoid, this cannot be assumed for each individual. Patients

dividual circumstances are such that potential febrile reactions following DTP might confound the man-
~~t of the patient. DT may be used. For inad-~~

have previously received at least two doses of tetanus toxoid.

Td is the preferred preparation for active tetanus immunization in wound management of patients 7 years old or older. This is to enhance diphtheria protection, since a large proportion of adults are susceptible. Thus, by taking advantage of acute health-care visits such as for wound management, some patients can be protected who otherwise would remain susceptible. For routine wound management in children under 7 years old who are not adequately immunized, DTP should be used instead of single antigen tetanus toxoid. If pertussis vaccine is contraindicated or in-

Table 35-8. Summary guide to tetanus prophylaxis in routine wound management—United States, 1985*

History of adsorbed tetanus toxoid (doses)	Clean, minor wounds		All other wounds†	
	Td (§)	TIG	Td (§)	TIG
Unknown or < three	Yes	No	Yes	Yes
> three	No (**)	No	No (††)	No

*Important details are in the text.

†Such as, but not limited to, wounds contaminated with dirt, feces, soil, saliva, etc.; puncture wounds; avulsions; and wounds resulting from missiles, crushing, burns and frostbite.

§For children less than 7 years old; DTP (DT, if pertussis vaccine is contraindicated) is preferred to tetanus toxoid alone. For persons 7 years old and older, Td is preferred to tetanus toxoid alone.

¶If only 3 doses of *fluid* toxoid have been received, then a fourth dose of toxoid, preferably an adsorbed toxoid, should be given.

**Yes, if more than 10 years since last dose.

††Yes, if more than 5 years since last dose. (More frequent boosters are not needed and can accentuate side effects.)

only adsorbed toxoid ~~in this~~

Pertussis prophylaxis for case contacts

Spread of pertussis can be limited by decreasing infectivity of the patient and by protecting close contacts of that patient. To reduce infectivity as quickly as possible, a course of oral erythromycin (children: 40 mg/kg/day; adults: 1 gm/day) or trimethoprim sulfamethoxazole (children: trimethoprim 8 mg/kg/day, —sulfamethoxazole 40 mg/kg/day; adults: trimethoprim 320 mg/day,—sulfamethoxazole 1600 mg/day) is recommended for patients with clinical pertussis. The antibiotic should be administered for 14 days to minimize any chance of antibiotic failure. Chemotherapy, however, probably does not affect the duration or severity of disease.

There are two approaches for protecting close contacts (such as children exposed in a household or day-care center) of patients with pertussis—active immunization and chemoprophylaxis. Close contacts under 7 years old who have not completed the 4-dose primary series of DTP injections or who have not received a dose of DTP within 3 years of exposure should be given a dose of vaccine and should complete a primary series with the minimal intervals (Table 1). While the usefulness of chemoprophylaxis has not been well demonstrated, it may be prudent to consider a 14-day course of erythromycin or trimethoprim-sulfamethoxazole for close contacts under 1 year old regardless of immunization status and for unimmunized close contacts under 7 years old.

Prophylactic postexposure passive immunization is not recommended. Studies have shown that use of human pertussis immune globulin neither prevents illness nor reduces its severity. This product is no longer available in the United States.

REFERENCES

1. ACIP. Diphtheria, tetanus, and pertussis: guidelines for vaccine prophylaxis and other preventive measures. MMWR 1981;30:392-6, 401-7(420).
2. ACIP. Supplementary statement of contraindications to receipt of pertussis vaccine. MMWR 1984;33:169-71.

3. Hinman AR, Koplan JP. Pertussis and pertussis vaccine: reanalysis of benefits, risks and costs. JAMA 1984;251:3109-13.
4. Linneman CC, Ramundo N, Perlstein PH, et al. Use of pertussis vaccine in an epidemic involving hospital staff. Lancet 1975;2:540-3.
5. Cody CL, Baraff LJ, Cherry JD, Marcy SM, Manclark CR. The nature and rate of adverse reactions associated with DTP and DT immunization in infants and children. Pediatrics 1981;68:650-60.
6. Miller DL, Ross EM, Alderslade R, Bellman MH, Rawson NSB. Pertussis immunization and serious acute neurological illness in children. Br Med J 1981;282:1595-9.
7. Baraff LJ, Cody CL, Cherry JD. DTP-associated reactions: an analysis by injection site, manufacturer, prior reactions and dose. Pediatrics 1984;73:31-6.
8. CDC. Adverse events following immunization surveillance. Surveillance report no. 1, 1979-1982, issued August 1984.
9. Hoffman HJ. SIDS and DTP. 17th Immunization Conference Proceedings, Atlanta, Georgia, May 1982. Atlanta: Centers for Disease Control, 1982;79-88.
10. Bellman MH, Ross EM, Miller DL. Infantile spasms and pertussis immunization. Lancet 1983;i:1031-4.
11. Barkin RM, Samuelson, JS, Gotlin LP. DTP reactions and serologic response with a reduced dose schedule. J Pediatr 1984;105:189-94.
12. British Medical Research Council. Vaccination against whooping-cough. Relation between protection in children and results of laboratory tests. Br Med J 1956;2:454-62.
13. Cameron J. The potency of whooping cough (pertussis) vaccines in Canada. J Biol Stand 1980;8:297-302.
14. Deforest A, Long SS, Lischner HW, Girone JAC, Srinivasan R, Bernier RH. Simultaneous administration of MMR, OPV and DTP vaccines. Presented at the 24th Interscience Conference on Antimicrobial Agents and Chemotherapy. October 9-10, 1984, Washington.
15. Bernbaum J, Anolik R, Polin RA, Douglas SD. Development of the premature infants host defense and its relationship to routine immunizations. Clinics in Perinatology 1984;11:73-84.
16. Gross PA, Lee H, Wolff JA et al. Influenza immunization in immunosuppressed children. J Pediatr 1978;92:30.
17. Jacobs RL, Lowe RS, Lanier BQ. Adverse reactions to tetanus toxoid. JAMA 1982;247:40-2.

Orenstein WA, Weisfeld JS, Halsey NA. Diphtheria and tetanus toxoids and pertussis vaccine, combined. In: Recent advances in immunization: a bibliographic review. (Scientific Pub No. 451). Washington, PAHO, 1983:30-51.
Strom J. Further experience of reactions especially of a cerebral nature in conjunction with triple vaccination: a study based on vaccinations in Sweden, 1959-1965. Br Med J 1967;4:320-3.
Taylor EM, Emery JL. Immunization and cot deaths. Lancet 1982;2:721.

Diphtheria and diphtheria toxoic

Crossley K, Irvine P, Warren JB, Lee BK, Mead K. Tetanus and diphtheria immunity in urban Minnesota adults. JAMA 1979;242:2298-300.
Brown GC, Volk VK, Gottshall RY, Kendrick PL, Anderson HD. Responses of infants to DTP-P vaccine used in nine injection schedules. Public Health Rep 1964;79:585-602.
Doull JA. Factors influencing selective distribution in diphtheria. J Prev Med 1930;4:371-404.
Edsall G, Altman JS, Gaspar AJ. Combined tetanus-diphtheria immunization of adults: use of small doses of diphtheria toxoid. Am J Public Health 1954;44:1537-45.
Ipsen J. Circulating antitoxin at onset of diphtheria in 425 patients. J Immunol 1946;54:325-47.
Gottlieb S, Martin M, McLaughlin FX, Panaro RJ, Levine L, Edsall G. Long-term immunity to diphtheria and tetanus: a mathematical model. Am J Epidemiol 1967;85:207-19.
Koopman JS, Campbell J. The role of cutaneous diphtheria infections in a diphtheria epidemic. J Infect Dis 1975;131:239-44.
Myers MG, Beckman CW, Vosdingh RA, Hankins WA. Primary immunization with tetanus and diphtheria toxoids: reaction rates and immunogenicity in older children and adults. JAMA 1982;248:2478-80.
Naiditch MJ, Bower AG. Diphtheria; a study of 1,433 cases observed during 10-year period at Los Angeles County Hospital. Am J Med 1954;17:229-45.
Scheibel I, Bentzon MW, Christensen PE, Biering A. Duration of immunity to diphtheria and tetanus after active immunization. Acta Pathol Microbiol Scand 1966;67:380-92.
Tasman A, Lansberg HP. Problems concerning the prophylaxis, pathogenesis, and therapy of diphtheria. Bull WHO 1957;16:939-73.
Volk VK, Gottshall RY, Anderson HD, Top FH, Bunney WE, Serfling RE. Antigenic responses to booster dose of diphtheria and tetanus toxoids. Seven to thirteen years after primary inoculation of noninstitutionalized children. Public Health Rep 1962;77:185-94.
Weiss BP, Strassburg MA, Feeley JC. Tetanus and diphtheria immunity in an elderly population in Los Angeles County. Am J Pub Health 1983;73:802-4.

Tetanus and tetanus toxoid

Blumstein GI, Kreithen H. Peripheral neuropathy following tetanus toxoid administration. JAMA 1966;198:1030-1.
Brown GC, Volk VK, Gottshall RY, Kendrick PL, Anderson HD. Responses of infants to DTP-P vaccine used in nine injection schedules. Public Health Rep 1964;79:585-602.

SELECTED BIBLIOGRAPHY
Combined diphtheria and tetanus toxoids and pertussis vaccine

Barkin RM, Pichichero ME. Diphtheria-pertussis-tetanus vaccine: reactogenicity of commercial products. Pediatrics 1979;63:256-60.
Bernier RH, Frank J, Dondero T. Diphtheria-tetanus toxoids-pertussis vaccination and sudden infant death syndrome in Tennessee. J Pediatr 1982;101:419-21.
Hirtz DG, Nelson KB, Ellenberg JH. Seizures following childhood immunizations. J Pediatr 1983;102:14-8.

Chen ST, Edsall G, Peel MM, Sinnathuray TA. Timing of antenatal tetanus immunization for effective protection of

Gordon J, Hood RL. Whooping cough and its epidemiological anomalies. Am J Med Sci 1951;222:333-61.

Henry RL, Dorman DC, Skinner JA, Mellis CM. Antimi-

207-19.

LaForce FM, Young LS, Bennett JV. Tetanus in the United States (1965-1966): epidemiologic and clinical features. N Engl J Med 1969;280:569-74.

MacLennan R, Schofield FD, Pittman M, Hardegree MC, Barile MF. Immunization against neonatal tetanus in New Guinea. Antitoxin response of pregnant women to adjuvant and plain toxoids. Bull WHO 1965;32:683-97.

Myers MG, Beckman CW, Vosdingh RA, Hankins WA. Primary immunization with tetanus and diphtheria toxoids: Reaction rates and immunogenicity in older children and adults. JAMA 1982;248:2478-80.

Peebles TC, Levine L, Eldred MC, Edsall G. Tetanus-toxoid emergency boosters: a reappraisal. N Engl J Med 1969;280:575-81.

Scheibel I, Bentzon MW, Christensen PE, Biering A. Duration of immunity to diphtheria and tetanus after active immunization. Acta Pathol Microbiol Scand 1966;67:380-92.

Volk VK, Gottshall RY, Anderson HD, Top FH, Bunney WE, Serfling RE. Antigenic response to booster dose of diphtheria and tetanus toxoids. Seven to thirteen years after primary inoculation of noninstitutionalized children. Public Health Rep 1962;77:185-94.

Weiss BP, Strassburg MA, Feeley JC. Tetanus and diphtheria immunity in an elderly population in Los Angeles County. Am J Pub Health 1983;73:802-4.

White WG, Barnes GM, Griffith AH, Gall D, Barker E, Smith JWG. Duration of immunity after active immunization against tetanus. Lancet 1969;2:95-6.

Pertussis and pertussis vaccine

Baraff LJ, Wilkins J, Wehrle PF. The role of antibiotics, immunizations, and adenoviruses in pertussis. Pediatrics 1978;61:224-30.

Berg JM. Neurologic complications of pertussis immunization. Br Med J 1958;2:24-7.

British Medical Research Council. The prevention of whooping-cough by vaccination. A Medical Research Council investigation. Br Med J 1951;1:1463-71.

British Medical Research Council. Vaccination against whooping-cough. A final report. Br Med J 1959;1:994-1000.

CDC. Pertussis—United States, 1982 and 1983. MMWR 1984;33:573-5.

Lambert HJ. Epidemiology of a small pertussis outbreak in Kent County. Michigan, Public Health Rep 1965;80:365-9.

Manclark CR, Hill JC, eds. International Symposium on Pertussis, 3rd. Bethesda, Md.: National Institutes of Health, 1979. (DHEW Publication no. (NIH) 79-1830).

Miller DL, Alderslade R, Ross EM. Whooping cough and whooping cough vaccine: The risks and benefits debate. Epidemiol Rev 1982;4:1-24.

Nelson JD. The changing epidemiology of pertussis in young infants. The role of adults as reservoirs of infection. Am J Dis Child 1978;132:371-3.

Pollard R. Relation between vaccination and notification rates for whooping cough in England and Wales. Lancet 1980;1:1180-2.

Pollock TM, Miller E, Lobb J. Severity of whooping cough in England before and after the decline in pertussis immunization. Arch Dis Child 1984;59:162-5.

Royal College of General Practitioners, Swansea Research Unit. Effect of a low pertussis vaccination uptake on a large community. Br Med J 1981;282:23-6.

Sato Y, Izumiyak K, Sato H, Cowell JL, Manclark CR. Role of antibody to leukocytosis-promoting factor hemagglutinin and to filamentous hemagglutinin in immunity to pertussis. Infect Immun 1981;31:1223-31.

Sato Y, Kimura M, Fukumi H. Development of a pertussis component vaccine in Japan. Lancet 1984;1:122-6.

Wilkins J, Williams FF, Wehrle PF, Portnoy B. Agglutinin response to pertussis vaccine. I. Effect of dosage and interval. J Pediatr 1971;79:197-202.

From MMWR 1985; 34:405-426.

POLYSACCHARIDE VACCINE FOR PREVENTION OF *HAEMOPHILUS INFLUENZAE* TYPE B DISEASE
Introduction

A polysaccharide vaccine* against invasive (bacteremic) disease caused by *Haemophilus influenzae* type b recently has been licensed in the United States. The purposes of this statement are to sum-

---

*Official name: Haemophilus b Polysaccharide Vaccine.

marize available information about this vaccine and to offer guidelines for its use in the prevention of invasive *H. influenzae* type b disease.

Haemophilus influenzae disease

H. influenzae is a leading cause of serious systemic bacterial disease in the United States. It is the most common cause of bacterial meningitis, accounting for an estimated 12,000 cases annually, primarily among children under 5 years of age. The mortality rate is 5%, and neurologic sequelae are observed in as many as 25%-35% of survivors. Virtually all cases of *H. influenzae* meningitis among children are caused by strains of type b (Hib), although this capsular type represents only one of the six types known for this species. In addition to bacterial meningitis, Hib is responsible for other invasive diseases, including epiglottitis, sepsis, cellulitis, septic arthritis, osteomyelitis, pericarditis, and pneumonia. Nontypeable (noncapsulated) strains of *H. influenzae* commonly colonize the human respiratory tract and are a major cause of otitis media and respiratory mucosal infection but rarely result in bacteremic disease. Hib strains account for only 5%-10% of *H. influenzae* causing otitis media.

Several population-based studies of invasive Hib disease conducted within the last 10 years have provided estimates of the incidence of disease among children under 5 years of age, the major age group at risk. These studies have demonstrated attack rates of meningitis ranging from 51 cases per 100,000 children to 77/100,000 per year and attack rates of other invasive Hib disease varying from 24/100,000 to 75/100,000 per year *(1)*. Thus, in the United States, approximately one of every 1,000 children under 5 years of age develops systemic Hib disease each year, and a child's cumulative risk of developing systemic Hib disease at some time during the first 5 years of life is about one in 200. Attack rates peak between 6 months and 1 year of age and decline thereafter. Approximately 35%-40% of Hib disease occurs among children 18 months of age or older, and 25% occurs above 24 months of age.

Incidence rates of Hib disease are increased in certain high-risk groups, such as Native Americans (both American Indians and Eskimos), blacks, individuals of lower socioeconomic status, and patients with asplenia, sickle cell disease, Hodgkin's disease, and antibody deficiency syndromes. Recent studies also have suggested that the risk of acquiring primary Hib disease for children under 5 years of age appears to be greater for those who attend day-care facilities than for those who do not *(2,3)*.

The potential for person-to-person transmission of systemic Hib disease among susceptible individuals has been recognized in the past decade. Studies of secondary spread of Hib disease in household contacts

of index patients have shown a substantially increased risk of disease among exposed household contacts under 4 years of age *(4)*. In addition, numerous clusters of cases in day-care facilities have been reported, and recent studies suggest that secondary attack rates in day-care classroom contacts of a primary case also may be increased *(5,6)*.

Haemophilus b polysaccharide vaccine

The Hib vaccine is composed of the purified, capsular polysaccharide of *H. influenzae* type b ([→3] ribose-β1 →1 ribitol-1 phosphate-5→). Antibodies to this antigen correlate with protection against invasive disease. The Hib vaccine induces an antibody response that is directly related to the age of the recipient; infants respond infrequently and with less antibody than do older children or adults *(7)*. Improved responses are observed by 18 months of age, although children 18-23 months of age do not respond as well as those 2 years of age or older. The frequency and magnitude of antibody responses reach adult levels at about 6 years of age *(8,9)*. Levels of antibodies to the capsular polysaccharide also decline more rapidly in immunized infants and young children than in adults.

In a manner similar to other polysaccharide antigens, revaccination with Hib vaccine results in a level of antibody comparable to that for a child of the same age receiving a first immunization *(10)*. Such polysaccharide antigens have been termed "T-cell independent" because of their failure to induce the T-cell memory response characteristic of protein antigens.

Limited data are available on the response to Hib vaccine in high-risk groups with underlying disease. By analogy to pneumococcal vaccine, patients with sickle cell disease or asplenia are likely to exhibit an immune response to the Hib vaccine. Patients with malignancies associated with immunosuppression appear to respond less well. Additional data on the immune response to Hib vaccine in these groups are needed.

A precise protective level of antibody has not been established. However, based on evidence from passive protection in the infant rat model and from experience with agammaglobulinemic children, an antibody concentration of 0.15 μg/ml correlates with protection *(7,8,11)*. In the Finnish field trial, levels of capsular antibody greater than 1 μg/ml in 3-week postimmunization sera correlated with clinical protection for a minimum of 1½ years *(9,12,13)*. Approximately 75% of children 18-23 months of age tested achieved a level greater than 1 μg/ml, as did 90% of 24-35 month old children *(9)*. Measurement of Hib antibody levels is not routinely available, however, and determination of antibody levels following vaccination is not indicated in the usual clinical setting.

Effectiveness of vaccine

In 1974, a randomized, controlled trial of clinical

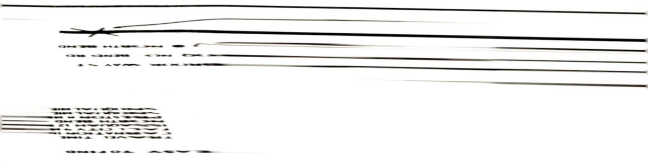

of vaccine may be necessary to ensure long-lasting immunity, routine revaccination is not recommended.

in the subgroup of children immunized at 18-23 months of age could not be evaluated statistically. The vaccine was not efficacious in children under 18 months of age.

Revaccination

Limited data regarding the potential need for revaccination are available at present. Current data show that children who have received the Hib vaccine 2-42 months previously have an immune response to the vaccine similar to that in previously unvaccinated children of the same age. No immunologic tolerance or impairment of immune response to a subsequent dose of vaccine occurs (10). As with other polysaccharide vaccines, the shorter persistence of serum antibodies in young children given Hib vaccine, compared with adults, suggests that a second dose of vaccine may be needed to maintain immunity throughout the period of risk, particularly for children in the youngest age group considered for vaccination (those 18-23 months of age). A second injection following the initial dose is likely to increase the protective benefit of vaccination for this high-risk group, because antibody titers 18 months after vaccination, although detectable in most vaccine recipients, are no longer significantly different from those in unvaccinated children of the same age.

Recommendations for vaccine use

Recently published data regarding vaccine efficacy and the risk of Hib disease among young children strongly support the use of Hib vaccine in the United States in high-risk persons for whom efficacy has been established. Specific recommendations are as follows:

1. **Immunization of all children at 24 months of age is recommended.** The precise duration of immunity conferred by a single dose of Hib vaccine at 24 months of age is not known, although, based on available data, protection is expected to last 1½-3½ years. Until further data are available to determine whether an additional dose

need a second dose of vaccine within 18 months following the initial dose to ensure protection. Additional data regarding the duration of the antibody response are needed to define the timing of a second dose more precisely.

Children who attend day-care facilities are at particular risk of acquiring systemic Hib disease. Initial vaccination at 18 months of age for this high-risk group should be considered.

Children with chronic conditions known to be associated with increased risk for Hib disease should receive the vaccine, although only limited data on immunogenicity and clinical efficacy in this group are available. These conditions include anatomic or functional asplenia, such as sickle cell disease or splenectomy (14), and malignancies associated with immunosuppression (15).

3. **Immunization of individuals over 24 months of age who have not yet received Hib vaccine should be based on risk of disease.** The risk of invasive Hib disease decreases with increasing age over the age of 2 years. Because the vaccine is safe and effective, however, physicians may wish to immunize previously unvaccinated healthy children between 2 years and 5 years of age to prevent the Hib disease that does occur in this age group. The potential benefit of this strategy in terms of cases prevented declines with increasing age of the child at the time of vaccination. Therefore, children 2-3 years of age who attend day-care facilities should be given a higher priority than day-care attendees who are 4-5 years old.

4. **Insufficient data are available on which to base a recommendation concerning use of the vaccine in older children and adults with the chronic conditions associated with an increased risk of Hib disease.**

5. **Vaccine is not recommended for children under 18 months of age.**
6. **Simultaneous administration of Hib and DTP vaccines at separate sites can be performed, because no impairment of the immune response to the individual antigens occurs under these circumstances.**

Side effects and adverse reactions

Polysaccharide vaccines are among the safest of all vaccine products. To date, over 60,000 doses of the Hib polysaccharide vaccine have been administered to infants and children, and several hundred doses have been given to adults (9,16). Only one serious systemic reaction has been reported thus far—a possible anaphylactic reaction that responded promptly to epinephrine. High fever (38.5 C [101.3 F] or higher) has been reported in fewer than 1% of Hib vaccine recipients. Mild local and febrile reactions were common, occurring in as many as half of vaccinated individuals in the Finnish trial. Such reactions appeared within 24 hours and rapidly subsided. Current preparations appear to result in fewer such local reactions. Simultaneous administration with DTP does not result in reaction rates above those expected with separate administration (17).

Precautions and contraindications

The Hib vaccine is unlikely to be of substantial benefit in preventing the occurrence of secondary cases, because children under 2 years old are at highest risk of secondary disease. Because the vaccine will not protect against nontypeable strains of *H. influenzae*, recurrent upper respiratory diseases, including otitis media and sinusitis, are not considered indications for vaccination.

New vaccine development

New vaccines, such as the Hib polysaccharide-protein conjugate vaccines, are being developed and evaluated and may prove to be efficacious for children under 18 months of age.

REFERENCES

1. Cochi SL, Broome CV, Hightower AW. Immunization of US children with *Hemophilus influenzae* type b polysaccharide vaccine: a cost-effectiveness model of strategy assessment. JAMA 1985;253:521-9.
2. Istre GR, Conner JS, Broome CV, Hightower A, Hopkins RS. Risk factors for primary invasive *Haemophilus influenzae* disease. Increased risk from day care attendance and school-aged household members. J Pediatr 1985;106:190-5.
3. Redmond SR, Pichichero ME. *Hemophilus influenzae* type b disease. An epidemiologic study with special reference to day-care centers. JAMA 1984;252:2581-4.
4. CDC. Prevention of secondary cases of *Haemophilus influenzae* type b disease. MMWR 1982;31:672-80.
5. Murphy TV, Breedlove JA, Fritz EH, Sebestyen DM, Hansen EJ. County-wide surveillance of invasive *Haemophilus* infections: risk of associated cases in child care programs (CCPs). Twenty-third Interscience Conference on Antimicrobial Agents and Chemotherapy 1983;229 (abstract #788).
6. Fleming D, Leibenhaut M, Albanes D, et al. *Haemophilus influenzae* b (Hib) disease—secondary spread in day care. Twenty-fourth International Conference on Antimicrobial Agents and Chemotherapy 1984;261 (abstract #967).
7. Smith DH, Peter G, Ingram DL, Harding AL, Anderson P. Responses of children immunized with the capsular polysaccharide of *Hemophilus influenzae*, type b. Pediatrics 1973;52:637-44.
8. Robbins JB, Parke JC Jr, Schneerson R, Whisnant JK. Quantitative measurement of "natural" and immunization-induced *Haemophilus influenzae* type b capsular polysaccharide antibodies. Pediatr Res 1973;7:103-10.
9. Peltola H, Käyhty H, Virtanen M, Mäkelä PH. Prevention of *Hemophilus influenzae* type b bacteremic infections with the capsular polysaccharide vaccine. N Engl J Med 1984;310:1561-6.
10. Käyhty H, Karanko V, Peltola H, Mäkelä PH. Serum antibodies after vaccination with *Haemophilus influenzae* type b capsular polysaccharide and responses to reimmunization: no evidence of immunological tolerance or memory. Pediatrics 1984;74:857-65.
11. Robbins JB, Schneerson R, Parke JC Jr. A review of the efficacy trials with *Haemophilus influenzae* type b polysaccharide vaccines. In: Sell SH, Wright PF, eds. *Haemophilus influenzae*. New York: Elsevier Science Publishing Co., 1982:255-63.
12. Käyhty H, Peltola H, Karanko V, Mäkelä PH. The protective level of serum antibodies to the capsular polysaccharide of *Haemophilus influenzae* type b. J Infect Dis 1983;147:1100.
13. Anderson P. The protective level of serum antibodies to the capsular polysaccharide of *Haemophilus influenzae* type b [Letter]. J Infect Dis 1984;149:1034-5.
14. Ward J, Smith AL. *Hemophilus influenzae* bacteremia in children with sickle cell disease. J Pediatr 1976;88:261-3.
15. Siber GR. Bacteremias due to *Haemophilus influenzae* and *Streptococcus pneumoniae*: their occurrence and course in children with cancer. Am J Dis Child 1980;134:668-72.
16. Parke JC Jr, Schneerson R, Robbins JB, and Schlesselman JJ. Interim report of a controlled field trial of immunization with capsular polysaccharides of *Haemophilus influenzae* type b and group C *Neisseria meningitidis* in Mecklenburg County, North Carolina (March 1974-March 1976) J Infect Dis 1977;136:S51-6.
17. Lepow ML, Peter G, Glode MP, et al. Response of infants to *Haemophilus influenzae* type b polysaccharide and diphtheria-tetanus-pertussis vaccines in combination. J Infect Dis 1984;149:950-5.

From MMWR 1985; 34:201

RECOMMENDATIONS FOR PROTECTION AGAINST VIRAL HEPATITIS

The following statement updates all previous recommendations on use of immune globulins for protection against viral hepatitis (MMWR 1981;30: 423-35) and use of hepatitis B vaccine and hepatitis B immune globulin for prophylaxis of hepatitis B (MMWR 1982;31:317-28 and MMWR 1984;33: 285-90).

Introduction

The term "viral hepatitis" is commonly used for several clinically similar diseases that are etiologically and epidemiologically distinct *(1)*. Two of these, hepatitis A (formerly called infectious hepatitis) and hepatitis B (formerly called serum hepatitis) have been recognized as separate entities since the early 1940s and can be diagnosed with specific serologic tests. The third, currently known as non-A, non-B hepatitis, is probably caused by at least two different agents, and lacking specific diagnostic tests, remains a disease diagnosed by exclusion. It is an important form of acute viral hepatitis in adults and currently accounts for most post-transfusion hepatitis in the United States. An epidemic type of non-A, non-B hepatitis, which is probably spread by the fecal-oral route and is different from the types seen in the United States, has been described in parts of Asia and North Africa *(2)*.

A fourth type of hepatitis, delta hepatitis, has recently been characterized as an infection dependent on hepatitis B virus. It may occur as a coinfection with acute hepatitis B infection or as superinfection of a hepatitis B carrier *(3)*.

Hepatitis surveillance

Approximately 21,500 cases of hepatitis A, 24,300 cases of hepatitis B, 3,500 cases of non-A, non-B hepatitis, and 7,100 cases of hepatitis type unspecified were reported in the United States in 1983. Most cases of each type occur among young adults. Since reporting from many localities is incomplete, the actual number of hepatitis cases occurring annually is thought to be several times the reported number.

Immune globulins

Immune globulins used in medical practice are sterile solutions of antibodies (immunoglobulins) from human plasma. They are prepared by cold ethanol fractionation of large plasma pools and contain 10%-18% protein. In the United States, plasma is primarily obtained from professional donors. Only plasma shown to be free of hepatitis B surface antigen (HBsAg) is used to prepare immune globulins.

Immune globulin (IG) (formerly called "immune serum globulin," ISG, or "gamma globulin") produced in the United States contains antibodies against the hepatitis A virus (anti-HAV) and the hepatitis B surface antigen (anti-HBs). Tests of IG lots prepared since 1977 indicate that both types of antibody have uniformly been present. Hepatitis B immune globulin (HBIG) is an IG prepared from plasma containing high titers of anti-HBs.

Neither IG nor HBIG commercially available in the United States transmits hepatitis or other viral infections. There is no evidence that the causative agent of AIDS (human T-lymphotropic virus type III/lymphadenopathy-associated virus [HTLV-III/LAV]) has been transmitted by IG or HBIG *(4)*.

Serious adverse effects from immune globulins administered as recommended have been exceedingly rare. Standard immune globulins are prepared for intramuscular use and should not be given intravenously. Two preparations for intravenous use in immunodeficient and other selected patients have recently become available in the United States but are not recommended for hepatitis prophylaxis. Immune globulins are not contraindicated for pregnant women.

Hepatitis A

Hepatitis A is caused by the hepatitis A virus (HAV), a 27-nm ribonucleic acid (RNA) agent that is a member of the picornavirus family. The illness caused by HAV characteristically has an abrupt onset with fever, malaise, anorexia, nausea, abdominal discomfort, and jaundice. Severity is related to age. In children, most infections are asymptomatic, and illness is usually not accompanied by jaundice. Most infected adults become symptomatically ill with jaundice. Fatality among reported cases is infrequent (about 0.6%).

Hepatitis A is primarily transmitted by person-to-person contact, generally through fecal contamination. Transmission is facilitated by poor personal hygiene, poor sanitation, and intimate (intrahousehold or sexual) contact. Common-source epidemics from contaminated food and water also occur. Sharing utensils or cigarettes or kissing are not believed to transmit the infection.

The incubation period of hepatitis A is 15-50 days (average 28-30). High concentrations of HAV (10^8 particles/g) are found in stools of infected persons. Fecal virus excretion reaches its highest concentration late in the incubation period and early in the prodromal phase of illness, and diminishes rapidly once jaundice appears. Greatest infectivity is during the 2-week period immediately before the onset of jaundice. Viremia is of short duration; virus has not been found in urine or other body fluids. A chronic carrier state with HAV in blood or feces has not been demonstrated. Transmission of HAV by blood transfusion has occurred but is rare.

The diagnosis of acute hepatitis A is confirmed by

finding IGM-class anti-HAV in serum collected during the acute or early convalescent phase of disease. IgG-class anti-HAV, which appears in the convalescent phase of disease and remains detectable in serum thereafter, apparently confers enduring protection against disease. Commercial tests are available to detect IgM anti-HAV and total anti/HAV in serum.

Although the incidence of hepatitis A in the United States has decreased over the last 15 years, it is still a common infection in older children and young adults. About 38% of reported hepatitis cases in this country are attributable to hepatitis A.

Recommendations for IG prophylaxis of hepatitis A. Numerous field studies conducted in the past 4 decades confirm that IG given before exposure or during the incubation period of hepatitis A is protective against clinical illness (5-7). Its prophylactic value is greatest (80%-90%) when given early in the incubation period and declines thereafter (7).

Preexposure prophylaxis. The major group for whom preexposure prophylaxis is recommended is international travelers. The risk of hepatitis A for U.S. citizens traveling abroad varies with living conditions, incidence of hepatitis A infection in areas visited, and length of stay (8,9). In general, travelers to developed areas of western Europe, Japan, and Australia are at no greater risk of infection than in the United States. In contrast, travelers to developing countries may be at significant risk of infection. In such areas, the best way to prevent hepatitis A and other enteric diseases is to avoid potentially contaminated water or food. Drinking water (or beverages with ice) of unknown purity and eating uncooked shellfish or uncooked fruits or vegetables that are not peeled (or prepared) by the traveler should be avoided.

IG is recommended for travelers to developing countries if they will be eating in settings of poor or uncertain sanitation (some restaurants or homes) or will be visiting extensively with local persons, especially young children, in settings with poor sanitary conditions. Persons who plan to reside in developing areas for long periods should receive IG regularly if they anticipate exposure as described above or will be living in rural areas with poor sanitation.

For such travelers, a single dose of IG of 0.02 ml/kg is recommended if travel is for less than 2 months. For prolonged travel, 0.06 ml/kg should be given every 5 months. For persons who require repeated IG prophylaxis, screening for total anti-HAV antibodies before travel may be useful to define susceptibility and eliminate unnecessary doses of IG in those who are immune.

Postexposure prophylaxis. A serologic test for the diagnosis of acute hepatitis A is now widely available. Since only 38% of acute hepatitis cases in the United States result from hepatitis A, serologic confirmation of hepatitis A in the index case is recommended before

treatment of contacts. Serologic screening of contacts for anti-HAV before giving IG is not recommended because screening is more costly than IG and would delay its administration.

IG should be given as soon as pobbible after exposure; giving IG more than 2 weeks after exposure is not indicated.

Specific recommendations for IG prophylaxis of hepatitis A depend on the nature of the HAV exposure.

1. *Close personal contact.* IG is recommended for all household and sexual contacts of persons with hepatitis A.

2. *Day-care centers.* Day-care facilities with children in diapers can be important settings for HAV transmission (10-12). IG should be administered to all staff and attendees of day-care centers or homes if: (a) one or more hepatitis A cases are recognized among children or employees; or (b) cases are recognized in two or more households of center attendees. When an outbreak (hepatitis cases in three or more families) occurs, IG should also be considered for members of households whose diapered children attend. In centers not enrolling children in diapers, IG need only be given to classroom contacts of an index case.

3. *Schools.* Contact at elementary and secondary schools is usually not an important means of transmitting hepatitis A. Routine administration of IG is not indicated for pupils and teachers in contact with a patient. However, when epidemiologic study clearly shows the existence of a school- or classroom-centered outbreak, IG may be given to those who have close personal contact with patients.

4. *Institutions for custodial care.* Living conditions in some institutions, such as prisons and facilities for the developmentally disabled, favor transmission of hepatitis A. When outbreaks occur, giving IG to residents and staff who have close contact with patients with hepatitis A may reduce the spread of disease. Depending on the epidemiologic circumstances, prophylaxis can be limited in extent or can involve the entire institution.

5. *Hospitals.* Routine IG prophylaxis for hospital personnel is not indicated. Rather, sound hygienic practices should be emphasized. Staff education should point out the risk of exposure to hepatitis A and emphasize precautions regarding direct contact with potentially infective materials (13).

   Outbreaks of hepatitis A among hospital staff occur occasionally, usually in association with an unsuspected index patient who is fecally incontinent. Large outbreaks have occurred among staff and family contacts of infected infants in neonatal intensive-care units. In outbreaks, prophylaxis of persons exposed to feces of infected patients may be indicated.

6. *Offices and factories.* Routine IG administration is not indicated under the usual office or factory conditions for persons exposed to a fellow worker with hepatitis A. Experience shows that casual contact in the work setting does not result in virus transmission.

7. *Common-source exposure.* IG might be effective in preventing foodborne or waterborne hepatitis A if exposure is recognized in time. However, IG is not recommended for persons exposed to a common source of hepatitis infection after cases have begun to occur in those exposed, since the 2-week period during which IG is effective will have been exceeded.

If a foodhandler is diagnosed as having hepatitis A, common-source transmission is possible but uncommon. IG should be administered to other foodhandlers but is usually not recommended for patrons. However, IG administration to patrons may be considered if (a) the infected person is directly involved in handling, without gloves, foods that will not be cooked before they are eaten; (b) the hygienic practices of the foodhandler are deficient; and (c) patrons can be identified and treated within 2 weeks of exposure. Situations where repeated exposures may have occurred, such as in institutional cafeterias, may warrant stronger consideration of IG use.

For postexposure IG prophylaxis, a single intramuscular dose of 0.02 ml/kg is recommended.

Hepatitis B

Hepatitis B virus (HBV) infection is a major cause of acute and chronic hepatitis, cirrhosis, and primary hepatocellular carcinoma worldwide. The frequency of HBV infection and patterns of transmission vary markedly in different parts of the world. In the United States, western Europe, and Australia, it is a disease of low endemicity, with only 0.1%-0.5% of the population being virus carriers and infection occurring primarily during adulthood. In contrast, HBV infection is highly endemic in China and Southeast Asia, sub-Saharan Africa, most Pacific islands, and the Amazon Basin; in these areas, 5%-15% of the population carry the virus, and most persons acquire infection at birth or during childhood. In other parts of the world, HBV is moderately endemic, and 1%-4% of persons are HBV carriers. Recommendations for prophylaxis of hepatitis B will vary in accordance with local patterns of HBV transmission. The recommendations that follow are intended for use in the United States.

Hepatitis B infection is caused by the HBV, a 42-nm, double-shelled deoxyribonucleic acid (DNA) virus. Several well-defined antigen-antibody systems have been associated with HBV infection (Table 35-9). HBsAg, formerly called "Australia antigen" or "hepatitis-associated antigen," is found on the surface of the virus and on accompanying 22-nm spherical and tubular forms. HBsAg can be identified in serum 30-60 days after exposure to HBV and persists for variable periods. The various subtypes (adr, adw, ayw, ayr) of HBsAg provide useful epidemiologic markers. Antibody against HBsAg (anti-HBs) develops after a resolved infection and is responsible for long term immunity. Anti-HBc, the antibody to the core antigen (an internal component of the virus), develops in all HBV infections and persists indefinitely. IgM anti-HBc appears early in infection and persists for 6 or more months; it is a reliable marker of acute or recent HBV infection. The hepatitis B e antigen (HBeAg) is a third antigen, presence of which correlates with HBV replication and high infectivity. Antibody to HBeAg (anti-HBe) develops in most HBV infections and correlates with lower infectivity.

The onset of acute hepatitis B is generally insidious. Clinical symptoms and signs include various combinations of anorexia, malaise, nausea, vomiting, abdominal pain, and jaundice. Skin rashes, arthralgias, and arthritis can also occur. Overall fatality rates for reported cases generally do not exceed 2%. The incubation period of hepatitis B is long—45-160 days (average 60-120).

HBV infection in the United States. The estimated lifetime risk of HBV infection in the United States varies from almost 100% for the highest-risk groups to approximately 5% for the population as a whole. An estimated 200,000 persons, primarily young adults, are infected each year. One-quarter become ill with jaundice; more than 10,000 patients require hospitalization; and an average of 250 die of fulminant disease each year. Between 6% and 10% of young adults with HBV infection become carriers. Chronic active hepatitis develops in over 25% of carriers and often progresses to cirrhosis. Furthermore, HBV carriers have a risk of developing primary liver cancer that is 12-300 times higher than that of other persons. It is estimated that 4,000 persons die from hepatitis B-related cirrhosis each year in this country and that more than 800 die from hepatitis B-related liver cancer.

The role of the HBV carrier is central in the epidemiology of HBV transmission. A carrier is defined as a person who is HBsAg-positive on at least two occasions at least 6 months apart. Although the degree of infectivity is best correlated with HBeAg-positivity, any person positive for HBsAg is potentially infectious. The likelihood of developing the carrier state varies inversely with the age at which infection oc-

Table 35.9. Hepatitis nomenclature

Abbreviation	Term	Comments
Hepatitis A		
HAV	Hepatitis A virus	Etiologic agent of "infectious" hepatitis; a picornavirus; single serotype.
Anti-HAV	Antibody to HAV	Detectable at onset of symptoms; lifetime persistence.
IgM anti-HAV	IgM class antibody to HAV	Indicates recent infection with hepatitis A, positive up to 4-6 months after infection.
Hepatitis B		
HBV	Hepatitis B virus	Etiologic agent of "serum" or "long-incubation" hepatitis; also known as Dane particle.
HBsAg	Hepatitis B surface antigen	Surface antigen(s) of HBV detectable in large quantity in serum; several subtypes identified.
HBeAg	Hepatitis B e antigen	Soluble antigen; correlates with HBV replication, high titer HBV in serum, and infectivity of serum.
HBcAg	Hepatitis B core antigen	No commercial test available.
Anti-HBs	Antibody to HBsAg	Indicates past infection with and immunity to HBV, passive antibody from HBIG, or immune response from HBV vaccine.
Anti-HBe	Antibody to HBeAg	Presence in serum of HBsAg carrier suggests lower titer of HBV.
Anti-HBc	Antibody to HBcAg	Indicates past infection with HBV at some undefined time.
IgM anti-HBc	IgM class antibody to HBcAg	Indicates recent infection with HBV; positive for 4-6 months after infection.
Delta hepatitis		
δ virus	Delta virus	Etiologic agent of delta hepatitis; may only cause infection in presence of HBV.
δ-Ag	Delta antigen	Detectable in early acute delta infection.
Anti-δ	Antibody to delta antigen	Indicates past or present infection with delta virus.
Non-A, non-B hepatitis		
NANB	Non-A, non-B hepatitis	Diagnosis of exclusion. At least two candidate viruses; epidemiology parallels that of hepatitis B.
Epidemic non-A, non-B hepatitis		
Epidemic NANB	Epidemic non-A, non-B hepatitis	Causes large epidemics in Asia, North Africa, fecal-oral or waterborne.
Immune globulins		
IG	Immune globulin (previously ISG, immune serum globulin, or gamma globulin)	Contains antibodies to HAV, low titer antibodies to HBV.
HBIG	Hepatitis B immune globulin	Contains high titer antibodies to HBV.

curs. During the perinatal period, HBV transmitted from HBeAg-positive mothers results in HBV carriage in up to 90% of infected infants, whereas 6%-10% of acutely infected adults become carriers.

Carriers and persons with acute infection have highest concentrations of HBV in the blood and serous fluids; less is present in other body fluids, such as saliva and semen. Transmission occurs via percutaneous or permucosal routes. Infective blood or body fluids can be introduced by contaminated needles or through sexual contact. Infection can occur in settings of continuous close personal contact, such as in households or among children in institutions for the mentally retarded, presumably via inapparent or unnoticed contact of infectious secretions with skin lesions or mucosal surfaces. Transmission of infection by transfusion of contaminated blood or blood products has been greatly reduced since the advent of routine screening with highly sensitive tests for HBsAg. HBV is not transmitted via the fecal-oral route or by contamination of food or water.

Serologic surveys demonstrate that, although HBV infection is uncommon among adults in the general population, it is highly prevalent in certain groups. Those at risk, based on the prevalence of serologic markers of infection, are described in Table 35-10. Immigrants/refugees and their descendants from areas of high HBV endemicity are at high risk of acquiring HBV infection. Homosexually active men and users of illicit injectable drugs are among the highest-risk groups, acquiring infection soon after adopting these lifestyles (10%-20%/year). Inmates of prisons have high prevalence of HBV markers usually because of prior parenteral drug abuse; actual risk of transmission in prisons is also associated with parenteral drug abuse in prisons. Patients and staff in custodial institutions for the mentally retarded are also at increased risk of having HBV infection. Classroom contacts, particularly teachers or instructors, of some deinstitutionalized carriers may also be at higher risk than the general population. Household contacts and sexual partners of HBV carriers are at increased risk, as are hemodialysis patients and recipients of certain pooled plasma products.

There is increased risk for medical and dental workers and related laboratory and support personnel who have contact with blood. Employment in a hospital without exposure to blood carries no greater risk than that for the general population.

Hepatitis B prophylaxis. Two types of products are available for prophylaxis against hepatitis B. Hepatitis B vaccine, licensed in 1981, provides active immunization against HBV infection, and its use is recommended for both pre- and postexposure prophylaxis, IG products provide temporary, passive protection and are indicated only in certain postexposure settings.

IG and HBIG. IG and HBIG contain different amounts of anti-HBs. IG is prepared from plasma that is not preselected for anti-HBs content. Since 1977, all lots tested have contained anti-HBs at a titer of at least 1:100 by radioimmunoassay (RIA). HBIG is pre-

Table 35-10. Prevalence of hepatitis B serologic markers in various population groups

Population group	Prevalence of serologic markers of HBV infection	
	HBsAg (%)	All markers (%)
High risk		
Immigrants/refugees from areas of high HBV endemicity	13	70-85
Clients in institutions for the mentally retarded	10-20	35-80
Users of illicit parenteral drugs	7	60-80
Homosexually active men	6	35-80
Household contacts of HBV carriers	3-6	30-60
Patients of hemodialysis units	3-10	20-80
Intermediate risk		
Health-care workers—frequent blood contact	1-2	15-30
Prisoners (male)	1-8	10-80
Staff of institutions for the mentally retarded	1	10-25
Low risk		
Health-care workers—no or infrequent blood contact	0.3	3-10
Healthy adults (first-time volunteer blood donors)	0.3	3-5

pared from plasma preselected for high-titer anti-HBs. In the United States, HBIG has an anti-HBs titer of higher than 1:100,000 by RIA. There is no evidence that the causative agent of AIDS (HTLV-III/LAV) has been transmitted by IG or HBIG *(4)*.

Hepatitis B vaccine. Hepatitis B vaccine licensed in the United States is a suspension of inactivated, alum-adsorbed 22-nm surface antigen particles that have been purified from human plasma by a combination of biophysical (ultracentrifugation) and biochemical procedures. Inactivation is a threefold process using 8M urea, pepsin at pH 2, and 1:4000 formalin. These treatment steps have been shown to inactivate representatives of all classes of viruses found in human blood, including the causative agent of AIDS (HTLV-III/LAV) *(14)*. HB vaccine contains 20 μg/ml of HBsAg protein.

After a series of three intramuscular doses of hepatitis B vaccine, over 90% of healthy adults develop protective antibody *(15,16)*. A course of three 10-μg doses induces antibody in virtually all infants and children from birth through 9 years of age. The deltoid (arm) is the recommended site for hepatitis B vaccination in adults; immunogenicity of vaccine in adults is significantly lower when injections are given in the buttock (81%) *(17)*. The immunogenicity of the intradermal route has not yet been clearly established.

Field trials of the U.S.-manufactured vaccine have shown 80%-95% efficacy in preventing infection or hepatitis among susceptible persons *(16,18)*. Protection against illness is virtually complete for persons who develop adequate antibody levels after vaccination. The duration of protection and need for booster doses are not yet defined. However, only 10%-15% of persons who develop adequate antibody after three vaccine doses will lose antibody within 4 years, and among those who lose antibody, protection against viremic infection and liver inflammation appears to persist. Immunogenicity and efficacy of the licensed vaccine in hemodialysis patients is much lower than in normal adults; protection may last only as long as adequate antibody levels persist *(19)*.

Vaccine usage. Primary vaccination consists of three intramuscular doses of vaccine, with the second and third doses given 1 and 6 months; respectively, after the first. Adults and older children should be given 20 μg (1.0 ml) per dose, while children under 10 years should receive 10 μg (0.5 ml) per dose. For patients undergoing hemodialysis and for other immunosuppressed patients, a 40-μg (2.0-ml) dose should be used. Vaccine doses administered at longer intervals provide equally satisfactory protection, but optimal protection is not conferred until after the third dose. Hepatitis B vaccine should only be given in the deltoid muscle in adults and children or in the anterolateral thigh muscle in infants and neonates. Since hepatitis B vaccine is an inactivated (noninfec-

tive) product, it is presumed that there will be no interference with other simultaneously administered vaccines.

Data are not available on the safety of the vaccine for the developing fetus. Because the vaccine contains only noninfectious HBsAg particles, there should be no risk to the fetus. In contrast, HBV infection in a pregnant woman may result in severe disease for the mother and chronic infection for the newborn. Pregnancy should not be considered a contraindication to the use of this vaccine for persons who are otherwise eligible.

Vaccine storage. Vaccine should be stored at 2 C-8 C (36 F-46 F) but not frozen. *Freezing destroys the potency of the vaccine.*

Side effects and adverse reactions. The most common side effect observed in prevaccination trials was soreness at the injection site. Among an estimated 750,000 vaccinees, approximately 100 episodes of severe illness have been reported after receipt of vaccine. These have included arthralgias, neurologic reactions (such as Guillain-Barré syndrome), and other illnesses. The rate of Guillain-Barré syndrome following HB vaccine does not appear to be significantly increased above that observed in normal adults. Such temporally associated illnesses are not considered to be etiologically related to hepatitis B vaccine.

Effect of vaccination on carriers and immune persons. The vaccine produces neither therapeutic nor adverse effects in HBV carriers *(20)*. Vaccination of individuals who possess antibodies against HBV from a previous infection is not necessary but will not cause adverse effects. Such individuals will have a postvaccination increase in their anti-HBs levels. Passively acquired antibody, whether from HBIG or IG administration or from the transplacental route, will not interfere with active immunization *(21)*.

Prevaccination serologic screening for susceptibility. The decision to screen potential vaccine recipients for prior infection depends on three variables: (1) the cost of vaccination; (2) the cost of testing for susceptibility; and (3) the expected prevalence of immune individuals in the group. Figure 35-1 shows the relative cost-effectiveness of screening, given different costs of screening tests and the expected prevalence of immunity. In constructing the figure, the assumption was made that the cost of three doses of vaccine is $100 and that there are additional costs for administration. For any combination of screening costs and immunity to hepatitis, the cost-effectiveness can be estimated. For example, if the expected prevalence of serologic markers for HBV is over 20%, screening is cost-effective if costs of screening are no greater than $30 per person. If the expected prevalence of markers is less than 8%, and if the costs of screening are greater than $10 per person, vaccination without screening is cost-effective.

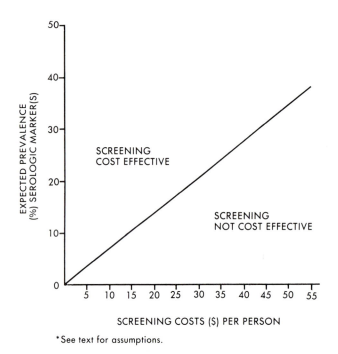

Fig. 35-1. Cost effectiveness of pre-vaccination screening of hepatitis B virus vaccine candidates (see text for assumptions).

Screening in groups with the highest risk of HBV infection (Table 35-10) will be cost-effective unless testing costs are extremely high. For groups at intermediate risk, cost-effectiveness of screening may be marginal, and vaccination programs may or may not utilize screening. For groups with a low expected prevalence of HBV serologic markers, such as health professionals in their training years, screening will not be cost-effective.

Revaccination of persons who do not respond to primary series (nonresponders) produces adequate antibody in only one-third when the primary vaccination has been given in the deltoid. Therefore, revaccination of nonresponders to deltoid injection is not recommended routinely. For persons who did not respond to a primary vaccine series given in the buttock, preliminary data from two small studies suggest that revaccination in the arm induces adequate antibody in over 75%. Revaccination should be strongly considered for such persons.

Preexposure vaccination. Persons at substantial risk of acquiring HBV infection who are demonstrated or judged likely to be susceptible should be vaccinated. They include:

1. *Health-care workers.* The risk of health-care workers acquiring HBV infection depends on the frequency of exposure to blood or blood products and on the frequency of needlesticks. These risks vary during the training and work-

ing career of each individual but are often highest during the professional training period. For this reason, it is recommended that vaccination be completed during training in schools of medicine, dentistry, nursing, laboratory technology, and other allied health professions.

The risk of HBV infection for hospital personnel can vary both among hospitals and within hospitals. In developing specific immunization strategies. hospitals should use available published data about the risk of infection (22-24) and may wish to evaluate their own clinical and institutional experience with hepatitis B. Studies in urban centers have indicated that occupational groups with frequent exposure to blood and/or needles have the highest risk of acquiring HBV infection, including (but not limited to) the following groups: medical technologists, operating room staff, phlebotomists and intravenous therapy nurses, surgeons and pathologists, and oncology and dialysis unit staff. Groups shown to be at increased risk in some hospitals include: emergency room staff, nursing personnel, and staff physicians.

Other health-care workers based outside hospitals who have frequent contact with blood or blood products are also at increased risk of acquiring HBV infection. These include (but are not limited to): dental professionals (dentists, oral surgeons, dental hygienists), laboratory and blood bank technicians, dialysis center staff, emergency medical technicians, and morticians.

2. *Clients and staff of institutions for the mentally retarded.* Susceptible clients and staff who work closely with clients of institutions for the mentally retarded should be vaccinated. Risks for staff are comparable to those for health-care personnel in other high-risk environments. However, the risk in institutional environments is associated, not only with blood exposure, but also with bites and contact with skin lesions and other infective secretions. Susceptible clients and staff who live or work in smaller (group) residential settings with known HBV carriers should also receive hepatitis B vaccine.

3. *Hemodialysis patients.* Numerous studies have established the high risk of HBV transmission in hemodialysis units. Although recent data have shown not only a decrease in the rate of HBV infection in hemodialysis units but also a lower vaccine efficacy in these patients, vaccination is recommended for susceptible patients. Environmental control measures and regular serologic screening (based on immune status) of patients should be maintained.

4. *Homosexually active men.* Susceptible homosexually active men should be vaccinated regardless of their ages or duration of their homosexual practices. It is important to vaccinate persons as soon as possible after their homosexual activity begins. Homosexually active women are not at increased risk of sexually transmitted HBV infection.

5. *Users of illicit injectable drugs.* All users of illicit injectable drugs who are susceptible to HBV should be vaccinated as early as possible after their drug use begins.

6. *Recipients of certain blood products.* Patients with clotting disorders who receive clotting factor concentrates have an elevated risk of acquiring HBV infection. Vaccination is recommended for these persons and should be initiated at the time their specific clotting disorder is identified. Screening is recommended for patients who have already received multiple infusions of these products.

7. *Household and sexual contacts of HBV carriers.* Household contacts of HBV carriers are at high risk of acquiring HBV infection. Sexual contacts appear to be at greatest risk. When HBV carriers are identified through routine screening of donated blood, diagnostic testing in hospitals, prenatal screening, screening of refugees, or other screening programs, they should be notified of their status and their susceptible household contacts vaccinated.

Families accepting orphans or unaccompanied minors from countries of high HBV endemicity should have the child screened for HBsAg, and if positive, family members should be vaccinated.

8. *Other contacts of HBV carriers.* Persons in casual contact with carriers at schools, offices, etc., are at minimal risk of acquiring HBV infection, and vaccine is not routinely recommended for them. However, classroom contacts of deinstitutionalized mentally retarded HBV carriers who behave aggressively or have special medical problems that increase the risk of exposure to their blood or serous secretions may be at risk. In such situations, vaccine may be offered to classroom contacts.

9. *Special high-risk populations.* Some American populations, such as Alaskan Eskimos, native Pacific islanders, and immigrants and refugees from areas with highly endemic disease (particularly eastern Asia and sub-Saharan Africa) have high HBV infection rates. Depending on specific epidemiologic and public health considerations, more extensive vaccination programs should be considered.

10. *Inmates of long-term correctional facilities.* The prison environment may provide a favorable setting for the transmission of HBV because of the frequent use of illicit injectable drugs and homosexual practices. Moreover, it provides an access point for vaccination of parenteral drug abusers. Prison officials should consider undertaking screening and vaccination programs directed at those who abuse drugs before or while in prison.

11. *Heterosexually active persons.* Heterosexually active persons with multiple sexual partners are at increased risk of acquiring HBV infection; risk increases with increasing sexual activity. Vaccination should be considered for persons who present for treatment of sexually transmitted diseases and who have histories of sexual activity with multiple partners.

12. *International travelers.* Vaccination should be considered for persons who plan to reside more than 6 months in areas with high levels of endemic HBV and who will have close contact with the local population. Vaccination should also be considered for short-term travelers who are likely to have contact with blood from or sexual contact with residents of areas with high levels of endemic disease. Hepatitis B vaccination of travelers ideally should begin 6

months before travel in order to complete the full vaccine series; however, partial series will offer some protection against HBV infection.

Postexposure prophylaxis for hepatitis B. Prophylactic treatment to prevent hepatitis B infection after exposure to HBV should be considered in the following situations: perinatal exposure of an infant born to an HBsAg-positive mother; accidental percutaneous or permucosal exposure to HBsAg-positive blood; or sexual exposure to an HBsAg-positive person.

Recent studies have established the relative efficacies of immune globulins and/or hepatitis B vaccine in various exposure situations. For perinatal exposure to an HBsAg-positive, HBeAg-positive mother, a regimen combining one dose of HBIG at birth with the hepatitis B vaccine series started soon after birth is 85%-90% effective in preventing development of the HBV carrier state (25,27). Regimens involving either multiple doses of HBIG alone, or the vaccine series alone, have 70%-75% efficacy, while a single dose of HBIG alone has only 50% efficacy (28).

For accidental percutaneous exposure or sexual exposure, only regimens including HBIG and/or IG have been studied. A regimen of two HBIG doses, one given after exposure and one a month later, is about 75% effective in preventing hepatitis B following percutaneous exposure; a single dose of HBIG has similar efficacy when used following sexual exposure (29-31). IG may have some effect in preventing clinical hepatitis B following percutaneous exposures and can be considered as an alternative to HBIG when it is not possible to obtain HBIG.

Recommendations on postexposure prophylaxis are based on the efficacy data discussed above and on the likelihood of future HBV exposure of the person requiring treatment. In perinatal exposure and percutaneous exposure of high-risk health-care personnel, a regimen combining HBIG with hepatitis B vaccine will provide both short- and long-term protection.

Perinatal exposure. One of the most efficient modes of HBV transmission is from mother to infant during birth. If the mother is positive for both HBsAg and HBeAg, about 70%-90% of infants will become infected, and up to 90% of these infected infants will become HBV carriers. If the HBsAg-positive carrier mother is HBeAg-negative, or if anti-HBe is present, transmission occurs less frequently and rarely leads to the HBV carrier state. However, severe acute disease, including fatal fulminant hepatitis in the neonate, has been reported (32,33). Prophylaxis of infants from all HBsAg-positive mothers is recommended, regardless of the mother's HBeAg or anti-HBe status.

The efficacy of a combination of HBIG plus the hepatitis B vaccine series has been confirmed in recent studies. Although the following regimen is recommended (Table 35-11), other schedules have also been effective (25-27,34). The major consideration for all these regimens is the need to give HBIG as soon as possible after delivery.

HBIG (0.5 ml [10 μg]) should be administered intramuscularly after physiologic stabilization of the infant and preferably within 12 hours of birth. Hepatitis B vaccine should be administered intramuscularly in three doses of 0.5 ml (10μg) each. The first dose should be given concurrently with HBIG but at a different site. If vaccine is not available at birth, the first vaccine dose may be given within 7 days of birth. The second and third doses should be given 1 month and 6 months, respectively, after the first. Testing for HBsAg and anti-HBs is recommended at 12-15 months to monitor the final success or failure of therapy. If HBsAg is not detectable, and anti-HBs is present, the child has been protected. Testing for anti-HBc is not useful, since maternal anti-HBc may persist for more than 1 year; the utility of testing for IgM anti-HBc is currently being evaluated. HBIG administered at birth should not interfere with oral polio and diphtheria-tetanus-pertussis vaccines administered at 2 months of age.

Maternal screening. Since efficacy of the treatment regimen depends on administering HBIG on the day of birth, it is vital that HBsAg-positive mothers be

Table 35-11. Hepatitis B virus postexposure recommendations

| Exposure | HBIG | | Vaccine | |
	Dose	Recommended timing	Dose	Recommended timing
Perinatal	0.5 ml IM	Within 12 hours	0.5 ml (10 μg) IM of birth	Within 1-2 hours of birth*; repeat at 1 and 6 months
Sexual	0.06 ml/kg IM	Single dose within 14 days of sexual contact	†	—

*The first dose can be given the same time as the HBIG dose but at a different site.
†Vaccine is recommended for homosexual men and for regular sexual contacts of HBV carriers and is optional in initial treatment of heterosexual contacts of persons with acute HBV.

identified before delivery. Mothers belonging to groups known to be at high risk of acquiring HBV infection (Table 35-12) should be tested routinely for HBsAg during a prenatal visit. If a mother belonging to a high-risk group has not been screened prenatally, HBsAg screening should be done at the time of delivery, or as soon as possible therafter, and the infant treated as above if the mother is HBsAg-positive. If the mother is identified as HBsAg-positive more than 1 month after giving birth, the infant should be screened for HBsAg, and if negative, treated with hepatitis B vaccine and HBIG.

The appropriate obstetric and pediatric staff should be notified directly of HBsAg-positive mothers, so the staff may take appropriate precautions to protect themselves and other patients from infectious material, blood, and secretions, and so the neonate may recieve therapy without delay after birth.

Acute exposure to blood that contains (or might contain) HBsAg. For accidental percutaneous or permucosal exposure to blood that is known to contain or might contain HBsAg, the decision to provide prophylaxis must take into account several factors: (1) the hepatitis B vaccination status of the exposed person; (2) whether the source of blood is known or unknown; (3) whether the HBsAg status of the source is known or unknown. Such exposures usually occur in persons who are candidates for hepatitis B vaccine; for any exposure in a person not previously vaccinated, hepatitis B vaccination is recommended.

The following outline and table summarize prophylaxis for percutaneous (needlestick or bite), ocular, or mucous-membrane exposure to blood according to the source of exposure and vaccination status of the exposed person (Table 35-9). For greatest effectiveness, passive prophylaxis with HBIG (or IG) should be given as soon as possible after exposure (its value beyond 7 days of exposure is unclear).

1. *Exposed person not previously vaccinated.* Hepatitis B vaccination should be considered the treatment of choice. Depending on the source of the exposure, HBsAg testing of the source and additional prophylaxis of the exposed person may be warranted (see below). Screening the exposed person for immunity should be considered if such screening is cost-effective (as discussed in preexposure prophylaxis) and if this will not delay treatment beyond 7 days.

   a. *Source known HBsAg-positive.* A single dose of HBIG (0.06 ml/kg) should be given as soon as possible after exposure and within 24 hours, if possible. The first dose of hepatitis B vaccine (20 μg) should be given intramuscularly at a separate site within 7 days of exposure, and the second and third doses given 1 month and 6 months later (Table 35-13).† If HBIG cannot be obtained, IG in an equivalent dosage (0.06 ml/kg) may provide some benefit.

   b. *Source known, HBsAg status unknown.* The following guidelines are suggested based on the relative probability that the source is HBsAg-positive and on the consequent risk of HBV transmission.

      (1) *High risk that the source is HBsAg-positive, such as patients with a high risk of HBV carriage (Table 35-13) or patients with acute or chronic liver disease (serologically undiagnosed).* The exposed person should be given the first dose of hepatitis B vaccine (20 μg) within 1 week of exposure and vaccination completed as recommended. The source person should be tested for HBsAg. If positive, the exposed person should be given HBIG (0.06 ml/kg) if within 7 days of exposure.

      (2) *Low risk that the source is positive for HBsAg.* The exposed person should be given the first dose of hepatitis B vaccine

---

†For persons who are not given hepatitis B vaccine, a second dose of HBIG should be given 1 month after the first dose.

Table 35-12. Women for whom prenatal HBsAg sceening is recommended

1.	Women of Asian, Pacific island, or Alaskan Eskimo descent, whether immigrant or U.S.-born.
2.	Women born in Haiti or sub-Saharan Africa
3.	Women with histories of:
	a. Acute or chronic liver disease.
	b. Work or treatment in a hemodialysis unit.
	c. Work or residence in an institution for the mentally retarded.
	d. Rejection as a blood donor.
	e. Blood transfusion on repeated occasions.
	f. Frequent occupational exposure to blood in medico-dental settings.
	g. Household contact with an HBV carrier or hemodialysis patient.
	h. Multiple episodes of venereal diseases.
	i. Percutaneous use of illicit drugs.

Table 35-13. Recommendations for hepatitis B prophylaxis following percutaneous exposure

	Exposed person	
Source	*Unvaccinated*	*Vaccinated*
HBsAg-positive	1. HBIG × 1 immediately* 2. Initiate HB vaccine† series.	1. Test exposed person for anti-HBs.§ 2. If inadequate antibody¶ HBIG (×1) immediately plus HB vaccine booster dose.

Known source
    High-risk
     HBsAg-positive
	1. Initiate HB vaccine series
	 2. Test source for HBsAg. If positive, HBIG × 1
		1. Test source for HBsAg only if exposed is vaccine nonresponder; if source is HBsAg-positive, give HBIG × 1 immediately plus HB vaccine booster dose

Low-risk HBsAg-positive	Initiate HB vaccine series.	Nothing required.
Unknown source	Initiate HB vaccine series.	Nothing required.

*HBIG dose 0.00 ml/kg IM.

†HB vaccine dose 20 µg IM for adults; 10 µg IM for infants or children under 10 years of age. First dose within 1 week; second and third doses, 1 and 6 months later.

§See text for details.

¶Less than 10 SRU by RIA, negative by EIA.

(20 µg) within 1 week of exposure and vaccination completed as recommended. Testing of the source person is not necessary.

   c. *Source unknown.* The exposed person should be given the first dose of hepatitis B vaccine (20 µg) within 7 days of exposure and vaccination completed as recommended.

2. *Exposed person previously vaccinated against hepatitis B.* For percutaneous exposures to blood in persons who have previously received one or more doses of hepatitis B vaccine, the decision to provide additional prophylaxis will depend on the source of exposure and on whether the vaccinated person has developed anti-HBs following vaccination.

   a. *Source known HBsAg-positive.* The exposed person should be tested for anti-HBs unless he/she has been tested within the last 12 months. If the exposed person has adequate§ antibody, no additional treatment is indicated.

    (1) If the exposed person has not completed vaccination and has inadequate levels of antibody, one dose of HBIG (0.06 ml/kg) should be given immediately and vaccination completed as scheduled.

    (2) If the exposed person has inadequate antibody on testing or has previously not responded to vaccine, one dose of HBIG

should be given immediately and a booster dose of vaccine (1 ml or 20 µg) given at a different site.

    (3) If the exposed person shows inadequate antibody on testing but is known to have had adequate antibody in the past, a booster dose of hepatitis B vaccine (1 ml or 20 µg) should be given.

   b. *Source known, HBsAg status unknown.*

    (1) *High risk that the source is HBsAg-positive.* Additional prophylaxis is necessary only if the exposed person is a known vaccine nonresponder. In this circumstance, the source should be tested for HBsAg and, if positive, the exposed person treated with one dose of HBIG (0.06 ml/kg) immediately and a booster dose of vaccine (1 ml or 20 µg) at a different site. In other circumstances, screening of the source for HBsAg and the exposed person for anti-HBs is not routinely recommended, because the actual risk of HBV infection is very low (less than 1 per 1,000).¶

    (2) *Low risk that the source is HBsAg-positive.* The risk of HBV infection is minimal. Neither testing of the source for

§Adequate antibody is 10 SRU or more by RIA or positive by EIA.

¶Estimated by multiplying the risk of vaccine nonresponse in the exposed person (.10) by the risk of the needle source being HBsAg-positive (.05) by the risk of HBV infection in a susceptible person having an HBsAg positive needle-stick injury (.20).

HBsAg, nor testing of the exposed person for anti-HBs, is recommended.

 c. *Source unknown*. The risk of HBV infection is minimal. No treatment is indicated.

Sexual contacts of persons with acute HBV infection. Sexual contact of HBsAg-positive persons are at increased risk of acquiring HBV infection, and HBIG has been shown to be 75% effective in preventing such infections (31). Because data are limited, the period after sexual exposure during which HBIG is effective is unknown, but extrapolation from other settings makes it unlikely that this period would exceed 14 days. Prescreening sexual partners for susceptibility before treatment is recommended if it does not delay treatment beyond 14 days after last exposure. Testing for anti-HBc is the most efficient prescreening test to use in this population group.

A single dose of HBIG (0.06 ml/kg) is recommended for susceptible individuals who have had sexual contact with an HBsAg-positive person, if HBIG can be given within 14 days of the last sexual contact, and for persons who will continue to have sexual contact with an individual with acute hepatitis B before loss of HBsAg in that individual. In exposures between heterosexuals, hepatitis B vaccination may be initiated at the same time as HBIG prophylaxis; such treatment may improve efficacy of postexposure treatment. However, since 90% of persons with acute HBV infection become HBsAg-negative within 15 weeks of diagnosis, the potential for repeated exposure to HBV is limited. Hepatitis B vaccine is, therefore, optional in initial treatment for such exposures. If vaccine is not given, a second dose of HBIG should be given if the index patient remains HBsAg-positive for 3 months after detection. If the index patient is a known carrier or remains positive for 6 months, hepatitis B vaccine should be offered to regular sexual contacts. For exposures among homosexual men, the hepatitis B vaccine series should be initiated at the time HBIG is given, since hepatitis B vaccine is recommended for all susceptible homosexual men. Additional doses of HBIG are unnecessary if vaccine is given. IG is an alternative to HBIG when it is not possible to obtain HBIG.

Household contacts of persons with acute HBV infection. Prophylaxis for other household contacts of persons with acute HBV infection is not indicated unless they have had identifiable blood exposure to the index case, such as by sharing toothbrushes or razors. Such exposures should be treated similarly to sexual exposures. If the index patient becomes a hepatitis B carrier, all household contacts should be given hepatitis B vaccine.

Delta hepatitis

The delta virus (also known as hepatitis D virus [HDV] by some investigators) is a defective virus that may only cause infection in the presence of active HBV infection. The delta virus has been characterized as a particle of 35–37 nm in size, consisting of RNA (mw 500,000) as genetic material and an internal protein antigen (delta-antigen), coated with HBsAg as the surface protein (3). Infection may occur as either coinfection with hepatitis B or superinfection of a hepatitis B carrier, each of which usually cause an episode of acute hepatitis. Coinfection usually resolves, while superinfection frequently causes chronic delta infection and chronic active hepatitis. Both types of infection may cause fulminant hepatitis.

Delta infection may be diagnosed by detection of delta-antigen in serum during early infection and by the appearance of delta antibody during or after infection. Routes of delta transmission appear to be similar to those of hepatitis B. In the United States, delta infection occurs most commonly among persons at high risk of acquiring HBV infection, such as drug addicts and hemophilia patients.

A test for detection of delta antibody is expected to be commercially available soon. Other tests (delta antigen, IgM anti-delta) are available only in research laboratories.

Since the delta virus is dependent on hepatitis B for replication, prevention of hepatitis B infection, either preexposure or postexposure, will suffice to prevent delta infection in a person susceptible to hepatitis B. Known episodes of perinatal, sexual, or percutaneous exposure to sera or persons positive for both HBV and delta virus should be treated exactly as such exposures to hepatitis B alone.

Persons who are HBsAg carriers are at risk of delta infection, especially if they participate in activities that put them at high risk of repeated exposure to hepatitis B (parenteral drug abuse, homosexuality). However, at present there are no products available that might prevent delta infection in HBsAg carriers either before of after exposure.

Non-A, non-B hepatitis

United States. Non-A, non-B hepatitis that presently occurs in the United States has epidemiologic characteristics similar to those of hepatitis B, occurring most commonly following blood transfusion and parenteral drug abuse. Multiple episodes of non-A, non-B hepatitis have been observed in the same individuals and may be due to different agents. Chronic hepatitis following acute non-A, non-B hepatitis infection varies in frequency from 20% to 70%. Experimental studies in chimpanzees have confirmed the existence of a carrier state, which may be present in up to 8% of the population.

Although several studies have attempted to assess the value of prophylaxis with IG against non-A, non-B hepatitis, the results have been equivocal, and no specific recommendations can be made (35,36). However, for persons with percutaneous exposure to blood from a patient with non-A, non-B hepatitis, it may be reasonable to administer IG (0.06 ml/kg) as soon as possible after exposure.

Epidemic (fecal-oral) non-A, non-B hepatitis. In recent years, epidemics of non-A, non-B hepatitis spread by water or close personal contact have been reported from several areas of Southeast Asia (Indian subcontinent, Burma) and North Africa (2). Such epidemics generally affect adults and cause unusually high mortality in pregnant women. The disease has been transmitted to experimental animals, and candidate viruses have been identified, however, no serologic tests have yet been developed (37).

Epidemic non-A, non-B hepatitis has not been recognized in the United States or western Europe, and it is unknown whether the causative agent is present in these areas.

Travelers to areas having epidemic non-A, non-B hepatitis may be at some risk of acquiring this disease by close contact or by contaminated food or water. The value of IG in preventing this infection is unknown. The best prevention of infection is to avoid potentially contaminated food or water, as with hepatitis A and other enteric infections.

REFERENCES

1. Francis DP, Maynard JE. The transmission and outcome of hepatitis A, B, and non-A, non-B: a review. Epidemiol Rev 1979;1:17-31.
2. Maynard JE. Epidemic non-A, non-B hepatitis. Seminars in Liver Disease 1984;4:336-9.
3. Rizzetto M. The delta agent. Hepatology 1983;3:729-37.
4. CDC. Provisional public health service inter-agency recommendations for screening donated blood and plasma for antibody to the virus causing acquired immunodeficiency syndrome. MMWR 1985;34:1-5.
5. Kluge T. Gamma-globulin in the prevention of viral hepatitis. A study on the effect of medium-size doses. Acta Med Scand 1963;174:469-77.
6. Stokes J Jr, Neefe JR. The prevention and attenuation of infectious hepatitis by gamma globulin. Preliminary note. JAMA 1945;127:144-5.
7. Mosley JW, Reisler DM, Brachott D, Roth D, Weiser J. Comparison of two lots of immune serum globulin for prophylaxis of infectious hepatitis. Am J Epidemiol 1968;87:539-50.
8. Woodson RD, Cahill KM. Viral hepatitis abroad. Incidence in Catholic missionaries. JAMA 1972;219:1191-3.
9. Woodson RD, Clinton JJ. Hepatitis prophylaxis abroad. Effectiveness of immune serum globulin in protecting Peace Corps volunteers. JAMA 1969;209:1053-8.
10. Storch G, McFarland LM, Kelso K, Heilman CJ, Caraway CT. Viral hepatitis associated with day-care centers. JAMA 1979;242:1514-8.
11. Hadler SC, Webster HM, Erben JJ, Swanson JE, Maynard JE. Hepatitis A in day-care centers. A community-wide assessment. N Engl J Med 1980;302:1222-7.
12. Hadler SC, Erbin JJ, Matthews D, Starko K, Francis DP, and Maynard JE. Effect of immunoglobulin on hepatitis A in day-care centers. JAMA 1983;249:48-53.
13. Favero MS, Maynard JE, Leger RT, Graham DR, and Dixon RE. Guidelines for the care of patients hospitalized with viral hepatitis. Ann Intern Med 1979;91:872-6.
14. ACIP. Hepatitis B vaccine: evidence confirming lack of AIDS transmission. MMWR 1984;33:685-7.
15. Krugman S, Holley HP Jr, Davidson M, Simberkoff MS, Matsaniotis N. Immunogenic effect of inactivated hepatitis B vaccine: comparison of 20 microgram and 40 microgram doses. J Med Virol 1981;8:119-21.
16. Szmuness W, Stevens CE, Harley EJ, et al. Hepatitis B vaccine: demonstration of efficacy in a controlled clinical trial in a high-risk population in the United States. N Engl J Med 1980;303:833-41.
17. CDC. Suboptimal response to hepatitis B vaccine given by injection into the buttock. MMWR 1985;34:105-13.
18. Francis DP, Hadler SC, Thompson SE, et al. The prevention of hepatitis B with vaccine. Report of the Centers for Disease Control multi-center efficacy trial among homosexual men. Ann Intern Med 1982;97:362-6,
19. Stevens CE, Alter HJ, Taylor PE, Zang EA, Harley EJ, and Szmuness W. Hepatitis B vaccine in patients receiving hemodialysis. Immunogenicity and efficacy. N Engl J Med 1984;311:496-501.
20. Dienstag JL, Stevens CE, Bhan AK, and Szmuness W. Hepatitis B vaccine administered to chronic carriers of hepatitis B surface antigen. Ann Intern Med 1982;96:576-9.
21. Szmuness W, Stevens CE, Oleszko WR, and Goodman A. Passive-active immunisation against hepatitis B: immunogenicity studies in adult Americans, Lancet 1981;1:576-7.
22. Pattison CP, Maynard JE, Berquist KR, Webster HM. Epidemiology of hepatitis B in hospital personnel. Am J Epidemiol 1975;101:59-64.
23. Dienstag JL, Ryan DM. Occupational exposure to hepatitis B virus in hospital personnel: infection or immunization? Am J Epidemiol 1982;115:26-39.
24. Maynard JE. Viral hepatitis as an occupational hazard in the health care profession. In: Vyas GN, Cohen SN, and Schmid R., eds.: Viral hepatitis. Philadelphia: Franklin Institute Press, 1978:321-31.
25. Beasley RP, Hwang LY, Lee GC, et al. Prevention of perinatally transmitted hepatitis B virus infections with hepatitis B immune globulin and hepatitis B vaccine. Lancet 1983;2:1099-102.
26. Wong VCW, Ip HMH, Reesink HW, et al. Prevention of the HBsAg carrier state in newborn infants of mothers who are chronic carriers of HBsAg and HBeAg by administration of hepatitis-B vaccine and hepatitis-B immunoglobulin: double-blind randomised placebo-controlled study. Lancet 1984;1:921-6.
27. Stevens CE, Toy PT, Tong MJ, et al. Perinatal hepatitis B virus transmission in the United States. Prevention by passive-active immunization. JAMA 1985;253:1740-5.

28. Beasley RP, Hwang LY, Stevens CE, et al. Efficacy of hepatitis B immune globulin for prevention of perinatal transmission of the hepatitis B virus carrier state: final report of a randomized double-blind, placebo-controlled trial. Hepatology 1983;3:135-41.

29. Seeff LB, Wright EC, Zimmerman HJ, et al. Type B hepatitis after needle-stick exposure: prevention with hepatitis B immune globulin. Final report of the Veterans Administration Cooperative Study. Ann Intern Med 1978;88:285-93.

30. Grady GF, Lee VA, Prince AM, et al. Hepatitis B immune globulin for accidental exposures among medical personnel: final report of a multicenter controlled trial. J Infect Dis 1978;138:625-38.

31. Redeker AG, Mosley JW, Gocke DJ, McKee AP, Pollack W. Hepatitis B immune globulin as a prophylactic measure for spouses exposed to acute type B hepatitis. N Engl J Med 1975;293:1055-9.

32. Sinatra FR, Shah P, Weissman JY, Thomas DW, Merritt RJ, Tong MJ. Perinatal transmitted acute icteric hepatitis B in infants born to hepatitis B surface antigen-positive and anti-hepatitis B between B e-positive carrier mothers. Pediatrics 1982;70:557-9.

33. Delaplane D, Yogev R, Crussi F, Shulman ST. Fatal hepatitis B in early infancy: the importance of identifying HBsAg-positive pregnant women and providing immunoprophylaxis to their newborns. Pediatrics 1983; 72:176-80.

34. Seeff LB, Koff RS. Passive and active immunoprophylaxis of hepatitis B. Gastroenterology 1984;86:958-81.

35. Seeff LB, Zimmerman JH, Wright EL, et al. A randomized, double-blind controlled trial of the efficacy of immune serum globulin for the prevention of post-transfusion hepatitis. A Veterans Administration cooperative study. Gastroenterology 1977;72:111-21.

36. Knodell RG, Conrad ME, Ginsburg AL, Bell CJ, and Flannery EP. Efficacy of prophylactic gammaglobulin in preventing non-A, non-B post-transfusion hepatitis, Lancet 1976;1:557-61.

37. Kane MA, Bradley DW, Shrestha SM, et al. Epidemic non-A, non-B hepatitis in Nepal. Recovery of a possible etiologic agent and transmission studies in marmosets. JAMA 1984;252:3140-5.

From MMWR 1985;34:313.

PREVENTION AND CONTROL OF INFLUENZA

These recommendations of the Immunization Practices Advisory Committee (ACIP) update for 1985-1986 the information on the vaccine and antiviral agent available for control of influenza (superseding MMWR 1984;33:253-66). Changes include addition of statements about: (1) the route of vaccine administration; (2) the use of amantadine in medical personnel during influenza A outbreaks; (3) the need to prepare contingency plans to expedite use of amantadine in aborting influenza A outbreaks among residents of institutions; and (4) reduction in the dosage of amantadine for older patients or persons with seizure disorders.

Introduction

Influenza viruses have continually demonstrated an ability to cause major epidemics of respiratory disease. Typical influenza illness is characterized by abrupt onset of fever, sore throat, and nonproductive cough, and unlike many other common respiratory infections, can cause extreme malaise lasting several days. More severe disease can result from invasion of the lungs by influenza virus (primary viral pneumonia) or by secondary bacterial pneumonia. High attack rates of acute illness and the frequent occurrence of lower respiratory tract complications usually result in dramatic rises in visits to physicians' offices and hospital emergency rooms. Furthermore, influenza frequently infects individuals who, because to their ages or underlying health problems, are poorly able to cope with the disease and often require medical attention, including hospitalization. Such persons are considered to be medically at "high risk" in epidemics. In one recent study, for example, hospitalization rates for adults with high-risk medical conditions increased during major epidemics by about twofold to fivefold in different age groups, reaching a maximum rate of about 800 excess hospitalizations per 100,000 high-risk persons.

A further indication of the impact of influenza epidemics is the significant increase that often occurs in mortality. Such excess mortality is attributed not only to the direct cause of influenza pneumonia but also to an increase in deaths from cardiopulmonary disease. Ten thousand or more excess deaths have been associated with epidemics 17 times from 1957 to 1984. Excess mortality again exceeded the epidemic threshold during the 1984-1985 influenza season. About 90% of the excess deaths attributed to pneumonia and influenza during epidemics occur among persons 65 years of age or older.

The greatest impact of influenza is normally seen when new strains appear against which most of the population lacks immunity. In these circumstances (e.g., 1957 and 1968), pandemics occur, and a quarter or more of the U.S. population was affected over 2-3 months.

Because of the increasing proportion of elderly persons in the U.S. population, and because age and its associated chronic diseases are risk factors for severe influenza illness, the future toll from influenza may increase, unless control measures are used more vigorously than in the past. Other populations at high risk for influenza-related complications are also increasing because of such factors as the success of intensive-care units for neonates, better management of diseases (such as cystic fibrosis), and better survival rates for organ transplant recipients. This statement discusses the presently available medical control measures, immunoprophylaxis with vaccines, and prophylaxis or therapy with the antiviral drug, amantadine.

Options for the control of influenza

For about 20 years, efforts to reduce the impact of influenza in the United States have been aimed primarily at immunoprophylaxis of persons at greatest risk of serious illness or death. Observations during influenza epidemics indicate that most influenza-related deaths occur among: (1) persons older than 65 years of age, and (2) persons with chronic underlying disorders of the cardiovascular, pulmonary, and/or renal systems, as well as those with metabolic diseases (including diabetes mellitus), severe anemia, and/or compromised immune function. Recommendations listed below apply primarily to these high-risk groups. In addition, measures are described that apply to other individuals or groups under special circumstances. Influenza control options should also be made available to individuals who wish to reduce their chances of acquiring influenza infection or to reduce the severity of disease.

Prophylaxis is likely to be achieved with greatest cost-effectiveness by vaccinating individuals for whom infection may have the most severe consequences and for whom there is a higher than average potential for infection. In addition, vaccination can best be organized when such high-risk individuals routinely have contact with the health-care delivery system for reasons other than acute respiratory infection before the influenza season, thereby permitting vaccine administration without special visits to doctors' offices or clinics. Other indications for prophylaxis (whether with vaccine or antiviral drugs) include the strong desire of any person to avoid a preventable illness.

The presently available specific therapy for influenza A, amantadine hydrochloride (Symmetrel®), is most likely to benefit individuals who seek medical attention promptly because of abrupt onset of an acute respiratory infection with troublesome symptoms during an influenza A epidemic. For high-risk individuals for whom influenza vaccine has not been used or has not prevented infection, amantadine therapy should be effective in reducing the severity of disease.

Inactivated influenza vaccine

Use of inactivated influenza vaccine is the single most important measure in preventing and/or attenuating influenza infection. Potency of present vaccines is such that nearly all vaccinated young adults develop hemagglutination-inhibition antibody titers that are likely to protect them against infection by strains like those in the vaccine and, often, by related variants that emerge. The elderly, the very young, and patients with certain chronic diseases may develop lower postvaccination antibody titers than

young adults. Under these circumstances, however, influenza vaccine may be more effective in preventing lower respiratory tract involvement or other complications of influenza than in preventing infection and involvement of the upper respiratory tract. Influenza vaccine will not prevent primary illnesses caused by other respiratory pathogens.

Annual vaccination against influenza has been recommended since 1963 for individuals at high risk of lower respiratory tract complications and death following influenza infection, i.e., the elderly and persons with chronic disorders of the cardiovascular, pulmonary, and/or renal systems, metabolic diseases, severe anemia, and/or compromised immune function. These groups have been identified primarily by reviews of death certificate data, supported by hospital-based or population-based studies. Each group encompasses patients along a continuum of underlying general health. In other words, within each broadly defined high-risk category, some persons may be more likely than others to develop severe complications from influenza infection.

Investigations of influenza outbreaks in nursing homes, for example, have demonstrated attack rates as high as 60%, with case-fatality ratios of 30% or more. Chronic diseases and other debilitating conditions are common among nursing home residents, and spread of infection can often be explosive in such relatively crowded and closed environments. Recent retrospective studies of noninstitutionalized patients also suggest that chronic underlying diseases, particularly those that affect the cardiovascular and pulmonary systems, may contribute more to the severity of illness than age alone. Since influenza infections are also known to invoke abnormalities in gas exchange and peripheral airways dysfunction in adults, children with compromised pulmonary function, including those with cystic fibrosis, chronic asthma, and bronchopulmonary dysplasia, as well as neonates in intensive-care units, may also be at higher risk of severe illness, although firm evidence is lacking. Children with congenital heart disease may also be considered at high risk, since respiratory viruses in general often produce severe infections in this population.

Target groups for vaccination

1. Based on the above observations, the previous, broadly defined high-risk group has been further classified on the basis of priority, so special efforts can be directed at providing vaccine to those who may derive the greatest benefit. Groups for which active, targeted vaccination efforts are most necessary are:
   a. Adults and children with chronic disorders of the cardiovascular or pulmonary systems that

are severe enough to have required regular medical follow-ups or hospitalization during the preceding year.

  b. Residents of nursing homes and other chronic-care facilities (e.g., institutions housing patients of any age with chronic medical conditions).

2. Although not proven, it is reasonable to believe that medical personnel can transmit influenza infections to their high-risk patients while they are themselves incubating infection, undergoing subclinical infection, or working despite the existence of mild symptoms. In many winters, nosocomial outbreaks of influenza are reported. The potential for introducing influenza to high-risk groups, such as patients with severely compromised cardiopulmonary or immune systems or infants in neonatal intensive-care units, should be reduced by vaccination programs targeted at medical personnel. Therefore, physicians, nurses, and other personnel who have extensive contact with high-risk patients (e.g., primary-care and certain specialty clinicians and staff of intensive care units) should receive influenza vaccination annually.

3. After considering the needs of the above two target groups, high priority should also be given to organizing special programs making vaccine readily available to persons at moderately increased risk of serious illness compared with the general population:

  a. Otherwise healthy individuals over 65 years of age.

  b. Adults and children with chronic metabolic diseases (including diabetes mellitus), renal dysfunction, anemia, immunosuppression, or asthma that are severe enough to require regular medical follow-ups or hospitalization during the preceding year.

Vaccine recommendations

Influenza vaccine is recommended for high-risk persons 6 months or older, for their medical-care personnel, and for other persons wishing to reduce their chances of acquiring influenza illness. Vaccine composition and doses are given in Table 35-14. Guidelines for use of vaccine are given below for different segments of the population. Although the 1985-1986 vaccine has the same formulation as the 1984-1985 vaccine, immunity declines in the year following vaccination. **Therefore, a history of vaccination for the 1984-1985 season does not preclude the need to be revaccinated for the 1985-1986 influenza season to provide optimal protection.**

Data on influenza vaccine immunogenicity and reactogenicity have generally been obtained when vaccine is administered by the intramuscular (deltoid) route. Because adequate evaluation of other routes in high-risk persons is lacking, the preferred route of vaccination is the deltoid muscle whenever possible.

High-priority target groups

Annual vaccination with inactivated influenza vaccine is considered the single most important measure in preventing or attenuating influenza infection and is strongly recommended for persons at high risk and

Table 35-14. Influenza vaccine* dosage by age of patient—United States, 1985-1986 season

Age group	Product†	Dosage§	No. doses	Route¶
6-35 mos.	Split virus only	0.25 ml	2**	IM
3-12 yrs.	Split virus only	0.5 ml	2**	IM
>12 years	Whole or split virus	0.5 ml	1	IM

*Contains 15 µg each of A/Chile/83(H1N1), A/Philippines/82(H3N2), and B/USSR/83 hemagglutinin antigens in each 0.5 ml. Manufacturers include Parke-Davis (Fluogen® split), Squibb-Connaught (Fluzone® whole or split), Wyeth Laboratories (Influenza Virus Vaccine, Trivalent split). Manufacturer's phone numbers to obtain further product information are: Parke-Davis—(800) 223-0432; Squibb-Connaught—(800) 822-2463; Wyeth—(800) 321-2304.

†Because of the lower potential for causing febrile reactions, only split (subvirion) vaccine should be used in children. Immunogenicity and reactogenicity of split and whole virus vaccines are similar in adults when used according to the recommended dosage.

§Pneumococcal vaccine and influenza vaccine can be given at the same time at different sites without an increase in side effects, but it should be emphasized that, whereas influenza vaccine is given annually, pneumococcal vaccine should be given only once to adults. Detailed immunization records should be provided to each patient to help ensure that additional doses of pneumococcal vaccine are not given.

¶The recommended site of vaccination is the deltoid muscle for adults and older children. The preferred site for infants and young children is the anterolateral aspect of the thigh musculature.

**Four weeks or more between doses, both doses recommended for maximum protection. However, if the individual received at least one dose of any influenza vaccine recommended from 1978-1979 to 1984-1985, one dose is sufficient.

for those providing their medical care. In most past years, only 20% of the groups defined as high-risk on the basis of medical condition or age received influenza vaccine in any given year. Increased efforts must be made to immunize persons in high-risk groups, particularly those in the highest-priority target groups (see target group 1 above).

As an initial step, the ACIP recommends that infection-control programs in institutions for the aged or chronically ill have as their goal the achievement of no less than 80% vaccination rates for the residents. Hospitals and physicians should have a similar objective for vaccinating patients with severe cardiopulmonary disorders and for vaccinating medical personnel who have the greatest potential to introduce influenza virus into high-risk hospital settings (see target group 2 above). Wherever possible, efforts should also be made to vaccinate persons at moderately increased risk (see target group 3 above). This latter objective often requires that active promotion of influenza vaccine be made by individual physicians who practice outside organizations that can set administrative guidelines and procedures for their professional staff. Establishing systems for influenza vaccination activities in physicians' offices and clinics is essential in providing vaccine.

General population. Physicians should administer vaccine to any persons in their practices who wish to reduce their chances of acquiring influenza infection. Persons who provide essential community services, such as fire and police department employees, and health-care personnel are not considered to be at increased occupational risk of serious influenza illness but may be considered for vaccination programs designed to minimize the possible disruption of essential activities that can occur during severe epidemics.

Pregnant women. Pregnancy has not been demonstrated to be a risk factor for severe influenza infection, except in the largest pandemics of 1918-1919 and 1957-1958. Influenza vaccine is considered generally safe for pregnant women. Nonetheless, when vaccine is given during pregnancy, waiting until after the first trimester is a reasonable precaution to minimize any concern over the theoretical possibility of teratogenicity.

Persons who should not be vaccinated. Inactivated influenza vaccine should not be given to persons who have an anaphylactic sensitivity to eggs (see SIDE EFFECTS AND ADVERSE REACTIONS below). Persons with acute febrile illnesses normally should not be vaccinated until their temporary symptoms have abated.

Strategies for implementing influenza vaccine recommendations

Influenza vaccine should normally be obtained to use during the fall. More effective programs for giving

influenza vaccine are needed in nursing homes and other chronic-care facilities, in physicians' offices, and in hospital settings. Adults and children in high-priority target groups who do not reside in nursing homes or other chronic-care facilities should be given influenza vaccine at the time of regular medical followups in the fall. Those not scheduled for regular medical appointments in the fall should be notified by their medical offices or clinics to come in specifically to receive influenza vaccine. During the fall, physicians responsible for care of hospitalized patients should consider administering influenza vaccine to patients with high-risk conditions before the patients are discharged.

These and other programs to annually vaccinate target groups require planning well in advance and should, whenever possible, be completed before the beginning of the influenza season. However, vaccine can be given right up to the time influenza virus activity is documented, and even thereafter, although temporary chemoprophylaxis may be indicated in these situations (see ANTIVIRAL AGENT: AMANTADINE below).

Vaccine composition

Influenza A viruses are classified into subtypes on the basis of two antigens: hemagglutinin (H) and neuraminidase (N). Three subtypes of hemagglutinin (H1, H2, H3) and two subtypes of neuraminidase (N1, N2) are recognized among influenza A viruses that have caused widespread human disease. Immunity to these antigens, especially hemagglutinin, reduces the likelihood of infection and the severity of disease if infection does occur. However, there may be sufficient antigenic variation (antigenic drift) within the same subtype over time, so that infection or vaccination with one strain may not induce immunity to distantly related strains of the same subtype. Although influenza B viruses have shown much more antigenic stability than influenza A viruses, antigenic variation does occur. As a consequence, the antigenic characteristics of current strains provide the basis for selecting virus strains included in the vaccine.

Based on the most recent epidemiologic and laboratory data (reported periodically in *MMWR* during the 1984-1985 influenza season), it is anticipated that strains prevalent in 1985-1986 will be closely related to A/Philippines/2/82(H3N2), A/Chile/1/83(H1N1), and B/USSR/100/83. Therefore, these strains will be included in the vaccine for use during the 1985-1986 season (Table 35-14). Although the components and their concentration in the 1985-1986 vaccine will be identical to those in the 1984-1985 vaccine, all 1984-1985 influenza vaccines released for civilian use have a June 30, 1985, expiration date. Remaining 1984-1985 vaccines should not be used beyond their expiration dates.

Side effects and adverse reactions

Vaccines used in recent years have generally been associated with only a few reactions; fewer than one-third of vaccinees have been reported to develop local redness or induration for 1 or 2 days at the site of injection.

Systemic reactions have been of two types:

1. Fever, malaise, myalgia, and other systemic symptoms of toxicity, although infrequent, most often affect children and others who have had no exposure to the influenza virus antigens contained in the vaccine. These reactions, which begin 6-12 hours after vaccination and persist for 1-2 days, are usually attributed to the influenza antigens (even though the virus is inactivated) and constitute most of the systemic side effects of influenza vaccination.

2. Immediate, presumably allergic, responses, such as flare and wheal or various respiratory tract symptoms of hypersensitivity, occur extremely rarely after influenza vaccination. These symptoms probably result from sensitivity to some vaccine component, most likely residual egg protein. Although current influenza vaccines contain only a small quantity of egg protein, on rare occasions, vaccine can induce hypersensitivity reactions. Individuals with anaphylactic hypersensitivity to eggs should *not* be given influenza vaccine. Such persons include those who, on eating eggs, develop swelling of the lips or tongue or experience acute respiratory distress or collapse. Unlike the 1976 swine influenza vaccine, subsequent vaccines have not been associated with an increased frequency of Guillain-Barré syndrome.

It has been reported that influenza vaccination may affect the clearances of warfarin and theophylline. Several studies, however, have failed to show any consistent adverse effect of influenza vaccination on patients taking these drugs.

Simultaneous pneumococcal vaccination

There is considerable overlap in the target groups for influenza vaccination and pneumococcal vaccine, Pneumococcal vaccine and influenza vaccine can be given at the same time at different sites without increased side effects, but it should be emphasized that, whereas influenza vaccine is given annually, pneumococcal vaccine should be given only once to adults. Detailed immunization records, which should be provided to each patient, will help ensure that additional doses of pneumococcal vaccine are not given.

Antiviral agent: amantadine

The only drug currently available for the specific prophylaxis and therapy of influenza virus infections is amantadine hydrochloride (Symmetrel®), which appears to interfere with the uncoating step in the virus replication cycle. The drug also reduces virus shedding. Amantadine is 70%-90% effective in preventing illnesses caused by circulating strains of type A influenza viruses (it is not effective against type B influenza). When administered within 24-48 hours after onset of illness, amantadine has been shown to reduce the duration of fever and other systemic symptoms with a more rapid return to routine daily activities and improvement in peripheral airway function. Since it may not prevent actual infection, persons who take the drug may still develop immune responses that will protect them when exposed to antigenically related viruses.

While considerable evidence shows that amantadine chemoprophylaxis is effective against influenza A, in most circumstances, it should not be used in lieu of vaccination, because it confers no protection against influenza B, and patient compliance could be a problem for continuous administration throughout epidemic periods, which generally last 6-12 weeks.

Amantadine prophylaxis recommendations. Specific circumstances for which amantadine prophylaxis is recommended include the following:

1. As short-term prophylaxis during the course of a presumed influenza A outbreak (e.g., in institutions for persons at high risk), particularly when the vaccine may be relatively ineffective (e.g., due to major antigenic changes in the virus). The drug should be given early in the outbreak in an effort to reduce the spread of the infection. Contingency planning for influenza outbreaks in institutions is needed to establish specific steps for rapid administration of amantadine when appropriate, including obtaining physicians' orders at short notice. When the decision to give amantadine for outbreak control is made, it is desirable to administer the drug to all residents of the affected institution, taking into account dosage recommendations and precautions given below and in the drug's package insert.

2. As an adjunct to late immunization of high-risk individuals. It is not too late to immunize even when influenza A is known to be in the community. However, since the development of a protective response following vaccination takes about 2 weeks, amantadine should be used in the interim. The drug is not known to interfere with antibody response to the vaccine.

3. To reduce disruption of medical care and to reduce spread of virus to high-risk persons when influenza A virus outbreaks occur. Amantadine prophylaxis is desirable for those physicians, nurses, and other personnel who have extensive contact with high-risk patients but who failed to receive the recommended annual influenza vaccination before the onset of influenza A activity. Such unprotected

health-care workers should be immediately offered vaccine and provided amantadine for the subsequent 2 weeks while a protective response to vaccination develops. If vaccine is not given, is unavailable, or is of low efficacy due to a major antigenic change in the virus, amantadine prophylaxis should be continued throughout the period of influenza A activity in the community. Other health-care workers in hospitals should also be offered amantadine as long as this does not jeopardize the availability of the drug for prophylaxis of staff having greatest contact with high-risk patients.

4. To supplement protection afforded by vaccination in those with impaired immune responses. Chemoprophylaxis may be considered for high-risk patients who may be expected to have a poor antibody response to influenza vaccine, e.g., those with severe immunodeficiency.

5. As chemoprophylaxis throughout the influenza season for those few high-risk individuals for whom influenza vaccine is contraindicated because of anaphylactic hypersensitivity to egg protein or prior severe reactions associated with influenza vaccination.

Amantadine can also be used prophylactically in other situations (e.g., unimmunized members of the general population who wish to avoid influenza A illness). This decision should be made on an individual basis.

Therapy. Since vaccine efficacy is less than 100%, amantadine should be considered for therapeutic use, particularly for persons in the high-risk groups if they develop illness compatible with influenza during a period of known or suspected influenza A activity in the community. The drug should be given within 24-48 hours of onset of illness and should be continued until 48 hours after resolution of signs and symptoms.

Persons who should not be given amantadine. Particular caution should be exercised for persons under 1 year of age, persons of any age with impaired renal function, or persons with an active seizure disorder (see below).

Dosage. The usual adult dosage of amantadine is 200 mg per day. Splitting the dose into 100 mg twice daily may reduce the frequency of side effects. Because renal function normally declines with age, and because side effects have been reported more frequently in older persons, a reduced dosage of 100 mg/day is generally advisable for persons aged 65 years and older to minimize the risk of toxicity. Dosages for children and for persons of any age with recognized renal disease are given in Table 35-15. Persons 10-64 years old without recognized renal disease but with

Table 35-15. Amantadine hydrochloride (Symmetrel®) dosage, by age of patient and level of renal function

Age group	Dosage*
No recognized renal disease	
1-9 yrs.†	4.4-8.8 mg/kg/day once daily or divided twice daily. Total dosage should not exceed 150 mg/day.
10-64 yrs.§	200 mg once daily or divided twice daily
≥65 yrs.	100 mg once daily¶
Recognized renal disease	
Creatinine clearance (ml/min 1.73m²)	
≥80	100 mg twice daily
60-79	200 mg/100 mg on alternate days
40-59	100 mg once daily
30-39	200 mg twice weekly
20-29	100 mg thrice weekly
10-19	200 mg/100 mg alternating every 7 days

*For prophylaxis, amantadine must be taken each day for the duration of influenza A activity in the community (generally 6-12 weeks). For therapy, amantadine should be started as soon as possible after onset of symptoms and should be continued for 24-48 hours after the disappearance of symptoms (generally 5-7 days).

†Use in children under 1 year has not been evaluated adequately in one study, a dose of 6.6 mg/kg/day was reportedly well-tolerated by children over 2 years of age.

§Reduction of dosage to 100 mg/day is also recommended for persons with an active seizure disorder, because such persons may be at risk of experiencing an increase in the frequency of their seizures when given amantadine at 200 mg/day.

¶The reduced dosage of 100 mg/day for person 65 years of age or older without recognized renal disease is recommended to minimize the risk of toxicity, because renal function normally declines with age and because side effects have been reported more frequently in the elderly.

an active seizure disorder may also be at risk of increased frequency of their seizures when given amantadine at 200 mg/day rather than 100 mg/day.

Side effects and adverse reactions. Five percent to 10% of otherwise healthy adults taking amantadine have reported side effects, such as insomnia, lightheadedness, irritability, and difficulty concentrating. These and other side effects (see package insert) may be more pronounced in patients with underlying disease, particularly those common among the elderly; *provisions for careful monitoring are needed for these individuals* so that adverse effects may be recognized promptly and the drug reduced in dosage or discontinued, if necessary. Since amantadine is not metabolized, toxic levels will occur when renal function is sufficiently impaired.

Other measures

Under special circumstances, supplementary control measures may be useful in further limiting the spread of influenza. Influenza is known to cause nosocomial infection; a number of measures, including isolation, cohorting of patients and personnel, limiting visitors, and avoiding elective admissions and surgery during an influenza outbreak, have all been suggested to limit further transmission. However, the effectiveness of most of these measures has not been conclusively demonstrated. Schools or classrooms have been closed occasionally when explosive outbreaks have occurred. The effect of this measure on virus transmission has not been established.

SELECTED BIBLIOGRAPHY

Barker WH, Mullooly JP. Influenza vaccination of elderly persons. Reduction in pneumonia and influenza hospitalizations and deaths. JAMA 1980;344:2547-9.

Barker WH, Mullooly JP. Impact of epidemic type A influenza in a defined adult population. Am J Epidemiol 1980;112:798-811.

Barker WH, Mullooly, J.P. Pneumonia and influenza deaths during epidemics: implications for prevention. Arch Intern Med 1982;142:85-9.

Bukowskyj M, Munt PW, Wigle R, Nakatsu K. Theophylline clearance. Lack of effect of influenza vaccination and ascorbic acid. Am Rev Resp Dis 1984;129:672-5.

Consensus Development Conference Panel. Amantadine: does it have a role in prevention and treatment of influenza? A National Institutes of Health Consensus Development Conference. Ann Intern Med 1980;92:256-8.

DeStefano F, Goodman RA, Noble GR, McClary GD, Smith SJ, Broome CV. Simultaneous administration of influenza and pneumococcal vaccines. JAMA 1982;247:2551-4.

Dolin R, Reichman RC, Madore HP, Maynard R, Linton PN, Webber-Jones J. A controlled trial of amantadine and rimantadine in the prophylaxis of influenza A infection. N Engl J Med 1982;307:580-4.

Dowdle WR, Coleman MT, Gregg MB. Natural history of influenza type A in the United States. 1957-1972. Prog Med Virol 1974;17:91-135.

Eickhoff T.C. Committee on immunization. Immunization against influenza: rationale and recommendations. J Infect Dis 1971;123:446-54.

Fedson DS, Kessler HA. A hospital-based influenza immunization program, 1977-78. Am J Public Health 1983;73:442-5.

Galasso GJ, Tyeryar FJ Jr, Cate TR, et al (eds.). Clinical studies of influenza vaccines—1976. J Infect Dis 1977; 136(Suppl):S341-S742.

Glezen WP. Serious morbidity and mortality associated with influenza epidemics. Epidemiol Rev 1982;4:25-44.

Hammond GW, Cheang M. Absenteeism among hospital staff during an influenza epidemic: implications for immunoprophylaxis. Can Med Assoc J 1984;131:449-52.

Horadam VW, Sharp JG, Smilack JD, Schonberger LB. Pharmacokinetics of amantadine hydrochloride in subjects with normal and impaired renal function. Ann Intern Med 1981;94:454-8.

Kaplan JE, Katona P, Hurwitz ES, Schonberger LB. Guillain-Barré syndrome in the United States, 1979-1980 and 1980-1981. Lack of an association with influenza vaccination. JAMA 1982;248:698-700.

Kilbourne ED. ed. The influenza viruses and influenza. New York: Academic Press, 1975.

La Montagne JR, Noble GR, Quinnan GV, et al. Summary of clinical trials of inactivated influenza vaccine-1978. Rev Infect Dis 1983;5:723-36.

Mufson MA, Kruase HE, Tarrant CJ, Schiffman G, Cano FR. Polyvalent pneumococcal vaccine given alone and in combination with bivalent influenza vaccine. Proc Soc Exp Biol Med 1980;163:498-503.

Nolan TF Jr, Goodman RA, Hinman AR, Noble GR, Kendal AP, Thacker SB. Morbidity and mortality associated with influenza B in the United States, 1979-1980. A report from the Center for Disease Control. J Infect Dis 1980;142:360-2.

Patriarca PA, Kendal AP, Stricof RL, Weber JA, Meissner MK, Dateno B. Influenza vaccination and warfarin or theophylline toxicity in nursing-home residents [Letter]. N Engl J Med 1983;308:1601-2.

Patriarca PA, Weber JA, Parker RA, et al. Efficacy of influenza vaccine in nursing homes. Reduction in illness and complications during an influenza A (H3N2) epidemic. JAMA 1985;253:1136-9.

Parkman PD, Galasso GJ, Top FH Jr, Noble GR. From the National Institute of Allergy and Infectious Diseases of the National Institutes of Health, the Center for Disease Control, and the Bureau of Biologics of the Food and Drug Administration. Summary of clinical trials of influenza vaccines. J Infect Dis 1976;134:100-7.

Wright PF, Dolin R, LaMontagne JR. From the National Institute of Allergy and Infectious Diseases of the National Institutes of Health, the Center for Disease Control, and the Bureau of Biologics of the Food and Drug Administration. Summary of clinical trials of influenza vaccines-II. J Infect Dis 1976;134:833-8.

Younkin SW, Betts RF, Roth FK, Douglas RG Jr. Reduction in fever and symptoms in young adults with influenza A/Brazil/78 H1N1 infection after treatment with aspirin or amantadine. Antimicrob Agents Chemother 1983; 23:577-82.

From MMWR 1985;34:261.

MEASLES PREVENTION

These revised ACIP Measles Prevention recommendations represent an update of the previous recommendations (MMWR 1978;27:427-30, 435-7) to include current information about vaccine effectiveness and measles elimination efforts. There are no basic changes in approach. Further discussion is included of atypical measles syndrome and of revaccination of prior recipients of killed measles virus vaccine. Recommendations for vaccination of persons with allergies are revised. As the incidence rate of measles declines, serologic confirmation becomes more important. New recommendations for international travel are included.

Introduction

Measles (rubeola) is often a severe disease, frequently complicated by middle ear infection or bronchopneumonia. Encephalitis occurs in approximately 1 of every 2,000 reported cases; survivors often have permanent brain damage and mental retardation. Death, predominantly from respiratory and neurologic causes, occurs in 1 of every 3,000 reported measles cases. The risk of death is known to be greater for infants and adults than for children and adolescents.

Measles illness during pregnancy increases fetal risk. Most commonly, this involves premature labor and moderately increased rates of spontaneous abortion and of low birth-weight infants. Results of 1 retrospective study in an isolated population suggest that measles infection in the first trimester of pregnancy was associated with an increased rate of congenital malformations.

Before measles vaccine was available, more than 400,000 measles cases were reported each year in the United States. Since the licensure of vaccine in 1963, the collaborative efforts of professional and voluntary medical and public health organizations in vaccination programs have resulted in a 99% reduction in the reported incidence of measles. In 1981, a provisional total of 3,032 cases were reported. In the pre-vaccine era, most measles cases affected preschool and young school-age children. In 1980, more than 60% of cases in which the age was known occurred among persons ≥10 years old. More than 25% of the cases were reported among the 10- to 14-year-old age group, and more than 20% were reported among the 15- to 19-year-old age group.

With the highly effective, safe measles vaccine now available, the degree of measles control that has been achieved in the United States has depended largely on the effectiveness of the continuing efforts to vaccinate all susceptible persons who can safely be vaccinated. An initiative to eliminate indigenous measles from the United States by fall of 1982 is proceeding satisfactorily.

Measles virus vaccine

Live measles virus vaccine[*] available in the United States is prepared in chick embryo cell culture. The vaccine virus strain has been attenuated beyond the level of the original Edmonston B strain and is therefore known as a further attenuated strain. Vaccine prepared with the further attenuated measles virus causes fewer reactions than its predecessor, Edmonston B vaccine, which is no longer distributed in the United States. Measles vaccine is available in monovalent (measles only) form and in combinations: measles-rubella (MR) and measles-mumps-rubella (MMR) vaccines. All vaccines containing measles antigen are recommended for use at about 15 months of age under routine conditions. MMR is the vaccine of choice for use in routine infant-child vaccination programs. In all situations where measles vaccine is to be used, a combination vaccine should be given if recipients are likely to be susceptible to rubella and/or mumps as well as to measles.

Measles vaccine produces a mild or inapparent, non-communicable infection. Measles antibodies develop in at least 95% of susceptible children vaccinated at about 15 months of age or older with the current further attenuated vaccine. Protection against measles has been assessed both by measuring serum antibodies and by evaluating clinical protection in epidemiologic studies. Evidence now extending through 16 years indicates that although the titers of vaccine-induced antibodies are lower than those following natural disease, the protection conferred appears to be durable.

The most commonly employed test for measurement of immunity to measles is the hemagglutination-inhibition (HI) test. Most, but not all, immune individuals will have measles HI antibody levels of ≥4. More sensitive methods to determine measles immunity are not widely available at present. Routine serologic screening to determine measles immunity is not recommended.

Asymptomatic measles reinfection can occur in persons who have previously developed antibodies, whether from vaccination or from natural disease. Symptomatic reinfections have been reported rarely. These individuals have had ≥4-fold rises in measles HI antibody titers but have not had detectable measles-specific IgM antibodies in appropriately timed serum specimens. These rare symptomatic reinfections do not appear to be epidemiologically important.

Vaccine shipment and storage

Failure of protection against measles may result from the administration of improperly stored vaccine. Since 1979 a new stabilizer has been added to the vaccine that makes it more resistant to inactivation

---

[*]Official name: Measles Virus Vaccine, Live. Attenuated.

by heat. However, during storage before reconstitution, measles vaccine must be kept at 2-8 C (35.6-46.4 F) or colder. It must also be protected from light, which may inactivate the virus. Vaccine must be shipped at 10 C (50 F) or colder and may be shipped on dry ice.

Vaccine usage

General recommendations

Persons can be considered immune to measles only if they have documentation of:

1. Physician-diagnosed measles,
2. Laboratory evidence of measles immunity, or
3. Adequate immunization with live measles vaccine on or after the first birthday.

Most persons born before 1957 are likely to have been infected naturally and generally need not be considered susceptible. All other children, adolescents, and adults are considered susceptible and should be vaccinated, if there are no contraindications. This includes persons who may be immune to measles but who lack adequate documentation of immunity.

Dosage. At least 95% of vaccine recipients develop measles antibody following a single dose of live vaccine administered around 15 months of age. Since evidence now extending through 16 years indicates that the protection conferred is durable, there is no need for a "booster" dose of vaccine.

Concern has been raised that the small percentage of persons who continue to be susceptible after receiving a single dose might be able to sustain measles transmission, and therefore a second dose has been suggested for all vaccinees in order to reduce the proportion of susceptible persons to below the 5% that remain after initial vaccination.

There is no evidence that measles transmission can be sustained among the small percentage of persons who remain susceptible after receiving 1 dose of vaccine. In fact, measles has been eliminated in most areas of the country using the single-dose recommendation. Since it is impractical and inefficient to attempt to identify the small percentage of remaining susceptible persons, efforts should be concentrated on extending initial vaccination to the greatest number of recipients.

After weighing the evidence, the Committee continues to recommend only a single dose of measles vaccine around 15 months of age.

A single dose of live measles vaccine (as a monovalent or combination product) should be given subcutaneously in the volume specified by the manufacturer. Immune globulin (IG) should NOT be given with further attenuated measles virus vaccine.

Age at vaccination. Measles vaccine is indicated for persons susceptible to measles, regardless of age, unless otherwise contraindicated (see below). Current evidence indicates that for a maximum rate of seroconversion, measles vaccine should preferably be given when children are about 15 months of age. Because cases continue to occur in preschool children, increased emphasis must be placed on vaccinating children promptly at 15 months of age. It is particularly important to vaccinate young children ≥ 15 months of age before they might encounter measles in day-care centers or other environments where young children cluster.

Because of the continuing occurrence of cases in older children and young adults, the immune status of all adolescents should be evaluated. Complete measles control will require protection of all susceptibles; therefore, increased emphasis must be placed on vaccinating susceptible adolescents and young adults. Susceptible persons include those who received inactivated vaccine or who were given live measles virus vaccine before their first birthday, as well as those who were never vaccinated or never had measles.

Revaccination of persons vaccinated according to earlier recommendations

Previous vaccination with live vaccine. Persons vaccinated with live measles vaccine before their first birthday should be identified and revaccinated.

There has been some confusion concerning the immunity of children vaccinated against measles at 12 months of age. Some recent data have indicated a slightly lower rate of protection among children vaccinated at 12 months of age than among those vaccinated at 13 months or later. The difference is not sufficient to warrant routinely revaccinating persons who were vaccinated at 12 months of age since the vast majority are fully protected. If, however, the parents of a child vaccinated when 12-14 months old request revaccination for the child, there is no immunologic or safety reason to deny the request.

Previous vaccination with killed vaccine or vaccine of unknown type. In the past, the Committee has recommended revaccination with live measles vaccine for persons vaccinated at any age with inactivated vaccine (available in the United States from 1963 to 1967) and for persons vaccinated with inactivated vaccine followed by live vaccine within 3 months. This recommendation was based on the knowledge that some persons who had received inactivated vaccine were at risk of developing severe atypical measles syndrome when exposed to the natural virus. Persons who developed atypical measles occasionally developed serious complications requiring hospitalization. The recommendation was also based on the belief that revaccination with live measles vaccine would usually protect such persons against atypical measles. Limited data suggest that a substantial percentage of persons revaccinated with live measles vaccine will be protected, although the duration of immunity and degree of protection are not known precisely.

A wide percentage range (4%-55%) of prior recipients of killed measles vaccine who were revaccinated with live measles vaccine have been reported to have had reactions to the live vaccine. Most of these reactions are mild and consist of local swelling and erythema with or without low-grade fever lasting 1-2 days. Rarely, more severe reactions, including prolonged high fevers and extensive local reactions, have been reported that have required hospitalization. Prior recipients of killed measles vaccine are more likely to have serious illness when exposed to natural measles than when given live measles virus vaccine.

The Committee has considered the risks and benefits of revaccination for prior recipients of inactivated measles vaccine and believes that if such persons are identified, they should be revaccinated with live measles virus vaccine to prevent atypical measles syndrome. Revaccination is particularly important when exposure to natural measles virus is considered likely.

These same recommendations apply to persons vaccinated between 1963 and 1967 with a vaccine of unknown type since their only vaccination may have been with inactivated vaccine. Since killed measles vaccine was not distributed in the United States after 1967, persons vaccinated after 1967 with a vaccine of unknown type need not be revaccinated.

Individuals exposed to disease

Use of vaccine. Exposure to measles is not a contraindication to vaccination. Available data suggest that live measles vaccine, if given within 72 hours of measles exposure, may provide protection. If the exposure did not result in infection, the vaccine should induce protection against subsequent measles infection.

Use of IG. IG can be given to prevent or modify measles in a susceptible person within 6 days of exposure. The recommended dose of IG is 0.25 ml/kg (0.11 ml/lb) of body weight (maximum dose—15 ml). IG may be especially indicated for susceptible household contacts of measles patients, particularly contacts under 1 year of age, for whom the risk of complications is highest. Live measles vaccine should be given about 3 months later when the passive measles antibodies should have disappeared, if the child is then at least 15 months old. *IG should not be used in an attempt to control measles outbreaks.*

Side effects and adverse reactions

Experience with approximately 131 million doses of measles vaccine distributed in the United States through 1981 indicates an excellent record of safety. About 5%-15% of vaccinees may develop a temperature of ≥ 103 F (≥ 39.4 C) beginning about the sixth day after vaccination and lasting up to 5 days. Reports generally indicate that most persons with fever are otherwise asymptomatic. Transient rashes have been reported in approximately 5% of vaccinees. Central nervous system conditions including encephalitis and encephalopathy have been reported once for approximately every million doses administered. The incidence rate of encephalitis or encephalopathy following measles vaccination is lower than the observed incidence rate of encephalitis of unknown etiology, suggesting that some or most of the reported severe neurologic disorders may be only temporally related to measles vaccination rather than due to vaccination. Limited data indicate that reactions to vaccine are not age-related.

Subacute sclerosing panencephalitis (SSPE) is a "slow virus" infection of the central nervous system associated with measles virus. Results from studies indicate that measles vaccine, by protecting against measles, significantly reduces the chance of developing SSPE. The recent decline in numbers of SSPE cases in the presence of careful surveillance is additional strong presumptive evidence of a protective effect of measles vaccination. However, there have been some reports of SSPE in children who did not have a history of natural measles but who did receive measles vaccine. Some of these cases may have resulted from unrecognized measles illness in the first year of life or possibly from the measles vaccine.

Revaccination risks

There is no evidence of enhanced risk from receiving live measles vaccine in persons who have previously received live measles vaccine or had measles. Specifically, there does not appear to be any enhanced risk of SSPE.

On exposure to natural measles, some children who had been given inactivated measles virus vaccine previously have developed atypical measles, sometimes with severe symptoms. Reactions, such as local edema and induration, lymphadenopathy, and fever, have at times been observed when live measles virus vaccine was administered to recipients of inactivated vaccine. However, despite the risk of local reaction, persons born since 1956 who have previously been given inactivated vaccine (whether administered alone or followed by a dose of live vaccine within 3 months) should be revaccinated with live vaccine to avoid the severe atypical form of natural measles and to provide full and lasting protection (see Previous Vaccination With Killed Vaccine or Vaccine of Unknown Type above).

Precautions and contraindications

Pregnancy. Live measles vaccine should not be given to women known to be pregnant. This precaution is based on the theoretical risk of fetal infection, which applies to the administration of any live virus vaccine to women who might be pregnant or who might become pregnant shortly after vaccination. No evidence exists to substantiate this theoretical risk from measles vaccine. Considering the importance of protecting adolescents and young adults against measles with its known serious risks, asking women if they are pregnant, excluding those who are, and explaining the theoretical risks to the others are the recommended precautions in a measles immunization program.

Febrile illness. Vaccination of persons with febrile illness should be postponed until recovery. However, susceptible children with minor illnesses such as upper respiratory infections should be vaccinated. Considering the importance of protecting against measles, medical personnel should use every opportunity to vaccinate susceptible children.

Allergies. Hypersensitivity reactions very rarely follow the administration of live measles vaccine. Most of these reactions are considered minor and consist of wheal and flare or urticaria at the injection site.

Live measles vaccine is produced in chick embryo cell culture. However, with over 131 million doses of measles vaccine distributed in the United States there have been 3 reported cases of immediate allergic reactions in children who had histories of anaphylactoid reactions to egg ingestion. These reactions to vaccine could potentially have been life threatening. Two children experienced difficulty breathing; 1 of these had hypotension. Persons with a history of anaphylactoid reactions (hives, swelling of the mouth and throat, difficulty breathing, hypotension and shock) subsequent to egg ingestion should be vaccinated only with extreme caution. Evidence indicates that persons are not at increased risk if they have egg allergies that are not anaphylactoid in nature. Such persons should be vaccinated in the usual manner. There is no evidence to indicate that persons with allergies to chickens or feathers are at increased risk of reaction to the vaccine.

Since measles vaccine contains trace amounts of neomycin (25 μg), persons who have experienced anaphylactoid reactions to topically or systemically administered neomycin should not receive measles vaccine. Most often, neomycin allergy is manifested as a contact dermatitis which is a delayed-type (cell-mediated) immune response rather than anaphylaxis. In such individuals, the adverse reaction, if any, to 25 μg of neomycin in the vaccine would be an erythematous, pruritic nodule or papule at 48-96 hours. A history of contact dermatitis to neomycin is not a contraindication to receiving measles vaccine.

Live measles virus vaccine does not contain penicillin.

Recent administration of IG. Vaccination should be deferred for 3 months after a person has received IG, whole blood, or other antibody-containing blood products because passively acquired antibodies might interfere with the response to the vaccine.

Tuberculosis. Tuberculosis may be exacerbated by natural measles infection. There is no evidence, however, that the live measles virus vaccine has such an effect. Therefore, tuberculin skin testing is not a prerequisite for measles vaccination. The value of protection against natural measles far outweighs the theoretical hazard of possibly exacerbating unsuspected tuberculosis. If there is a need for tuberculin skin testing, it can be done on the day of vaccination and read 48 to 72 hours later. If a recent vaccinee proves to have evidence of tuberculous infection, prompt investigation and, if indicated, preventive treatment or treatment for tuberculous disease should be initiated. It is prudent to wait 4-6 weeks after measles immunization before administering a tuberculin skin test since measles vaccination may temporarily suppress tuberculin reactivity.

Altered immunity. Replication of the measles vaccine virus may be potentiated in patients with immune deficiency diseases and by the suppressed immune responses that occur with leukemia, lymphoma, or generalized malignancy, or with therapy with corticosteroids, alkylating drugs, antimetabolites, or radiation. Patients with such conditions should not be given live measles virus vaccine. Since vaccinated persons do not transmit vaccine virus, the risk to these patients of being exposed to measles may be reduced by vaccinating their close susceptible contacts. Management of such persons, should they be exposed to measles, can be facilitated by prior knowledge of their immune status. If susceptible, they should receive IG following exposure (see below).

Management of patients with contraindications to measles vaccine

If immediate protection against measles is required for persons for whom live measles virus vaccine is contraindicated, passive immunization with IG, 0.25 ml/kg (0.11 ml/lb) of body weight, should be given as soon as possible after known exposure (maximum dose—15 ml). It is important to note, however, that IG, which will usually prevent measles in normal children, may not be effective in children with acute leukemia or other conditions associated with altered immunity.

Simultaneous administration of vaccines

The simultaneous administration of MMR and OPV has resulted in seroconversion rates and rates of side effects that are similar to those observed when the vaccines are administered separately. Field experience and antibody data regarding simultaneous administration of DTP and measles vaccine indicate that the protective response is satisfactory and the incidence of side effects is not increased. Because of the limited accessibility of some population subgroups, the Committee recommends taking maximal advantage of each clinic visit to promptly vaccinate susceptible persons ≥15 months of age, including, if necessary, administering MMR, OPV, and DTP simultaneously. See ACIP statement, "General Recommendations on Immunization."

Measles elimination

High priority is being placed on the elimination of indigenous measles transmission from the United States in 1982. The Measles Elimination Program was launched in 1978, and reported measles incidence rates reached record low levels in 1980 and 1981. The major components of the strategy to eliminate measles are achieving and maintaining high immunization levels, surveillance of disease, and prompt outbreak-control measures. The following recommendations are presented to help preserve the level of measles control already achieved, and to bring about the further reductions in morbidity that will be required to achieve elimination of indigenous measles transmission.

Ongoing programs. The best means of reducing the incidence of measles is by having an immune population. Universal immunization as part of good health care should be accomplished through routine and intensive programs carried out in physicians' offices and public health clinics. Programs aimed at vaccinating children against measles at about 15 months of age should be established and maintained in all communities. In addition, all other persons thought to be susceptible, regardless of age, should be vaccinated when they are identified, unless vaccine is otherwise contraindicated.

Official health agencies should take whatever steps are necessary, including development and enforcement of school immunization requirements, to assure that all persons in schools (at all grade levels) and day-care settings are protected against measles. Enforcement of such requirements has been correlated with reduced measles incidence rates. Adequate evidence of immunity to measles should consist of either (1) a physician-documented history of measles disease, (2) laboratory evidence of measles immunity, or (3) a documented history of vaccination with live measles virus vaccine on or after the first birthday. Evidence of measles vaccination should be considered adequate only if the date of vaccination is provided.

Measles outbreaks have been and continue to be reported from places where young adults are concentrated, such as colleges. Measles control in these places may require careful evaluation of susceptibility and vaccination of those who are susceptible.

Measles outbreaks also have been and continue to be reported from places where preschool children are concentrated, such as day-care centers. Most states currently require evidence of immunity to measles for children enrolled in day-care centers. Measles control in preschool children requires careful evaluation of susceptibility and vaccination of those who are susceptible.

Concern is often expressed because of observations during outbreaks that cases occur in persons with a history of proper vaccination. Even under optimal conditions of storage and use, measles vaccine may have a 5% failure rate. A 90% or greater reduction in attack rates has been demonstrated consistently in appropriately vaccinated persons when compared with unvaccinated persons at risk. As greater numbers of susceptibles become vaccinated and as the measles incidence rate is further reduced, there will be a relative increase in the proportion of cases seen among appropriately vaccinated persons.

Outbreak control. All reports of suspected measles cases should be investigated rapidly. A measles outbreak exists in a community whenever a case is confirmed as measles. Once an outbreak occurs, preventing dissemination of measles depends on promptly vaccinating susceptible persons. Ideally, they will have been identified before the outbreak (by school record reviews, for example); if not, they must be quickly identified.

Speed in implementing control programs is essential in preventing the spread of measles. Control activities should not be delayed until laboratory results on suspected cases are received. All persons who cannot readily provide: (1) a physician-*documented* history of measles, (2) laboratory evidence of measles immunity, or (3) a *documented* history of vaccination with live measles virus vaccine on or after the first birthday should be vaccinated or excluded from school. Documentation of vaccination should be considered adequate only if the date of vaccination is provided. If a person's measles immunity is in doubt, he/she should be vaccinated.

An effective means of terminating school outbreaks and increasing rates of immunization quickly is to exclude all children or adolescents who cannot present valid evidence of immunity through vaccination or prior disease. Experience with outbreak control indicates that almost all students who are excluded from school because they lack evidence of immunity to measles quickly comply with requirements and are promptly readmitted to school. Exclusion should include pupils who have been exempted from measles vaccination because of medical, religious, or other reasons. Exclusion should continue until at least 2 weeks after the onset of rash of the last case of measles in the community. Less rigorous approaches such as voluntary appeals for vaccination have not been effective in terminating outbreaks.

Recent studies have indicated that some persons vaccinated before 11 months of age may have a less predictable immune response to measles vaccine when revaccinated on or after the first birthday. Approximately 50% of infants who failed to seroconvert initially will, after revaccination, develop HI antibody that is persistent; the remaining 50% will not develop sustained levels of HI antibody. Evaluations in one study showed that all these children, whether HI antibody negative or positive, had antibody detectable by a sensitive neutralization test. There is no evidence to indicate that these children are susceptible to measles.

The risk of measles complications resulting from measles is high among infants less than 1 year of age. Therefore, considering the benefits and risks, the Committee recommends that infants as young as 6 months of age may be vaccinated as pre-exposure prophylaxis when exposure to natural measles is considered likely. Because infants vaccinated before the first birthday have a significantly lower rate of seroconversion, they should be revaccinated when they are about 15 months old to ensure protection.

IG should not be used in an attempt to control measles outbreaks.

Importations. Measles importations are a continuing source of reported measles cases in the United States. With the recent substantial decline in measles incidence, the proportion of reported cases that are due to importations has increased. Although most imported measles cases result in limited transmission, several large outbreaks have occurred recently. Because of the possibility of multistate outbreaks if exposure of susceptible persons to a patient occurs on a common carrier, such as an airplane, rapid reporting of such imported cases to state and local health departments is important so that other state health departments can be notified to identify exposed contacts as well as to initiate surveillance and control measures.

International travel. Persons born after 1956 who travel abroad should be protected against measles, since measles is endemic in many countries throughout the world. No immunization or record of immunization is required for entry into the United States. However, it is recommended that international travelers should have immunity to measles consisting of physician's verification of prior measles disease, laboratory evidence of measles immunity, or verified measles vaccination on or after the first birthday. Since the risk of serious complications and death is greater for adults, it is especially important to protect young adults who have escaped measles disease and have not been vaccinated. Most persons born before 1957 need not be considered susceptible.

Surveillance

As the incidence rate of measles declines in the United States, aggressive surveillance becomes increasingly important. Known or suspected measles cases should be reported immediately to local health departments. Serologic confirmation should be attempted for every suspected case of measles that cannot be linked to a confirmed case. Measles infection can be serologically confirmed by a 4-fold rise in CF or HI antibody titer. The acute-phase serum specimen should be drawn as soon after rash onset as possible, preferably within the first 7 days after rash onset. The convalescent-phase serum specimen should be drawn 10 or more days after the acute-phase serum specimen. If the acute-phase specimen is drawn more than 7 days after rash onset, a 4-fold rise in antibody titer may not be apparent. Occasionally 4-fold rises may not be detected even if the first specimen is drawn within the first 7 days after rash onset. Measles infection may also be serologically confirmed by demonstrating measles-specific IgM antibody. A single serum specimen should be drawn between 1 and 2 weeks after rash onset. Although measles-specific IgM antibody may be detected shortly after rash onset, false negative results may occur if the specimen is drawn earlier than 1 week or later than 2 weeks following rash onset. Reporting of suspect cases and implementation of outbreak-control activities should not be delayed while awaiting laboratory results.

Effective surveillance of measles and its complications can delineate inadequate levels of protection, further define groups needing special attention, and assess the effectiveness of control activities. Continuous and careful review of adverse events following measles vaccination is also important. All adverse events following vaccination should be evaluated and reported in detail to local and state health officials as well as to the manufacturer.

SELECTED BIBLIOGRAPHY

Barkin RM. Measles mortality. Analysis of the primary cause of death. Am J Dis Child 1975;129:307-9.

CDC. School exclusion in two measles outbreaks—Wisconsin. MMWR 1979;28:488,493-4.

CDC. Measles importations—United States. MMWR 1981; 30:455-6,461-2.

CDC. Measles surveillance report No. 11, 1977-1981 (in press).

Halsey NA, Modlin JF, Jabbour JT, Dubey L, Eddins DL, Ludwig DD. Risk factors in subacute sclerosing panencephalitis: a case-control study. Am J Epidemiol 1980; 111:415-24.

Hayden GF. Measles vaccine failure. A survey of causes and means of prevention. Clin Pediatr 1979;18:155-67.

Hinman AR, Brandling-Bennett AD, Nieburg PI. The opportunity and obligation to eliminate measles from the United States. JAMA 1979;242:1157-62.

Hinman AR, Eddins DL, Kirby CD, Orenstein WA, Bernier RH, Turner PM, Bloch AB. Progress in measles elimination. JAMA 1982;247:1592-5.

Jespersen CS, Littauer J, Sagild U:. Measles as a cause of fetal defects. Acta Paediatr Scand 1977;66:367;72.

Karnin PB, Fein BT, Britton HA. Use of live, attenuated measles virus vaccine in children allergic to egg protein. JAMA 1965;193:1125-6.

Krause PJ, Cherry JD, Carney JM, Naiditch MJ, O'Connor K. Measles-specific lymphocyte reactivity and serum antibody in subjects with different measles histories. Am J Dis Child 1980;134:567-71.

Krugman RD, Rosenberg R, McIntosh K, Herrmann K, Witte JJ, Ennis FA, Meyer BC. Further attenuated measles vaccines: the need for revised recommendations. J Pediatr 1977;91:766-7.

Krugman S. Further attenuated measles vaccine: characteristics and use. Rev Infect Dis (in press).

Landrigan PJ, Witte JJ. Neurologic disorders following live measles vaccination. JAMA 1973;223:1459-62.

Langmuir AD. Medical importance of measles. Am J Dis Child 1962;103:224-6.

Linnemann CC, Dine MS, Roselle GA, Askey PA. Measles immunity after revaccination: results in children vaccinated before 10 months of age. Pediatrics 1982;69:332-5.

Marks JS, Halpin TJ, Orenstein WA. Measles vaccine efficacy in children previously vaccinated at 12 months of age. Pediatrics 1978;62:955-60.

McAleer WJ, Markus HZ, McLean AA, Buynak EB, Hilleman MR. Stability on storage at various temperatures of live measles, mumps and rubella vaccines in a new stabilizer. J Biol Stand 1980;8:281-7.

Modlin JF, Jabbour JT, Witte JJ, Halsey NA. Epidemiologic studies of measles, measles vaccine, and subacute sclerosing panencephalitis. Pediatrics 1977;59:505-12.

Shasby DM, Shope TC, Downs H, Herrmann KL, Polkowski J. Epidemic measles in a highly vaccinated population. N Engl J Med 1977;296:585-9.

Siegel M, Fuerst HT. Low birth weight and maternal virus diseases: a prospective study of rubella, measles, mumps, chickenpox, and hepatitis. JAMA 1966;197:680-4.

Weibel RE, Buynak EB, McLean AA, Hilleman MR. Follow-up surveillance for antibody in human subjects following live attenuated measles, mumps, and rubella vaccines. Proc Soc Exp Biol Med 1979; 162:328-32.

Wilkins J, Wehrle PF. Evidence for reinstatement of infants 12 to 14 months of age into routine measles immunization programs. Am J Dis Child 1978;132:164-6.

Wilkins J, Wehrle PF. Additional evidence against measles vaccine administration to infants less than 12 months of age: altered immune response following active/passive immunization. J Pediatr 1979;94:865-9.

Yaeger AS, Davis JH, Ross LA, Harvey B. Measles immunization: successes and failures. JAMA 1977;237:347-51.

From MMWR 1982;31:217-224, 229-231.

MENINGOCOCCAL VACCINES
Introduction

A polysaccharide vaccine against disease caused by *Neisseria meningitidis* serogroups A, C, Y, and W-135 is currently licensed in the United States. This statement updates the previous statement (*MMWR* 1978;27:327-9), summarizes available information on the vaccine, and offers guidelines for its use in the civilian population of the United States.

Meningococcal disease

N. meningitidis causes both endemic and epidemic disease, principally meningitis and meningococcemia. It is the second most common cause of bacterial meningitis in the United States (approximately 20% of all cases), affecting an estimated 3,000-4,000 people each year. The case-fatality rate is approximately 10% for meningococcal meningitis and 20% for meningococcemia, despite therapy with antimicrobial agents, such as penicillin, to which all strains remain highly sensitive.

No major epidemic of meningococcal disease has occurred in the United States since 1946, although localized community outbreaks have been reported. The incidence of endemic meningococcal disease peaks in the late winter to early spring. Attack rates are highest among children aged 6-12 months and then steadily decline; by age 5 years, the incidence approximates that for adults. Serogroup B, for which a vaccine is not yet available, accounts for 50%-55% of all cases; serogroup C, for 20%-25%; and serogroup W-135, for 15%. Serogroups Y (10%) and A (1%-2%) account for nearly all remaining cases. Serogroup W-135 has emerged as a major cause of disease only since 1975 (1). While serogroup A causes only a small proportion of endemic disease in the United States, it is the most common cause of epidemics elsewhere. Less commonly, serogroups C and B can also cause epidemic disease.

People with certain chronic conditions appear to be at increased risk of developing meningococcal infection. Meningococcal disease is particularly common among individuals with component deficiencies in the final common complement pathway (C3, C5-C9), many of whom experience multiple episodes of infection (2). Asplenic persons seem also to be at increased risk of developing meningococcal disease and experience particularly severe infections (3). It is uncertain whether individuals with other diseases associated with immunosuppression are at higher risk of acquiring meningococcal disease, as they are for disease caused by other encapsulated bacteria. In the past, new military recruits were at especially high risk, particularly for serogroup C disease; however, since routine vaccination of recruits with the bivalent A/C vaccine began in 1971, disease caused by those serogroups has been uncommon. Military recruits currently receive the A,C,Y,W-135 vaccine.

Meningococcal polysaccharide vaccines

The recently licensed quadrivalent A,C,Y,W-135 vaccine (Menomune®—A/C/Y/W-135, manufactured by Squibb-Connaught) is the formulation currently available in the United States. The vaccine consists of 50 μg each of the respective purified bacterial·capsular polysaccharides.

Vaccine efficacy. Numerous studies have demonstrated the immunogenicity and clinical efficacy of the A and C vaccines. The serogroup A polysaccharide induces antibody in some children as young as 3 months of age, although a response comparable to that seen in adults is not achieved until 4 or 5 years of age; the serogroup C component does not induce a good antibody response before age 18-24 months (4,5). The serogroup A vaccine has been shown to have a clinical efficacy of 85%-95% and to be of use in controlling epidemics. A similar level of clinical efficacy has been demonstrated for the serogroup C vaccine, both in American military recruits and in an epidemic. The group Y and W-135 polysaccharides have been shown to be safe and immunogenic in adults (6-9) and in children over 2 years of age; clinical protection has not been demonstrated directly, but is assumed, based on the production of bactericidal antibody, which for group C has been correlated with clinical protection. The antibody responses to each of the four polysaccharides in the quadrivalent vaccine are serogroup-specific and independent.

Duration of efficacy. Antibodies against the group A and C polysaccharides decline markedly over the first 3 years following a single dose of vaccine (5,10-13). This antibody decline is more rapid in infants and young children than in adults. Similarly, while vaccine-induced clinical protection probably persists in schoolchildren and adults for at least 3 years, a recent study in Africa has demonstrated a marked decline in the efficacy of the group A vaccine in young children over time. In this study, efficacy declined from greater than 90% to less than 10% over 3 years in those under 4 years of age at the time of vaccination; in older children, efficacy was still 67% 3 years after vaccination (14).

Recommendations for vaccine use

Routine vaccination of civilians with meningococcal polysaccharide vaccine is not recommended for the following reasons: (1) the risk of infection in the United States is low; (2) a vaccine against serogroup B, the major cause of meningococcal disease in the United States, is not yet available; and (3) much of the meningococcal disease in the United States occurs among children too young to benefit from the vaccine. However, the vaccine has been shown to be of use in aborting outbreaks due to serogroups represented in the vaccine and should be used in their control. In an outbreak, the serogroup should be determined and the population at risk delineated by neighborhood, school, dormitory, or other reasonable boundary. Although endemic disease is very uncommon above age 5 years, older children, adolescents, and young adults constitute a higher proportion of cases during epidemics and may warrant vaccination during an outbreak (15).

Routine immunization with the quadrivalent vaccine is recommended for particular high-risk groups, including individuals with terminal complement component deficiencies and those with anatomic or functional asplenia. Persons splenectomized because of trauma or nonlymphoid tumors and those with inherited complement deficiencies have acceptable antibody responses to meningococcal vaccine, although clinical efficacy has not been documented (2,16). It should be recognized that such individuals frequently have preexisting antibody against *N. meningitidis* and may not be protected by vaccination.

Vaccination with the A-C vaccine may benefit some travelers to countries recognized as having hyperendemic or epidemic disease and Americans living in these areas, particularly those who will have prolonged contact with the local populace. One area of the world recognized as having recurrent epidemics of meningococcal disease is the part of sub-Saharan Africa known as the "meningitis belt," which extends from Mauritania in the west to Ethiopia in the east. Epidemics have been recognized in other parts of the world, and updated information can be obtained from travelers' clinics, state health departments, and CDC.

Primary immunization. For both adults and children, vaccine is administered subcutaneously as a single 0.5-ml dose. The vaccine can be given at the same time as other immunizations, if needed. Good antibody levels are achieved within 10-14 days after vaccination.

Precautions and contraindications

Reactions. Adverse reactions to meningococcal vaccine are mild and infrequent, consisting principally of localized erythema lasting 1-2 days. Up to 2% of young children develop fever transiently after vaccination (13).

Pregnancy. On theoretical grounds, it is prudent not to immunize pregnant women unless there is a substantial risk of infection. However, evaluation of the vaccine in pregnant women during an epidemic in Brazil demonstrated no adverse effects. Further, antibody studies in these women showed good antibody levels in maternal and cord blood following vaccination during any trimester; antibody levels in the infants declined over the first few months and did not affect their subsequent response to immunization (17).

Revaccination

Revaccination may be indicated for individuals at high risk of infection, particularly children who were first immunized under 4 years of age; such children should be considered for revaccination after 2 or 3 years if they remain at high risk. The need for revaccination in older children and adults remains unknown.

Prospects for future meningococcal vaccines

Work is continuing on a serogroup B meningococcal vaccine, as well as on improved A and C vaccines. Candidate vaccines include capsular polysaccharides complexed with meningococcal outer-membrane proteins or covalently linked to carrier proteins. Clinical efficacy data for these vaccines are not available.

Antimicrobial chemoprophylaxis

Antimicrobial chemoprophylaxis of intimate contacts remains the chief preventive measure in sporadic cases of *N. meningitidis* disease in the United States. Intimate contacts include (1) household members, (2) day-care-center contacts, and (3) anyone directly exposed to the patient's oral secretions, such as through mouth-to-mouth resuscitation or kissing. The attack rate for household contacts is 0.3%-1%, 300-1,000 times the rate in the general population.

Unless the causative organism is known to be sensitive to sulfadiazine, the drug of choice is rifampin, given twice daily for 2 days (600 mg every 12 hours to adults; 10 mg/kg every 12 hours to children 1 month of age or older; 5 mg/kg every 12 hours to children under 1 month of age). Rifampin has been shown to be 90% effective in eradicating nasopharyngeal carriage. No serious adverse effects have been noted. However, rifampin prophylaxis is not recommended for pregnant women, as the drug is teratogenic in laboratory animals. Also, as well as turning urine orange, rifamin is excreted in tears, resulting in staining of contact lenses; thus, they should not be used during the course of therapy.

Because systemic antimicrobial therapy of meningococcal disease does not reliably eradicate nasopharyngeal carriage of *N meningitidis*, it is also important to give chemoprophylaxis to the index patient before a discharge from the hospital *(18)*.

Nasopharyngeal cultures are not helpful in determining who warrants chemoprophylaxis and unnecessarily delay institution of this preventive measure.

REFERENCES

1. Band JD, Chamberland ME, Platt T, Weaver RE, Thornsberry C, Fraser DW. Trends in meningococcal disease in the United States, 1975-1980. J Infect Dis 1983;148:754-8.
2. Ross SC, Densen P. Complement deficiency states and infection: epidemiology, pathogenesis and consequences of neisserial and other infections in an immune deficiency. Medicine 1984;63:243-73.
3. Francke EL, Neu HC. Postsplenectomy infection. Surg Clin North Am 1981;61:135-55.
4. Peltola H, Kayhty H, Kuronen T, Haque N, Sarna S, Mäkelä PH. Meningococcus group A vaccine in children three months to five years of age. Adverse reactions and immunogenicity related to endotoxin content and molecular weight of the polysaccharide. J Pediatr 1978;92:818-22.
5. Gold R, Lepow ML, Goldschneider I, Draper TF, Gotschlich EC. Kinetics of antibody production to group A and group C meningococcal polysaccharide vaccines administered during the first six years of life: prospects for routine immunization of infants and children. J Infect Dis 1979;140:690-7.
6. Griffiss JM, Brandt BL, Altieri PL, Pier GB, Berman SL. Safety and immunogenicity of group Y and group W135 meningococcal capsular polysaccharide vaccines in adults. Infect Immun 1981;34:725-32.
7. Armand J, Arminjon F, Mynard MC, Lafaix C. Tetravalent meningococcal polysaccharide vaccine groups A,C,Y,W 135: clinical and serological evaluation. J Biol Stand 1982;10:335-9.
8. Ambrosch F, Wiedermann G, Crooy P, George AM. Immunogenicity and side-effects of a new tetravalent meningococcal polysaccharide vaccine. Bull WHO 1983; 61:317-23.
9. Vodopija I, Baklaic Z, Hauser P, Roelants P, Andre FE, Safary A. Reactivity and immunogenicity of bivalent (AC) and tetravalent (ACW135Y) meningococcal vaccines containing O-acetyl-negative or O-acetyl-positive group C polysaccharide. Infect Immun 1983;42:599-604.
10. Artenstein MS. Meningococcal infections: 5. Duration of polysaccharide-vaccine-induced antibody. Bull WHO 1971;45:291-3.
11. Lepow ML, Goldschneider I, Gold R, Randolph M, Gotschlich EC. Persistence of antibody following immunization of children with groups A and C meningococcal polysaccharide vaccines. Pediatrics 1977;60: 673-80.
12. Greenwood BM, Whittle HC, Bradley AK, Fayet MT, Gilles HM. The duration of the antibody response to meningococcal vaccination in an African village. Trans R Soc Trop Med Hyg 1980;74:756-60.
13. Käyhty H, Karanko V, Peltola H, Sarna S, Mäkelä PH. Serum antibodies to capsular polysaccharide vaccine of group A *Neisseria meningitidis* followed for three years in infants and children. J Infect Dis 1980;142:861-8.
14. CDC. Unpublished data.
15. Peltola H. Meningococcal disease: still with us. Rev Infect Dis 1983;5:71-91.
16. Ruben FL, Hankins WA, Zeigler Z, et al. Antibody responses to meningococcal polysaccharide vaccine in adults without a spleen. Am J Med 1984;76:115-21.
17. McCormick JB, Gusmao HH, Nakamura S, et al. Antibody response to serogroup A and C meningococcal polysaccharide vaccines in infants born of mothers vaccinated during pregnancy. J Clin Invest 1980;65: 1141-4.
18. Abramson JS, Spika JS. Persistence of *Neisseria meningitidis* in the upper respiratory tract after intravenous antibiotic therapy for systemic meningococcal disease. J Infect Dis 1985;151:370-1.

From MMWR 1985;34:255.

MUMPS VACCINE

This revised ACIP recommendation on mumps vaccine represents an updating of the 1980 recommen-

dation.* Changes include an expanded statement on allergic reactions. There are no major changes in approach.

Introduction

There has been a steady decrease in the incidence rate of reported mumps cases in the United States since the introduction of the live mumps virus vaccine. In 1981, there was a record low of 4,729 cases, which represents a 97% decline from the 185,691 cases reported in 1967, the year of live mumps virus vaccine licensure. Mumps is still primarily a disease of young schoolage children; only about 15% of reported cases occur among adolescents and adults.

Mumps disease is generally self-limited, but it may be moderately debilitating. Benign meningeal signs appear in up to 15% of cases, but permanent sequelae are rare. Nerve deafness if one of the most serious of the rare complications involving the central nervous system (CNS).

Orchitis (usually unilateral) has been reported as a complication in up to 20% of clinical mumps cases in postpubertal males, although sterility is a rare sequela. Symptomatic involvement of other glands and organs has been observed less frequently.

There are limited experimental, clinical, and epidemiologic data that pancreatic damage may result from injury caused by direct viral invasion. However, further research is indicated to determine whether mumps infection contributes to the pathogenesis of diabetes mellitus.

Mumps infection during the first trimester of pregnancy may increase the rate of spontaneous abortion. There is no evidence that mumps during pregnancy causes congenital malformations.

Naturally acquired mumps infection, including the estimated 30% of cases that are subclinical, confers longlasting immunity.

Mumps virus vaccine

Live mumps virus vaccine† is prepared in chick-embryo cell culture. From its introduction in December 1967, through 1981, more than 55 million doses have been distributed in the United States. The vaccine produces a subclinical, non-communicable infection with very few side effects. Mumps vaccine is available both in monovalent (mumps only) form and in combinations: mumps-rubella and measles-mumps-rubella (MMR) vaccines. The combined MMR vaccine is the vaccine of choice. In all situations where mumps vaccine is be to used, MMR vaccine should be given if recipients are likely to be susceptible to

measles and/or rubella as well as to mumps. There is a positive benefit-ratio for mumps immunization that is more marked when mumps vaccine is administered as MMR. All vaccines containing measles antigen should be used at about 15 months of age under routine conditions.

Following vaccination, more than 90% of persons susceptible to mumps develop measurable antibody, which, although of considerably lower titer than that following natural infection, is protective and long-lasting. The duration of vaccine-induced immunity is unknown, but observations over 15 years of live vaccine use indicate both the persistence of anitbody and continuing protection against infection. Reported clinical vaccine efficacies have ranged from 75%-90%.

A killed mumps virus vaccine was licensed for use in the United States from 1950 through 1978. This vaccine induced antibody, but the immunity was transient. From 1967, the year of licensure of live mumps vaccine, until 1978, the number of doses of killed mumps vaccine administered is unknown, but appears to have been limited.

Vaccine shipment and storage

Failure of protection against mumps may result from the administration of improperly stored vaccine. During storage before reconstitution, mumps vaccine must be kept at 2-8 C (35.6-46.4 F) or colder. It must also be protected from light, which may inactivate the virus. Vaccine must be shipped at 10 C (50 F) or colder and may be shipped on dry ice. After reconstitution, the vaccine should be stored in a dark place at 2-8 C and discarded if not used within 8 hours. Temperature measuring devices should be available at all sites of vaccine storage and monitored daily.

Vaccine usage

(See also the current ACIP statement, "General Recommendations on Immunization," MMWR 1980; 29:76, 81-3.)

General recommendations. Susceptible children, adolescents, and adults should be vaccinated against mumps, unless vaccination is contraindicated. Mumps vaccine can be of particular value for children approaching puberty and for adolescents and adults, especially males, who have not had mumps. Persons who previously received killed mumps vaccine might benefit from revaccination with live mumps vaccine. Persons can be considered susceptible to mumps unless they have documentation of (1) physician-diagnosed mumps or laboratory evidence of immunity, or (2) adequate immunization with live mumps virus vaccine when 12 or more months of age. Most adults are likely to have been infected naturally and generally may be considered immune, even if they did not have clinically recognizable disease.

---

*Replaces previous recommendation on this subject published in MMWR 1980;29:87-8, 93-4.

†Official name: Mumps Virus Vaccine, Live.

Because there is no evidence that persons who have previously either received the vaccine or had mumps are at any risk of local or systemic reactions from receiving live mumps vaccine, testing for susceptibility before vaccination is unnecessary. Furthermore, such testing may be unreliable (e.g., mumps skin test and the complement-fixation antibody test). Those tests that have demonstrated reliability (neutralization, ELISA, and radial hemolysis antibody tests) are not readily available.

Dosage. A single dose of vaccine in the volume specified by the manufacturer should be administered subcutaneously.

Age. Live mumps virus vaccine is recommended for all children at any age after 12 months. It should not be administered to younger infants because persisting maternal antibody may interfere with seroconversion. Persons vaccinated before the first birthday might benefit from revaccination after reaching one year of age.

Individuals exposed to disease

Use of vaccine. When given after exposure to mumps, live mumps virus vaccine may not provide protection. However, if the exposure did not result in infection, the vaccine should induce protection against subsequent infection.

Use of immune globulin (IG). Immune globulin has not been demonstrated to be of established value in postexposure prophylaxis and is not recommended.

Adverse effects. Parotitis after vaccination has been reported rarely. Allergic reactions including rash, pruritus, and purpura have been associated temporally with mumps vaccination but are uncommon and usually mild and of brief duration. Very rarely, manifestations of CNS involvement, such as febrile seizures, unilateral nerve deafness, and encephalitis within 30 days of mumps vaccination, are reported. No deaths have been reported among patients with such complications, and almost all have recovered completely. It should be emphasized that reports of nervous system illness following mumps vaccination do not necessarily denote an etiologic relationship between the illness and the vaccine. The frequency of reported CNS dysfunction following mumps vaccination is lower than the observed background incidence rate of CNS dysfunction in the normal population.

Precautions and contraindications

Pregnancy. Although mumps virus is capable of infecting the placenta and fetus, there is no good evidence that it causes congenital malformations in humans. Mumps vaccine virus also has been shown to infect the placenta, but the virus has not been isolated from the fetal tissues from susceptible women who were vaccinated and underwent elective abor-

tions. However, because of the theoretical risk of fetal damage, it is prudent to avoid giving mumps vaccine to pregnant women.

Allergies. Live mumps vaccine is produced in chick-embryo cell culture. Persons with a history of anaphylactic reactions (hives, swelling of the mouth and throat, difficulty breathing, hypotension, or shock) subsequent to egg ingestion should be vaccinated only with extreme caution. Evidence indicates that persons are not at increased risk if they have egg allergies that are not anaphylactic in nature. Such persons may be vaccinated in the usual manner. There is no evidence to indicate that persons with allergies to chickens or feathers are at increased risk of reaction to the vaccine.

Since mumps vaccine contains trace amounts of neomycin (25 μg) persons who have experienced anaphylactic reactions to topically or systemically administered neomycin should not receive mumps vaccine. Most often, neomycin allergy is manifested as a contact dermatitis which is a delayed-type (cell-mediated immune response rather than anaphylaxis. In such individuals, the adverse reaction, if any, to 25 μg of neomycin in the vaccine would be an erythematous, pruritic nodule or papule at 48-96 hours. A history of contact dermatitis to neomycin is not a contraindication to receiving mumps vaccine. Live mumps virus vaccine does not contain penicillin.

Recent administration of immune globulin. Passively acquired antibody can interfere with the response to live, attenuated-virus vaccines. Therefore, administration of mumps vaccine should be deferred until approximately 3 months after the administration of immune globulin.

Altered immunity. Replication of the mumps vaccine virus may be potentiated in patients with immune deficiency diseases and by the suppressed immune responses that occur with leukemia, lymphoma, generalized malignancy, or with therapy with corticosteroids, alkylating drugs, antimetabolites, or radiation. Patients with such conditions should not be given live mumps virus vaccine. Since vaccinated persons do not transmit mumps vaccine virus, the risk of mumps exposure for those patients may be reduced by vaccinating their close susceptible contacts.

Other. There is no proven association between mumps vaccination and pancreatic damage or subsequent development of diabetes mellitus.

Mumps control

The principal strategy to remove the burden of mumps illness is through achieving and maintaining high immunization levels. Universal immunization as a part of good health care should be routinely carried out in physicians' offices and public health clinics. Programs aimed at vaccinating children with MMR should be established and maintained in all communities. In addition, all other persons thought to be susceptible should be vaccinated unless otherwise contraindicated. Because of limited accessibility to some population subgroups, the Committee recommends taking maximal advantage of clinic visits to vaccinate susceptible persons 15 months of age or older by administering MMR, DTP, and OPV simultaneously if all are needed. Health agencies should take necessary steps, including the development and enforcement of school immunization requirements, to assure that all persons in schools at all grade levels and in day-care settings are protected against mumps.

Surveillance

There is a continuing need to improve the reporting of mumps cases and mumps complications and to document the duration of vaccine effectiveness. Continuous and careful review of adverse reactions is also important. All severe reactions in vaccinated individuals should be evaluated and reported in detail to local or state health officials and to the manufacturer. Even though there are no data to raise concern about a teratogenic effect of mumps vaccine, the Centers for Disease Control would like to collect prospective data on mumps vaccination of women in early pregnancy. Therefore, administration of mumps vaccine to a woman within 3 months of conception should be reported through state health departments to the Immunization Division, Centers for Disease Control, (404/329-3747).

SELECTED BIBLIOGRAPHY

Drash AL. The etiology of diabetes mellitus. N Engl J Med 1979;300:1211-3. Editorial.

Ennis FA, Hopps HE, Douglas RD, Meyer HM Jr. Hydrocephalus in hamsters: Induction by natural and attenuated mumps viruses. J Infect Dis 1969;119:75-9.

Harris RW, Turnbull CD. Isacson P, Karzon DT, Winkelstein W Jr. Mumps in a northeast metropolitan community. I. Epidemiology of clinical mumps. Am J Epidemiol 1968;88:224-33.

Hayden GF, Preblud SR, Orenstein WA, Conrad JL. Current status of mumps and mumps vaccine in the United States. Pediatrics 1978;62:965-9.

Hilleman MR, Buynak EB, Weibel RE, Stokes J Jr. Live, attenuated mumps-virus vaccine. N Engl J Med 1968; 278:227-32.

Koplan JP, Preblud SR. A benefit-cost analysis of mumps vaccine. Am J Dis Child 1982;136:362-4.

Sinaniotis CA, Daskalopoulou E, Lapatsanis P, Doxiadis S. Diabetes mellitus after mumps vaccination. Arch Dis Child 1975;50:749-50. Letter.

Weibel RE, Buynak EB, McLean AA, Hilleman MR. Followup surveillance of antibody in human subjects following live attenuated measles, mumps, and rubella virus vaccines. Proc Soc Exp Biol Med 1979;162:328-32.

Witte JJ, Karchmer AW. Surveillance of mumps in the United States as background for use of vaccine. Public Health Rep 1968;83:95-100.

Yamauchi T, Wilson C, St. Geme JW Jr. Transmission of live, attenuated mumps virus to the human placenta. N Engl J Med 1974;290:710-2.

From MMWR 1982;31:617.

PLAGUE VACCINE
Introduction

Plague is a natural infection of rodents and their ectoparasites and occurs in many parts of the world, including the western United States, where a few human cases develop each year following exposure to infected wild rodents or their fleas. Epidemic plague may result when domestic rat populations and their fleas become infected. Recently the areas of the most intensive epidemic and epizootic infection have been some countries in Africa, Asia, and South America.

Plague vaccine

Plague vaccines* have been used since the late 19th century, but their effectiveness has never been measured precisely. Extensive field experience indicates that immunization with plague vaccine reduces the incidence and severity of disease.

The plague vaccine licensed for use in the United States is prepared from *Yersinia pestis* organisms grown in artificial media, inactivated with formaldehyde, and preserved in 0.5% phenol.

Vaccine usage

General recommendations. Because human plague is rare in most parts of the world, there is no need to vaccinate persons other than those at particularly high risk of exposure. Routine vaccination is not needed for persons living in plague-enzootic areas like those in the western United States. It is not indicated for most travelers to countries reporting cases,[†] particularly if their travel is limited to urban areas with modern hotel accommodations.

In most countries of South America, Asia, and Africa where plague is reported, the risk of exposure exists primarily in rural mountainous or upland areas. Following natural disasters and at times when regular sanitary practices are interrupted, plague can extend from its usually endemic areas into urban centers. Rarely, pneumonic plague has been reported in conjunction with outbreaks of bubonic plague, and tourist travel to those specific locations should be avoided.

Routine bacteriologic precautions are sufficient to prevent accidental infection with plague; therefore, immunization of clinical laboratory workers is unnecessary.

---

*Official name: Plague Vaccine.

†For a current listing, consult the most recent issue of the World Health Organization's *Weekly Epidemiological Record*.

Ecologists and other field workers who might come in contact with wild animals and their ectoparasites in areas where plague has been known to occur should be made aware of the potential risks of plague and told how to minimize direct contact with potentially infective animals and their tissues or parasites. These precautionary measures are generally sufficient to prevent infection.

Vaccine recipients. Vaccination should be a routine requirement for:

1. All laboratory and field personnel who are working with *Y. pestis* organisms resistant to antibiotics

2. Persons engaged in aerosol experiments with *Y. pestis;* and

3. Persons engaged in field operations in plague-enzootic areas where preventing exposure cannot be observed (such as some disaster areas).

Selective plague vaccination might be considered for:

1. Laboratory personnel regularly working with *Y. pestis* or plague-infected rodents;

2. Workers (for example, Peace Corps volunteers and agricultural advisors) who reside in plague-enzootic or plague-epidemic rural areas where avoidance of rodents and fleas is impossible; and

3. Persons whose vocation brings them into regular contact with wild rodents or rabbits in plague-enzootic areas.

Primary immunization. All injections should be given intramuscularly.

Adults and children over 10 years old. The primary series consists of 3 doses of vaccine. The first 2 doses, 0.5 ml each, should be administered 4 or more weeks apart, followed by a third dose, 0.2 ml, 4-12 weeks after the second injection. When less time is available, satisfactory but less than optimal results can be obtained with 3 injections of 0.5 ml administered at least 1 week apart.

Children less than 10 years old. The primary series also is 3 doses of vaccine, but the doses are smaller. The manufacturer's guide to proportionate dosages is: infants under 1 year—one-fifth adult dose; 1-4 years—two-fifths adult dose; 5-10 years—three-fifths adult dose. The intervals between injections are the same as for adults.

Booster doses. When needed because of continuing exposure, boosters should be given at approximately 6-month intervals to a total of 5 doses (3 primary vaccination doses plus 2 boosters). More than 90% of vaccinees should then have a passive hemagglutination (PHA) antibody titer of 1:128 or more. Thereafter, booster doses at 1-2 year intervals, depending on the degree of continuing exposure, should provide good protection.

Booster dosages for children and adults is the same as the third dose in the primary series. The primary series need never be repeated for booster doses to be effective.

Table 35-16. Recommended doses, by volume (ml), for immunization against plague

Dose number	Age (years)			
	<1	*1-4*	*5-10*	*>10*
1 and 2	0.1 ml	0.2 ml	0.3 ml	0.5 ml
3 and Boosters	0.04 ml	0.08 ml	0.12 ml	0.2 ml

Summary

The recommended doses for primary and booster vaccination are shown in Table 35-16.

Precautions and contraindications

Mild pain, erythema, and side effects such as induration at the injection site occur frequently. With repeated doses, fever, headache, and malaise are more common and also tend to be more severe. Sterile abscesses occur, but rarely. No fatal or disabling complications have been reported.

SELECTED BIBLIOGRAPHY

Bartelloni PJ, Marshall JD Jr, Cavanaugh DC. Clinical and serological responses to plague vaccine U.S.P. Milit Med 1973;138:720-722.

Burmeister RW, Tigertt WD, Overholt EL. Laboratory-acquired pneumonic plague. Ann Intern Med 1962; 56:789-800.

Cavanaugh DC, Elisberg BL, Llewellyn CH, et al. Plague immunization. V. Indirect evidence for the efficacy of plague vaccine. J Infect Dis 1974;129(Suppl):S37-S40.

Chen TH, Meyer KF. An evaluation of *Pasteurella pestis* fraction-1-specific antibody for the confirmation of plague infections. Bull WHO 1966;34:911-918.

Marshall JD Jr, Bartelloni PJ, Cavanaugh DC, et al. Plague immunization. II. Relation of adverse clinical reactions to multiple immunizations with killed virus. J Infect Dis 1974;129(Suppl):S19-S25.

Marshall JD Jr, Cavanaugh DC, Bartelloni PJ, et al. Plague immunization. III. Serologic response to multiple inoculations of vaccine. J Infect Dis 1974;129(Suppl):S26-S29.

Published in MMWR 1978;27:255.

PNEUMOCOCCAL POLYSACCHARIDE VACCINE

These revised recommendations of the Immunization Practices Advisory Committee (ACIP) on pneumococcal polysaccharide vaccine update the previous recommendations (MMWR 1981;30:410-2, 417-9) to include current information and practices.

Introduction

A 23-valent polysaccharide vaccine against disease caused by *Streptococcus pneumoniae* (pneumococcus) was licensed in the United States in 1983. It replaces the 14-valent polysaccharide vaccine licensed in 1977. This statement includes new data that have become available about pneumococcal vaccine and its effec-

Table 35-17. Current estimated occurrence of serious pneumococcal disease—United States

Pneumococcal disease	Estimated cases (1,000s/yr)	Estimated incidence (per 100,000 pop/yr)	Estimated case-fatality ratio (%)
Pneumonia	150-570	68-260	5
Bacteremia	16-55	7-25	20
Meningitis	2.6-6.2	1.2-2.8	30

tiveness and new recommendations regarding its use for selected persons and groups.

Pneumococcal disease

Pneumococcal disease is important, because it is responsible for a substantial number of cases and deaths in the United States each year. Although pneumococcal pneumonia accounts for less than 25% of all pneumonia, it is, nevertheless, a common disease. Pneumococcal pneumonia occurs in all age groups. In adults, its incidence increases gradually among those over 40 years old, with a twofold increase in incidence among those over 60 years old. Estimates on the occurrence of serious pneumococcal diseases in the United States are based on surveys, research reports, and several community-based studies (Table 35-17).

Mortality from pneumococcal disease is highest among patients with bacteremia or meningitis, patients with underlying medical conditions, and older persons. In some high-risk patients, mortality has been reported as high as 40% for bacteremic disease and 55% for meningitis. These rates occur despite therapy with antibiotics, such as penicillin, to which most (97%) clinically significant pneumococci isolated in the United States are exquisitely sensitive.

Patients with certain chronic conditions are clearly at increased risk of developing pneumococcal infection, as well as experiencing more severe pneumococcal illness. These conditions include: sickle cell anemia, Hodgkin's disease, multiple myeloma, cirrhosis, alcoholism, nephrotic syndrome, renal failure, chronic pulmonary disease, splenic dysfunction, and history of splenectomy or organ transplant. Other patients may be at greater risk of developing pneumococcal infection or having more severe illness because of diabetes mellitus, congestive heart failure, or conditions associated with immunosuppression. Patients with cerebrospinal fluid (CSF) leakage complicating skull fractures or neurosurgical procedures can have recurrent pneumococcal meningitis.

Pneumococcal polysaccharide vaccines

The new pneumococcal vaccine is composed of purified, capsular polysaccharide antigens of 23 types of *S. pneumoniae* (Danish types 1, 2, 3, 4, 5, 6B, 7F, 8, 9N, 9V, 10A, 11A, 12F, 14, 15B, 17F, 18C, 19A, 19F, 20, 22F, 23F, and 33F). Each polysaccharide is

extracted separately and combined into the final product. Each dose of the new vaccine contains 25 μg of each polysaccharide antigen.

The 23 bacterial types represented in the current vaccine are responsible for 87% of bacteremic pneumococcal disease in the United States reported to CDC in 1983, compared with 71% for the previous 14-valent formulation (1). Studies of the cross-reactivity of human antibodies against related types suggest that cross-protection may occur among some of these types (e.g., 6A and 6B) (2).

Although the new polysaccharide vaccine contains only 25 μg of each antigen, compared with 50 μg of antigen in the old 14-valent vaccine, a study of 53 adults reveals comparable levels of immunogenicity of the two vaccines (3). Most healthy adults show a twofold or greater rise in type-specific antibody, as measured by radioimmunoassay, within 2-3 weeks after vaccination. In contrast, the vaccine is generally less antigenic for children under 2 years old than for other vaccinees. However, because the precise protective titers of antibody for any of these serotypes have not been established, measuring antibody levels in vaccinated persons is not indicated.

Effectiveness of pneumococcal polysaccharide vaccines

In the 1970s, two randomized, controlled trials were conducted in populations with a high incidence of disease in South Africa and New Guinea using newly formulated pneumococcal vaccine (4,5). Both studies demonstrated significant reductions in the occurrence of pneumonia in these young, healthy populations.

It should be noted, however, that two randomized, controlled trials of pneumococcal vaccine in older-aged U.S. adults showed less satisfactory results (6). One was of outpatients over 45 years old; the other, of inpatients of a chronic-care psychiatric facility. In neither study was there any difference in the occurrence of respiratory morbidity and mortality between those vaccinated with a polyvalent pneumococcal vaccine and those given a placebo. In the first study, data suggested some vaccine protection against bacteremic pneumococcal disease, but the incidence of pneumococcal disease was low and may not have enabled a valid assessment of vaccine efficacy. In the other study, there were no fewer cases of radiologically diagnosed pneumonia among vaccinees than among controls.

Another method for estimating the efficacy of pneumococcal vaccine compares the distribution of serotypes of pneumococci isolated from the blood of vaccinated and unvaccinated persons (9). Recent data obtained by this method are based on comparing 210 *S. pneumoniae* isolates from the blood of persons who received the 14-valent vaccine with 1,475 blood isolates from unvaccinated persons. These data show that among persons over 60 years old with no underlying illness or no chronic pulmonary disease, chronic heart disease, or diabetes mellitus, the estimated efficacy ranges between 60% and 80%. However, among persons with cirrhosis or renal failure, the estimated efficacy appears to be lower.

In another recent study, controls were matched to 90 patients with systemic evidence of pneumococcal infection (isolates from blood, CSF, and other normally sterile body fluids) (10). Although vaccine efficacy was 0% for patients with severe immunocompromising conditions, it was 70% for all patients over 55 years of age and 77% for patients at moderately increased risk of pneumococcal infection.

Only a few studies of pneumococcal vaccine efficacy in children have been conducted. In a small, nonrandomized study of children and young adults 2-25 years old who had sickle cell anemia or had had splenectomy, the occurrence of bacteremic pneumococcal disease was significantly reduced by immunization with an 8-valent vaccine (7). Pneumococcal vaccine has shown no significant benefit in preventing otitis media in children (8).

The duration of protection induced by vaccination is unknown. While elevation of antibody titers has been shown 5 years after immunization, studies of persistence of elevated titers are ongoing.

Recommendations for vaccine use

Newly available data regarding vaccine efficacy support the broader use of pneumococcal vaccine in the United States. Vaccination is particularly recommended for the following:

Adults

1. Adults with chronic illnesses, especially cardiovascular disease and chronic pulmonary disease, who sustain increased morbidity with respiratory infections.
2. Adults with chronic illnesses specifically associated with an increased risk for pneumococcal disease or its complications. These include splenic dysfunction or anatomic asplenia, Hodgkin's disease, multiple myeloma, cirrhosis, alcoholism, renal failure, CSF leaks, and conditions associated with immunosuppression.
3. Older adults, especially those aged 65 and over, who are otherwise healthy.

Children

1. Children aged 2 years and older with chronic illnesses specifically associated with increased risk for pneumococcal disease or its complications. These include anatomic or functional asplenia, such as sickle cell disease or splenectomy, nephrotic syndrome, CSF leaks, and conditions associated with immunosuppression.
2. Recurrent upper respiratory diseases, including otitis media and sinusitis, are *not* considered indications for vaccine use in children.

General considerations. When elective splenectomy is being considered, pneumococcal vaccine should be given at least 2 weeks before the operation, if possible. Similarly, when immunosuppressive therapy is being planned, as in patients who are candidates for organ transplants, the interval between vaccination and initiation of immunosuppressive therapy should be as long as possible.

Although vaccine failures have been reported in some of these groups, especially those who are immunocompromised, vaccination is still recommended for such persons because they are at high risk of developing severe disease.

Strategies for vaccine delivery

Programs for vaccine delivery to these high-risk groups need to be developed further to achieve maximum immunization rates in such groups. More effective programs are needed for giving vaccine in nursing homes and other chronic-care facilities, in physicians' offices, and in hospitals, as only a small proportion of severe pneumococcal disease occurs in previously healthy individuals.

Two-thirds of persons with serious pneumococcal disease have been hospitalized within 5 years before the pneumococcal illness (11). Vaccine can be given to hospitalized patients—including at time of discharge—to prevent future admissions for pneumococcal disease. In addition, persons who visit physicians frequently and have chronic conditions are likely to be at higher risk of pneumococcal infection than those who require infrequent visits. Office-based programs to identify and immunize the frequent user of medical care should help prevent pneumococcal illness. Furthermore, pneumococcal vaccine and influenza vaccine can be given at different sites at the same time without an increase in side effects (12).

Medicare has partially reimbursed the cost of pneumococcal vaccination since 1981. It has been determined that hospitals may be reimbursed for pneumococcal immunization of Medicare recipients independent of reimbursement based on systems of prospective payments.

Adverse reactions

About half of those given pneumococcal vaccine develop mild side effects, such as erythema and pain at the injection site. In less than 1% of those given pneumococcal vaccine, fever, myalgias, and severe local reactions have been reported *(6,13,14)*. Severe adverse effects, such as anaphylactoid reactions, have rarely been reported—about 5 per million doses administered. For additional information, the package insert should be reviewed.

Revaccination

It should be emphasized that pneumococcal vaccine should be given *only once* to adults. Arthus reactions and systemic reactions have been common among adults given second doses *(15)* and are thought to result from localized antigen-antibody reactions involving antibody induced by previous vaccination. Therefore, second or "booster" doses are *not* recommended, at least at this time. Data on revaccination of children are not yet sufficient to provide a basis for comment.

Persons who have received the 14-valent pneumococcal vaccine should *not* be revaccinated with the 23-valent vaccine, as the modest increase in coverage does not warrant the possible increased risk of adverse reactions. However, when there is doubt or no information on whether a person has ever received pneumococcal vaccine, the vaccine should be given. Complete records of vaccination can help to avoid repeat doses.

Precautions

The safety of pneumococcal vaccine for pregnant women has not been evaluated. It should not be given to otherwise healthy pregnant women. Women at high risk of pneumococcal disease ideally should be vaccinated before pregnancy.

REFERENCES

1. Broome CV, Facklam RR. Epidemiology of clinically significant isolates of *Streptococcus pneumoniae* in the United States. Rev Infect Dis 1981;3:277-81.
2. Robbins JB, Austrian R, Lee C-J, et al. Considerations for formulating the second-generation pneumococcal capsular polysaccharide vaccine with emphasis on the cross-reactive types within groups. J Infect Dis 1983; 148:1136-59.
3. Pankey G, Schiffman G. The immunogenicity and reactogenicity of a 22 valent pneumonococcal vaccine [Abstract]. Clin Research 1982;30:376A.
4. Austrian R, Douglas RM, Schiffman G, et al. Prevention of pneumococcal pneumonia by vaccination. Trans Assoc Am Physicians 1976;89:184-94.
5. Riley ID, Tarr PI, Andrews M, et al. Immunisation with a polyvalent pneumococcal vaccine. Reduction of adult respiratory mortality in a New Guinea Highlands community. Lancet 1977;I:1338-41.
6. Austrian R. Surveillance of pneumococcal infection for field trials of polyvalent pneumococcal vaccines. Report DAB-VDP-12-84, National Institutes of Health, 1980.
7. Ammann AJ, Addiego J, Wara DW, Lubin B, Smith WB, Mentzer WC. Polyvalent pneumococcal-polysac-charide immunization of patients with sickle-cell anemia and patients with splenectomy. N Engl J Med 1977; 297:897-900.
8. Klein JO, Teele DW, Sloyer JL, et al. Use of pneumococcal vaccine for prevention of recurrent episodes of otitis media. In: Weinstein L, Fields BN, eds. Seminars in infectious disease. New York: Thieme-Stratton Inc: 1982:305-10.
9. Broome CV, Facklam RR, Fraser DW. Pneumococcal disease after pneumococcal vaccination: an alternative method to estimate the efficacy of pneumococcal vaccine. N. Engl J Med 1980;303:549-52.
10. Shapiro ED, Clemens JD. A controlled evaluation of the protective efficacy of pneumococcal vaccine for patients at high risk for serious pneumococcal infections. Ann Intern Med (in press).
11. Fedson DS, Chiarello LA. Previous hospital care and pneumococcal bacteremia: importance for pneumococcal immunization. Arch Intern Med 1983;143:885-9.
12. DeStefano F, Goodman RA, Noble GR, McClary GD, Smith SJ, Broome CV. Simultaneous administration of influenza and pneumococcal vaccines. JAMA 1982;247: 2551-4.
13. Semel JD, Seskind C. Severe febrile reaction to pneumococcal vaccine [Letter]. JAMA 1979;241:1792.
14. Schwartz JS. Pneumococcal vaccine: clinical efficacy and effectiveness. Ann Intern Med 1982;96:208-20.
15. Borgono JM, McLean AA, Vella PP, et al. Vaccination and revaccination with polyvalent pneumococcal polysaccharide vaccines in adults and infants (40010). Proc Soc Exp Biol Med 1978;157:148-54.

From MMWR 1984;33:273-281.

POLIOMYELITIS PREVENTION

This revised ACIP recommendation* on poliomyelitis prevention addresses issues important in poliomyelitis control in the United States today. Specifically, situations that constitute increased risk are defined, and alternatives for protection are outlined. Recommendations for immunization of adults are presented, clarifying the role of inactivated polio vaccine in immunizing adults. These recommendations also address the problems of interrupted immunization schedules and completion of primary immunization. Oral polio vaccine remains the vaccine of choice for primary immunization of children.

Introduction

Poliovirus vaccines, used widely since 1955, have dramatically reduced the incidence of poliomyelitis in the United States. The annual number of reported cases of paralytic disease declined from more than 18,000 in 1954 to an average annual number of less than 13 in 1973-1980. The risk of poliomyelitis is generally very small in the United States today, but epidemics are likely to occur if the immunity of the

---

*This recommendation supersedes the recommendation on poliomyelitis published in MMWR 1979;28:510-20.

population is not maintained by immunizing children beginning in the first year of life. Small outbreaks have occurred in 1970, 1972, and 1979 as a result of introduction of virus into susceptible populations in communities with low immunization levels.

As a result of the Childhood Immunization Initiative efforts, 1977-1979, immunization levels in children are now higher than ever before. The School Enterer Assessments in kindergarten and first-grade levels have indicated that the percentage of these children who have completed primary vaccination against poliomyelitis reached 95% in the 1980-81 school year. Immunization levels in preschool children and in those who are in higher grades may be substantially lower than the levels at school entry.

Laboratory surveillance of enteroviruses shows that the circulation of wild polioviruses has diminished markedly. Inapparent infection with wild strains no longer contributes significantly to establishing or maintaining immunity, making universal vaccination of infants and children even more important.

Poliovirus vaccines

Two types of poliovirus vaccines are currently licensed in the United States: Oral Polio Vaccine (OPV)* and Inactivated Polio Vaccine (IPV).†

Oral polio vaccine (OPV). Within several years after it was licensed in the United States in 1963, trivalent OPV, the live attenuated vaccine combining all 3 strains of poliovirus, almost totally supplanted the individual monovalent OPV antigens used earlier. Full primary vaccination with OPV will produce long-lasting immunity to all 3 poliovirus types in more than 95% of recipients: Most recipients are protected after a single dose.

OPV consistently induces intestinal immunity that provides resistance to reinfection with polioviruses. Administration of OPV may interfere with simultaneous infection by wild polioviruses, a property which is of special value in epidemic-control campaigns. In rare instances (once in approximately 3.2 million doses distributed), OPV has been associated with paralytic disease in vaccine recipients or their close contacts. In the 12-year period 1969-1980, approximately 290 million doses of OPV were distributed, and 92 cases of paralysis associated with vaccine were reported. Twenty-five cases of paralysis occurred in otherwise healthy vaccine recipients, 55 cases in healthy close contacts of vaccine recipients, and 12 cases in persons (recipients or contacts) with immune-deficiency conditions.

Inactivated polio vaccine (IPV). Licensed in 1955, IPV has been used extensively in this country and many other parts of the world. It is given by subcutaneous injection. Where extensively used, IPV has brought about a great reduction in paralytic poliomyelitis cases. Approximately 428 million doses have been administered in the United States, mostly before 1962. Although IPV has not been widely used in this country for more than a decade, a Canadian product licensed for use in the United States is now available.

It is generally accepted that primary vaccination with 4 doses of IPV produces immunity to all 3 poliovirus types in more than 95% of recipients. Additional experience with the IPV product available since 1968 is necessary to establish whether the duration of immunity is comparable to that induced by OPV. Experience in other countries forms the basis for the present recommendations on booster doses.

There is considerable evidence from epidemiologic studies that immunizing with IPV diminished circulation of wild poliovirus in the community, although it is known that persons vaccinated with IPV can subsequently be infected with and excrete in feces either wild strains or attenuated vaccine virus strains. No paralytic reactions to IPV are known to have occurred since the 1955 cluster of poliomyelitis cases caused by vaccine that contained live polioviruses that had escaped inactivation. Serious adverse reactions are not anticipated with the current IPV product.

An improved IPV product with higher potency has been developed in Europe. Studies in Africa and Europe have revealed essentially 100% seroconversion following 2 doses. Duration of protection is under study. Preliminary studies are now under way in a U.S. population to compare this product with OPV.

Routine immunization

Rationale for choice of vaccine. Although IPV and OPV are both effective in preventing poliomyelitis, OPV is the vaccine of choice for primary immunization of children in the United States when the benefits and risks for the entire population are considered. OPV is preferred because it induces intestinal immunity, is simple to administer, is well accepted by patients, results in immunization of some contacts of vaccinated persons, and has a record of having essentially eliminated disease associated with wild polioviruses in this country. The choice of OPV as the preferred polio vaccine in the United States has also been made by the Committee on Infectious Diseases of the American Academy of Pediatrics (1) and a special expert committee of the Institute of Medicine, National Academy of Sciences (2).

Some poliomyelitis experts contend that greater use of IPV in the United States for routine vaccination would provide continued control of naturally occurring poliovirus infections and simultaneously reduce the problem of OPV-associated disease. They argue

---

*Official name: Poliovirus Vaccine, Live, Oral, Trivalent.
†Official name: Poliomyelitis Vaccine.

that there is no substantial evidence that OPV and currently available IPV differ in their ability to protect individuals from disease. They question the public health significance of higher levels of gastrointestinal immunity achieved with OPV, and they question whether the transmission of vaccine virus to close contacts contributes substantially to the level of immunity achieved in the community.

Some countries successfully prevent poliomyelitis with IPV. However, because of many differences between these countries and the United States, particularly with respect to risks of exposure to wild polioviruses and the ability to achieve and maintain very high vaccination rates in the population, their experiences with IPV may not be directly applicable here.

Prospective vaccinees or their patients should be made aware of the polio vaccines available and the reasons why recommendations are made for giving specific vaccines at particular ages and under certain circumstances. Furthermore, the benefits and risks of the vaccines for individuals and the community should be stated so that vaccination is carried out among persons who are fully informed.

Recommendations for infants, children, and adolescents
Primary immunization (Table 35-18)

OPV. For infants, children, and adolescents through secondary school age (generally up to age 18) the primary series of OPV consists of 3 doses. In infancy the primary series is integrated with DTP vaccination, and the first dose is commonly given at 6-12 weeks of age. At all ages the first 2 doses should be separated by at least 6, and preferably 8, weeks. The third dose is given at least 6 weeks, customarily 8-12 months, after the second dose. In high-risk areas, an additional dose of OPV is often given within the

first 6 months of life. Breast feeding does not interfere with successful immunization.

IPV. The primary series consists of 4 doses of vaccine; volume and route of injection are specified by the manufacturer. In infancy, the primary schedule is usually integrated with DTP vaccination, as with OPV. Three doses can be given at 4- to 8-week intervals; the fourth dose should follow 6-12 months after the third.

All children should complete primary immunization before entering school, preferably with all OPV or all IPV. If, however, a combination of IPV and OPV is used, a total of 4 doses constitutes a primary series.

Supplementary immunization

OPV. Before entering school, all children who previously received primary immunization with OPV (3 doses) in early childhood should be given a fourth dose. However, if the third primary dose is administered on or after the fourth birthday, a fourth (supplementary) dose is not required. The additional dose will increase the likelihood of complete immunity in the small percentage of children who have not previously developed serum antibodies to all 3 types of polioviruses. The need for supplementary doses after 4 doses of OPV has not been established, but children considered to be at increased risk of exposure to poliovirus (as noted below under Recommendations for Adults) may be given a single additional dose of OPV.

IPV. Before entering school, all children who previously received primary immunization with either IPV alone or a combination of IPV and OPV (a total of 4 doses) in early childhood should be given at least 1 dose of OPV or 1 additional dose of IPV. However, if the fourth primary dose is administered on or after the fourth birthday, a fifth (supplementary) dose is not required at school entry. Use of a primary series

Table 35-18. Routine poliomyelitis immunization schedule summary, 1981*

Dose	OPV age/interval	IPV age/interval
Primary 1	Initial visit, preferably 6-12 weeks of age	Initial visit, preferably 6-12 weeks of age
Primary 2	Interval of 6-8 weeks	Interval of 4-8 weeks
Primary 3	Interval of ≥6 weeks, customarily 8-12 months	Interval of 4-8 weeks
Primary 4		Interval of 6-12 months
Supplementary	4-6 years of age† (school entry)	4-6 years of age† (school entry)
Additional supplementary		Interval of every 5 years§

*Important details are in the text.
†If the third primary dose of OPV is administered on or after the fourth birthday, a fourth (supplementary) dose is not required. If the fourth primary dose of IPV is administered on or after the fourth birthday, a fifth (supplementary) dose is not required at school entry.
§Supplementary doses are recommended every 5 years after the last dose until the 18th birthday or unless a complete primary series of OPV has been completed.

of OPV would eliminate the need for subsequent booster doses of IPV. Children who received primary immunization with IPV should obtain a booster dose of IPV every 5 years until the age of 18 years, unless a primary series of OPV is given. The need for such supplementary doses after the 5 basic doses of the currently available IPV product has not been firmly established. Further experience may lead to alteration of this recommendation.

Children incompletely immunized. Polio vaccination status should be reevaluated periodically, and those who are inadequately protected should complete their immunizations.

OPV. To help assure seroconversion to all 3 serotypes of poliovirus, completion of the primary series of 3 doses of OPV is recommended. Time intervals between doses longer than those recommended for routine primary immunization do not necessitate additional doses of vaccine. Individuals who received only 1 dose of each of the monovalent OPVs in the past should receive 2 doses of trivalent OPV at least 6 weeks apart. One dose of each monovalent OPV (poliovirus types 1, 2, and 3) is at least equivalent to 1 dose of trivalent OPV.

IPV. Regulations for vaccine licensure adopted since 1968 require a higher potency IPV than was previously manufactured. Four doses of IPV administered after 1968 are considered a complete primary series. As with OPV, time intervals between doses longer than those recommended for routine primary immunization do not necessitate additional doses.

Incompletely immunized children who are at increased risk of exposure to poliovirus (as noted below under Recommendations for Adults) should be given the remaining required dose or, if time is a limiting factor, at least a single dose of OPV.

Recommendations for adults

Routine primary poliovirus vaccination of adults (generally those 18 years old or older) residing in the United States is not necessary. Most adults are already immune and also have a very small risk of exposure to poliomyelitis in the United States. Immunization is recommended for certain adults who are at greater risk of exposure to wild polioviruses than the general population, including:

1. Travelers to areas or countries where poliomyelitis is epidemic or endemic.
2. Members of communities or specific population groups with disease caused by wild polioviruses.
3. Laboratory workers handling specimens which may contain polioviruses.
4. Health-care workers in close contact with patients who may be excreting polioviruses.

For individuals in the above categories, polio vaccination is recommended as detailed below.

Unvaccinated adults. For adults at increased risk of exposure to poliomyelitis, primary immunization with IPV is recommended whenever this is feasible. IPV is preferred because the risk of vaccine-associated paralysis following OPV is slightly higher in adults than in children. Three doses should be given at intervals of 1-2 months, a fourth dose should follow 6-12 months after the third.

In circumstances where time will not allow at least 3 doses of IPV to be given before protection is required, the following alternatives are recommended:

1. If less than 8, but more than 4, weeks are available before protection is needed, 2 doses of IPV should be given at least 4 weeks apart.
2. If less than 4 weeks are available before protection is needed, a single dose of OPV is recommended.

In both instances, the remaining doses of vaccine should be given later at the recommended intervals, if the person remains at increased risk.

Incompletely immunized adults. Adults who are at increased risk of exposure to poliomyelitis and who have previously received less than a full primary course of OPV or IPV should be given the remaining required doses of either vaccine, regardless of the interval since the last dose and the type of vaccine previously received.

Adults previously given a complete primary course of OPV or IPV. Adults who are at increased risk of exposure to poliomyelitis and who have previously completed a primary course of OPV may be given another dose of OPV. The need for further supplementary doses has not been established. Those adults who previously completed a primary course of IPV may be given a dose of either IPV or OPV. If IPV is used exclusively, additional doses may be given every 5 years, but their need also has not been established.

Unimmunized or inadequately immunized adults in households in which children are to be given OPV

Adults who have not been adequately immunized against poliomyelitis with OPV or IPV are at a very small risk of developing OPV-associated paralytic poliomyelitis when children in the household are given OPV. About 4 such cases have occurred annually among contacts since 1969, during which time about 24 million doses of OPV were distributed yearly (see Adverse Reactions).

Because of the overriding importance of ensuring prompt and complete immunization of the child and the extreme rarity of OPV-associated disease in contacts, the Committee recommends the administration of OPV to a child regardless of the poliovirus-vaccine status of adult household contacts. This is the usual practice in the United States. The responsible adult should be informed of the small risk involved. An acceptable alternative, if there is strong assurance that ultimate, full immunization of the child will not be jeopardized or unduly delayed, is to immunize adults according to the schedule outlined above before giving OPV to the child.

Precautions and contraindications

Pregnancy. Although there is no convincing evidence documenting adverse effects of either OPV or IPV on the pregnant woman or developing fetus, it is prudent on theoretical grounds to avoid vaccinating pregnant women. However, if immediate protection against poliomyelitis is needed, OPV is recommended.

Immunodeficiency. Patients with immune-deficiency diseases, such as combined immunodeficiency, hypogammaglobulinemia, and agammaglobulinemia, should not be given OPV because of their substantially increased risk of vaccine-associated disease. Furthermore, patients with altered immune states due to diseases such as leukemia, lymphoma, or generalized malignancy, or with immune systems compromised by therapy with corticosteroids, alkylating drugs, antimetabolites, or radiation should not receive OPV because of the theoretical risk of paralytic disease. OPV should not be used for immunizing immunodeficient patients and their household contacts; IPV is recommended. Many immunosuppressed patients will be immune to polioviruses by virtue of previous immunization or exposure to wild-type virus at a time when they were immunologically competent. Although these persons should not receive OPV, their risk of paralytic disease is thought to be less than that of naturally immunodeficient individuals. Although a protective immune response to IPV in the immunodeficient patient cannot be assured, the vaccine is safe and some protection may result from its administration. If OPV is inadvertently administered to a household-type contact of an immunodeficient patient, close contact between the patient and the recipient of OPV should be avoided for approximately 1 month after vaccination. This is the period of maximum excretion of vaccine virus. Because of the possibility of immunodeficiency in other children born to a family in which there has been 1 such case, OPV should not be given to a member of a household in which there is a family history of immunodeficiency until the immune status of the recipient and other children in the family is documented.

Adverse reactions

OPV. In rare instances, administration of OPV has been associated with paralysis in healthy recipients and their contacts. Other than efforts to identify persons with immune-deficiency conditions, no procedures are currently available for identifying persons likely to experience such adverse reactions. Although the risk of vaccine-associated paralysis is extremely small for vaccinees and their susceptible, close, personal contacts, they should be informed of this risk.

IPV. No serious side effects of currently available IPV have been documented. Since IPV contains trace amounts of streptomycin and neomycin, there is a possibility of hypersensitivity reactions in individuals sensitive to these antibiotics.

Case investigation and epidemic control

Each suspected case of poliomyelitis should prompt an immediate epidemiologic investigation, including an active search for other cases. If evidence implicates wild poliovirus and there is a possibility of transmission, a vaccination plan designed to contain spread should be developed. If evidence implicates vaccine-derived poliovirus, no vaccination plan need be developed, as no outbreaks associated with vaccine virus have been documented to date. Within an epidemic area, OPV should be provided for all persons over 6 weeks of age who have not been completely immunized or whose immunization status is unknown, with the exceptions noted above under Immunodeficiency.

REFERENCES

1. American Academy of Pediatrics. Report of the Committee on Infectious Diseases. 18th ed. Evanston, Illinois: AAP, 1977.
2. Nightingale E. Recommendations for a national policy on poliomyelitis vaccination. N Engl J Med 1977;297:249-53.

SELECTED BIBLIOGRAPHY

CDC. Poliomyelitis surveillance summary 1979. Atlanta: CDC, 1981.

Fite-Wassilak SG, Hinman AR. Is there a need for "catch-up" polio vaccination preadolescence? JAMA 1981;246: 1239.

Hardy GE, Hopkins CC, Linnenman CC Jr, et al. Trivalent oral poliovirus vaccine: a comparison of two infant immunization schedules. Pediatrics 1970;45:444-8.

International symposium on reassessment of inactivated poliomyelitis vaccine. Bilthoven 1980. Dev Biol Stand 47 (S. Karger, Basel 1981).

Krugman S, Katz SL. Childhood immunization procedures. JAMA 1977;237:2228-30.

Mayer TR, Balfour HH. Prevalence of poliovirus neutralizing antibodies in young adult women. JAMA 1981; 246:1207-9.

Nightingale E. Recommendations for a national policy on poliomyelitis vaccination. N Engl J Med 1977;297:249-53.

Salk J, Salk D. Control of influenza and poliomyelitis with killed virus vaccines. Science 1977;195:834-47.

Sanders DY, Cramblett HG. Antibody titers to polioviruses in patients ten years after immunization with Sabin vaccine. J Pediatr 1974;84:406-8.

Schonberger LB, McGowan JE, Gregg MB. Vaccine-associated poliomyelitis in the United States. 1961-1972 Am J Epidemiol 1976;104:202-11.

World Health Organization. The relation between acute persisting spinal paralysis and poliomyelitis vaccine (oral): results of a WHO enquiry. Bull WHO 1976;53:319-31.

From MMWR 1982;31:22-26, 31-34.

RABIES PREVENTION—UNITED STATES, 1984

These revised recommendations of the Immunization Practices Advisory Committee (ACIP) on rabies prevention update the previous recommendations (MMWR 1980;29:65-72, 277-80) to reflect the current status of rabies and antirabies biologics in the United States. For assistance on problems or questions about rabies prophylaxis, call local or state health departments.*

Introduction

Although rabies rarely affects humans in the United States, every year, approximately 25,000 persons receive rabies prophylaxis. Appropriate management of those who may have been exposed to rabies infection depends on the interpretation of the risk of infection and the efficacy and risk of prophylactic treatment. All available methods of systemic prophylactic treatment are complicated by instances of adverse reactions. These are rarely severe. Decisions on management must be made immediately; the longer treatment is postponed, the less likely it is to be effective.

Data on the efficacy of active and passive immunization after rabies exposure have come from both human and animal studies. Evidence from laboratory and field experience in many areas of the world indicates that postexposure prophylaxis combining local wound treatment, vaccine, and rabies immune globulin, is uniformly effective when appropriately used. However, rabies has occasionally developed in humans who had received postexposure antirabies prophylaxis with vaccine alone.

In the United States, rabies in humans has decreased from an average of 22 cases per year in 1946-1950 to zero to five cases per year since 1960. The number of rabies cases among domestic animals has decreased similarly. In 1946, more than 8,000 rabies cases were reported among dogs; 153 cases were reported in 1982. Thus, the likelihood of human exposure to rabies in domestic animals has decreased greatly, although bites by dogs and cats continue to be the principal reasons given for antirabies treatments.

The disease in wildlife—especially skunks, foxes, raccoons, and bats—has become more prevalent in recent years, accounting for approximately 85% of all reported cases of animal rabies every year since 1976. Wild animals now constitute the most important potential source of infection for both humans and domestic animals in the United States. Rabies among animals is present throughout the United States; only Hawaii remains consistently rabies-free.

Four of the six rabies fatalities in U.S. citizens occurring between 1980 and 1983 were related to exposure to rabid dogs outside the United States. In much of the world, including most of Asia and all of Africa and Latin America, the dog remains the major source of human exposure.

Rabies immunizing products

There are two types of immunizing products: (1) vaccines that induce an active immune response, which requires about 7-10 days to develop but may persist for as long as a year of more, and (2) globulins that provide rapid passive immune protection, which persists for a short period of time, with a half-life of about 21 days. Both types of products should be used concurrently for rabies postexposure prophylaxis.

Vaccines for use in the United States. Human diploid cell rabies vaccine (HDCV)* is an inactivated virus vaccine prepared from fixed rabies virus grown in WI-38 or MRC-5 human diploid cell culture. The vaccine grown on WI-38 cells and developed in the United States is inactivated with tri-n-butyl phosphate and β-propiolactone (Wyeth Laboratories' WYVAC®), while that grown in MRC-5 cells and developed in Europe is inactivated with β-propiolactone (Merieux Institute's RABIES VACCINE®). Both vaccines are supplied as 1.0 ml, single-dose vials of lyophilized vaccine with accompanying diluent.

Globulins

Rabies immune globulin, human (RIG). RIG (Cutter Laboratories' HYPERAB® and Merieux Institutes' IMOGAM®) is antirabies gamma globulin concentrated by cold ethanol fractionation from plasma of hyperimmunized human donors. Rabies neutralizing antibody content is standardized to contain 150 international units (IU) per ml. It is supplied in 2-ml (300 IU) and 10-ml (1,500 IU) vials for pediatric and adult use, respectively.

Antirabies Serum, Equine (ARS). ANTIRABIES SERUM® (Sclavo) is a refined, concentrated serum obtained from hyperimmunized horses. Neutralizing antibody content is standardized to contain 1,000 IU

---

*If these are unavailable, call the Division of Viral Diseases, Center for Infectious Diseases, CDC ([404] 329-30095 during working hours, or [404]329-2888 nights, weekends, and holidays).

---

*Official name: Rabies Vaccine. The duck embryo vaccine which was used from 1957-1982 is no longer available in the United States.

per vial. Volume is adjusted by the manufacturer on the basis of antibody potency in each lot. Currently, a 1,000-IU vial contains approximately 5 ml.

Rationale for choice of rabies immunizing products

Both types of HDCV rabies vaccines are considered equally efficacious and safe when used as indicated on the labels. Only the Merieux Institute vaccine has been evaluated by the intradermal (ID) dose/route for preexposure immunization. No data are available on ID use with the Wyeth Laboratories vaccine. RIG is preferred over ARS, because the latter has a much higher risk of adverse reactions.

Vaccines. The effectiveness of rabies vaccines is measured by their ability to protect persons exposed to rabies and to induce antibodies to rabies virus. HDCV has been used concurrently with RIG or ARS to treat 45 persons bitten by rabid dogs or wolves in Iran, 31 persons bitten by a variety of rabid animals in Germany, and 511 persons bitten by a variety of rabid animals in the United States. In these studies, no person contracted rabies after receiving HDCV in combination with RIG.

All persons treated with RIG and five 1.0-ml intramuscular (IM) doses of HDCV and tested have developed a rabies antibody titer. The definition of a minimally acceptable antibody titer varies between laboratories and is influenced by the type of test conducted. CDC currently specifies a 1:5 titer by the rapid fluorescent-focus inhibition test (RFFIT) as acceptable. The World Health Organization (WHO) specifies a titer of 0.5 I.U.

Serious adverse reactions associated with rabies vaccines include systemic, anaphylactic, and neuroparalytic reactions. Serious adverse reactions occur at lower rates in the HDCV vaccine than with previously available types of rabies vaccine.

Globulins. RIG and ARS are both effective; however, ARS causes serum sickness in over 40% of adult recipients. RIG rarely causes adverse reactions and should be the product of choice when available.

Rationale of treatment

Physicians must evaluate each possible rabies exposure. Local or state public health officials should be consulted if questions arise about the need for prophylaxis.

In the United States, the following factors should be considered before specific antirabies treatment is initiated:

Species of biting animal. Carnivorous wild animals (especially skunks, raccoons, foxes, coyotes, and bobcats) and bats are the animals most commonly infected with rabies and have caused most of the indigenous cases of human rabies in the United States since 1960. Unless an animal is tested and shown not to be rabid,

postexposure prophylaxis should be initiated upon bite or nonbite exposure to the animals. (See definition in Type of Exposure below.) If treatment has been initiated and subsequent testing in a competent laboratory shows the exposing animal is not rabid, treatment can be discontinued.

The likelihood that a domestic dog or cat is infected with rabies varies from region to region; hence, the need for postexposure prophylaxis also varies.

Rodents (such as squirrels, hamsters, guinea pigs, gerbils, chipmunks, rats, and mice) and lagomorphs (including rabbits and hares) are rarely found to be infected with rabies and have not been known to cause human rabies in the United States. In these cases, the state or local health department should be consulted before a decision is made to initiate postexposure antirabies prophylaxis.

Circumstances of biting incident. An unprovoked attack is more likely than a provoked attack to indicate the animal is rabid. Bites inflicted on a person attempting to feed or handle an apparently healthy animal should generally be regarded as provoked.

Type of exposure. Rabies is transmitted by introducing the virus into open cuts or wounds in skin or via mucous membranes. The likelihood of rabies infection varies with the nature and extent of exposure. Two categories of exposure should be considered.

Bite: Any penetration of the skin by teeth.

Nonbite: Scratches, abrasions, open wounds, or mucous membranes contaminated with saliva or other potentially infectious material, such as brain tissue, from a rabid animal. Casual contact, such as petting a rabid animal (without a bite or nonbite exposure as described above), does not constitute an exposure and is not an indication for prophylaxis. There have been two instances of airborne rabies acquired in laboratories and two probable airborne rabies cases acquired in a bat-infested cave in Texas.

The only documented cases of rabies from human-to-human transmission occurred in four patients in the United States and overseas who received corneas transplanted from persons who died of rabies undiagnosed at the time of death. Stringent guidelines for acceptance of donor corneas should reduce this risk.

Bite and nonbite exposures from humans with rabies theoretically could transmit rabies, although no cases of rabies acquired this way have been documented. Each potential exposure to human rabies should be carefully evaluated to minimize unnecessary rabies prophylaxis.

Management of biting animals

A healthy domestic dog or cat that bites a person should be confined and observed for 10 days and evaluated by a veterinarian at the first sign of illness during confinement or before release. Any illness in the animal should be reported immediately to the local health department. If signs suggestive of rabies develop, the animal should be humanely killed and its head removed and shipped, under refrigeration, for examination by a qualified laboratory designated by the local or state health department. Any stray or unwanted dog or cat that bites a person should be killed immediately and the head submitted, as described above, for rabies examination.

Signs of rabies in wild animals cannot be interpreted reliably; therefore, any wild animal that bites or scratches a person should be killed at once (without unnecessary damage to the head) and the brain submitted, as described above, for examination for evidence of rabies. If the brain is negative by fluorescent-antibody examination for rabies, the saliva can be assumed to contain no virus, and the bitten person need not be treated. If the biting animal is a particularly rare or valuable specimen and the risk of rabies small, consideration may be given to initiating post exposure treatment to the bitten person and delaying killing the animal for rabies testing.

Postexposure prophylaxis

The essential components of rabies postexposure prophylaxis are local treatment of wounds and immunization, including administration, in most instances, of both globulin and vaccine (Tables 35-19 and 35-20).

Local treatment of wounds. Immediate and thorough washing of all bite wounds and scratches with *soap and water* is perhaps the most effective measure for preventing rabies. In experimental animals, simple local wound cleansing has been shown to reduce markedly the likelihood of rabies.

Tetanus prophylaxis and measures to control bacterial infection should be given as indicated.

Immunization. Postexposure antirabies immunization should always include administration of both antibody (preferably RIG) and vaccine, with one exception: persons who have been previously immunized with the recommended preexposure or postexposure regimens with HDCV or who have been immunized with other types of vaccines and have a history of documented adequate rabies antibody titer (See Rationale for Choice of Rabies Immunizing Products) should receive only vaccine. The combination of globulin and vaccine is recommended for both bite exposures and nonbite exposures (as described under Rationale of Treatment), regardless of the interval between exposure and treatment. The sooner treatment is begun after exposure, the better. However, there have been instances in which the decision to

Table 35-19. Rabies postexposure prophylaxis guide—July 1984*

Animal species	Condition of animal at time of attack	Treatment of exposed person†
Domestic dogs and cats	Healthy and available for 10 days of observation	None, unless animal develops rabies§
	Rabid or suspected rabid	RIG¶ and HDCV
	Unknown (escaped)	Consult public health officials. If treatment is indicated, give RIG¶ and HDCV
Wild Skunk, bat, fox, coyote, raccoon, bobcat, and other carnivores	Regard as rabid unless proven negative by laboratory tests**	RIG¶ and HDCV
Other Livestock, rodents, and lagomorphs (rabbits and hares)	Consider individually. Local and state public health officials should be consulted on questions about the need for rabies prophylaxis. Bites of squirrels, hamsters, guinea pigs, gerbils, chipmunks, rats, mice, other rodents, rabbits, and hares almost never call for antirabies prophylaxis.	

*These recommendations are only a guide. In applying them, take into account the animal species involved, the circumstances of the bite or other exposure, the vaccination status of the animal, and presence of rabies in the region. Local or state public health officials should be consulted if questions arise about the need for rabies prophylaxis.
†*All bites and wounds should immediately be thoroughly cleansed with soap and water*. If antirabies treatment is indicated, both rabies immune globulin (RIG) and human diploid cell rabies vaccine (HDCV) should be given as soon as possible, *regardless* of the interval from exposure. Local reactions to vaccines are common and do not contraindicate continuing treatment. Discontinue vaccine if fluorescent-antibody tests of the animal are negative.
§During the usual holding period of 10 days, begin treatment with RIG and HDCV at first sign of rabies in a dog or cat that has bitten someone. The symptomatic animal should be killed immediately and tested.
¶If RIG is not available, use antirabies serum, equine (ARS). Do not use more than the recommended dosage.
**The animal should be killed and tested as soon as possible. Holding for observation is not recommended.

Table 35-20. Rabies immunization—June 1984

I. PREEXPOSURE IMMUNIZATION. Preexposure immunization consists of three doses of HDCV, 1.0 ml, IM (i.e., deltoid area), one each on days 0, 7, and 28. (See text for details on use of 0.1 ml HDCV ID as an alternative dose/route.) Administration of routine booster doses of vaccine depends on exposure risk category as noted below. Preexposure immunization of immunosuppressed persons is not recommended.

Criteria for Preexposure Immunization			
Risk category	Nature of risk	Typical populations	Preexposure regimen
Continuous	Virus present continuously, often in high concentrations. Aerosol, mucous membrane, bite, or nonbite exposure possible. Specific exposures may go unrecognized.	Rabies research lab workers.* Rabies biologics production workers.	Primary preexposure immunization course. Serology every 6 months. Booster immunization when antibody titer falls below acceptable level.*
Frequent	Exposure usually episodic, with source recognized, but exposure may also be unrecognized. Aerosol, mucous membrane, bite, or nonbite exposure.	Rabies diagnostic lab workers,* spelunkers, veterinarians, and animal control and wildlife workers in rabies epizootic areas.	Primary preexposure immunization course. Booster immunization or serology every 2 years.†
Infrequent (greater than population-at-large)	Exposure nearly always episodic with source recognized. Mucuous membrane, bite, or nonbite exposure.	Veterinarians and animal control and wildlife workers in areas of low rabies endemicity. Certain travelers to foreign rabies epizootic areas. Veterinary students.	Primary preexposure immunization course. No routine booster immunization or serology.
Rare (population-at-large)	Exposure always episodic, mucous membrane, or bite with source recognized.	U.S. population-at-large, including individuals in rabies-epizootic areas.	No preexposure immunization.

II. POSTEXPOSURE IMMUNIZATION. All postexposure treatment should begin with immediate thorough cleansing of all wounds with soap and water.

Persons not previously immunized:	RIG, 20 I.U./kg body weight, one half infiltrated at bite site (if possible), remainder IM; 5 doses of HDCV, 1.0 ml (i.e., deltoid area), one each on days 0, 3, 7, 14 and 28.
Persons previously immunized§:	Two doses of HDCV, 1.0 ml, IM (i.e., deltoid area), one each on days 0 and 3. RIG should not be administered.

*Judgment of relative risk and extra monitoring of immunization status of laboratory workers is the responsibility of the laboratory supervisor (see U.S. Department of Health and Human Service's *Biosafety in Microbiological and Biomedical Laboratories*, 1984).

†Preexposure booster immunization consists of one dose of HDCV, 1.0 ml/dose. IM (deltoid area). Acceptable antibody level is 1:5 titer (complete inhibition in RFFIT at 1:5 dilution). Boost if titer falls below 1:5.

§Preexposure immunization with HDCV; prior postexpsoure prophylaxis with HDCV; or persons previously immunized with any other type of rabies vaccine *and* a documented history of positive antibody response to the prior vaccination.

begin treatment was made as late as 6 months or longer after the exposure due to delay in recognition that an exposure had occurred.

HDCV. HDCV is the only type of vaccine currently available in the United States and should be administered in conjunction with RIG at the beginning of postexposure therapy, as described below. In 1977, WHO established a recommendation for six IM doses of HDCV based on studies in Germany and Iran of a regimen of RIG or ARS and six doses of HDCV. When used in this way, the vaccine was safe and effective in protecting 76 persons bitten by proven rabid animals. The vaccine also induced an excellent antibody response in all recipients. Studies conducted by CDC in the United States have shown that a regimen of one dose of RIG and five doses of HDCV was safe and induced an excellent antibody response in all recipients. Of 511 persons bitten by proven rabid animals and so treated, none developed rabies.

Five 1-ml doses of HDCV should be given intramuscularly (for example, in the deltoid region). Other routes of administration, such as the ID route, have not been adequately evaluated for postexposure prophylaxis and should not be used. The first dose should be given as soon as possible after exposure; an additional dose should be given on days 3, 7, 14, and 28 after the first dose. (WHO currently recommends a sixth dose 90 days after the first dose.) Because the antibody response following the recommended vaccination regimen with HDCV has been so satisfactory, routine postvaccination serologic testing is not recommended. In unusual instances, as when the patient is known to be immunosuppressed, serologic testing is indicated. Contact state health department or CDC for recommendations.

RIG (or ARS if RIG is not available). RIG is administered only once, at the beginning of antirabies prophylaxis, to provide immediate antibodies until the patient responds to HDCV by active production of antibodies. If RIG was not given when vaccination was begun, it can be given up to the eighth day after the first dose of vaccine was given. From about the eighth day on, RIG is not indicated, since an antibody response to the vaccine is presumed to have occurred. The recommended dose of RIG is 20 IU/kg or approximately 9 IU/lb of body weight. (When ARS must be used, the recommended dose is 40 IU/kg, approximately 18 IU/lb or 1,000 IU/55 lb body wieght.) If anatomically feasible, up to half the dose of RIG should be thoroughly infiltrated in the area around the wound, the rest should be administered intramuscularly. Because RIG may partially suppress active production of antibody, no more than the recommended dose of RIG should be given.

Treatment outside the United States

If postexposure is begun outside the United States with locally produced biologics, it may be desirable to provide additional treatment when the patient reaches the United States. State health departments should be contacted for specific advice in such cases.

Preexposure immunization

Preexposure immunization may be offered to persons in high-risk groups, such as veterinarians, animal handlers, certain laboratory workers, and persons spending time (e.g., 1 month or more) in foreign countries where rabies is a constant threat. Persons whose vocational or avocational pursuits bring them into contact with potentially rabid dogs, cats, foxes, skunks, bats, or other species at risk of having rabies should also be considered for preexposure prophylaxis.

Preexposure prophylaxis is given for several reasons. First, it may provide protection to persons with inapparent exposures to rabies. Second, it may protect persons whose postexposure therapy might be expected to be delayed. Finally, although it does not eliminate the need for additional therapy after a rabies exposure, it simplifies therapy by eliminating the need for globulin and decreasing the number of doses of vaccine needed. This is of particular importance for persons at high risk of being exposed in countries where the available rabies immunizing products may carry a higher risk of adverse reactions.

Preexposure immunization does not eliminate the need for prompt postexposure prophylaxis following an exposure; it only reduces the postexposure regimen.

Human diploid cell rabies vaccine. Three 1.0 ml injections of HDCV should be given intramuscularly (for example, in the deltoid area), one on each of days 0, 7, and 28. In a study in the United States, more than 1,000 persons received HDCV according to this regimen; antibody was demonstrated in the sera of all subjects when tested by the RFFIT. Other studies have produced comparable results. Because the antibody response following the recommended vaccination regimen with HDCV has been so satisfactory, routine postvaccination serology is not recommended.

Booster doses of vaccine. Persons who work with live rabies virus in research laboratories or vaccine production facilities and are at risk of inapparent exposure should have the rabies antibody titer of their serum determined every 6 months; booster doses of vaccine should be given, as needed, to maintain an adequate titer (see Rationale for Choice of Rabies Immunizing Products). Other laboratory workers, such as those doing rabies diagnostic tests, spelunkers, and those veterinarians, animal control and wildlife officers in areas where animal rabies is epizootic should have boosters every 2 years or have their serum tested for rabies antibody every 2 years and, if the titer is inadequate, have a booster dose. Veterinarians and animal control and wildlife officers, if working in areas of low rabies endemicity, do not require routine booster doses of HDCV after completion of primary preexposure immunization (Table 35-14).

Postexposure therapy of previously immunized persons. When an immunized person who was vaccinated by the recommended regimen with HDCV or who had previously demonstrated rabies antibody is exposed to rabies, that person should receive two IM doses (1.0 ml each) of HDCV, one immediately and one 3 days later. RIG should not be given in these cases. If the immune status of a previously vaccinated person who did not receive the recommended HDCV regimen is not known, full primary postexposure antirabies treatment (RIG plus five doses of HDCV) may be necessary. In such cases, if antibody can be demonstrated in a serum sample collected before vaccine is given, treatment can be discontinued after at least two doses of HDCV.

Intradermal use of HDCV. HDCV produced by the Merieux Institute has been used for preexposure immunization in a regimen of three 0.1 ml doses given ID in the lateral aspect of the upper arm over the deltoid area, one dose each on days 0, 7, and 28. Experience gained with over 2,000 persons vaccinated in the United States by the ID route has shown that antibody was produced in all recipients, although the mean response was somewhat lower and may be of shorter duration than with comparable IM immunization. Antibody response in some groups vaccinated outside the United States has been found to be inadequate for reasons not yet determined.

Current data provide a sufficient basis to recommend the 0.1 ml ID dose/route as an alternative to the 1.0 ml IM dose/route for preexposure immunization in the United States. Postvaccination serology is not necessary following ID (or IM) immunization, except for persons suspected of being immunosuppressed. The manufacturer has not yet met the packaging and labeling requirements necessary to obtain approval by the U.S. Food and Drug Administration for the ID route. Since the 1.0-ml vial presently available is intended for IM use and contains no preservatives, the reconstituted vaccine must be used immediately. Data on ID immunization are not available for Wyeth Laboratories' vaccine, and it should not be used for ID vaccination.

Accidental inoculation with modified live rabies virus

Individuals may be accidentally exposed to attenuated rabies virus while administering modified live rabies virus (MLV) vaccines to animals. While there have been no reported human rabies cases resulting from exposure to needlesticks or sprays with licensed MLV vaccines, vaccine-induced rabies has been observed in animals given MLV vaccines. Absolute assurance of a lack of risk for humans, therefore, cannot

be given. The best evidence for a low risk, however, is the absence of recognized cases of vaccine-associated disease in humans despite frequent accidental exposures.

Currently available MLV animal vaccines are made with one of two attenuated strains of rabies virus: high egg passage (HEP) Flury strain or Street Alabama Dufferin (SAD) strain. The HEP Flury and SAD virus strains have been used in animal vaccines for over 10 years without evidence of associated disease in humans; therefore, postexposure treatment is not recommended following exposure to these types of vaccine by needlesticks or sprays.

Because the data are insufficient to assess the true risk associated with any of the MLV vaccines, preexposure immunization, and periodic boosters are recommended for all persons dealing with potentially rabid animals or frequently handling animal rabies vaccines.

Adverse reactions

Human diploid cell rabies vaccine. Reactions after vaccination with HDCV are less common than with previously available vaccines. In a study using five doses of HDCV, local reactions, such as pain, erythema, and swelling or itching at the injection site, were reported in about 25% of recipients of HDCV, and mild systemic reactions, such as headache, nausea, abdominal pain, muscle aches, and dizziness were reported in about 20% of recipients. Two cases of neurologic illness resembling Guillain-Barré syndrome that resolved without sequelae in 12 weeks, and a focal subacute central nervous system disorder temporally associated with HDCV vaccine, have been reported.

Recently, a significant increase has been noted in "immune complex-like" reactions in persons receiving booster doses of HDCV. The illness, characterized by onset 2-21 days postbooster, presents with a generalized urticaria and may also include arthralgia, arthritis, angioedema, nausea, vomiting, fever, and malaise. In no cases were the illnesses life-threatening. Preliminary data suggest this "immune complex-like" illness may occur in up to 6% of persons receiving booster vaccines and much less frequently in persons receiving primary immunization. Additional experience with this vaccine is needed to define more clearly the risk of these adverse reactions.

Vaccines in other countries. Many developing countries use inactivated nerve tissue vaccines (NTV) or inactivated suckling mouse brain vaccine (SMBV). NTV is reported to provoke neuroparalytic reactions at a rate of about 1/2,000 vaccinees; the rate for SMBV is about 1/8,000.

Rabies immune globulin, human. Local pain and low-grade fever may follow receipt of RIG. Although not reported specifically for RIG, angioneurotic edema, nephrotic syndrome, and anaphylaxis have been reported after injection of immune serum globulin (ISG). These reactions occur so rarely that the causal relationship between ISG and these reactions is not clear.

Antirabies serum, equine. ARS produces serum sickness in at least 40% of adult recipients; reaction rates for children are lower. Anaphylactic reactions may occur. When RIG is not available, and ARS must be used, the patient should be tested for sensitivity to equine serum. (See package circular for details.)

Because adverse reactions are associated more frequently with ARS than with RIG, and ARS might sensitize recipients to equine protein, ARS should be used only when RIG cannot be obtained.

Management of adverse reactions. Once initiated, rabies prophylaxis should not be interrupted or discontinued because of local or mild systemic adverse reactions to rabies vaccine. Usually such reactions can be successfully managed with anti-inflammatory and antipyretic agents (aspirin, for example).

When a person with a history of hypersensitivity must be given rabies vaccines, antihistamines may be given; epinephrine should be readily available to counteract anaphylactic reactions, and the person should be carefully observed immediately after immunization.

Serious systemic anaphylactic or neuroparalytic reactions occurring during the administration of rabies vaccines pose a serious dilemma for the attending physician. A patient's risk of developing rabies must be carefully considered before deciding to discontinue vaccination. Moreover, the use of corticosteroids to treat life-threatening neuroparalytic reactions carries the risk of inhibiting the development of active immunity to rabies. It is especially important in these cases that the serum of the patient be tested for rabies antibodies. Advice and assistance on the management of serious adverse reactions in persons receiving rabies vaccines may be sought from the state health department or CDC.

All serious systemic neuroparalytic or anaphylactic reactions to a rabies vaccine should be immediately reported to the state health department or the Division of Viral Diseases, Center for Infectious Diseases, CDC ([404] 329-3095 during working hours, or [404] 329-2888 at other times).

Precautions and contraindications

Immunosuppression. Corticosteroids, other immunosuppressive agents, and immunosuppressive illnesses can interfere with the development of active immunity and predispose the patient to developing rabies. Immunosuppressive agents should not be administered during postexposure therapy, unless essential for the treatment of other conditions. When rabies postexposure prophylaxis is administered to persons receiving steroids or other immunosuppres-

sive therapy, it is especially important that serum be tested for rabies antibody to ensure that an adequate response has developed.

Pregnancy. Because of the potential consequences of inadequately treated rabies exposure and limited data that indicate that fetal abnormalities have not been associated with rabies vaccination, pregnancy is not considered a contraindication to postexposure prophylaxis. If there is substantial risk of exposure to rabies, preexposure prophylaxis may also be indicated during pregnancy.

Allergies. Persons with histories of hypersensitivity should be given rabies vaccines with caution. When a patient with a history suggesting hypersensitivity to HDCV must be given that vaccine, antihistamines can be given; epinephrine should be readily available to counteract anaphylactic reactions, and the person should be carefully observed.

SELECTED BIBLIOGRAPHY

Anderson LJ, Nicholson KG, Tauxe RV, Winkler WG. Human rabies in the United States, 1960 to 1979: epidemiology, diagnosis, and prevention. Ann Intern Med 1984;728-35.

Anderson LJ, Sikes RK, Langkop CW, et al. Postexposure trial of a human diploid cell strain rabies vaccine. J Infect Dis 1980;142:133-8.

Baer, GM, ed. The natural history of rabies. New York: Academic Press, 1975.

Bahmanyar M, Fayaz A, Nour-Salehi S, Mohammadi M, Koprowski H. Successful protection of humans exposed to rabies infection: postexposure treatment with the new human diploid cell rabies vaccine and antirabies sérum. JAMA 1976;236:2751-4.

Bernard KW, Smith PW, Kader RJ, Moran MJ. Neuroparalytic illness and human diploid cell rabies vaccine. JAMA 1982;248:3136-8.

Boe E, Nyland H. Guillain-Barré syndrome after vaccination with human diploid cell rabies vaccine. Scand J Infect Dis 1980;12:231-2.

CDC. Systemic allergic reactions following immunization with human diploid cell rabies vaccine. MMWR 1984; 33:185-7.

Corey L, Hattwick MAW. Treatment of persons exposed to rabies. JAMA 1975;232:272-6.

Greenberg M, Childress J. Vaccination against rabies with duck-embryo and Semple vaccines. JAMA 1960;173: 333-7.

Helmick CG: The epidemiology of human rabies postexposure prophylaxis, 1980-1981. JAMA 1983;250:1990-6.

Hattwick MAW. Human rabies. Public Health Rev 1974; 3:229-74.

Hattwick MAW, Rubin RH, Music S, Sikes RK, Smith JS, Gregg MM. Postexposure rabies prophylaxis with human rabies immune globulin. JAMA 1974;227:407-10.

Reck FM Jr, Powell HM, Culbertson CG. A new antirabies vaccine for human use. J Lab Clin Med 1955;45:679-83.

Rubin RH, Hattwick MAW, Jones S, Gregg MB, Schwartz VD. Adverse reactions to duck embryo rabies vaccine. Range and incidence. Ann Intern Med 1973;78:643-9.

Tierkel ES, Sikes RK. Preexposure prophylaxis against rabies. Comparison of regimens. JAMA 1967;201:911-4.

Tint H, Rosanoff EI. Clinical responses to T(n)BP-disrupted HDCS (WI-38) rabies vaccine. Dev Biol Stand 1976;37:287-9.

Wiktor TJ, Plotkin SA, Koprowski H. Development and clinical trials of new human rabies vaccine of tissue culture (human diploid cell) origin. Dev Biol Stand 1978;40:3-9.

World Health Organization. Sixth report of the Expert Committee on Rabies. Geneva, Switzerland: World Health Organization, 1973 (WHO technical report no. 523).

Sinnecker H, Atanasiu P, Bahmanyar M, Selimov M, Wandeler AI, Bogel K (Working Group 2, World Health Organization). Vaccine potency requirements for reduced immunization schedules and preexposure treatment. Dev Biol Stand 1978;40:268-70.

From MMWR 1984;33:393-402.

SYSTEMIC ALLERGIC REACTIONS FOLLOWING IMMUNIZATION WITH HUMAN DIPLOID CELL RABIES VACCINE

Human diploid cell rabies vaccine (HDCV) has been licensed for use since June 9, 1980. Approximately 400,000 doses have been administered to an estimated 100,000 persons in the United States since that time. The majority of these were for postexposure treatments. Information on possible adverse reactions to HDCV has been collected by CDC from individual physicians and from medical personnel in charge of providing rabies preexposure and postexposure prophylaxis to large cohorts of persons, such as veterinary students and animal-control workers. During the past 46 months, 108 clinical reports of systemic allergic reactions ranging from hives to anaphylaxis were reported to CDC (11 per 10,000 vaccinees). Few patients required hospitalization, and no deaths secondary to the reactions were reported.

The reports of systemic allergic reactions included nine cases of presumed Type I immediate hypersensitivity (1/10,000), 87 cases of presumed Type III hypersensitivity reactions (9/10,000), and 12 cases of allergic reactions of indeterminate type (Table 35-21). These reactions were classified on the basis of clinical observations only. Type I hypersensitivity reactions refer to immunoglobulin E (IgE)-mediated immediate reactions, such as anaphylaxis and atopy, whereas Type III hypersensitivity refers to immunoglobulin G (IgG)- or immunoglobulin M (IgM)-mediated immune complex disease characterized by antigen-antibody complex deposition in tissues, complement activation, and inflammation (1).

Hypersensitivity reactions presumed to be Type III occurred 2-21 days after a dose or doses of HDCV; patients presented with a generalized or pruritic rash or urticaria, sometimes accompanied by arthralgias, angioedema, fever, nausea, vomiting, and malaise. All nine of the presumed immediate hypersensitivity reactions occurred during either primary preexposure immunization (vaccine administered on days 0, 7, and 21 or 28) or postexposure immunization (vaccine on days 0, 3, 7, 14, and 28 and rabies immune globulin on day 0). However, 81 (93%) of 87 of the presumed Type III hypersensitivity reactions were observed following booster immunization. Although the presumed Type III reactions occurred in six persons during primary immunization series, none were observed following the first dose of the primary series.

Routine boosters of HDCV at 2-year intervals have been recommended for persons with continuing risks

Table 35-21. Reports of systemic allergic reactions following immunization with human diploid cell rabies vaccine—United States, June 1980-March 1984

| | Preexposure | | | | Postexposure | | |
| | Primary series | | Booster dose | | Primary series | Booster dose | |
Reaction type*	ID	IM	ID	IM	IM	IM	Total
Type I (immediate hypersensitivity)	1	0	0	0	8	0	9
Type III (immune complex disease)	1	0	42	34	5	5	87
Indeterminate (Type I or Type III)	0	0	0	0	11	1	12
Total	2	0	42	34	24	6	108

*Characterization of reactions is based on clinical definition, not immunopathologic changes:

Type I: Immediate hypersensitivity, as used here, refers to an immunologic illness occurring within minutes to hours after a dose of HDCV and characterized with either bronchospasm, laryngeal edema, generalized pruritic rash, urticaria, or angioedema.

Type III: Presumed immune complex disease, as used here, refers to an immunologic illness occurring 2-21 days after a dose or doses of HDCV and characterized by a generalized pruritic rash or urticaria; the patient may also have arthralgias, arthritis, angioedema, nausea, vomiting, fever, and malaise.

Key: ID, intradermal; IM, intramuscular.

Table 35-22. Signs and symptoms in three cohorts reporting presumed immune complex-type hypersensitivity reactions* after booster immunization with human diploid cell rabies vaccine

	Cohort A	Cohort B	Cohort C
No. with reaction/total persons given boosters (%)	23/226 (10%)	22/123 (18%)	6/29 (21%)
Vaccine	Merieux	Wyeth	Merieux
Route of booster	ID†	IM§	IM
No. with sign or symptom (%)¶			
Pruritic rash	16 (70%)	5 (18%)	1 (17%)
Urticaria	20 (87)	20 (91%)	6 (100%)
Edema	10 (43%)	10 (45%)	4 (67%)
Joint pain	4 (17%)	3 (14%)	0
Fever	1 (4%)	0	0
Difficulty breathing	1 (4%)	2 (9%)	0
Mean delay after booster before reaction (range)	9.4 days (3-13)	8.6 days (2-11)	10.5 days (8-11)

*Coombs and Gell Type III.
†Intradermal.
§Intramuscular.
¶Total in each cohort greater than 100%, because multiple signs and symptoms could be reported in each person.

of exposure. As increasing numbers of persons received their first routine 2-year boosters, reports of presumed Type III hypersensitivity reactions increased in frequency. In approximately half of known cohorts who received booster immunizations between January 1982 and March 1984, some recipients had presumed Type III hypersensitivity reactions. Sixty-seven (7%) of 962 persons in these cohorts fit the above case description for presumed Type III hypersensivity reactions.

Table 35-22 illustrates the clinical features in three of the cohorts reporting presumed Type III reactions following booster immunization with HDCV. When performed, urinalyses, blood urea nitrogen (BUN), and serum creatinine determinations have been normal. Elevated white blood cell counts ranging from 14,000 to 24,000 (predominantly polymorphonuclear leukocytes) were reported in two cases. Serum complement levels (C-3, C-4, and CH-50) were depressed in two patients when serum was drawn at the time of most active clinical symptoms; one of these also had detectable cryoglobulins. Serum-complement levels were normal in five other patients whose sera were collected at other times. Respiratory distress was infrequently seen. Most patients' symptoms improved within 2-3 days when treated with antihistamines, but a few required systemic corticosteroids and epinephrine.

Preliminary analysis of epidemiologic features of the illness in several cohorts revealed a male/female relative risk of 2.3 (95% confidence limits, 1.2-4.4). No significant associations have been demonstrated between persons who reported presumed Type III

hypersensitivity reactions and age, route of primary or booster immunization (intramuscular or intradermal), timing of booster after primary immunization, history of other allergies, or history of previous immunization with rabies vaccines other than HDCV. HDCV produced by both Merieux Institute and Wyeth Laboratories has been associated with reactions. In two groups for which serologic data were available, no difference was shown in pre-booster antibody titers between reactors and nonreactors, but post-booster titers were significantly higher in those who developed reactions. Most presumed Type III reactions were reported to have occurred following booster doses, but six occurred following two or more doses of HDCV given for primary immunization.

Reported by P Schnurrenberger, DVM, School of Veterinary Medicine, Auburn University, Auburn, Alabama; D Dreesen, DVM, J Brown, DVM, PhD, School of Veterinary Medicine, University of Georgia; A Deutsch, MD, Athens, Georgia; M Burridge, PhD, College of Veterinary Medicine, University of Florida, Gainesville; D Howard, PhD, School of Veterinary Medicine, Kansas State University, Manhattan; JT Bell, DVM, College of Veterinary Medicine, Mississippi State University, Mississippi State; G Quinnan, MD, Director, Div of Virology, Center for Drug and Biologics, US Food and Drug Administration; Div of Host Factors, Div of Viral Diseases, Center for Infectious Diseases, CDC.

Editorial Note: Primary immunization with HDCV appears to sensitize some recipients to an, as yet, unidentified component of the vaccine. When booster doses of HDCV are then administered, these persons develop a hypersensitivity reaction clinically consistent with Type III immune complex disease. Until this reaction problem can be resolved, it would be prudent to carefully assess each use of rabies vaccine for routine booster immunization. Persons who have experienced Type III hypersensitivity reactions should receive no further doses of HDCV unless: (1) they are exposed to rabies* or (2) they are truly likely to be inapparently and/or unavoidably exposed to rabies virus and have unsatisfactory antibody titers. The routine use of booster immunization in persons without histories of hypersensitivity reactions is clearly indicated only in those subjected to inapparent and/or unavoidable exposures to rabies virus. All available data suggest an anamnestic antibody response will occur in any person who previously received primary preexposure immunization with HDCV, even when the antibody titer at the time of the booster was low or undetectable.

Individuals with histories of presumed Type III hypersensitivity to HDCV may be at higher risk of subsequent hypersensitivity reactions, and vaccine should be administered under appropriate medical supervision.

REFERENCE

1. Coombs RRA, Gell PGH. Classification of allergic reactions responsible for clinical hypersensitivity and disease. In: Gell PGH, Coombs RRA, Lachmann PJ, eds. Clinical aspects of immunology. 3rd ed. Oxford: Blackwell Scientific Publications, 1975: 761-81.

From MMWR 1984;33:185-187.

RUBELLA PREVENTION

These revised Immunization Practices Advisory Committee (ACIP) recommendations for the prevention of rubella update the previous recommendations (MMWR 1981;30:37-42, 47) to include current information about vaccine effectiveness, duration of immunity, vaccination in pregnancy, and progress in controlling congenital rubella syndrome.

While there are no basic changes in approach, the available epidemiologic data indicate that the elimination of congenital rubella syndrome can be achieved and even hastened by focusing particular attention on more effective delivery of vaccine to older individuals—particularly women of childbearing age. The importance of vaccinating preschool-aged children is also emphasized. As the incidence of rubella declines, serologic confirmation of cases becomes more important. Recommendations for international travel are included.

Introduction

Rubella is a common childhood rash disease. It is often overlooked or misdiagnosed because its signs and symptoms vary. The most common—postauricular and suboccipital lymphadenopathy, arthralgia, transient erythematous rash, and low fever—may not be recognized as rubella. Similar exanthematous illnesses are caused by adenoviruses, enteroviruses, and other common respiratory viruses. Moreover, 25%-50% of infections are subclinical. Transient polyarthralgia and polyarthritis sometimes accompany or follow rubella. Among adults, and particularly among women, joint manifestations occur so frequently (up to 70%), they may be considered an expected manifestation of adult infection. Central nervous system complications and thrombocytopenia have been reported at rates of 1/6,000 cases and 1/3,000 cases, respectively. The former is more likely to occur among adults; the latter, among children.

By far the most important consequences of rubella are the abortions, miscarriages, stillbirths, and fetal anomalies that result from rubella infection in early pregnancy, especially in the first trimester. Preventing fetal infection and consequent congenital rubella syndrome (CRS) is the objective of rubella immunization programs.

The most commonly described anomalies associated with CRS are ophthalmologic (cataracts, microphthalmia, glaucoma, chorioretinitis), cardiac (patent ductus arteriosus, pulmonary artery stenosis, atrial or ventricular septal defects), auditory (sensorineural deafness), and neurologic (microcephaly, meningoencephalitis, mental retardation). In addition, infants with CRS frequently are retarded in growth and have radiolucent bone disease, hepatosplenomegaly, thrombocytopenia, and purpuric skin lesions (blueberry-muffin appearance). Moderate and severe cases of CRS are readily recognizable at birth; mild cases (e.g., those with only slight cardiac involvement or deafness) may not be detected for months or even years after birth. Although CRS has been estimated to occur among 20%-25% or more of infants born to women who acquire rubella during the first trimester, the actual risk of infection and subsequent defects may be considerably higher. If infected infants are followed for at least 2 years, up to 80% of infants will be found to be affected. The risk of any defect falls to approximately 10%-20% by the 16th week, with defects rarely occurring after infection beyond the 20th week. However, fetal infection without clinical stigmata of CRS can occur at any stage of pregnancy. Inapparent maternal rubella infection can also result in malformations.

The average life-time expenditure associated with a CRS infant has recently been estimated to be in excess of $220,000, which includes costs associated with institutionalization of the retarded, blind, and/

---

*Postexposure prophylaxis in previously immunized persons consists of two 1-ml intramuscular doses of HDCV, one each on days 0 and 3.

or deaf and the education of hearing- and sight-impaired teenagers and adolescents.

Postinfection immunity appears to be long-lasting. However, as with other viral diseases, reexposure to natural rubella occasionally leads to reinfection without clinical illness or detectable viremia. Because many rash illnesses may mimic rubella infection, and because many rubella infections are unrecognized, the only reliable evidence of immunity to rubella is the presence of specific antibody. Laboratories that regularly perform antibody testing are generally the most reliable, because their reagents and procedures are strictly standardized (see below).

Before rubella vaccines became available in 1969, most rubella cases occurred among school-aged children. Since control of rubella in the United States was based on interrupting transmission, the primary target group for vaccine was children of both sexes. Secondary emphasis was placed on vaccinating susceptible adolescents and young adults, especially women. By 1977, vaccination of children 12 months of age and older had resulted in a marked decline in the reported rubella incidence among children and had interrupted the characteristic 6- or 9-year rubella epidemic cycle. However, this vaccination strategy had less effect on reported rubella incidence among persons 15 years of age and older (i.e., childbearing ages for women) who subsequently accounted for more than 70% of reported rubella patients with known ages. Approximately 10%-20% of this latter population continued to be susceptible, a proportion similar to that of prevaccine years, and reported CRS continued at a low but constant endemic level (an annual average of 32 reported confirmed and compatible cases* between 1971 and 1977).

Increased efforts were made to effectively vaccinate junior and senior high school students and to enforce rubella immunization requirements for school entry. All susceptible military recruits began to receive rubella vaccine. Published accounts of rubella outbreaks in hospitals caused concern about the need to screen and/or vaccinate susceptible personnel. A number of states stressed the need for ensuring proof of rubella immunity (i.e., documentation of vaccination or seropositivity) for college entrance. These factors, combined with the 1977 Childhood Immunization Initia-

tive and the 1978 Measles Elimination effort (which encouraged use of combined vaccines containing measles and rubella antigens), have led to decreases in reported rubella in all age groups.

The number of rubella vaccine doses administered in the public sector to persons 15 years of age and older doubled between 1978 and 1981. By 1980, reported incidence among adolescents and young adults was lower than that among young children. Children under 5 years of age had the highest overall incidence and accounted for approximately one-fourth of all rubella patients with known ages. Compared with prevaccine years, by 1981 the overall reported rate of rubella had declined by 96%, with a 90% or greater decrease in cases in all age groups. Predictably, the number of reported confirmed and compatible CRS cases started to decline further (provisional totals of 14 cases for 1980 and 10 for 1981).

By 1982, more than 118 million doses of rubella virus vaccine had been distributed in the United States. However, the reported incidence of rubella rose slightly between 1981 and 1982 due to isolated outbreaks in adolescent and young adult populations and particularly in hospitals and universities. As expected, the reported number of confirmed and compatible CRS cases had increased slightly (a provisional total of 11 for 1982). While children under 5 years of age had the highest reported incidence of rubella, they accounted for only half as many cases in 1982 as in 1981 (20% compared with 38%). In contrast, persons 15 years of age or older accounted for almost twice as many cases in 1982 as in 1981 (62% compared with 36%) and had a twofold increase in their estimated rate (from 0.4 cases/100,000 population in 1981 to 0.8/100,000 in 1982). The greatest increase in reported rates within this age group occurred in those 25-29 years of age.

The provisional data for 1983 indicate a record low number of rubella cases (934) was reported to CDC; the reported confirmed and compatible CRS total is only four. However, assuming the slight increase in reported rubella among older individuals between 1981 and 1982 was real, it indicates that rubella in postpubertal populations is still a problem in this country and continues to deserve particular attention.

Rubella serology testing and immunity

Until recently, hemagglutination-inhibition (HI) antibody testing has been the most frequently used method of screening for the presence of rubella antibodies. However, the HI test is now being supplanted by a number of equally or more sensitive assays to determine rubella immunity. These include latex agglutination, fluorescence immunoassay, passive hemagglutination, hemolysis-in-gel, and enzyme immunoassay (EIA) tests. When adults who have failed to produce detectable HI antibodies following

---

*A confirmed case has at least one defect in categories A or B and laboratory confirmation of rubella infection. A compatible case has any two complications listed in A or one from A and one from B without laboratory confirmation.
  A. Cataracts/congenital glaucoma (either or both count as one); congenital heart disease, loss of hearing, pigmentary retinopathy.
  B. Purpura, splenomegaly, jaundice, microcephaly, mental retardation, meningoencephalitis, radiolucent bone disease.

vaccination have been examined more closely, almost all have had detectable antibody by a more sensitive test. Similarly, a small number of children who initially seroconverted has lost detectable HI antibody over 10 years of followup. However, almost all have had detectable antibody by more sensitive tests. Immunity was confirmed in a number of these children by documenting a booster response (i.e., no immunoglobulin M [IgM] antibody and a rapid rise and fall in immunoglobulin G [IgG] antibody) following revaccination.

Although it is recognized that some individuals possess antibody levels following previous vaccination or infection that are below the detectable level of the reference HI test, the clinical significance of such low level antibody has not been well documented outside the study setting. Limited data suggest that, on rare occasions, viremia has occurred in persons with low antibody levels. Further study is warranted to assess the appropriate interpretation of antibodies detectable only by these more sensitive tests. Use of an internationally accepted standard would greatly facilitate resolution of this uncertainty. The available data continue to support the fact that any level of detectable antibody should be considered presumptive evidence of immunity.

Live rubella virus vaccine

The live rubella virus vaccine* currently distributed in the United States is prepared in human diploid cell culture. In January 1979, this vaccine (RA 27/3) replaced the HPV-77:DE-5 vaccine grown in duck embryo cell culture. Although both subcutaneous and intranasal administration of the vaccine have been studied, it is licensed only for subcutaneous administration. The vaccine is produced in monovalent form (rubella only) and in combinations: measles-rubella (MR), rubella-mumps, and measles-mumps-rubella (MMR) vaccines.

In clinical trials, 95% or more of susceptible persons who received a single dose of rubella vaccine when they were 12 months of age or older developed antibody. Clinical efficacy and challenge studies have shown that more than 90% of vaccinees can be expected to have protection against both clinical rubella and asymptomatic viremia for a period of at least 15 years. Based on available follow-up studies, vaccine-induced protection is expected to be life-long. Therefore, a history of vaccination is presumptive evidence of immunity.

Although vaccine-induced titers are generally lower than those stimulated by rubella infection, vaccine-induced immunity usually protects against both clinical illness and viremia after natural exposure. There have been, however, a small number of reports

---

*Official name: Rubella Virus Vaccine, Live.

indicating that viremic reinfection following exposure may occur in vaccinated individuals with low levels of detectable antibody. The frequency and consequences of this phenomenon are currently unknown, but its occurrence is believed rare. Such reports are to be expected, since there are also rare reports of clinical reinfection and fetal infection following natural immunity.

Some vaccinees intermittently shed small amounts of virus from the pharynx 7-28 days after vaccination. However, studies of more than 1,200 susceptible household contacts and experience gained over 15 years of vaccine use have yielded good evidence that vaccine virus is not transmitted. These data indicate that vaccinating susceptible children, whose mothers or other household contacts are pregnant, does not present a risk. Rather, vaccination of such children provides protection for these pregnant women.

Vaccine shipment and storage

Administering improperly stored vaccine may result in lack of protection against rubella. During storage, before reconstitution, rubella vaccine must be kept at 2 C-8 C (35.6 F-46.4 F) or colder. It must also be protected from light, which may inactivate the virus. Reconstituted vaccine should be discarded if not used within 8 hours. Vaccine must be shipped at 10 C (50 F) or colder and may be shipped on dry ice.

Vaccine use

General recommendations. Persons 12 months of age or older should be vaccinated, unless they are immune. Persons can be considered immune to rubella only if they have documentation of:
1. Laboratory evidence of rubella immunity or
2. Adequate immunization with rubella vaccine on or after the first birthday.

The clinical diagnosis of rubella is unreliable and should not be considered in assessing immune status.

All other children, adolescents, and adults—particularly women—are considered susceptible and should be vaccinated if there are no contraindications (see below). This includes persons who may be immune to rubella but who lack adequate documentation of immunity. Vaccinating children protects them against rubella and prevents their spreading the virus. Vaccinating susceptible postpubertal females confers individual protection against rubella-induced fetal injury. Vaccinating adolescent or adult females and males in high-risk population groups, such as those in colleges, places of employment, or military bases, protects them against rubella and reduces the chance of epidemics. This is exemplified by the experience with vaccinating all military recruits, which has virtually eliminated rubella from military bases. Similar results could be achieved by ensuring proof of immunity of all employees, all college students and staff, and all hospital personnel, including physicians, nurses, health-profession students, technicians, dietary workers, etc.

As discussed above, it is generally believed that any detectable antibody titer specific for rubella (whether resulting from vaccination or from naturally acquired rubella), even if very low, should be considered evidence of protection against subsequent viremic infection—including the reported "reinfection" of persons with low levels of antibody demonstrated by boosts in antibody titer. This suggests that immune females reinfected during pregnancy would be unlikely to infect their fetuses. Moreover, because there is very little pharyngeal excretion, there appears to be no risk to susceptible contacts in such reinfection settings. In view of the data on reinfection accumulated during the past decade, the ACIP sees no reason to revaccinate persons with low levels of rubella antibody. Rather, more attention should be directed toward vaccinating the truly susceptible population.

Dosage. A single dose of 0.5 cc of reconstituted vaccine (as a monovalent or preferably a combination product such as MR or MMR) should be administered subcutaneously.

Age at vaccination. Live rubella virus is recommended for all children 12 months of age or older. It should not be given to younger infants, because persisting maternal antibodies may interfere with seroconversion. When the rubella vaccine is part of a combination that includes the measles antigen, the combination vaccine should be given to children at 15 months of age or older to maximize measles seroconversion. Older children who have not received rubella vaccine should be vaccinated promptly. Because a history of rubella illness is not a reliable indicator of immunity, all children should be vaccinated unless there are contraindications (see below).

Vaccination of women of childbearing age. The ACIP has weighed several factors in developing recommendations for vaccinating women of childbearing age against rubella. Although there may be theoretical risks in giving rubella vaccine during pregnancy, available data on previously and currently available rubella vaccines indicate that the risk, if any, of teratogenicity from live rubella vaccines is quite small. As of December 31, 1983, CDC has followed to term 214 known rubella-susceptible pregnant females who had been vaccinated with live rubella vaccine within 3 months before or 3 months after conception. Ninety-four received HPV-77 or Cendehill vaccines, one received vaccine of unknown strain, and 119 received RA 27/3 vaccine. None of the 216 babies (two of the mothers receiving RA 27/3 vaccine delivered twins) has malformations compatible with congenital rubella infection. This finding includes the four infants born to these susceptible women who had serologic evidence of subclinical infection. (Three of the infants were exposed to HPV-77 or Cendehill vaccine; one was exposed to RA 27/3 vaccine.)

Based on the experience to date, the maximum estimated theoretical risk of serious malformations attributable to RA 27/3 rubella vaccine, derived from the binomial distribution, is 3%. (If the 95 susceptible infants exposed to other rubella vaccines are included, the maximum theoretical risk is 1.7%.) However, the observed risk with both the HPV-77 or Cendehill and RA 27/3 strains of vaccine is zero. In either case, this risk is far less than the 20% or greater risk of CRS associated with maternal infection during the first trimester of pregnancy.

Although experience with the RA 27/3 vaccine is more limited than that with the other rubella vaccines, rubella vaccine virus has been isolated from abortion material from one (3%) of 32 susceptible females who had been given RA 27/3 vaccine while pregnant, whereas virus was isolated from abortion material from 17 (20%) of 85 susceptible females who had been given HPV-77 or Cendehill vaccines while pregnant. This provides additional evidence that the RA 27/3 vaccine does not pose any greater risk of teratogenicity than did the HPV-77 or Cendehill vaccines.

Therefore, the ACIP believes that the risk of vaccine-associated defects is so small as to be negligible and should not ordinarily be a reason to consider interruption of pregnancy. However, a final decision about interruption of pregnancy must rest with the individual patient and her physician.

The continuing occurrence of rubella among women of childbearing age and the lack of evidence for teratogenicity from the vaccine indicate strongly that increased emphasis should continue to be placed on vaccinating susceptible adolescent and adult females of childbearing age. However, because of the theoretical risk to the fetus, females of childbearing age should receive vaccine only if they say they are not pregnant and are counseled not to become pregnant for 3 months after vaccination. In view of the importance of protecting this age group against rubella, reasonable practices in a rubella immunization program include: (1) asking females if they are pregnant, (2) excluding those who say they are, and (3) explaining the theoretical risks to the others.

Use of vaccine following exposure. There is no conclusive evidence that giving live rubella virus vaccine after exposure will prevent illness. Additionally, there is no evidence that vaccinating an individual incubating rubella is harmful. Consequently, since a single exposure may not cause infection and postexposure vaccination will protect an individual exposed in the future, vaccination is recommended, unless otherwise contraindicated.

Use of human immune globulin following exposure. Immunoglobulin (IG) given after exposure to rubella will not prevent infection or viremia, but it may modify or suppress symptoms and create an unwarranted sense of security. The routine use of IG for postexposure prophylaxis of rubella in early pregnancy is not recommended. Infants with congenital rubella have been born to women given IG shortly after exposure. IG might be useful only when a pregnant woman who has been exposed to rubella would not consider termination of pregnancy under any circumstances.

Recent administration of IG. Vaccine should be administered about 2 weeks before or deferred for about 3 months after receipt of IG, because passively acquired antibodies might interefere with the response to the vaccine. On the other hand, previous administration of anti-Rho (D) immune globulin (human) or blood products does not generally interfere with an immune response and is not a contraindication to postpartum vaccination. However, in this situation, 6- or 8-week postvaccination serologic testing should be done on those who have received the globulin or blood products to assure that seroconversion has occurred. Obtaining laboratory evidence of seroconversion in other vaccinees is not necessary.

Side effects and adverse reactions

Children sometimes have vaccine side effects, such as low-grade fever, rash and lymphadenopathy. Up to 40% of vaccinees in large-scale field trials have had joint pain, usually of the small peripheral joints, but frank arthritis has generally been reported for fewer than 2%. Arthralgia and transient arthritis occur more frequently and tend to be more severe in susceptible women than in children. While up to 3% of susceptible children have been reported to have arthralgia, arthritis has rarely been reported in these vaccinees. By contrast, up to 10%-15% of susceptible female vaccinees have been reported to have arthritis-like signs and symptoms. Transient peripheral neuritic complaints, such as paresthesias and pain in the arms and legs, have also very rarely occurred.

When joint symptoms or nonjoint-associated pain and paresthesias do occur, they generally begin 3-25 days (mean 8-14 days) after immunization, persist for 1-11 days (mean 2-4 days) and rarely recur. Adults with joint problems usually have not had to disrupt work activities. The occasional reports of persistent or recurrent joint signs and symptoms probably represent a rare phenomenon. No joint destruction has been reported. While the presence of immune complexes following vaccination has been reported to be associated with arthralgia and arthritis, the available data are still inconclusive. Comparable studies on naturally infected persons have not been conducted.

Likewise, there is no clear association between joint symptoms and persistence of rubella virus in lymphocytes.

The vast majority of published data indicate that only susceptible vaccinees have side effects of vaccination. There is no conclusive evidence of an increased risk of these reactions for persons who are already immune when vaccinated.

Although vaccine is safe and effective for all persons 12 months of age or older, its safety for the developing fetus is not fully known. Therefore, though the risk, if any, appears to be minimal, rubella vaccine should not be given to women known to be pregnant because of the theoretical risk of fetal abnormality caused by vaccine virus (see above).

Precautions and contraindications

Pregnancy. Pregnant women should not be given rubella vaccine. If a pregnant woman is vaccinated or if she becomes pregnant within 3 months of vaccination, she should be counseled on the theoretical risks to the fetus. As noted above, rubella vaccination during pregnancy should not ordinarily be a reason to consider interruption of pregnancy. Instances of vaccination during pregnancy should be reported through state health departments to the Division of Immunization, Center for Prevention Services, CDC.

Because of the increasing number of cases reported to CDC, the experience with known susceptibles is becoming well defined. Therefore, CDC now encourages reporting only cases involving women known to be susceptible at the time of vaccination.

Febrile illness. Vaccination of persons with severe febrile illness should be postponed until recovery. However, susceptible children with mild illnesses, such as upper respiratory infection, should be vaccinated. Considering the importance of protecting against rubella, medical personnel should use every opportunity to vaccinate susceptible individuals.

Allergies. Hypersensitivity reactions very rarely follow the administration of live rubella vaccine. Most of these reactions are considered minor and consist of wheal and flare or urticaria at the injection site.

Live rubella vaccine is produced in human diploid cell culture. Consequently, a history of anaphylactic reactions to egg ingestion needs to be taken into consideration only if measles or mumps antigens are to be included with rubella vaccine.

Since rubella vaccine contains trace amounts of neomycin (25 µg), persons who have experienced anaphylactic reactions to topically or systemically administered neomycin should not receive rubella vaccine. Most often, neomycin allergy is manifested as a contact dermatitis, which is a delayed-type (cell-mediated) immune response, rather than anaphylaxis. In such individuals, the adverse reaction, if any, to 25 μg of neomycin in the vaccine would be an erythematous, pruritic nodule or papule at 48-96 hours. A history of contact dermatitis to neomycin is not a contraindication to receiving rubella vaccine. Live rubella vaccine does not contain penicillin.

Altered immunity. Replication of live rubella vaccine virus may be potentiated in patients with immune deficiency diseases and by the suppressed immune responses that occur with leukemia, lymphoma, generalized malignancy, and therapy with corticosteroids, alkylating drugs, antimetabolites, and radiation. Patients with such conditions should not be given live rubella virus vaccine. Since vaccinated persons do not transmit vaccine virus, the risk to these patients of being exposed to rubella may be reduced by vaccinating their close susceptible contacts. Management of such patients, should they be exposed to rubella, can be facilitated by prior knowledge of their immune status.

Patients with leukemia in remission whose chemotherapy has been terminated for at least 3 months may receive live virus vaccines for infections to which they are still susceptible (i.e., have neither had the disease nor the vaccine before developing leukemia). The exact interval after discontinuing immunosuppression that coincides with the ability to respond to individual vaccines is not known. Experts vary in their judgments from 3 months to 1 year.

Short-term (less than 2 weeks) corticosteroid therapy, topical steroid therapy (e.g., nasal, skin), and intra-articular, bursal, or tendon injection with corticosteroids should not be immunosuppressive and do not necessarily contraindicate live virus vaccine administration. However, live vaccines should be avoided if systemic immunosuppressive levels are reached by topical application.

Simultaneous administration of certain live virus vaccines. See General Recommendations on Immunization, (MMWR 1983;32:2-8, 13-17).

Elimination of CRS

Widespread vaccination of school-aged children since 1969 has effectively prevented major epidemics of rubella and congenital rubella in this country. With continued vaccination of children at levels approaching 100%, an immune birth cohort will eventually replace the 10%-15% of persons of childbearing age currently susceptible to rubella, and rubella can be expected to disappear. Since this process will take 10-30 years, cases of CRS can still be expected to occur.

Elimination of CRS can be hastened by intensifying and expanding existing efforts to vaccinate susceptible adolescents and young adults, particularly women of childbearing age, along with continuing routine vaccination of children. Effective vaccination of all susceptible children in junior and senior high schools can be expected to contribute greatly to the elimination

of CRS. Over the last 3 years, such efforts have resulted in decreases in the reported incidence of rubella in all persons and in the incidence of reported CRS. In 1982, the rubella cases that occurred were largely in older, postschool-aged populations, clearly indicating that rubella in postpubertal populations is still a problem in this country.

The major components of a strategy to eliminate CRS are achieving and maintaining high immunization levels, accurate surveillance of rubella and CRS, and prompt outbreak-control measures. The following recommendations are presented to help preserve the level of rubella and CRS control already achieved and to bring about the further reduction in susceptibility that will be required to achieve elimination of CRS.

Ongoing programs. The primary strategy for eliminating CRS in the United States is to interrupt rubella transmission by achieving and maintaining high immunization levels in all children. Official health agencies should take steps, including developing and enforcing immunization requirements, to assure that all students in grades kindergarten through 12 are protected against rubella, unless vaccination is contraindicated. School entry laws should be vigorously enforced. States that do not require proof of immunity of students at all grade levels should consider expanding existing laws or regulations to include the age groups not yet protected.

Recent age-specific data indicate that preschool-aged children account for an important proportion of reported rubella cases. Proof of rubella immunity for attendance at day-care centers should be required and enforced. Licensure should depend on such requirements.

To hasten the elimination of CRS, new emphasis will have to be directed towards vaccinating susceptible females of childbearing age—the group at highest risk. A multifaceted approach is necessary. A number of approaches are discussed below.

Premarital screening and vaccination. Routine premarital testing for rubella antibody identifies many susceptible women before pregnancy. Documented histories of rubella vaccination or serologic evidence of immunity should be considered acceptable proof of immunity. To ensure a significant reduction in susceptibles through premarital screening, more aggressive follow-up of women found to be susceptible will be required.

Postpartum vaccination. Prenatal screening should be carried out on all pregnant women not known to be immune. Women who have just delivered babies should be vaccinated before discharge from the hospital, unless they are known to be immune. Although such women are unlikely to become pregnant, counseling to avoid conception for 3 months following vaccination is still necessary. It is estimated that postpartum vaccination of all women not known to be immune could prevent one-third to one-half of current CRS cases. Breast-feeding is not a contraindication to vaccination, even though virus may be excreted in breast milk, and infants may be infected. Vaccination should be extended to include all post-abortion settings.

Routine vaccination in any medical setting. Vaccination of susceptible women of childbearing age should be part of routine general medical and gynecologic outpatient care, should take place in all family-planning settings, and should become routine before discharge from a hospital for any reason, if there are no contraindications (see above). Vaccine should be offered to adults, especially women of childbearing age, any time contact is made with the health-care system, including when children are undergoing routine examinations or immunizations.

Vaccination of medical personnel. Medical personnel, both male and female (volunteers, trainees, nurses, physicians, etc.), who might transmit rubella to pregnant patients or other personnel, should be immune to rubella. Consideration should be given to making rubella immunity a condition for employment.

Vaccination of workers. Ascertainment of rubella immune status and availability of rubella immunization should be components of the health-care program in places where women of childbearing age congregate or represent a significant proportion of the work force. Such settings include day-care centers, schools, colleges, companies, government offices, and industrial sites.

Vaccination for college entry. Colleges are high-risk areas for rubella transmission because of large concentrations of susceptible persons. Proof of rubella, as well as measles immunity, should be required for attendance for both male and female students.

General principles. Voluntary programs have generally been less successful than mandatory programs. The military services require rubella immunity of susceptible recruits and have essentially eliminated rubella from military bases. In all settings where young adults congregate, males as well as females should be included, since males may transmit disease to susceptible females.

When practical, and when reliable laboratory services are available, potential female vaccinees of childbearing age can have serologic tests to determine susceptibility to rubella. However, with the exception of premarital and prenatal screening, routinely performing serologic tests for all women of childbearing age to determine susceptibility so that vaccine is given only to proven susceptible women is expensive and has been ineffective in some areas. Two visits to the health-care provider are necessary—one for screening and one for vaccination. Accordingly, the ACIP

believes that rubella vaccination of a woman who is not known to be pregnant and has no history of vaccination is justifiable without serologic testing and may be preferable, particularly when costs of serology are high and follow-up of identified susceptibles for vaccination is not assured. Vaccinated women should avoid becoming pregnant for a 3-month period following vaccination. In addition, vaccine should be administered in the above-mentioned settings only if there are no contraindications to vaccination.

Routine serologic screening of male vaccinees is not recommended. There are no conclusive data indicating the vaccination of immune individuals carries an increased risk of joint or other complications.

Health-care providers are encouraged to use MMR in routine childhood vaccination programs and whenever rubella vaccine is to be given to persons likely to be susceptible to measles and/or mumps as well as to rubella.

Outbreak control. Outbreak control will play an important role in CRS elimination. Aggressive responses to outbreaks may interrupt chains of transmission and will increase immunization levels in persons who might otherwise not be vaccinated. Although methods for controlling rubella outbreaks are evolving, the major strategy should be to define target populations, ensure that susceptible individuals are vaccinated rapidly (or excluded from exposure if a contraindication exists), and maintain active surveillance to modify control measures if the situation changes.

Since a simple, accurate clinical case definition for rubella has not yet been developed, laboratory confirmation of cases is important. However, control measures should be implemented *before* serologic confirmation. This approach is especially important in any outbreak setting involving pregnant women (e.g., in obstetric-gynecologic and prenatal clinics). All persons who cannot readily provide laboratory evidence of immunity or a documented history of vaccination on or after the first-year birthday should be considered susceptible and vaccinated if there are no contraindications.

An effective means of terminating outbreaks and increasing rates of immunization quickly is to exclude from possible contact individuals who cannot provide valid evidence of immunity. Experience with measles-outbreak control indicates that almost all students who are excluded from school because they lack evidence of measles immunity quickly comply with requirements and are promptly readmitted to school. Exclusion should include all persons who have been exempted from rubella vaccination because of medical, religious, or other reasons. Exclusion should continue until 3 weeks after the onset of rash of the last reported case in the outbreak setting. Less rigorous approaches, such as voluntary appeals for vaccination, have not been effective in terminating outbreaks.

Mandatory exclusion and vaccination of adults should be practiced in rubella outbreaks in medical settings where large numbers of pregnant women may be exposed. This approach may be successful in terminating, or at least limiting, outbreaks. Vaccination during an outbreak has not been associated with significant personnel absenteeism. However, it is clear that vaccination of susceptible persons before an outbreak occurs is preferable, since vaccination causes far less absenteeism and disruption of routine work activities and schedules than rubella infection.

Surveillance

Surveillance of rubella and CRS has three purposes: (1) to provide important data on program progress and long-term trends; (2) to help define groups in greatest need of vaccination and in turn provide information for formulation of new strategies; and (3) to evaluate vaccine efficacy, duration of vaccine-induced immunity, and other issues related to vaccine safety and efficacy.

As the rates of rubella and CRS decline in the United States, effective surveillance becomes increasingly important. Known or suspected rubella cases should be reported immediately to local health departments. Since an accurate assessment of CRS elimination can be made only through aggressive case finding, surveillance of CRS will have to be intensified.

Surveillance of rubella is complicated by the fact that the clinical disease is not characteristic and can be confused with a number of other illnesses. Thus, there is a need for laboratory confirmation of cases, particularly in nonoutbreak settings. Similarly, laboratory confirmation of suspected cases of CRS is also necessary, since the constellation of findings of CRS may not be specific.

Laboratory diagnosis

Rubella. Rubella infection can be serologically confirmed by a fourfold rise in HI or complement fixation (CF) antibody titer. Kits using EIA or latex agglutination assays are also becoming available for diagnostic use. The acute-phase serum specimen should be drawn as soon after rash onset as possible, preferably within the first 7 days. The convalescent-phase serum specimen should be drawn 10 or more days after the acute-phase serum specimen. If the acute-phase serum specimen is drawn more than 7 days after rash onset, a fourfold rise in HI antibody titer may not be detected. In this case, CF testing may be especially useful, since CF antibodies appear in serum later than HI antibodies. Both the acute and convalescent specimens should be tested simultaneously in the same laboratory.

Occasionally, fourfold rises may not be detected, even if the first specimen is drawn within the first 7 days after rash onset. Rubella infection may also be serologically confirmed by demonstrating rubella-specific IgM antibody. If IgM is to be determined, a single serum specimen should be drawn between 1 week and 2 weeks after rash onset. Although rubella-specific IgM antibody may be detected shortly after rash onset, false-negative results may occur if the specimen is drawn earlier than 1 week or later than 3 weeks following rash onset.

In the absence of rash illness, the diagnosis of subclinical cases of rubella can be facilitated by obtaining the acute-phase serum specimen as soon as possible after *exposure*. The convalescent-phase specimen should then be drawn 28 or more days after exposure. If acute- and convalescent-phase sera pairs provide inconclusive results, rubella-specific IgM antibody testing can be performed, but negative results should be interpreted cautiously. Expert consultation may be necessary to interpret the data.

Confirmation of rubella infection in pregnant women of unknown immune status following rash illness or exposure can frequently be difficult. A serum specimen should be obtained as soon as possible. Unfortunately, serologic results are often nonconfirmatory. Such situations can be minimized by performing prenatal serologies routinely. In addition, health providers should request that laboratories performing prenatal screening retain such specimens until delivery so that retesting, if necessary, can be done.

Congenital rubella. Suspected cases of CRS should be managed with contact isolation (see CDC "Guidelines for Isolation Precautions in Hospitals") and, while diagnostic confirmation is pending, should be cared for only by personnel known to be immune. Confirmation by attempting virus isolation can be done using nasopharyngeal and urine specimens. Serologic confirmation can be obtained by testing cord blood for the presence of rubella-specific IgM antibodies. An alternative, but less rapid serologic method, is to document persistence of rubella-specific antibody in a suspected infant for more than 3 months of age at a level beyond that expected from passive transfer of maternal antibody (i.e., a rubella HI titer in the infant that does not decline at the expected rate of one twofold dilution per month). If CRS is confirmed, precautions will need to be exercised through the first year of life, unless nasopharyngeal and urine cultures are negative for rubella virus.

Adverse events. Continuous and careful review of adverse events following rubella vaccination is important. All adverse events following rubella vaccination should be evaluated and reported in detail through local and state health officials to CDC, as well as to the manufacturer.

International travel

Persons without evidence of rubella immunity who travel abroad should be protected against rubella, since rubella is endemic and even epidemic, in many countries throughout the world. No immunization or record of immunization is required for entry into the United States. However, it is recommended that international travelers have immunity to rubella consisting of laboratory evidence of rubella antibodies or verified rubella vaccination on or after the first-year birthday. It is especially important to protect susceptible women of childbearing age, particularly those planning to remain out of the country for a prolonged period of time.

SELECTED BIBLIOGRAPHY

Baba K, Yabuuchi H, Okuni H, et al. Rubella epidemic in an institution: protective value of live rubella vaccine and serological behavior of vaccinated, revaccinated, and naturally immune groups. Biken J 1978;21:25-31.

Balfour HH Jr, Groth KE, Edelman CK, Amren DP, Best JM, Banatvala JE. Rubella viraemia and antibody responses after rubella vaccination and reimmunization. Lancet 1981;1:1078-80.

Buimovici-Klein E, Hite RL, Bryne T, Cooper LZ. Isolation of rubella virus in milk after postpartum immunization. J Pediatr 1977;91:939-41.

CDC. Rubella in universities—Washington, California. MMWR 1982;32:394-5.

CDC. Rubella outbreak among office workers—New York City. MMWR 1983;32:349-52.

CDC. Rubella vaccination during pregnancy—United States, 1971-1982. MMWR 1983;32:429-432, 437.

CDC. Rubella and congenital rubella—United States, 1983. MMWR 1984;33:237-42, 247.

Chappell JA, Taylor MA. Implications of rubella susceptibility in young adults. Am J Public Health 1979;69:279-81.

Cooper LZ, Krugman S. The rubella problem. DM 1969; Feb:3-38.

Coyle PK, Wolinsky JS, Buimovici-Klein E, Moucha R, Cooper LZ. Rubella-specific immune complexes after congenital infection and vaccination. Infect Immun 1982;36:498-503.

Crawford GE, Gremillion DH. Epidemic measles and rubella in air force recruits: impact of immunization. J Infect Dis 1981;144:403-10.

Dales LG, Chin J. An outbreak of congenital rubella. West J Med 1981;135:266-70.

Dales LG, Chin J. Public health implications of rubella antibody levels in California. Am J Public Health 1982;72:167-72.

Greaves WL, Orenstein WA, Hinman AR, Nersesian WS. Clinical efficacy of rubella vaccine. Pediatr Infect Dis 1983;2:284-6.

Greaves WL, Orenstein WA, Stetler WC, Preblud SR, Hinman AR, Bart KJ. Prevention of rubella transmission in medical facilities. JAMA 1982;248:861-4.

Herrmann KL, Halstead SB, Wiebenga NH. Rubella antibody persistence after immunization. JAMA 1982;247:193-6.

Hillary IB, Griffith AH. Persistence of antibody 10 years after vaccination with Wistar RA27/3 strain live attenuated rubella vaccine. Br Med J 1980;280:1580-1.

Horstmann DM. Controlling rubella: problems and perspectives. Ann Intern Med 1975;83:412-7.

International conference on rubella immunization. Am J Dis Child 1969;118:1-410.

International Symposium on the Prevention of Congenital Rubella Infection, Washington, D.C., March 13-15, 1984, Rev Infect Dis (in press).

Klein EB, Byrne T, Cooper LZ. Neonatal rubella in a breast-fed infant after postpartum maternal infection. J Pediatr 1980;97:774-5.

Landes RD, Bass JW, Millunchick EW, Oetgen WJ. Neonatal rubella following postpartum maternal immunization. J Pediatr 1980;97:465-7.

Koplan JP, White CC. An update of the benefits and costs of measles and rubella immunization. In: Proceedings of the Symposium "Conquest of Agents that Endanger the Brain," Baltimore, Maryland, October 28-29, 1982 (in press).

Landrigan PJ, Stoffels MA, Anderson E, Witte JJ. Epidemic rubella in adolescent boys. Clinical features and results of vaccination. JAMA 1974;227:1283-7.

Lamprecht C, Schauf V, Warren D, Nelson K, Northrop R, Christiansen M. An outbreak of congenital rubella in Chicago. JAMA 1982;247:1129-33.

Lerman SJ, Nankervis GA, Heggie AD, Gold E. Immunologic response, virus excretion, and joint reactions with rubella vaccine. A study of adolescent girls and young women given live attenuated virus vaccine (HPV-77: DE-5). Ann Intern Med 1971;74:67-73.

Lieberman E, Faich GA, Simon PR, Mullan RJ. Premarital rubella screening in Rhode Island. JAMA 1981;245:1333-5.

Mann JM, Preblud SR, Hoffman RE, Brandling-Bennet AD, Hinman AR, Herrmann KL. Assessing risks of rubella infection during pregnancy. A standardized approach. JAMA 1981;245:1647-52.

McLaughlin MC, Gold LH. The New York rubella incident; a case for changing hospital policy regarding rubella testing and immunization. Am J Public Health 1979;69:287-9.

Miller E, Cradock-Watson JE, Pollock TM. Consequences of confirmed maternal rubella at successive stages of pregnancy. Lancet 1982;II:781-4.

Miller KA, Zager TD. Rubella susceptibility in an adolescent female population. Mayo Clin Proc 1984;59:31-4.

Nelson DB, Layde MM, Chatton TB. Rubella susceptibility in inner-city adolescents: the effect of a school immunization law. Am J Public Health 1982;72:710-3.

Orenstein WA, Bart KJ, Hinman AR, et al. The opportunity and obligation to eliminate rubella from the United States. JAMA 1984;251:1988-94.

O'Shea S, Best JM, Banatvala JE. Viremia, virus excretion, and antibody responses after challenge in volunteers with low levels of antibody to rubella virus. J Infect Dis 1983;148:639-47.

O'Shea S, Best JM, Banatvala JE, Marshall WC, Dudgeon JA. Rubella vaccination: persistence of antibodies for up to 16 years. Br Med J 1982;285:253-5.

Polk BF, Modlin JF, White JA, DeGirolami PC. A controlled comparison of joint reactions among women receiving one of two rubella vaccines. Am J Epidemiol 1982;115:19-25.

Polk BF, White JA, DeGirolami PC, Modlin JF. An outbreak of rubella among hospital personnel. N Engl J Med 1980;303:541-5.

Preblud SR, Gross F, Halsey NA, Hinman AR, Herrmann KL, Koplan JP. Assessment of susceptibility to measles and rubella. JAMA 1982;247:1134-7.

Preblud SR, Serdula MK, Frank JA Jr, Brandling-Bennett AD, Hinman AR. Rubella vaccination in the United States: a ten-year review. Epidemiol Rev 1980;2:171-94.

Preblud SR, Stetler HC, Frank JA Jr, Greaves WL, Hinman AR, Herrmann KL. Fetal risk associated with rubella vaccine. JAMA 1981;246:1413-7.

Recommendations for the control of rubella within hospitals. The Advisory Committee on Infections within Hospitals of the American Hospital Association. Infect Control 1981;2:410-1, 424.

Robinson RG, Dudenhoeffer FE, Holroyd HJ, Baker LR, Bernstein DI, Cherry JD. Rubella immunity in older children, teenagers, and young adults: a comparison of immunity in those previously immunized with those unimmunized. J Pediatr 1982;101:188-91.

Serdula MK, Halstead SB, Wiebenga NH, Herrmann KL. Serological response to rubella revaccination. JAMA 1984;251:1974-7.

Storch GA, Myers N. Latex-agglutination test for rubella antibody: validity of positive results assessed by response to immunization and comparison with other tests. J Infect Dis 1984;149:459-64.

Tingle AJ, Yang T, Allen M, Kettyls GD, Larke RPB, Schulzer M. Prospective immunological assessment of arthritis induced by rubella vaccine. Infect Immun 1983;40:22-8.

Weibel RE, Buynak EB, McLean AA, Roehm RR, Hilleman MR. Persistence of antibody in human subjects for 7 to 10 years following administration of combined live attenuated measles, mumps, and rubella virus vaccines. Proc Soc Exp Biol Med 1980;165:260-3.

Weibel RE, Villarejos VM, Klein EB, Buynak EB, McLean AA, Hilleman MR. Clinical and laboratory studies of live attenuated RA 27/3 and HPV 77-DE rubella virus vaccines (40931). Proc Soc Exp Biol Med 1980;165:44-9.

From MMWR 1984;33:301-318.

RUBELLA VACCINATION DURING PREGNANCY—UNITED STATES, 1971-1983

From January 1971 to December 1983, 1,096 pregnant women who received rubella vaccine either within 3 months before or 3 months after their presumed dates of conception were reported to CDC. These women were followed prospectively to determine the risk of fetal abnormalities following exposure to the vaccine.

Cendehill and HPV-77 vaccines

Before April 1979, data were collected on 538 women vaccinated during pregnancy with either Cendehill or HPV-77 rubella vaccines (1). The outcomes of conception—live birth, stillbirth, or spontaneous or induced abortion—were known for 143 (96%) of the 149 women known to be susceptible at the time of vaccination. Ninety-four (66%) of these 143 women carried their infants to term. All gave birth to infants free of defects compatible with congenital rubella syndrome (CRS) (2), although eight infants had serologic evidence of intrauterine infection (1,3). These eight children were all followed for at least 2 years, at which time all were growing and developing normally. The longest follow-up is for a child who is now 8½ years old who had both an elevated rubella-specific immunoglobulin M (IgM) titer at birth and persistence of hemagglutination inhibition (HI) antibodies. Although he is still HI-antibody positive (he has not been vaccinated), he continues to grow and develop normally.

An additional 196 infants born to women who either were immune (22) or of unknown immune status (174) at the time of vaccination were also free of CRS-associated defects. Three other women (one susceptible, one immune, and one of unknown immune status) received unknown strains of rubella vaccine. All three delivered normal-appearing, healthy infants.

RA 27/3 Vaccine

Since licensure of the RA 27/3 rubella vaccine in 1979, 555 women who received this vaccine during pregnancy have been reported to CDC (Table 35-23). One hundred fifty-seven of these 555 women were known to be susceptible at the time of vaccination. Outcomes of pregnancy are known for 147 (94%) of these women. Of the 147 women, 119 (81%) delivered 121 living infants. An additional 28 immune women and 309 women of unknown immune status delivered 338 living infants. All of these 459 infants were free of defects compatible with CRS.

The dates of vaccination and estimated dates of confinement were known for all of the 119 susceptible women who had full-term pregnancies (Figure 35-2). Forty-four women (37%) were vaccinated within 1 week before to 4 weeks after conception, the period of presumed highest risk.

Serologic evaluations (rubella HI titers and specific IgM on cord or neonatal blood specimens) were performed on 104 (86%) of the 121 infants whose mothers were susceptible. One normal-appearing infant had a rubella-specific IgM antibody titer of 1:8 in cord blood and a corresponding HI titer of 1:128. The maternal titer was also 1:128. Retesting of cord blood and testing of a 2-month follow-up specimen run simultaneously showed an expected decrease in maternally derived HI antibody over the 2-month period from a titer of 1:64 to 1:16, suggesting that subclinical infection may not have occurred. The infant had no evidence of defects compatible with CRS at birth or at the 18-month and 29-month follow-up examinations. Further follow-up sera could not be obtained to document persistence or disappearance of HI antibodies.

Table 35-23. Pregnancy outcomes for 555 recipients of RA 27/3 vaccine—United States, January 1979 through December 1983

Prevaccination immunity status	Total women	Live births	Spontaneous abortions and stillbirths	Induced abortions	Outcome unknown
Susceptible	157	121*	3	25	10
Immune	30	28	1	0	1
Unknown	368	310†	8	23	28
Total	555	459	12	48	39

*Includes two twin births.
†Includes one twin birth.

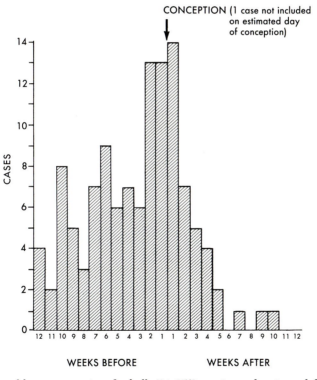

Fig. 35-2. Interval between receipt of rubella RA 27/3 vaccine and estimated date of conception. In weeks, among susceptible women with live births—United States, January 1979 through December 1983.

Blood studies were also obtained on 150 of the 241 infants born to mothers whose immune statuses were unknown at the time of vaccination. Subclinical infection was documented in two infants. One infant had a rubella-specific IgM antibody titer of 1:16 in cord blood. Both mother and infant had HI titers of 1:32 at the time of birth; the infant had a persistent HI titer of 1:32 at 4 months of age. This infant had no evidence of defects compatible with CRS at birth or at the 10-month and 17-month examinations. A serum specimen was not obtained at the follow-up visits. The second infant had a persistent HI titer of 1:8 at 3 months of age, suggesting that there had been subclinical infection. This infant was diagnosed as normal at the 3-month follow-up visit.

While none of the 121 infants born to susceptible women had defects compatible with CRS, two infants did have asymptomatic glandular hypospadias. However, both had negative rubella-specific IgM titers (less than 1:4) in cord blood at birth. A 6-month follow-up serum was available for one of the infants; he had a rubella HI antibody titer of less than 1:8.

Twenty-five susceptible women elected to have induced abortions (Table 35-23). Thus, rubella virus has now been isolated from the products of conception in one (3%) of 32 cases involving susceptible women (19 cases reported to CDC and 13 from the literature) (4-6).

Reported by Surveillance and Investigations Section, Surveillance, Investigations, and Research Br, Div of Immunization, Center for Prevention Svcs, CDC.

Editorial Note: Since 1971, CDC has maintained a register to monitor and quantitate the risks to the fetus following exposure to attenuated rubella vaccine virus. Data are obtained through reports from physicians and from state and local health departments, as well as directly from women vaccinated either within 3 months before or 3 months after conception. The patients are followed prospectively to determine the outcome of pregnancy. In 1979, when RA 27/3 rubella vaccine replaced the other rubella vaccines, concern was raised that it might have greater fetotropic and teratogenic potential than earlier vaccines. As with the other vaccines, data collected so far show no evidence that the RA 27/3 rubella vaccine can cause defects compatible with CRS.

Forty-four (37%) of the 119 susceptible mothers were vaccinated with RA 27/3 vaccine during the highest risk period for viremia and fetal defects (1 week before to 4 weeks after conception) (7,8). Neither those infants nor any others were born with CRS; therefore, the observed risk of CRS following rubella vaccination continues to be zero. The theoretical maximum risk for the occurrence of CRS in this group of 121 children, however, based on the 95% confidence limits of the binomial distribution, may be as high as 3.0%. (If the 95 infants exposed to other rubella vaccines are included, the maximum theoretical risk is 1.7%.) This overall maximum risk remains far less than the 20% or greater risk of CRS associated with maternal infection with wild rubella virus during the first trimester of pregnancy (3) and is no greater than the 4%-5% rate of birth defects in the absence of exposure to rubella vaccine (9,10).

These favorable data are consistent with the German experience cited at the International Symposium on the Prevention of Congenital Rubella Infection recently held at the Pan American Health Organization.* A total of 91 susceptible women vaccinated with either the Cendehill or RA 27/3 strain of vaccine gave birth to normal-appearing infants. Limited data presented at the symposium from the United Kingdom also support the CDC observations.

The occurrence of any congenital defect following maternal vaccination deserves careful analysis and follow-up. Two infants born to susceptible mothers had asymptomatic glandular hypospadias. While hypospadias has been noted in CRS cases (11,12), there are no data to suggest that glandular hypospadias should be considered a CRS-associated defect. In any case, neither of the two infants in question had serologic evidence of rubella virus infection. Ten other infants born to mothers of unknown immune status (eight) or known to be immune (two) at the time of vaccination had some type of defect (13). However, none of the defects were compatible with CRS and serologic testing, when done, did not confirm rubella virus infection.

While no CRS-like defects have been noted, it is clear that rubella vaccine viruses, including the RA 27/3 strain, can cross the placenta and infect the fetus. Approximately 1%-2% of infants born to susceptible vaccinees had serologic evidence of subclinical infection, regardless of vaccine strain (3). On the other hand, while the rubella virus isolation rate from the products of conception for the RA 27/3 vaccine is only 3% (1/32), the rate of virus isolation for Cendehill and HPV-77 vaccines is 20% (17/85) (3). These data indicate that the risk of placental or fetal infection from RA 27/3 vaccine is minimal.

In view of the data collected through 1983, the Immunization Practices Advisory Committee (ACIP) continues to state that: (1) pregnancy remains a contraindication to rubella vaccination because of the theoretical, albeit small, risk of CRS; (2) reasonable precautions should be taken to preclude vaccination of pregnant women, including asking women if they are pregnant, excluding those who say they are, and ex-

---

*These proceedings are to be published in *Reviews of Infectious Diseases*.

plaining the theoretical risks to the others; and (3) if vaccination does occur within 3 months of conception, the risk of CRS is so small as to be negligible; thus, rubella vaccination of a pregnant woman should not ordinarily be a reason to consider interruption of pregnancy. The patient and her physician, however, should make the final decision (14).

Since the inception of its vaccine-in-pregnancy register, CDC has encouraged reporting of all such cases. Because of the increasing number of cases reported to CDC, the experience with known susceptibles is becoming well defined. Therefore, CDC now encourages reporting only cases involving women known to have been susceptible at the time of vaccination. Laboratory services for serologic determination and culture of placental and fetal tissue will continue to be available at CDC for susceptible cases that are reported.

REFERENCES

1. CDC. Rubella vaccination during pregnancy—United States, 1971-1981. MMWR 1982:31:477-81.
2. CDC. Rubella and congenital rubella—United States, 1983. MMWR 1984;33:237-42, 247.
3. Preblud SR, Stetler HC, Frank JA Jr, Greaves WL, Hinman AR, Herrmann KL. Fetal risk associated with rubella vaccine JAMA 1981:246:1413-7.
4. Banatvala JE, O'Shea S, Best JM, Nicholls MWN, Cooper K. Transmission of RA 27/3 rubella vaccine strain to products of conception [Letter]. Lancet 1981; 1:392.
5. Furukawa T, Miyata T, Kondo K, Kuno K, Isomura S, Takekoshi T. Clinical trials of RA 27/3 (Wistar) rubella vaccine in Japan. Am J Dis Child 1969;118:262-3.
6. Bernstein DI, Ogra PL. Fetomaternal aspects of immunization with RA 27/3 live attenuated rubella virus vaccine during pregnancy. J Pediatr 1980;97:467-70.
7. O'Shea S, Parsons G, Best JM, Banatvala JE, Balfour HH Jr. How well do low levels of rubella antibody protect? [Letter]. Lancet 1981;II:1284.
8. Balfour HH Jr, Groth KE, Edelman CK, Amren DP, Best JM, Banatvala JE. Rubella viraemia and antibody responses after rubella vaccination and reimmunization. Lancet 1981;I:1078-80.
9. CDC. Congenital malformations surveillance report January-December 1980. Atlanta, Georgia, Centers for Disease Control, 1982:24.
10. CDC. Unpublished data.
11. Desmond MM, Montgomery JR, Melnick JL, Cochran GG, Verniaud W. Congenital rubella encephalitis. Effects on growth and early development. Am J Dis Child 1969;118:30-1.
12. Ziring PR. Congenital rubella: the teenage years. Pediatr Ann 1977;6:762-70.
13. CDC. Rubella vaccination during pregnancy—United States, 1971-1982. MMWR 1983;32:429-32, 437.
14. ACIP. Rubella prevention. MMWR 1984;33:301-10, 315-18.

From MMWR 1984;33:365-368.

SMALLPOX VACCINE

These revised ACIP recommendations on smallpox vaccine update the previous recommendations (MMWR 1980;29:417-20) to include current information on the changes in the International Health Regulations and the ending of distribution of smallpox vaccine to civilians. The basic recommendation is unchanged—smallpox vaccine is only indicated for civilians who are laboratory workers occupationally exposed to smallpox or other closely related orthopox viruses.

Smallpox vaccine

Smallpox vaccine (vaccinia virus) is a highly effective immunizing agent against smallpox. The judicious use of smallpox vaccine has eradicated smallpox. At the World Health Assembly in May 1980, the World Health Organization (WHO) declared the world free of smallpox (1-4). Smallpox vaccination of civilians is now indicated *only* for laboratory workers directly involved with smallpox (variola virus) or closely related orthopox viruses (e.g., monkeypox, vaccinia, and others).

Surveillance of suspected cases of smallpox

There is no evidence of smallpox transmission anywhere in the world. WHO has coordinated the investigation of 173 rumors of smallpox between 1979 and 1984 (5-7). All have been diseases other than smallpox, most commonly chickenpox or other rash illnesses. Even so, a suspected case of smallpox is a public health emergency and must be promptly investigated. Assistance in the clinical evaluation, collection of laboratory specimens, and preliminary laboratory diagnosis is available from state health departments and CDC (telephone: (404) 329-3145 during the day and (404) 329-2888 outside usual working hours).

Misuse of smallpox vaccine

There is no evidence that smallpox vaccination has any value in the treatment or prevention of recurrent herpes simplex infection, warts, or any disease other than those caused by orthopox viruses (8). Misuse of smallpox vaccine to treat herpes infections has been associated with severe complications (9-11). Smallpox vaccine should never be used therapeutically.

Smallpox vaccination not required for international travel

Smallpox vaccination is no longer required for international travel. In January 1982, the International Health Regulations were changed deleting smallpox from the Regulations (12). The International Certificates of Vaccination no longer include a smallpox vaccination certificate.

Smallpox vaccine no longer available for civilians

In May 1983, the only active, licensed producer of smallpox vaccine in the United States discontinued distribution of smallpox vaccine to civilians *(13)*. As a result, smallpox vaccine is no longer available to civilians.

Smallpox vaccine available to protect at-risk laboratory workers

CDC provides smallpox vaccine to protect laboratory workers occupationally exposed to smallpox virus and other closely related orthopox viruses *(14)*. Vaccine will be provided *only* for the protection of personnel of such laboratories. The vaccine should be administered to eligible employees under the supervision of a physician selected by the laboratory. Vaccine will be shipped to physicians responsible for vaccinating at-risk workers. Requests for vaccine should be sent to:

Drug Immunobiologic and Vaccine Service
Center for Infectious Diseases
Building 1, Room 1259
Centers for Disease Control
Atlanta, Georgia 30333
(404) 329-3356

Smallpox vaccination of military personnel

U.S. military personnel are routinely vaccinated against smallpox.

Consultation for complications of smallpox vaccination

CDC can assist physicians in the diagnosis and management of patients with suspected complications of smallpox vaccination. Vaccinia immune globulin (VIG) is available when indicated. Physicians should call (404) 329-3145 during the day and (404) 329-2888 evenings and weekends.

The majority of persons with such complications are likely to be recently vaccinated mulitary personnel or their contacts infected through person-to-person spread of vaccinia virus *(15-17)*. Such person-to-person spread can be extremely serious if the person infected has eczema or is immunocompromised.

Health-care workers are requested to report complications of smallpox vaccination to CDC through state and local health departments.

REFERENCES

1. WHO. Smallpox eradication. Weekly Epidemiological Record 1980;55:33-40.
2. WHO. Smallpox eradication. Weekly Epidemiological Record 1980;55:121-8.
3. WHO. Delcaration of global eradication of smallpox. Weekly Epidemiological Record 1980;55:145-52.
4. WHO. Smallpox vaccination policy. Weekly Epidemiological Record 1980;55:153-60.
5. CDC. Investigation of a smallpox rumor—Mexico. MMWR 1985 1985;34:343-4.
6. WHO. Orthopox virus surveillance: post-smallpox eradication policy. Weekly Epidemiological Record 1983;58:149-56.
7. WHO. Smallpox Eradication Unit. Personal communication.
8. Kern AB, Schiff, BL. Smallpox vaccinations in the management of recurrent herpes: a controlled evaluation. J Invest Dermatol 1959;33:99-102.
9. CDC. Vaccinia necrosum after smallpox vaccination—Michigan. MMWR 1982;31:501-2.
10. U.S. Food and Drug Administration. Inappropriate use of smallpox vaccine. FDA Drug Bulletin 1982;12:12.
11. Freed ER, Duma RJ, and Escobar, MR. Vaccinia necrosum and its relationship to impaired immunologic responsiveness. Am J Med 1972;52:411-20.
12. WHO. Smallpox vaccination certificates. Weekly Epidemiological Record 1981;39:305.
13. CDC. Smallpox vaccine no longer available for civilians—United States. MMWR 1981;32:387.
14. CDC. Smallpox vaccine available for protection of at-risk laboratory workers. MMWR 1983;32:543.
15. CDC. Contact spread of vaccinia from a recently vaccinated marine—Louisiana. MMWR 1984;33:37-8.
16. CDC. Contact spread of vaccinia from a National Guard vaccinee—Wisconsin. MMWR 1985;34:182-3.
17. Urdahl P, Rosland JH. Vaccinia genitalis. Tidsskr Nor Laegeforen 1982;102:1453-4.

From MMWR 1985;34:341.

TYPHOID VACCINE
Introduction

The incidence of typhoid fever has declined steadily in the United States in the last half century, and in the recent years fewer than 400 cases have been reported annually. The continuing downward trend is due largely to better sanitation and other control measures; vaccine is not deemed to have played a significant role. An increasing proportion of cases reported in the United States (about 50% in 1976) were acquired by travelers in other countries.

Typhoid and paratyphoid A and B vaccines

Although typhoid vaccines* have been used for many decades, only recently has definitive evidence of their effectiveness been observed in well controlled field investigations. Several different preparations of typhoid vaccine have been shown to protect 70-90 percent of recipients, depending in part on the degree of their subsequent exposure.

The effectiveness of paratyphoid A vaccine has never been established, and field trials have shown that usually small amounts of paratyphoid B antigens contained in "TAB" vaccines (vaccines combining typhoid and paratyphoid A and B antigens) are not effective.

---

*Official name: Typhoid Vaccine.

Knowing this and recognizing that combining paratyphoid A and B antigens with typhoid vaccine increases the risk of vaccine reaction, one should use typhoid vaccine alone.

Vaccine usage

Routine typhoid vaccination is no longer recommended for persons in the United States. Selective immunization is, however, indicated for:

1. Persons with intimate exposure to a documented typhoid carrier, such as would occur with continued household contact.

2. Travelers to areas where there is a recognized risk of exposure to typhoid because of poor food and water sanitation. It should be emphasized, however, that even after typhoid vaccination there should be careful selection of foods and water in these areas.

There is no evidence that typhoid vaccine is of value in the United States in controlling common-source outbreaks. Furthermore, there is no reason to use typhoid vaccine for persons in areas of natural disaster such as floods or for persons attending rural summer camps.

Primary immunization. On the basis of the field trials referred to above, the following dosages of vaccines available in the USA are recommended:

Adults and children over 10 years old. 0.5 ml subcutaneously on 2 occasions, separated by 4 or more weeks.

Children less than 10 years old.* 0.25 ml subcutaneously on 2 occasions, separated by 4 or more weeks.

In instances where there is not sufficient time for 2 doses to be administered at the interval specified, it has been common practice to give 3 doses of the same volumes listed above at weekly intervals recognizing that this schedule may be less effective. When vaccine is to be administered for travel overseas under constraint of time, a second dose may be administered en route at a more suitable interval.

Booster doses. Under conditions of continued or repeated exposure, a booster dose should be given at least every 3 years. Even when more than 3 years have elapsed since the prior immunization, a single booster injection is sufficient.

The following alternative routes and dosages of booster immunization can be expected to produce comparable antibody responses; generally less reaction follows vaccination by the intradermal route (except when acetone killed and dried vaccine is used. This vaccine should not be given intradermally).

Adults and children over 10 years old. 0.5 ml subcutaneously or 0.1 ml intradermally.

---

*Since febrile reactions to typhoid vaccine are common, an antipyretic may be indicated.

Children 6 months to 10 years. 0.25 ml subcutaneously or 0.1 ml intradermally.

SELECTED BIBLIOGRAPHY

Ashcroft, MT, Singh B, Nicholson CC, et al. A seven-year field trial of two typhoid vaccines in Guyana. Lancet 1967;2:1056-1059.

Cvjetanovic B, Uemura K. The present status of field and laboratory studies of typhoid and paratyphoid vaccine: with special reference to studies sponsored by the World Health Organization. Bull WHO 1965;32:29-36.

Hejfec LB, Levina LA, Kuz'minova ML, et al. Controlled field trials of paratyphoid B vaccine and evaluation of the effectiveness of a single administration of typhoid vaccine. Bull WHO 1968;38:907-915.

Hornick RB, Woodward TE, McCrumb FR, et al. Typhoid fever vaccine—yes or no? Med Clin North Am 1967; 51:617-623.

Hornick RB, Greisman SE, Woodward TE, et al. Typhoid fever: pathogenesis and immunologic control. N Engl J Med 1970;283:686-691, 739-746.

Mallory A, Belden EA, Brachman PS. The current status of typhoid fever in the United States and a description of an outbreak. J Infect Dis 1969;119:673-676.

Polish Typhoid Committee: Controlled field trials and laboratory studies on the effectiveness of typhoid vaccines in Poland, 1961-64: final report. Bull WHO 1966;34:211-222.

Schroeder S. The interpretation of serologic tests for typhoid fever. JAMA 1968;206:839-840.

Typhoid vaccines. Lancet 1967;2:1075-1076.

Yugoslav Typhoid Commission: A controlled field trial of the effectiveness of acetone-dried and inactivated and heat-phenol-inactivated typhoid vaccines in Yugoslavia: report. Bull WHO 1964;30:623-630.

Published in MMWR 1978;27:231.

TYPHUS VACCINE
Introduction

The United States has not experienced an outbreak of louse-borne (epidemic) typhus since 1922. The last reported case, 1950, did not result from an indigenous source of infection.

Louse-borne typhus was widespread in many countries affected by World War II. Since 1945, reported cases have declined steadily. Effective insecticides and generally improved standards of living have permitted many populations to free themselves of louse infestation. A human reservoir of latent infections persists in many parts of the world, and resurgence of the disease might occur under conditions of war or disaster. Vaccination of any civilian population in the United States, however, is unwarranted.

Typhus vaccine

Typhus vaccines* of the type available today were first used widely in World War II. Although no controlled studies of typhus vaccine have been carried out in human populations, experience from the field and the laboratory suggests that the incidence and severity of typhus cases are diminished among the vaccinated, especially if booster doses have been received.

Typhus vaccine is prepared from formaldehyde inactivated *Rickettsia prowazekii* grown in embryonated eggs. This vaccine provides protection against only louse-borne (epidemic) typhus; it does not protect against murine or scrub typhus.

Vaccination usage

General recommendations. The rarity of epidemic typhus minimizes the need for vaccination. Typhus is at present no threat to United States residents visiting most other countries. This is true even in places still reporting large numbers of cases if travel is limited to urban areas with modern hotel accommodations. It is only in mountainous, highland, or areas where a cold climate and other local conditions favor louse infestation that a potential threat exists.

Vaccination may be indicated for travelers to rural or remote highland areas of Ethiopia, Rwanda, Burundi, Mexico, Ecuador, Bolivia, or Peru, and mountainous areas of Asia. Even there, however, the risk of typhus for U.S. travelers is extremely low. No typhus case in an American traveler is known to have occurred in recent years. Vaccination against typhus is not required by any country as a condition for entry.

Vaccine recipients. Typhus vaccination is suggested only for the following special-risk groups:

1. Such persons as scientific investigators (e.g., anthropologists, archaeologists, or geologists), oilfield and construction workers, missionaries, and some government workers who live in or visit areas where the disease actually occurs and who will be in close contact with the indigenous population in such areas.

2. Medical personnel, including nurses and attendants, providing care for patients in areas in which louse-borne (epidemic) typhus occurs.

3. Laboratory personnel working with *Rickettsia prowazekii*.

Primary immunization. Two subcutaneous injections of vaccine 4 or more weeks apart using the dose volume indicated by the manufacturer for adults or for children.

Booster doses. A single subcutaneous injection of vaccine at intervals of 6-12 months for as long as opportunity for exposure exists using the dose volume indicated by the manufacturer for adults or for children. The primary series need never be repeated for booster doses to be effective.

Precautions and contraindications

Reactions. A day or more of pain, tenderness, induration, and erythema at the site of vaccine injection

---

*Official name: Typhus Vaccine.

is relatively common. Severe systemic reactions are infrequent, but transient fever and malaise may occur.

Contraindications. As is the case for all vaccines propagated in eggs, typhus vaccine should not be administered to anyone who is hypersensitive to eggs.

SELECTED BIBLIOGRAPHY

Donovick R, Wyckoff RWG. The comparative potencies of several typhus vaccines. Public Health Rep 1945;60:605-612.

Ecke RS, Gilliam AG, Snyder JC, et al. The effect of Cox-type vaccine on louse-borne typhus fever. an account of 61 cases of naturally occurring typhus fever in patients who had previously received one or more injections of Cox-type vaccine. Am J Trop Med 1945;25:477-462.

Gilliam AG. Efficacy of Cox-type vaccine in the prevention of naturally acquired louse-borne typhus fever. Am J Hyg 1945;44:401-410.

Sadusk JF. Typhus fever in the United States Army following immunization. Incidence, severity of disease, modification of the clinical course and serologic diagnosis. JAMA 1947;133:1192-1199.

Smadel JE, Jackson EB, Campbell JM. Studies on epidemic typhus vaccine. Arch Inst Past Tunis 1959;36:481-499.

Topping NH. Typhus fever. A note on the severity of the disease among unvaccinated and vaccinated laboratory personnel at the National Institutes of Health. Am J Trop Med 1944;24:57-62.

Wisseman CL Jr. The present and future of immunization against the typhus fevers. In First International Conference on Vaccines Against Viral and Rickettsial Diseases of Man. Pan American Health Organization, Scientific Publication No. 147, 1967, pp. 523-527.

Published in MMWR 1978;27:189.

YELLOW FEVER VACCINE
Introduction

At present, cases of yellow fever are reported from only Africa and South America. Two forms of yellow fever—urban and jungle—are distinguishable epidemiologically. Clinically and etiologically, they are identical.

Urban yellow fever is an epidemic viral disease of man transmitted from infected to susceptible persons by a vector, the *Aedes aegypti* mosquito. With the elimination or suppression of *A. aegypti*, urban yellow fever has disappeared from previously epidemic foci.

Jungle yellow fever is an enzootic viral disease transmitted among non-human hosts by a variety of mosquito vectors. It is currently observed only in the jungles of South America and Africa, but in the past it extended into parts of Central America as well. Human cases are rare. The disease can ostensibly disappear from an area for years and then reappear. Delineation of affected areas depends upon surveillance of animal reservoirs and vectors, accurate diagnosis, and prompt reporting of all cases.

Urban yellow fever can be prevented by eradicating *A. aegypti* mosquitoes or by suppressing their numbers to the point that they no longer perpetuate infection. At the present time, jungle yellow fever can most effectively be prevented in humans by immunization.

Yellow fever vaccine

Yellow fever vaccine* is a live, attenuated virus preparation made from 1 or 2 strains of virus: 17D and Dakar (French neurotropic). The Dakar strain has been associated with a significant (0.5 percent) incidence of meningoencephalitic reactions and is not recommended. The 17D strain has caused no significant complications.

Licensed vaccine available in the United States is prepared from the 17D strain, which is grown in chick embryo inoculated with a fixed passage level seed virus. The vaccine is freeze-dried supernate of centrifuged embryo homogenate.

Vaccine should be stored at the temperature recommended by the manufacturer (<5 C) until it is reconstituted by the addition of sterile physiologic saline. Unused vaccine should be discarded within approximately 1 hour of reconstitution.

Vaccine usage
Vaccine recipients

1. Persons 6 months of age or older traveling or living in areas where yellow fever infection exists, currently parts of Africa and South America. (These are listed in the Weekly Summary of Countries with Areas Infected with Quarantinable Diseases—available in most health departments.)

2. Laboratory personnel who might be exposed to virulent yellow fever virus.

Vaccination for international travel. For purposes of international travel, yellow fever vaccines must be approved by the World Health Organization and administered at an approved Yellow Fever Vaccination Center. Vaccines should have an International Certificate of Vaccination filled in, signed, and validated with the stamp of the Center where the vaccination is administered. (Yellow Fever Vaccination Centers in the United States are designated by the Foreign Quarantine Program of the Public Health Service. They can be identified by contacting State and local health departments.)

Vaccination for international travel may be required under circumstances other than those specified herein. Some countries in Africa require evidence of vaccination from all entering travelers; some may waive the requirements for travelers coming from noninfected areas and staying less than 2 weeks. These

---

*Official name: Yellow Fever Vaccine.

requirements may change, so all travelers should seek current information from health departments and travel agencies.

Some countries require an individual, even if only in transit, to have a valid International Certificate of Vaccination if he or she has been in countries either known or thought to harbor yellow fever virus.

Primary immunization. For both adults and children a single subcutaneous injection of 0.5 ml of reconstituted vaccine is used.

Booster doses. Yellow fever immunity following vaccination with 17D strain virus persists for more than 10 years; the International Health Regulations do not require revaccination more often than every 10 years.

Precautions and contraindications

Reactions to 17D yellow fever vaccine are generally mild. Five to 10 percent of vaccinees have mild headache, myalgia, low-grade fever, or other minor symptoms 5-10 days after vaccination. Symptoms cause less than 0.2 percent to curtail regular activities. Although more than 34 million doses of vaccine have been distributed, only 2 cases of encephalitis have been reported in the United States.

Contraindications

Pregnancy. Although specific information is not available concerning adverse effects of yellow fever vaccine on the developing fetus, it is prudent on theoretical grounds to avoid vaccinating pregnant women and to postpone travel until after delivery.

The morbidity and mortality from yellow fever disease are not altered by pregnancy. Therefore, pregnant women who MUST travel to areas where the risk of yellow fever is high should be vaccinated. It is believed that under these circumstances, the small theoretical risk for mother and fetus from vaccination is far outweighed by the risk from yellow fever infection.

Altered immune states. Infection with the yellow fever vaccine virus could pose excessive risk to patients with leukemia, lymphoma, or generalized malignancy or to those whose immunologic responses are suppressed by steroids, alkylating drugs, antimetabolites, or radiation.

Hypersensitivity. Live yellow fever vaccine is produced in chick embryos and should not be given to persons clearly hypersensitive to eggs. Furthermore, it should not be given to persons hypersensitive to other vaccine components such as trace amounts of particular antibiotics. (See the manufacturer's label.)

If international regulations are the only reason to vaccinate a person hypersensitive to eggs, efforts should first be made to obtain a waiver. A physician's letter which clearly states the contraindication to vaccination has been acceptable to some governments. (Ideally, it should be written under his letterhead and bear the authenticating stamp used by health departments and official immunization centers to validate International Certificates of Vaccination.) Because this is not uniformly true, however, it is prudent for the traveler to obtain specific and authoritative advice from the country or countries he plans to visit. Their embassies or consulates may be contacted. Subsequent waiver of requirements should be documented by appropriate letters.

SELECTED BIBLIOGRAPHY

Burruss HW, Hargett MV. Yellow fever vaccine inactivation studies. Public Health Rep 1947;62:940-956.

Groot H, Ribeiro RB. Neutralizing and hemagglutination-inhibition antibodies to yellow fever 17 years after vaccination with 17D vaccine. Bull WHO 1962;27:669-707.

Hargett MV, Burruss HW, Donovan A. Aqueous-base yellow fever vaccine. Public Health Rep 1943;58:505-512.

Rosenzweig EC, Babione RW, Wisseman CL Jr. Immunological studies with group B arthropod-borne viruses. IV. Persistence of yellow fever antibodies following vaccination with 17D strain yellow fever vaccine. Am J Trop Med 1963;12:230-235.

Smith HH, Calderon-Cuervo H, Leyva JP. A comparison of high and low subcultures of yellow fever vaccine (17D) in human groups. Am J Trop Med 21:579-587, 1941;21:579-587.

Smithburn KC, Durieux C, Koerber R, et al. Yellow fever vaccination. WHO Monograph Series No. 30, Geneva, 1956.

Strode GK (ed): Yellow fever. 1st Edition, New York: McGraw Hill, 1951.

Tauraso NM, Myers MG, Nau EV, et al. Effect of interval between inoculation of live smallpox and yellow-fever vaccines on antigenicity in man. J Infect Dis 1972;126:362-371.

Wisseman CL, Sweet BH. Immunological studies with group B arthropod-borne viruses. III. Response of human subjects to revaccination with 17D strain yellow fever vaccine. Am J Trop Med 1962;11:570-575.

Published in MMWR 1978;27:268.

APPENDIXES

APPENDIX 1

In the following tables are listed the currently recommended doses of various antimicrobial drugs, selected from among those in common use. These recommendations are separated into two tables: one applies to older infants and children, the other to newborn infants. This separation is necessary because the immaturity of the newborn infant often results in decreased excretion and/or detoxification of drugs, thus requiring alterations in dosage regimens to reduce the likelihood of toxicity. The table for older infants and children provides different recommendations for mild and severe infection; that for newborn infants is not divided because infections in this age group, with some exceptions, must be considered to be severe. All pediatric doses are in milligrams per kilogram of body weight per day, unless otherwise noted. Adult doses are given as the total daily dose, with the intervals assumed to be the same as those for children.

The recommended doses are not absolute; they are only intended as a guide. Individual clinical judgment about the problem, alterations in renal function, patient response, laboratory results, and other factors may dictate modification of these recommendations.

Package insert information should be consulted for such details as diluent for reconstitution of injectable preparations, steps taken to avoid incompatibilities, and similar precautions.

Antimicrobial drugs for newborn infants

Agent, generic (trade)	Route	Dosage/kg/24 hours	
		<7 days of age	*7 to 28 days of age*
Penicillin G, crystalline (numerous)	IV, IM	50,000 to 150,000 units in 2 doses	100,000 to 250,000 units in 3 doses
Penicillinase-resistant penicillins			
Methicillin (Staphcillin, Celbenin)	IV, IM	50 to 100 mg in 2 doses	100 to 200 mg in 3 doses
Oxacillin (Prostaphlin, Bactocill)	IV, IM	50 to 100 mg in 2 doses	100 to 200 mg in 3 doses
Nafcillin (Unipen)	IV, IM	50 mg in 2 doses	75 mg in 3 doses
Broad-spectrum penicillins			
Ampicillin (numerous)	IV, IM	100 mg in 2 doses	200 mg in 3 doses
Carbenicillin (Geopen, Pyopen)	IV	200 to 300 mg in 2 doses	400 mg in 4 doses
Mezlocillin (Mezlin)	IV	150 mg in 2 doses	<2 kg: 225 mg in 3 doses >2 kg: 300 mg in 4 doses
Aminoglycosides			
Kanamycin (Kantrex)	IV,* IM	15 mg in 2 doses	25 mg in 2 doses
Neomycin (Mycifradin)	PO	100 mg in 3 to 4 doses	100 mg in 3 to 4 doses
Gentamicin (Garamycin)	IV,* IM	6 mg in 2 doses	7.5 mg in 3 doses
Tobramycin (Nebcin)	IV,* IM	4 mg in 2 doses	5 mg in 3 doses
Amikacin (Amikin)	IV,* IM	15 mg in 2 doses	15 mg in 2 doses
Chloramphenicol (Chloromycetin)	IV	Premature: 25 mg in 2 doses Term: 25 mg in 2 doses	Premature: 25 mg in 2 doses Term: 50 mg in 2 doses
Cephalosporins			
Cephalothin (Keflin)	IV	40 mg in 2 doses	60 mg in 3 doses
Cefazolin (Kefzol, Ancef)	IV, IM	40 mg in 2 doses	40 mg in 2 doses
Cefotaxime (Claforan)	IV, IM	100 mg in 2 doses	150 mg in 3 doses
Moxalactam (Moxam)	IV, IM	100 mg in 2 doses	150 mg in 3 doses
Clindamycin (Cleocin)	IV, IM, PO	Term: 15 mg in 3 doses†	Premature: <28 days and/or <3.5 kg: 15 mg in 3 doses Premature: >28 days and/or >3.5 kg: 20 mg in 4 doses Term: 20 mg in 4 doses
Metronidazole (Flagyl)	IV, PO	15 mg/kg loading dose, then 15 mg in 2 doses	15 mg/kg loading dose, then 15 mg in 2 doses
Vancomycin (Vancocin)	IV*	30 mg in 2 doses	45 mg in 3 doses
Nystatin (Mycostatin)	PO	200,000 to 400,000 units in 4 doses	200,000 to 400,000 in 4 doses
Amphotericin B (Fungizone)	IV‡	0.25 to 1 mg in 1 dose	0.25 to 1 mg in 1 dose

*Intravenous administration over 30 to 60 minutes.
†Limited data on clindamycin in term infants less than 7 days old.
‡See p. 566 under "Comments."

Antimicrobial drugs for pediatric patients beyond the newborn period

Agent, generic (trade)	Route	Dosage/kg/24 hours		Comments
		Mild-moderate infections	Severe infections	
Penicillin G, crystalline, K, or Na (numerous)	IV, IM	50,000 to 100,000 units in 4 doses	100,000 to 400,000 units in 4 to 6 doses	1.68 mEq K or Na per 1,000,000 units; use Na salt for large IV doses
Penicillin G, procaine (numerous)	IM	25,000 to 50,000 units in 1 to 2 doses	Inappropriate	Contraindicated in procaine allergy
Penicillin G, benzathine (Bicillin, Permapen)	IM	<30 lbs: 600,000 units 30 to 60 lbs: 1,200,000 units >60 lbs: 2,400,000 units	Inappropriate	Major use, prevention of rheumatic fever by treatment and prophylaxis of streptococcal infections
Penicillin G, potassium (numerous)	PO	25,000 to 50,000 units in 4 doses	Inappropriate	Absorption variable: administer unbuffered penicillin G at least 1 hour before or 2 hour after meals
Penicillin V, phenoxymethyl penicillin (numerous)	PO	25 to 50 mg in 4 doses	Inappropriate	1600 units = 1 mg
Penicillinase-resistant penicillins Methicillin (Staphcillin, Celbenin)	IV, IM	100 to 200 mg in 4 doses (daily adult dose, 4 to 8 gm)	200 to 300 mg in 4 to 6 doses (daily adult dose, 8 to 12 gm)	All antistaphylococcal penicillins: primarily of benefit in the treatment of penicillin G–resistant staphylococcal infections; methicillin-resistant staphylococci are usually resistant to all other semisynthetic antistaphylococcal penicillins as well as all cephalosporins
Oxacillin (Prostaphlin, Bactocill)	IV, IM	50 to 100 mg in 4 doses (daily adult dose, 2 to 4 gm)	100 to 200 mg in 4 to 6 doses (daily adult dose, 4 to 12 gm)	Absorption of oral preparations variable: administer at least 1 hour before or 2 hour after meals
	PO	50 to 100 mg in 4 doses (daily adult dose, 2 to 4 gm)		
Nafcillin (Unipen, Nafcil)	IV, IM	50 to 100 mg in 4 doses (daily adult dose, 2 to 4 gm)	100 to 200 mg in 4 to 6 doses (daily adult dose, 4 to 12 gm)	
	PO	50 to 100 mg in 4 doses (daily adult dose, 2 to 4 gm)	Inappropriate	

Antimicrobial drugs for pediatric patients beyond the newborn period—cont'd

Agent, generic (trade)	Route	Dosage/kg/24 hours		Comments
		Mild-moderate infections	Severe infections	
Cloxacillin (Tegopen)	PO	50 to 100 mg in 4 doses (daily adult dose, 2 to 4 gm)	Inappropriate	Ineffective against penicillin G–resistant staphylococci
Dicloxacillin (Dynapen, Pathocil, Veracillin)	PO	25 to 50 mg in 4 doses (daily adult dose, 2 to 4 gm)	Inappropriate	High incidence of skin rash in patients with infectious mononucleosis
Broad-spectrum penicillins				
Ampicillin (numerous)	IV, IM	50 to 100 mg in 4 doses (daily adult dose, 2 to 4 gm)	200 to 400 mg in 4 doses (daily adult dose, 8 to 12 gm)	
	PO	50 to 100 mg in 4 doses (daily adult dose, 2 to 4 gm)	Inappropriate	
Amoxicillin (Amoxil, Larotid, Polymox)	PO	20 to 40 mg in 3 doses (daily adult dose, 750 mg to 1.5 gm)	Inappropriate	
Mezlocillin (Mezlin)	IV, IM	200 to 300 mg in 4 to 6 doses (daily adult dose, 16 to 24 gm)	200 to 300 mg in 4 to 6 doses (daily adult dose, 16 to 24 gm)	
Piperacillin (Piperacil)	IV, IM	200 to 300 mg in 4 to 6 doses (daily adult dose, 16 to 24 gm)	200 to 300 mg in 4 to 6 doses (daily adult dose, 16 to 24 gm)	
Carbenicillin (Geopen, Pyopen)	IV	100 to 200 mg in 4 doses (daily adult dose, 4 to 8 gm)	400 to 600 mg in 4 to 6 doses (daily adult dose, 20 to 30 gm)	Carbenicillin contains 4.7 mEq and ticarcillin contains 5.2 mEq Na/gm. Emergence of bacterial resistance is a major problem
Ticarcillin (Ticar)	IV	50 to 100 mg in 4 doses (daily adult dose, 4 to 8 gm)	200 to 300 mg in 4 to 6 doses (daily adult dose, 12 to 24 gm)	

	Route			
Cephalosporins				
Cephalothin (Keflin)	IV, IM	40 to 80 mg in 4 doses (daily adult dose, 2 to 4 gm)	100 to 150 mg in 4 to 6 doses (daily adult dose, 8 to 12 gm)	
Cephazolin (Kefzol, Ancef)	IV, IM	50 mg in 4 doses (daily adult dose, 2 gm)	100 mg in 4 doses (daily adult dose, 4 to 6 gm)	
Cephalexin (Keflex)	PO	25 to 50 mg in 4 doses (daily adult dose, 1 to 2 gm)	Inappropriate	
Cefaclor (Ceclor)	PO	40 to 60 mg in 3 to 4 doses	Inappropriate	
Cefuroxime (Zinacef)	IV, IM	50 to 100 mg in 3 doses (daily adult dose, 3 gm)	200 to 240 in 3 or 4 doses (daily adult dose, 6 gm)	
Cefotaxime (Claforan)	IV, IM	50 to 100 mg in 4 doses (daily adult dose, 4 gm)	200 mg in 4 to 6 doses (daily adult dose, 8 gm)	
Cefoperazone (Cefobid)	IV	100 mg in 2 to 3 doses (daily adult dose, 2 to 4 gm)	150 mg in 3 doses (daily adult dose, 8 to 12 gm)	
Moxalactam (Moxam)	IV, IM	150 in 3 to 4 doses (daily adult dose, 4-8 gm)	200 in 4 doses (daily adult dose, 8 to 10 gm)	
Macrolides				
Erythromycin (numerous)	PO	20 to 50 mg in 3 to 4 doses (daily adult dose, 1 to 2 gm)	Inappropriate	
	IV	Inappropriate	20 to 40 mg in 3 to 4 doses (daily adult dose 1 to 4 gm)	Continuous drip preferred but may be given in 4 doses
Clindamycin (Cleocin)	IV, IM	10 to 25 mg in 4 doses (daily adult dose, 600 to 1200 mg)	25 to 40 mg in 4 doses (daily adult dose, 1200 to 2700 mg)	Use only when specifically indicated because of side effects of diarrhea and pseudomembranous enterocolitis
	PO	8 to 16 mg in 4 doses (daily adult dose, 600 to 1200 mg)	Inappropriate	

Antimicrobial drugs for pediatric patients beyond the newborn period—cont'd

Agent, generic (trade)	Route	Dosage/kg/24 hours		Comments
		Mild-moderate infections	Severe infections	
Aminoglycosides				
Streptomycin (numerous)	IM	Inappropriate	20 to 40 mg in 3 doses (daily adult dose, 1 to 2 gm)	Aminoglycosides enter CSF poorly; when used intravenously administer over 30 to 60 minutes
Kanamycin (Kantrex)	IM, IV	15 mg in 2 to 3 doses	25 mg in 2 to 3 doses (daily adult dose, 1 to 2 gm)	
Gentamicin (Garamycin)	IV, IM	Inappropriate	5 to 7 mg in 3 doses (daily adult dose, 3 to 7 mg/kg/day)	
Netilmycin (Netromycin)	IV, IM	Inappropriate	5 to 7 mg in 3 doses (daily adult dose, 3 to 7 mg/kg/day)	
Tobramycin (Nebcin)	IV, IM	Inappropriate	3 to 5 mg in 3 doses (daily adult dose, 3 to 5 mg/kg/day)	
Amikacin (Amikin)	IV, IM	Inappropriate	15 mg in 2 doses (daily adult dose, 15 mg/kg/day; maximum 1.5 gm)	
Neomycin (Mycifradin)	PO	100 mg in 4 doses	100 mg in 4 doses	
Metronidazole (Flagyl)	IV, PO	IV dose: 30 mg in 4 doses (adult dose, 15 mg/kg loading dose then 30 mg/kg in 4 doses) PO dose: 15 to 35 mg in 3 doses (daily adult dose, 2250 mg)	IV dose: 30 mg in 4 doses (adult dose, 15 mg/kg loading dose then 30 mg/kg in 4 doses) PO dose: 15 to 35 mg in 3 doses (daily adult dose, 2250 mg)	
Vancomycin (Vancocin)	IV, PO	IV dose: 40 mg in 4 doses (daily adult dose, 2 gm) PO dose: 50 mg in 4 doses (daily adult dose, 500 mg)	IV dose: 40 mg in 4 doses (daily adult dose, 2 gm) PO dose: 50 mg in 4 doses (daily adult dose, 500 mg)	

Drug	Route			
Tetracycline (numerous)	IV	Inappropriate	20 to 30 mg in 2 to 3 doses (daily adult dose, 1 to 2 gm)	Infuse IV over a 2-hour period
	PO	20 to 40 mg in 4 doses (daily adult dose, 1 to 2 gm)	Inappropriate	Responsible for staining of developing teeth; use only in children over 8 years of age and only when specifically indicated
Chloramphenicol Succinate	IV	Inappropriate	50 to 100 mg in 3 to 4 doses (daily adult dose, 2 to 4 gm)	Not recommended for intramuscular administration
Palmitate	PO	Inappropriate	50 to 75 mg in 3 to 4 doses (daily adult dose, 2 to 4 gm)	
Sulfonamides Sulfadiazine	IV, SC	120 mg in 4 doses	120 mg in 4 doses	The first dose of sulfadiazine, sulfisoxazole, and triple sulfonamides should be doubled; daily adult dose PO 2 to 4 gm; IV, SC—same as children
Sulfisoxazole (Gantrisin)	IV, SC	120 mg in 4 doses	120 mg in 4 doses	
	PO	120 mg in 4 doses	Inappropriate	
Triple sulfonamides	IV, SC	120 mg in 4 doses	120 mg in 4 doses	
Trimethoprim-sulfamethoxazole (Bactrim, Septra)	PO	8 mg trimethoprim, 40 mg sulfamethoxazole in 2 doses	20 mg trimethoprim, 100 mg sulfamethoxazole in 2 doses	
Urinary antiseptic agents Methenamine mandelate (Mandelamine)	PO	50 to 75 mg in 3 to 4 doses (daily adult dose, 2 to 4 gm)	Inappropriate	Should not be used for infants; urine pH must be adjusted to 5 to 5.5
Nitrofurantoin (Furadantin, Macrodantin)	PO	5 to 7 mg in 4 doses (daily adult dose, 200 to 400 mg)	Inappropriate	Should not be used for infants

Antimicrobial drugs for pediatric patients beyond the newborn period—cont'd

Agent, generic (trade)	Route	Dosage/kg/24 hours		Comments
		Mild-moderate infections	Severe infections	
Antifungal agents				
Nystatin (Mycostatin, Nilstat)	PO	600,000 to 2,000,000 units; total daily dose in 3 to 4 doses		
Amphotericin B (Fungizone)	IV	0.25 to 1 mg in 1 dose	0.25 to 1 mg in 1 dose	Use a slow infusion; begin with a relatively low dose, then increase the dose over several days; do not allow the IV solution to mix with other drugs, since the agent is in an easily disturbed colloid
Flucytosine (Ancobon)	PO	50 to 150 mg in 4 doses (daily adult dose, 50 to 150 mg/kg/day in 4 doses)	50 to 150 mg in 4 doses (daily adult dose, 50 to 150 mg/kg/day in 4 doses)	Note: "Flucytosine is rarely used alone because of the rapidity with which fungi develop resistance."
Griseofulvin (many)	PO	11 mg in 1 dose (daily adult dose, 250 to 500 mg)	11 mg in 1 dose (daily adult dose, 250 to 500 mg)	
Ketoconazole (Nizoral)	PO	5 to 10 mg in 1 or 2 doses (daily adult dose, 200 to 400 mg in 1 dose)	5 to 10 mg in 1 or 2 doses (daily adult dose, 200 to 400 mg in 1 dose)	

APPENDIX 2

PREVENTION OF ACQUIRED IMMUNE DEFICIENCY SYNDROME (AIDS): REPORT OF INTER-AGENCY RECOMMENDATIONS*

Since June 1981, over 1,200 cases of acquired immune deficiency syndrome (AIDS) have been reported to CDC from 34 states, the District of Columbia, and 15 countries. Reported cases of AIDS include persons with Kaposi's sarcoma who are under age 60 years and/or persons with life-threatening opportunistic infections with no known underlying cause for immune deficiency. Over 450 persons have died from AIDS, and the case-fatality rate exceeds 60% for cases first diagnosed over 1 year previously (1,2). Reports have gradually increased in number. An average of one case per day was reported during 1981, compared with three to four daily in late 1982 and early 1983. Current epidemiologic evidence identifies several groups in the United States at increased risk for developing AIDS (3-7). Most cases have been reported among homosexual men with multiple sexual partners, abusers of intravenous (IV) drugs, and Haitians, especially those who have entered the country within the past few years. However, each group contains many persons who probably have little risk of acquiring AIDS. Recently, 11 cases of unexplained, life-threatening opportunistic infections and cellular immune deficiency have been diagnosed in patients with hemophilia. Available data suggest that the severe disorder of immune regulation underlying AIDS is caused by a transmissible agent.

A national case-control study and an investigation of a cluster of cases among homosexual men in California indicate that AIDS may be sexually transmitted among homosexual or bisexual men (8,9). AIDS cases were recently reported among women who were steady sexual partners of men with AIDS or of men in high-risk groups, suggesting the possibility of heterosexual transmission (10). Recent reports of unexplained cellular immunodeficiencies and opportunistic infections in infants born to mothers from groups at high risk for AIDS have raised concerns about in utero or perinatal transmission of AIDS (11). Very little is known about risk factors for Haitians with AIDS.

The distribution of AIDS cases parallels that of hepatitis B virus infection, which is transmitted sexually and parenterally. Blood products or blood appear responsible for AIDS among hemophilia patients who require clotting factor replacement. The likelihood of blood transmission is supported by the occurrence of AIDS among IV drug abusers. Many drug abusers share contaminated needles, exposing themselves to blood-borne agents, such as hepatitis B virus. Recently, an infant developed severe immune deficiency and an opportunistic infection several months after receiving a transfusion of platelets derived from the blood of a man subsequently found to have AIDS (12). The possibility of acquiring AIDS through blood components or blood is further suggested by several cases in persons with no known risk factors who have received blood products or blood within 3 years of AIDS diagnosis (2). These cases are currently under investigation.

No AIDS cases have been documented among health care or laboratory personnel caring for AIDS patients or processing laboratory specimens. To date, no person-to-person transmission has been identified other than through intimate contact or blood transfusion.

---

*From MMWR 1983; 32:101-103.

Several factors indicate that individuals at risk for transmitting AIDS may be difficult to identify. A New York City study showed that a significant proportion of homosexual men who were asymptomatic or who had nonspecific symptoms or signs (such as generalized lymphadenopathy) had altered immune functions demonstrated by in vitro tests (2,13,14). Similar findings have been reported among patients with hemophilia (2,15,16). Although the significance of these immunologic alterations is not yet clear, their occurrence in at least two groups at high risk for AIDS suggests that the pool of persons potentially capable of transmitting an AIDS agent may be considerably larger than the presently known number of AIDS cases. Furthermore, the California cluster investigation and other epidemiologic findings suggest a "latent period" of several months to 2 years between exposure and recognizable clinical illness and imply that transmissibility may precede recognizable illness. Thus, careful histories and physical examinations alone will not identify all persons capable of transmitting AIDS but should be useful in identifying persons with definite AIDS diagnoses or related symptoms, such as generalized lymphadenopathy, unexplained weight loss, and thrush. Since only a small percentage of members of high-risk groups actually has AIDS, a laboratory test is clearly needed to identify those with AIDS or those at highest risk of acquring AIDS. For the above reasons, persons who may be considered at increased risk of AIDS include those with symptoms and signs suggestive of AIDS; sexual partners of AIDS patients; sexually active homosexual or bisexual men with multiple partners; Haitian entrants to the United States; present or past abusers of IV drugs; patients with hemophilia; and sexual partners of individuals at increased risk for AIDS.

Statements on prevention and control of AIDS have been issued by the National Gay Task Force, the National Hemophilia Foundation, the American Red Cross, the American Association of Blood Banks, the Council of Community Blood Centers, the American Association of Physicians for Human Rights, and others. These groups agree that steps should be implemented to reduce the potential risk of transmitting AIDS through blood products, but differ in the methods proposed to accomplish this goal. Public health agencies, community organizations, and medical organizations and groups share the responsibility to rapidly disseminate information on AIDS and recommended precautions.

Although the cause of AIDS remains unknown, the Public Health Service recommends the following actions:

1. Sexual contact should be avoided with persons known or suspected to have AIDS. Members of high risk groups should be aware that multiple sexual partners increase the probability of developing AIDS.

2. As a temporary measure, members of groups at increased risk for AIDS should refrain from donating plasma and/or blood. This recommendation includes all individuals belonging to such groups, even though many individuals are at little risk of AIDS. Centers collecting plasma and/or blood should inform potential donors of this recommendation. The Food and Drug Administration (FDA) is preparing new recommendations for manufacturers of plasma derivatives and for establishments collecting plasma or blood. This is an interim measure to protect recipients of blood products and blood until specific laboratory tests are available.

3. Studies should be conducted to evaluate screening procedures for their effectiveness in identifying and excluding plasma and blood with a high probability of transmitting AIDS. These procedures should include specific laboratory tests as well as careful histories and physical examinations.

4. Physicians should adhere strictly to medical indications for tranfusions, and autologous blood transfusions are encouraged.

5. Work should continue toward development of safer blood products for use by hemophilia patients.

The National Hemophilia Foundation has made specific recommendations for management of patients with hemophilia (17).

The interim recommendation requesting that high-risk persons refrain from donating plasma and/or blood is especially important for donors whose plasma is recovered from plasmapheresis centers of other sources and pooled to make products that are not inactivated and may transmit infections, such as hepatitis B. The clear intent of this recommendation is to eliminate plasma and blood potentially containing the putative AIDS agent from the supply. Since no specific test is known to detect AIDS at an early stage in a potential donor, the recommendation to discourage donation must encompass all members of groups at increased risk for AIDS, even though it includes many individuals who may be at little risk of transmitting AIDS.

As long as the cause remains unknown, the ability to understand the natural history of AIDS and to undertake preventive measures is somewhat compromised. However, the above recommendations are prudent measures that should reduce the risk of acquiring and transmitting AIDS.

Reported by the Centers for Disease Control, the Food and Drug Administration, and the National Institutes of Health.

REFERENCES

1. CDC. Update on acquired immune deficiency syndrome (AIDS)—United States. MMWR 1982;31:507-8, 513-4.
2. CDC. Unpublished data.
3. CDC. Update on Kaposi's sarcoma and opportunistic infections in previously healthy persons—United States. MMWR 1982;31:294, 300-1.
4. CDC. Opportunistic infections and Kaposi's sarcoma among Haitians in the United States. MMWR 1982;31: 353-4, 360-1.
5. CDC. *Pneumocystis carinii* pneumonia among persons with hemophilia A. MMWR 1982;31:365-7.
6. CDC. Update on acquired immune deficiency syndrome (AIDS) among patients with hemophilia A. MMWR 1982;31:644-6, 652.
7. Vieira J, Frank E, Spira TJ, Landesman SH. Acquired immune deficiency in Haitians: opportunistic infections in previously healthy Haitian immigrants. N Engl J Med 1983;308:125-9.
8. CDC. Unpublished data.
9. CDC. A cluster of Kaposi's sarcoma and *Pneumocystis carinii* pneumonia among homosexual male residents of Los Angeles and Orange Counties, California. MMWR 1982;31:305-7.
10. CDC. Immunodeficiency among female sexual partners of males with acquired immune deficiency syndrome (AIDS)—New York. MMWR 1983;31:697-8.
11. CDC. Unexplained immunodeficiency and opportunistic infections in infants—New York, New Jersey, California. MMWR 1982;31:665-7.
12. CDC. Possible transfusion-associated acquired immune deficiency syndrome (AIDS)—California. MMWR 1982; 31:652-4.
13. CDC. Persistent, generalized lymphadenopathy among homosexual males. MMWR 1982;31:249-51.
14. Kornfield H, Vande Stouwe RA, Lange M, Reddy MM, Grieco MH. T-lymphocyte subpopulations in homosexual men. N Engl J Med 1982;307:729-31.
15. Lederman MM, Ratnoff OD, Scillian JJ, Jones PK, Schacter B. Impaired cell-mediated immunity in patients with classic hemophilia. N Engl J Med 1983;308: 79-83.
16. Menitove JE, Aster RH, Casper JT, et al. T-lymphocyte subpopulations in patients with classic hemophilia treated with cryoprecipitate and lyophilized concentrates. N Engl J Med 1983;308:83-6.
17. Medical and Scientific Advisory Council. Recommendations to prevent AIDS in patients with hemophilia. New York: National Hemophilia Foundation, January 14, 1983.

PROVISIONAL PUBLIC HEALTH SERVICE INTER-AGENCY RECOMMENDATIONS FOR SCREENING DONATED BLOOD AND PLASMA FOR ANTIBODY TO THE VIRUS CAUSING ACQUIRED IMMUNODEFICIENCY SYNDROME*

In March 1983, the U.S. Public Health Service issued inter-agency recommendations on the prevention of acquired immunodeficiency syndrome (AIDS) *(1)*. Included was the recommendation that members of groups at increased risk for AIDS should refrain from donating plasma and/or blood. That recommendation was made to decrease the risk of AIDS associated with the administration of blood or blood products, which accounts for about 2% of all reported AIDS cases in the United States.

Evidence has shown that a newly recognized retrovirus is the cause of AIDS. Although this virus has been given several names, including human T-lymphotropic virus type III (HTLV-III) *(2)*, lymphadenopathy-associated virus (LAV) *(3)*, and AIDS-associated retrovirus (ARV) *(4)*, it is referred to as HTLV-III in this discussion. Tests to detect antibody to HTLV-III will be licensed and commercially available in the United States in the near future to screen blood and plasma for laboratory evidence of infection with the virus. The antibody tests are modifications of the enzyme-linked immunosorbent assay (ELISA), which uses antigens derived from whole disrupted HTLV-III *(5)*.

There is considerable experience with the ELISA test in research laboratories, but much additional information will be gathered following its widespread application. In the early phases of testing, a number of false-positive tests may be encountered. Adjustments in interpretation are anticipated as more is learned about the performance of the test in an individual laboratory and about the specific proportion of falsely positive or falsely negative tests in the screening setting where the test is used.

The present recommendations concern the use of these tests to screen blood and plasma collected for transfusion or manufactured into other products. They are intended to supplement, rather than replace, the U.S. Food and Drug Administration's recently revised recommendations to blood and plasma collection facilities and the earlier inter-agency recommendations *(1)*. Additional public health applications of these tests in the understanding and control of AIDS will be described in a subsequent report.

---

*From MMWR 1985;34:1-5.

BACKGROUND
Antibody detection studies

The ELISA test has been used in many research programs for detecting antibodies to HTLV-III in patients with AIDS and with AIDS-related conditions. In different studies, HTLV-III antibody was found to range from 68% to 100% of patients with AIDS, and in 84%-100% of persons with related conditions, such as unexplained generalized lymphadenopathy (5-7). Serologic surveys have yielded variable seropositivity rates in groups at increased risk for AIDS: 22%-65% of homosexual men (8-11), 87% of intravenous-drug abusers admitted to a detoxification program in New York City (12), 56%-72% of persons with hemophilia A (13,14), and 35% of women who were sexual partners of men with AIDS (15). In contrast to the above groups, HTLV-III antibody has been detected in fewer than 1% of persons with no known risks for AIDS (4-10).

The time needed to develop a positive antibody test following infection is not known. Data regarding the interval between infection with HTLV-III and seroconversion are limited. A nurse who sustained a needle-stick injury while caring for an AIDS patient developed antibody between 4 and 7 weeks following exposure (16). Additionally, a recent study described several asymptomatic individuals infected with HTLV-III for more than 6 months in the absence of detectable antibody (17,18). Nonetheless, currently available ELISA tests can be expected to identify most persons with HTLV-III infection.

Virus isolation studies

HTLV-III has been isolated from blood, semen, and saliva and has been recovered from many individuals in the presence of antibody (19,20). HTLV-III has been isolated from the blood of 85% or more of seropositive individuals with AIDS (21), lymphadenopathy, or other AIDS-associated conditions (2) and from three of four mothers of infants with AIDS (2). The virus has also been isolated from asymptomatic seropositive homosexual men and hemophiliacs, and has been recovered from 95% of seropositive high-risk blood donors who had been implicated in the transmission of AIDS through transfusion (21). The recovery of HTLV-III from these high-risk donors 2 or more years after their initial donation provides evidence that viremia may persist for years in both asymptomatic and symptomatic individuals. HTLV-III has also been isolated from some asymptomatic seronegative persons, but this is the exception (17).

Modes of transmission

Epidemiologic data suggest that the virus has been transmitted through intimate sexual contact; sharing contaminated needles; transfusion of whole blood, blood cellular components, plasma, or clotting factor concentrates that have not been heat treated; or from infected mother to child before, at, or shortly after the time of birth. No other products prepared from blood (e.g., immunoglobulin, albumin, plasma protein fraction, hepatitis B vaccine) have been implicated, nor have cases been documented to occur through such common exposures as sharing meals, sneezing or coughing, or other casual contact.

Natural history of infection

Information about the course of infection with HTLV-III is incomplete, but the majority of infected adults will not acquire clinically apparent AIDS in the first few years after infection. In some studies 5%-19% of seropositive homosexual men developed AIDS within 2-5 years after a previously collected serum sample was retrospectively tested and found to be seropositive. An additional 25% developed generalized lymphadenopathy, oral candidiasis, or other AIDS-associated conditions within the same interval (11,22). The long-term prognosis for most persons infected with HTLV-III is unknown.

SCREENING BLOOD AND PLASMA
Initial testing

Persons accepted as donors should be informed that their blood or plasma will be tested for HTLV-III antibody. Persons not wishing to have their blood or plasma tested must refrain from donation. Donors should be told that they will be notified if their test is positive and that they may be placed on the collection facility's donor deferral list, as is currently practiced with other infectious diseases, and should be informed of the identities of additional deferral lists to which the positive donors may be added.

All blood or plasma should be tested for HTLV-III antibody by ELISA. Any blood or plasma that is positive on initial testing must not be transfused or manufactured into other products capable of transmitting infectious agents.

When the ELISA is used to screen populations in whom the prevalence of HTLV-III infections is low, the proportion of positive results that are falsely positive will be high. Therefore, the ELISA should be repeated on all seropositive specimens before the donor is notified. If the repeat ELISA test is negative, the specimen should be tested by another test.

Other testing

Other tests have included immunofluorescence and radioimmunoprecipitation assays, but the most extensive experience has been with the Western blot technique (22), in which antibodies can be detected to HTLV-III proteins of specific molecular weights.

Based on available data, the Western blot should be considered positive for antibody to HTLV-III if band p24 or gp41 is present (alone or in combination with other bands).

Notification of donors

If the repeat ELISA test is positive or if other tests are positive, it is the responsibility of the collection facility to ensure that the donor is notified. The information should be given to the donor by an individual especially aware of the sensitivities involved. At present, the proportion of these seropositive donors who have been infected with HTLV-III is not known. It is, therefore, important to emphasize to the donor that the positive result is a preliminary finding that may not represent true infection. To determine the significance of a positive test, the donor should be referred to a physician for evaluation. The information should be given to the donor in a manner to ensure confidentiality of the results and of the donor's identity.

Maintaining confidentiality

Physicians, laboratory and nursing personnel, and others should recognize the importance of maintaining confidentiality of positive test results. Disclosure of this information for purposes other than medical or public health could lead to serious consequences for the individual. Screening procedures should be designed with safeguards to protect against unauthorized disclosure. Donors should be given a clear explanation of how information about them will be handled. Facilities should consider developing contingency plans in the event that disclosure is sought through legal process. If donor deferral lists are kept, it is necessary to maintain confidentiality of such lists. Whenever appropriate, as an additional safeguard, donor deferral lists should be general, without indication of the reason for inclusion.

Medical evaluation

The evaluation might include ELISA testing of a follow-up serum specimen and Western blot testing, if the specimen is positive. Persons who continue to show serologic evidence of HTLV-III infection should be questioned about possible exposure to the virus or possible risk factors for AIDS in the individual or his/her sexual contacts and examined for signs of AIDS or related conditions, such as lymphadenopathy, oral candidiasis, Kaposi's sarcoma, and unexplained weight loss. Additional laboratory studies might include tests for other sexually transmitted diseases, tests of immune function, and where available, tests for the presence of the virus, such as viral culture. Testing for antibodies to HTLV-III in the individual's sexual contacts may also be useful in establishing whether the test results truly represent infection.

RECOMMENDATIONS FOR THE INDIVIDUAL

An individual judged most likely to have an HTLV-III infection should be provided the following information and advice:

1. The prognosis for an individual infected with HTLV-III over the long term is not known. However, data available from studies conducted among homosexual men indicate that most persons will remain infected.
2. Although asymptomatic, these individuals may transmit HTLV-III to others. Regular medical evaluation and follow-up is advised, especailly for individuals who develop signs or symptoms suggestive of AIDS.
3. Refrain from donating blood, plasma, body organs, other tissue, or sperm.
4. There is a risk of infecting others by sexual intercourse, sharing of needles, and possibly, exposure of others to saliva through oral-genital contact or intimate kissing. The efficacy of condoms in preventing infection with HTLV-III is unproven, but the consistent use of them may reduce transmission.
5. Toothbrushes, razors, or other implements that could become contaminated with blood should not be shared.
6. Women with a seropositive test, or women whose sexual partner is seropositive, are themselves at increased risk of acquiring AIDS. If they become pregnant, their offspring are also at increased risk of acquiring AIDS.
7. After accidents resulting in bleeding, contaminated surfaces should be cleaned with household bleach freshly diluted 1:10 in water.
8. Devices that have punctured the skin, such as hypodermic and acupuncture needles, should be steam sterilized by autoclave before reuse or safely discarded. Whenever possible, disposable needles and equipment should be used.
9. When seeking medical or dental care for intercurrent illness, these persons should inform those responsible for their care of their positive antibody status so that appropriate evaluation can be undertaken and precautions taken to prevent transmission to others.
10. Testing for HTLV-III antibody should be offered to persons who may have been infected as a result of their contact with seropositive individuals (e.g., sexual partners, persons with whom needles have been shared, infants born to seropositive mothers).

Revised recommendations will be published as additional information becomes available and additional experience is gained with this test.

Reported by Centers for Disease Control; Food and Drug Administration; Alcohol, Drug Abuse, and Mental Health Administration; National Institutes of Health; Health Resources and Services Administration.

REFERENCES

1. CDC. Prevention of acquired immune deficiency syndrome (AIDS): Report of inter-agency recommendations. MMWR 1983;32:101-3.
2. Gallo RC, Salahuddin SZ, Popovic M, et al. Frequent detection and isolation of cytopathic retroviruses (HTLV-III) from patients with AIDS and at risk for AIDS. Science 1984;224:500-3.
3. Barré-Sinoussi F, Chermann JC, Rey F, et al. Isolation of a T-lymphotropic retrovirus from a patient at risk for acquired immune deficiency syndrome (AIDS). Science 1983;220:868-71.
4. Levy JA, Hoffman AD, Kramer SM, Landis JA, Shimabukuro JM, Oschiro LS. Isolation of lymphocytopathic retroviruses from San Francisco patients with AIDS. Science 1984;225:840-2.
5. Sarngadharan MG, Popovic M, Bruch L, Schüpbach J, Gallo RC. Antibodies reactive with human T-lymphotropic retroviruses (HTLV-III) in the serum of patients with AIDS. Science 1984;224:506-8.
6. Safai B, Sarngadharan MG, Groopman JE, et al. Seroepidemiological studies of human T-lymphotropic retrovirus type III in acquired immunodeficiency syndrome. Lancet 1984;1:1438-40.
7. Laurence J, Brun-Vezinet F, Schutzer SE, et al. Lymphadenopathy associated viral antibody in AIDS. N Engl J Med 1984;311:1269-73.
8. Melbye M, Biggar RJ, Ebbesen P, et al. Seroepidemiology of HTLV-III antibody in Danish homosexual men; prevalence, transmission, and disease outcome. Brit Med J 1984;289:573-5.
9. CDC. Antibodies to a retrovirus etiologically associated with acquired immunodeficiency syndrome (AIDS) in populations with increased incidences of the syndrome. MMWR 1984;33:377-9.
10. Weiss SH, Goedert JJ, Sarngadharan MB, et al. Screening test for HTLV-III (AIDS agent) antibodies: specificity, sensitivity, and applications. JAMA 1985;253:221-5
11. Goedert JJ, Sarngadharan MG, Biggar RJ, et al. Determinants of retrovirus (HTLV-III) antibody and immunodeficiency conditions in homosexual men. Lancet 1984;2:711-6.
12. Spira TJ, Des Jarlais DC, Marmor M, et al. Prevalence of antibody to lymphadenopathy-associated virus among drug-detoxification patients in New York. N Engl J Med 1984;311:467-8.
13. Ramsey RB, Palmer EL, McDougal JS, et al. Antibody to lymphadenopathy-associated virus in hemophiliacs with and without AIDS. Lancet 1984;2:397-8.
14. Tsoukas C, Gervais F, Shuster J, Gold P, O'Shaughnessy M, Robert-Guroff M. Association of HTLV-III antibodies and cellular immune status of hemophiliacs. N Engl J Med 1984;311:1514-15.
15. Harris CA, Cabradilla C, Klein RS, et al. Antibodies to a core protein (p25) of lymphadenopathy associated virus (LAV) and immunodeficiency in heterosexual partners of AIDS patients. Presentation at 24th Interscience Conference on Antimicrobial Agents and Chemotherapy. Washington, D.C., 1984.
16. Anonymous. Needlestick transmission of HTLV-III from a patient infected in Africa. Lancet 1984;2:1376-7.
17. Salahuddin SZ, Groopman JE, Markham PD, et al. HTLV-III in symptom-free seronegative persons. Lancet 1984;2:1418-20.
18. Groopman JE. Unpublished data.
19. Groopman JE, Salahuddin SZ, Sarngadharan MG, et al. HTLV-III in saliva of people with AIDS-related complex and healthy homosexual man at risk for AIDS. *Science* 1984, 226:447-9.
20. Zagury, D, Bernard J, Leibowitch J, et al. HTLV-III in cells cultured from semen of two patients with AIDS, Science 1984;226:449-51.
21. Feorino PM, Jaffe HW, Palmer E, et al. Transfusion-associated acquired immunodeficiency syndrome: evidence for persistent infection in blood donors. Submitted for publication.
22. Darrow WW, Jaffe HW, Braff E, et al. Acquired immunodeficiency syndrome (AIDS) in a cohort of homosexual men. Presentation at 24th Interscience Conference on Antimicrobial Agents and Chemotherapy, Washington, D.C., 1984.
23. Tsang, VCW, Peralta JM, Simons AR. Enzyme-linked immunoelectrotransfer blot techniques (EITB) for studying the specificities of antigens and antibodies separated by gel electrophoresis. Methods Enzymol 1983; 92:377-91.

INDEX